THIRD EDITION

A Comprehensive Guide to Geriatric Rehabilitation

Edited by

TIMOTHY L. KAUFFMAN, PT, PhD
Kauffman Physical Therapy, Lancaster, Pennsylvania; Adjunct Assistant Professor of Rehabilitation Medicine, Physical Therapy Department, Columbia University, New York, New York, USA

RON SCOTT, PT, EdD, JD, LLM
Health Law Attorney-Mediator, Private Practice, San Antonio, Texas; Associate Professor, Rocky Mountain University of Health Professions, Provo, Utah, USA

JOHN O. BARR, PT, MA, PhD, FAPTA
Professor, Physical Therapy Department, St Ambrose University, Davenport, Iowa, USA

MICHAEL L. MORAN, PT, DPT, ScD
Professor, Physical Therapy Department, Misericordia University, Dallas, Pennsylvania, USA

Foreword by

STEVEN L. WOLF, PT, PhD, FAPTA, FAHA
Professor, Department of Rehabilitation Medicine, Professor of Geriatrics, Department of Medicine, Associate Professor, Department of Cell Biology, Emory University School of Medicine; Professor of Health and Elder Care, Nell Hodgson Woodruff School of Nursing at Emory University; Senior Research Scientist, Atlanta VA Center of Excellence in Vision and Cognitive Neurorehabilitation, Atlanta, Georgia, USA

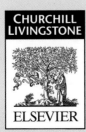
CHURCHILL LIVINGSTONE

ELSEVIER

Edinburgh • London • New York • Oxford • Philadelphia • St Louis • Sydney • Toronto • 2014

**CHURCHILL
LIVINGSTONE
ELSEVIER**

First edition 1999
Second edition 2007
  Reprinted 2014

ISBN 978-0-7020-4588-2

Notices

Knowledge and best practice in this field are constantly changing. As new research and experience broaden our understanding, changes in research methods, professional practices, or medical treatment may become necessary.

Practitioners and researchers must always rely on their own experience and knowledge in evaluating and using any information, methods, compounds, or experiments described herein. In using such information or methods they should be mindful of their own safety and the safety of others, including parties for whom they have a professional responsibility.

With respect to any drug or pharmaceutical products identified, readers are advised to check the most current information provided (i) on procedures featured or (ii) by the manufacturer of each product to be administered, to verify the recommended dose or formula, the method and duration of administration, and contraindications. It is the responsibility of practitioners, relying on their own experience and knowledge of their patients, to make diagnoses, to determine dosages and the best treatment for each individual patient, and to take all appropriate safety precautions.

To the fullest extent of the law, neither the Publisher nor the authors, contributors, or editors, assume any liability for any injury and/or damage to persons or property as a matter of products liability, negligence or otherwise, or from any use or operation of any methods, products, instructions, or ideas contained in the material herein.

 your source for books, journals and multimedia in the health sciences

www.elsevierhealth.com

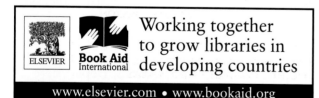 Working together to grow libraries in developing countries

www.elsevier.com • www.bookaid.org

The Publisher's policy is to use **paper manufactured from sustainable forests**

Printed in China

Contents

UNIT THREE

Neuromuscular and neurological disorders   179

UNIT FOUR

Neoplasms   243

UNIT FIVE

Cardiopulmonary disease   265

Dedications

To my wife, Brenda, and to our parents, Walter and Lillian, Bob and Lois. To our son Ben and his wife Beth with whom I share the joys and challenges of daily patient care and who wrote the Aquatic Therapy chapter. To our daughter Emily and her husband Brian West for their loving support. To the students all over the world who will learn from this book and provide the best possible care in all settings. To all of our patients who teach us so much. To our world class contributors, may our combined effort make life better for millions of people.

Timothy L. Kauffman

To my wonderful wife of 40 years, Pepi; our two sons, Ron Jr. and Paul; our super grandchildren – Isabel, Jonas and Marlee; and our sweet daughter-in-law, Amanda, with love.

Ron Scott

To my wife Jeanne and our children Katie and Mike Jr. To our grandchildren Adelynn and Gwendolynn and our son-in-law Kyle. To my parents Jack and Jane. To colleagues and students over the many years. Thank you all!

Michael L. Moran

My mother
Who attained one hundred years
Is our oldest book

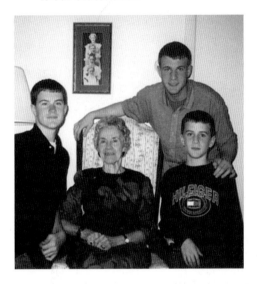

Dedicated to the memory of Norma Schumacher Barr with grandsons (L to R) Tom, Greg & Evan Barr (11/28/1911 to 1/11/2012)

John O. Barr

Contributors

MARTHA ACOSTA, PT, PhD
Assistant Professor, Department of Physical Therapy, UT Health Center, San Antonio, Texas, USA

CHERYL L. ANDERSON, PT, PhD, MBA
Adjunct Professor, Physical Therapy Department, The College of St Scholastica, Duluth, Minnesota, USA

SUSAN BARKER, PT, PhD
Professor and Chair, Physical Therapy Department, Misericordia University, Dallas, Pennsylvania, USA

JOHN O. BARR, PT, MA, PhD, FAPTA
Professor, Physical Therapy Department, St Ambrose University, Davenport, Iowa, USA

DARCI BECKER, PhD, CCC-SLP, BCS-S
Assistant Professor, Master of Speech-Language Pathology Program, St Ambrose University, Davenport, Iowa, USA

SHERRI R. BETZ, PT, GCS, CEEAA, PMA®-CPT
TheraPilates® Physical Therapy, Santa Cruz, California, USA

RICHARD W. BOHANNON, PT, EdD, NCS, FAPTA, FAHA
Professor, University of Connecticut, Storrs; Principal, Physical Therapy Consultants, West Hartford, Connecticut, USA

MICHELLE A. BOLTON, PT, DPT
Physical Therapist, Kauffman Physical Therapy, Lancaster, Pennsylvania, USA

JENNIFER M. BOTTOMLEY, PT, MS, PhD
Associate Professor, Simmons College, Boston, Massachusetts, USA; President, International Association of Physical Therapists working with Older Persons (IPTOP), World Confederation for Physical Therapy

MARK A. BRIMER, PT, PhD
Florida Fall Prevention & Rehabilitation LLC, Satellite Beach, Florida, USA

STEPHEN BRUNTON, MD
Director of Faculty Development, Cabarrus Family Medicine Residency Program, Concord, North Caroline; Adjunct Clinical Professor, Department of Family Medicine, University of North Carolina, Chapel Hill, North Carolina, USA

BLAINE CARMICHAEL, PA-C, MPAS, DFAAPA
Senior Physician Assistant, Alamo City Medical Group, San Antonio, Texas, USA

RONNI CHERNOFF, PhD, RD
Professor and Director, Geriatric Research Education and Clinical Center (GRECC), Central Arkansas Geriatric Education Center, Little Rock, Arkansas, USA

CHARLES D. CICCONE, PT, PhD
Professor, Department of Physical Therapy, Ithaca College, Ithica, New York, USA

MERYL COHEN, PT, MS, DPT, CCS
Assistant Professor, Department of Physical Therapy, Miller School of Medicine, University of Miami, Florida, USA

ANITA CRAIG, DO
Assistant Professor, Department of Physical Medicine and Rehabilitation, University of Michigan Hospital and Health Systems, Ann Arbor, Michigan, USA

CAROL M. DAVIS, DPT, EdD, FAPTA
Professor Emerita, Department of Physical Therapy, University of Miami School of Medicine, Coral Gables, Florida, USA

GORDON DICKINSON, MD
Professor of Medicine, Division of Infectious Diseases, University of Miami Miller School of Medicine; Chief, Infectious Diseases Section, Miami Veterans Affairs Medical Center, Miami, Florida, USA

DOUGLAS J. DIGIROLAMO, PhD
Assistant Professor, Johns Hopkins University Center for Musculoskeletal Research, Department of Orthopedic Surgery, Baltimore, Maryland, USA

BRIAN J. ECKENRODE, PT, DPT, MS, OCS
Assistant Professor, Department of Physical Therapy, Arcadia University, Glenside, Pennsylvania, USA

JOAN E. EDELSTEIN, PT, MA, FISPO
Special Lecturer, Physical Therapy Department, Steinhardt School of Culture, Education and Human Development, New York University, New York, New York, USA

BARBARA J. EHRMANN, PT, DPT, MBA
Clinical Assistant Professor, Physical Therapy Department, St Ambrose University, Davenport, Iowa, USA

TERI ELLIOTT-BURKE, PT, MHS, BCIA-PMDB
Co-owner, WoMen's Physical Therapy Institute, Lake Zurich, Illinois, USA

NICOLE L. EVANOSKY, PT, DPT
Assistant Professor and Director of Clinical Education, Physical Therapy Department, Misericordia University, Dallas, Pennsylvania, USA

MICHAEL FISCHER, OD, FAAO
Director, Vision Services, Northport VA Medical Center, Northport, New York; Adjunct Assistant Clinical Professor, SUNY College of Optometry, New York; Low Vision Clinical Consultant, Lighthouse Guild International, New York, New York, USA

WALTER R. FRONTERA, MD, PhD
Professor and Chair, Department of PM&R, Vanderbilt University School of Medicine & Medical Director of Rehabilitation Services, Vanderbilt University Medical Center, Nashville, Tennesse, USA

EMILY L. GERMAIN-LEE, MD
Director of Albright Clinic, Director of Bone Research, Associate Director, Osteogenesis Imperfecta Program, Kennedy Krieger Institute; Associate Professor, Pediatric Endocrinology, Johns Hopkins University School of Medicine, Baltimore, Maryland, USA

DEBORAH GOLD, PhD
Associate Professor of Medical Sociology, Departments of Psychiatry & Behavioral Sciences, Sociology, and Psychology, Duke University Medical Center, Durham, North Carolina, USA

RANDY GORDON, DNP, FNP-BC
Instructor, MSN Department, Chamberlain College of Nursing, Downers Grove, Illinois, USA

EDWARD JAMES R. GORGON, MPHYSIO, PTRP
Assistant Professor & Chairperson, Department of Physical Therapy, University of the Philippines, Phillippines

STEPHEN A. GUDAS, PT, PhD
Associate Professor, Director of Gross Anatomy Laboratory, Department of Anatomy and Neurobiology, VCU/Medical College of Virginia, Richmond, Virginia, USA

BRENDA L. HAGE, PhD, DNP, CRNP
Professor, Department of Nursing, Misericordia University, Dallas, Pennsylvania, USA

JUNE E. HANKS, PT, PhD, DPT, CWS, CLT
Associate Professor, Doctor of Physical Therapy Program, Bellarmine University, Louisville, Kentucky, USA

RICHARD HAYDT, PT, DPT, OCS, MTC, FAAOMPT
Associate Professor, Department of Physical Therapy, Misericordia University, Dallas, Pennsylvania, USA

SARAH HAYES, BSc Physiotherapy, PGDip Statistics, PhD
Postdoctoral Research Fellow, Centre for Pain Research & School of Psychology, National University of Ireland, Galway, Ireland

BARRY HULL, MD, FAAFP
Medical Director, A New Start Medical Center, Fayetteville, Georgia, USA

BENJAMIN W. KAUFFMAN, PTA
Physical Therapist Assistant, Facilities Manager, Kauffman Physical Therapy, Lancaster, Pennsylvania, USA

BETH E. KAUFFMAN, MPT, ATC
Physical Therapist, Kauffman Physical Therapy, Lancaster, Pennsylvania, USA

TIMOTHY L. KAUFFMAN, PT, PhD
Owner, Kauffman Physical Therapy, Lancaster, Pennsylvania; Adjunct Assistant Professor of Rehabilitation Medicine, Physical Therapy Department, Columbia University, New York, New York, USA

KAREN KEMMIS, PT, DPT, CDE, CEEAA
Clinician and Adjunct Professor, SUNY Upstate Medical University, Syracuse, New York, USA

DENNIS W. KLIMA, PT, MS, PhD, GCS, NCS
Assistant Professor, University of Maryland Eastern Shore, Princess Anne, Maryland, USA

BARBARA KOEHLER, PT, MPTSc
Lecturer, Department of Health, Zurich University of Applied Sciences, Winterthur, Switzerland

EDMUND M. KOSMAHL, PT, EdD
Professor, Physical Therapy Department, The University of Scranton, Pennsylvania, USA

KEVIN J. LAWRENCE, PT, DHS, OCS
Associate Professor, Department of Physical Therapy, Tennessee State University, Nashville, Tennessee, USA

ROLANDO T. LAZARO, PT, PhD, DPT, GCS
Associate Professor, Samuel Merrit University, Oakland, Calilfornia, USA

SANDRA J. LEVI, PT, PhD
Associate Program Director, Physical Therapy Department, Midwestern University, Illinois, USA

DAVID LEVINE, PT, PhD, DPT, OCS, CCRP
Professor and Walter M. Cline Chair of Excellence, Department of Physical Therapy, The University of Tennessee at Chattanooga, Tennessee, USA

CARLEEN LINDSEY, PT, MScAH, CEEAA
Partner, Bristol Physical Therapy, Bristol, Connecticut, USA

MARK LOMBARDI, PT, DPT, ATC
Director of Rehabilitation, Scranton Orthopedic
Specialists, Dickson City, Pennsylvania, USA

MICHELLE M. LUSARDI, PT DPT, PhD
Professor Emerita, Department of Physical Therapy,
Department of Physical Therapy, Sacred Heart
University, Fairfield, Conneticut, USA

DIANE MADRAS, PT, PhD
Associate Professor, Physical Therapy Department,
Misericordia University, Dallas, Pennsylvania, USA

KATIE L. MCARTHUR, AuD
Audiologist, Clermont, Florida, USA

**NIALL MCGRANE, BSc Physio, BA Psychol, BSc Health
Sciences**
PhD Candidate, Discipline of Physiotherapy, School of
Medicine, Trinity College, Dublin, Ireland

P. CHRISTOPHER METZGER, MD, FACS
Orthopaedic Surgeon, Scranton Orthopaedic Specialists,
Scranton, Pennsylvania, USA

MOLLY MIKA, MS, OTR/L

MARILYN E. MILLER, PT, PhD, GCS
Assistant Professor, Physical Therapy Department,
California State University Fresno, Fresno, California, USA

STEPHEN E. MOCK, PhD
Senior Partner, Phido Audiology & Hearing Aids,
Gettysburg, Pennsylvania, USA

MICHAEL L. MORAN, PT, DPT, ScD
Professor, Department of Physical Therapy, Misericordia
University, Dallas, Pennsylvania, USA

RICHARD MOWRER, PTA, CSCS
Physical Therapist Assistant, Drayer Physical Therapy
Institute, Harrisburg, Pennsylvania, USA

JENNIFER NITZ, PhD, MPhty, BPhty, FACP
Division of Physiotherapy, School of Heath and
Rehabilitation Sciences, The University of Queensland,
St Lucia, Australia

**CAROLINE O'CONNELL, BSc (HONS) Physio,
Dip Stats, MISCP**
School of Physiotherapy, The University of Dublin,
Trinity College, Dublin, Ireland

ALEXANDRA PAPAIOANNOU, MD, MSc, FRCP(C), FACP
Professor, Department of Medicine, McMaster University,
Hamilton, Ontario, Canada

MAUREEN ROMANOW PASCAL, PT, DPT, NCS
Associate Professor, Department of Physical Therapy,
Misericordia University, Dallas, Pennsylvania, USA

DAVID PATRICK, PT, MS, CPT
Keystone Prosthetics and Orthotics, Dickson City,
Pennsylvania, USA

CLIVE PERRY, MBBS, FRANZCR, FRCR
Radiologist, Department of Radiology, Lancaster General
Hospital, Lancaster, Pennsylvania, USA

STEVEN PHEASANT, PT, PhD
Associate Professor, Department of Physical Therapy,
Misericordia University, Dallas, Pennsylvania, USA

RANDOLPH RASCH, PhD, RN, FNP-BC, FAANP
Professor and Chair, Department of Community Practice,
School of Nursing, University of North Carolina at
Greensboro, Greensboro, North Carolina, USA

KANWAL RAZZAQ, MD
Infectious Diseases Consultant, Bluefield Regional
Hospital, Blufield, West Virginia, USA

PAMELA REYNOLDS, PT, PhD, MS, GCS
Associate Professor, Gannon University, Erie,
Pennsylvania, USA

JAMES K. RICHARDSON, MD
Associate Professor, Department of Physical Medicine
and Rehabilitation, University of Michigan Medical
School, Michigan, USA

NATIVDAD RODRIGUEZ, MT, MS
Department of Physiology, University of Puerto Rico
School of Medicine, San Juan, Puerto Rico

WENDY ROMNEY, PT, DPT, NCS
Clinical Assistant Professor, Department of Physical
Therapy, Sacred Heart University, Fairfield,
Conneticut, USA

BRUCE P. ROSENTHAL, OD, FAAO
Chief of the Low Vision Service, Lighthouse Guild
International, New York; Adjunct Professor, Mount
Sinai Hospital, New York; Adjunct Clinical Professor,
State College of Optometry, State University of New
York, New York, USA

JOHN SANKO, PT, EdD
Associate Professor, Physical Therapy Department, The
University of Scranton, Scranton, Pennsylvania, USA

ADRIAN M. SCHOO, PT, PhysioD, MHHScPT
Professor of Rural Allied Health Education, Rural Clinical
School of Medicine, Flinders University, Adelaide,
South Australia

RON SCOTT, PT, EdD, JD, LLM
Health Law Attorney-Mediator, Private Practice, San
Antonio, Texas; Associate Professor, Rocky Mountain
University of Health Professions, Provo, Utah, USA

JAY SHAPIRO, MD
Director, Osteogenesis Imperfecta Program, Kennedy
Kreiger Institute, Baltimore, Maryland, USA

JAMES SIBERSKI, MS
Coordinator, Gerontology Education, College
Misericordia University, Dallas, Pennsylvania, USA

CHRISTINE STABLER, MD
Family Practice Resident Program, Lancaster General
Hospital, Lancaster, Pennsylvania, USA

WILLIAM H. STAPLES, PT, DPT, DHSc, GCS, CEEAA
Assistant Professor, Krannert School of Physical Therapy,
University of Indianapolis, Indianapolis, Indiana, USA

CHRISTI STEWART, MD
Physician, LGHP Geriatrics, Lancaster General Hospital,
Lancaster, Pennsylvania, USA

EMMA K. STOKES, BSc, MSC, PhD
Lecturer, School of Physiotherapy, The University of
Dublin, Trinity College, Dublin, Ireland

HILMAR H.G. STRACKE, MD, PhD
University Hospital Giessen, Giessen, Germany

LISA TEWS, MA, CCC/SLP
Speech-language Pathologist, Genesis Medical Center,
Davenport, Iowa, USA

EERIC TRUUMEES, MD
Orthopedics Department, William Beaumont Hospital,
Royal Oak, Michigan; Bioengineering Department,
Wayne State University, Detroit, Michigan, USA

DARCY A. UMPHRED, PT, PhD, FAPTA
Professor Emeritus, Dept of Physical Therapy, University
of the Pacific, Stockton, California, USA

KRISTIN von NIEDA, PT, MEd, DPT
Associate Professor, Department of Physical Therapy,
Arcadia University, Glendale, Pennsylvania, USA

CHRIS L. WELLS, PT, PhD, CCS, ATC
Associate Professor, School of Medicine, Department
of Physical Therapy and Rehabilitation Science,
University of Maryland, Baltimore, Maryland; Clinical
Specialist, Department of Rehabilitation Services,
University of Maryland Medical Center, Baltimore,
Maryland, USA

MARY ANN WHARTON, PT, MS
Associate Professor of Physical Therapy and
Curriculum Coordinator, Department of Physical
Therapy, Saint Francis University, Loretto,
Pennsylvania; Adjunct Associate Professor, Physical
Therapist Assistant Program, Community College
of Allegheny County, Boyce Campus, Monroeville,
Pennsylvania, USA

SUSAN L. WHITNEY, PT, PhD, NCA, ATC
Associate Professor, Physical Therapy Department,
University of Pittsburg, Pittsburg, Pennsylvania,
USA

RITA A. WONG, PT, EdD, FAPTA
Professor of Physical Therapy; Assistant Dean for
Graduate and Professional Studies, Marymount
University, Arlington, Virginia, USA

MICHELLE E. WORMLEY, PT, MPT, PhD, CLT
Clinical Assistant Professor, Department of Physical
Therapy, Sacred Heart University, Fairfield,
Connecticut, USA

DIANE M. WRISLEY, PT, PhD, NCS
Associate Professor, Physical Therapy Department,
Lynchburg College, Lynchburg, Virginia, USA

ANA RODRIGUEZ ZAYAS, PhD
Department of Physiology, University of Puerto Rico
School of Medicine, San Juan, Puerto Rico

Foreword

The beginning of wisdom is the recognition of how little one knows.

ARISTOTLE

Why is it that the notion of wisdom is so often associated with age? Have we ever heard of a 'wise young owl' or 'a wise child'? Perhaps, the infrequent 'wise beyond his/her years' but that is about it! There seems to be something synonymous about age and wisdom. Now beginning its third edition, what was the *Geriatric Rehabilitation Manual* has expanded its content and adopted the name *Comprehensive Guide to Geriatric Rehabilitation* and with this transformation has taken on an aura of perspicacity... for would we not associate a comprehensive guide with being more omnipotent than a 'manual'? And what better topic to foster guidance than being led through managing and treating the aging process, by editors who, undeniably, have acquired more wisdom befitting their own maturation.

Part of that maturation is manifest in an expansion of topical areas and of contributing authors to include those from 8 other countries, a collective unique to this book. This effort toward becoming more encompassing brings with it the distinctive opportunity to gain multiple perspectives. To see treatment issues through the eyes of others and to embrace such opportunities can only expand our own knowledge. This insight is born from experience and a combination of wisdom and courage to do so. While the total number of chapters has not changed, the composition of 102 contributors holds a collection of 21 different degrees. This assembly of experts has focused on updating their bibliographies as well as cross referencing concepts and chapters. The breadth of contributors and topics fosters an opportunity for rehabilitation clinicians and students from multiple countries to best study the provision of care amongst an internationally aging community. While most of the previous contributors continue their loyalty and dedication to this text, 28 of the 102 authors are new and bring with them fresh perspectives. Indeed, the chapters on joints and ligaments (Chapter 4), senile dementia and cognitive impairment (Chapter 28), multiple sclerosis (Chapter 29), skin disorders (50), considerations in elder patient communication (Chapter 53), dysphagia (Chapter 54), function of the aging hand (Chapter 63), and gait training (Chapter 68) contain very new materials with contributions from first-time authors to this book writing either independently or in collaboration with previous authors.

The content is cleverly arranged in units comparable to the previous edition but not only separates problem areas into unique entities but also integrates them into components that truly reflect the complexity of care and intervention often required to successfully treat older adults.

The text also presents quick access to important information regarding problems encountered by providers when evaluating geriatric clients. Part of this assimilation is seen in the chapter on healthcare of older persons (Chapter 74). Chapters on treating the geriatric spine (Chapter 24), frailty (Chapter 65), Pilates (Chapter 72), considerations of healthcare issues for older adults (Chapter 76), and multidisciplinary entry level professional competencies for health providers working with older adults (Chapter 78) represent several of the additions to this edition. The chapter on imaging of geriatric tissues (Chapter 14) is outstanding and represents one of the most comprehensive reviews and instructional efforts ever directed toward students and clinicians. The units that cover vision (Chapter 51), hearing (Chapter 52), and communication (Chapter 53) collectively comprise much of Unit 7 and are unique to this book in that this constellation of information about pathologies in the aging sensorium is not typically provided elsewhere.

If students, clinicians and educators with a vested commitment to improving the quality of life for those of us bolstering the ranks, and tilting the aging distribution to the right, take a moment to reflect upon friends or family members who are aging in front of them at a rate that often seems to be accelerating, and then ask the question, 'If I was not a healthcare provider for that person, but had to work with one who was, what would I want them to know in order to assure me that the best and most comprehensive care could be extended?', I would imagine that the answer might be, 'I would want them to know everything!' Such a request is a tall order to fill. Now, if one examines the comprehensive nature of this text, can one safely conclude that its content indeed serves as a guide for the understanding and delivery of such comprehensive care? I believe that the answer is a resounding 'yes!' What lies beyond these first few pages is an international perspective on the understanding and treatment of virtually every physiological and behavioral aspect of geriatric care. The collective wisdom of those who have penned these chapters will serve us well, whether we be student, clinician, investigator and, of course, knowledgeable caregiver.

Steven L. Wolf, PT, PhD, FAPTA, FAHA
Professor, Department of Rehabilitation Medicine,
Professor of Geriatrics, Department of Medicine,
Associate Professor, Department of Cell Biology,
Emory University School of Medicine;
Professor of Health and Elder Care,
Nell Hodgson Woodruff School of
Nursing at Emory University;
Senior Research Scientist,
Atlanta VA Center of Excellence in Vision
and Cognitive Neurorehabilitation

Preface

Please read the Prefaces from the first and second editions of the *Geriatric Rehabilitation Manual*. They present the organizational structure and the philosophical foundation for this third edition. For the third edition's Preface, I am taking the liberty, as a clinician and author, to share a few defining milestones in my experience as a therapist that led to a lifetime of studying, teaching and providing the best possible care.

Why have I toiled for almost five years, spending hours and hours communicating with thousands of care providers, researchers and professors to produce this book? The answer is that this work represents a life's journey that started when I was a physical therapy student, over four decades ago. Each of the co-editors has experienced parallel life and career paths.

Hip fractures are serious injuries that far too often precipitate the downward spiral that ends in death. This was especially true in 1971 when not all hip fractures were treated with open reduction internal fixation. Having entered the physical therapy profession from the perspective of a young athlete, I was upset when my patients with hip fractures died. As a student I agonized over my failure to get my patients up and walking which might have prevented the urinary tract or respiratory track infections that led to their deaths.

Six years after my graduation from physical therapy school, when I was taking my first gerontology class, I learned of the Orgel hypothesis (see Theoretical perspectives, Chapter 1) which posits that errors in protein synthesis occur: thus, making faulty proteins. In my mind, I immediately thought: 'Aha! That is why I could not build the strength in my patients and why they died.'

With these experiences and perspectives in mind, I designed a research project to examine strength training for young and older women using an identical training stimulus for both age groups. At the time, other researchers had an age bias and did not exercise older subjects with intensity because of the potential risk of injury. This was the same reasoning that my human research committee applied to my proposal. I was not allowed to exercise a large muscle group or anyone over 75 years of age. I chose to exercise the small finger abductor digiti minimi.

My results were outstanding with both the young and older females improving at the statistical significance level of $P < 0.0001$. Also, there was no significant difference in strength gains when comparing the young and the old (Kauffman, 1985).

I presented my research as a poster at the 1979 Gerontological Society of America meeting. Nathan Shock and Arthur Norris, from the Baltimore Longitudinal Study, viewed my work and asked questions; I recognized them because I referred to their work in my thesis. They said that if my results hold up with other muscle groups, then thinking about aging would change dramatically.

Three years later in 1982, I presented a paper at the World Confederation of Physical Therapy meeting in Stockholm. My title was *The Hypokinetic Model: A New Look at the Effect of Age on Neuromuscular Function*. Our daughter was born three weeks before the meeting and, thus, I struggled with a major decision: to leave my baby or to withdraw the paper? I went to the meeting and dedicated my paper to our newborn daughter and to people all over the world so that they may 'live well' based on what we were learning at the time. Gunar Grimby, a renowned researcher, was in the audience and he asked how I could present all of those age-related declines because he was finding that hypokinesis was a real factor in what is labeled as aging. I explained that I agreed and that his research was part of the purpose behind my presentation. Hypokinesis is a significant factor in aging changes.

Since these career path experiences took place, time has passed and new research has filled the gaps in our knowledge. Concomitantly, demographics on aging have changed dramatically (see Chapter 76).

Going back to the original question posed in this preface, the answer why we, the editors and all of our contributors, have worked so hard to make this the best possible comprehensive guide to geriatric rehabilitation is that we want people to age well and to recover from life's diseases and injuries. For people to age well, healthcare providers must have access to knowledge and information that will enable them to provide the best possible care for the aging patient.

The readers of this book must realize that the 91-year-old woman or the 79-year-old man in front of them, waiting to be treated, is someone's spouse, mother/father, grandmother/grandfather and probably even great grandmother/grandfather. Their loved ones want them to receive the best possible and compassionate care. This book hopefully will enable care providers all over the world to do just that.

By rehabilitating aging persons and compressing morbidity (decreasing the debilitating effects of diseases to the shortest time before death) we are enriching and enhancing the quality of life for our patients, their families and ourselves.

After all, working with aging persons is working with living history. During my career, I have treated a soldier who fought in the Spanish–American War at the

Battle of San Juan, a negotiator for the United States, at Panmunjom, to end the Korean War, a man who saw Babe Ruth hit home runs, women who survived concentration camps, a woman who guarded the coastline of Suriname (formerly Dutch Guiana) against enemy intruders, a German night-fighter pilot and the generations that survived WWI, the Great Depression, and WWII. The contact we have with these people is a gift. It puts us in touch with our living history and enriches us as people and as healthcare providers. That is why seemingly endless hours and energy went into this book by world-class contributors.

Respectfully,
Timothy L. Kauffman

REFERENCE

Kauffman TL 1985 Strength training in young and aged women. Arch Phys Med Rehabil 66:223–226

Preface to the second edition

Aging ... the passage of time ... brings with it an abundance of experiences within the psychosocial, economic and medical milieu that our patients and we healthcare practitioners face every day. In order to provide quality healthcare for the older person, given the constraints of time and healthcare payment systems, one must have easily accessible, concise, and yet comprehensive, information. This book will enable the busy healthcare provider to review, or to learn quickly about, a range of pathologies/conditions, examinations/diagnostic procedures and interventions that can be effectively used in the physical rehabilitation of older persons.

No two individuals experience the passage of time in identical fashion. Thus, one hallmark of aging is the uniqueness of each person. Because aging may be viewed as an accumulation of 'microinsults' that present as a collection of chronic diseases affecting multiple body systems, interactive relationships must be considered in patient evaluation and treatment. These interactive, multi-system relationships are emphasized in this book.

One of the challenges encountered in geriatric patient care is that the symptoms and signs, and responses to treatment, may not be clear-cut. There is professional reward in recognizing this and in determining an appropriate course of patient care in a manner that supports each aging patient so that he or she has a sense of control and worth in the presence of physical losses and illnesses. We hope that this textbook and its readers acknowledge this challenge and reward.

This book is written for both practicing clinicians and students who are practicing to become clinicians. It is appropriate for entry-level practitioners in geriatric rehabilitation settings, including physicians, nurses, physical therapists, occupational therapists, speech pathologists, respiratory therapists and social workers. We believe that the seasoned practitioner will also benefit from the broad review of information that this book provides and by recognizing that he or she is giving proper care according to today's standards.

For the healthcare provider who is newly entering the field of geriatric rehabilitation, this text will prove to be truly invaluable. In this second edition of the *Geriatric Rehabilitation Manual*, we updated evidence to support the use of specific examination and evaluation procedures, as well as interventions. However, we clearly acknowledge that not every suggestion provided in this book has been subjected to rigorous clinical research. Nonetheless, a range of suggestions are offered because they represent wisdom from the field of rehabilitation and are concepts that can be further investigated.

Throughout the text, the reader should appreciate that the different writing styles employed by our authors also reflect different evaluation and intervention approaches. The authors were encouraged to discuss the science of geriatric rehabilitation and to infuse the art of humane patient care for older persons.

This book is organized into eleven distinct, but interrelated, units. The first unit is concerned with key anatomical and physiological considerations seen with aging and having significant impact on the older individual. Also included are overviews of laboratory and imaging procedures, and pharmacologic considerations for older persons. The second and third units review important aging-related conditions and disorders of the musculoskeletal and neuromuscular/neurological systems respectively. Neoplasms commonly encountered in older persons are the focus of the fourth unit. Aging-related conditions of the cardiovascular, pulmonary, integumentary and sensory systems are presented in units five through seven. Unit eight highlights a range of specific clinical problems and conditions commonly encountered with older patients. Critically, all of these units emphasize important examination and diagnostic procedures needed for a thorough evaluation and stress interventions that can be of significant benefit to the older patient. The ninth unit presents select physical therapeutic interventions that are especially important in managing rehabilitative care. Key societal issues related to aging are discussed in the tenth unit. The concluding unit focuses on the successful rehabilitation team that includes both professional and non-professional caregiver members.

We sincerely hope that students and colleagues who utilize the *w* will appreciate that:

1. Aging is not stagnant, dull or unattractive.
2. Aging is dynamic and fluctuating, with a wide range of responses.
3. Aging is diverse – its hallmark is the variability of individuals.
4. Aging is challenging.
5. Aging is complex.
6. The study of aging is the study of life – our assessments and interventions must be lifelong.
7. Aging and living are synonymous.

ABOVE ALL ELSE, AGING IS TO BE VALUED AND VENERATED.

Respectfully, the Editors:
Timothy L. Kauffman PT, PhD
John O. Barr PT, PhD
Michael L. Moran PT, ScD

Preface to the first edition

The passage of time ... aging ... brings a plethora of experiences that constitute the psychosocial, economic and medical milieu that our patients and we as healthcare practitioners face every day. To provide quality healthcare for the older person in this robust arena, given the constraints of time and healthcare payment systems, one must have easily accessible, comprehensive, and concise information. This text is written to enable the healthcare provider to review or to learn quickly the pathology of a diagnosis or condition and to present treatment ideas, especially for rehabilitation, prevention (maintenance) care and prognosis.

No two individuals experience life in identical fashion; thus, one hallmark of aging is the 'uniqueness' of each person. Because aging may be viewed as an accumulation of microinsults that present as a collection of chronic diseases and one or more acute problems, the interactive relationships must be considered. This perspective is different from the isolated computerized model of labeling geriatric patients with the clean number listed in the *International Classification of Diseases*, 9th edition, *Clinical Modifications*. We as healthcare providers must remain constantly vigilant to avoid this lure of simplification.

One of the issues encountered in geriatric patient care is that the symptoms and signs or responses to treatment may not be as clear as might be expected. The reward is recognizing this and determining an appropriate course of patient care in order to support each aging patient so that he or she has a sense of worth and control even in the presence of physical losses and illnesses. This textbook and, we hope, its readers will acknowledge the challenge and reward.

This book is for clinicians. Although not specifically designed to be a textbook for classroom instruction, students become practitioners; thus, it is also appropriate for the entry-level practitioner in the geriatric rehabilitation setting, including physicians, nurses, physical therapists, occupational therapists, speech pathologists, respiratory therapists and social workers.

The text is written with a dual purpose for the seasoned practitioner who will benefit from reviewing the information and recognizing that he or she is giving proper care according to today's standards. Furthermore, the seasoned practitioner will also learn because of the breadth of information presented in this text.

For the healthcare provider who is newly entering the field of geriatric care, this text will prove to be invaluable. It is clearly acknowledged that not every suggestion offered within the chapters has been put to the rigors of clinical research in order to validate efficacy; however, the suggestions are offered nonetheless because they represent potential treatment ideas, and they are the standard wisdom of the rehabilitation field at this time. Although some of the ideas have not been proven, they have not been refuted. If they had been refuted, they would no longer represent the standard wisdom that defines the ambits of care. These treatment ideas should be employed by thinking practitioners for individual patients.

Throughout the text, the reader should recognize different writing styles that also reflect different treatment approaches. The authors were encouraged to discuss the science of geriatric rehabilitation and to infuse the art of patient care, the soft underbelly of humane medical care for persons who are undergoing involution and are closing out a life. Some of the chapters in this text have references within the material presented. Other chapters have only selected readings at the end of the chapter. The editorial board encouraged each of the writers to minimize the references so that more treatment ideas, graphs and clinical forms could be included. Readers are strongly encouraged to seek out further information from the lists of suggested readings.

The text is organized into seven separate areas. The first unit deals with some overview of geriatric care and the review of systems as they relate to aging. This should be helpful for classroom instruction and review of age-related changes. Chapter 1 specifically deals with the complexity of aging, pathology and healthcare.

The second unit deals with aging pathokinesiology and is clearly directed at specific clinical conditions. It also parallels a rudimentary systems review, since the unit is subdivided into topics pertaining to musculoskeletal involvement, neuromuscular and neurological involvement, neoplasms, cardiopulmonary diseases, and finally blood vessel, circulatory and skin disorders.

The third unit deals with the aging and pathological sensorium, especially as it relates to vision, hearing and communication. The following unit (Unit IV) presents a potpourri of common specific conditions, complaints and problems and is followed by special considerations or physical therapeutic intervention techniques (Unit V). The sociopolitical, legal and ethical considerations are addressed in Unit VI because they also impact on geriatric rehabilitation. It is important to recognize that the paradigm shifts at the end of life from the medical model to the dying model, which is more culture based. There is less concern about traditional rehabilitation constructs and greater emphasis on value of life and palliation to minimize suffering and to maintain quality for the dying patient and the family.

Unit VII, the final unit, elucidates the prominent members of the geriatric rehabilitation healthcare team. I hope that healthcare providers and others who use this manual will understand that:

1. Aging is not stagnant, dull, and/or unattractive.
2. Aging is very dynamic, perhaps too fluctuating, with a wide range of responses.
3. Aging is very diverse – a hallmark is the variability of individuals.
4. Aging is very challenging.
5. Aging is very complex.
6. The study of aging is the study of life – it starts in the uterus and our intervention must be lifelong.
7. Aging and living are synonymous.
8. ABOVE ALL ELSE, AGING IS VENERABLE AND VALUED.

Respectfully,
Timothy L. Kauffman PT, PhD

Acknowledgments

A book of this breadth cannot be conceived, nurtured, and published without a host of persons making significant contributions. First, I want to acknowledge the commissioning editor, Rita Demetriou-Swanwick, for nurturing this project along. Additionally, Clive Hewat, the development editor, and Anne Collett, the project manager, for wrestling with the constant effort to manage the details and reach a final product, as well as Elaine Leek and Rajakumar Murthy. Also, I say thanks to all of the persons from Elsevier who have helped to complete this book but have never sent me an email and thus remain anonymous.

I must express immeasurable gratitude to my wife, Brenda, daughter, Emily, son, Ben, and daughter-in-law, Beth, who have contributed significantly through their support as well as administratively by collating information, assisting with editing, and allowing me the time to stay on track. Special recognition goes to Janine Eyster, Jamie Perrone, Michelle Bolton, Marty McKeon, Julie Sostack and Krystle Groff who have backed me up and allowed time to work on this project. Special recognition goes to Lynn Sterkenberg for her administrative support and Karen King. Finally, this book would not have been completed without the sharing, reflecting, and tireless contributions from my co-editors, John Barr, Mike Moran and Ron Scott, and their wives, Rhonda, Jeanne and Pepi, and their families.

Also, I want to acknowledge my professors at the University of Pennsylvania who taught me the requisite skills to use both the science and the art of healthcare. These professors include Dorothy Baetke, Jane Carlin, Eugene Michaels, Elsa Ramsden, Rose Myers, Mary Day and Risa Granick.

TIMOTHY L. KAUFFMAN

Anatomical and physiological considerations

UNIT.CONTENTS

Chapter 1
Wholeness of the individual

TIMOTHY L. KAUFFMAN

CHAPTER CONTENTS

INTRODUCTION

Aging is a wonderful and unique experience. The word 'wonderful' should not imply that aging includes only good things, but rather that it is extraordinary and remarkable. Aging starts in the uterus at the time of conception. It represents the passage of time, not pathology. By the age of 1 year, each individual's uniqueness is evident, and by the age of 5 years the personality is well formed. Multiply the first 5 years of life by 15 and expand the environmental and life experiences, and one of the hallmarks of aging becomes clear – individual uniqueness. No two people age identically. Idiosyncrasy is the norm, and it is important that the healthcare provider looks at the wholeness of the individual geriatric patient as well as the chief presenting complaint or primary diagnosis.

In the healthcare arena of the United States of America today, the wholeness of the patient is compressed into an electronic number taken from the International Classification of Diseases (ICD), with the 10th coding revision being implemented in 2014. Its requisite use for reimbursement often fails to portray the wholeness of the individual patient's clinical presentation, which typically involves multimorbidity. Over 50% of older persons in the US have three or more chronic conditions (Boyd et al., 2012). Medical care must be given to the whole patient and the record should document that.

The importance of the whole person and multimorbidities is supported by the findings of White et al. (2013). They studied well-functioning persons, 70–79 years old, and measured decline of gait speed over 8 years. The mortality risk was highest among those with the fastest decline of speed. This loss was more likely in older persons with knee pain, muscle weakness, physical inactivity and higher body mass index.

Age alone is a factor to consider; however, chronological age based on date of birth is not always similar to physiological age, which is based on cross-sectional measurements and comparisons with age-estimated or established norms. For example, a specific 70-year-old man may have an aerobic capacity that is similar to that of the average 60-year-old; the older man is said to have a 10-year physiological age advantage. In Chapter 15 there is a photograph of three individuals ranging in age from 60 to 93; it clearly shows differences among the three, although generalizations can be cautiously extrapolated. But far too often such an age span is grouped together as if aging changes are monolithic: they are not. It is not common to compare a 10-year-old with a 43-year-old, which also represents an age span of 33 years. When dealing with a patient who has lived for seven decades or more, the person's individuality must be acknowledged by providers, administrators and health delivery systems if optimal care is to be rendered.

VARIOUS MEDICAL MODELS OR PERSPECTIVES

The standard medical model of signs and symptoms equaling a diagnosis of disease does not fit well with the geriatric population (Fig. 1.1). Fried et al. (1991) found that this medical model was able to fit actual cases in fewer than half of the geriatric patients they studied. They developed several other models: the synergistic morbidity model, the attribution model, the causal chain model and the unmasking event model (Fried et al., 1991).

The *synergistic morbidity model* uses a scenario in which the patient presents with a history of multiple, generally chronic diseases (represented by A, B and C in Fig. 1.2) that result in cumulative morbidity. When this hypothetical patient loses functional capacity, medical attention is sought. This may also be viewed as a cascading effect.

The *attribution model* uses a scenario in which a patient attributes declining capacity to the worsening of a previously diagnosed chronic health condition (see Fig. 1.2). However, physical examination and workup reveal a new, previously unrecognized condition that

Medical

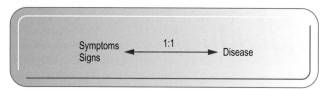

Figure 1.1 Diagnosis of illness presentation in the elderly: diagrammatic representation of the medical model. *(From Fried et al., 1991, with permission of Blackwell.)*

Synergistic morbidity

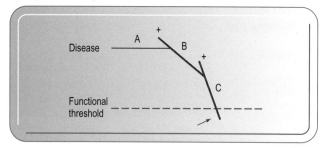

Attribution

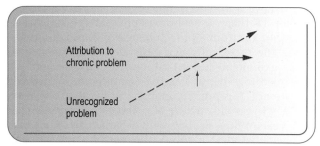

Figure 1.2 Diagrammatic representations of the synergistic morbidity model and the attribution model for diagnosis of illness presentation in a geriatric population. The description of each model is provided in the text. The arrow indicates the usual time of presentation for medical evaluation. *(From Fried et al., 1991, with permission of Blackwell.)*

is causing the declining health status. This possibility is especially important to consider when evaluating or caring for a patient labeled with a chronic disease such as multiple sclerosis, arthritis or postpolio syndrome. Not all new complaints are attributable to the chronic condition.

The *causal chain model* (Fig. 1.3) uses a scenario in which one illness causes another illness and functional decline. In this case, disease A causes disease B, which precipitates a chain of additional conditions that may worsen the present medical problems and/or lead on to further medical problems. For example, a patient who has severe arthritis (Fig. 1.3, disease A') is unable to maintain good cardiovascular health, which leads to heart disease (disease B'). The cardiac condition leads to peripheral vascular disease (disease C' and C''), which may reflect back to disease B and/or lead to amputation (disease D').

The final model is the *unmasking event model* (see Fig. 1.3). In this situation, a patient has an unrecognized

Causal chain

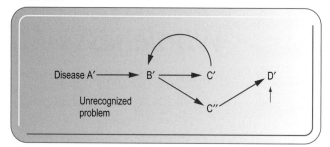

Unmasking event

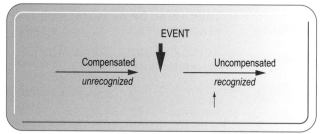

Figure 1.3 Diagrammatic representations of the causal chain model and the unmasking event model for diagnosis of illness presentation in a geriatric population. The description of each model is provided in the text. The arrow indicates the usual time of presentation for medical evaluation. *(From Fried et al., 1991, with permission of Blackwell.)*

and subclinical or compensated condition. When the compensating factor is lost, the condition becomes apparent and is often viewed as an acute problem. For example, a patient who suffers from vertigo may have functional balance because the visual and proprioceptive systems compensate for the deficient vestibular system. However, when walking on soft carpet or in a darkened room, this individual may have marked balance dysfunction, which may lead to a fracture resulting from a fall.

Coming from a similar perspective, Besdine (1990) presented several important concepts that relate to the complexity of geriatric care in his introduction to the first edition of the *Merck Manual of Geriatrics*. First, he states that 'the restriction of independent functional ability is the final common outcome for many disorders in the elderly'. Like Fried et al. (1991) in their attribution and unmasking event models, Besdine warns that 'deterioration of functional independence in active, previously unimpaired elders is an early subtle sign of untreated illness characterized by the absence of typical symptoms and signs of disease'. Additionally, he suggests that in geriatric medicine there is a 'poor correlation between type and severity of problem (functional disability) and the disease problem list'. Besdine warns further that finding a diseased organ or diseased tissue does not necessarily determine the degree of functional impairment that will be found. Another lesson he points out is that 'the severity of illness as measured by objective data does not necessarily determine the presence or severity of functional dependency'.

Recent research validates the need to consider the wholeness of each patient because of the complexity of treating the aging patient. Boyd et al. (2005a) studied clinical practice guidelines (CPGs) as they might apply to a hypothetical 79-year-old woman with chronic obstructive pulmonary disease, chronic heart failure, hypertension, stable angina, atrial fibrillation, hypercholesterolemia, diabetes mellitus, osteoarthritis and osteoporosis. They reported that most CPGs did not present modifications for these common geriatric comorbidities. Using the relevant CPGs, this hypothetical woman would have been prescribed 12 medications, with a high cost for the drugs and a risk of adverse drug interactions. In another study, Boyd et al. (2005b) reported that hospitalization for an acute illness in moderately disabled, community-dwelling older women led to increased dependence in daily living activities that persisted for up to 18 months after hospitalization and the resolution of the acute problem. They advocate improved interventions during *and* after hospitalization.

Because of the uniqueness of each aging patient, these authors advocate an interdisciplinary team approach to effectively treat the common multiple comorbidities. The whole person must be considered and rehabilitation services should be consulted in the majority of geriatric cases.

AGING CONSIDERATIONS AND REHABILITATION

PHYSICAL EXERCISE

Exercise, Fitness and Aging

From a philosophical point of view, one might consider movement to be the most fundamental feature of the animal kingdom in the biological world. Thus, life is movement. Movement is crucial not only for securing basic needs such as food, clothing and shelter but also for obtaining fulfillment of higher psychosocial needs that involve quality of life. Maintaining independence in thought and mobility is a universal desire that is, unfortunately, not achieved by all individuals.

The value of exercise and fitness is that they help to maintain the fullest vigor possible as time ages everyone. By exercising, it is hoped that one may enhance the quality of life, decrease the risk of falls and maintain or improve function in various activities. Fitness, however, is more than aerobic capacity. It is a state of mind and it involves endurance (physical work capacity determined by oxygen consumption, V_{O_2}), strength, flexibility, balance, coordination and agility.

The benefits of exercise are systemic and may be viewed as being favorable for all body systems and functions provided the phenomena of overuse are abated before causing irreparable damage to the organism. The opposite is also true; the deleterious effects of hypomobility (less than normal mobility) are profound (see Chapter 56). Box 1.1 presents a number of the beneficial effects of exercise on the actions of various cells, tissues and systems and on the organism as a whole, as judged by comparing the findings with those of sedentary people.

The beneficial effects of the systemic response to aerobic exercise by the cardiopulmonary and cardiovascular

---

Box 1.1 *Aging markers, risks and diseases modified by exercise*

- Aerobic capacity
- All cause of mortality
- Breast cancer
- C-reactive protein, inflammatory markers
- Chronic renal failure
- Cognitive function
- Colon cancer
- Congestive heart disease
- Coronary artery disease
- Depression
- Disability
- Falls
- Hyperlipidemia
- Hypertension
- Melanoma
- Obesity
- Osteoporosis
- Pancreatic cancer
- Peripheral vascular disease
- Prostate cancer
- Quality of life
- Sarcopenia
- Stroke
- Total adipose tissue
- Type 2 diabetes
- Walking speed

From Anand et al. (2008); Chodzko-Zajko et al. (2009); Fiatarone Singh (2004); Kokkinos (2012).

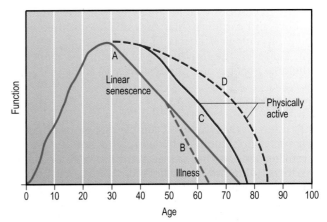

Figure 1.4 The age-related effects of exercise and illness on function. The age-related declines have been described as linear senescence and are shown in curve A. Illness such as heart disease or cancer may accentuate the decline, as shown in curve B. Physically active people benefit by delaying the declines in function, as shown in curve C. Curve D represents a higher level of fitness and the absence of misfortune.

systems as well as by the musculoskeletal system are fairly well recognized (Chodzko-Zajko et al., 2009; Kokkinos, 2012). These are presented hypothetically in Figure 1.4, which compares typical linear senescence, disease and levels of physical activity. Less well recognized is the association between fitness and mortality. A higher level of fitness is associated with a lower mortality rate (Fiatarone Singh, 2004). However, many exercise enthusiasts do not extol the benefits of exercise in order to lengthen lives. Rather, the emphasis is placed on experiencing a better quality of life by maintaining robust health and physical competence.

Exercise and Cancer

Over the past few decades, the death rate from heart disease has been decreasing and the incidence of cancer deaths increasing. A favorable relationship is now being shown between exercise and a lower risk of cancer (Kushi et al., 2012). The exact mechanism is not clear; however, it is possible that aerobic exercise enhances immune function, which reduces cancer risk. Aoi et al. (2010) showed in laboratory animals that exercise disrupted tumorigenesis and tumor necrosis factor alpha was decreased. It appears that the favorable effect of exercise on cancer risk is found in melanoma, breast, colon, prostate and pancreas cancers (Anand et al., 2008). Conversely, the risk of skin cancer increases for those who work and play in the sun without proper protection but exercise reduces risk for melanoma.

The benefits of exercise for cancer rehabilitation are not to be overlooked. Exercise may control or reduce nausea during chemotherapy. It reduces muscle loss and fatigue, enhances satisfaction with life and improves psychosocial adjustment (Ferrar et al., 2011). Immune function may also be maintained or enhanced. The full relationship between exercise and cancer remains to be defined.

Exercise is extremely diverse, ranging from passive range of motion to strength training in order to enhance muscle hypertrophy, and includes balance and gait mobility and cardiovascular fitness. The multiple interactive physiological effects of exercise require recognition. However, the importance of looking at the whole individual goes beyond physical activity alone.

CONFUSION

Only a few decades ago, the simple symptom of confusion was synonymous with aging and senility. Now it is well recognized that acute confusion may be caused by drugs (diuretics, tricyclic antidepressants, antihistamines, barbiturates, sleep-inducing hypnotic drugs); sleep deprivation; infection (typically respiratory or urinary tract infections that are not always febrile); diet; dehydration; sunset syndrome; cardiac arrhythmia; environmental influences (heat, cold); and stress (psychosocial factors, depression, anxiety). Thus, when working with an acutely confused patient, one must look at a variety of potential interactive causes (*Merck Manual*, 2011).

ADDITIONAL CONSIDERATIONS

In addition to a lifetime of experience yielding individual variations, other gerontological considerations influence rehabilitation care. For example, integrative functions decline to a greater degree than can be communicated by simple measurements. Nerve conduction velocity may show a small decline in a 65-year-old when compared with a 25-year-old, but integrative activities such as responding to postural perturbation are likely to show a greater decline. This is one reason why the etiology of falls in the elderly is complex, involving intrinsic factors (age-related changes in neuromusculoskeletal integrity) and extrinsic factors such as environmental challenges (*Merck Manual*, 2011).

Within the aging individual, the physiological range of homeostasis is sometimes greater than in younger individuals. As shown in Figure 1.5, the mean skin temperature of various body parts is similar when young and old adults are compared; however, the physiological range of measurements is greater in aging individuals (Kauffman, 1987).

When rehabilitating the geriatric patient, it is vital to remember that multiple chronic diseases are common and many systems may be involved. Because of the greater physiological range of homeostasis, and the multiple systems and diseases that may be involved, the aging individual is more vulnerable to the stresses of rehabilitation and presentation of illnesses may be unusual or ambiguous (see Box 1.2).

A comprehensive functional assessment is crucial if treatment is to be effective. Because of the many concomitant conditions and diseases, improvement may manifest more slowly and with a greater variety of responses during the rehabilitation process. This uniqueness is not always acceptable within the scope of the present healthcare delivery system and the classic medical model, as shown by Fried et al. (1991) in Figure 1.1.

THEORETICAL PERSPECTIVES

Since antiquity, humans have developed models and theories about the causes of aging. It is not the intent of this text to explore all of these causes; however, it may be helpful to perceive them at work in the fields of gerontology, which is the study of aging, and geriatrics, which is the medical treatment of aging persons. The intention of this book is to combine gerontology and geriatrics. For more extensive reviews of different theories of aging, the reader is referred to Weinert and Timiras (2003).

Hippocrates, at some time around 400 BC, and Aristotle, in approximately 350 BC, were in agreement when they wrote about health, medicine and old age. They reasoned that the human body consists of many structures that deal with the four conditions of heat, coldness, moistness and dryness. The following statement is attributed to Hippocrates in his work *On Ancient Medicine*: 'Whoever pays no attention to these things or paying attention does not comprehend them, how can he understand the diseases which befall a man?' Humankind was seen 'in relation to the articles of food and drink, and to his other occupations'. Aristotle, in his short physical treatise *On Youth and Old Age, On Life and Death, On Breathing*, wrote: 'Hence, of necessity, life must be coincident with the maintenance of heat, and what we call death is its destruction'. These perspectives remain viable today because we know that the loss of moistness (dehydration) and loss of heat (hypothermia) are serious conditions for all human beings.

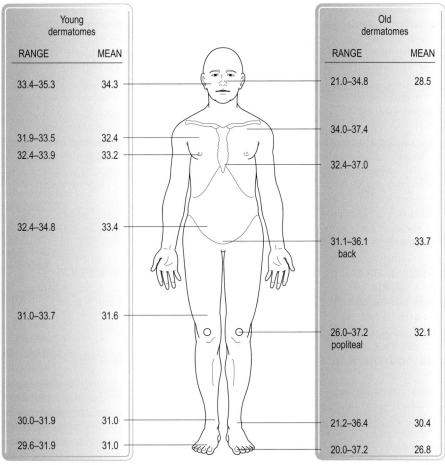

Figure 1.5 A sample of skin temperatures of young and old adults. Measurements of skin temperature were made by various investigators with different instruments under resting conditions without extreme ambient temperatures or humidity. When possible, range and mean temperatures (°C) are reported. *(From Kauffman, 1987, with permission.)*

Box 1.2   *Unusual presentations of illness in aging persons*

- **Acute bowel infarction:** confusion, may be no abdominal pain or tenderness.
- **Appendicitis:** may be diffuse abdominal pain, but tenderness should be right lower quadrant.
- **Bacteremia:** low grade fever may be absent. May manifest with general malaise, anorexia, night sweats.
- **Heart failure:** confusion, agitation, anorexia, weakness, fatigue, weight loss, lethargy.
- **Hyperparathyroidism:** fatigue, cognitive changes, anorexia, constipation, emotional instability.
- **Hyperthyroidism:** common signs may be absent. May present with tachycardia, weight loss, fatigue, weakness, tremors, palpitations, atrial fibrillation and apathetic affect.

- **Meningitis:** possibly no headache or nuchal rigidity but may be fever and cognitive change.
- **Myocardial infarction:** may be no chest pain but present with diaphoresis, dyspnea, epigastric distress, syncope, weakness, vomiting, confusion or upper extremity pain.
- **Peptic ulcer:** pain may be absent, possible presentations are painless gastrointestinal bleeding, severe anemia, bloating, nausea, early satiety.
- **Pneumonia:** malaise, anorexia, confusion, fever may be absent, cough without significant production.
- **Urinary tract infections:** confusion, dizziness, anorexia, fatigue, weakness possibly without fever.

Modified from Unusual presentations of illness in the elderly, in The Merck Manual of Geriatrics, 3rd edn, 2011.

Montaigne, the French philosopher of the 16th century, may be seen as arguing for the present day progressive decline model, or wear and tear theory. In his *Book One*, Essay 1.19, he notes 'how nature deprives us of light and sense of our own bodily decay. What remains to an old man of the vigour of his youth and better

day?' He saw withered bodies with decrepit motion. In his Essay 1.57, Montaigne noted that few people live to the age of 40 years and, 'To die of old age is a death rare, extraordinary, and singular, and, therefore, so much less natural than the others … and the more remote, the less to be hoped for.' He believed it to be 'an idle conceit to expect to die as a decay of strength which is the effect of extremist age'. Death, rather, was the result of everyday occurrences such as injuries, accidents, pleurisy or the plague and, hence, he calls these natural deaths.

More contemporary theories can be divided into social theories and biological theories. One social theory that created a tremendous amount of research is called the disengagement theory. Basically, this holds that the relationship between an aging person and society is changed because of the inevitable events within our life cycle and eventually ends with death, which is universal. This can easily be seen as life's central roles change, such as employment for men and motherhood for women. Disengagement for males and females is different and may be the result of individual ego changes or changes imposed by society, such as mandatory retirement. This theory has mostly been rejected by research; however, it provided a foundation for the study of the social process of aging, including changing roles (Achenbaum & Bengtson, 1994).

The activity theory is another social perspective that has been criticized but which has nonetheless provided a stimulus for research into a valid theory of aging. In essence, this theory states that, as people age, life satisfaction will be greater in those with activities. Those who maintain activities or add new activities, especially social activities, seem to have better morale, satisfaction, happiness and reduced mortality (Menec, 2003). It is important to note that, as presented earlier, there are many benefits to physical exercise; however, a rehabilitation specialist should not forget the importance of social activity as well.

There are several biological theories of aging that have generated considerable interest. The first and probably most widely accepted by general society is the progressive decline model. This indicates that the longer we live, the more wear and tear there is; everything progressively declines. From a gerontological perspective, it is well recognized that there are indeed changes with the passage of time. The research model of 40–50 years ago fits this perspective well, as most aging research was based on cross-sectional data in an attempt to define the age-related diminutions in nearly all measurements.

Another theory is the biological time clock, which postulates that aging is directed by biological time and, specifically, cell replication. Research has demonstrated that, in some cells, there are a finite number of replications after which apoptosis or programmed cell death occurs. This theory is used to support the concept that the human lifespan (the maximum number of years an individual can live) has not changed. In other words, we have a biological clock that says the maximum number of years a human being can live is somewhere between 120 and 130 years.

The free radical theory posits that, during the normal biological process of oxidative phosphorylation, free radicals are generated. This oxidative damage increases with age and can cause changes in cell function and tissues. Oxygen radicals contribute to the pathophysiological changes associated with aging and thus may be a factor in determining the lifespan of a species (Weinert & Timiras, 2003).

The cross-linkage theory suggests that aging takes place because of chemical reactions that create irreparable damage to DNA and cause subsequent cell death. This concept is easily used to explain the clinical complaint of increased stiffness that is common among elderly people.

The immune theory of aging indicates that a breakdown in the immune system leads to a greater risk of disease and cancer. As the body ages, it becomes less able to recognize itself, so the immune system produces antibodies that are detrimental to the host organism.

The error catastrophe theory of aging, sometimes referred to as the Orgel hypothesis, postulates that there are errors in cellular RNA transcription leading to faulty structures, especially proteins (Weinert & Timiras, 2003; Giampapa et al., 2012). This was considered to be a plausible explanation as to why earlier research demonstrated poor potential for muscle hypertrophy with increasing age. However, research by Fiatarone Singh (2004) and others (see Chapter 16) has indicated that the potential for muscle hypertrophy is sustained with increasing age and is achievable through proper exercise stimulus.

CONCLUSION

Aging is life's journey, leading to changes, uniqueness and, usually, multiple diagnoses. It ends in death. It is incumbent upon healthcare providers to recognize these complexities and thus, when rendering care, the whole patient must be considered, including societal and cultural implications. Each patient is more than a number or code.

REFERENCES

Achenbaum W, Bengtson V 1994 Re-engaging the disengagement theory of aging: on the history and assessment of theory development gerontology. Gerontologist 34:756–763
Anand P, Kunnumakara A, Sundaram C et al 2008 Cancer is a preventable disease that requires major lifestyle changes. Pharm Res 25:2097–2116
Aoi W, Naito Y, Takagi T et al 2010 Regular exercise reduces colon tumorigenesis associated with suppression on iNOS. Biochem Biophys Res Commun 399:14–19
Besdine R 1990. In: Abrams EB, Berkow R et al (eds) Introduction to The Merck Manual of Geriatrics. Merck & Co., Inc., Rahway, NJ, pp. 2–4
Boyd C, Darer J, Boult C et al 2005a Clinical practice guidelines and quality of care for older patients with multiple comorbid diseases. J Am Med Assoc 294:716–724
Boyd C, Xue Q, Guralnik J et al 2005b Hospitalization and development of dependence in activities of daily living in a cohort of disabled older women: The Women's Health and Aging Study I. J Gerontol Biol Sci 60A:888–893
Boyd C, McNabney M, Brandt N et al 2012 Guiding principles for the care of older adults with multimorbidity: an approach for clinicians: American Geriatrics Society Expert Panel on the Care of Older Adults with Multimorbidity. J Am Geriatr Soc 60:E1–E25
Giampapa V, Burzynski S, Pero R 2012 Theories of aging. Old and new concepts of the aging process. In: Giampapa V (ed) The Principles and Practice of Antiaging Medicine for the Clinical Physician, River Publishers, Aalborg, Denmark
Chodzko-Zajko W, Proctor D, Fiatarone Singh M et al 2009 Exercise and physical activity for older adults. Med Sci Sport Exer 41:1510–1530
Ferrar R, Huedo-Medina T, Johnson B et al 2011 Exercise interventions for cancer survivors: a meta-analysis of quality of life outcomes. Ann Behav Med 41:32–47

Fiatarone Singh M 2004 Exercise and aging. Clin Geriatr Med 20:201–221

Fried LP, Storer D, King D et al 1991 Diagnosis of illness presentation in the elderly. J Am Geriatr Soc 39:117–123

Kauffman T 1987 Thermoregulation and the use of heat and cold. In: Jackson O (ed) Therapeutic Considerations for the Elderly, Churchill Livingstone, New York, pp. 72

Kokkinos P 2012 Physical activity, health benefits, and mortality risk. International Scholarly Research Network Cardiology, Article ID 718789. http://dx.doi.org/10.5402/2012/718789

Kushi L, Doyle C, McCullough M et al 2012 American Cancer Society guidelines on nutrition and physical activity for cancer prevention. CA Cancer J Clin 62:30–67

Menec V 2003 The relationship between everyday activities and successful aging: a 6-year longitudinal study. J Gerontol Soc Sci 58B:S74–S82

The Merck Manual of Geriatrics (Beers MH, Berkow R, eds) 2011 3rd edn. [Online]. Merck & Co. Inc., Whitehouse Station, NJ. (Accessed at www.merckmanuals.com/professional/geriatrics.html December 2013)

Weinert B, Timiras P 2003 Invited review: theories of aging. J Appl Physiol 95:1706–1716

White D, Neogi T, Nevitt M et al 2013 Trajectories of gait speed predict mortality in well-functioning older adults: the health, aging and body composition study. J Gerontol A Biol Sci Med Sci 68:456–464

Chapter 2

Skeletal muscle function in older people

WALTER R. FRONTERA • ANA RODRIGUEZ ZAYAS • NATIVIDAD RODRIGUEZ

CHAPTER CONTENTS

INTRODUCTION

Impairments such as muscle weakness, slowing of movement, loss of muscle power, and early muscle fatigue are prominent features of old age in humans. Further, aging is often accompanied by inactivity and chronic diseases (such as diabetes) that will further impair neuromuscular performance. As a result, many elderly men and women have functional limitations on walking, lifting, maintaining postural balance and recovering from impending falls. This leads to reduced activity and limited participation in recreation and work. The independence associated with mobility is critical in achieving a longer lifespan and, especially, a high quality of life.

The increasing number and overall percentage of the elderly population, and the social and economic consequences of this increase, underline the importance of understanding neuromotor performance in elderly people. The mechanisms underlying these changes are complex (Stackhouse et al., 2001), but alterations in the components of the motor units play a central role. By the age of 80, 40–50% of muscle strength, muscle mass (sarcopenia), alpha motoneurons, and muscle cells are lost. In this chapter we will briefly discuss the age-associated changes in the motor unit, skeletal muscle functional properties and skeletal muscle structural characteristics (Table 2.1).

MOTOR UNIT

In the elderly there is a decrease in the number of functional motor units associated with a concomitant enlargement of the cross-sectional area of the remaining units. This motor unit remodeling is achieved by selective denervation of muscle fibers, especially type IIb fibers, followed by reinnervation by axonal sprouting from juxtaposed innervated units. This process leads not only to a net loss of fibers and functional motor units but also to an increase in motor unit size (fibers dispersed throughout a larger territory) and, therefore, the amplitude and duration of the motor unit potential. Other changes in the motor unit that could contribute to the development of sarcopenia (defined as the loss of muscle mass associated with aging) are: (i) a decrease in the number of nerve terminals; (ii) fragmentation of the neuromuscular junction; (iii) a decrease in neurotransmitter release; and (iv) a lower number of acetylcholine receptors.

MUSCLE STRENGTH

Muscle strength is an important determinant of functional capacity in older people. In general, the decline in strength starts during the third decade of life and accelerates during the sixth and seventh decades. The overall rate of decline is approximately 8–12% per decade (Schiller et al., 2000), although there is significant variation and some individuals seem to better preserve their strength over time (Hughes et al., 2001). Because of this decline in maximal force-generating capacity (strength), older people may be performing many activities while generating force closer to their maximal capacity. Under these conditions, acute or chronic diseases, hospitalization resulting from trauma or surgery, and inactivity may accelerate the decline in strength and result in disability. This concept of 'close to maximal capacity' is important during rehabilitation when the aim is not only to regain muscle strength but also to enhance functional reserve.

It may be possible to modify these age-related alterations with behavioral and pharmacological interventions, including exercise training, nutritional interventions and, in some cases, hormonal supplementation. Strength and

Table 2.1 **The effects of aging at different levels of the human motor unit**	
Motor unit	↓ Number and ↑ size
Contractile properties	↑ Contraction and 50% relaxation times
Anterior horn	↓ Number of cells
Peripheral nerves	↓ Motor nerve conduction velocity
Neuromuscular junction	↓ More complex and irregular
Muscle	
Strength	↓ Upper and lower extremities
Contractility	Slower velocity
Mass	↓ Segmental and whole body
Fiber number	↓ Types I and II (mainly)
Fiber area	↓ Type II fiber area
Fiber type	No change; increased co-expression of myosin isoforms
Local muscular endurance	↑ Endurance; earlier onset of fatigue

↑ = increase; ↓ = decrease.

power training in frail older people is accompanied by improvements in physical function (Bean et al., 2009).

PHYSIOLOGY OF MUSCLE WEAKNESS

Physiologically, muscle weakness may result from a decrease in the ability to activate the existing muscle mass, a reduction in the quantity of muscle tissue and therefore in the number of force-generating cross-bridges, a decrease in the force developed by each cross-bridge, or a combination of all three factors. Several studies have reported changes in neural mechanisms, including central nervous system drive, a delay in the conduction velocity of motor nerve fibers and a delay in transmission at the level of the neuromuscular junction. The ability to maximally activate the remaining motor unit pool is relatively preserved in the aged, although some reports show a significant reduction (Reid et al., 2012).

On the other hand, muscle atrophy is associated with a reduction in the number of motor neurons in the spinal cord and an incomplete reinnervation of denervated muscle cells leading to a decrease in the number and size of muscle fibers. Alterations in the proportions of motor units and myofibers of different types, particularly a decrease in the number or the relative cross-sectional area of type II fast fibers, are also noticeable. Finally, losses in the ability of the sarcoplasmic reticulum to handle calcium within the fibers, changes in the myosin molecule, an increased passive resistance of the connective tissue structures and/or a combination of factors may contribute to altered contractile behavior.

SPEED OF CONTRACTION AND MUSCLE POWER

An important characteristic of neuromuscular performance is the time course of muscle actions. This characteristic can be studied *in vivo* with measurements of the speed of contraction of individual muscles or muscle groups and *in vitro* by measuring the maximal shortening velocity of single muscle fibers (Larsson & Moss, 1993). This property is important because the velocity of movement (and thus power generation) can have greater relevance than absolute muscle strength in the ability to perform a number of the activities of daily living and in fall prevention (Foldvari et al., 2000).

In the elderly, the *in vivo* muscle twitch (evoked by electrical stimulation) is characterized by prolonged contraction and 50% relaxation times. Thus, fused tetanic forces occur at lower stimulation frequencies, an adaptation that increases muscle efficiency. However, this adaptation also lengthens the time for muscle relaxation, thus impairing the ability to perform rapid powerful alternating movements. Human studies have shown that the time to produce the same absolute and relative forces during voluntary contractions is lengthened in the elderly and, therefore, the ability to generate explosive force (power) and to accelerate a limb is reduced (Frontera et al., 2000; Bean et al., 2009). These alterations have a negative effect on the protective reactions used before or during a fall. Several studies have shown that, in the elderly, differences in skeletal muscle power could explain more of the variability in function and disability, particularly during lower intensity tasks such as walking compared with higher intensity activities such as climbing stairs or rising from a chair.

MUSCLE ENDURANCE

Muscle fatigability is another important component of performance. Fatigue is typically measured as a loss of force during repeated or continuous activation. Alterations in muscles with advanced adult age that may contribute to a decrease in muscle endurance include reduced blood supply and capillary density, impairment of glucose transport and therefore substrate availability, lower mitochondrial density, decreased activity of oxidative enzymes, decreased rate of phosphocreatine repletion, reduced maximal motor unit discharge rates, and a general shift toward a greater type I fiber composition. The extent of these age-related alterations appears to vary by muscle group and level of habitual physical activity.

The effect of age on local muscular endurance is controversial and probably reflects different experimental approaches. The results of some investigations suggest that older men and women fatigue more than younger subjects, which is consistent with studies in animal models. Other investigators, however, have demonstrated similar fatigability in young and old subjects, whereas still others have observed that older adults fatigue less than younger. Even less clear than the effect of old age on the magnitude of fatigue is its effect on the potential mechanisms that contribute to fatigue.

MUSCLE MASS AND QUALITY

Lower muscle mass or sarcopenia has been correlated with poor physical function. The likelihood of physical disability (measured as ability to perform activities of daily living) increases when the skeletal muscle index (SMI, determined by estimating whole body muscle mass and dividing by height in meters squared) values are lower than $5.75\,kg/m^2$ in women and $8.50\,kg/m^2$ in men (Melton et al., 2000). In that study, these cut-off points were used to determine the degree of sarcopenia.

The factors contributing to the loss of muscle mass with age seem to be a reduction in the numbers of both type I and type II muscle fibers and a decline in cross-sectional area, predominantly of type II fibers; the cross-sectional area of type I fibers seems to be well maintained. As mentioned above, the relative area (percentage of type II fibers divided by the mean fiber area of type II fibers) occupied by type II fibers is significantly reduced with age. Because of the differences in mechanical properties among muscle fiber types, the reduction in relative area of a fiber type may contribute to the changes in whole muscle contractile behavior. In addition to the loss of muscle mass, recent studies show that the quality of muscle fibers (force-generating capacity adjusted for muscle size) is impaired in older men (Frontera et al., 2008, 2012).

PROTEIN METABOLISM

Age-related changes in the processes that regulate muscle protein mass contribute to sarcopenia as protein is the primary structural and functional macromolecule in muscle. Muscle protein content is determined by the balance between protein synthesis and breakdown and some studies in humans have shown that postabsorptive muscle protein synthesis declines with age. Although not all studies concur, it seems that mixed muscle and myofibrillar protein synthesis rates decline with advanced adult age (Welle et al., 1993; Toth et al., 2005) and increase in response to exercise training (Hasten et al., 2000). It is also possible that a failure to degrade damaged proteins and replacing them with newly synthesized proteins contribute to age-related decline in muscle mass and quality of muscle proteins (Irving et al., 2011).

Specific skeletal muscle proteins and groups of proteins, with important structural and functional roles, have different rates of metabolism. From both quantitative and functional perspectives, myosin heavy chain (MyHC) is the most important protein in skeletal muscle and its synthesis is reduced with age. In addition to the overall mass of MyHC protein, the type of MyHC isoforms expressed has relevance for both the metabolism and functionality of aging muscle. Because the isoforms are synthesized at different rates, a change in MyHC isoform distribution with age could contribute to altered MyHC protein synthesis rates. Additionally, a shift in MyHC isoform distribution can alter muscle performance given the different functional properties of each isoform (Hasten et al., 2000; Marx et al., 2002).

INFLAMMATION

Aging is associated with increased cytokine levels/production and reduced circulating insulin-like growth factor-1 (IGF-1) concentrations. Studies in cultured myocytes and animal models have demonstrated the catabolic effects of cytokines and the anabolic effects of IGF-1 on skeletal muscle. Because aging is associated with increased levels of inflammatory markers, it is thought that immune activation may contribute to the development of sarcopenia. There is a growing body of evidence suggesting that chronic inflammation is one of the most important biological mechanisms underlying the decline in physical function that is often observed over the aging process. The plasma concentration of interleukin 6 (IL-6), a cytokine that plays a central role in inflammation, tends to increase with age and high serum levels of IL-6 predict disability in the elderly (Taaffe et al., 2000). Also, some preliminary data suggest that IL-6 is associated with accelerated sarcopenia (Taaffe et al., 2000). Resistance exercise training reduces the levels of inflammatory markers and increases muscle mass and function. IGF-1 is an important modulator of muscle mass and function across the entire lifespan and recent findings show that low plasma IGF-1 levels are associated with poor knee extensor muscle strength, slow walking speed and self-reported difficulties with mobility tasks. These findings suggest a role for IGF-1 in the causal pathway leading to disability in the elderly. IL-6 inhibits the secretion of IGF-1 and its biological activity, and higher plasma IL-6 levels and lower plasma IGF-1 levels have been associated with lower muscle strength and power (Hasten et al., 2000). Thus, the balance between the catabolic effect of cytokines and the anabolic effect of IGF-1 may play an important role in the development of sarcopenia (Barbieri et al., 2003).

MUSCLE FAT

Fat infiltration of skeletal muscle is common among the elderly and has been associated with a greater incidence of mobility limitations. Muscle attenuation (indicative of fat infiltration) is an independent determinant of incident mobility limitations. People in the lowest quartile of muscle attenuation (with the greatest amount of fat infiltration into the muscle) were 50–80% more likely to develop mobility limitations during follow-up, which was independent of muscle area, muscle strength or total body fat mass.

REFERENCES

Barbieri M, Ferrucci L, Ragno E et al 2003 Chronic inflammation and the effect of IGF-1 on muscle strength and power in older persons. Am J Physiol 284:E481–487

Bean JF, Kiely DK, LaRose S et al 2009 Increased velocity exercise specific to task (InVEST) training vs. the National Institute on Aging's (NIA) strength training program: changes in limb power and mobility. J Gerontol A Biol Sci Med Sci 64:983–991

Foldvari M, Clark M, Laviolette LC et al 2000 Association of muscle power with functional status in community-dwelling elderly women. J Gerontol A Biol Sci Med Sci 55:M192–199

Frontera WR, Hughes VA, Fielding RA et al 2000 Aging of skeletal muscle: a 12-year longitudinal study. J Appl Physiol 88:1321–1326

Frontera WR, Reid KF, Phillips EM et al 2008 Muscle fiber size and function in elderly humans: a longitudinal study. J Appl Physiol 105:637–642

Frontera WR, Rodriguez Zayas A, Rodriguez N 2012 Aging of human muscle: understanding sarcopenia at the single muscle cell level. Phys Med Rehab Clin N Am 23:201–207

Hasten DL, Pak-Loduca J, Obert KA et al 2000 Resistance exercise acutely increases MyHC and mixed muscle protein synthesis rates in 78–84 and 23–32 year olds. Am J Physiol 278:E620–626

Hughes VA, Frontera WR, Wood M et al 2001 Longitudinal muscle strength changes in older adults: influence of muscle mass, physical activity and health. J Gerontol A Biol Sci Med Sci 56:B209–17

Irving BA, Robinson MM, Sreekumaran Nair K 2011 Age effect on myocellular remodeling: Response to exercise and nutrition in humans. Ageing Res Rev 11:374–389

Larsson L, Moss RL 1993 Maximum velocity of shortening in relation to myosin isoform composition in single fibres from human skeletal muscles. J Physiol 472:595–614

Marx JO, Kraemer WJ, Nindl BC et al 2002 Effects of aging on human skeletal muscle myosin heavy-chain mRNA content and protein isoform expression. J Gerontol A Biol Sci Med Sci 57:B232–238

Melton III JL, Khosla S, Crowson C et al 2000 Epidemiology of sarcopenia. J Am Geriatr Soc 48:6215–6230

Reid KF, Doros G, Clark DJ et al 2012 Muscle power failure in mobility-limited older adults: preserved single fiber function despite lower whole muscle size, quality and neuromuscular activation. Eur J Appl Physiol 112:2289–2301

Schiller B, Casas Y, Tarcy B et al 2000 Age-related declines in knee extensor strength and physical performance in healthy Hispanic and Caucasian women. J Gerontol A Biol Sci Med Sci 55:B563–569

Stackhouse SK, Stevens JE, Lee SC et al 2001 Maximum voluntary activation in nonfatigued and fatigued muscle of young and elderly individuals. Phys Ther 81:1102–1109

Taaffe DR, Harris TB, Ferrucci L et al 2000 Cross-sectional and prospective relationships of interleukin-6 and C-reactive protein with physical performance in elderly person: MacArthur studies of successful aging. J Gerontol A Biol Sci Med Sci 55:M706–708

Toth MJ, Matthews DE, Tracy RP et al 2005 Age-related differences in skeletal muscle protein synthesis: relation to markers of immune activation. Am J Physiol 288:E883–891

Welle S, Thornton C, Jozefowicz R et al 1993 Myofibrillar protein synthesis in young and old men. Am J Physiol 264:E693–698

Chapter 3
Effects of aging on bone

DOUGLAS J. DIGIROLAMO • EMILY L. GERMAIN-LEE • JAY SHAPIRO

CHAPTER CONTENTS

INTRODUCTION

Bone is a tissue that gives form to the body, supporting its weight, protecting organs and facilitating movement by providing attachments for muscles so that they can act as levers in the musculoskeletal system. Bone also plays a major role in mineral homeostasis, serving as a reservoir for calcium to allow for its precisely controlled levels, critical to proper nerve and muscle function. In addition to these classically defined roles of the skeleton, recent research suggests the skeleton may play an unanticipated role in other aspects of metabolism as well, namely, glucose homeostasis (DiGirolamo et al., 2012). The skeleton consists of a mineralized organic matrix in which highly specialized cells, including osteoblasts (bone-forming cells), osteoclasts (bone-resorbing cells) and osteocytes (a terminally differentiated subset of osteoblasts that reside in the bone matrix) produce and maintain this mineralized matrix through their concerted actions (Marks & Popoff, 1988). Although the basic cellular processes involved in the modeling and remodeling of the skeleton remain the same throughout life, their relative activity – and ultimately skeletal strength and shape – can be influenced by a variety of factors, including hormones, physical activity, pharmacologic agents and nutrition, which guide both the growth and involution of the skeleton with age.

BONE STRUCTURE

MACROSCOPIC ANATOMY

Bones vary widely in their shape but can be broadly divided into two categories: flat bones (skull bones, scapula, mandible etc.) and long bones (tibia, femur, humerus etc.). These two categories are based largely upon the method of bone formation by which these bones develop. The bones of the appendicular skeleton, as well as the bones of the vertebral column and base of the skull, are formed by endochondral ossification. In this process, bone forms through a cartilage intermediate that is produced by chondrocytes, providing a template upon which osteoblasts can form new bone. By contrast, flat bones, including most of the bones of the face, the vault of the skull and the pelvis, are formed by intramembranous ossification. In intramembranous ossification, osteoblasts form bone matrix *de novo*, without a cartilage anlage (Olsen et al., 2000). These two methods of bone formation are present, not only during development, but in adult life as well. For example, a fracture heals via endochondral bone formation, where a cartilage callus is first formed, followed by bone formation in the callus, and finally, remodeling to repair the fracture site to its original anatomic state. Intramembranous bone formation is less common in adult life, but it can be observed in such clinical settings as distraction osteogenesis for limb lengthening. In this procedure, an osteotomy is performed on a long bone and the two ends of bone are separated by a defined distance and externally fixed. This distance is then increased at regular intervals by turning a screw on the external fixator, stimulating bone formation between the bone ends and, thus, lengthening the limb. In the space between the two cut bone ends, known as the distraction gap, osteoblasts form new bone directly, without a cartilage template.

Gross inspection of the skeleton reveals that there are two types of bone tissue found in all bones: cortical (compact) bone and trabecular (cancellous) bone. Cortical and trabecular bone have the same matrix composition (predominantly collagen with hydroxyapatite mineral), but the mass of the cortical bone matrix per unit volume is considerably greater due to higher mineral content. Much of the difference between cortical and trabecular bone is secondary to the dual function of bone as both a structural element and a reservoir for calcium in the body. Cortical bone forms the dense outer shell (cortex) of long bones, such as the femur, and bears the majority of mechanical force exerted on the skeleton. This dense (generally 90% by volume calcified) cortical tissue is the predominant type of bone in the diaphysis (midshaft) of long bones, where little or no trabecular bone is present. Moving toward the end of the femur, the thick cortical walls of the diaphysis become thinner and increase in diameter. This region, the metaphysis, is where spicules of trabecular bone emerge, formed from the cartilage template produced by chondrocytes in the epiphyseal growth plate. Still further toward the end of the femur and nearing the knee, atop the epiphysis, is a thin shell of subchondral bone that underlies articular cartilage. As well as occupying the ends of long bones as described above, trabecular bone forms the greater part of each vertebral body and is present at other sites such as the iliac crest. Interestingly, despite accounting for nearly 60% of the surface area of bone in the body, trabecular bone represents only 25% of the total skeletal mass (Fernandez-Tresguerres-Hernandez-Gil et al., 2006). This allows a large surface area for osteoclasts to resorb bone mineral and release calcium rapidly when necessary, while the dense cortical bone remains relatively unaffected and capable of bearing the mechanical loads applied to the skeleton. Trabecular bone is the most metabolically active compartment of the skeleton, with a high rate of turnover and a blood supply that is much greater than that of cortical bone (Banse, 2002).

MICROSCOPIC ANATOMY

To carry out the diverse functions of bone formation and bone resorption, as well as maintain mineral homeostasis, bone cells assume specialized forms categorized by function, morphology and characteristic location. Bone cells derive from two distinct progenitor cell types: mesenchymal stem/stromal cells (MSCs) and hematopoietic stem cells (HSCs). The mesenchymal cells give rise to bone-lining cells, pre-osteoblasts, osteoblasts and osteocytes. Hematopoietic stem cells, which are also residents of the bone marrow and reside within specialized 'niches', give rise to monocyte/macrophage precursors (as well as many other immune cell lineages not immediately relevant to the discussion of bone cells) that ultimately differentiate into pre-osteoclasts and osteoclasts.

Undifferentiated MSCs that have the potential to become osteoblasts reside in bone canals, along the endosteum (inner lining of the cortex), periosteum (outer lining of the cortex), trabeculae and within the marrow. These cells, under the control of numerous growth factors and hormones – like sex steroids, growth hormone (GH) and insulin-like growth factor-1 (IGF-1) – will undergo proliferation, differentiate into pre-osteoblasts, and finally become mature osteoblasts to form new bone. Mature, bone-forming osteoblasts never appear or function individually but are always found in clusters along the bone surface where they produce osteoid – bone matrix composed predominantly of highly ordered collagen fibrils, upon which hydroxyapatite mineral forms. Upon completing bone formation, active osteoblasts follow one of three courses: they may remain on the surface of the bone, decrease their synthetic activity and assume the flatter form of bone-lining cells; they may surround themselves with matrix, further differentiate to become osteocytes and continue

mineralizing bone (roughly 10–20%); or they may undergo programmed cell death and disappear from the site of bone formation.

Osteoclasts are large, multinucleated cells found on bone surfaces that are responsible for bone resorption. Specific hormones and growth factors produced by osteoblasts and osteocytes (as well as other cell types in pathological conditions) influence their development from monocyte/macrophage precursors. These precursors differentiate and fuse together to form osteoclasts on the surface of bone, where they are very efficient at destroying bone matrix. They begin by binding to the surface of the bone and creating a sealed space between the cell membrane and the bone matrix. Osteoclasts then use membrane bound proton pumps to transport protons into, and acidify, the sealed space, decreasing the pH from ~7 to 4. This acidic environment solubilizes the hydroxyapatite mineral found in bone, releases calcium and phosphate, and allows access to the organic matrix, which is degraded by osteoclast-secreted acid proteases. Growth factors bound in the organic matrix are also released during this process, which stimulates osteoblast formation and, thus, couples the two processes to ensure proper maintenance of bone mass (Fernandez-Tresguerres-Hernandez-Gil et al., 2006).

Osteocytes, as mentioned previously, differentiate from a subset of mature osteoblasts and become entombed within lacunae in the newly formed, mineralizing bone matrix. During this process, they form an extensive network of neuron-like cell projections, connecting them to other osteocytes, osteoblasts, bone-lining cells, blood vessels and nerves through a vast canalicular network in bone. Unlike the relatively short-lived osteoclasts (~3 weeks) and osteoblasts (~3 months), osteocytes have an estimated life span of 10–20 years in humans and comprise 90–95% of bone cells. Although their precise function has yet to be clearly established, osteocytes are widely assumed to play a role in transducing mechanical forces into anabolic signals within bone, allowing bone to adapt to increased or decreased activity. More recently, they have been demonstrated to produce factors that can regulate both osteoblast and osteoclast development, implicating them as a possible 'conductor' in orchestrating bone remodeling. In addition, osteocytes secrete a growth factor known as fibroblast growth factor 23 (FGF23), which regulates phosphate homeostasis through endocrine actions in the kidney (Bonewald, 2011). Despite their populous nature and obvious importance in bone physiology, many aspects of osteocyte function remain undefined due to their highly specialized microenvironment in bone and the inherent technical difficulty in generating faithful model systems.

BONE REMODELING

Throughout life, physiological remodeling (removal and replacement) of bone occurs without affecting the shape or density of the bone. In fact, bone is far more dynamic than many people appreciate, with the entire human skeleton being replaced through the process of normal remodeling approximately every 10 years. A complete remodeling cycle includes osteoclast activation, resorption of bone, osteoblast activation, formation of new bone at the site of resorption and reversion to a resting state. Skeletal remodeling takes place in response to a number of growth factors, hormones and mechanical signals, some of which have already been discussed. This continual remodeling serves to repair micro-damage that accumulates in the bone over time (or major damage in the case of fracture) and ensures the mechanical integrity of bone (Cardoso et al., 2009; Herman et al., 2010), as well as maintains calcium and phosphate homeostasis (Quarles, 2008). It should be noted that this process is distinct from bone modeling, in which osteoblasts form bone continuously without a resorptive cycle. One such example of modeling is periosteal apposition during pubertal growth, in which periosteal osteoblasts continuously deposit new bone on the periosteal surface to increase the cross-sectional area of long bones, dramatically increasing their strength (Bachrach & Asbmr, 2009).

Remodeling occurs both on the surface of trabecular and cortical bone, as well as within cortical bone. Internal, or osteonal, remodeling begins when osteoclasts create a tunnel through bone. These cutting cones of osteoclasts create large resorption cavities. Immediately behind the cutting cones, groups of osteoblasts follow the advancing osteoclasts. Layers of osteoblasts arrange themselves along the surface of the resorption cavity behind the osteoclast and deposit successive lamellae of new bone matrix, which then mineralize and fill the canal. In normal adult bone, remodeling is usually a tightly controlled process in which bone resorption equals bone formation, achieved through teams of osteoblasts and osteoclasts forming tightly regulated basic multicellular units (BMUs) or bone remodeling units (BRUs) (Dempster, 2003; Kular et al., 2012).

Unfortunately, this delicate balance inherently favors the destruction of bone, as the resorptive portion of a remodeling cycle takes ~3 weeks, compared to the ~3 months required for complete bone formation. The nature of this inherent imbalance between formation and resorption time can be easily appreciated if one imagines a packet of bone as a moving truck. Unpacking a moving truck (resorption) is relatively quick and easy, as one simply has to pull out the contents and put them elsewhere. By contrast, packing a moving truck (formation) requires careful attention to packing the items into boxes, carefully arranging those boxes to fit into the cargo space and then securing them all for the move (in the case of our metaphor – producing collagen, secreting and aligning collagen fibrils, and mineralizing the newly formed matrix). Primary osteoporosis is defined as a pathological unbalancing of bone resorption and formation that leads to persistent deficits of bone mass, which ultimately translates into increased fracture susceptibility. Changes in bone homeostasis may also result secondary to a number of other pathological conditions (e.g. cancer, kidney disease, endocrine disorders etc.).

AGE-RELATED CHANGES IN BONE

SEX STEROIDS

The peak bone mass attained in adult life is governed by a combination of genetic, hormonal (predominantly estrogen, GH and IGF-1), nutritional and mechanical factors (Bonjour et al., 1994). In humans, this peak bone mass is attained in the third decade of life and is a large determinant of one's susceptibility to fractures later in life regardless of sex, race etc. This is because a slow loss of bone mass (~0.5% per year) begins around age 40 in both sexes and continues for the rest of life (Mazess, 1982; Clarke & Khosla, 2010). Thus, the greater the peak bone mass, the longer it will take to reach the threshold of bone density at which fracture risk begins to rise. At all ages, however, women have a lower bone mass than men and, with increasing age, this gap widens. This widening gap is largely the result of an accelerated period of bone loss in women around the time of menopause, when bone loss rates of 5–6% per year for up to 10 years are not unusual. This accelerated loss is associated with the withdrawal of estrogen (Dempster, 2003; Downey & Siegel, 2006; Clarke & Khosla, 2010), which results in a dramatic increase in bone resorption – as much as 90% as indicated by biochemical markers. Bone formation markers are also increased during menopause (although formation decreases later), but only by 45%, thus favoring the high turnover bone loss that decimates bone density in postmenopausal women.

Men do not suffer the sudden drop in sex steroid levels and concomitant rapid bone loss observed in women, and they are, therefore, less susceptible to fracture than females with age because they retain a greater percentage of their bone mass. The slow bone loss that is observed in men was long assumed to result from reduced serum testosterone, as it predominates in many other aspects of male physiology. In recent years, however, numerous studies have proved this not to be the case. In fact, reduced estrogen – converted by aromatase from testosterone – is responsible for age-related bone loss in men. Further, estrogen actually appears to be critical for proper bone growth in men earlier in life. Thus, throughout life in both genders (even into the eighth and ninth decades), estrogen has significant anabolic effects on bone, and its reduction accounts for a large portion of age-related bone loss (Raisz, 2005; Clarke & Khosla, 2010).

SECONDARY HYPERPARATHYROIDISM

In both genders, levels of parathyroid hormone (PTH) tend to gradually increase with age (Ledger et al., 1995). Parathyroid hormone is responsible for maintaining calcium balance in the body, in concert with vitamin D, by regulating bone resorption, calcium reabsorption in the kidney and calcium absorption in the small intestine (Quarles, 2008). Although this gradual rise in PTH level is certainly multifactorial, vitamin D deficiency is common among the elderly and likely contributes to bone loss by disturbing this PTH–vitamin D endocrine loop. Thus, as blood calcium would drop from reduced vitamin D (thereby less intestinal calcium absorption and renal reabsorption of calcium), PTH would stimulate additional bone resorption to maintain healthy blood calcium levels, thereby further contributing to age-related bone loss. Although the cause of vitamin D deficiency with age remains unclear, recent studies have identified an inverse correlation between BMI and vitamin D levels (Wortsman et al., 2000; Vimaleswaran et al., 2013). It has been suggested that the reduction in vitamin D may result from the increased fat mass capable of storing vitamin D and thus sequestering it from the circulation, providing a possible explanation for reduced vitamin D levels in the elderly since body fat, much to our chagrin, unavoidably increases with age.

GH/IGF-1 AXIS

As mentioned previously, bone formation rates decline in both sexes with increasing age. This drop in osteoblast function and bone formation parallels the reduction in GH and IGF-1 levels observed in aging (Perrini et al., 2010). These two factors have been demonstrated, in numerous studies, to be critical for osteoblast proliferation, survival and function, particularly mineralization. The GH/IGF-1 axis is also intimately linked to the positive effects exerted by sex steroids on bone, particularly during pubertal growth (Olson et al., 2011). Thus, it is likely that the decline of GH and IGF-1 levels also contributes significantly to age-related bone loss by failing to sufficiently stimulate bone formation.

OTHER FACTORS

Immobility (Fox et al., 2000), systemic acidosis (as might be seen with poor kidney function) (Arnett, 2003) and some pharmaceutical agents (e.g. glucocorticoids and corticosteroids) (Weinstein, 2012) can also impact on bone mass in a negative fashion. Unfortunately, it is not uncommon for an individual to encounter one or more of these negative modifiers with increasing age. In this regard, reduced activity and/or immobility due to injury pose an especially significant risk for exacerbating frailty and increasing fracture risk in an elderly population. Muscle mass and function also suffer significant loss with disuse and aging (Jang & Van Remmen, 2011; Marimuthu et al., 2011), leading to an increased propensity for falls and, with concomitant bone loss, even greater risk of fracture. Other factors that can impair osteoblast function and stimulate osteoclast formation/activity include chronic inflammation – possibly associated with cellular senescence (Freund et al., 2010) – and accumulated oxidative damage (Almeida et al., 2007), as might be observed with long-term obesity. Finally, nutrition also contributes to bone loss with age, beyond simply vitamin D and calcium intake, since appetite decreases. This decrease in appetite results in a reduction of both macro- and micronutrients across the board. For example, reduced protein intake has been linked to

poorer bone mass in the elderly (Bonjour, 2011). This observation is not surprising when one considers that the vast majority of bone is organic collagen matrix, which requires adequate protein building blocks to produce and maintain.

FUTURE DIRECTIONS

Recent advances in our understanding of the molecular signals regulating bone and muscle growth have identified new strategies to enhance bone mass, either directly or indirectly. Of course, the most effective strategy to prevent bone loss and reduce fracture risk begins much earlier in life by attaining the highest peak bone mass possible and raising the 'starting point' for inevitable bone decline. Maintaining high activity levels with age is also critical to help reduce the rate at which bone mass declines as a result of the many factors described above. Higher activity levels with age also help to avoid frailty by maintaining greater muscle mass and function, which helps to maintain balance and coordination. Unfortunately, these proactive measures may not be sufficient if genetics happen not to be on one's side in the fight against bone loss. In such a case, a number of pharmaceutical interventions are also available to help stave off age-related bone loss. Bisphosphonates are the current standard therapy for bone loss and help spare bone mass by blocking osteoclasts from resorbing bone, although they cannot replace lost bone mass. By contrast, intermittent administration of PTH can replace lost bone mass (and is currently the only pharmaceutical available that is capable of this action), although the mechanism by which it does so remains elusive. Novel biologics are emerging as well, which exploit our knowledge of the bone remodeling pathways to help tip the balance back in favor of formation. One example of such a biologic is denosumab (marketed under the trade name Prolia), which is an antibody that binds and inhibits a factor that promotes osteoclast formation, known as RANKL.

In addition to such strategies that directly target aspects of the bone remodeling process, recent studies have demonstrated a viable alternative to enhance bone mass indirectly by increasing the mechanical load on bone, via increased muscle. One example of such a strategy is to increase muscle mass by targeting pathways that would normally suppress muscle growth, such as myostatin (McPherron et al., 1997). Myostatin is produced by skeletal muscle cells, circulates in the blood and acts to limit muscle cell hypertrophy. When the activity of myostatin is lost by naturally occurring mutations in the gene, this suppressive force is relieved and muscles attain striking size and mass. Perhaps not surprisingly, given the known effects of muscle force to promote maintenance or increase of bone mass, animals with myostatin mutations also have markedly increased bone mineral density (Hamrick et al., 2003). Although the precise mechanisms by which myostatin is normally regulated and exerts these effects in muscle are still being elucidated, its activity can be blocked artificially by a variety of both naturally occurring and engineered myostatin-binding proteins (reviewed in Lee, 2004, 2012). It is not hard to envision how beneficial such a therapy could be in addressing age-related frailty, as the improved muscle mass would not only help to improve bone mass indirectly, but also improve balance, coordination and mobility to further reduce risk of falls and fractures.

CONCLUSION

The rapid increase in the understanding of the mechanisms that control the development and regulation of the musculoskeletal system has led to many advances in our approach to treating age-related bone loss. The ability to manipulate formation and resorption of bone, both directly and indirectly, will substantially improve the treatment of musculoskeletal disorders. Further, interventions that exploit this knowledge of bone cell function offer the potential to treat numerous other diseases with skeletal involvement.

REFERENCES

Almeida M, Han L, Martin-Millan M et al 2007 Skeletal involution by age-associated oxidative stress and its acceleration by loss of sex steroids. J Biol Chem 282:27285–27297

Arnett T 2003 Regulation of bone cell function by acid-base balance. Proc Nutr Soc 62:511–520

Bachrach LK, ASBMR 2009 Skeletal development in childhood and adolescence In: Primer on the Metabolic Bone Diseases and Disorders of Mineral Metabolism. John Wiley & Sons, New York, pp. 74–79.

Banse X 2002 When density fails to predict bone strength. Acta Orthop Scand Suppl 73:1–57

Bonewald LF 2011 The amazing osteocyte. J Bone Miner Res 26:229–238

Bonjour JP 2011 Protein intake and bone health. Int J Vitam Nutr Res 81:134–142

Bonjour JP, Theintz G, Law F et al 1994 Peak bone mass. Osteoporos Int 4(suppl1):7–13

Cardoso L, Herman BC, Verborgt O et al 2009 Osteocyte apoptosis controls activation of intracortical resorption in response to bone fatigue. J Bone Miner Res 24:597–605

Clarke BL, Khosla S 2010 Physiology of bone loss. Radiol Clin North Am 48:483–495

Dempster DW 2003 The pathophysiology of bone loss. Clin Geriatr Med 19:259–270, v–vi

DiGirolamo DJ, Clemens TL, Kousteni S 2012 The skeleton as an endocrine organ. Nat Rev Rheumatol 8:674–683

Downey PA, Siegel MI 2006 Bone biology and the clinical implications for osteoporosis. Phys Ther 86:77–91

Fernandez-Tresguerres-Hernandez-Gil I, Alobera-Gracia MA, del-Canto-Pingarron M et al 2006 Physiological bases of bone regeneration II. The remodeling process. Med Oral 11:E151–E157

Fox KM, Magaziner J, Hawkes WG et al 2000 Loss of bone density and lean body mass after hip fracture. Osteoporos Int 11:31–35

Freund A, Orjalo AV, Desprez PY et al 2010 Inflammatory networks during cellular senescence: causes and consequences. Trends Mol Med 16:238–246

Hamrick MW, Pennington C, Byron CD 2003 Bone architecture and disc degeneration in the lumbar spine of mice lacking GDF-8 (myostatin). J Orthop Res 21:1025–1032

Herman BC, Cardoso L, Majeska RJ et al 2010 Activation of bone remodeling after fatigue: differential response to linear microcracks and diffuse damage. Bone 47:766–772

Jang YC, Van Remmen H 2011 Age-associated alterations of the neuromuscular junction. Exp Gerontol 46:193–198

Kular J, Tickner J, Chim SM 2012 An overview of the regulation of bone remodelling at the cellular level. Clin Biochem 45:863–873

Ledger GA, Burritt MF, Kao PC et al 1995 Role of parathyroid hormone in mediating nocturnal and age-related increases in bone resorption. J Clin Endocrinol Metab 80:3304–3310

Lee S-J 2004 Regulation of muscle mass by myostatin. Ann Rev Cell Dev Biol 20:61–86

Lee S-J 2012 Myostatin: regulation, function, and therapeutic applications. In: Hill JA, Olson EN (eds) Muscle: Fundamental Biology and Mechanisms of Disease. Academic Press, London, pp. 1077–1084

McPherron AC, Lawler AM, Lee S-J 1997 Regulation of skeletal muscle mass in mice by a new TGF-beta superfamily member. Nature 387:83–90

Marimuthu K, Murton AJ, Greenhaff PL 2011 Mechanisms regulating muscle mass during disuse atrophy and rehabilitation in humans. J Appl Physiol 110:555–560

Marks Jr. SC, Popoff SN 1988 Bone cell biology: the regulation of development, structure, and function in the skeleton. Am J Anat 183:1–44

Mazess RB 1982 On aging bone loss. Clin Orthop Relat Res 165:239–252

Olsen BR, Reginato AM, Wang W 2000 Bone development. Annu Rev Cell Dev Biol 16:191–220

Olson LE, Ohlsson C, Mohan S 2011 The role of GH/IGF-I-mediated mechanisms in sex differences in cortical bone size in mice. Calcif Tissue Int 88:1–8

Perrini S, Laviola L, Carreira MC 2010 The GH/IGF1 axis and signaling pathways in the muscle and bone: mechanisms underlying age-related skeletal muscle wasting and osteoporosis. J Endocrinol 205:201–210

Quarles LD 2008 Endocrine functions of bone in mineral metabolism regulation. J Clin Invest 118:3820–3828

Raisz LG 2005 Pathogenesis of osteoporosis: concepts, conflicts, and prospects. J Clin Invest 115:3318–3325

Vimaleswaran KS, Berry DJ, Lu C et al 2013 Causal relationship between obesity and vitamin D status: bi-directional Mendelian randomization analysis of multiple cohorts. PLoS Med 10:e1001383

Weinstein RS 2012 Glucocorticoid-induced osteoporosis and osteonecrosis. Endocrinol Metab Clin North Am 41:595–611

Wortsman J, Matsuoka LY, Chen TC 2000 Decreased bioavailability of vitamin D in obesity. Am J Clin Nutr 72:690–693

Chapter 4

Effects of age on joints and ligaments

BRIAN J. ECKENRODE

INTRODUCTION

The older adult exhibits specific joint and ligamentous changes, which ultimately can affect an individual's function. All joints and ligaments in the body undergo age-related changes; in addition, they are susceptible to age-related diseases and injury. This can result in the loss of joint mobility and have impact on activities of daily living, occupational demands, and restrict community participation and recreation. Changes to these tissues have been theorized to be a result of multiple factors, including age, history of trauma, and local or systemic pathology. Clinicians should appreciate these alterations in the joints and ligaments of older individuals and understand how this may impact on rehabilitation.

JOINTS AND LIGAMENTS

The joints of the skeletal system function to provide for movement of bones and absorb shock through the cushioning provided by joint fluid and cartilage (Levangie & Norkin, 2011). Three main types of joints are found in the human body: immovable, slightly movable, or freely movable joints. Immovable joints function to provide support between bones and will fuse to provide added support and strength. Slightly movable joints contain either hyaline cartilage (i.e. ribs to sternum) or fibrocartilage (i.e. intervertebral discs). With age, hyaline cartilage becomes stiffer from a decrease in water content and an increase in calcium which can lead to and increase in joint stiffness and less elasticity (Levangie & Norkin, 2011). Fibrocartilage also has been shown to lose water during aging, which also stiffens these joints and decreases movement. Collagen in the ligaments of these joints becomes shorter, stiffer and less elastic (Levangie & Norkin, 2011).

Freely movable joints are the most common type of joint in the body; they connect the appendicular skeleton to the axial skeleton. These joints have a synovial membrane that is responsible for the secretion and maintenance of synovial fluid, providing nutrition to articular cartilage and lubricating the joint space through loading and compression (Ahmed et al., 2005). With age, the synovial membrane becomes stiffer and is less able to produce and remove synovial fluid (Levangie & Norkin, 2011). Ligaments and tendons surround these joints, providing additional support and controlling movement. The capsule, ligaments and tendons of the synovial joint are all made up of fibrous connective tissue that provides stability and strength to the joint (Ahmed et al., 2005). There is an increased formation of cross-links and loss of elastic fibers of the capsule and ligaments with age, which increases joint stiffness and decreases the joint's ability to provide cushioning and movement (Levangie & Norkin, 2011). The loss of mobility of joints can have a significant impact in overall function of an individual (Box 4.1).

CARTILAGE

Articular cartilage functions to provide the articulating surfaces with a load-bearing and force-distribution structure, and also serves to lower the friction between the joint surfaces (Ahmed et al., 2005). Articular cartilage is absent of vascular elements but is in contact with synovial fluid on the articular surface of joints (Carrington, 2005). It consists of an extracellular matrix, made up of primarily type II collagen, water and proteoglycans, and chondrocytes. Chondrocytes function to maintain

---

Box 4.1 *Summary of age-related changes in synovial joints and ligaments*

- Decreased flexibility of the joint capsule
- Decreased quality and quantity of synovial fluid
- Increased cross-link formation in ligaments
- Increased stiffness of ligaments
- Decreased amount of elastic fibers
- Decreased quality of information from joint receptors

Adapted from Amundsen, 2007.

Box 4.2 *Summary of age-related changes in articular cartilage*

- Decreased cartilage thickness and stiffness
- Increased cartilage defect severity and prevalence
- Decreased quality and content of proteoglycans
- Decreased content of glycosaminoglycans
- Decreased water content
- Decreased synovial fluid perfusion
- Increased resistance to gliding

Adapted from Amundsen, 2007.

cartilage homeostasis through the production of extracellular matrix component (Leong & Sun, 2011). The extracellular matrix makes up the majority of the cartilage volume and is highly hydrated to allow for the diffusion of nutrients from the surrounding synovium, underlying bone, or perichondrium. Water contributes up to 80% of the wet weight of articular cartilage, some of which moves freely in and out of the tissue (Buckwalter et al., 2005). Articular cartilage is dependent on the repetitive compression and release from weight-bearing for nutrition as it allows for the drawing in and exudation of water from the matrix.

The risk of progressive degeneration of cartilage increases with time in individuals older than 40 years of age (Buckwalter et al., 2000); see Box 4.2. Due to its avascular nature, articular cartilage has low metabolic activity and poor regenerative capacity (Pearle et al., 2005). The relative immobility of chondrocytes and limited proliferation of mature chondrocytes contribute to the limited repair capacity (Buckwalter & Mankin, 1997). The concentration of glycosaminoglycans found in cartilage can vary with patient age, cartilage injury and disease (Buckwalter et al., 2005). With aging there is an overall decrease in proteoglycan synthesis and content (DeGroot et al., 2004), in addition the proteoglycans produced are smaller and more irregular (Leong & Sun, 2011). A decrease in water content and decrease in the ability of proteoglycans to absorb and hold water result in a decreased ability to dissipate joint forces.

Previously, it has been thought that the degenerative changes seen with osteoarthritis (OA) were considered a natural part of aging (Ahmed et al., 2005). However, these changes may not be an inevitable consequence of aging; rather changes in the aging joint may make it more susceptible to degeneration (Ahmed et al., 2005). Aging is the most influential risk factor for developing OA (Leong & Sun, 2011), in conjunction with other risk factors (Loeser, 2010). Structural, compositional and mechanical alterations to cartilage with age have been shown to vary from changes of degenerative diseases such as OA (Roth & Mow, 1980; Buckwalter et al., 1993; Buckwalter et al., 1994; Martin & Buckwalter, 2002). With aging, the decline of the chondrocytes increases the risk of articular cartilage degeneration and limits the ability of the cells to repair the tissue once degenerative changes occur (Martin & Buckwalter, 2002) and may predispose the joint to damage when exposed to mechanical loads (Leong & Sun, 2011).

Evidence for changes in cartilage with aging comes primarily from radiographs, magnetic resonance imaging (MRI) studies or *in vitro* experiments. MRI studies have shown that with increasing age, cartilage thickness decreases for some joints (Karvonen et al., 1994). Karvonen et al. (1994) found significant cartilage thinning in the weight-bearing aspect of the femoral condyles, but not in the posterior femoral condyles, tibia or patella in individuals without OA. Hudelmaier et al. (2001) found a significant reduction of cartilage thickness in the femur of elderly women and men, and in the patella of elderly women. Ding et al. (2005) reported that the most consistent knee structural changes with increasing age are an increase in cartilage defect severity and prevalence, cartilage thinning and an increase in bone size, with inconsistent change in cartilage volume (Ding et al., 2005).

In vitro experiments have revealed that the compressive (Armstrong et al., 1979; Armstrong & Mow, 1982) and tensile (Kempson, 1991) stiffness of articular cartilage decreases with age. These studies suggest that, with age, individuals exhibit a larger amount of cartilage deformation under a given load (Hudelmaier et al., 2001). This increase in cartilage deformation may initiate or accelerate the OA process (Hudelmaier et al., 2001). Other *in vitro* studies have shown that an increase in pentosidine levels may increase cartilage stiffness (Bank et al., 1998). Pentosidine is a product of non-enzymatic glycation in healthy human articular cartilage. This biomarker has been shown to increase 50-fold from age 20 years to age 80 years, indicating a slower turnover of collagen after maturity (Bank et al., 1998; DeGroot et al., 2004). The increase in pentosidine levels may lead to less deformation of cartilage and cause faster degeneration. Many other mechanisms for causes of cartilage changes over time have been studied including chondrocyte senescence, chondrocyte apoptosis, accumulation of advanced glycation end products and chondrocyte death due to oxidative stress (Carrington, 2005).

One final theory for changes in cartilage with aging is that individuals may utilize different motor strategies during functional tasks (Papa & Cappozzo, 2000), which may adversely affect joint cartilage. Changes in one tissue of the musculoskeletal system are likely to affect interacting tissues (Carrington, 2005). This is an important factor to consider when working with older individuals.

CONCLUSION

In summary, the thinning of knee joint cartilage occurs physiologically with aging, in the absence of cartilage disease (Hudelmaier et al., 2001). Changes to the joints and ligaments may result in the development of OA. The loss of muscle mass and a gain in fat mass may also contribute to the progression of OA, as this may change forces of joint loading (Loeser, 2010). Rehabilitation interventions, such as manual techniques, therapeutic exercise, neuromuscular re-education and gait training aimed at specific joint impairments and general functional limitations, may help to address the deficits and achieve the goals of the older patient.

REFERENCES

Ahmed MS, Matsumura B, Cristian A 2005 Age-related changes in muscles and joints. Phys Med Rehabil Clin North Am 16(1):19–39

Amundsen LR 2007 Effects of age on joints and ligaments. In: Kauffman TL, Barr JO, Moran ML (eds) Geriatric Rehabilitation Manual, 2nd edn. Churchill Livingstone, Philadelphia, PA, pp. 17–20

Armstrong CG, Bahrani AS, Gardner DL 1979 In vitro measurement of articular cartilage deformations in the intact human hip joint under load. J Bone Joint Surg Am 61(5):744–755

Armstrong CG, Mow VC 1982 Variations in the intrinsic mechanical properties of human articular cartilage with age, degeneration, and water content. J Bone Joint Surg Am 64(1):88–94

Bank RA, Bayliss MT, Lafeber FP et al 1998 Ageing and zonal variation in post-translational modification of collagen in normal human articular cartilage. The age-related increase in non-enzymatic glycation affects biomechanical properties of cartilage. Biochem J 330:345–351

Buckwalter JA, Mankin HJ 1997 Articular cartilage. Part I: Tissue design and chondrocyte-matrix interactions. J Bone Joint Surg 79(4):600–611

Buckwalter JA, Woo SL, Goldberg VM et al 1993 Soft-tissue aging and musculoskeletal function. J Bone Joint Surg Am 75(10):1533–1548

Buckwalter JA, Roughley PJ, Rosenberg LC 1994 Age-related changes in cartilage proteoglycans: quantitative electron microscopic studies. Microsc Res Tech 28(5):398–408

Buckwalter JA, Martin J, Mankin HJ 2000 Synovial joint degeneration and the syndrome of osteoarthritis. Am Acad Orthop Surg Instr Course Lect 49:481–489

Buckwalter JA, Mankin HJ, Grodzinsky AJ 2005 Articular cartilage and osteoarthritis. Am Acad Orthop Surg Instr Course Lect 54:465–480

Carrington JL 2005 Aging bone and cartilage: cross-cutting issues. Biochem Biophys Res Commun 328(3):700–708

DeGroot J, Verzijl N, Wenting-van Wijk MJ et al 2004 Accumulation of advanced glycation end products as a molecular mechanism for aging as a risk factor in osteoarthritis. Arthritis Rheum 50(4):1207–1215

Ding C, Cicuttini F, Scott F et al 2005 Association between age and knee structural change: a cross sectional MRI based study. Ann Rheum Dis 64(4):549–555

Hudelmaier M, Glaser C, Hohe J et al 2001 Age-related changes in the morphology and deformational behavior of knee joint cartilage. Arthritis Rheum 44(11):2556–2561

Karvonen RL, Negendank WG, Teitge RA et al 1994 Factors affecting articular cartilage thickness in osteoarthritis and aging. J Rheumatol 21(7):1310–1318

Kempson GE 1991 Age-related changes in the tensile properties of human articular cartilage: a comparative study between the femoral head of the hip joint and the talus of the ankle joint. Biochim Biophys Acta 1075(3):223–230

Leong DJ, Sun HB 2011 Events in articular chondrocytes with aging. Curr Osteoporos Rep 9(4):196–201

Levangie PK, Norkin CC 2011 Joint Structure and Function: A Comprehensive Analysis, 5th edn. FA Davis, Philadelphia, PA

Loeser RF 2010 Age-related changes in the musculoskeletal system and the development of osteoarthritis. Clin Geriatr Med 26(3):371–386

Martin JA, Buckwalter JA 2002 Aging, articular cartilage chondrocyte senescence and osteoarthritis. Biogerontology 3(5):257–264

Papa E, Cappozzo A 2000 Sit-to-stand motor strategies investigated in able-bodied young and elderly subjects. J Biomech 33(9):1113–1122

Pearle AD, Warren RF, Rodeo SA 2005 Basic science of articular cartilage and osteoarthritis. Clin Sports Med 24(1):1–12

Roth V, Mow VC 1980 The intrinsic tensile behavior of the matrix of bovine articular cartilage and its variation with age. J Bone Joint Surg Am 62(7):1102–1117

Chapter 5

Aging and the central nervous system

EDWARD JAMES R. GORGON • ROLANDO T. LAZARO • DARCY A. UMPHRED

INTRODUCTION

Changes that occur in the central nervous system (CNS) with aging can be discussed at a cellular level such as mitochondrial function, at a system level such as the size of a nuclear mass, at a functional level such as the ability to stand up, or at a social level in terms of the capacity to interact and communicate. These changes, however, do not necessarily translate into limitations in the ability to engage in preferred activities and meaningful participations among healthy older people. Maintaining good health and independent function is possible in advanced age. It has been established, however, that activity limitations and participation restrictions are common among older people (Wilkie et al., 2006). Multiple-system physiological decline in old age and the complex effects of chronic pathologies and significant acute diseases interact and result in diminished functional capacity in this population (Fried & Guralnik, 1997). It is therefore important to differentiate changes in the CNS that occur with healthy aging from those that are caused by disease or pathology (Woodford & George, 2011). Recent work investigating CNS changes in aging suggests that neuroplasticity is a strong driver in the variability of functional performance in older people. This will be discussed in more detail in the latter portion of this chapter.

As humans age, their activity level changes and their activity choices, nutritional intake and general health vary tremendously. Genetic predisposition as well as environmental factors account for how the CNS acts and reacts in an aging individual, so it becomes difficult to compare one individual with another. The accumulation of minor and major traumas, exposure to toxins and other environmental factors, and overuse and disuse of major body systems affect the function of the CNS. Therefore, difficulties arise when asking, 'What is expected with normal aging?' Yet, when one looks specifically at the CNS, certain changes are observed with aging. These changes may not immediately result in disease, impairments, activity limitations or participation restrictions. However, the cumulative effects of these changes may dramatically influence an aging adult's ability to compensate and relearn once a specific pathology has created functional loss and a decrease in quality of life.

NERVOUS SYSTEM CHANGES WITH AGING

Multiple cross-sectional and longitudinal studies have established that in the brain there is a decrease in regional volume and gyral thickness with an increase in ventricular size in advanced age (Long et al., 2012). Substantial changes in brain regional volumes have been demonstrated, especially for the caudate and cerebellum, and, to a similar extent, the prefrontal and inferior parietal cortices and hippocampus (Raz et al., 2005). However, in the healthy aging human, there is no conclusive research showing that these and other changes, such as those in neurotransmitters, are related to impairment in function. Loss of conduction velocity in sensory and motor nerves within the central and peripheral nervous systems as well as loss of myelin sheaths and the large myelinated fibers with advancing age have also been reported (Werner et al., 2012). Although these losses might appear to explain a propensity for falling as a result of delays in sensory information processing and motor response, a connection between a deficiency in one part of the system and the overall function of an individual has not been proven. Further, it is not understood why some individuals can function well into very old age without severe functional loss whereas others cannot.

CHANGES IN SENSATION

Changes that occur in both the visual and auditory systems with aging have been documented (Stephen et al., 2010). As noted in Chapter 51, visual acuity may decline gradually from middle age onward and may decrease rapidly in the eighth decade of life (Sjöstrand et al., 2011). Traditional testing of acuity is valid for reading but not for functional tasks such as observing walking surface variations in a darkened room. Other common changes, such as altered color discrimination and light adaptation, can translate to impaired vision and may add to any visual acuity deficit. For an individual to respond appropriately, it requires receiving an input, processing that input both perceptually and cognitively at an intellectual level or automatically at a motor level, and finally selecting the motor response that best matches the environmental requirements. An individual who wears bifocal or trifocal lenses and glances down for visually augmented feedback may see a distorted image, so inaccurate information is sent to the CNS. Thus, the motor response may be appropriate for the input being received but inappropriate for the actual environment. Conversely, an individual with visual impairment may respond adequately to environmental demands and show no signs of motor limitation. The nervous system functions on consensus and will always use other sensory systems and prior learning, if available, to determine how to respond to visual information.

As discussed in Chapter 52, hearing loss is also common among older people, the causes of which are either peripheral or central deficits generally associated with disease or biological aging (Chisolm et al., 2003). Loss of auditory acuity translates to difficulty in hearing and word recognition, or difficulty carrying on a normal conversation within a noisy environment, which may result in isolation and self-exclusion from participation in group activities. Although hearing loss itself does not impair movement, often, when the auditory portion of the eighth cranial nerve is involved, the vestibular portion is also affected (Møller, 2000). This can potentially result in vertigo and impaired balance, and increase an individual's risk of falling (Ishiyama, 2009).

CHANGES IN COGNITIVE FUNCTION AND THE LIMBIC SYSTEM

The processing of information in the cognitive and emotional areas of the CNS cannot be ignored when considering CNS changes with aging, with or without pathology. Subtle non-pathological declines do occur with aging in key cognitive domains and correlate with, but not necessarily impair, the ability to carry out daily function (Vance et al., 2010). Changes across cognitive domains and across older individuals are not uniform, with some cognitive functions demonstrating greater extents of change than others (Glisky, 2007). This underscores the need to consider the complexity of cognitive decline in clients undergoing rehabilitation. Healthcare providers must remember that when the processing or learning of cognitive materials becomes a problem, procedural learning of motor programs will become the only avenue to regain functional control over movement. Principles of motor learning then become paramount in optimizing the therapeutic environment for client improvement (Umphred et al., 2013: 69).

The healthcare provider must consider the emotional (limbic) system in all clients, especially when looking at CNS function. Emotions are controlled and modified by the limbic system. This system has extensive connections to the hypothalamus, so emotion is often expressed through regulation of the autonomic nervous system and in the tone of the striated muscle system (Groenewegen & Uylings, 2000). The hypothalamus regulates the areas of the brainstem that control the heart, lungs, internal organs and immune system.

Many behavioral syndromes have been attributed to this area of the brain. The most pertinent to older people, the 'general adaptive syndrome' (GAS), was described by Hans Selye in 1956 (Stojanovich, 2010; Umphred et al., 2013: 111). Today, it is considered a response to stress and can be observed in any frail individual, including older persons with fragile bodily systems. The GAS response is paradoxical to the anticipated response. Under stress, an individual generally has a sympathetic response, with an increase in heart rate and blood pressure and a fight–flight reaction. In the GAS, the same environmental conditions initially cause a sympathetic response but, over time and sometimes quickly, individuals may experience a switch to a parasympathetic reaction. Blood pressure drops, heart rate decreases, blood pools in the periphery and level of consciousness can drop. The GAS is a survival response to stress because, without such a response, the increase in heart rate and blood pressure would cause heart failure or vascular rupture. Treatment based on the GAS signs and symptoms may be aimed at increasing the sympathetic response, which may cause an even greater paradoxical reaction.

Research since 1956 has shown that hormone levels increase with stress (Lupien et al., 2009) and the amount of hormones elicited increases with age (McEwen, 2002). By virtue of advanced age, a client may be very close to multiple-system failure and would be considered frail. A client may have recently developed a disease that adds stress to an already frail system. If the corresponding treatment creates more stress in the individual, it may result in a GAS, which has the potential of evolving into a life-threatening situation. The client's response may be to withdraw while the healthcare provider's reaction might be to increase the level of input to motivate or heighten arousal in the client. With further withdrawal, the client can potentially die from heart failure from diminished heart rate and blood pressure. The healthcare provider should thus evaluate the client's emotional response to the environment and try to keep a homeostatic autonomic balance. This requires being sensitive to body functions controlled by the limbic system such as respiration, blood pressure and level of alertness, as well as specific motor responses to interventions (Umphred et al., 2013: 111).

CHANGES IN THE MOTOR SYSTEM

The motor system, with the guidance of prior learning and experience as well as analysis by the CNS of current needs, modulates the state of the motor pools in the brainstem and spinal cord. This modulation drives peripheral nerves and orchestrates synergistic interactions of muscle groups to create functional behavior. Ultimate control of human behavior is the result of the consensus of a variety of areas within the motor system. Understanding how this motor system controls movement is the key to identifying motor impairments and understanding activity limitations.

The areas typically considered to be part of the motor system are the premotor and motor areas of the frontal lobes, basal ganglia, cerebellum, brainstem, spinal cord and all the interneurons that link these systems. The thalamus plays a key role as a relay station and modulator whereas the limbic system has the ability to alter the state of motor responses both directly and indirectly (Kandel et al., 2012). The sensory areas guide and alter existing motor programs. Where the motor system begins and ends is not clear because there are so many interdependent systems that loop between one area and another. Therefore, a linear analysis is not appropriate. There is not one specific area that controls motor output, yet certain nuclear masses are responsible for specific aspects of motor function. When any one of these areas is impaired, specific clinical symptoms manifest. Motor control over base tone in striated muscles is regulated by many areas, so a deficit does not automatically reflect the involvement of a specific area. A deficit in one loop of many interconnected neuronal loops might present a clinical problem that would make it appear as if a nuclear mass or system was damaged.

Research does show that the motor system changes with age (Mora et al., 2007), although such changes cannot account entirely for the functional changes observed in older people (Mahncke et al., 2006). For example, it is accepted that there is an age differential when looking at modulation of the H-reflex which may be due to the aging neuromuscular system (Koceja & Mynark, 2000). Similarly, control over the Ia fibers as a readiness state for spontaneous movement decreases with aging (Mankovsky et al., 1982) and may be associated with a decrease in the ability to modulate inhibitory function (Fujiyama et al., 2009). Moreover, proprioceptive input has less influence on the motor cortex excitability (Degardin et al., 2011). These suggest that an aging CNS no longer has the refined regulating ability over preprogrammed synergistic patterning. Comparing performance of younger adults to older adults indicates that older people possibly begin to lose some movement automaticity and compensate through increased brain network activity (Wu & Hallett, 2005). Whether these changes are due to disuse or aging is not clear. As there are central, muscle and mechanical changes with aging, a decrease in functional ability is considered multifactorial (Degardin et al., 2011). The significance of these changes may be more meaningful following injury or disease. If the aging CNS loses some of its plasticity or ability to adapt, then it may take more time to learn new programs or alter existing ones. This might explain why aging adults seem to exhibit synergistic patterns very quickly following injury, whereas younger adults may take more time to develop the same abnormal patterns, given appropriate conditions.

A complete explanation of the specifics of the motor control system (Shumway-Cook & Woollacott, 2012) is not within the scope of this chapter, but a brief overview of the system might help the reader to understand and appreciate its complexity. The frontal lobe of the brain not only helps process the motivation to move (prefrontal) but also modulates information that travels between primary motor centers such as the basal ganglia and cerebellum (Kandel et al., 2012). In addition, it plays a primary role in regulating, but not dictating, fine and gross motor function through the corticospinal and corticobulbar systems. Normal movement results from the coordinated work of multiple areas that influence the final common pathways of motor neurons. After summating and modulating messages from other areas of the CNS, the frontal lobe sends messages concurrently to the basal ganglia and cerebellum (Kandel et al., 2012). In turn, these centers formulate new motor plans or draw upon existing plans to correctly modulate the motor system. If either a center or the loops connecting the centers is damaged or diseased, then motor function may be incoordinated and unsuited to the environmental context of the activity. The cerebellum, unlike the basal ganglia, is simultaneously aware of the peripheral kinematics through input from proprioceptors in the limbs and trunk, and from the vestibular system based on the position of the head in space. Similarly, the cerebellum is constantly updated on the existing states of the motor pool through ascending tracts that send that information directly to the anterior cerebellar lobes. Thus, the cerebellum is considered a synergistic programmer and plays a key role in feed-forward regulation of movement.

The role of the cerebellum in higher-center regulation of motor programming interfaces with the limbic system as well as the frontal lobe and basal ganglia. Deficits within the frontal lobe, limbic system or basal ganglia can affect cerebellar function and have been shown to trigger, what appears to be, cerebellar neuronal damage (Umphred et al., 2013: 601, 631–7). The cerebellum is not only responsible for helping write new programs, it also ensures that the programs being used at any one moment match the environmental context. If there is a mismatch between the desired movement sequence and environmental stimuli, the cerebellum will try to readjust the synergistic patterns and run the program that matches the environmental demands. For example, if an individual is walking on a level cement surface and suddenly the surface changes because of a crack or a hole, the cerebellum will adjust balance strategies in order to regain the center of gravity and hence allow the person to keep walking. If the perturbation created is too large, such that the cerebellum cannot correct the patterns being run, consensus of the CNS will determine what new program should be initiated.

The basal ganglia are responsible for changing the plan of movement and initiating new programs, whereas the cerebellum, in preparation for the changes to take place, regulates the state of the motor generators (base tone) and controls the force, speed and direction of movement. For example, if an individual is rising to a standing position and goes beyond vertical and starts to fall, the basal ganglia change the motor setting from rising to vertical to falling. Both the basal ganglia and cerebellum play roles in modulating posture but the specific roles are different. The basal ganglia and aspects of the cerebellum contribute in the development of new motor programs and refinement of existing ones. Both relay specific motor programming to the frontal lobes through the thalamus and down to the motor generators of the cranial and spinal neurons through the brainstem. Therefore, changes in any of these structures or in the pathways between them that occur with aging could have critical effects on normal movement. Along with pathology, such changes can become cumulative and eventually result in altered motor performance and loss of function. For example, a reported loss with age of Purkinje cells in the cerebellum has not been related to movement impairment (Rajput et al., 2011). However, this change along with cerebellar degeneration or a cerebellar stroke would be cumulative and the result might be a greater deficit than would occur in a young adult without Purkinje cell loss who develops a similar pathology.

HEALTHY AGING AND PATHOLOGICAL AGING IN THE CNS

Various studies have endeavored to describe changes in the CNS that occur with healthy aging by differentiating those with changes that mark pathological aging. Longitudinal studies have reported brain loss and multiple-domain cognitive decline over time in healthy older people, with significantly extensive changes observed on follow-up measurement in those who eventually developed mild cognitive impairment or dementia, compared to those who did not (Johnson et al., 2009). Evidence suggests that in healthy aging, brain shrinkage can be minimal and does not appear to correlate with any important limitation in functional ability. In terms of neuropathologic changes, such as the development of senile plaques or neurofibrillary tangles, even in the 'oldest old', or people who were at least 85 years of age, such change can be minimal and cognitive ability can remain stable (Green et al., 2000). These normal aging-related changes are in stark contrast to the severe neuronal loss found in people with neurodegenerative conditions such as Alzheimer's disease, frontotemporal dementia and Parkinson's disease (Yankner et al., 2008), and the extensive neuropathologic changes and steep cognitive decline seen in oldest old people with Alzheimer's dementia (Green et al., 2000). Literature supports the concept that older people can be healthy and functionally stable into advanced age, and pathological conditions precede and determine functional loss. The aging process may affect the potential of the nervous system to adapt, but age is only one factor that influences that potential. Aging should never be considered the primary cause of functional limitations or restrictions in normal life activities.

MODELS OF REHABILITATION FOR OLDER PEOPLE

It is important for clinicians to follow a rehabilitation model that allows them to understand the relationship between the health condition, consequent abnormalities in body structure and function, and the impact of these on, as well as interactions with, an individual's physical and societal functioning. In this chapter, the International Classification of Functioning, Disability and Health (the ICF model) will be briefly discussed and supplemented by the Behavioral model for evaluation and intervention of human movement performance.

INTERNATIONAL CLASSIFICATION OF FUNCTIONING, DISABILITY AND HEALTH (ICF) MODEL

The ICF model (Fig. 5.1) is the second World Health Organization (WHO) model, introduced in 2001 in the hope of forging a universal language for functioning, disability and health (WHO, 2001). This model is considered to be an empowerment model and based on the strengths of the individual. It replaces the previous disablement model (the International Classification of Impairments, Disabilities and Handicaps, or ICIDH), which identified the healthy individual from one who had a disability associated with a health condition. The new model replaces the terminology of impairment, disability and handicap with positive words that define bodily functions and structures, activities and participation, and highlights the impact of personal factors and of the environment and society on disablement (Guralnik & Ferrucci, 2009). The ICF is underpinned by concepts similar to those of the Nagi model and, by virtue of support from a worldwide consensus, this model is expected to be used universally (Jette, 2009).

In this model, the identification of functional bodily structures and functions relates to those systems and subsystems that are normal; abnormalities in these systems are also called impairments. The ICF defines activities as tasks, functional behaviors and activities of daily life that can be executed by the individual as well as those activities that are limited ('activity limitations'). Participation in life identifies the social or family engagements of the individual and the restrictions in those engagements ('participation restrictions'). Often therapists begin their examination at either an activity or life participation entry point. The client presents with changes in normal activities and the desire to return to a better quality of life motivates participation in the rehabilitation process. The therapist conducts a comprehensive assessment covering the multiple relevant body functions and structures

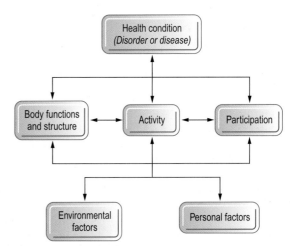

Figure 5.1 The International Classification of Functioning, Disability and Health (ICF) model. *(From WHO, 2001, with permission from the World Health Organization.)*

that contribute and interact to produce the activity limitations. As the therapist examines the functional activities category, environmental and personal variables that may affect activity and function must be considered within the framework of the whole person (Gordon et al., 2006). Intervention might include strategies aimed at ameliorating impairments and activity limitations, and addressing personal and contextual barriers, to optimize functioning and participation. However, as the client starts to re-engage in valued activities and participations, positive changes in body functions and structures as well as activities may also be driven by such engagement. Thus, the arrows within Figure 5.1 can go in either direction and the model posits that an improvement in participation can have a positive impact on the other dimensions of health (Guralnik & Ferrucci, 2009).

The use of the ICF as a client-oriented problem-solving model has been described previously through frameworks and instruments developed for analyzing client problems, identifying specific rehabilitation goals and establishing links between disabilities and relevant and modifiable variables that form the basis for intervention and outcome measurement (Rauch et al., 2008). The ICF shifts focus from the cause to the impact of disease and disability (Jette, 2006). The deleterious effects of health conditions on older people pervades beyond activities and extends

into household, community, leisure or sports participations (Alma et al., 2011) and quality of life (Marengoni et al., 2011). Participation restrictions are common among community-dwelling older people and onset and persistence increase with age (Wilkie et al., 2008; Wilkie et al., 2006). The goal for therapists therefore is always to guide the client toward the desired participations and therefore an enhanced quality of life. Interventions need not always be aimed at the level of impairments and activity limitations. Using the ICF can provide therapists with a broader view of how clients live with disease and disability, which, in turn, can be the basis for more holistic interventions.

THE BEHAVIORAL MODEL

Therapists are expected to identify the specific components that have led to functional problems, predict how long it will take to correct or develop compensation for the problem, and establish a plan of care that will allow the client to become functional in the shortest time possible. This responsibility of differential diagnosis is closely interrelated with the ICF concepts of specific system impairments, functional strengths or activity limitations, and adaptation that allows for participation in life and retention of the highest quality of life possible, as shown in Figure 5.2. The relationships are multifactorial and do

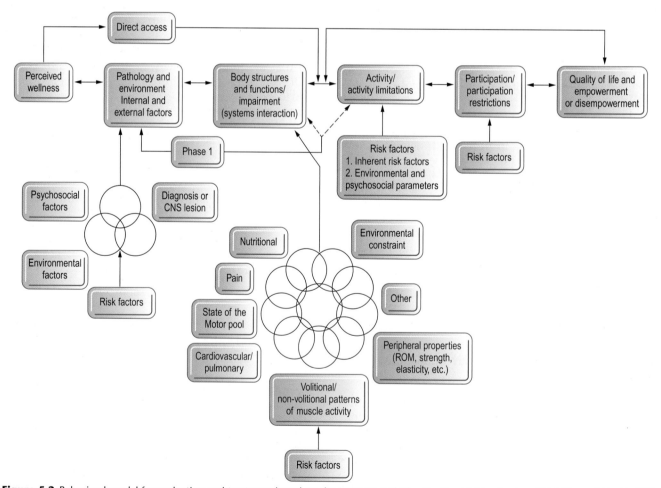

Figure 5.2 Behavioral model for evaluation and treatment based on the International Classification of Functioning, Disability and Health (ICF) enablement schema. ROM, range of motion. (*From Umphred et al., 2013, Fig 1.1, p. 6 by permission of Elsevier.*)

not necessarily proceed in a linear or unidirectional fashion. Many risk factors both inherent and external to the individual need to be considered as part of this diagnostic process. Inherent risk factors include all bodily systems that may be changing due to age, such as the nervous or cardiopulmonary systems, and may or may not have anything to do with pathology or disease. External risk factors are environmental and can be based on structural limitations, such as stairs or tri-level dwellings, or more socially driven, such as family beliefs regarding aging. As movement specialists, therapists need to look at motor behaviors and how those movement patterns assist in creating the ability to perform functional activities and independence that leads to life participation. Similarly, therapists need to simultaneously recognize how movement limitations restrict performance of both function and participation and determine whether those limitations can be reduced, corrected or adapted to give the individual a higher quality of life. The consumer determines what he or she wants to participate in and defines what quality of life is. The therapist always needs to remember and not assume that all individuals regain function similarly or that the function the therapist values is the same as the client's. These movement diagnoses are behavior driven and not disease or pathology driven, as is a medical diagnosis.

Therapists usually evaluate functional skills first, assessing both attainable and identifiable limitations, by looking at daily living activities. What allows an individual to demonstrate normal functional skills are the interactions of many body systems and their abilities to function adequately to allow for a normal motor response to a specific task. A breakdown in any part of one of these systems or subsystems can lead to movement limitations. Not all system problems lead to functional limitations and often it is the summation of system and subsystem impairments that create the greatest problems. Therapists need to evaluate how the different bodily systems are affecting movement and whether the central and/or peripheral central nervous systems have the potential to be corrected. This conclusion will guide the therapist in the direction of either creating a learning environment that allows the individual to regain normal function or teaching the client to compensate for the problem(s), which again should lead to functional control. Working on complex activities that the client values, such as golfing, can simultaneously work on many bodily system problems such as balance, endurance and strengthening, while creating a plan of care that will lead to the individual's future participation in life.

THEORIES OF MOTOR LEARNING, MOTOR CONTROL AND NEUROPLASTICITY

Physical and occupational therapists are specialists who are concerned with movement problems that affect quality of life, including both activities of daily living and activities of life participation, or any skill that is valued by the client. Three distinct categories must be differentiated when analyzing motor behavior as an expression of CNS response to environmental demands or task-specific goals: motor control, motor learning and neuroplasticity.

Motor control as a system includes components that are differentiated into biomechanical, musculoskeletal (power, strength and muscle elasticity), and central (state of the motor pool, availability of synergistic programming, postural integrity, balance, force, speed, trajectory, and automatic versus anticipatory programming). All of these components interact and must be evaluated within the context of the environment in which the activity is occurring. That context will determine whether the CNS can adapt or must be accommodated by changes in the external environment. Movement should never be analyzed by considering only one variable such as the biomechanical, musculoskeletal or central basis. If only one part is considered, the person is forgotten and this will have important implications on both prognosis and treatment (Umphred et al., 2013: 77).

Movement is always a combination of interactions of all of the variables that determine the motor patterns observed. These patterns assist a therapist in determining whether the movement expressions are caused by degeneration due to age, disuse over time, or disease. Box 5.1 illustrates the variables under motor control that are considered to originate within the nervous system and those that do not. Thus, the study of motor control involves keen assessment of how an individual controls movements already acquired.

To understand the distinctions between a system or subsystem function and a physiological mechanism problem (impairment) and a functional activity or activity limitation, it is necessary to analyze how the various systems function together in the healthy older person. The human body has large physiological reserves; a deficit in a portion of one system may have little or no effect on the whole organism because the reserves in other areas can substitute for small deficiencies.

It has been postulated that, with aging, many areas of physiological reserve may be close to a critical level of maximal adaptation (Fried & Guralnik, 1997) and hence the older person's body systems find it increasingly difficult to maintain homeostasis (Fulop et al., 2010). In this scenario, the whole organism functions normally, using all its capability to adapt until the occurrence of an acute problem in one area (Fried et al., 2000). Similar to a domino or cascading effect, one small problem forces the entire motor system beyond its capability to adapt or learn, and the end result is loss of function in specific activities affected by the given pathology or disease. For example, an aging individual who chooses to become more sedentary over time may no longer need to keep the vestibular system at a high level of sensitivity. The lack of movement may lead to joint limitation in the ankles and hips, which may decrease the limits of stability for balance and develop a fear of falling. As the individual ages, the visual system may also become compromised. None of these minor impairments necessarily leads to balance dysfunction or falls. If, however, this same person then suffers a vascular insult with acute residual motor impairments, the additional pre-existing impairments become compounded and interact with the new problem.

In some instances there can be improvement within systems or subsystems as a result of impairment-focused training, functional training and environmental

---

Box 5.1 *Motor control components and system interactions: classification of system and subsystem impairments*

IMPAIRMENTS WITHIN THE CENTRAL NERVOUS SYSTEM

1. Tone, reflexes and abnormal state of the motor neuron pool (hypotonicity, hypertonicity, rigidity, tremor).
2. Synergies, either volitional or reflexive (pattern of motor program, flexibility over programming).
3. Sensory integration and organization (somatosensory, visual and vestibular).
4. Balance and postural control (limits of stability; interaction with ankle, hip and stepping strategies; sensory integration; interaction with postural function, and with task/environmental context).
5. Speed of movement (ability to alter rate of movement throughout entire task, movement responses to speed demands).
6. Timing (ability to start, stop and change a motor plan; interaction with environmental context; muscle sequencing in relation to task).
7. Reciprocal movement (ability to change direction, rotatory components present/absent, turnaround time/delay, smoothness of agonist/antagonist).
8. Trajectory or pattern of movement (trajectory, velocity, acceleration curve; smoothness throughout range).
9. Accuracy (placement of entire body or a component part at a specific point in space; changes with demand for speed, difficulty of task, direction or distance).
10. Emotional influences (value placed on activity, differentiation of procedural and declarative learning, fear, motivation).
11. Perception (interaction of sensory organization with perceptual processing).
12. Cognition, levels of consciousness and memory (ability to use cognition to assist with motor learning, short, intermediate and long-term cognitive abilities).

IMPAIRMENTS OUTSIDE OF THE CENTRAL NERVOUS SYSTEM AND INTERACTION WITH THE ENVIRONMENT

1. Range of motion (specific joint limitation).
2. Muscle performance (strength, power and endurance).
3. Endurance (cardiovascular and pulmonary; differentiation from disuse from system failure or inefficiency).
4. Cardiac function (output, pacing, endurance, interaction with respiratory system).
5. Circulatory function (ability to supply muscles with oxygen, minerals, etc.).
6. Respiratory function (input/output and exchange; interaction with the cardiac system).
7. Other organ system interactions (skin integrity; kidney, liver, intestinal function).
8. Hormonal and nutritional factors (daily biorhythms, drug and nutritional interactions on central and peripheral functions).
9. Psychosocial factors (family demands; ethnicity, cultural or religious beliefs; past experiences and role identification; individual's belief in and acceptance of healthcare system and expectations).
10. Task content (new learning versus old learning).
11. Environmental construct (specific task or functional activity; familiarity with existing task or environment).

Adapted from Umphred et al., 2013, p. 181.

---

manipulations. This is especially true if some reserve is still available and the client is motivated to learn and regain function. If the clinician correctly relates specific impairments to functional movement problems and creates an optimal environment for relearning, then function may still be improved even with depleted reserves (Rossini & Dai, 2004). In other instances, the therapist cannot change the impairment but can find an alternative way for the client to use intact systems and, concurrently, for task and environment to be configured, so that the client may perform the desired function.

Motor learning is the study of how an individual acquires, modifies and retains motor memory patterns so that programs can be used, reused and modified during functional activities. Therefore, it does not only involve motor processes, but also the sensory (perceptual) and cognitive processes that are critical in the creation of permanent change in motor behavior. The critical elements of motor learning deal with the stages of learning, practice context that optimizes the learning, practice schedule used and reinforcement strategies employed to optimize that learning (Shumway-Cook & Woollacott, 2012).

Neuroplasticity can be defined as the lifelong ability of the nervous system to undergo structural, functional and connective reorganization, whether in an adaptive process resulting in a beneficial gain in function or a maladaptive process resulting from an adverse event such as injury or loss of function (Cramer et al., 2011). These changes occur in response to a variety of both external and internal demands placed upon the CNS as part of development and learning; in interacting with the environment; or in relation to disease or therapeutic intervention. Neuroplasticity does not stop once an individual reaches old age. The CNS internally adapts to occurrences in life whether they result from normal changes or from chronic disease, trauma, metabolic imbalances, dietary or external demands. Table 5.1 differentiates motor control, motor learning and neuroplasticity concepts.

Until the more recent scientific discoveries regarding neuroplasticity, the medical and research environments believed that, once a neuron was damaged or died, the only mechanism able to replace the function of that specific cell was adaptation of other neurons. Further, it was thought that adaptation ultimately led to a decrease in the function of the CNS. As observant clinicians, therapists have recognized that clients learn following CNS damage and that the potential for learning cannot be determined through a medical protocol even when the client is of advanced age and has incurred an injury to the CNS. Neuroplasticity literature has shown that change and cellular growth can occur, especially when the external and internal environments nurture that change and the activity has some novelty (May, 2011). In older people without dementia or other significant cognitive pathologies, experimental evidence suggests that aerobic physical activity can drive positive changes in the aged brain that include neurogenesis and increased volume in prefrontal and hippocampal areas of the brain as well as enhanced

Table 5.1	**Differentiation between motor control, motor learning and neuroplasticity**	
	Control Function	**Neuromechanism**
Motor control	Using existing synaptic connections and existing programming	*Neurotransmitters*: 10ths to 100ths of millisecond to respond *Neuropeptides*: hours or days for transmission to synapse; response can be hours, days, months, or lifetimes (in the case of certain drugs)
Motor learning	Modification of existing motor programs and synaptic firing patterns	Repetition of practice of new program takes days, weeks or months and needs continual practice to ensure permanent learning. Practice must continue from site to site as the client's skills improve. Variation of practice within the program is critical for adaptability. Motor control must be established before new learning can occur
Neuroplasticity	Modification of surviving cellular structure to reform primary function, assume a different function, and regain control of sensory processing and motor programming	Based on environmental demands placed on the organism and potential for neuroplasticity. Repetition of practice takes weeks, months, or years and continual environmental demands. Internal motivation to regain function is paramount to this type of neurofunction. Thus, never say never because the never is up to the client's internal motivation and potential

Modified from Umphred and Arce, 2013.

functional connectivity (Erickson et al., 2012). Animal models of brain injury have demonstrated that task-specific training and aerobic exercise can activate molecular pathways for neurogenesis and learning and memory, as well as induce neural sprouting, synaptogenesis and dendritic branching (Dimyan & Cohen, 2011). Thus, current literature provides evidence to contradict previously held beliefs about the aged and injured CNS, and suggests a positive outlook for clients given appropriately designed and well-timed therapeutic conditions.

For intervention to drive brain plasticity, it must promote participation of older people in sufficiently complex and intensive sensory, cognitive and motor activities that can engage and strengthen neural substrates underpinning motor learning (Mahncke et al., 2006). Attention and motivation of the individual, mental practice, environmental tasks that allow the motor functions of the CNS to succeed, and optimizing the potential change by focusing and integrating aspects of motor learning and client engagement create the best environment to encourage neuroplasticity (Danzl et al., 2012). Box 5.2 lists several principles of neural plasticity that have key ramifications on therapeutic interventions for optimized recovery in the damaged CNS (Umphred et al., 2013: 87). As clinicians, educators and researchers, the authors have always believed that 'If a motor behavior looked right to us or other people, was easy and enjoyable for the client, then somehow the intervention was creating change in the direction of normality and functional recovery no matter the theory.' Neuroplasticity has given the basic scientific validity to that statement.

SYSTEM INTERACTIONS AND REHABILITATION

It is the total interaction of all systems that the therapist must consider when establishing goals with a client. Some systems that have changed over a long period of time may not readapt quickly, such as joint contractures in the musculoskeletal system. Sometimes the body gives up an aspect of a system, such as range of motion, to compensate for another system problem, such as power. If range is regained but power is not available, then the

therapist has merely shifted to a new impairment, which may create an even greater functional problem.

Some systems that have changed may no longer have the ability to adapt, such as vision. Still others, for example the CNS itself, may have undergone both chronic and acute injury, such as disuse prior to a stroke. The therapist will have to assess which systems are trying to compensate for the deficient systems and are thereby obscuring the dysfunction, and which systems are permanently damaged and no longer have the ability to compensate and learn.

Loss of primary sensory input from peripheral damage and diminution of that sensory information on the primary somatosensory parietal receiving lobes are more devastating to the nervous system than loss of associative areas, which can be replaced by other areas. The difficulty therapists have with assessment is determining whether the primary system is non-functional or whether the amount of incoming sensory information is not at a level that awareness is recognized. This same phenomenon exists within the motor system. If a system is overpowered by the tone of another system, the initial behavior will be masked. For example, if an individual experiences a stroke and has residual hypotonia within the involved upper extremity, the natural inclination of a therapist is to try to increase proximal tone for better stabilization. But, if the tone is increased without functional control of fluid and relaxed movement patterns, the tone is often asymmetrical and hypertonic. This increase of proximal tone through the ventral medial and lateral descending tracts often overpowers the descending corticospinal tract and, thus, hand function is minimal if present.

If the visual system is deficient and compensation is not available, increasing awareness of the vestibular and somatosensory systems will allow for retention of motor programs for balance. If this specific training is not a focus, then balance impairments and a potential for falls exist. Disuse, fear of falling or falling itself can lead to functional movement problems and a decrease in social participation. Although disuse and muscle weakness, affective fear and reinforced fear following a fall are not permanently damaged physiological mechanisms, they can certainly lead to chronic motor problems.

Box 5.2   *Basic principles of neuroplasticity that could guide clinical practice*

1. *Use it or lose it* – Maintenance of neural mechanisms is dependent upon use and thus lack of biological activity to stimulate such mechanisms can lead to functional degradation.
2. *Use it and improve it* – Use and training can drive enhancement in the function and structure of specific neural mechanisms.
3. *Be specific* – The training experience must match the desired outcome; the nature of neural plasticity is dictated by the nature of the training.
4. *Repetition is essential* – Learning requires repetition, progressed in difficulty and spaced over time.
5. *Intensity matters* – Plasticity changes require a sufficient training intensity to ensure durability of pathways.
6. *Time matters* – Different forms of plasticity occur at different times during training; timing of training onset and training duration influence the course of neural plasticity.
7. *Salience is important* – Training must be sufficiently salient (i.e. purposeful and behavior-specific) to support change in neural mechanisms.
8. *Age must be addressed* – Training-induced plasticity occurs most readily in a young brain, but neural adaptation continues across the life span with learning-based training. With aging, greater efforts at variety, integration and discovery may be needed.
9. *Transference* – Neural plasticity that results from training a specific motor behavior can also enhance acquisition of similar behaviors and adaptation in other experiences and other parts of the body.
10. *Interference* – Plastic changes after one training experience may interfere with the acquisition of changes in similar systems.
11. *Patient expectation* – Patient expectation can facilitate the outcomes of training; patients who expect to get better can enhance their learning.
12. *Reward or feedback* – Feedback allows modification of training behaviors, correcting errors and improving accuracy of learning.
13. *Environment* – Enriching the environment, by providing sufficient sensory and motor stimulation as well as opportunities for enhanced memory and social interaction, can maximize learning and modulate plastic changes in the nervous system.
14. *Fun* – Learning is greatest when it is associated with discovery and fun.
15. *Helping others* – Maintaining the fitness of the brain is best when individuals look beyond themselves to help and involve others.

Adapted from Umphred et al., 2013, Box 4.1, p. 87.

The acute physiological reason for a fall, such as a stroke, heart attack or acute hypotension, needs to be addressed by a medical team. The prognosis of impairments resulting from disuse or fear can be integrated into intervention for the acute CNS damage (Chen et al., 2005) and falls within the functional diagnosis identified by the movement specialists. All three (visual, vestibular and somatosensory) impairments individually and collectively alter balance and the end result is a high risk of falls and fall-related impairments. If sensory deprivation in any one or more of the sensory systems responsible for balance is also present, that system is also considered deficient in a physiological mechanism. Central impairments may include problems in the state of the motor pool, synergistic patterning, postural control, perceptual distortion of position in space, anxiety, or other deficits in systems that work for consensus when controlling movement. Each mechanism can be evaluated as it is identified and quantitatively measured. The number and magnitude of impairments within bodily systems will determine prognosis of movement functions and clearly direct intervention strategies toward desired outcomes.

When the therapist introduces the activity and motor learning becomes necessary, the specific stage of learning must be identified: acquisition, refinement or retention. The first stage, acquisition, requires extra reinforcement, which can be internally driven through normal sensory feedback systems or externally driven through augmented feedback from someone else. As the individual increases his or her skill in the activity (refinement), less feedback is necessary and internal self-correction should become more observable. Similarly, the type of practice schedule selected by the therapist can range from mass practice (daily and structured) to distributed practice (scheduled by the therapist or client with larger gaps between treatment),

or random practice (part of an activity of daily living). Finally, for an individual who needs to retain skills, practice is organized using functional goal-directed tasks in variable environments to promote problem-solving in 'real world' contexts. Acquisition of a skill requires mass practice whereas retention depends more on random practice (Shumway-Cook & Woollacott, 2012).

When the therapist introduces the activity, another concept must be considered. The task itself will determine whether it will be practiced as a cohesive activity, taught in separate parts and then put together as a whole, or taught as a progressive sequence of parts. This is the practice context. Discrete tasks like reaching overhead with the upper extremity and continuous tasks like walking are more easily taught as whole activities, whereas serial tasks like getting up from a wheelchair into a standing position is generally learned best as an activity that is broken into parts and then practiced progressively. Therapists need to look at prior learning before dividing activities into their respective parts. If the individual has a coming to stand program, then there is little need to teach the person to move the weight forward within the chair, center the base of support over the feet and then shift the weight forward and stand up. In fact, teaching that four-step process may be much more difficult than asking the client to stand up and recognizing a power or balance problem that can be corrected with training.

If new learning is impossible, then the need to create an environment that optimizes old learning should be clearly identified and used in the therapeutic setting to achieve optimal functioning. The challenge with older people is that change can create confusion and stress, and may limit new learning, whereas novelty, motivation and repetitive practice will enhance the brain's ability to learn and respond appropriately to functional demands.

As a team, the client, therapist and caregiver first need to identify outcomes relevant to the client and the client's functional desires. Such is key to organizing task-specific and purposeful practice to stimulate biological activity in neural substrates that support the functional skills, in keeping with principles of adaptive plasticity. Second, practice of those functional activities is critical but variance within that environment is crucial to allow for correction of errors within the movement itself. Maintenance of novelty to motivate attention and learning of the task is also important. Both variance and novelty in the practice structure can provide the necessary impetus for greater flexibility in neural mechanisms and hence increase the potential for transference of training. For example, if the client is reaching for an object within a cabinet while standing at a sink, the exact standing position in relation to the sink will result in challenges to stability and, simultaneously, the level of reaching while standing will shift the center of gravity. Both of these factors can be used to create challenges to the task, vary the activity and specific muscle and joint range interactions, and introduce novelty. Reaching for objects of varied dimensions and weights, placing those from one shelf level to another, or doing additional activities such as picking up soap and washing the hands are all variations on the original motor activities that allow environmental dimensions to change and novelty to remain.

Much of the previous research regarding aging, changes within the nervous system and motor control identified that, as humans age, they lose cognitive function, memory and motor skills. These results, which were statistically significant from a research perspective, did not necessarily prove significant when functional behaviors such as sit to stand, eating using utensils and standing balance were analysed. Whether the CNS changes progress to neuroplasticity or functional loss has more to do with the novelty of the task, motivation of the learner, environmental variables and state (e.g. healthy or not) of the components of the body.

Current research suggests that changes in function are almost always related to disease or pathology (Marengoni et al., 2011; Woodford & George, 2011). Disuse is another variable that drives decline. Older people who have maintained their health, who stay physically and mentally active, who participate in life activities and engage in new, novel learning should not show functionally significant changes in motor behavior. The brain will engage in neuroplasticity under normal healthy environments when cellular change is occurring. Variables that help to nurture neuroplasticity and learning are motivation, attention to the task, maintenance of metabolic health, ability to successfully use multiple sensory input systems as part of maintaining and relearning motor function, and challenging the CNS both physically and mentally on a consistent level. Thus, declines in motor skills, executive functioning and memory may be better correlated with a long pattern of disuse over decades rather than chronological age. Older people show declines in many abilities but the cause of those declines are multifactorial and should not be labeled as 'aging' (Rossini & Dai, 2004).

CLINICAL EXAMPLES

As mentioned previously, functional training may improve impairments. In other instances, when the impairment cannot be changed, a therapist may be able to find alternatives that allow the client to compensate and use intact systems to perform the desired function, giving the individual increased control and opportunities to participate in life.

In the first scenario, the client has a high probability of going beyond skill acquisition through refinement and may even retain and carry the skill learned into other functional activities. In the second scenario, compensation is being taught and thus the skill learned is activity-specific and may have little carryover to other functional behaviors. Given the plasticity of the CNS, there is usually untapped potential within the client and empowering that person with hope will play a key role in unlocking the limbic aspect of neuroplasticity. As soon as hope is taken away, the CNS loses its drive to change and thus the likelihood of neuroplasticity becomes low.

An example of the first instance might be Mr Smith, who recently had a stroke with residual motor problems in both his right upper and lower extremities. The therapist worked with him, putting him into postures and situations or activities involving sitting, which demanded that his trunk and hip muscles respond with balance and weight shifting. These responses activated existing neurological mechanisms to regain power, strength, balance and movement range that might have been lost because of hospitalization or disuse at home. The therapist also used a partial body weight support system to allow the client to practice walking and meet the need for normal power in walking, posture and co-activation during walking. Initially, the therapist placed the client's right foot on each step but within 2 weeks the client was able to bring the right foot through during the swing phase of gait and walk short distances using a quad cane for balance. The CNS was learning to regain and control all the mechanisms at the level that allowed for normal ambulation without generating abnormal gait patterns. The use of the cane was to make sure his balance stayed within his limits of stability and created greater safety within the client's emotional system. Motor learning was occurring because, although it had taken weeks, walking was progressively improving over time without the presence of abnormal movement patterns. The client, through whole–part learning, was able to stand–pivot–transfer from bed to chair to toilet to shower to chair independently before leaving rehabilitation. Although the client had motor control over the upper extremities, his power was poor. Initially, the therapist supported the shoulder during reaching and hand-to-mouth activities to prevent the development of an abnormal shoulder pattern. The client practiced effortless reaching with his shoulder supported over a ball, again to reduce the need for power while encouraging functional arm movement with controlled hand dexterity.

Once it was determined that Mr Smith had hand and arm function, the therapist, with consent from the client, encouraged him to use only his right limb. This might be considered constraint-induced therapy but the client was volitionally making the decision, which encouraged emotional buy-in and increased the possibility of neuroplasticity. Although he was discharged from the rehabilitation program, he returned for a follow-up visit 6 months later. At that time, his right upper extremity function was still not normal but he could use his hand to write his name and the entire extremity to assist in any upper extremity functional activity of his choice. This follow-up improvement probably resulted from neuroplasticity within the CNS due to repetitive practice by the client at home.

For a clinician, whether the change was due to learning, spontaneous recovery or neuroplasticity is irrelevant. Both the therapist and client's goal is functional recovery and, as long as that was the outcome, the exact neuromechanism seems unimportant. It is up to researchers to help determine how the CNS adapts and changes so that future therapeutic programs can be more effective and efficacious. In this example, it is important for the therapist to identify by early testing what previously learned motor programs are intact within the neuromusculoskeletal loop systems. Initially, that determination may be identified by eliciting responses or guiding movement and discerning the programs as they come in to assist in a functional movement. If alternative loops or synaptic sensitivities exist, recovery potential is high and prognosis is good, as long as the treatments are consistent with appropriate environmental contexts, practice scheduling, practice context and the goals and expectations of the client.

An example of the second scenario might be Mrs Jones, who was an older person with a recent amputation following prolonged diabetic instability and eventual gangrene. The therapist was never going to change the physiological mechanism that caused the limb amputation or medical condition of diabetes. The amputation had, by itself, altered the state of the CNS. The sensory system had changed, as had the posture, balance and motor programming needed to ambulate with a prosthetic device. The inherent sensory feedback necessary to create new programs had to be evaluated. The sensory physiological mechanisms might have been progressively deteriorating because of the diabetes. However, if new learning could occur and new programs be written, this older individual might be able to run the programs, even with progressive sensory deterioration. Thus, the therapist had to work with the client in using a prosthetic device to regain normal gait programming. Strengthening the residual limb muscles would not necessarily translate into a smooth and normal gait using a prosthesis.

To match the context of the environment with the task, programming necessary and client-specific impairments, the therapist worked on standing and walking. Additional considerations such as skin integrity, pain and range of motion had to be interfaced with the practice environment. The therapist was potentially optimizing the environment for early and maximal function. Knowing that the gait training would be considered a new learning situation allowed the therapist to guard for error while the client walked.

The old programs for walking that were learned by the client as a small child and practiced for decades would function with the remaining muscle groups but not as a total program that encompassed the prosthesis. In this situation, the therapist wanted the client to concentrate on the task at first to bring in somatosensory awareness and sensory–motor planning. Once the client demonstrated that the program was present, the therapist needed to distract the client's attention on the walking motor activity and allow the motor system to practice the program. For the client to be truly successful in this new variation of ambulation, she had to practice it as a feedforward automatic task. At first, the practice had to be performed on a mass-practice level before it was performed as an activity of daily living, in which walking was part of life and practiced on a random schedule. As Mrs Jones began to regain her participation in life, with walking as an expected outcome, she started to challenge herself in many environments, which further increased her ability to adapt and change. Varying the lighting or surface, increasing walking speed and distance, or distracting with conversation or movement in the environment are examples of challenges a therapist might use and eventually recommend to a caregiver. Gait is a pre-programmed pattern that develops variability in relationship to different contexts, so practicing the gait pattern as a whole would be the context of choice. In this example, the therapist has created an environment that has changed the CNS, even though the original physiological mechanism that was damaged was not centrally induced.

CONCLUSION

The CNS is a complex conglomerate of nuclear masses that communicate with all bodily systems and expresses thoughts, feelings and desires to the world through motor behaviors. This function, or the goals it represents, does not change with advancing age, nor does a specific age imply that the CNS is no longer functioning adequately or has a diminished ability to adapt. Yet, through life's experiences, age itself does potentially affect all bodily functions, including that of the nervous system. Life's physical traumas, habits and environmental stressors can all become additive and cause slow progressive deterioration of one or all of the body's anatomical systems over time. The CNS has the capability to adapt depending upon internal and external environmental demands. Change and novelty can create neuroplasticity. However, change and novelty, when beyond the system's capabilities to adapt, can cause functional motor problems. The nervous system adapts more easily when change occurs slowly. Unfortunately, many older people experience a variety of CNS trauma or pathologies that dramatically affect functional movement. Whether these problems cause specific impairments, activity limitations or participation restrictions is often client-specific and directly correlates more with the health condition than age. Therapists should evaluate the interactions of the various physiological body mechanisms or impairments and relate them to functional behaviors in order to identify the intervention protocols that will lead to optimal performance in the shortest time frame. Application and generation of knowledge regarding motor control, motor learning and neuroplasticity play key roles in the effectiveness of a clinician and, ultimately, the quality of life of the individuals who receive clinical services.

REFERENCES

Alma MA, van der Mei SF, Melis-Dankers BJM et al 2011 Participation of the elderly after vision loss. Disabil Rehabil 33:63–72

Chen KM, Chen WT, Wang JJ et al 2005 Frail elders' views of Tai Chi. J Nurs Res 13:11–20

Chisolm TH, Willott JH, Lister JJ 2003 The aging auditory system: anatomic and physiologic changes and implications for rehabilitation. Int J Audiol 42:2S3–10

Cramer SC, Sur M, Dobkin BH et al 2011 Harnessing neuroplasticity for clinical applications. Brain 134:1591–1609

Danzl MM, Etter NM, Andreatta RO 2012 Facilitating neurorehabilitation through principles of engagement. J Allied Health 41:35–41

Degardin A, Devos D, Cassim F et al 2011 Deficit of sensorimotor integration in normal aging. Neurosci Lett 12:208–212

Dimyan MA, Cohen LG 2011 Neuroplasticity in the context of motor rehabilitation after stroke. Nat Rev Neurol 7:76–85

Erickson KI, Weinstein AM, Lopez OL 2012 Physical activity, brain plasticity, and Alzheimer's disease. Arch Med Res 43:615–621

Fried LP, Bandeen-Roche K, Chaves PH et al 2000 Preclinical mobility disability predicts incident mobility disability in older women. J Gerontol A Biol Sci Med Sci 55:M43–M52

Fried L, Guralnik J 1997 Disability in older adults: evidence regarding significance, etiology, and risk. J Am Geriatr Soc 45:92–100

Fujiyama H, Garry MI, Levin O et al 2009 Age-related differences in inhibitory processes during interlimb coordination. Brain Res 25: 38–47

Fulop T, Larbi A, Witkowski JM et al 2010 Aging, frailty and age-related diseases. Biogerontology 11:547–563

Glisky EL 2007 Changes in cognitive function in human aging. In: Riddle DR (ed) Brain Aging: Models, Methods, and Mechanisms. CRC Press, Boca Raton, FL

Gordon J, Hodges P, Jette AM 2006 Models for neurological rehabilitation. III STEP: Symposium on Translating Evidence into Practice, July 15–21, 2005, Salt Lake City, Utah. APTA, Alexandria, VA

Green MS, Kaye JA, Ball MJ 2000 The Oregon Brain Aging Study: neuropathology accompanying healthy aging in the oldest old. Neurology 54:105–113

Groenewegen HJ, Uylings HB 2000 The prefrontal cortex and the integration of sensory, limbic and autonomic information. Prog Brain Res 126:3–28

Guralnik JM, Ferrucci L 2009 The challenge of understanding the disablement process in older persons. J Gerontol A Biol Sci Med Sci 64A:1169–1171

Ishiyama G 2009 Imbalance and vertigo: the aging human vestibular periphery. Semin Neurol 29:491–499

Jette AM 2006 Toward a common language for function, disability, and health. Phys Ther 86:726–734

Jette A 2009 Toward a common language of disablement. J Gerontol A Biol Sci Med Sci 64A:1165–1168

Johnson DK, Storandt M, Morris JC et al 2009 Longitudinal study of the transition from healthy aging to Alzheimer disease. Arch Neurol 66:1254–1259

Kandel ER, Schwartz JH, Jessell TM et al 2012 Principles of Neural Science, 5th edn. McGraw Hill, New York

Koceja DM, Mynark RG 2000 Comparison of heteronymous monosynaptic Ia facilitation in young and elderly subjects in supine and standing positions. Int J Neurosci 103:1–17

Long X, Liao W, Jiang C et al 2012 Healthy aging: an automatic analysis of global and regional morphological alterations of human brain. Acad Radiol 19:785–793

Lupien SJ, McEwen BS, Gunnar MR et al 2009 Effects of stress throughout the lifespan on the brain, behaviour and cognition. Nat Rev Neurosci 10:434–445

McEwen BS 2002 Sex, stress and the hippocampus: allostasis, allostatic load and the aging process. Neurobiol Aging 23:921–939

Mahncke HW, Bronstone A, Merzenich MM 2006 Brain plasticity and functional losses in the aged: scientific bases for a novel intervention. Prog Brain Res 157:81–109

Mankovsky NB, Mints AY, Lisenyuk VP 1982 Age peculiarities of human motor control in aging. Gerontology 28:314–322

Marengoni A, Angleman S, Melis R et al 2011 Aging with multimorbidity: a systematic review of the literature. Ageing Res Rev 10:430–439

May A 2011 Experience-dependent structural plasticity in the adult human brain. Trends Cogn Sci 15:475–482

Møller AR 2000 Hearing: Its Physiology and Pathophysiology. Academic Press, St Louis, MO, p 239

Mora F, Segovia G, del Arco A 2007 Aging, plasticity and environmental enrichment: structural changes and neurotransmitter dynamics in several areas of the brain. Brain Res Rev 55:78–88

Rajput AH, Robinson CA, Rajput ML et al 2011 Cerebellar Purkinje cell loss is not pathognomonic of essential tremor. Parkinsonism Relat Disord 17:16–21

Rauch A, Cieza A, Stucki G 2008 How to apply the International Classification of Functioning, Disability and Health (ICF) for rehabilitation management in clinical practice. Eur J Phys Rehabil Med 44:329–342

Raz N, Lindenberger U, Rodriguez KM et al 2005 Regional brain changes in aging healthy adults: general trends, individual differences and modifiers. Cereb Cortex 15:1676–1689

Rossini PM, Dai FG 2004 Integration technology for evaluation of brain function and neural plasticity. Phys Med Rehabil Clin North Am 15:263–306

Shumway-Cook A, Woollacott MH 2012 Motor Control: Translating Research into Clinical Practice, 4th edn. Lippincott Williams & Wilkins, Philadelphia, PA

Sjöstrand J, Laatikainen L, Hirvelä H et al 2011 The decline in visual acuity in elderly people with healthy eyes or eyes with early age-related maculopathy in two Scandinavian population samples. Acta Ophthalmol 89:116–123

Stephen JM, Knoefel JE, Adair J et al 2010 Aging-related changes in auditory and visual integration measured with MEG. Neurosci Lett 484:76–80

Stojanovich L 2010 Stress and autoimmunity. Autoimmun Rev 9:A271–A276

Umphred DA, Arce F 2013 Motor control, motor learning and neuroplasticity. In: Umphred DA, Lazaro RT (eds) Neurological Rehabilitation for Physical Therapist Assistant, 2nd edn. Slack Inc., Thorofare, NJ

Umphred DA, Lazaro RT, Roller ML et al (eds) 2013 Umphred's Neurological Rehabilitation, 6th edn. Elsevier, St Louis, MO

Vance DE, Heaton K, Fazeli PL et al 2010 Aging, speed of processing training, and everyday functioning: implications for practice and research. Activities Adapt Aging 34:276–279

Werner RA, Franzblau A, D'Arcy HJS et al 2012 Differential aging of median and ulnar sensory nerve parameters. Muscle Nerve 45:60–64

WHO (World Health Organization) 2001 International Classification of Functioning, Disability and Health: ICF. WHO, Geneva. Available at: www.who.int/classifications/icf/en. Accessed December 2012

Wilkie R, Peat G, Thomas E et al 2006 The prevalence of person-perceived participation restriction in community-dwelling older adults. Qual Life Res 15:1471–1479

Wilkie R, Thomas E, Mottram S et al 2008 Onset and persistence of person-perceived participation restriction in older adults: a 3-year follow-up study in the general population. Health Qual Life Outcomes 6:92

Woodford HJ, George J 2011 Neurological and cognitive impairments detected in older people without a diagnosis of neurological or cognitive disease. Postgrad Med J 87:199–206

Wu T, Hallett M 2005 The influence of normal human ageing on automatic movements. J Physiol 562:605–615

Yankner BA, Lu T, Loerch P 2008 The aging brain. Annu Rev Pathol Mech Dis 3:41–66

Chapter 6

Cardiac considerations in the older patient

MERYL COHEN

CHAPTER CONTENTS

INTRODUCTION

Determination of health and wellness among young individuals is relative, varying from person to person. Similarly, the effects of an aging cardiovascular system vary among the elderly. Controversies exist in the literature regarding the application of a single model to the influence of aging on heart function. Structural changes that occur with aging are more consistent and more easily identifiable than are physiological changes. The latter findings are difficult to distinguish for several reasons, including the interrelatedness of dynamic variables contributing to myocardial performance, the pathophysiology and symptomatology of heart disease, and the concept of hypokinesis in American society, to which the older person is, to an extent, considered to be entitled (Lakatta, 1993; Susic, 1997). In addition, comparison of studies is limited because of measurement inconsistencies and varying definitions of 'elderly' and 'heart disease'. Many of the pioneering studies of the 1950s and 1960s continue to be reproduced using new definitions of 'old' and paying more deliberate attention to the presence of heart disease in study populations. Recent studies have been more effective at teasing out consequences of aging that are independent of disease, fitness and environment (Kaye & Esler, 2008).

There is general consensus regarding the effects of aging on several factors that influence cardiac performance. These factors have been studied in older individuals who are healthy and in those with heart disease, both at rest and during various levels of exertion. This chapter presents these findings as a model of declining cardiac performance with increasing age. Comparison is made to the baseline 'young' model in an attempt at defining a 'healthy older' model. The unique influences of exercise and disease on this model are then discussed, with an emphasis on the clinical implications of these physiological changes.

CARDIOVASCULAR STRUCTURE

Age-related changes in cardiovascular tissue can be found in cardiac contractile fibers, conducting tissue and valvular structure (Lakatta & Levy, 2003a). Although the actual number of myocytes decreases, the myocyte volume per nucleus increases in both ventricles. Commonly, the coronary microvasculature is unable to accommodate this increase in tissue volume, which raises the likelihood of myocardial ischemia. In addition there is an increase in nondistensible fibrous tissue and an accumulation of senile amyloid deposits (see Box. 6.1). The loss of pacemaker cells (sinoatrial node tissue) and the increase in fibrous tissue in conducting pathways combine to increase the risk of cardiac arrhythmias in the elderly.

Simultaneous age-related changes occur in coronary arteries and systemic vasculature. These changes tend to increase the stiffness of the vessel walls (see Table 6.1; Fig. 6.1) (Priebe, 2000). Typically, proximal portions of the arteries change first, and the left coronary artery changes before the right. Together, the locations of the changes and the increased vessel rigidity cause an increase in peripheral vascular resistance. The heart attempts to adapt to this increased afterload (see discussion below) with myocellular hypertrophy, which probably accounts for the increase in myocyte volume previously mentioned. Alterations found in endothelial cells lining the arterial lumen cause a decrease in laminar blood flow, possibly establishing sites for lipid deposition and further increase cardiac afterload. In addition, decreased nitric oxide release from the coronary endothelium further reduces vasodilator capacity in the older individual (Susic, 1997; Lakatta & Levy, 2003b).

Recent advances in genetic and stem cell research have provided further insight into aging cardiac mitochondria and chromosome structure. Cardiac function, which relies heavily on ATP-generating properties of mitochondria,

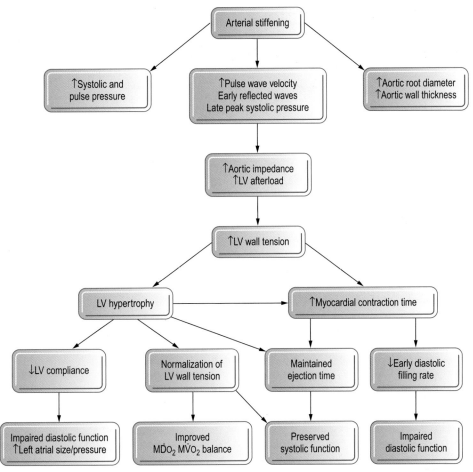

Figure 6.1 Cardiac adjustments to arterial stiffening during aging. L, left; LV, left ventricular. $M\dot{D}O_2$, myocardial oxygen supply; $M\dot{V}O_2$, myocardial oxygen demand. *(Reproduced with permission from Priebe, 2000. © The Board of Management and Trustees of the British Journal of Anaesthesia. Reproduced by permission of Oxford University Press/British Journal of Anaesthesia.)*

is negatively affected by the significant decline in mitochondria biogenesis and function seen with normal aging (Moslehi et al., 2012).

CARDIOVASCULAR PHYSIOLOGY

The job of the heart is to pump blood rich with oxygen to body tissues. The ability of the heart to do this work efficiently is closely affected by three other systems: the lungs, the vasculature and the blood. Age- or disease-related changes occurring in these systems will directly affect cardiac function.

Cardiac output (CO), or the volume of blood pumped to body tissues each minute, depends on the frequency of cardiac contractions (heart rate) and the volume of blood ejected with each contraction (stroke volume). Heart rate (HR) can be influenced by many external factors; however, intrinsically, the HR depends on pacemaker tissue function and autonomic nervous system stimulation. In addition to the loss of pacemaker cells in older people, there is also a decreased sensitivity to beta-adrenergic stimulation (see Box 6.2). These two age-associated changes in HR control may or may not affect the resting HR, but they do typically decrease the

maximal exercise HR (Fleg et al., 1994). CO is maintained in the older individual if the stroke volume (SV) is able to increase and compensate for any blunted HR response. This is the case if the individual remains physically fit, but usually the resting and submaximum CO tend to decrease with aging owing to a decrease in SV. This reduction in SV may be a result of alterations in a number of variables (see Box 6.2).

SV is influenced by ventricular filling (preload), ventricular contractility and peripheral vascular resistance (afterload). Ventricular filling occurs early during diastole and is rapid and mostly passive, with the last portion of filling attributed to atrial contractions. However, with aging, a prolonged contraction relaxation time and decreased myocardial compliance (due to increased nondistensible fibrous tissue) cause a greater dependency on slower, active atrial contraction for the majority of diastolic filling (see Fig. 6.2).

Myocardial contractility is directly affected by sympathetic nervous system stimulation, specifically, beta-adrenergic receptors. Older individuals are less responsive to catecholamine stimulation, which results in a blunted inotropic response. Alteration in blood pressure control may result. This is further evidenced by

Table 6.1 **Age-related cardiovascular responses to exercise**

Response	Effects of Aging	After Exercise Training
Resting		
Oxygen consumption	↔	↔
Heart rate	↔	↔
Stroke volume	↔	↔
Arteriovenous oxygen difference	↑	?
Submaximal exercise		
Oxygen consumption	↔	
Heart rate	↔	↓
Stroke volume	↔	?
Arteriovenous oxygen difference	↑	?
Maximal exercise		
Oxygen consumption	↓	↑
Heart rate	↓	↔
Stroke volume	↓ or ↑	↑
Arteriovenous oxygen difference	↓ or ↔	↑ or ↔
Cardiac output	↔ (?) or ↑	↔

↑=increased; ↓=decreased; ↔=no change; ?=insufficient data on elderly subjects.
Reprinted from Protas E 1993 Physiological change and adaptation to exercise in the older adult. In: Guccione A (ed) Foundation of Geriatric Physical Therapy, 2nd edn. Mosby-Year Book St Louis, MO, with permission from Elsevier.

Box 6.1 *Age-related changes in cardiovascular tissue*

CARDIAC

↓ Number of myocytes (myofibrils and pacemaker cells)
↑ Size of myocytes (myocellular hypertrophy)
↑ Lipid deposition in myocytes
↑ Lipofuscin deposition in myocytes
↓ Mitochondria
↓ Mitochondrial oxidative phosphorylation
↑ Oxidative damage
↑ Amyloid deposition in the heart
↓ Rate of protein synthesis in internodal tracts
↑ Fribrosis and calcification of valves (especially the mitral annulus and aortic valve)

VASCULAR

↑ Endothelial cell heterogeneity (size, shape, axial orientation)
↑ Nondistensible collage, fibrous tissues and calcium in media
↑ Thickness of smooth-muscle cells in media
↓ Release of nitric oxide by coronary endothelium

↑=increase; ↓=decrease.

Box 6.2 *Age-related changes in cardiovascular function*

↓ Beta-adrenergic responsiveness
↓ Cardiovagal baro-receptor sensitivity (↑ SNS tone)
↑ Afterload (vascular impedance)
↓ Early diastolic filling
↑ Dependency on atrial contraction
↓ Contraction–relaxation time (prolonged)
↑ Left ventricular end-diastolic pressure (rest and exercise)
↓ Ability to adjust to rapid volume shifts
↑ Vascular tone
Left ventricular hypertrophy

↑=increase; ↓=decrease. SNS, sympathetic nervous system

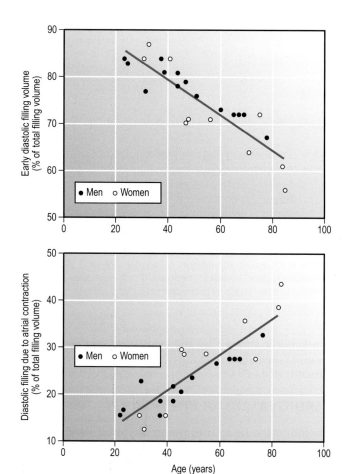

Figure 6.2 Age-associated decrease in early diastolic filling rate is compensated for by an increase in filling due to atrial contraction. *(Reproduced from Swinne CJ, Shapiro EP, Lima SD et al 1992 Age-associated changes in left ventricular diastolic performance during isometric exercise in normal subjects. Am J Cardiol 69:823–6, with permission from Excerpta Medica.)*

decreased baro-receptor reflex sensitivity and reduced HR variability (see Fig. 6.3). The latter measure is a marker of cardiac autonomic nervous system modulation; less HR variability indicates less vagal influences on the heart (De Meersman & Stein, 2007; Monahan, 2007; Kaye & Esler, 2008). In addition, if diastolic filling volumes are inadequate, contractile tension can be diminished due to the Frank Starling law of the heart, which states that the *energy of contraction is proportional to the initial length of the cardiac muscle fiber.*

The final component of SV determination is cardiac afterload (opposition to left ventricular ejection). As discussed above, afterload increases with aging due to increased vascular rigidity. Vascular stiffness is a result not only of loss of elastic elements but also of decreased responsiveness to catecholamine stimulation, which enables prolonged vasoconstriction.

It is important to note that in the aging heart's attempt to maintain CO, the consequent left ventricular hypertrophy can account for the onset of

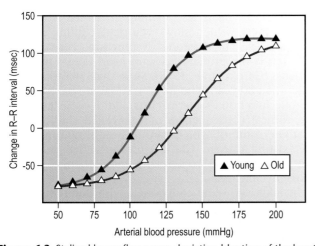

Figure 6.3 Stylized baroreflex curves depicting blunting of the heart rate response to changes in blood pressure in older individuals compared to younger subjects. *(Reproduced from Kaye & Esler, 2008: 184, Figure 3, with permission from Springer Science and Business Media.)*

myocardial ischemia independent of coronary atherosclerosis (see Fig. 6.4). On a purely physiological basis, several factors may contribute to the older heart's increased predisposition to developing ischemia (and sudden cardiac death):

- a disproportionate increase in myocyte size relative to the available circulation, resulting in demand by tissue for more oxygen than the blood can supply;
- an inability of aging coronary vessels to dilate due to increasing stiffness and prolonged sympathetic-mediated vasoconstriction, resulting in an inadequate blood supply for cardiac demand;
- the prolonged time for ventricular relaxation, which utilizes more energy and oxygen than a rapid relaxation period, thus creating a supply–demand imbalance;
- myocardial ischemia caused by any of these physiological processes of aging, which further decreases myocardial compliance and worsens ischemia, ventricular filling and, finally, systolic function *potentially resulting in heart failure.*

AGE-RELATED CARDIOVASCULAR CHANGES AND EXERCISE

The decline in cardiac performance that occurs with aging reduces cardiac reserves. The healthy older individual is less able to accommodate to the added stress of exertion and fatigues more easily than does the healthy younger individual with comparable workloads. Maximal oxygen consumption (Vo_2 max), a measure of total body oxygen intake at exhaustion and an index of overall cardiovascular and pulmonary fitness, tends to decrease with aging (Dehn & Bruce, 1972; Christou

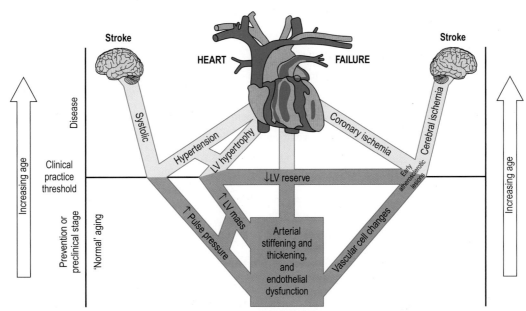

Figure 6.4 Changes in the vasculature and heart associated with aging. Changes below the bisecting line tend to occur with 'normal' aging and without clinical symptoms. Above a certain aging threshold, these changes tend to produce clinical symptoms. LV, left ventricular. *(Reproduced from Lakatta & Levy, 2003b, with permission from Lippincott Williams & Wilkins.)*

& Seals, 2008). Oxygen consumption (V_{O_2}) can be expressed by the following formula (the Fick equation):

$$V_{O_2} = CO \times A - V_{O_2} \text{ difference}$$
$$\text{Oxygen consumption} = \text{Cardiac output} \times \text{Arteriovenous oxygen difference}$$

The decline in V_{O_2} max may be partially attributed to a decrease in CO. The age-related decrease in skeletal muscle mass and consequent decrease in oxygen extraction may also contribute to the decrease in V_{O_2} max (see Table 6.1).

Elderly individuals who exercise regularly show less of a decrease in V_{O_2} max and may be able to reverse a number of age-associated changes in cardiovascular function (see Table 6.1). It is of interest to note that many of the benefits of exercise training enjoyed by older persons are similar to those found in the younger population. For example, compared to sedentary elderly individuals, older persons who are exercise-conditioned tend to have a lower resting HR and blood pressure, improved diastolic function, lower peripheral vascular resistance, and improved peripheral oxygen utilization. Autonomic function and baro-receptor reflex sensitivity also improve (De Meersman & Stein, 2007; Monahan, 2007). In addition, 'trained' elderly demonstrate lower rates of myocardial infarction, heart failure and overall morbidity and mortality due to disease. Strength training also contributes to improved endurance and efficiency in daily activities (Nied & Franklin, 2002).

AGE-RELATED CARDIOVASCULAR CHANGES AND DISEASE

Increased morbidity is associated with advancing age. More than 50% of all individuals over 60 years of age have heart disease. The combination of age-related changes in the cardiovascular system and the impact heart disease has on cardiac performance make physiological responses during rest and exercise difficult to anticipate. Isolation of the effects of aging on the heart is inconclusive in the presence of heart disease. For example, myocardial scarring due to the chronic ischemia of coronary artery disease decreases ventricular compliance and slows ventricular filling, eventually promoting diastolic dysfunction. As discussed previously, the senescent heart also exhibits increased myocardial wall stiffness, which slows ventricular filling and can similarly lead to diastolic dysfunction. Diastolic dysfunction is the primary cause of heart failure in elderly patients (Gardin et al., 1998). More than 50% of patients older than 80 years who have heart failure have 'normal' systolic function. Table 6.2 lists additional examples of the clinical consequences of age-related cardiovascular changes, some of which cannot be distinguished from pre-existing disease. Clinical measures that may assist the practitioner in recognizing these changes are also listed in Table 6.2.

In addition, older individuals with comorbidities of the lung or circulation can show significantly reduced exercise capacities. Failure of the lungs to diffuse oxygen into the blood effectively or failure of the blood to transport oxygen and exchange it in the tissue creates a

---

Table 6.2 Clinical consequences of age-related cardiovascular changes and clinical measurements

Age-Related Change[a]	Clinical Consequences	Clinical Measure/Symptom[b]
↓ Beta-adrenergie responsiveness	Blunted heart rate response to exercise	HR, BP, RR, RPE
	Orthostatic hypotension	HR, BP, lightheadedness, change in color
	Longer to reach steady state	HR, RR
	Longer to recover from exercise	HR, RR
↑ Vascular tone;	Systolic hypertension	BP
↑ vascular stiffness	Signs of ventricular hypertrophy	Laterally placed PMI
(↑ Afterload)	Symptoms of myocardial ischemia	RPP, ECG, chest pain, change in color
	Arrhythmias (e.g. sss[c])	HR, BP, ECG, rhythm
↓ Pacemaker and conducting tissue cells	Conduction blocks	HR, BP, ECG, rhythm
↓ Ventricular compliance	Diastolic dysfunction, heart failure	S4, BP (may be normal)
↓ Early diastolic filling	Left atrial hypertrophy, atrial arrhythmias	HR, ECG, rhythm
Prolonged relaxation time	Symptoms of ischemia	RPP, ECG, chest pain, change in color
↓ Vagal control of HR (↓ variability)	Arrhythmias, ischemia, sudden caradiac death	ECG, HR[d], BP symptoms, 24 hour Holter monitor

[a]↑ =increase; ↓=decrease.
[b]HR, heart rate; BP, blood pressure; RR, respiratory rate; RPE, rating of perceived exertion; PMI, point of maximal impulse; RPP, rate-pressure product; S4, fourth heart sound
[c]sss, sick sinus syndrome
[d]5 minute HR (Voss, 2012).

greater demand on cardiac efficiency. The older individual may not have the reserve capacity to increase either the HR or the SV to meet this demand. This may stimulate compensatory mechanisms in cardiac performance such as ventricular hypertrophy or it may result in relatively premature fatigue.

It is worth noting that the older individual typically takes medication for the management of heart disease or other illnesses. Many of these agents directly alter the physiological performance of the heart at rest or during exercise or both. Oftentimes, the prescribed dosage of a drug does not achieve the desired therapeutic outcome or the polypharmacy of the older person increases the risk of drug toxicity. For example, digoxin, a drug prescribed for the management of congestive heart failure and atrial arrhythmias, can be toxic to an older individual. Digoxin tends to accumulate in the blood because of the reduced glomerular filtration rate through the kidneys, a common finding with aging. When quinidine, an antiarrhythmic drug, is taken in combination with digoxin, the serum digoxin level may double, further increasing the risk of digoxin toxicity, a potentially fatal condition. Hence, knowledge of the indications and pharmacokinetics of commonly prescribed drugs is essential for caregivers working with a geriatric population.

Dehydration is a common finding in an older individual. The direct cardiovascular effects of dehydration, including reduced ventricular filling volume, can impair cardiac performance and result in hypotension. The combination of dehydration and the delay in autonomic responses to position change that is commonly seen in the older individual, often results in orthostatic hypotension.

CONCLUSION

Cardiac performance is a dynamic interplay of compensatory mechanisms, some of which may not be available to the older individual. The senescent cardiovascular system, stressed by the presence of disease of the heart or other organs and commonly supported by pharmacological agents, appears vulnerable to decompensation.

Although the aging process cannot be stopped, healthcare providers are challenged not only to help the healthy older individual to safely slow or reverse the progressive decline but also to consider these changes when implementing a demanding rehabilitation program. The value of an exercise program for older individuals should not be underestimated. Minimal improvements in cardiovascular and pulmonary fitness can enable an older person to continue to live independently.

REFERENCES

Christou DD, Seals DR 2008 Decreased maximal heart rate with aging is related to reduced beta-adrenergic responsiveness but is largely explained by a reduction in intrinsic heart rate. J Appl Physiol 105:24–29

De Meersman RE, Stein PK 2007 Vagal modulation and aging. Biol Psychol 74:165–173

Dehn MM, Bruce RA 1972 Longitudinal variations in maximal oxygen intake with age and activity. J Appl Physiol 33:805–807

Fleg JL, Schulman S, O'Connor F et al 1994 Effects of acute beta-adrenergic receptor blockade on age-associated changes in cardiovascular performance during dynamic exercise. Circulation 90:2333–2341

Gardin JM, Arnold AM, Bild ED 1998 Left ventricular diastolic filling in the elderly: Cardiovascular Health Study. Am J Cardiol 82:345–351

Kaye DM, Esler MD 2008 Autonomic control of the aging heart. Neuromol Med 10:179–186

Lakatta EG 1993 Cardiovascular regulatory mechanisms in advanced age. Physiol Rev 73(32):413–467

Lakatta EG, Levy D 2003a Arterial and cardiac aging: major shareholders in cardiovascular disease enterprises. Part I: Aging arteries: A 'set up' for vascular disease. Circulation 107:139–146

Lakatta EG, Levy D 2003b Arterial and cardiac aging: major shareholders in cardiovascular disease enterprises. Part II: The aging heart in health: Links to heart disease. Circulation 107:346–354

Monahan KD 2007 Effect of aging on baroreflex function in humans. Am J Physiol Regul Integr Comp Physiol 293:R3–R12

Moslehi J, DePinho RA, Sahin E 2012 Telomeres and mitochondria in the aging heart. Circ Res 110:1226–1237

Nied RI, Franklin B 2002 Promoting and prescribing exercise for the elderly. Am Fam Phys 65:419–427

Priebe HJ 2000 The aged cardiovascular risk patient. Br J Anaesth 85:763–778

Susic D 1997 Hypertension, aging and atherosclerosis: the endothelial interface. Med Clin North Am 81(5):1231–1240

Voss A, Heitmann A, Schroeder R et al 2012 Short-term heart rate variability – age dependence in healthy subjects. Physiol Meas 33:1289–1311

Chapter 7

Pulmonary considerations in the older patient

MERYL COHEN

INTRODUCTION

Age-related changes in the pulmonary system of a healthy individual are slow and progressive. Often, the decline in pulmonary function is not noticed until the person reaches 60, 70, or even 80 years of age. Unlike the cardiovascular system, the pulmonary system has large ventilatory reserves available to compensate for the structural and physiological consequences of aging. However, in the presence of pulmonary disease, these reserves are often inadequate and can impose severe limitations on the performance of physical activities. In addition, exposure to environmental toxins over a lifetime can contribute to a more rapid decline in pulmonary function in the older person.

The age-related changes that occur in lung tissue and in the 'musculoskeletal pump' are discussed in this chapter. A clear distinction among the effects of aging, subclinical disease and prolonged exposure to air pollutants on the pulmonary system is difficult to establish, as all three cause similar structural and physiological abnormalities (Chan & Welsh, 1998; Wu and Shephard, 2011). General observations regarding the senescent lung and the effects of exercise and pulmonary disease on age-related changes in pulmonary function are also discussed. The clinical effects of aging on the pulmonary system and the implications for caregivers of older individuals are identified.

PULMONARY STRUCTURE

Age-associated changes can be found in the anatomical structures of the pulmonary system. Both the gas-exchanging organ – the lung tissue – and the musculoskeletal pump – the thoracic cage and its muscular attachments – show decline in the older individual when they are compared to the organs of a healthy younger person (see Box 7.1).

Box 7.1 *Age-related changes in pulmonary system structure*

AIRWAYS
- ↑ Rigidity of trachea and bronchi (↑ calcification)
- ↓ Elasticity of bronchiolar walls
- ↓ Cilia
- Replacement of smooth muscle fibers in bronchioles with noncontractile tissue

LUNGS
- ↑ Mucus layer (thickening) and ↑ mucus glands
- ↑ Thinning of alveolar walls (↓ alveolar collagen)
- ↓ Functional respiratory surface resulting from destruction of alveolar septa (loss of fibrous supporting network)
- ↑ Alveolar diameter with a ↓ in alveolar surface area
- ↓ Alveolar–capillary interface (due to ↑ alveolar size and ↓ capillary bed)
- ↑ Lung compliance
- ↓ Lung parenchymal weight
- Vascular walls stiffen as media and intima thicken
- Probable ↓ surfactant-producing cells

RESPIRATORY MUSCLES
- ↓ Contractile protein
- ↑ Noncontractile protein
- ↑ Connective tissue
- ↓ Capillary numbers relative to muscle fibers
- ↑ Contraction and relaxation times
- Alteration in diaphragm position and efficiency

SKELETON
- ↓ Loss of bone mineralization
- ↓ Disc spaces
- ↓ Costal movements resulting from reduced sternal and costovertebral motion (↑ stiffness of joints and calcification)
- ↑ Anterior–posterior thorax diameter
- ↑ Kyphosis resulting from a decrease in thoracic length

↑ = increase; ↓ = decrease.

THE LUNG

Changes in the alveolar membrane, including loss of the alveolar–capillary interface, and increase in alveolar size due to the destruction of the walls of individual alveoli, are the major forms of damage found in the aging lung (Brandstetter & Kasemi, 1983). The general disintegration of the supporting fibrous network of the lung and of the septa of the alveoli is considered a consequence of aging, but these changes can also result from repeated inflammatory injuries caused by life-long exposure to environmental oxidants and cigarette smoke. However, Pelkonen and colleagues have demonstrated that when older individuals stop smoking, the rate of alveolar membrane destruction is slower when alveolar tissue is compared to that of older individuals who continue to smoke (Pelkonen et al., 2001).

THE MUSCULOKELETAL PUMP

Many of the age-related changes in the thoracic cage result from the loss of mineral and bone matrix and the increased cross-linking of collagen fibers which contribute to the characteristic thoracic kyphosis and barrel chest of the older individual. The decreased mobility of the bony thorax and the less efficient resting position of the muscles of respiration alter lung performance and further contribute to the decline in pulmonary function with age (Polkey et al., 1997; Janssens et al., 1999) (see also Chapter 23, The Aging Bony Thorax).

PULMONARY PHYSIOLOGY

The primary functions of the pulmonary system are to exchange gas between the blood and the atmospheric air and to protect the body from airborne invaders. Resting lung function results from a balance of elastic tissue forces pulling inward and musculoskeletal-pump forces pulling outward. This dynamic and mostly involuntary interplay between lung tissue and chest wall musculoskeletal components depends on the compliance of both. Age-related changes in lung tissue compliance result from structural changes in the alveoli. The decrease in efficiency of pulmonary function is not generally perceived in normal elderly people because compromise of other systems with less reserve usually accounts for the alterations in their activity patterns.

The decline in alveolar structure and the pulmonary capillary bed contributes to the changes seen in ventilation (movement of gas to and from the alveoli) and gas distribution. Effective diffusion of oxygen and carbon dioxide into and out of the bloodstream depends on the integrity of the alveolar membrane and on adequate vascularity. Because alveolar membranes and capillary interfaces are compromised in the older individual, the ventilation–perfusion mismatching that is normally found in young individuals worsens with advancing age (Chan & Welsh, 1998; Janssens et al., 1999). As a result, there are larger ventilated areas relative to perfused portions of the lung (physiological dead space) which leads to a noticeable reduction in diffusing capacity (see Box 7.2).

Box 7.2 Age-related changes in pulmonary function

- ↑ Ventilation–perfusion mismatch (less homogenous)
- ↓ Diffusing capacity
- ↑ Physiological dead space
- ↓ Lung emptying
- ↑ Respiratory muscle oxygen consumption (rest)
- ↑ Minute ventilation (rest)
- ↓ Inspiratory muscle strength

↑ = increase; ↓ = decrease.

Box 7.3 Age-related changes in pulmonary function measures

- ↑ Residual volume (RV)
- ↑ Functional residual capacity (FRC)
- ↓ or ↔ Total lung capacity (TLC)
- ↑ Closing volume
- ↓ Maximal voluntary ventilation (MVV); ↓ 30% between 30 and 70 years of age
- ↓ Vital capacity (VC); ↓ 25% between 30 and 70 years of age
- ↓ Forced expiratory volume (FEV_1)
- ↓ Arterial pressure of oxygen (PaO_2); 75 mmHg is normal for 70 years of age
- ↓ Oxygen saturation
- ↓ Diffusing capacity of carbon monoxide (DLCO)

↑ = increase; ↓ = decrease; ↔ = no change.

The loss of elastic recoil in alveolar and conducting tissue and the disintegration of the fibrous supporting network also contribute to an increase in ventilation–perfusion imbalance. Smaller airways are unable to stay patent at low lung volumes (with expiration), leading to early airway closure. The resulting collapse of distal airways creates an imbalance in ventilation–perfusion. In addition, the excessive decrease in ventilation as compared to circulation causes a lowering of arterial oxygen pressure (PaO_2) (See Box 7.3 and Fig. 7.1.).

An increase in closing volume due to small airway collapse and poor lung emptying due to increased alveolar compliance and decreased elastic recoil help to account for the increase in functional residual capacity (FRC). This is the volume at which the lung comes to rest at the end of quiet expiration. Residual volume (RV), the volume that remains in the lung after maximal expiration, increases as well. The increases in lung volume tend to flatten the diaphragm, the major muscle responsible for inspiration, as it is unable to return to its original resting position. The altered diaphragm mechanics cause an increase in the anterior–posterior diameter of the rib cage. Changes in the position of the diaphragm and in the dimensions of the thorax increase the work of breathing, and the muscle primarily responsible for inspiration is at a mechanical disadvantage when it comes to performing the increased work (Fig. 7.2).

The progressive decrease in chest wall compliance and the consequent stiffness also increase the energy expended when breathing. More oxygen is consumed by the respiratory muscles, and the minute ventilation (the amount of air moved into or out of the lungs per unit of

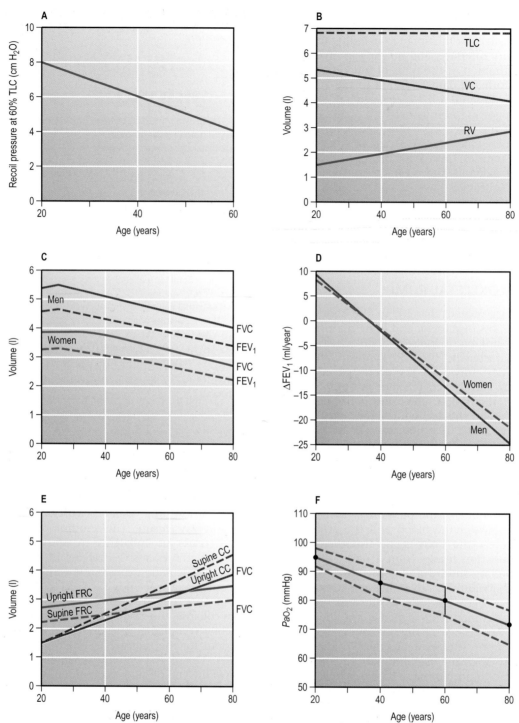

Figure 7.1 Representative changes in respiratory function with age. Curves show mean or generalized changes, and there may be consider-able variation among individuals. Note the varying age scales on the horizontal axes. **(A)** Changes in lung elastic recoil with age; **(B)** changes in static lung volume with age; **(C)** changes in FVC (solid lines) and FEV_1 (dashed lines) with age in men and women; **(D)** changes in the rate of loss of FEV_1 with age in men (solid line) and women (dashed line); **(E)** changes in CC (defined as RV plus CV) and in FRC with age: solid lines, upright posture; dashed lines, supine posture; **(F)** changes in PaO_2 (at sea level) with increasing age: dashed lines represent 62SD from the mean for the subjects studied. CC, closing capacity; CV, closing volume; FEV_1, forced expiratory volume; FRC, functional residual capacity; FVC, forced vital capacity; PaO_2, arterial oxygen pressure; RV, residual volume; TLC, total lung capacity; VC, vital capacity. *(From Pierson DJ 1992 Effects of aging on the respiratory system. In: Pierson DJ, Kacmarek RM (eds) Foundations of Respiratory Care. Churchill Livingstone, New York, with permission from the publishers.)*

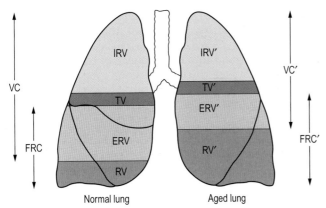

Figure 7.2 Schematic representation of lung volume changes associated with aging. Note that with senescence, there is a decrease in the inspiratory reserve volume (IRV), the expiratory reserve volume (ERV) and the vital capacity (VC). There is a corresponding increase in residual volume (RV) and functional residual capacity (FRC) such that the total lung capacity remains about the same. TV, tidal volume. *(Chan & Welsh, 1998.)*

Table 7.1 **Age-related pulmonary changes with exercise**		
	Effects of Aging	After Endurance Exercise Training
Submaximal exercise		
Minute ventilation ($\dot{V}_E$)	↑	↓
Carbon dioxide production	↑	↓
Blood lactate	↑	↓
Maximal exercise		
Maximal exercise ventilation [$\dot{V}_{E(max)}$]	↓	↑
Maximal voluntary ventilation (MVV)	↓	↑
$\dot{V}_{E(max)}$/MVV	↓	↑

↑ = increase; ↓ = decrease.
Source: Protas E 1993 Physiological change and adaptation to exercise in the older adult. In: Guccione A (ed) Geriatric Physical Therapy. Mosby, St Louis, MO, p. 42, with permission from Elsevier.

time) increases to meet this demand. In addition, there are age-related decreases in the strength and endurance of ventilatory muscles that are similar to those seen in skeletal muscle (Lowman, 2011). Inspiratory and abdominal muscle weakness can also compromise cough efficacy. This becomes more significant with aging as the mucous layer of lung tissue thickens and a more forceful cough is required to mobilize secretions.

The decrease in thoracic mobility also results in decreased vital capacity (the maximum amount of air that can be exhaled following a maximum inhalation) and decreased maximal voluntary ventilation (the volume of air breathed when an individual breathes as fast and as deeply as possible for a given time). This decline in pulmonary function can negatively impact on an older individual's ability to exercise.

AGE-RELATED PULMONARY CHANGES AND EXERCISE

In general, pulmonary responses to low and moderate exercise are the same in people of all ages. The pulmonary system can respond to the increased demands of exercise by increasing the minute ventilation, which is dependent on the tidal volume (the volume of air normally inhaled and exhaled with each breath during quiet breathing) and the frequency of breathing (respiratory rate). In the older individual, initial increases in minute ventilation are achieved by increases in tidal volume. Increases in tidal volume are due to greater abdominal excursion in the older individual since the decreased compliance of the musculoskeletal pump limits significant thorax movement. Dyspnea is perceived when the increase in tidal volume reaches 55% to 60% of vital capacity (Altose et al., 1985; Janssens et al., 1999). As already discussed, vital capacity decreases with advancing age. Hence, the ability to increase minute ventilation may be reduced at higher intensities of exercise.

In addition, the older individual tends to perform work less efficiently, generating more blood lactate. The resultant acidosis is compensated for by an increased ventilatory effort to expire more carbon dioxide. Often this results in early fatigue and a higher rating of perceived exertion (RPE) for a given workload by comparison to a younger or more fit older individual.

At low exercise workloads, an older individual continues to demonstrate ventilation–perfusion mismatching and decreased diffusing capacity. However, during vigorous exercise, pulmonary artery pressure increases. This tends to increase the alveolar capillary blood flow throughout the lungs. With improved perfusion, the ventilation–perfusion imbalance lessens and lung function and exercise tolerance improves (Zadai, 1992).

With exercise training, an older individual is able to show some improvement in the pulmonary response to exercise (see Table 7.1). Most of the improved pulmonary function results from greater efficiency of ventilatory and skeletal muscle performance (Pelkonen et al., 2003; Watsford et al., 2005). This is evidenced by the decreased production of lactate and carbon dioxide when undertaking a given workload. The individual is able to work at a lower percentage of maximal voluntary ventilation and has an increased ventilatory response for a given oxygen uptake (V_E/V_{O_2}) and less perceived dyspnea. Improved pulmonary function may also be attributed to the increase in thoracic mobility typically seen after exercise training. Individuals who are initially sedentary show the greatest improvement in function. Measurements commonly used in the clinic to monitor pulmonary response to exercise are found in Box 7.4.

Exercise can also help to mobilize secretions by way of increasing minute ventilation. Secretion retention can predispose an older individual to disease, hence exercise may further prevent decline of pulmonary function.

AGE-RELATED PULMONARY CHANGES AND DISEASE

The weakening of pulmonary structure and the decline in performance that occur with advancing age tend to have minimal impact on the functional ability of the healthy older individual. In the presence of chronic lung disease, pulmonary performance may be the limitation to exercise. Although the physiological changes in chronic obstructive pulmonary disease (COPD) are similar to those observed with aging, any lung disease that alters alveolar cell function or thoracic cage mobility can negatively impact on lung function.

The cumulative effects of COPD on the pulmonary changes normally seen with aging include a range of physiological outcomes. During rest, an individual may or may not show an increase in minute ventilation. At low workloads, an early increase in minute ventilation is observed as the lungs attempt to improve the ventilation–perfusion imbalance. Clinically, the older individual with COPD may be chronically short of breath but accepts it as a normal part of aging. As the intensity of work increases or as the disease progresses, the growing work of breathing causes an increase in the relative percentage of oxygen delivered to the respiratory muscles. Often, in the presence of thoracic cage rigidity and a significant loss of diffusing capacity, the extra energy required for pulmonary muscle function is obtained from inefficient anaerobic processes. This is seen clinically as a significant increase in dyspnea and heart rate and a decrease in arterial oxygen tension, which creates an even greater minute ventilation. In an attempt to meet this increased demand for oxygen, the heart tries to increase its performance. In some patients with compromised heart reserve, a decline in heart function can occur and, when combined with increased performance efforts, this can lead to heart failure and further compromise of the oxygen delivery system.

Age-related changes in the lungs may increase an older person's risk of developing pulmonary disease. The thickening of the mucous layer, the loss of cilia and ciliary function within airways, decreased cough effectiveness due to muscle weakness, and early airway closure combined with increased closing volume may contribute to the increased risk of pneumonia that is seen in the older population (Puchelle et al., 1979). In addition, the age-associated decline in the physiological performance of the immune system, the decline of antioxidant defenses, and reduced cellular reparatory processes may further predispose senescent lungs to infection (Lowman, 2011).

Importantly, it has been noted that changes found on radiographic chest imaging that appear to be disease-related may in reality be a 'normal' age-related finding (Copley et al., 2009; Wu & Shephard., 2011). When compared to healthy 55-year-old individuals, healthy individuals over 75 years of age, irrespective of smoking history, were found to have evidence of bronchial dilatation, bronchial wall thickening, small cysts and subpleural basal reticular pattern on computerized tomography (CT). These 'normal' age-related CT findings might otherwise result in extensive medical testing and unnecessary treatment, highlighting the need for additional clinical research to assist healthcare providers in distinguishing age-related changes from disease.

CONCLUSION

Age-related changes occur in lung tissue and in the musculoskeletal pump. Pathological conditions potentiate the effects of these changes.

Although the objective benefits of exercise training are difficult to measure, older individuals with pulmonary disease are able to recognize an improved physical work capacity and sense of wellbeing. Respiratory and peripheral muscle conditioning and increased thoracic cage mobility improve the mechanical efficiency of the musculoskeletal pump and of oxygen extraction by the tissues. This may interrupt the declining cycle of dyspnea, inactivity and worsening dyspnea, and enable an individual to remain independent and active. In addition, the improved strength and endurance of respiratory and abdominal muscles can facilitate cough effectiveness and assist in the management of retained secretions, thus decreasing the risk of pulmonary infections.

REFERENCES

Altose MD, Leitner J, Cherniak NS 1985 Effects of age and respiratory efforts on the perception of resistive ventilatory loads. J Gerontol 40:147–153

Brandstetter RD, Kasemi H 1983 Aging and the respiratory system. Med Clin North Am 67:419–431

Chan ED, Welsh CH 1998 Geriatric respiratory medicine. Chest 114:1704–1733

Copley SJ, Wells AU, Hawtin KE et al 2009 Lung morphology in the elderly: comparative CT study of subjects over 75 years old versus those under 55 years old. Radiology 251:566–573

Janssens JP, Pache JC, Nicod LP 1999 Physiological changes in respiratory function associated with ageing. Eur Respir J 13:197–205

Lowman JD 2011 The aging pulmonary system. In: Hardage J (ed) Focus: Physical Therapist Practice in Geriatrics, Issue 4, pp. 1–26

Pelkonen M, Notkola IL, Tukianinen H et al 2001 Smoking cessation, decline in pulmonary function and total mortality: a 30 year follow up study among Finnish cohorts of the Seven Countries Study. Thorax 56:703–707

Pelkonen M, Notkla IL, Lakka T et al 2003 Delaying decline in pulmonary function with physical activity: a 25-year follow-up. Am J Respir Crit Care Med 168:494–499

Polkey MI, Harris ML, Hughes PD et al 1997 The contractile properties of the elderly human diaphragm. Am J Respir Crit Care Med 155:1560–1564

Puchelle E, Zahm JM, Bertrand A 1979 Influence of age on bronchial mucociliary transport. Scand J Respir Dis 60:307–313

Watsford M, Murphy AJ, Pine MJ et al 2005 The effect of habitual exercise on respiratory-muscle function in older adults. J Aging Phys Act 13:34–44

Wu CC, Shephard JO 2011 Imaging features of the normal aging chest. In: Katlic MR (ed) Cardiothoracic Surgery in the Elderly. Springer, New York, pp. 143–156

Zadai CC (ed) 1992 Pulmonary Management in Physical Therapy. Churchill Livingstone, New York

Chapter 8

Effects of aging on the digestive system

RONNI CHERNOFF

CHAPTER CONTENTS

INTRODUCTION

There is little change that can be attributed to age in gastrointestinal (GI) function in the absence of disease due to the large reserve capacity of this multiorgan system. The GI tract serves two major functions in the body, the first is the ingestion, digestion, absorption and excretion of nutrients and their byproducts; the functional reserve is greatest in the midgut, pancreas and liver. Intestinal segments may adapt, and functional reserve tends to buffer change so that only long-term observation may uncover abnormalities. This is less true for the proximal (esophagus) and distal (large colon) portions of the gut. The second major function of the gut is as an organ that filters and defends against pathogens.

The ingestion, digestion and absorption of nutrients are essential processes that are part of the maintenance of nutritional status. The function of the GI tract is, therefore, intricately involved in nutrition and a factor in an individual's nutritional status. Because of the physiological changes that occur with advancing age, older people may have difficulties in meeting their nutritional requirements and fighting microorganisms. Common GI symptoms are often nonspecific and do not indicate the exact nature or severity of disease (Ravindran et al., 2014).

The physiological changes associated with advancing age include the loss of lean body mass and body protein compartments, a decrease in total body water, reduction in bone density and a proportional gain in total body fat. Loss of lean body mass and muscle integrity, as well as a decrease in vagal sensitivity, may impact peristalsis and the ability to move a bolus through the GI tract. In an older individual, adequate nutrition is an important factor for the maintenance of health and recovery from disease. It is important to note that many studies that describe changes in the GI tract with aging are conducted on subjects who have chronic conditions that may affect GI physiology or function (Ravindran et al., 2014).

NUTRITIONAL REQUIREMENTS IN AGING

ENERGY

The maintenance of health status and the provision of adequate nutrition in elderly people requires an understanding of the impact of age on nutritional requirements. The most well-documented change that occurs over time is the decrease in energy metabolism. This reduction in energy requirements is related to a decrease in total protein mass rather than a reduction in the metabolic activity of aging tissue.

Basal energy requirements reflect the energy needed for all of the metabolic processes that are involved in maintaining cell function and keeping the brain and vital organs functioning; the reduction of active metabolic mass will result in lowered energy needs.

PROTEIN

Protein requirements in elderly individuals might be expected to decrease to accommodate a lower total lean body mass. However, studies appear to indicate that protein requirements may be slightly higher in older subjects. One explanation is that a lower calorie intake contributes to reduced retention of dietary nitrogen, therefore requiring more dietary protein to achieve nitrogen balance (Campbell et al., 2014). It has been reported that ingestion of 25–30 g of high-quality protein at each meal may help older adults maintain muscle mass, although longitudinal research is needed to assess this notion (Paddon-Jones & Rasmussen, 2009).

Protein needs are also affected by immobility, which contributes to negative nitrogen balance. Elderly people who are bed-bound, wheelchair-bound or otherwise immobilized will require higher levels of dietary protein to achieve nitrogen equilibrium. Surgery, sepsis, long-bone fractures and unusual losses, such as those that occur with burns or GI disease, increase the need for dietary protein.

Some clinicians have been wary of providing high levels of protein for fear of precipitating renal disease in elderly individuals. Research has shown that there is no evidence that dietary protein induces deterioration of renal function in individuals who have no pre-existing evidence of renal disease. For elderly patients who have a measurable decline in renal function, therapeutic regimens should be followed.

FAT

The major contribution of fat in the diet is energy, essential fatty acids and fat-soluble vitamins. Because only small amounts of fat are needed to provide essential fatty acids, and fat-soluble vitamins are available from other dietary sources, the primary contribution from dietary fat is the provision of calories. For older people, restricting dietary fat, thereby reducing caloric intake, is a reasonable strategy to maintain caloric balance without restricting intake of other nutrients; however, in some individuals, too rigid restrictions on dietary fat may contribute to energy deficits.

Altering the type and amount of dietary fat in the diet of older adults is somewhat controversial. As a controllable variable in the reduction of the risk of heart disease, there are major differences in opinion regarding the need for dietary fat alteration in adults over 65. One approach to lowering risk in older adults is to reduce the intake of saturated fat and simultaneously increase the intake of polyunsaturated and monounsaturated fat, keeping the total fat intake about the same. In one study cited by deLorgeril and Salen (2011) in their review, subjects who had previously suffered a myocardial infarction were put on a Mediterranean-style diet with more complex carbohydrate, fruit, green vegetables and fish with less beef, lamb, or pork, and monounsaturated cooking oils. The group on this type of diet had fewer cardiac events and deaths at 2-year follow-up than did a control group who made no dietary modifications. Even on this modified diet, there was no change in total cholesterol or low-density lipoprotein cholesterol levels. The Mediterranean diet is recommended routinely as secondary prevention of coronary heart disease.

CARBOHYDRATES

Carbohydrate (CHO) intake in the diets of elderly people should be approximately 55–60% of the total caloric intake, with an emphasis on complex CHOs. The ability to metabolize CHO appears to decline with advancing age. Nevertheless, glucose is an efficient energy substrate that can be used by all body tissues but is necessary for energy production in brain and red blood cells (Kohlmeier, 2003; Keim et al., 2014).

It is important to encourage complex CHO intake in elderly people because foods in this group provide fiber, a constituent of the diet that enhances bowel motility, which tends to decrease over time. Bowel disorders that can be managed by a diet high in fiber include constipation and diverticular disease. Dietary fiber intake also

decreases total cholesterol, LDL-cholesterol and triglycerides levels (Clemens et al., 2012). Fresh fruits and vegetables are difficult to chew if oral health status is not optimal or dentures do not fit properly, and these foods are expensive when they are out of season. Cereal fibers should be encouraged as an alternative; however, it is difficult to obtain adequate fiber from cereal foods alone.

VITAMINS

Vitamin requirements for adults over 65 are mostly speculative, although there is much ongoing research. Vitamin deficiencies may exist subclinically in the elderly, particularly for some of the water-soluble vitamins. In times of stress, after illness or injury, a depleted reserve capacity may not be able to compensate for rapid depletion of tissue stores and the individual may become overtly deficient. Subclinical deficiencies may exist in people who have adequate but not excess dietary intake, because the absorption and utilization of these vitamins may be compromised by the use of multiple medications or single nutrient supplements or by the declining efficiency of the small bowel to absorb micronutrients.

The water-soluble vitamins that are often the focus of attention are vitamin C and vitamin B_{12}. Although there appears to be no age-related alteration in vitamin C (ascorbic acid) absorption, deficiency in this vitamin is often linked with wound-healing problems or a tendency to bruise easily. Vitamin C is an essential factor needed to make collagen, the protein matrix that holds cells together, and is therefore required when new tissue is being made. The recommended daily allowance (RDA) for vitamin C is 60 mg/day, a level that is far exceeded in most American diets. With large doses of supplemental vitamin C, tissue saturation is reached rapidly and the excess vitamin is excreted in urine. Very large doses (greater than 1 g/day) may contribute to some serious side-effects, such as the formation of kidney stones or chronic diarrhea in sensitive individuals. There is little evidence that massive doses of vitamin C aid in wound healing, ward off the common cold or cure cancer.

Vitamin B_{12} is a vitamin for which many older adults may be at risk for deficiency. The major dietary source of vitamin B_{12} is red meat and organ meats, which many elderly people have eliminated from their diets because of the fat and cholesterol content. In addition to dietary inadequacy, some older adults have a condition called atrophic gastritis, in which gastric acid production is decreased. Gastric acid is necessary for the release of vitamin B_{12} from a series of protein carriers; it is then linked to an intrinsic factor that forms a complex with the vitamin, allowing it to be absorbed. Production of intrinsic factor is also decreased with atrophic gastritis. Symptoms of vitamin B_{12} deficiency are generally nonspecific but include irritability, lethargy and mild dementia.

It is less likely that elderly people will be deficient in fat-soluble vitamins (A, D, E, K) because of the ability to store these vitamins in liver tissue. The greatest risk is for deficiency of vitamin D, particularly for homebound or institutionalized elderly people. Limited exposure to sunlight, the use of sunscreens and an inadequate intake of dairy products contribute to this risk. It is also known that the amount of vitamin D precursor in skin, which is stimulated by sunlight, particularly ultraviolet rays, decreases with age. Dietary vitamin D goes through several conversions in the liver and kidney, resulting in production of the active form of the vitamin; the kidney becomes less efficient at the final step of conversion with advanced age. Because vitamin D is an important nutrient in bone mineralization and immune function, it is wise to encourage the inclusion of foods rich in vitamin D in the diets of elderly individuals who may be at risk of deficiency.

For vitamin A, the risk of vitamin toxicity is greater than the risk of deficiency. This is especially true of older people who are taking over-the-counter vitamin supplements, many of which have very high levels of vitamin A. Beta-carotene, a vitamin A precursor, has received a great deal of attention in recent years because of its apparent protective effect against various types of neoplasms. The long-term effects of high doses of beta-carotene have not been adequately explored.

MINERALS

The requirements for most minerals do not change with age. An exception is iron, for which there is a decreased requirement because of a tendency to increase tissue iron stores with advancing age and a cessation of menstrual blood loss in women. Calcium requirements have attracted much attention in recent years. Investigators have suggested that the recommendations for dietary calcium intake increase from 800 mg/day to 1200 or 1500 mg/day to reduce the risk of osteoporosis. However, the controversy surrounding calcium requirements in older people has not yet been settled, with many investigators believing that the recommendations should not be changed.

For most other major minerals, such as sodium and potassium, requirements are not changed by the aging process but are affected by the presence of acute or chronic diseases and their treatment (medications).

WATER

Water is an important nutrient for older people. Inadequate fluid intake may lead to rapid dehydration and precipitate associated problems: hypotension, elevated body temperature, constipation, nausea, vomiting, mucosal dryness, decreased urine output and mental confusion. It is particularly noteworthy that these problems are rarely attributed to fluid imbalances, which can be easily corrected.

Fluid intake should be adequate to compensate for normal losses (through kidneys, bowel, lungs and skin) and for unusual losses associated with increased body temperature, vomiting, diarrhea or hemorrhage. A reasonable estimate of fluid needs is approximately 1 ml of fluid/kcal ingested or 30 ml/kg actual body weight. The minimum intake for all older adults regardless of their size or caloric intake should be approximately 1500 ml/ day. Fluid needs can be met with water, juices, beverages such as tea or coffee, gelatin desserts and other foods that are liquid at room temperature. Tube-feeding formulas contain approximately 750 ml water per liter of solution; it is wise to compensate for the solid displacement by adding 25% of the volume of the tube feeding as additional free water.

Meeting all of these changes is often challenging. Encouraging older adults to consume an adequate diet may be linked to a functional and healthy GI tract. Age does have an impact on GI structure and function and it is worth assessing GI function in older adults.

AGE AND THE GI TRACT

THE AGING ORAL CAVITY

The changes associated with the aging process affect the structures of the mouth. Bone loss is a common problem and, in the oral cavity, where the alveolar bone is more prone to brittleness and fragility, there is an increased likelihood of tissue damage occurring because of oral trauma, periodontal disease and loss of teeth. Nutritional deficiencies are also manifested in periodontal and perioral tissue, which can impair chewing and normal ingestion of food.

As lean body mass decreases, gum tissue may be lost because of disease and atrophy. This process, along with bone resorption, leads to an increased risk of root caries, periodontal disease and loss of structure to support dentures. These changes, along with others in oral musculature and the mucous membranes, contribute to difficulty in chewing food adequately. Many individuals alter their dietary intake to compensate for their diminished efficiency in chewing, thereby putting themselves at risk for malnutrition. Malnutrition is associated with negative outcomes and adds an additional burden to the challenge of rehabilitation.

Other changes that may occur in the mouth and affect nutritional status include decreased taste and smell sensitivity, loss of taste and smell, and decreased salivary flow, which may be associated with disease conditions or the effects of medications. In chronically ill patients, the possibility that this condition may be present should be investigated. It is important to assess the ability of an individual to consume adequate nutrients to restore or maintain nutritional status through a period of rehabilitation.

THE ESOPHAGUS

The esophagus is the conduit that serves to transport food from the mouth to the stomach. Although it may not seem to be a very important part of the GI tract, esophageal dysfunction may have a profound impact on nutritional status and, therefore, on the recovery from an illness or other physiological problem.

The most common dysfunction of the esophagus is swallowing disorders (Robbins & Banaszynski, 2014). Swallowing problems may be characterized by pain, choking, spitting or vomiting. These symptoms are usually associated with an obstruction, cerebrovascular accident, neurological disease or degenerative muscular disease. Gastroesophageal reflux may be a secondary problem resulting from weakness in the lower esophageal sphincter, failure of peristalsis, or an injury or illness in the stomach (Katz et al., 2013).

Diagnosis and correction of esophageal problems are key to safe ingestion of food and liquids. Depending on the etiology and severity of the dysfunction, dietary modification may be the appropriate treatment. More severe problems require medical, pharmacological or surgical interventions. In either case, ensuring adequate nutritional intake is important to maintaining nutritional status.

THE STOMACH

The stomach serves several functions in the digestive process: its mechanical action breaks up food; it digests food through chemical and enzymatic actions; and it serves as a reservoir to hold partially digested food until it can be released into the small intestine. There is no evidence that age has a significant effect on gastric function; however, age-related conditions and diseases may result in altered gastric function.

The gastric conditions most commonly seen in elderly individuals are atrophic gastritis, peptic ulcer disease and gastroesophageal reflux disease. Atrophic gastritis may contribute to a perception of food intolerance but, more importantly, it may be a major factor in vitamin B_{12} deficiency because gastric acid is required for the digestion process that allows this vitamin to be absorbed. Folic acid may also be malabsorbed with this condition (Johnson et al., 2010).

Peptic ulcer disease is increasing among the elderly, although the incidence in the general population appears to be declining (Wang & Peura, 2011). Medications, such as H_2 (histamine) antagonists and antacids, may have multiple side-effects, which could lead to other problems, including constipation, obstruction, osteomalacia, diarrhea, dehydration and electrolyte disturbances.

Gastroesophageal reflux disease is usually associated with the incompetence of the lower esophageal sphincter. There is no evidence that this is an age-related condition but some older individuals do experience this condition.

THE PANCREAS

There is no strong evidence that age affects the pancreas in any significant way; however, glucose intolerance seems to increase and insulin secretion tends to decrease with advanced age and there appears to be a reduction in secretory output (Scheen, 2005). This reduction is not considered clinically significant until pancreatic output is less than 10% of normal or these changes become symptomatic.

Diseases of the pancreas do commonly occur in older people. Acute pancreatitis occurs in older patients and may have severe consequences, resulting in sepsis and shock. An uncomplicated course may have a brief period of pain, nausea and vomiting, and tends to occur in individuals who have biliary tract disease. A more severe occurrence may result in abscesses, other septic symptoms or shock, and may require surgery and stress metabolic management.

Chronic primary inflammatory pancreatitis is a disease of older people. Symptoms include steatorrhea, diabetes, pancreatic calcification and weight loss. This is often a pain-free condition with an unpredictable response to therapy.

THE AGING LIVER

The liver tends to get smaller in mass with advancing age, which can lead to changes in structure and function. This may be important because many of the functions of the liver (synthesis, excretion and metabolism) are crucial for the maintenance of health. These functions are more affected by systemic disease and liver disease, both of which are common in elderly people.

The changes that occur which are important considerations in elderly people include alterations in drug metabolism and a decrease in the rate of protein synthesis. Both of these factors contribute to a diminished ability to respond appropriately to drug therapy, to adequately clear drugs through the liver or to tolerate the physiological burden associated with disease. In elderly people, who often are receiving multiple prescription medications, this clearance ability may be a major factor in drug-related symptoms (McLachlan & Pont, 2012)

THE SMALL BOWEL

The GI tract, beginning at the mouth and ending at the anus, is a large muscle that propels food and its digested products through the body. Food is ingested and almost immediately acted upon by digestive enzymes, chemicals and mechanical actions. Many of the critical digestion and absorption functions occur in the small bowel. Age and disease can have an impact on the normal function of the small bowel.

The most common disorder of CHO metabolism is the disaccharidase deficiency of lactase. Lactase deficiency occurs with age and with common GI diseases such as viral gastroenteritis, Crohn's disease, bacterial infections and ulcerative colitis. Symptoms are associated with the ingestion of milk and milk products, and occur when the ingestion of lactose exceeds the production of lactase in the small bowel.

Another disorder with vague symptoms is celiac disease; this involves sensitivity to gluten, a protein commonly found in wheat products. It frequently results from an injury to the small bowel from exposure to gluten, which contributes to malabsorption and steatorrhea. The treatment is to eliminate gluten, found in wheat, rye or barley-based products, from the diet and replace it with products made from corn, rice or potato. Replacement of malabsorbed nutrients (iron, folic acid, calcium, vitamin D) should be part of the therapy.

Another source of malabsorption in older individuals is bacterial overgrowth. This may be associated with the decrease in gastric acid production by the stomach and the age-related decrease in bowel motility. Generalized malabsorption may result from this condition; vitamin B_{12} is a nutrient that is at risk of being malabsorbed.

Other conditions that may damage the small bowel and impair its ability to digest and absorb essential nutrients include radiation enteritis and inflammatory bowel diseases. Radiation enteritis is often a consequence of treatment for cancer of the cervix, uterus, prostate, bladder or colon. Because of their rapidly dividing characteristics, the cells in the small intestine are vulnerable to damage from radiation. Symptoms of diarrhea, nausea, cramping and distension often occur years after the period of therapy and may go unreported. Malabsorption and dehydration are potential nutritional consequences. Inflammatory bowel disease may occur, with its symptoms attributed to other conditions because it is less common in older adults.

Along with the digestive and absorptive bowel functions is a mucosal immune system that exists independently of the peripheral immune system and functions separately from the nutritional functions of the bowel mucosa. Age-related deterioration of immune function has been well recognized in older adults; the incidence of infection, autoimmune diseases and cancer is higher among older adults. Although immunosenescence in both host and cell-mediated systems is well described, mucosal immunity is less well understood (Spencer & Belkaid, 2012).

THE LARGE INTESTINE

The primary function of the large intestine is the absorption of water, electrolytes, bile salts and short-chain fatty acids. The major conditions related to the large intestine that are experienced by older people are colon cancer, diverticulosis and constipation. If diagnosed early enough, colon cancer is treatable with surgery and radiation therapy. Diverticular disease may be asymptomatic in elderly patients until an infection occurs and the individual becomes symptomatic. Dietary treatment is the same for older patients as it is for younger patients.

Constipation is a common complaint among older adults. It may occur as a result of many conditions: neurological disease, drug effects, systemic disease, inadequate fluid intake, lack of dietary bulk and physical inactivity. However, the primary issue may be aging smooth muscle; there has been very little exploration of this physiological process and extensive research is needed. Treatment should be based on the etiology of the condition and include adequate hydration, dietary fiber and physical activity (Bitar & Patil, 2004; Toner & Claros, 2012; Cherniak, 2013).

DIETARY MANAGEMENT OF MALNUTRITION

As with other nutritional problems, the patient who is in rehabilitation should be encouraged to eat as much as possible. Underlying disease conditions should be treated first with nutritional adequacy encouraged as appropriate. Smaller, frequent meals may be accepted more readily by elderly patients with smaller appetites and early satiety. Oral liquid supplements can be added to solid food if fluid overload is not a contraindication. The goal of refeeding should be to provide 35 kcal/kg of the patient's actual weight and at least 1 g of protein/kg.

Experience has demonstrated that only 10% of elderly people who have protein energy malnutrition can consume adequate calories orally to correct their nutritional deficiencies; most patients therefore require more aggressive nutritional intervention, such as enteral or parenteral feeding.

CONCLUSION

The impact of aging on GI tract function happens slowly over time but will often contribute to nutritional challenges that may affect the ingestion, digestion and absorption of nutrients. In older individuals, the ability to maintain nutritional status will also be affected by chronic conditions and episodes of acute illness that require adequate nutritional reserve. For most of the changes encountered, nutritional solutions can be devised; the greatest challenge is to recognize that there is a problem and to start interventions as soon as possible.

REFERENCES

Bitar KN, Patil SB 2004 Aging and gastrointestinal smooth muscle. Mech Aging Dev 125:907–910

Campbell WW, Carnell NS, Thalacker AE 2014 Protein metabolism and requirements. In: Chernoff R (ed) Geriatric Nutrition: The Health Professional's Handbook, 4th edn. Jones & Bartlett, Boston, MA

Cherniak EP 2013 Use of complementary and alternative medicine to treat constipation in the elderly. Geriatr Gerontol Int 13:815–816

Clemens R, Kranz S, Mobley AR et al 2012 Filling America's fiber intake gap: summary of a roundtable to probe realistic solutions with a focus on grain-based foods. J Nutr 142:1390s–1401s

de Lorgeril M, Salen P 2011 Mediterranean diet in secondary prevention of CHD. Pub Health Nutr 14(12A):2333–2337

Johnson MA, Hausman DB, Davey A et al 2010 Vitamin B$_{12}$ deficiency in African American and White octogenarians and centenarians in Georgia. J Nutr Health Aging 14(5):339–345

Katz PO, Gerson LB, Vela MF 2013 Guidelines for the diagnosis and management of gastroesophageal reflux disease. Am J Gastroenterol 108(3):308–328

Keim NL, Levin RJ, Havel PJ 2014 Carbohydrates. In: Ross CA, Caballero B, Cousins RJ (eds) Modern Nutrition in Health and Diseases. Lippincott Williams & Wilkins, Philadelphia, PA

Kohlmeier M 2003 Carbohydrates, alcohols, and organic acids. In: Nutrient Metabolism. Academic Press, Boston, MA

McLachlan AJ, Pont LG 2012 Drug metabolism in older people – a key consideration in achieving optimal outcomes with medicines. J Gerontol A Biol Sci Med Sci 67(2):175–180

Paddon-Jones D, Rasmussen BB 2009 Dietary protein recommendations and the prevention of sarcopenia. Curr Opin Clin Nutr Metab Care 12:86–90

Ravindran NC, Moskovitz DN, Kim Y-I 2014 The aging gut. In: Chernoff R (ed) Geriatric Nutrition: The Health Professional's Handbook, 4th edn. Jones & Bartlett, Boston, MA

Robbins J, Banaszynski K 2014 Swallowing problems in older adults. In: Chernoff R (ed) Geriatric Nutrition: The Health Professional's Handbook, 4th edn. Jones & Bartlett, Boston, MA

Scheen AJ 2005 Diabetes mellitus in the elderly: insulin resistance and/or impaired insulin secretion? Diabetes Metab 31:27–34

Spencer SP, Belkaid Y 2012 Dietary and commensal derived nutrients: shaping mucosal and systemic immunity. Curr Opin Immunology 24:379–384

Toner F, Claros E 2012 Preventing, assessing and managing constipation in older adults. Nursing 42(12):32–39

Wang AY, Peura DA 2011 The prevalence and incidence of *Heliobacter pylori*-associated peptic ulcer disease and upper gastrointestinal bleeding throughout the world. Gastrointest Endosc Clin North Am 21(4):613–635

Chapter 9

Effects of aging on vascular function

KRISTIN VON NIEDA

CHAPTER CONTENTS

INTRODUCTION

The study of aging has grown significantly in recent years. Several factors, such as increase in the aging population, the increase in life expectancy and the increase in health expenditure, contribute to growth. Studies concerned with aging have also evolved in scope. Earlier studies focused on identifying a single cause or explanation for aging. More recently, aging has been viewed as a complex process in which many factors and processes interrelate. Thus, a single cause or process is no longer sufficient to address the intricacies of the vascular aging process (Weinert & Timiras, 2003; Kovacic et al., 2011a).

Age-associated changes occur in the musculoskeletal, neuromuscular, cardiovascular, pulmonary and integumentary systems. This chapter addresses a subset of the cardiovascular and pulmonary systems and focuses on the effects of aging on the vascular system. Just as these systems function interdependently, it is impossible to isolate and limit aging effects to the vascular system without having an awareness of concomitant age-associated changes in other systems.

REVIEW OF THE STRUCTURE AND FUNCTIONS OF THE VASCULAR SYSTEM

The oxygen transport system is the biological system responsible for (i) bringing oxygen into the body from the ambient environment; (ii) circulating oxygen throughout the body; (iii) supplying oxygen at the tissue level; and (iv) ultimately removing the waste products created as a result of utilizing oxygen. The vascular system is the means by which oxygen and nutrients are delivered to the working tissues, and by which the metabolic byproducts are removed from the tissues. The vascular network supplies a steady stream of oxygen-rich blood that allows working tissues and muscles to function at optimal levels. The ability to shunt blood preferentially and to deliver oxygen to the areas of greatest metabolic demand makes the vascular system an essential component of the oxygen transport system.

The vascular system is made up of three basic types of blood vessel: the arteries, capillaries and veins. The thickness of each layer of the vessels varies throughout the vascular system depending on the location and function of the specific vessel (see Fig. 9.1).

The arterial system functions to accommodate the large volume of blood received as cardiac output and to propel it forward using the property of elastic recoil. The presence of smooth muscle in the arterial system allows it to control and direct the flow of blood throughout the vascular system via autonomic and endothelial controls and in response to local metabolic demand.

The normal structure of the arteries includes three layers. The adventitia is the outermost layer and attaches the vessel to the surrounding tissue. It consists of longitudinally oriented connective tissue with varying amounts of elastic and collagenous fibers. The middle layer or the media is usually the thickest and is a highly elastic, circumferentially oriented fibromuscular layer. Its function is to provide vascular support and to regulate blood flow and blood pressure by facilitating changes in

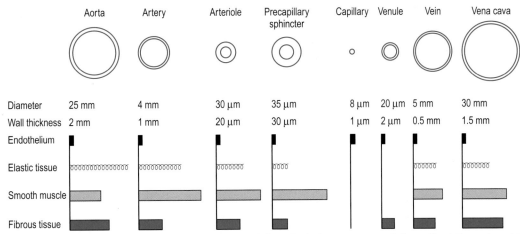

Figure 9.1 Internal diameter, wall thickness and relative amounts of the principal components of the walls of the various blood vessels that compose the circulatory system. Cross-sections of the vessels are not drawn to scale because of the huge range in size from aorta and vena cava to capillary. *(From Berne RM, Levy MN 1981 Cardiovascular Physiology, 4th edn. CV Mosby, St Louis, MO, p. 2, with permission.)*

diameter. The intima, the innermost layer, is composed of a single, continuous layer of endothelial cells that separates blood from the vessel wall. The endothelium serves as a barrier between the circulating blood and the underlying interstitium and cells, allowing selective transport on macromolecules in the blood to meet metabolic demands in surrounding tissues. The endothelium responds to regulatory substances released by physical and chemical stimuli and has many important functions, including regulation of vascular tone and growth, thrombosis and thrombolysis, and interaction with platelets and leukocytes.

The capillaries are the smallest and most numerous of the blood vessels, forming the connection between the arteries and the veins. The capillaries are thin and fragile in comparison to arteries and veins, and there is little resistance to the diffusion of oxygen and other metabolic products. The capillary wall is one endothelial cell thick, which allows for the exchange of nutrients and waste products at the tissue level.

The veins have the same three layers as the arteries; however, the walls are thinner and less rigid because there is less smooth muscle and connective tissue. The veins are capacitance vessels, which serve as collecting tubules for blood as it exits the capillary beds. At any given time, the majority of the blood volume is located in the venous circulation. The maintenance of a larger reservoir of venous blood allows for adequate venous return as well as a necessary reserve during periods of increased oxygen demand.

Venous return is the principle determinant of cardiac preload, and sufficient venous return is necessary to ensure sufficient cardiac output. This function is accomplished by a combination of venous smooth muscle contraction, external muscle compression and a series of unidirectional internal venous valves.

AGE-ASSOCIATED VASCULAR CHANGES

Advancing age and associated vascular changes are recognized as a major risk factor for cardiac disease. Aging in the presence of cardiovascular disease accelerates structural and physiological changes, and the presence of other risk factors further influences the rate at which the changes occur. Hence, physiological aging and chronological aging cannot be considered equivalent.

In addition to the alteration of the underlying cardiovascular structures and functions, the increase in life expectancy also lengthens the exposure time to certain risk factors. In this sense, age-associated cardiovascular changes in structure and function are 'partners' with cardiovascular disease mechanisms. More specifically, it is the interaction between age, disease and several additional factors, such as lipid levels, diabetes, sedentary lifestyle and genetics, that determines the threshold, severity and prognosis of the disease in older people (Lakatta & Levy, 2003). The presence of risk factors such as abdominal obesity, which is associated with metabolic risk factors, such as insulin resistance, metabolic syndrome and impaired glucose tolerance, compounds the effects of aging on the vascular system (Scuteri et al., 2005).

Age-related cardiovascular changes occur in healthy, unhealthy and seemingly healthy older people. Lakatta and Levy (2003) differentiated between 'successful' and 'unsuccessful' aging. 'Successful' aging refers to healthy individuals, for whom the age-associated changes pose little or no threat to the development of disease. 'Unsuccessful' aging encompasses individuals who do not have or have not yet experienced clinical cardiovascular disease, but whose age-related cardiovascular changes put them at risk for future disease.

STRUCTURAL CHANGES ASSOCIATED WITH AGING

Structural changes associated with aging occur throughout the vascular system. Significant changes occur within the walls of the large elastic arteries, in which the intimal medial thickness increases two- to three-fold between the ages of 20 and 90 years (Nagai et al., 1998). The adventitia is most affected by a decrease in the number of elastic fibers and an increase in collagen, resulting in a loss of distensibility and a reduction in elastic recoil, essential for accommodating blood volume and propelling the blood into the vascular system. Both within the intima and the media, there is increased calcification, loss of elastin content, fragmentation of the elastin and an increase in collagen. These changes lead to increased systolic blood pressure, decreased diastolic blood pressure and widened pulse pressure, which in turn may affect ventricular hypertrophy, renal impairments and adverse cerebrovascular events (Kovacic et al., 2011b). Lipid deposits in the intima further contribute to vascular wall thickening. These structural changes appear to be similar to the atherosclerotic changes seen in disease states, but occur even in the absence of occult disease and within populations with a low incidence of atherosclerosis (Moore et al., 2003).

Recently, telomere shortening was implicated in vascular aging and cardiovascular disease (Kovacic et al., 2011a). A telomere is a region of repetitive nucleotide sequences at each end of a chromosome, which makes it possible for cells to divide and protects the ends of the chromosome from deteriorating. Telomeres shorten with each cell division, and cells are generally unaffected until the telomeres become too short. When this occurs, cellular division ceases and cellular senescence or cell death ensues. Kovacic et al. (2011) reported on several studies linking increased incidence of coronary artery disease or atherosclerotic disease and shortened telomere length in peripheral blood leukocytes. Further, leukocyte telomere length was found to decrease by 6–9% per decade, and there was a predictive value for cardiovascular events associated with shortened telomeres. To some extent physical activity has a positive effect on the maintenance of telomere length (Werner et al., 2009).

Aging is linked to significant changes in the microcirculation, resulting in age-associated endothelial dysfunction. The endothelial cells become irregularly shaped and are no longer longitudinally oriented along the vessels. Endothelial permeability is increased (Ferrari et al., 2003), disrupting the selective transport system and resulting in concentrations of macromolecular materials and proinflammatory substances that further contribute to plaque formation or atherosclerosis. Within the media, vascular smooth muscle cells proliferate, migrate and infiltrate into the subendothelial space (Lakatta & Levy, 2003). The irregular alignment and the increase in intimal medial thickness affect the dynamics of and resistance to blood flow, thereby affecting the transport of oxygen and other nutrients.

Lakatta and Levy (2003) also reported that arterial stiffness may be influenced by endothelial regulation of vascular smooth muscle tone. The age-associated changes in endothelial function further contribute to vascular stiffness in both the large and peripheral arteries, thereby hindering the normal contractile capability of vascular smooth muscle.

The age-associated increase in vascular wall thickness is accompanied by dilatation of the large arteries, loss of compliance and an increase in arterial stiffness, which may not be uniform throughout the vascular system (D'Alessio, 2004; Ungvari et al., 2010). In peripheral vessels there is less of an increase in diameter of the vessels and more of an increase in wall thickening. In large arteries there is an age-dependent loss of capacitive compliance, whereas the reduction in small artery

compliance is oscillatory or reflective (McVeigh et al., 1999). Both types of compliance changes contribute to modifications in the generation, propulsion and reflection of pulse waves in the aging vascular system.

Pulse wave velocity (PWV), a noninvasive measure of vascular stiffness, increases with age in populations with little or no atherosclerosis, indicating that the increase in stiffness can develop independent of atherosclerotic changes (Lakatta & Levy, 2003; Strait & Lakatta, 2012). The increase in PWV is associated with changes in vascular structure, most notably the increased collagen, decreased elastin, increased elastin fragments and calcification in the media. When a forward pulse wave reaches an area of mismatch in the vascular structure, the wave is reflected back through the artery to the central aorta. Whereas in young subjects the reflected wave arrives at the proximal aorta in diastole, the reflected wave in older vessels travels faster and arrives during late systole, causing an increased load for the ventricle and a potential adverse affect on coronary blood flow (Strait & Lakatta, 2012).

Age-associated changes also affect the venous vessels. There is an overall increase in stiffness and a decrease in venous compliance Hernandez and Frank (2004). The venous valves begin to lose their integrity and the efficiency of unidirectional flow is lessened. It becomes more difficult to maintain venous return, and there exists the potential for venous stasis and retrograde flow. In a study of cross-sectional area (CSA) of the femoral and long saphenous veins, CSA was found to be associated with body mass index, gender and the presence of varicose veins but not necessarily with age (Kroeger et al., 2003).

Varicose veins are more commonly found in the lower extremities and are characterized by tortuous dilatation and changes in the smooth muscle composition and extracellular matrix in the vessel walls, resulting in the venous stasis and venous back flow (Jacob, 2003). Peripheral edema formation is common. The incidence of varicose veins increases with age and is also affected by body mass index, prior or family history, and the presence of the disease during pregnancy. The estimated incidence of varicose veins in women increases from 41% to 73% between the fifth and seventh decades. For the same time span, the incidence for men increases from 24% to 73% (Statistics from Varicose Veins, 2006). Although recognized as the most common vascular disease, the presence of varicose veins is not clearly linked to disease development. Results from the Normative Aging Study population, taken over more than 35 years of follow-up, showed that men with varicose veins were less likely to develop symptomatic congestive heart failure than men without varicose veins (Scott et al., 2004).

PHYSIOLOGICAL CHANGES ASSOCIATED WITH AGING

The age-associated structural alterations in blood vessels are further influenced by physiological changes that have a significant impact on the cardiovascular system. It is difficult to elucidate the intricacies of all of the interrelationships, and this section addresses only some of the interactions between the systems.

Systolic blood pressure (SBP) is known to increase with age. Blood pressure analysis of 2036 subjects over a period of 30 years in the Framingham Heart Study indicated age-related increases in SBP, pulse pressure (PP) and mean arterial pressure (MAP), with an early rise (until 50 years of age) and a late fall (after 60 years of age) in diastolic blood pressure (DBP) (Franklin et al., 1997). The increase in MAP is attributed to the progressive increase in vascular resistance associated with aging, but vascular change in PP is a function of left ventricular ejection, large artery stiffness, early pulse wave reflection and heart rate. The rise in SBP is a result of both the increase in vascular resistance and increased stiffness in the large arteries. Under normal conditions and when arterial tone and PWV are normal (before the influence of age-associated changes on the vascular system), the reflected pulse wave reaches the heart after the aortic valve closes, thereby enhancing DBP. With the age-associated increases in arterial stiffness and PWV, the reflected pulse wave reaches the heart before the aortic valve closes, resulting in an increase in SBP and the loss of the diastolic pressure enhancement. The late fall in DBP is associated with large artery stiffness. Franklin et al. (1997) concluded that large artery stiffness rather than vascular resistance becomes the predominant factor for blood pressure changes as aging progresses. As the arterial walls become stiffer, they also become less distensible, and the lumen diameter of large central arteries increases to help accommodate blood volume as it is ejected from the left ventricle.

The loss of the elastic recoil together with the increased stiffness precipitates a decrease in the ability of the vessel to compress and propel the blood forward through the vascular system. A higher PP must then be generated to move a given volume of blood through a vessel. Because the heart is the pump that generates the initial propelling force, a decrease in the compliance of the arterial system results in an increase in the workload being placed on the heart.

At the level of the arterioles, capillaries and endothelium, alterations in structure result in alterations in function. Endothelial dysfunction has an enormous impact on the vascular system because the actions of endothelial cells are complex and involve several systems. With aging, the integrity of the endothelium is damaged and there is decreased activity of endothelium-derived relaxed factors (EDRF) including nitric oxide (NO), bradykinin and hyperpolarizing factor. Release of EDRF normally results in vasodilatation and serves to counter the actions of endothelium-derived constricting factors (EDCF) (e.g. endothelin, angiotensin II), both on vascular tone and on the stimulation of growth factors derived from endothelial cells. With the decrease in EDRF activity, the vessels remain more narrowed, thus contributing to the increase in resistance to flow and the increase in PP and SBP. NO is essential for endothelial health and factors in the control of vascular tone, inhibition of platelet function and reduction in the proliferation of the intima. Oxidative stress is associated with aging and results in inactivation or reduction of NO synthesis. The age-related alteration in NO activity results in an increase in the growth and proliferation of these cells, which accumulate and add to vascular wall thickening and platelet formation (Taddei et al., 2001). The effect on areas of the vascular system include severe impairment of blood flow and stress-induced vasodilatation, which limit necessary minute adjustments in blood supply in response to demand (Ungvari et al., 2010).

Another important function of the endothelium that changes with aging is the mediation of proinflammatory and anti-inflammatory responses through a complex series of reactions to changes in EDRF and EDCF activity, growth factors, adhesion molecules, monocytes, cytokines, lipids and enzymes. Proinflammatory substances are no longer adequately inhibited, resulting in local inflammation, plaque formation, thrombosis and plaque rupture. With endothelial dysfunction there is an increase in plasma C-reactive protein, which is both a mediator and a marker of inflammation.

A variable pattern in the distribution of blood flow at rest is noted. Much of this decrease may be attributed to the diminished ability of the smaller arteries and arterioles to vasodilate. The net change toward vasoconstriction in these vessels also increases the turbulence of the blood flow. The endothelium responds to mechanical forces, such as the shear force of turbulent blood flow, promoting inflammation and its related sequelae. The shear forces from normal laminar flow act in a protective manner against atherogenesis. Turbulent flow is significantly more resistive than laminar flow, and the work required by the cardiovascular system to overcome the increased resistance intensifies.

Age-associated hormonal changes play a role in the development of vascular changes. Vascular aging differs in men and women. In men, circulating testosterone levels decrease with age. Low testosterone is associated with arterial stiffness and is recognized as a cardiovascular risk factor (Hougaku et al., 2006). Circulating testosterone aids in the synthesis and bioavailability of NO essential for vascular health. Endothelial dysfunction occurs earlier in men than in women, because the decline in testosterone levels begins in early adulthood (Lopes et al., 2012). Lopes et al. reported after a thorough review of studies related to testosterone and aging, that age-associated decline of testosterone levels is associated with age-related metabolic and cardiovascular diseases, insulin resistance and atherosclerosis. Estrogen appears to have a protective effect on the endothelium, and there is an abrupt and sharp decline in endothelial function after the onset of the menopause (Taddei et al., 1996). Menopause and the associated decline in natural estrogen often occurs at a time when age-related vascular changes occur, making it difficult to determine age-related changes from lack of estrogen (Novella et al., 2012).

Given the structural and functional changes in aging blood vessels, it is not surprising to recognize aging as a major risk factor for cardiovascular disease.

AUTONOMIC SYSTEM CHANGES WITH AGING

Autonomic control declines with age, primarily reflecting an enhancement of sympathetic nervous system activity and a suppression of parasympathetic nervous system activity (Harris & Matthews, 2004). Because of changes in the interplay between the autonomic nervous system and the cardiovascular system, it becomes more difficult to maintain hemodynamic stability. There is a decrease in beta-adrenoreceptor responsiveness in the vasculature. The vascular responses of alpha-1-adrenoreceptors are either unaltered or may be increased with age (Priebe, 2000). The loss of responsiveness to beta-adrenergic stimuli with or without an increase in alpha-1-adrenoreceptor stimulation results in a predominance of alpha-1-adrenergic-mediated responses. Without sufficient vasodilatory input from beta-adrenoreceptors, the autonomically mediated vasoconstriction compounds the vasoconstriction resulting from the previously described mechanisms.

A significant decrease in the reactivity of cardiopulmonary reflexes, especially the reflex mediated by the baroreceptors, occurs with advancing age. Baroreceptor activity is directed by the stretch demand of vascular walls in the aorta and the carotid arteries by the blood flowing through the vessels. A decrease in the required stretch, and thus in baroreceptor activity, normally results in signals ordering restoration of cardiac output to increase blood pressure. This reflex activity is essential to prevent the orthostatic hypotensive response that can occur when moving from the reclining to the upright position. The pressor effect on SBP and PP, which normally occurs when moving into an upright position, changes with aging. The reduction in autonomic control may result in orthostatic hypotension if the elevated PPs do not adequately compensate (Cleophas & Van Marum, 2003). A decrease in overall baroreceptor activity coupled with the decreased compliance of the vessel wall hinders the short-term regulation that normally occurs in the cardiac and vascular systems as a result of body position changes.

Deconditioning is another physiological state that results in an exaggerated orthostatic response. Many elderly individuals are sedentary and therefore deconditioned. This state results in less efficient oxygen transport and poorly functioning skeletal muscles. A deconditioned person needs more energy to perform tasks and is less able to adapt quickly and efficiently to alterations in the body's homeostasis. Thus, the exaggeration of the orthostatic response during body position changes can be great. Any health professional working with an elderly patient must be aware of this potential for an increased orthostatic response and know how to monitor and treat it.

TYPICAL ALTERATIONS IN THE VASCULAR RESPONSE TO EXERCISE WITH AGING

The ability to adapt and respond to the changing needs of the body during exercise is an essential function of the vascular system. One of the primary differences in the response to exercise in the elderly is the more rapid onset of fatigue, resulting from the demands placed on the cardiovascular system. The structural and functional changes in the vascular system impede the ability of the vasculature to supply the tissues with the increased oxygen needed during exercise. Maximal aerobic power refers to the body's ability to transport and use oxygen ($\dot{V}o_2$ max). Oxygen consumption increases linearly with the intensity and magnitude of exercise. With aging, $\dot{V}o_2$ max decreases as a function of body weight and age-related changes in the oxygen transport system, including the reduced ability to use oxygen and to shunt blood flow to active muscles. This deficit often causes an older individual to reach fatigue more quickly when exercising (see Chapter 6).

In a study comparing the responses of young and old adults to peak exercise, Stratton et al. (1994) reported differences in several measured variables. There was a lower heart rate response and a smaller increase in ejection fraction. Systolic, diastolic and mean blood pressures were higher in the old than in the young. During submaximal exercises, there were no differences in ejection fraction between the young and the old.

Under normal circumstances, exercise or any other period of increased activity is sympathetically mediated and results in an increased release of the adrenergic mediators. This in turn raises the activity level in most body systems and triggers an increase in cardiac output and oxygen transport during exercise. The age-associated changes in beta-adrenergic receptors in the vascular system lessen the ability to facilitate the increased need for oxygen delivery during exercise (Stratton et al., 1994).

At a more local level, the peripheral vessels are less responsive to alterations in metabolic activity. Normally, increased metabolic activity in skeletal muscle results in vasodilatation to meet the oxygen demand of the tissue. The stimulation of skeletal muscle vascular adrenergic receptors during exercise also results in vasodilatation. Vessels in older individuals have less ability to vasodilate in response to increased metabolic activity. Older individuals also demonstrate decreased activity mediated through the adrenergic receptors. The inability to increase blood supply quickly coupled with a decrease in structural ability to vasodilate prevents blood from being shunted rapidly from areas of low metabolic activity to areas of more active muscle metabolism. Loss of this mechanism decreases an older individual's ability to do skeletal muscle work (Evans, 1999).

When exercising, older individuals have been shown to have a higher percentage of their cardiac output shunted to the skin and viscera and a lower percentage directed toward working muscle. Thermoregulation is decreased in the elderly as a function of the loss of muscle mass associated with age and inactivity (Marks, 2002). Normal thermoregulation relies on the processes of conduction, convection and evaporation. Sweating decreases with aging (Marks, 2002). Evaporation, which is sympathetically mediated, is the predominant mechanism for heat loss during exercise. Older individuals attempt to compensate for this loss by shunting more cardiac output to the skin to regulate heat loss via conduction and convection, which are not efficient mechanisms for adequate heat loss at rest or during exercise. This shunting also prevents the delivery of an adequate blood volume to skeletal muscle (see Chapter 10 Thermoregulation).

With aging, muscle capillary density decreases and further limits the blood supply available to working muscle. An important measure of the oxygen transport function is the arteriovenous oxygen difference, which is a measure of the utilization of oxygen by working muscles. Changes in skeletal muscle tissue structure, mitochondria and metabolic enzymes result in a decreased arteriovenous oxygen difference, which indicates that less oxygen is being extracted from the capillary bed for use during exercise.

TYPICAL ALTERATIONS IN THE VASCULAR RESPONSE TO EXERCISE TRAINING WITH AGING

Stratton et al. (1994) showed that exercise training had significant effects on all vascular variables except end-systolic volume index. They also showed that the increase in maximal oxygen consumption and workload, and the percentage increases, were not significantly different between old and young. They concluded that, despite differences in the response to a single episode of exercise, similar changes in cardiovascular functions in old and young men occurred as a result of endurance exercise training.

Marks (2002) reported a decrease in $\dot{V}o_2$ max associated with aging, specifically a loss of 9–15% between the ages of 45 and 55, with accelerations in losses between the ages of 65 and 75 and further accelerations from 75 to 85. This decline in aerobic power can be improved by 10–25% in older individuals who participate regularly in aerobic exercise. The loss of $\dot{V}o_2$ max in women is greater than in men. Marks (2002) reported on studies indicating that an increase in walking of 2 miles per day may be as effective as traditional exercise for lowering blood pressure in women.

In a cross-sectional study of healthy men, DeSouza et al. (2000) concluded that regular aerobic exercise can prevent age-associated loss of endothelium-dependent vasodilatation (EDV). Aerobic exercise can also restore EDV in previously sedentary middle-aged and older healthy men. The aerobic exercise intervention consisted primarily of walking.

Carotid artery compliance decreases by 40–50% in healthy sedentary men and women between the ages of 25 and 75 years. Regular aerobic exercise attenuates the loss and was shown to restore compliance to some degree (Seals, 2003).

In a case controlled study of 17 patients with chronic obstructive pulmonary disease (COPD), Vivodtzev et al. (2010) investigated whether exercise training reduces arterial stiffness. The results indicated an improvement in arterial stiffness in patients in the training group, as evidenced by a reduction in PWV proportional to changes in exercise capacity measured as changes in maximal heart rate and oxygen consumption.

CONCLUSION

Age-associated changes occur in all of the various components of the oxygen transport system, including the vasculature. In rehabilitation, it is important to note that strength and fitness training programs in the elderly have been shown to decrease the amount of decline in function of many bodily systems, including the vascular system. Although training will not entirely eliminate the inevitable decline that occurs with advancing age, the severity of the decline will be lessened.

REFERENCES

Cleophas TJ, Van Marum R 2003 Age-related decline in autonomic control of blood pressure: implications for the pharmacological management of hypertension in the elderly. Drugs Aging 20:313–319

D'Alessio P 2004 Aging and the endothelium. Exp Gerontol 39:165–171

DeSouza CA, Shapiro LF, Clevenger CM et al 2000 Regular aerobic exercise prevents and restores age-related declines in endothelium-dependent vasodilation in healthy men. Circulation 102:1351–1357

Evans WJ 1999 Exercise training guidelines for the elderly. Med Sci Sports Exerc 31:12–17

Ferrari AU, Radaelli A, Centola M 2003 Invited review: aging and the cardiovascular system. J Appl Physiol 95:2591–2597

Franklin SS, Gustin 4th W, Wong ND ct al 1997 Hemodynamic patterns of age-related changes in blood pressure. The Framingham Heart Study. Circulation 96:308–315

Harris KF, Matthews KA 2004 Interactions between autonomic nervous system activity and endothelial function: a model for the development of cardiovascular disease. Psychosom Med 66:153–164

Hernandez JP, Frank WD 2004 Age and fitness differences in limb venous compliance do not affect tolerance to maximal lower body negative pressure in men and women. J Appl Physiol 97:925–929

Hougaku H, Fleg JR, Najjar SS et al 2006 Relationship between androgenic hormones and arterial stiffness, based on longitudinal hormone measurements. Am J Physiol Endocrinol Metab 290:E234–E242

Jacob MP 2003 Extracellular matrix remodeling and matrix metalloproteinases in the vascular wall during aging and pathological conditions. Biomed Pharmacother 57:195–202

Kovacic JC, Moreno P, Hachinski V et al 2011a Cellular senescence, vascular disease, and aging: Part 1 of a 2-part review. Circulation 123:1650–1660

Kovacic JC, Moreno P, Nabel EG et al 2011b Cellular senescence, vascular disease, and aging: Part 2 of a 2-part review. Circulation 123:1900–1910

Kroeger K, Rudofsky G, Roesner J et al 2003 Peripheral veins: influence of gender, body mass index, age and varicose veins in cross-sectional area. Vascular Med 8:249–255

Lakatta EG, Levy D 2003 Arterial and cardiac aging: major shareholders in cardiovascular disease enterprises. Part I: aging arteries: a 'set-up' for vascular disease. Circulation 107:139–146

Lopes RA, Neves KB, Carneiro FS et al 2012 Testosterone and vascular function in aging. Front Physiol 3:89

McVeigh GE, Bratelli CW, Morgan DJ et al 1999 Age-related abnormalities in arterial compliance identified by pressure pulse contour analysis: aging and arterial compliance. Hypertension 33:1392–1398

Marks BL 2002 Physiologic responses to exercises in older women. Top Geriatr Rehabil 18:9–20

Moore A, Mangoni AA, Lyon D, Jackson SH 2003 The cardiovascular system. Br J Clin Pharmacol 56:254–260

Nagai Y, Metter EJ, Earley CJ et al 1998 Increased carotid artery intimal-medial thickness in asymptomatic older subjects with exercise-induced myocardial ischemia. Circulation 98:1504–1509

Novella S, Dantas AP, Segarra G et al 2012 Vascular aging in women: is estrogen the fountain of youth? Front Physiol 3:165

Priebe HJ 2000 The aged cardiovascular risk patient. Br J Anaesth 85:763–768

Scott TE, Mendez MV, LaMorte WW et al 2004 Are varicose veins a marker for susceptibility to coronary artery disease in men? Results from the Normative Aging Study. Ann Vascular Surg 18:459–464

Scuteri A, Najjar SS, Morrell CH et al 2005 The metabolic syndrome in older individuals: prevalence and prediction of cardiovascular events: the Cardiovascular Health Study. Diabetes Care 28:882–887

Seals DR 2003 Habitual exercise and the age-associated decline in large artery compliance. Exerc Sport Sci Rev 31:68–72

Strait JB, Lakatta EG 2012 Age associate cardiovascular changes and their relationship to heart failure. Heart Fail Clin 8:143–164

Stratton JR, Levy WC, Cerquireira MD et al 1994 Cardiovascular responses to exercise. Effects of aging and exercise training in healthy men. Circulation 89:1648–1655

Taddei S, Virdis A, Ghiadoni L et al 1996 Menopause is associated with endothelial dysfunction in women. Hypertension 28:576–582

Taddei S, Virdis A, Ghiadoni L et al 2001 Age-related reduction of NO availability and oxidative stress in humans. Hypertension 38:274–279

Ungvari Z, Kaley G, de Cabo R et al 2010 Mechanisms of aging: new perspectives. J Gerontol A Biol Sci Med Sci 65:1028–1041

Varicose Veins 2006 Statistics available at: www.cureresearch.com/v/varicose_veins/stats_printer.htm. Accessed November 2013

Vivodtzev I, Minet C, Wuyam B et al 2010 Significant improvement in arterial stiffness after endurance training in patients with COPD. Chest 137:1270–1275

Weinert BT, Timiras PS 2003 Physiology of aging. Invited review: theories of aging. J Appl Physiol 95:1706–1716

Werner C, Furster T, Widman T et al 2009 Physical exercise prevents cellular senescence in circulating leukocytes and in the vessel wall. Circulation 120:2438–2447

Chapter 10

Thermoregulation: considerations for aging people

JOHN SANKO

Chapter Contents

INTRODUCTION

Core body temperature is a relatively stable physiological function and one of the most frequently measured vital signs. Core temperature normally does not vary by more than ±0.55°C (±1°F) unless a febrile illness develops (Gonzalez et al., 2001). Humans like other mammals are warm-blooded homeotherms, which means they must maintain their internal temperature within a narrow range, which in humans hovers near 37°C (98.6°F). Life-sustaining biochemical processes are altered if the internal environment deviates from the optimal. Internal temperatures above 45–50°C (113–122°F) denature the protein structure of various enzymes, which results in biochemical breakdown, tissue destruction, severe illness and death (Fig. 10.1). Body temperatures below 33.9°C (93°F) slow metabolism to dangerously low levels and disrupt nerve conduction, which, in turn, results in decreased brain activity. Life-threatening cardiac arrhythmias begin to appear at temperatures near 30°C (86°F) (see Fig. 10.1).

All warm-blooded animals, including humans, live only a few degrees away from death (Astrand et al., 2003). Core temperatures falling outside the normal range are indicative of some pathology or the failure of the thermoregulatory system to maintain homeostatic thermal balance. The complexity of the physiological mechanisms involved in thermoregulation is shown in Figure 10.2. The effect of aging and the interaction of normal aging with and lifestyle changes on an individual's ability to regulate body temperature are not fully understood. Changes in body composition, decreased aerobic capacity, sedentary lifestyle and the increased prevalence of chronic diseases such as heart disease, diabetes and decreased kidney function along with the increased use of prescription drugs makes it difficult to determine the true impact aging has on thermoregulation (Kenney & Munce, 2003). It is clear, however, that the fitter, more active and healthy an older individual, the more able they will be able to withstand a thermoregulatory challenge.

HYPERTHERMIA

Hyperthermia is the condition in which internal core temperature exceeds the normal range. Hyperthermia can be caused by infections, brain lesions, environmental conditions or heavy exercise. When caused by an infection, the responsible microorganisms release toxins called pyrogens into the bloodstream; they reach the temperature control centers of the brain and raise the thermal set point. This state, known as fever, is actually beneficial and is part of the immune system's response (see Chapter 11). Higher core temperatures adversely affect the invading microorganism's ability to replicate. This generally limits the extent of the infection and leads to its suppression.

In the older adult, the fever response is often diminished or absent, which may explain the increased morbidity and mortality rates associated with infections in the elderly (Blatteis, 2011). When the ambient temperature rises above 30°C (86°F), progressive vasodilatation of the cutaneous vasculature commences and is followed by sweating and evaporation (Gonzalez et al., 2001). Factors such as high humidity and physical activity magnify the effects of ambient temperature, taxing the thermoregulatory mechanisms. This is an

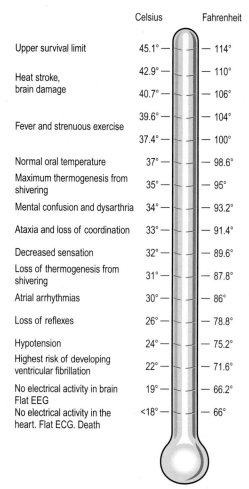

Figure 10.1 Physiological consequences of variations in core temperature. Core temperature has a direct effect on physiological function. Extreme core temperature will seriously challenge homeostasis, which can have fatal consequences. *(Data from Guyton AC, Hall JE 2000 Textbook of Medical Physiology, 10th edn, Elsevier Saunders, St Louis, MO, and Rhodes RA, Tanner GA (eds) 2003 Medical Physiology, 2nd edn, Lippincott, Williams & Wilkins, Baltimore, MD.)*

especially important factor in home healthcare when treating debilitated patients. Unlike fever, non-febrile rises in body temperature are not beneficial and threaten homeostasis. If normal thermal regulation is in any way impaired, these increases can reach dangerous levels. With core temperatures above 40.7°C (106°F), heat stroke and irreversible brain damage becomes imminent (see Fig. 10.1).

If the internal core temperature drops below 34.1°C (94°F), the ability of the hypothalamus to regulate body temperature is also severely impaired (Gonzalez et al., 2001). If the body temperature continues to fall unchecked, loss of motor control, sensation and consciousness will be followed by ventricular fibrillation and death see (Fig. 10.1).

HYPOTHALAMUS AND THERMAL REGULATION

The hypothalamus normally acts as the body's thermostat, initiating heat-dissipating, heat-conserving, or heat-generating mechanisms in relation to internal core and body surface temperatures (Gonzalez et al., 2001). The temperature-reduction mechanisms include vasodilatation, sweating, inhibition of shivering, and decreased chemical thermogenesis. When body temperature begins to rise, sympathetic outflow from the hypothalamus to the cutaneous vasculature is inhibited, allowing for vasodilatation and increased heat transfer from the skin to the external environment. This mechanism is capable of increasing heat dissipation through the skin by as much as 800%. Sweating and evaporative loss further enhance the skin's ability to dissipate heat. When the challenge of cold is presented to the body, the hypothalamus conserves or generates body heat by measuring sympathetic tone, which results in vasoconstriction of the cutaneous circulation, piloerection, shivering and increased metabolism through the secretion of thyroxine (Gonzalez

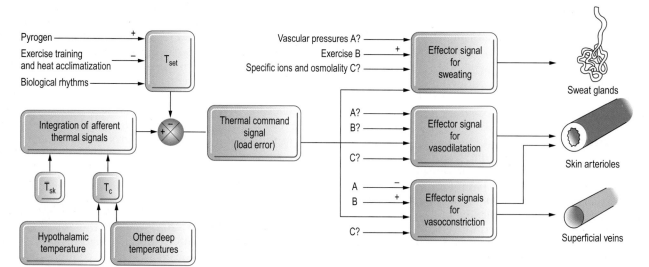

Figure 10.2 Physiological mechanisms for maintaining thermoregulatory homeostasis. Breakdown or impairment in any of the thermoregulatory mechanisms can lead to serious problems in maintaining homeostasis. T_c, core temperature; T_{set}, body's set temperature and the factors that affect it; T_{sk}, skin temperature. *(From Pandolf KB, Sawka MN, Gonzalez RR (eds) 1988 Human Performance Physiology and Environmental Medicine at Terrestrial Extremes. Benchmark, Indianapolis, p 106, with permission from the McGraw-Hill Companies.)*

et al., 2001; Hall, 2010). The efficiency of these mechanisms may be altered by skin atrophy, diminished vascular tree and reduced muscle mass, which are discussed in greater detail below.

MOBILITY AND PSYCHOSOCIAL FACTORS

In spite of the exquisite physiological mechanisms for dealing with temperature change, behavioral modification may be human beings' greatest defense against environmental challenges to thermoregulatory homeostasis. When our surroundings become too warm or too cold we try to avoid such conditions by moving to a more comfortable location or changing the thermostat or control for the heating or air conditioning. In addition, we may add or remove clothing as conditions warrant. The very young, the elderly and those physically or mentally unable to take care of themselves are at the greatest risk when exposed to extremes of environmental conditions. This may be due in part to their inability to recognize the magnitude of the situation and take appropriate action.

Older adults often find themselves dependent upon others for their wellbeing, commonly as a result of deficits in physical or cognitive function. The incidence of chronic disease increases dramatically with age. Over 50% of those beyond 65 years of age report some limitation in mobility due to arthritis and a significant number have other orthopedic problems that limit their ability to carry out the normal activities of daily living (ADLs) (Guccione, 2011). Musculoskeletal and neurological conditions often reduce the older adult's functional level to a point where he or she becomes partially, if not fully, dependent upon others to carry out the ADLs. Thermoregulatory stress may be one of many reasons why elderly people who are dependent on others for help with ADLs have a four times greater chance of dying within a 2-year period than those who are totally independent. In addition, approximately 15% of the population over 65 years of age are in some way cognitively impaired. The incidence of cognitive impairment rises rapidly with age. Some deterioration in mental function is seen in nearly 50% of those individuals 85 years of age and older (Guccione, 2011). These physical and mental impairments, as well as others, combined with a reduction in the functional capacity of various organ systems make the older adult particularly vulnerable to thermoregulatory stress. Thermoregulation and aging has been studied from a physiological basis for some time, but added emphasis has recently focused on the area of behavioral thermoregulation. A great deal of research needs to be done on the relationship between thermal comfort and thermal sensation. Thermal comfort is defined as a state of mind of whether the individual feels satisfaction or dissatisfaction with ambient conditions while thermal sensation is the perception resulting from the stimulation of the body's thermoreceptors (Flouris, 2010). Autonomic response to temperature change, although essential, may not be as powerful and important to our survival as behavioral thermoregulation (Romanovsky, 2007; Van Someren, 2007).

THERMAL INJURY

Heat stroke, heat exhaustion and hypothermia are most prevalent among the elderly population and are inversely related to socioeconomic status. A study in Hong Kong showed an increase in mean environmental temperature of 1°C above 28.2°C (82.76°F) resulted in a 1.5% increase in mortality over a 2-week period. Those affected most were individuals over 75 years of age, the unmarried and women (Chan et al., 2011). Similarly, a study of ambulance calls, emergency department visits and mortality in Australia during a 12-day heatwave in 2011 once again showed those over 75 years of age to be the most impacted (Schaffer et al., 2012). When elderly individuals on fixed incomes turn the heat down in the winter because they cannot pay high heating bills, they are certainly predisposing themselves to hypothermia. Conversely, elderly people unable to afford air conditioning are 50 times more likely to die of heat stroke than those who have access to air conditioning (Wongsurawat, 1994). Although it has been stated that numerous predisposing physiological factors share responsibility, many temperature-related threats to health could undoubtedly be prevented if elderly individuals just stayed indoors, turned the heat or air conditioning up or down, and dressed more appropriately (Gonzalez et al., 2001). In cases in which economic status or physical or mental condition makes these actions impossible, those involved should be referred to the appropriate agencies for their protection, safety and welfare.

PHYSIOLOGICAL FACTORS

SKIN RECEPTORS AND CIRCULATORY RESPONSE

Even when they are healthy and mentally alert, the elderly are less able to sense changes in skin temperature, and this makes them more susceptible to thermoregulatory problems (Gonzalez et al., 2001). Thermoreceptors for both hot and cold are found in the skin, the spinal cord and the hypothalamus itself. Skin temperature, unlike core temperature, is extremely variable. Receptors in the skin provide the hypothalamus with important feedback regarding the need to dissipate, conserve, or generate heat. Numerous bare nerve endings just below the skin are sensitive to heat and cold. They are classified as warm or cold receptors, depending on their rate of discharge when exposed to variations in temperature. It is not known whether the effectiveness of these thermoreceptors declines with age. However, because their function depends on an adequate oxygen supply, it seems reasonable to assume that any age-associated impairments in cutaneous circulation would reduce the effectiveness of thermoreceptors. It is known that the dermis becomes thinner and less vascularized with age (Farage et al., 2010).

The changes in skin thickness and circulation along with reduced autonomic nervous system function alter the effectiveness of the vasomotor response. The vasomotor mechanism can alter cutaneous blood flow from near zero when exposed to extreme cold to increases of 500–1000% when exposed to vigorous warming. The evaporative loss of sweat from the skin surface helps to dissipate heat in the cutaneous circulation. A study that compared men aged 45–57 years with men aged 18–23 years indicated that the older men required twice as long before the onset of sweating during moderate intensity exercise. Subsequent studies of older women showed even greater impairments in the sweating mechanism. The number of sweat glands does not appear to change significantly with aging. Therefore, it is reasonable to assume that the decline in autonomic nervous system function reduces the performance of sweat glands and alters the body's ability to dissipate excess heat. In addition, the hypothalamus appears to become less sensitive to temperature variations, and there is evidence of age-correlated reductions in autonomic nervous system function (Hall, 2010).

It is unclear how much of the thermoregulatory impairment seen in the elderly is age-related and how much is the result of chronic disease processes and a sedentary lifestyle. The efficiency of the cardiovascular system's ability to dissipate body heat is enhanced by aerobic fitness. Resistive exercise has been found to be particularly beneficial in maintaining or retarding muscle loss in the elderly and should be considered when not contraindicated. Muscle is a significant tissue not only for heat generation, but also for the mobility needed for thermoregulation.

OTHER PHYSIOLOGICAL FACTORS

The ingestion of food, alcohol and medications to control blood pressure, cardiac function, depression and pain all exert influence on thermal balance and regulation. A sufficient, well-balanced diet is essential to provide the calories needed to generate heat and maintain adequate levels of metabolically active muscles. Muscle, which is the major organ of metabolism and heat generation, can decrease by 10–12% in the older adult. One-third of the US population over 65 has some form of nutritional deficit, often eating inappropriate quantities of foods low in nutritional values. Reduced caloric intake, lower basal metabolic rate, reduced lean body mass and lower cardiac output may all contribute to thermoregulatory changes in the aging adult (Novieto & Zhang, 2010). Because 80% of the calories consumed go toward the maintenance of body temperature, this deficit can further contribute to the thermoregulatory inadequacies experienced by some older adults. The shivering mechanism, which can increase metabolism and heat generation by 300–500%, is also adversely affected by the loss of muscle tissue (Gonzalez et al., 2001).

POSSIBLE EFFECTS OF MEDICATION

Although there is still a great deal to be learned regarding the effects of aging on the thermoregulatory function, it appears that physical conditioning and adequate nutrition help to preserve this function in healthy older adults. All older individuals are, however, not healthy or physically fit. Many have chronic conditions that interfere with their abilities to deal with even mild variations in temperature (Kenny et al., 2010). In addition, various medications can interfere with the normal physiological responses necessary to maintain thermal homeostasis. Dehydration may occur in individuals taking diuretics for the management of congestive heart failure or hypertension. Beta-antagonists are another category of medication commonly prescribed for elderly individuals with heart disease and hypertension. Because they slow the heart rate and affect circulation they can have an effect on thermoregulation.

Although the use of illicit drugs is lowest among the elderly, the misuse of prescription drugs is a major problem for this group. In one survey of elderly persons living independently in the community, 83% reported they were using two or more prescription drugs, with an average of 3.8 medications per person (Hooyman & Kiyak, 2010). Many elderly people have been found to misuse prescription and nonprescription over-the-counter drugs. Surveyed individuals reported taking two to three times the recommended dosages of aspirin, laxatives and sleeping pills. Misuse of laxatives could further increase the rate and severity of dehydration and sedatives defeat the autonomic nervous system's ability to react to environmental conditions. In addition, psychotropic drugs are often prescribed for depression in the elderly. Several studies have demonstrated that the inhibition of the sweating reflex by these drugs increases the risk of death during prolonged heatwaves (Nordon et al., 2009).

Alcohol also inhibits the body's ability to regulate temperature by interfering with the vasomotor system and altering cutaneous blood flow, which impairs the body's ability to dissipate or conserve heat. The dehydrating effects of alcohol can also contribute to an inadequate thermoregulatory response by reducing plasma volume and decreasing the sweat response. Combined with prescription and nonprescription medications, alcohol can create serious problems for any individual.

POSTSURGICAL CONSIDERATIONS

A number of geriatric patients receiving physical therapy in acute and extended care facilities are postsurgical patients. The tremendous advancements and successes in joint replacement surgery have made these procedures relatively commonplace. Plasma lost during surgery may result in some degree of dehydration, but anesthetics present the greater challenge to thermoregulation for these patients. Most anesthetics and sedatives impair the body's ability to maintain core temperature by blocking the normal heat-generating activity. There are some benefits of mild hypothermia for the surgical patient, but there are also increased risks for the elderly. A 2°C (3.6°F) drop in core temperature has been shown to substantially increase blood loss during hip arthroplasty surgery. The incidence of ischemic myocardial events increases for a 24-hour period following intraoperative hypothermia. Higher rates of wound infections, delayed healing and immunosuppression are also seen following anesthesia-induced hypothermia. The elderly appear to be at the greatest risk for developing one or more of these complications because of their predisposition to hypothermia, even when exposed to only moderately cold conditions (Mayer & Sessler, 2004).

CLINICAL CONSIDERATIONS

In spite of the fact that numerous age-correlated alterations in thermoregulation have been identified, the ability to regulate internal core temperature appears to remain within acceptable limits in the healthy, fit older adult. Furthermore, few of the changes seen in autonomic, circulatory and thermal function are solely the result of biological aging. Reduced physical work capacity, body composition changes, chronic illness, the use and misuse of various medications, and alterations in cognitive function become more prevalent with advancing age and influence the function of various body systems involved with thermoregulation. Studies on thermoregulation and aging have generally shown that aging reduces sweat gland output, skin blood flow, cardiac output, peripheral vasoconstriction and reduced muscle mass. In spite of these changes, healthy older individuals seem to be able to handle most variations in ambient temperature. Gender may also play an important role. Although both males and females lose muscle mass as they age, females tend to have a greater increase in percentage body fat, which may account for their ability to better maintain core temperature when exposed to cooler ambient temperatures (Kenney & Munce, 2003).

Whenever treating any individual with exercise or thermal modalities, age should be a consideration. Ideally, the ambient temperature in exercise areas should be 19.8–22°C (68–72°F) with a relative humidity of 60% or less. When exercise is to be performed outdoors, appropriate clothing is a necessity. Planning outdoor activities during moderate weather is also important. It would not be prudent to exercise in mid-afternoon on a hot summer day or late in the evening on a cold winter day. Because older adults may build up heat more quickly and take longer to dissipate it than their younger counterparts, frequent rest periods in well-ventilated areas should be incorporated into any exercise regimen.

CONCLUSION

The safe and effective use of exercise, heat, cold, or hydrotherapy requires thorough assessment of the individual's condition, medical history, and ability to withstand thermal or cryogenic stress. A past medical history of hypersensitivity to heat or cold, Raynaud's disease, urticaria, wheals, diabetes or heart disease requires further consideration prior to intervention. Pain and temperature sensation should be assessed.

The normal effects of direct heating and cooling of the tissue may be altered in some elderly individuals (Fig. 10.3). Vital signs should be monitored along with skin temperature, sensation, color, sweat rate, and rate of perceived exertion (RPE). Additional care should be taken with individuals on medication and those who have impaired cognitive and mental function.

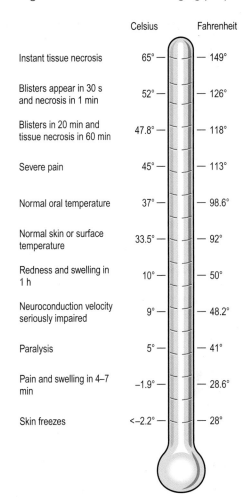

Figure 10.3 Effect on body tissues of direct exposure to heat and cold. Surface temperature may be very different from core temperature. Extremes in local tissue temperature will lead to cell death and tissue necrosis, regardless of core temperature. Local thermoregulatory impairments can lead to systemic consequences if not corrected. *(Data from Guyton AC, Hall JE 2000 Textbook of Medical Physiology, 10th edn, St Louis, MO, Elsevier Saunders, and Rhodes RA, Tanner GA (eds) 2003 Medical Physiology, 2nd edn, Lippincott, Williams & Wilkins, Baltimore, MD.)*

Physiologically elderly individuals will have changes in their ability to regulate the internal temperature that will be magnified by a host of comorbidities and other factors, so ensuring appropriate thermoregulation behaviors may become the responsibility of the caregiver.

Should a thermoregulatory crisis occur, standard emergency and medical procedures should be followed (Tables 10.1 and 10.2). A few simple precautions can help to prevent many of these crises (Boxes 10.1 and 10.2). Additional research in the area of thermoregulation and aging is needed to resolve the many contradictory findings. Until these questions have been answered, the clinician must carefully consider the use of modalities and exercises with people of various ages, based on the current body of knowledge and experience, and common sense.

Table 10.1	**Heat-related emergencies**	
Condition	Signs and Symptoms	Treatment
Heat edema	Swollen feet and ankles	Elevate the lower extremities and wear support stockings. If symptoms are a consequence of a cardiovascular condition, drug therapy may be required
Heat cramps	Severe muscle spasm, particularly in the lower extremities	Allow patient to rest in a cool place, cool with moist towels and drink electrolyte replacement fluids
Heat syncope	Pooling of blood in veins resulting in decreased cardiac output; symptoms ranging from lightheadedness to loss of consciousness; typically cool and wet skin	Allow patient to lie down, rest and drink electrolyte fluids. This condition is caused by physical exertion in a warm environment by an individual not acclimatized to that environment
Heat exhaustion	Loss of volume in the circulatory system as a result of excessive sweating; cool and clammy skin; nausea, headache, confusion, weakness and low blood pressure	Rest and fluid replacement; fluids with electrolytes may be necessary. Unconsciousness occurs rarely
Heat stroke	High skin and core body temperature; loss of consciousness; possible convulsions; dry skin, indicating loss of the sweating mechanism for cooling	This is the most severe heat-related condition. Cool the body as rapidly as possible. Seek immediate medical care

Data from Pollak AN (ed) 2005 Emergency Care and Transportation of the Sick and Injured, 9th edn. Jones & Bartlett, Boston, MA.

Table 10.2	**Cold-related emergencies**	
Condition	Signs and Symptoms	Treatment
Chilblains	Skin lesions that occur after prolonged exposure of the skin to temperatures below 15.4°C (60°F)	Protect the injured area and prevent re-exposure
Trench foot	Swollen body part (usually foot); waxy, mottled appearance of skin; complaints of numbness; caused by prolonged exposure to cool water	Remove wet shoes and socks. Gently rewarm. Cover any blisters with sterile dressings
Frostnip	Reddened skin that becomes blanched; numbness or tingling; ears, nose, lips, fingers and toes most commonly affected	Gently warm the involved area. If the condition does not resolve itself, treat the individual for frostbite
Frostbite	Waxy appearance of skin; may turn mottled	Gently warm but do not rub or squeeze the injured part. Transport patient immediately for advanced medical treatment
Hypothermia	Shivering in early stages; drowsiness and lethargy; slow breathing and bradycardia; possible loss of consciousness	Gently rewarm the individual in mild cases. Immediately transport for advanced medical care in moderate to severe cases
Cold allergy	Urticaria, erythema, itching and edema; systemic reactions, including hypotension, tachycardia, syncope and gastrointestinal dysfunction	Gently warm and acclimatize the individual

Data from Pollak AN (ed) 2005 Emergency Care and Transportation of the Sick and Injured, 9th edn. Jones & Bartlett, Boston, MA.

Box 10.1 *How to avoid hyperthermia*

- Wear loose-fitting, light clothing during periods of high heat and humidity.
- Take cool baths or showers during periods of high heat and humidity.
- Drink adequate amounts of fluids, even when not thirsty.
- Use air conditioning or fans to cool and circulate the air.
- Avoid excessive exercise during peak temperatures of the day, especially when humidity is high and fans and air conditioning are not available. This is particularly important in the home healthcare setting.
- When performing physical activity or exercise outdoors, use caution. Avoid working in direct sunlight on hot days. Take frequent breaks in cool or shady areas.

Box 10.2 *How to avoid hypothermia*

- Wear several layers of loose-fitting clothing and a hat.
- Stay dry.
- Maintain an adequate balanced diet.
- Drink adequate amounts of fluids, but limit alcohol consumption.
- Turn up the heating when the weather is cool.
- When performing physical activities or exercise outdoors, use caution. A great deal of heat loss can occur even when the temperatures are only moderately cool. Always consider windchill.
- Frequent checks should be made on elderly individuals in the community who live alone.

REFERENCES

Astrand PO, Rodahl K, Dahl HA et al 2003 Textbook of Work Physiological Basis of Exercise, 4th edn. Human Kinetics Publishers, Champaigne, IL

Blatteis CM 2011 Age-dependent changes in temperature regulation. Gerontology 58:289

Chan EYY, Goggins W, Kim JJ et al 2011 Help-seeking behavior during elevated temperature in Chinese population. J Urban Health 88:637

Farage MA, Miller KW, Berardesca E et al (eds) 2010 Textbook of Aging Skin. Springer, New York

Flouris AD 2010 Functional architecture of behavioural thermoregulation. Eur J Appl Physiol 111:1

Gonzalez EG, Myers SJ, Edelstein JE et al (eds) 2001 Downey and Darling's: The Physiological Basis of Rehabilitation Medicine, 3rd edn. Elsevier Mosby, St Louis, MO

Guccione AA (ed) 2011 Geriatric Physical Therapy, 2nd edn. Elsevier Mosby, St Louis, MO

Hall JE 2010 Guyton and Hall Textbook of Medical Physiology, 12th edn. Saunders Elsevier, Philadelphia, PA

Hooyman NR, Kiyak HA 2010 Social Gerontology: A Multidisciplinary Perspective, 9th edn. Pearson, Upper Saddle River, NJ

Kenney WL, Munce TA 2003 Invited review: Aging and human temperature regulation. J Appl Physiol 95:2598

Kenny GP, Yardley J, Braun C et al 2010 Heat stress in older individuals and patients with common chronic diseases. CMAJ 182:1053

Mayer SA, Sessler DI et al (eds) 2004 Therapeutic Hypothermia. Marcel Dekker, New York

Nordon C, Martin-Latry K, de Roquefeuil L et al 2009 Risk of death related to psychotropic drug use in older people during the European 2003 heatwave. Am J Geriatr Psychiatry:1059–1067

Novieto DT, Zhang Y 2010 Thermal comfort implications of the aging effects on metabolism, cardiac output and body weight. Proceedings NCEUB Conference on Adapting to Change: New Thinking on Comfort, Windsor, April 2010. Available at http://nceub.org.uk. Accessed November 2010

Romanovsky AA 2007 Thermoregulation: some concepts have changed. Functional architecture of the thermoregulatory system. Am J Physiol Regul Interact Compar Physiol 292:R37

Schaffer A, Muscatello D, Broome R et al 2012 Emergency department visits, ambulance calls, and mortality associated with an exceptional heat wave in Sidney, Australia, 2011: a time series. Environ Health 11:3

Van Someren EJW 2007 Thermoregulation and aging. Am J Physiol Regul Integr Compar Physiol 292:R99

Wongsurawat N 1994 Temperature regulation in the aged. In: Felsenthal G, Garrison SJ, Steinberg FU (eds) Rehabilitation of the Aging and Elderly Patient. Williams & Wilkins, Baltimore, MD

Chapter 11

The aging immune system

KANWAL RAZZAQ • GORDON DICKINSON

CHAPTER CONTENTS

INTRODUCTION

Humans possess an elaborate array of host defenses against the many potential pathogens in their environment. Among these protective mechanisms are important mechanical and physiological guards such as skin and mucosal barriers, valvular structures like the epiglottis and the urethral valves, cleansing fluids (tears and respiratory tract mucus) and involuntary activities such as coughing. These defenses are, however, frequently breached and it is the immune response that is the final and most potent form of protection. 'Immune response' generally refers to internal cellular and humoral defense mechanisms, especially those that are acquired.

INNATE AND ACQUIRED IMMUNITY

Immunity can be categorized as innate or acquired. The components of innate immunity are generally present from birth and do not require exposure to a pathogen for their development. Innate immunity includes the macrophage/phagocyte cell lines, which act as nonspecific scavengers within the body, engulfing and killing invaders that have breeched the skin or mucosal barriers. To assist the macrophages, there are substances in the serum called complement and acute-phase reactants that facilitate the attachment and ingestion of pathogens. The macrophages, as well as the complement and acute-phase reactants, are poised to function as an immediate response system against virtually all bacteria; however, even in the presence of complement and acute-phase reactants, phagocytic cells often have difficulty promptly and efficiently ingesting pathogens. Some bacteria, for example *Streptococcus pneumoniae* and *Haemophilus influenzae*, form a polysaccharide capsule that shields them from these defenses. Moreover, many pathogens are either too large for ingestion by macrophages (e.g. parasites) or thrive in an intracellular location (e.g. viruses, mycobacteria and an assortment of other pathogens). To bolster these defenses, an acquired immune system has evolved, which is extremely potent and pathogen-specific, but which must be primed by a first-time exposure to the pathogen. Once in place, acquired immunity is permanent. The term 'immunity' generally refers to the activity of the acquired immune system.

T AND B LYMPHOCYTES

The principal components of the acquired immune system are the T and B lymphocytes. All lymphocytes originate from progenitors in the bone marrow. Some evolve into B lymphocytes, so-called because in birds these cells originate in the bursa of Fabricius. The B lymphocytes become antibody factories when activated by helper/inducer T lymphocytes. T lymphocytes circulate through the thymus gland and develop the ability to recognize foreign matter (an antigen), retain memory of the antigen and influence B lymphocytes to produce antibodies against this antigen. These highly specific antibodies attach themselves to the invader, either killing it directly or facilitating the process of phagocytosis, and ultimately cause the destruction and clearance of the invader from the body. Because the lymphocytes retain a memory of the invader, the next exposure to this invader prompts a specific and immediate response. This ability of the immune system to develop and maintain a highly effective and specific response is the basis of vaccination.

When activated, natural killer cells, another subset of lymphocytes, have the ability to select and destroy abnormal host cells (i.e. malignant cells) and destroy intracellular pathogens such as viruses by destroying the cells harboring them. Other T lymphocytes, the T-suppressor lymphocytes, have the ability to downregulate and turn off the immune response once an invader is repelled. The macrophages and lymphocytes interact with one another by secreting soluble products known as cytokines. There are many unique cytokines, and presumably others remain to be discovered.

IMMUNE FUNCTION CHANGES AND RISKS OF INFECTION

The aging process is associated with changes in immune function, particularly in those functions directed or carried out by the lymphocyte system. Although some research has suggested that the aging process itself may be the result of the immune system turning against the body, at present such a theory remains speculative. Most observations of age-associated altered immune function concern failure of or deficiency in function. The increased incidence of malignancies results partly from a loss of the immune system's surveillance and eradication of abnormal cells as they arise. Aging is also associated with increased activity or loss of control of some aspects of the immune system. For example, the incidence of monoclonal gammopathies (multiple myeloma) rises in the older population and the frequency of both anti-idiotypic (antibodies directed against other antibodies) and autoimmune antibodies increases as a person ages. Long before our understanding of the intricacies of the cellular immune system and the specialized properties of its various components began, it was known that the thymus gland progressively atrophies until it becomes virtually a vestigial organ in later life. Investigation of immune function suggests that the most dramatic changes occur within the cellular arm of the immune system (Akbar & Fletcher, 2005; Gomez et al., 2005; Goronzy & Weyand, 2005). B lymphocytes, the cells involved in the production of antibodies ('humoral immunity'), function relatively well, even in the very old (Chen et al., 2009; Siegrist & Aspinall, 2009). Specific changes in immune function that have been described as being associated with aging are listed in Box 11.1.

Box 11.1 *Changes in immune function associated with aging*

- Atrophy of the thymus with decreased production of thymic hormones
- Decreased *in vitro* responsiveness to interleukin-2
- Decreased cell proliferation in response to mitogenic stimulation
- Decreased cell-mediated cytotoxicity
- Enhanced cellular sensitivity to prostaglandin E2
- Increased synthesis of anti-idiotypic antibodies
- Increase in autoimmune antibodies
- Increased incidence of serum monoclonal immunoproteins
- Decreased representation of peripheral blood B lymphocytes in men
- Diminished delayed hypersensitivity
- Enhanced ability to synthesize interferon gamma, interleukin 6, tumor necrosis factor alpha

---

Clinically, the aging individual is at an increased risk both for infection and for a negative outcome of infection. The origin of some of this risk may be in diminished immune function. For example, the incidence and mortality rate of pneumococcal pneumonia, low throughout adolescence and most of the adult years, rises dramatically in people over the age of 65. The consequences of influenza are also enhanced in the elderly, with a dramatically increased risk of death. Primary varicella (chickenpox) is a dreaded infection in older people because of the potential for severe pneumonitis and encephalitis, which often have fatal outcomes in this population. The elderly are also at risk for reactivation of latent infections. For example, varicella zoster and reactivation tuberculosis are seen with increased frequency in older people. Conversely, there is some evidence that the senescence of the immune system correlates more closely with the quantity of comorbid diseases rather than with chronological age (Castle et al., 2005).

RISKS OF INFECTION RELATED TO OTHER PATHOLOGIES

Not all of the increased risks of infection are attributable to changes in immune function. Indeed, many diseases afflicting the elderly result in increased vulnerability to infection that is unrelated to changes in the immune system. For example, the pulmonary edema of congestive heart failure is frequently a contributing factor to the development of pneumonia, presumably because the edema enhances bacterial growth and compromises clearance mechanisms. Peripheral vascular disease causes ischemic breakdown of skin and soft tissue, allowing direct invasion of microbes while impairing the blood flow necessary to carry host defenses to the site of invasion. Another example is a cerebrovascular accident, which leaves the patient with an impaired cough mechanism and malfunctioning epiglottic closure, with an attendant risk for aspiration. What is usually transient colonization with aspirated oral bacterial flora may progress, if not cleared, to cause bronchitis or pneumonia. Malignancies, which occur more frequently in the elderly, increase the risk of infection by a number of mechanisms. They can interfere with the cleansing effects of body fluids by interrupting normal flow – as seen with endobronchial carcinoma or laryngeal carcinoma, for example – thereby setting the stage for entrapment of bacteria normally swept away by mucus flow. Malignancies also frequently erode normal cutaneous or mucosal barriers, providing a direct invasion route into soft tissues and body cavities. The inanition that frequently accompanies metastatic malignancy is, moreover, associated with impaired cellular immunity.

All of these diseases may contribute indirectly to the risk of infection simply because the patient is hospitalized in a facility where the opportunity of acquiring a virulent multidrug-resistant pathogen is much increased.

IMPLICATIONS OF IMMUNE DYSFUNCTION

As noted above, the major clinical significance of immune dysfunction in the elderly is an increased risk

Box 11.2 *Infections that occur with increased frequency among the elderly*

- Pneumonia
- Tuberculosis
- Bacteremia
- Infectious diarrhea
- Septic arthritis
- Urinary tract infection
- Skin and soft-tissue infections
- Infective endocarditis
- Meningitis

of infection and, all too frequently, severe morbidity when an infection occurs. A number of infections are recognized to occur more frequently in the elderly (Box 11.2). The implications for health professionals are obvious. Because infections may rapidly overwhelm the immune defenses and initiate an irrevocable course, clinicians must monitor patients closely. Early warning signals may be subtle: a sensation of being unwell, a change in mentation (lethargy, confusion), a decrease in appetite or a diminution of physical activity. Such clinical signs and symptoms of infection may be muted in the older patient; crucial clues may be easily overlooked or attributed to other conditions. Fever, the hallmark of infection, may be subdued or even replaced by a drop in temperature in the older patient and chills may be absent. Caregivers should pay attention to subtle clinical hints and investigate by questioning and examining the patient followed by the use of laboratory and radiographic studies as appropriate. Because the elderly patient frequently has other diseases that may cause these signs and symptoms, a timely and accurate diagnosis is often difficult to establish.

THERAPEUTIC INTERVENTION

Because bacteriological analysis to detect the causative pathogen takes hours or days, empiric treatment is frequently necessary to avoid undue morbidity and mortality associated with serious infections. The decision to initiate empiric antimicrobial treatment is often problematic when the presence of an infection has not yet been proven and the causative organism is not known. To diagnose and choose treatment, the clinician must weigh all available evidence, searching carefully for clues at typical sites of infection: respiratory tract, urinary tract, pressure sores on the skin, catheter insertion sites, and the biliary and gastrointestinal tracts. If a decision is taken to initiate empiric treatment, knowledge of a patient's prior infections and recent experiences with nosocomial pathogens within the facility will help the physician choose appropriate antibiotics. This process of determining the probable causative organism and starting empiric treatment is particularly difficult in the extended-care facility and the homecare setting and when the patient is being transferred between different treatment facilities. Effective and timely communication among the healthcare team members is a necessity if patients in such circumstances are to receive optimal

care. As in all areas of healthcare, prevention is greatly preferred to treatment. Of primary importance is attention to the seemingly mundane details of daily care to avoid situations that are known to place a patient at risk for infection. Malnutrition exacerbates the frailty of the elderly, so monitoring the patient's nutritional needs and intervening to ensure that they are met are important. Such nutritional intervention may require no more than assistance with meals. Although nutritional supplements are commercially available, balanced meals prepared to accommodate the patient's taste and any impairment of mastication are usually sufficient. Measures to avoid skin breakdown should also be followed meticulously: for example, frequent turning of the immobile patient, cleaning of skin soiled by incontinence and attending to bowel and urinary habits to minimize incontinence. Discontinuation of unnecessary medical devices such as intravenous catheters and urinary catheters also eliminates two of the greatest iatrogenic sources of serious infection.

Basic to the prevention of nosocomial infections is strict attention to good infection control practices that are universally recommended but seldom scrupulously followed. In many centers, the problem of nosocomial spread of pathogens has been exacerbated by the emergence of multidrug-resistant pathogens, a phenomenon likely to continue in the future. Outbreaks of infection within hospitals and nursing homes caused by methicillin-resistant *Staphylococcus aureus* (MRSA) and multidrug-resistant enterobacteriaceae, streptococci and even *Mycobacterium tuberculosis* have been documented. However, most, if not all, outbreaks are avoidable.

EXERCISE AND THE IMMUNE SYSTEM

It is clear that appropriate physical exercise is of benefit to the elderly, and there are data to suggest that exercise is beneficial to immune function (Kohut et al., 2005). What is not clear is whether this is a direct benefit of exercise or an indirect benefit through psychosocial factors (Kohut et al., 2005). The exercise stimulus is clearly an important factor to consider. Natural killer cell activity has been shown to increase with 10 weeks of resistance training using three sets of 10 repetitions. The graded weight training, involving 10 different exercises, was performed on machines and used an intensity of one repetition maximum (1 RM) (McFarlin et al., 2005). Regardless, it is easy to suggest that regular exercise, consistent with the cardiovascular and musculoskeletal constraints of the individual, is beneficial for the aging immune system as well as the global health of the elderly (Simpson et al., 2012).

VACCINES

Vaccinations are an important component of preventive medicine, especially for the elderly. The aging immune system, however, may pose a challenge to vaccine effectiveness. In general the levels of antibodies elicited are less than levels in younger adults. Also, the failure of recommended vaccines to prevent an event is higher in the elderly. But it should be noted that even when a vaccine failure occurs, the disease is often ameliorated. The major cause of vaccine failure is the failure to administer. The Advisory Committee on Immunization Practices (ACIP) is the body that promulgates vaccine guidelines for the public health in the United States of America. The ACIP regularly updates these guidelines based upon the best scientific information available. All adults should be encouraged to be vaccinated according to these recommendations. At the time of writing, pneumococcal, zoster, tetanus–diphtheria–acellular pertussis (Tdap) and influenza vaccines are recommended for adults (CDC, 2013).

CONCLUSION

Changes in the immune systems of elderly people add to the complexity and challenge of providing appropriate healthcare. Comorbidities further complicate this problem. Because an elevation in body temperature is not always seen, clinicians and care providers must be aware of the subtle manifestations of infection such as a sense of being unwell, lethargy, confusion and diminished appetite or physical activity. The choice of medical intervention is not always obvious, but good nutrition and infection control are necessary. Vaccinations are helpful, although their use is not without controversy.

REFERENCES

Akbar AN, Fletcher JM 2005 Memory T cell homeostasis and senescence during aging. Curr Opin Immunol 17:480–485

Castle SC, Uyemura K, Rafi A et al 2005 Comorbidity is a better predictor of impaired immunity than chronological age in older adults. J Am Geriatr Soc 53:1565–1569

CDC (Centers for Disease Control and Prevention) 2013 ACIP Recommendations and Reports. Available at: www.CDC.gov/vaccines/pubs. Accessed November 2013

Chen WH, Kozlovsky BF, Effros RB et al 2009 Vaccination in the elderly: an immunological perspective. Trends in Immunology 30:351–359

Gomez CR, Boehmer ED, Kovacs EJ 2005 The aging innate immune system. Curr Opin Immunol 17:457–462

Goronzy JJ, Weyand CM 2005 T-cell development and receptor diversity during aging. Curr Opin Immunol 17:468–475

Kohut ML, Lee W, Martin A et al 2005 The exercise-induced enhancement of influenza immunity is mediated in part by improvements in psychosocial factors in older adults. Brain Behav Immun 19:357–366

McFarlin BK, Flynn M, Phillips M et al 2005 Chronic resistance training improves natural killer cell activity in older women. J Gerontol A Biol Sci Med Sci 60:1315–1318

Siegrist C, Aspinall R 2009 B-cell responses to vaccination at the extremes of age. Nat Rev Immunol 9:185–194

Simpson RJ, Lowder TW, Spielmann G et al 2012 Exercise and the aging immune system. Age Res Rev 11:404–420

Chapter 12

Pharmacology considerations for the aging individual

CHARLES D. CICCONE

CHAPTER CONTENTS

INTRODUCTION

Older adults receiving physical rehabilitation services are commonly taking medications to help resolve acute and chronic ailments. These medications are intended to improve the patient's health but they frequently cause side-effects that can have a negative impact on the patient's response to physical rehabilitation. The elderly are more susceptible to adverse effects of drugs owing to many factors, including excessive drug use, declining function in various physiological systems, and altered drug metabolism and excretion.

In particular, age-related physiological changes in liver and kidney function can profoundly affect drug metabolism and excretion (Shi & Klotz, 2011). Many medications are metabolized and inactivated to some extent in the liver, and age-related decreases in liver size, hepatic blood flow and enzymatic capacity can impair the body's ability to metabolize these medications. Likewise, the kidneys are the primary site of drug excretion, and progressive decreases in renal mass, renal blood flow, filtration capacity and nephron function can reduce the body's ability to remove various drugs and their metabolites from the bloodstream. Because of these age-related physiological changes, the body is not able to eliminate drugs in a timely and predictable manner, thus leading to drug accumulation and an increased risk of adverse drug reactions.

Deficiencies in other physiological systems may also increase the likelihood of adverse drug reactions in older adults (Petrovic et al., 2012). For example, an older adult with impaired balance reactions will be more likely to fall when taking benzodiazepines (i.e., Valium-like drugs) and other drugs that impair balance. An older patient who has cognitive deficits might become more confused when taking opioids and other medications that affect cognition. Hence, problems related to a decline in any physiological system will almost certainly be magnified by drugs that adversely affect that system.

Nonetheless, older adults often rely on medications to help improve their health and quality of life. It follows that health professionals should be aware of the primary medications being taken by their elderly clients and how those medications can affect patients' participation in rehabilitation.

Some of the primary medications used to treat conditions commonly seen in older adults are addressed here. This discussion is not meant to be all-inclusive but should help clinicians to recognize and understand how medications taken by the elderly can affect their response to rehabilitation.

TREATMENT OF PAIN AND INFLAMMATION

OPIOID ANALGESICS

Opioid (narcotic) medications such as morphine and meperidine (Table 12.1) are powerful analgesics that bind to neuronal receptors in the spinal cord and brain. These medications reduce synaptic activity in pain-transmitting pathways, thereby decreasing pain perception. Common side-effects of opioids include sedation, respiratory depression, constipation and orthostatic hypotension. Practitioners should also be aware that older adults are more susceptible to opioid-induced psychotropic reactions such as confusion, anxiety, hallucinations and euphoria/dysphoria (Papaleontiou et al., 2010). Opioids can also increase the risk of falls in older adults, by either increasing sedation or causing dizziness from orthostatic hypotension. These reactions are especially common in elderly patients recovering from surgery, perhaps because of opioid side-effects being magnified by the residual effects of the general anesthetic, and because of the disorientation and wooziness that often occur after surgery.

NON-OPIOID ANALGESICS

Nonsteroidal anti-inflammatory drugs (NSAIDs) are the primary group of non-opioid analgesics. NSAIDs

Table 12.1	**Analgesic and anti-inflammatory medications**	
Category	**Common Examples**	
	Generic Name	**Trade Name**
Opioid analgesics	Hydromorphone	Dilaudid, others
	Meperidine (pethidine)	Demerol
	Morphine	Many trade names
	Oxycodone	OxyContin, others
	Propoxyphene	Darvon
Non-opioid analgesics	Aspirin	Many trade names
NSAIDs	Ibuprofen	Advil, Motrin, others
	Ketoprofen	Orudis, others
	Ketorolac	Toradol
	Meloxican	Mobic
	Naproxen	Aleve, others
	Piroxicam	Feldene, others
COX-2 inhibitors	Celecoxib	Celebrex
Acetaminophen	–	Tylenol, others
Glucocorticoids	Betamethasone	Celestone
	Dexamethasone	DexPak
	Hydrocortisone	Cortef, others
	Methylprednisolone	Medrol, others
	Prednisolone	Prelone, others
	Prednisone	Sterapred

COX-2, cyclooxygenase type 2; NSAIDs, nonsteroidal anti-inflammatory drugs

include aspirin, ibuprofen and similar agents (see Table 12.1), and these drugs are often effective in treating mild to moderate pain. These medications actually produce four clinically important effects: decreased pain, decreased inflammation, decreased fever and decreased blood coagulation. There is also considerable evidence that NSAIDs may decrease the risk of certain cancers, including colorectal cancer. All of these effects are mediated through inhibition of the biosynthesis of lipid compounds called prostaglandins. Certain prostaglandins mediate painful sensations by increasing the nociceptive effects of bradykinin. NSAID-mediated inhibition of prostaglandin synthesis therefore helps reduce painful sensations in a variety of clinical conditions. The primary problem associated with NSAIDs is gastrointestinal distress, including gastric irritation and ulceration. These medications may also cause damage to the liver and kidneys, especially in older adults who have preexisting hepatic or renal dysfunction.

In addition to traditional NSAIDs, newer drugs known as COX-2 inhibitors have been developed (Gatti & Adami, 2010). These drugs are so named because they inhibit the cyclooxygenase (COX)-2 enzyme that synthesizes prostaglandins during pathological conditions. The COX-2 enzyme synthesizes prostaglandins that cause pain, inflammation and other harmful effects, whereas the COX-1 enzyme synthesizes prostaglandins that are beneficial and often help protect various tissues and organs. Whereas traditional NSAIDs (e.g. aspirin, ibuprofen) inhibit both isoforms of the COX enzyme, the COX-2 drugs are designed to inhibit only the production of harmful prostaglandins (reducing pain and inflammation) while sparing the production of beneficial prostaglandins in the stomach, kidneys, and other organs and tissues. Indeed, the incidence of gastric problems is lower with COX-2 drugs, and some older adults have used these drugs successfully for extended periods to treat osteoarthritis and similar problems with minimal side-effects. The COX-2 drugs, however, may also produce serious cardiovascular problems including heart attack and stroke in susceptible patients. Hence, these drugs should be avoided in those at risk for cardiovascular disease (Gatti & Adami, 2010). Currently, celecoxib (Celebrex) is the only COX-2 drug that remains on the market, and this drug must be used cautiously when treating pain in older adults.

Acetaminophen (paracetamol), the active ingredient in Tylenol and other products, is another type of non-opioid analgesic. This agent is different from the NSAIDs in that it does not produce any appreciable anti-inflammatory or anticoagulant effects. Likewise, acetaminophen does not produce gastrointestinal irritation, but this medication can cause severe hepatotoxicity in those with liver disease or after an overdose.

ANTI-INFLAMMATORY MEDICATIONS

Treatment of inflammation consists primarily of the NSAIDs and anti-inflammatory steroids. As indicated earlier, NSAIDs inhibit the synthesis of prostaglandins, and this inhibition reduces the proinflammatory effects of certain prostaglandins. NSAIDs tend to be effective in treating a variety of conditions that exhibit mild to moderate inflammation. More severe inflammatory conditions often require the use of anti-inflammatory steroids known as glucocorticoids. Medications such as hydrocortisone and prednisolone (see Table 12.1) inhibit a number of the cellular and chemical aspects of the inflammatory response, often producing a dramatic decrease in the symptoms of inflammation. However, glucocorticoids cause many severe side-effects including breakdown of collagenous tissues, hypertension, glucose intolerance, gastric ulcer, glaucoma and adrenocortical suppression. Tissue breakdown (catabolism) can cause severe muscle wasting and osteoporosis, especially in older people who may already be somewhat debilitated.

PSYCHOTROPIC MEDICATIONS

ANTIANXIETY DRUGS

Treatment of anxiety has traditionally consisted of benzodiazepines, including diazepam and similar agents (Table 12.2) (Rheinhold et al., 2011). These drugs work by increasing the inhibitory effects of

Table 12.2 **Psychotropic medications**		
Category	**Common Examples**	
	Generic Name	**Trade Name**
Antianxiety drugs		
Benzodiazepines	Alprazolam	Xanax
	Chlordiazepoxide	Librium, others
	Diazepam	Valium
	Lorazepam	Ativan
	Oxazepam	Serax, others
Azapirones	Buspirone	Buspar
Antidepressants		
Tricyclics	Amitriptyline	Elavil, others
	Amoxapine	Asendin
	Doxepin	Sinequan, others
	Imipramine	Tofranil, others
	Nortriptyline	Pamelor, others
	Trimipramine	Surmontil
MAO inhibitors	Isocarboxazid	Marplan
	Tranylcypromine	Parnate
Second-generation drugs	Buproprion	Wellbutrin
	Citalopram[a]	Celexa
	Desvenlafaxine[b]	Pristiq
	Escitalopram[a]	Lexapro
	Duloxetine[b]	Cymbalta
	Fluoxetine[a]	Prozac
	Maprotiline	Ludiomil
	Paroxetine[a]	Paxil
	Sertraline[a]	Zoloft
	Venlafaxine[b]	Effexor
Antipsychotics		
	Aripiprazole[c]	Abilify
	Chlorpromazine	Thorazine
	Clozapine[c]	Clozaril
	Haloperidol	Haldol
	Olanzapine[c]	Zyprexa
	Prochlorperazine	Compazine, others
	Quetiapine[c]	Seroquel
	Risperdone[c]	Risperdal
	Thioridazine	Mellaril

MAO, monoamine oxidase
[a]Selective serotonin-reuptake inhibitors.
[b]Norepinephrine serotonin-reuptake inhibitors.
[c]Atypical antipsychotics.

gamma-aminobutyric acid (GABA), an endogenous neurotransmitter, in areas of the brain that control mood and behavior. The primary side-effect of benzodiazepine agents is sedation. These drugs may also cause tolerance and physical dependence when used continually for prolonged periods (more than 6 weeks). Benzodiazepines also have extremely long metabolic half-lives in older adults, which means that it takes a very long time to metabolize and eliminate these drugs. As a result, benzodiazepines can accumulate in older patients and reach toxic levels, shown by symptoms of confusion, slurred speech, dyspnea, incoordination and pronounced weakness.

A non-benzodiazepine antianxiety medication known as buspirone (Buspar) may also be effective in some older patients (Rheinhold et al., 2011). This agent, chemically classified as an azapirone, increases serotonin activity in the brain, thus decreasing symptoms of anxiety. Buspirone is often prescribed for older adults because this agent does not appear to produce sedation or cause tolerance and physical dependence. However, it may take longer to exert its antianxiety effects, and may not be as effective in treating severe anxiety compared with the benzodiazepines.

Finally, certain antidepressants such as paroxetine (Paxil) and venlafaxine (Effexor) may reduce anxiety even in people who are not depressed (Rheinhold et al., 2011). These drugs affect the function of amine neurotransmitters that are important for mood and behavior (see below), and they may provide an effective alternative for older adults who do not respond adequately to more traditional antianxiety agents.

ANTIDEPRESSANTS

Several different types and categories of antidepressant medication exist (see Table 12.2) (Bottino et al., 2012). These drugs all share the common goal of trying to increase activity at synapses in the brain that use amine neurotransmitters, including catecholamines (norepinephrine), 5-hydroxytryptamine (serotonin) and dopamine. Although the details remain unclear, depression is thought to be caused by a defect in the release of, sensitivity to, or postsynaptic signals of these amine neurotransmitters in specific areas of the brain that control mood (i.e. the limbic system). Traditional antidepressants are nonselective and cause increased activity at synapses that use norepinephrine, serotonin and dopamine. However, certain newer antidepressants are more selective for serotonin and norepinephrine pathways (see Table 12.2). These drugs include the selective serotonin-reuptake inhibitors (SSRIs) such as fluoxetine (Prozac) and sertraline (Zoloft), and the serotonin-norepinephrine reuptake inhibitors (SNRIs) such as duloxetine (Cymbalta) and venlafaxine (Effexor). There is still considerable debate about which drugs are most effective in treating depression, but newer, more selective drugs may be preferred in older adults because their side-effects are better tolerated (see below).

The primary side-effects of traditional (nonselective) antidepressants are sedation, orthostatic hypotension and the results of decreased acetylcholine function (anticholinergic effects), such as dry mouth, urinary retention, constipation, tachycardia and confusion. These side-effects are often much more pronounced in older people because of age-related declines in various physiological systems combined with the fact that some of these drugs have much longer metabolic half-lives in older adults. For example, the elimination half-life of amitriptyline (a traditional nonselective antidepressant) is normally around 16 hours in young individuals, whereas it may be twice as long (31 hours) in healthy older adults. More selective agents such as the SSRIs and SNRIs tend to have fewer sedative, hypotensive and anticholinergic effects, and these drugs may therefore be used preferentially in older adults. Another primary concern about antidepressants is that there is typically a 1- to 2-week time lag between initiation of drug treatment and improvement of depression, and some patients may need up to 6 weeks before receiving the full benefit from these drugs. Depression may actually worsen in some patients during this period, and clinicians should be especially careful to note any increase in depressive symptoms while waiting for these drugs to take effect.

ANTIPSYCHOTICS

Schizophrenia and other psychotic disorders are associated with increased activity in certain dopamine pathways of the brain, which in turn cause imbalances in serotonin and other neurotransmitters (Shin et al., 2011). As a result, antipsychotic medications block specific dopamine receptors in these pathways to help normalize dopaminergic influence and resolve the neurochemical imbalances that underlie psychosis. Common antipsychotics are listed in Table 12.2. These agents typically cause side-effects such as sedation, orthostatic hypotension, anticholinergic effects and movement disorders including tardive dyskinesia, pseudoparkinsonism, severe restlessness (akathisia) and various other dystonias and dyskinesias. Tardive dyskinesia is characterized by oral–facial movements such as extending the tongue, grinding the jaw, puffing the cheeks, and various other fragmented movements of the neck, trunk and extremities. This problem is often regarded as the most serious side-effect of antipsychotic medications because symptoms of tardive dyskinesia may take several months to disappear or may remain indefinitely after the antipsychotic drug is discontinued. Some of the newer antipsychotics are regarded as 'atypical' because they are as effective as traditional agents but pose a lower risk of tardive dyskinesia and other side-effects; hence these atypical antipsychotics may be used preferentially in older adults (Shin et al., 2011). Nonetheless, therapists should be cognizant of any aberrant movement patterns in patients taking antipsychotic medications, especially symptoms of tardive dyskinesia.

NEUROLOGICAL DISORDERS

PARKINSON'S DISEASE

The motor symptoms of Parkinson's disease (bradykinesia, rigidity, resting tremor) are related to the loss of dopaminergic neurons in the basal ganglia (Singer, 2012). The primary method of drug treatment is levodopa (L-dopa), which is the metabolic precursor to dopamine. Although dopamine will not cross the blood–brain barrier, levodopa will enter brain tissues where it is subsequently converted to dopamine, thus helping to restore the influence of dopamine in the basal ganglia. Levodopa is often administered with carbidopa, a drug that prevents premature conversion of levodopa to dopamine in the peripheral circulation. Combining levodopa with carbidopa in preparations such as Sinemet allows levodopa to reach the brain before undergoing conversion to dopamine.

Levodopa is associated with several side-effects, including gastrointestinal irritation, hypotension and psychotic-like symptoms. Other movement problems, including dyskinesias and dystonias, may also occur, especially at higher dosages. However, the most devastating problems are typically related to a decrease in long-term effectiveness; patients who respond well to levodopa initially, commonly experience progressively diminishing benefits after 4–5 years of continual use. This phenomenon is probably related to a progressive increase in the severity of Parkinson's disease; that is, drug therapy cannot adequately resolve the motor symptoms because of the advanced degeneration of dopaminergic neurons in the basal ganglia. Helping patients and their families to deal with the physical as well as psychological impact of decreased levodopa effectiveness is one of the more difficult tasks that therapists face.

Several other types of medications are also indicated in Parkinson's disease (Table 12.3). These agents are often used to supplement levodopa therapy, but they can also serve as the primary agent when levodopa is poorly tolerated or no longer effective. A common strategy is to combine several agents in low to moderate doses to obtain optimal benefits while avoiding the excessive side-effects that would occur with large amounts of any single drug.

SEIZURES

Some of the medications commonly used to control seizure activity are listed in Table 12.3. These agents act on the brain to selectively reduce excitability in neurons that initiate seizures (Jankovic & Dostic, 2012); however, it is often difficult to reduce excitation in these neurons without producing some degree of general inhibition throughout the brain. This is especially true in the older patient who has had a previous cerebral injury such as a cerebrovascular accident or closed head injury. As a result, older patients taking antiseizure medications are especially prone to side-effects such as sedation, fatigue, weakness, incoordination, ataxia and visual disturbances (e.g. blurred vision and diplopia). Therapists should pay particular attention to patients taking antiseizure medication because they are in a position to help determine whether dosages are too high (as indicated by excessive side-effects) or too low (as evidenced by an increase in seizure activity).

ALZHEIMER'S DISEASE

Donepezil (Aricept), tacrine (Cognex) and several other medications (see Table 12.3) were developed to help improve cognition and intellectual function in patients with Alzheimer's disease (Atri, 2011). These drugs are cholinergic stimulants; they decrease acetylcholine breakdown at synapses in the brain, thereby helping to maintain acetylcholine influence in areas of the brain that are undergoing the neuronal degeneration associated with Alzheimer's disease. Memantine (Namenda) was also developed as a complementary strategy to treat Alzheimer's disease. This drug blocks the N-methyl-D-aspartate receptor in the brain, thereby reducing the potentially damaging effects of excitatory amino acids such as glutamate. None of the currently available drugs cures Alzheimer's disease, but they may help patients retain more intellectual and functional ability during the early stages of the disease. The primary side-effects associated with these drugs include loss of appetite and gastrointestinal distress (diarrhea, nausea and vomiting).

Table 12.3   Neurological medications

Category	Examples	Rationale for Use
Treatment of Parkinson's disease		
Dopamine precursors	Levodopa (Sinemet[a])	Converted to dopamine in the brain; helps resolve dopamine deficiency
Anticholinergic drugs	Benztropine (Cogentin), biperiden (Akineton), diphenhydramine (Benadryl)	Normalize acetylcholine imbalance caused by dopamine loss
COMT inhibitors	Entacapone (Comtan), tolcapone (Tasmar)	Prevent levodopa breakdown in bloodstream
Dopamine agonists	Bromocriptine (Parlodel), cabergoline (Dostinex), pramipexole (Mirapex), ropinirole (Mirapex), rotigotine (Neupro)	Directly stimulate dopamine receptors in brain
MAO-B inhibitors	Rasagiline (Azilect), selegiline (Eldepryl)	Decrease dopamine breakdown in brain
Antiseizure medications		
Barbiturates	Phenobarbital (Solfoton), pentobarbital (Nembutal)	Increase inhibitory effects of GABA in brain; may also inhibit release of glutamate
Benzodiazapines	Clonazepam (Klonopin), clorazepate (Tranxene)	Increase inhibitory effects of GABA in brain
Carboxylic acids	Valproic acid (Depakene)	May increase GABA concentrations in brain
Hydantoins	Phenytoin (Dilantin)	Decrease sodium entry into hyperexcitable neurons
Iminostilbenes	Carbamazepine (Tegretol), oxcarbazepine (Trileptal)	Similar to hydantoins
Succinimides	Ethosuximide (Zarontin)	May decrease calcium entry into hyperexcitable neurons
Second generation antiseizure drugs	Felbamate (Felbatol), gabapentin (Neurontin), lamotrigine (Lamictal), gabapentin (Neurontin), lacosamide (Vimpat), levetiracetam (Keppra), pregabalin (Lyrica), rufinamide (Banzel), tiagabine (Gabitril), topiramate (Topamax), zonasamide (Zonegran)	Various effects; generally either increase effects of inhibitory neurotransmitters (e.g. GABA) or decrease the effects of excitatory neurotransmitters (e.g. glutamate, aspartate)
Treatment of Alzheimer's dementia		
Cholinergic stimulants	Donepezil (Aricept), galantamine (Reminyl), rivastigmine (Exelon), tacrine (Cognex)	Increase acetylcholine influence in the brain
NMDA antagonists	Memantine (Namenda)	Blocks effects of excitatory neurotransmitters (glutamate)

COMT, catechol-O-methyltransferase; GABA, gamma-aminobutyric acid; MAO-B, monoamine oxidase type B; NMDA, N-methyl-D-aspartate
[a]Sinemet is the trade name for levodopa combined with carbidopa.

CARDIOVASCULAR DRUGS

ANTIHYPERTENSIVE MEDICATIONS

Several drug categories (Table 12.4) are used to treat high blood pressure in older adults and reduce the chance of hypertensive-related incidents such as stroke, myocardial infarction and kidney disease (Aronow, 2012). Angiotensin-converting enzyme (ACE) inhibitors prevent the formation of angiotensin II, which is a powerful vasoconstrictor and stimulant of vascular smooth muscle growth. Agents such as alpha blockers, beta blockers and other sympatholytic drugs decrease sympathetic nervous system stimulation of the heart and vasculature, thereby decreasing myocardial contraction force and peripheral vascular resistance. Calcium-channel blockers reduce myocardial contractility and vascular smooth muscle contraction by limiting calcium entry into these tissues. Diuretics increase sodium and water excretion, thereby decreasing blood pressure by reducing fluid volume in the vascular system. Certain direct-acting vasodilators (see Table 12.4) reduce vascular resistance by inhibiting vascular smooth muscle contraction.

Elderly people with hypertension are treated routinely with diuretic agents because these drugs are fairly safe and well tolerated. ACE inhibitors have also been used increasingly in older patients because these agents reduce blood pressure and prevent adverse structural changes in the heart and vasculature. In contrast, sympatholytics and vasodilators tend to produce many unfavorable side-effects in older patients, so these drugs should be used only in severe cases. Calcium-channel blockers can also be used to treat hypertension in older adults, but the short-acting forms of these drugs should be avoided because they may decrease blood pressure too rapidly and increase the risk of myocardial infarction in certain patients. Hence, sustained- or continuous-release versions of the calcium-channel blockers should be used preferentially in older patients with hypertension.

Antihypertensive drugs produce various side-effects, depending on the specific agent; however, it is important that clinicians are aware that hypotension and orthostatic hypotension are always possible whenever blood pressure is reduced pharmacologically. Blood pressure may fall by more than 10–20 mmHg, especially when an older patient sits or stands up suddenly. Likewise, physical therapy interventions that cause extensive peripheral vasodilation (e.g. warm water in the Hubbard tank or therapeutic pool) must be used very

Table 12.4 Cardiovascular medications

Category	Examples	Rationale for Use
Antihypertensive drugs		
ACE inhibitors	Captopril (Capoten), enalapril (Vasotec), lisinopril (Prinivil)	Decrease angiotensin II synthesis; promote vasodilation and increases vascular compliance
Alpha blockers	Doxazosin (Cardura), prazosin (Minipress), terazosin (Hytrin)	Promote vasodilation by decreasing sympathetic stimulation of vasculature
Beta blockers	Atenolol (Tenormin), metoprolol (Lopressor), nadolol (Corgard), propranolol (Inderal)	Decrease myocardial contractility by decreasing sympathetic stimulation of the heart
Calcium-channel blockers	Diltiazem (Cardizem), nifedipine (Procardia, others), verapamil (Calan, others)	Promote vasodilation and decreased myocardial contractility by limiting calcium entry into vasculature and heart
Diuretics	Chlorothiazide (Diuril), furosemide (Lasix), spironolactone (Aldactone)	Decrease intravascular fluid volume; reduce workload on heart
Vasodilators	Hydralazine (Apresoline), minoxidil (Loniten)	Promote vasodilation by inhibiting contraction of vascular smooth muscle
Treatment of congestive heart failure		
Digitalis glycosides	Digoxin (Lanoxin)	Increases myocardial contractility by increasing calcium concentration in heart muscle
Others	Diuretics, ACE inhibitors, beta blockers, vasodilators	See above
Treatment of hyperlipidemia		
Statins	Atorvastatin (Lipitor), fluvastatin (Lescol), lovastatin (Mevachor), pravastatin (Pravachol), rosuvastatin (Crestor), simvastatin (Zocor)	Decrease total cholesterol, LDL-cholesterol and triglyceride levels
Fibric acids	Fenofibrate (Tricor), gemfibrozil (Lopid)	Primarily decrease triglyceride levels; may also increase LDL breakdown
Others	Cholestyramine (Questran), ezetimibe (Zetia), niacin (Nicotinex, others)	Decrease total cholesterol

LDL, low-density lipoprotein

cautiously because these interventions add to the hypo-tensive drug effects and produce dangerously low blood pressure in older adults. Finally, some antihypertensive agents, for example beta blockers, blunt the cardiac response to exercise and this effect may limit physical work capacity during activities that require high cardiac output, such as climbing stairs and exercise training.

TREATMENT OF CONGESTIVE HEART FAILURE

Congestive heart failure (CHF) occurs commonly in older adults and is characterized by a progressive decline in myocardial pumping ability (Morrissey et al., 2011). Digitalis glycosides such as digoxin are often used to treat CHF (see Table 12.4). These agents increase calcium entry into myocardial tissues, thereby increasing con-tractile force. Digitalis drugs often produce temporary hemodynamic improvements that decrease the symp-toms of CHF, but these agents do not alter the progres-sion of the disease or decrease the rather high morbidity and mortality rates associated with heart failure. These agents have a small safety margin and can accumulate rapidly in the bloodstream causing toxicity in older patients. Digitalis toxicity is associated with symptoms such as gastrointestinal distress, confusion, blurred vision and cardiac arrhythmias. Clinicians should be alert for these symptoms because digitalis-induced arrhythmias can be quite severe or fatal.

Because of the problems related to digitalis, other medications have been used alone or with digitalis drugs to help treat patients with CHF. Diuretics and vasodi-lators have been used to decrease the workload on the failing heart by reducing fluid volume or decreasing vascular resistance, respectively. More importantly, ACE inhibitors can decrease angiotensin II-mediated vasocon-striction and vascular hypertrophy so that cardiac work-load is reduced. Unlike digitalis drugs, ACE inhibitors appear to improve the prognosis of patients with heart failure and decrease the morbidity and mortality associ-ated with CHF. ACE inhibitors are tolerated fairly well by older adults, and have relatively minor side-effects such as a mild allergic reaction (skin rash) or a dry persistent cough. As a result, ACE inhibitors are now considered as the primary treatment for many older patients with CHF.

TREATMENT OF HYPERLIPIDEMIA

Several drugs have been introduced to the market to help improve plasma lipid profile and reduce the adverse effects of atherosclerosis on the cardiovascular system (Last et al., 2011). The primary category of lipid-low-ering drugs is the statins (see Table 12.4). Statin drugs inhibit an enzyme known as 3-hydroxy-3-methylgluta-ryl coenzyme A (HMG-CoA) that is responsible for syn-thesizing cholesterol in the body. This effect reduces endogenous cholesterol biosynthesis and also facilitates a number of other beneficial effects on plasma lipids (reduced low-density lipoproteins, reduced triglycerides). A second category of antihyperlipidemia agents is the fibric acids. Although the exact mechanism of their action is not known, fibric acids can reduce triglyceride

levels and increase low-density lipoprotein breakdown. An eclectic group of other agents (e.g. ezetimibe, niacin) is also available, and these agents work in various ways to treat hyperlipidemia.

Drugs used to treat hyperlipidemia produce various side-effects including gastrointestinal disturbances (nau-sea, cramping, diarrhea). Statins can also produce mus-cular pain, weakness and inflammation. This so-called 'statin-induced myopathy' can be quite severe in some people and even lead to breakdown of skeletal mus-cle tissues (rhabdomyolysis). Therefore, if muscle pain occurs spontaneously in older adults or any individual taking lipid-lowering drugs, clinicians should refer the patient back to the physician immediately to determine the source of the pain. If statin-induced myopathy is the suspected cause, the drug is usually discontinued and the patient is allowed several weeks to recover from the muscle damage before resuming exercise or other vigor-ous activities.

CONCLUSION

Medications often produce favorable as well as adverse responses in elderly patients receiving rehabilitation. Therapists and other clinicians must be aware of the types of medication commonly taken by older adults and of the possible side-effects associated with these medications. Geriatric patients are more susceptible to adverse drug effects, and clinicians often play an important role in helping to identify problematic drug responses in the elderly. Likewise, therapists must be able to plan and modify rehabilitation strategies to capi-talize on beneficial drug effects while minimizing or avoiding adverse effects.

References

Aronow WS 2012 Current approaches to the treatment of hyperten-sion in older persons. Postgrad Med 124:50–59
Atri A 2011 Effective pharmacological management of Alzheimer's disease. Am J Manag Care 17(suppl13):S346–S355
Bottino CM, Barcelos-Ferreira R, Ribeiz SR 2012 Treatment of depres-sion in older adults. Curr Psychiatry Rep 14:289–297
Gatti D, Adami S 2010 Coxibs: a significant therapeutic opportunity. Acta Biomed 81:217–224
Jankovic SM, Dostic M 2012 Choice of antiepileptic drugs for the elderly: possible drug interactions and adverse effects. Expert Opin Drug Metab Toxicol 8:81–91
Last AR, Ference JD, Falleroni J 2011 Pharmacologic treatment of hyperlipidemia. Am Fam Physician 84:551–558
Morrissey RP, Czer L, Shah PK 2011 Chronic heart failure: cur-rent evidence, challenges to therapy, and future directions. Am J Cardiovasc Drugs 11:153–171
Papaleontiou M, Henderson Jr CR, Turner BJ et al 2010 Outcomes associated with opioid use in the treatment of chronic noncancer pain in older adults: a systematic review and meta-analysis. J Am Geriatr Soc 58:1353–1369
Petrovic M, van der Cammen T, Onder G 2012 Adverse drug reactions in older people: detection and prevention. Drugs Aging 29:453–462
Rheinhold JA, Mandos LA, Rickels K et al 2011 Pharmacological treat-ment of generalized anxiety disorder. Expert Opin Pharmacother 12:2457–2467
Shi S, Klotz U 2011 Age-related changes in pharmacokinetics. Curr Drug Metab 12:601–610
Shin JK, Malone DT, Crosby IT et al 2011 Schizophrenia: a systematic review of the disease state, current therapeutics and their molecular mechanisms of action. Curr Med Chem 18:1380–1404
Singer C 2012 Managing the patient with newly diagnosed Parkinson disease. Cleve Clin J Med 79(suppl2):S3–S7

Chapter 13

Laboratory assessment considerations for the aging individual

CHRISTINE STABLER

CHAPTER CONTENTS

INTRODUCTION

Of all people who have ever lived to the age of 65, over half are alive today. This striking statement has significant implications for the ongoing care of the elderly. Until now, little research has been conducted to evaluate the specific differences seen in the laboratory assessment of the older individual.

The Human Genome Project has finally been completed and the genetic basis of many biological functions has been identified; however, there is still much to learn about the biology of aging. It is known that cells and tissues have finite lifespans, and that growth and replication slows with age. However, it seems that many metabolic and biological functions remain constant over the lifetime of humans. Extrapolating these data from tissue to human is somewhat risky but it is accurate to do so in that aging itself is not marked by predictable biochemical changes. As people age they become more dissimilar, belying any stereotype of aging. Abrupt declines in system functions or marked changes in laboratory values should be attributed to the effects of disease, not normal aging. Finally, in the absence of disease or modifiable risk factors, the concept of healthy old age is absolutely valid. This chapter will review the laboratory differences between the well young adult and the well older individual and identify the known variations that occur in the absence of disease.

AGE-RELATED CONSIDERATIONS

Certain basic tenets apply when evaluating the elderly patient. In the process of aging, there is a decline in metabolic reserves in most organ systems, particularly in the cardiovascular, central nervous, gastrointestinal, hematopoietic and endocrine systems. Disease states will affect these vulnerable systems and become evident through laboratory value changes more rapidly than in younger adults. The fragile renal and hepatic systems of older adults are more susceptible to the effects of pharmacological agents and less tolerant of their side-effects.

Normal laboratory values are derived from analyses of what are considered to be disease-free healthy populations (Huber et al., 2006). Normal ranges are based on plus or minus 2 standard deviations (SD) from the mean value. The populations analyzed are heterogeneous for age and assume that aging individuals are the same as young adults. In many cases this may be true, but adequate reference ranges for laboratory testing in the elderly are generally lacking (Brigden & Heathcote, 2000). Specific differences may be caused by the loss of certain biological reserves in those aged over 75, ironically the fastest-growing segment of the elderly population. There are some predictable changes in laboratory values that occur with age which can be attributed to the normal aging process and not to disease states. Although there is significant variation from one individual to the next, these changes begin in the fourth decade of life and continue in a linear fashion into old age. With these exceptions, it is important to understand that most laboratory values in the elderly are similar to those of the healthy young (Coresh et al., 2003).

In blood chemistry, the level of serum alkaline phosphatase, an enzyme found in bone and liver, increases with age. In men, it increases by up to 20% between the ages of 40 and 80. In women, slightly greater increases (0–37%) are seen. Serum albumin, traditionally a marker of nutrition, decreases slightly with age, despite adequate nutrition. Levels of serum prealbumin, a marker of current nutrition, should be equivalent to those of healthy young individuals (16–35 mg/dl) (Kubota et al., 2012). In healthy individuals, serum magnesium decreases by about 15% between the ages of 30 and 80. Uric acid, a metabolic product of purine metabolism, increases slightly in normal aging individuals without disease. Other chemistries, such as serum electrolytes, serum bilirubin, liver enzymes and total proteins, remain unchanged with age (Feld & Schwabbauer, 2000).

Lipid values also change with aging. In both women and men, total cholesterol levels increase by 30–40 mg/dl from 30 to 80 years of age. High-density lipoprotein (HDL), which is thought to be protective against atherosclerosis, increases by approximately 30% in men, but falls by up to 30% in women after menopause. This is attributed to the fact that, during the reproductive years, women have significantly higher levels of HDL than men because of the positive effect of estrogen on lipid production in the liver. Triglycerides, or blood fats, increase by 30–50% in both men and women from age 30 to 80. Serum levels of low-density lipoprotein (LDL), cholesterol molecules associated with accelerated atherosclerosis, are unchanged by age (Kubota et al., 2012).

Fasting blood glucose levels increase by 2 mg/dl for each decade over the age of 30. Glucose metabolism, as measured by postprandial glucose levels, increases by up to 10 mg/dl for each decade over the age of 30. The risk of developing diabetes mellitus in individuals with insulin resistance caused by either genetic predilection or obesity increases with age.

Thyroid function is measured by serum triiodothyronine (T3) and thyroxine (T4) levels as well as levels of the pituitary hormone thyroid-stimulating hormone (TSH). Both TSH and T3 levels may decrease slightly with age; a marked or progressive development of abnormal values indicates a disease state in the elderly. Serum T4 levels remain unchanged in healthy elderly individuals.

Levels of serum creatinine do not change with age but less creatinine is produced and serum creatinine clearance, a measurement of renal function, declines by approximately 10 ml/min/1.73 m^2 for each decade over the age of 40. This phenomenon is explained by an age-related reduction in muscle mass in older individuals and by a decrease in protein byproducts like creatinine being delivered to the kidney. It is exacerbated by the age-related loss of renal tissue, parenchyma, that begins in the fifth decade (Coresh et al., 2003). Creatinine clearance can be calculated using a simple formula including the patient's serum creatinine value, gender, weight and age. Therefore, a normal serum creatinine level does not necessarily indicate normal renal function. Like creatinine, many drugs require renal clearance during metabolism; the age-related decline in renal function therefore necessitates adjustments in the dosing of these drugs. If too large a dose of medication is delivered to an even minimally impaired kidney, incomplete clearance occurs leaving potentially toxic metabolites in the kidney tissue (parenchyma). This can build up and further damage the kidney in a process called interstitial nephritis. This can be reversed with immediate withdrawal of the drug but, occasionally, permanent impairment can occur. The most common drugs responsible for this phenomenon are nonsteroidal anti-inflammatory agents and antibiotics (Mantha, 2005).

Hematological assessment of the elderly is achieved by white blood cell, hemoglobin, hematocrit, platelet and red blood cell counts. White blood cell counts may decrease slightly in the healthy older individual, whereas it is thought that hemoglobin, hematocrit and platelet counts should remain constant with aging.

However, anemia is quite common in the elderly. It can be associated with many chronic diseases of aging such as arthritis, diabetes, renal impairment and bone marrow suppression by drugs and environmental chemicals. The World Health Organization has established norms of 13 g/dl or more for men and 12 g/dl for women for hemoglobin levels. In the elderly, some experts accept slightly lower values as normal (11.5 g/dl in men and 11 g/dl in women); if they remain constant, these values should not trigger extensive investigations (Thein et al., 2009).

Serum vitamin B$_{12}$ levels may decrease with age (Park & Johnson, 2006). Normal values in young adults are >190 pg/ml; levels of >150 pg/ml are acceptable in older adults in the absence of macrocytic changes to the red blood cells. Levels of vitamins C, E, D and B$_6$ also show a slight age-related decrease.

The erythrocyte sedimentation rate (ESR) increases with age by approximately 22 mm/h from a norm of 20–25 mm/h to acceptable rates of up to 40 mm/h (in men) and 45 mm/h (in women) in the elderly. Levels greater than these are indicative of inflammatory or neoplastic conditions, which commonly occur in the geriatric population. Isolated increases in ESR are associated with increases in all causes of mortality. By definition, those with elevated ESRs have a higher death rate than age-matched individuals, regardless of the cause of death. Increases in ESR mandate workup for disease states. Normal values for serum C-reactive protein (CRP), another measurement of overall inflammation, remain unchanged, regardless of age.

The assessment of nutritional status has been studied extensively. In normal healthy ambulatory elderly individuals, serum protein and albumin levels are relatively unchanged with age. Nutritional status is assessed by the measurement of serum prealbumin and albumin levels, and indirectly by the numbers of white blood cells known as lymphocytes. Nutritional deficiencies, however, are common in the elderly and are caused by a multitude of factors including poor intake, a reduction in the acuity of taste, loss of appetite, depression, malabsorption from intestinal surgery or disease, and interactions with medications. It is important to consider nutritional status when caring for the elderly to maximize the potential for rehabilitation.

INDICATIONS FOR LABORATORY ASSESSMENT

When is laboratory assessment necessary? Routine laboratory testing should be determined by a patient's presentation, history and current use of medication. For example, a patient who must use diuretics requires a regular assessment of serum electrolytes, especially serum potassium. Simple alterations in diet, such as increased sodium levels, may cause potassium wasting in the elderly kidney and precipitate hypokalemia, a cause of muscle weakness. A patient on anticholesterol medication such as the 3-hydroxy-3-methylglutaryl coenzyme A (HMG-CoA) reductase inhibitors requires initial assessment of liver functions, whereas a patient receiving ticlopidine (Ticlid), a platelet inhibitor used in patients with transient ischemic attacks and stroke, requires a regular blood count.

Laboratory assessment is especially important in the evaluation of a patient who presents with new physical findings. The workup for dementia and delirium is particularly vital. Neurosyphilis, vitamin B_{12} and folic acid deficiencies, and acute infection can be detected by laboratory assessment and are precipitants of acute delirium and dementia. Radiological findings and other physical diagnostic tests such as lumbar puncture can quickly identify reversible causes for a patient's neurological changes.

Lethargy and altered levels of consciousness may also be presenting symptoms in a patient with abnormal laboratory values. Hypoglycemia, hyponatremia, acidosis, hypoxia and hypocalcemia are direct causes of central nervous system depression and can be identified through commonly used laboratory tests. Neuromuscular irritability, tetany and muscle spasms may present in severe cases of hypocalcemia.

A patient who presents with peripheral, sensory or motor deficits may be suffering from a disease that is identifiable by analysis of blood chemistries. Peripheral neuropathies are caused by diabetes mellitus (hyperglycemia), heavy metal ingestion and medication toxicities, Vitamin B_{12} deficiency and biochemical assessment can identify these problems.

Deteriorating renal function as indicated by an elevation in the levels of serum creatinine and blood urea nitrogen may place the patient at a greater risk of medication toxicity. Frequent assessment of drug serum levels and adjustment of doses is the hallmark of safe continued usage in the face of renal insufficiency. Abnormalities in thyroid hormone levels may present differently in the elderly than in younger adults. Cardiac arrhythmias and weight loss may be the presenting symptoms of hyperthyroidism in the elderly, whereas hypothyroidism may present more insidiously,

with the typical symptoms of myxedema occurring less frequently. Alterations in mental status, lethargy, weight gain and thought disorders may be caused by hypothyroidism in the elderly.

Table 13.1 indicates the normal values of routinely used laboratory assessments and Box 13.1 shows the possible age-related effects on these values. Significant deviations from these values may indicate the presence of disease or deterioration of organ systems.

Table 13.1 **Selected normal laboratory values**	
	Normal Values
Serum electrolytes	
Carbon dioxide	23–31 mEq/l
Chloride	98–107 mEq/l
Potassium	3.5–5.1 mEq/l
Sodium	136–145 mEq/l
Metabolic indicators	
Calcium	8.6–10.0 mg/dl
Cholesterol	240 mg/dl
Creatinine	0.8–1.5 mg/dl
Free thyroxine (T_4)	0.8–2.3 mg/dl
Glucose, fasting	80–110 mg/dl
Glucose, 2 h postprandial	80–110 mg/dl
Protein	
Total	6.0–8.0 g/dl
Albumin	3.5–5.5 g/dl
Globulin	2.0–3.5 g/dl

Box 13.1 *Effect of aging on laboratory values*

INCREASED	UNCHANGED	DECREASED
Serum copper	Hemoglobin	Creatinine clearance
Serum ferritin	RBC count	Serum calcium
Serum immunoreactive	WBC count	Serum iron parathormone
Parathormone	Serum vitamin A	Serum phosphorus
Serum cholesterol	Leukocyte zinc	Serum thiamine
Serum uric acid	Serum pantothenate	Serum zinc
Serum fibrinogen	Serum riboflavin	Serum 1,25-dihydroxycholecalciferol
Serum norepinephrine	Serum carotene	Serum vitamin B_6
Serum triglycerides	Erythrocyte sedimentation rate	Serum vitamin B_{12}
Serum glucose	Serum IgM, IgG, IgA	Plasma vitamin C
Prostate-specific antigen (PSA)	Blood urea nitrogen	Serum selenium
	Serum creatinine[a]	Plasma gammatocopherol (vitamin E)
	Serum alkaline phosphatase	Triiodothyronine (T_3)
		Serum testosterone
		Dihydroepiandrosterone

From Beers MH, Berkow R (eds) 2000 The Merck Manual of Geriatrics, p. 1384. © 2000 by Merck & Co, Inc., Whitehouse Station, NJ, with permission.

[a]Serum creatinine may be normal even though creatinine clearance is decreased with aging as a result of an age-related decrease in creatinine production.

CONCLUSION

In summary, the clinical use of laboratory testing for the assessment of geriatric patients is a useful tool when combined with physical assessment. Laboratory values, although traditionally derived from middle-aged populations, can be applied to elderly populations, with rare exceptions. Abnormal laboratory values should not be attributed to age alone but be investigated for the presence of disease states. Perioperative laboratory assessment should be guided by history and exam as well as medication use, not age alone. Reductions in physiological reserves account for the earlier presence of abnormal values in asymptomatic disease states in the elderly.

REFERENCES

Brigden M, Heathcote J 2000 Problems in interpreting laboratory tests. What do unexpected results mean? Postgrad Med 107(7):145–162

Coresh J, Astor BC, Greene T et al 2003 Prevalence of chronic kidney disease and decreased kidney function in the adult US population: Third National Health and Nutrition Examination Survey. Am J Kidney Dis 41(1):1

Feld R, Schwabbauer M 2000 Clinical Chemistry in the Physician's Office. Peer Review. University of Iowa College of Medicine, Iowa City, IA

Huber K, Mostafaie N, Strangl G et al 2006 Clinical chemistry reference values for 75-year-old apparently healthy persons. Clin Chem Lab Med 44:1355–1360

Kubota K, Kadomura T, Ohta K et al 2012 Analyses of laboratory data and establishment of reference values and intervals for healthy elderly people. J Health Aging 16(4):412

Mantha S 2005 The usefulness of preoperative laboratory screening. J Clin Anaesthesiol 17(1):51–57

Park S, Johnson M 2006 What is an adequate dose of vitamin B12 in older people with poor vitamin B12 status? Nutr Rev 64:373–378

Thein M, Ershler WB, Artz AS et al 2009 Diminished quality of life and physical function in community-dwelling elderly with anemia. Medicine (Baltimore) 88(2):107

Chapter 14

Imaging

CLIVE PERRY

INTRODUCTION

This chapter will review the current position of medical imaging, the general principles of imaging and the way it can be used to solve clinical questions.

With the discovery of X-rays by Wilhelm Conrad Roentgen in 1895, the age of medical imaging was born. With the advent of the technological age, new discoveries have added other modalities, providing unique information regarding anatomy, pathology and the function of living organs. The relatively low cost and power of modern computers has allowed very large image data sets to be generated quickly. New software allows multiple display formats including three-dimensional, multiplanar, real-time, fused and functional images. This has enabled imaging to remain a relevant and essential part of modern clinical decision-making, resulting in increased efficiencies and better outcomes. The digital nature of modern images allows the efficient storage and dissemination of information to the referring physician and radiologist via local networks and the internet.

BASIC PRINCIPLES

All medical imaging has the same basic requirements. The first is an energy source that interacts benignly with biological tissue and is capable of representing the structure and/or function of this tissue. The second is an ability to capture and store the energy or data that result from this interaction and display them as an image. As an example, let us look at the photograph. The energy source, light, is reflected from the subject and captured on photographic film or digitally to produce an image, the photograph (Fig. 14.1).

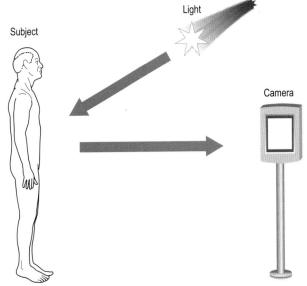

Figure 14.1 Basic principles of imaging. Light is reflected from the subject and the energy (light) enters the camera where it is captured by the photographic film to produce an image – the photograph.

IMAGING MODALITIES

X-RAYS

X-rays, like light, are part of the electromagnetic spectrum but have a higher energy and shorter wavelength, which allows them to pass into and through the human body (Fig. 14.2). Different tissue types absorb different amounts of the X-ray beam: bone, a very dense tissue, absorbs most of the beam whereas lungs, consisting mainly of air, do not. As a result, varying amounts of

Chest stand

Patient

X-ray tube

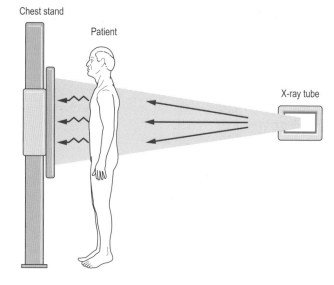

Figure 14.2 X-rays (radiography). X-rays are produced by the X-ray tube. X-rays have a higher energy than light and pass through the patient; the X-ray film contained within the chest stand captures them. The X-rays are absorbed to a different degree by different tissues as explained in the text. The end result is a chest radiograph, as seen in Figure 14.3A. Note the X-rays enter the patient posteriorly and exit anteriorly. This orientation produces the best image and is a posterior to anterior radiograph, better known as PA, chest X-ray (CXR).

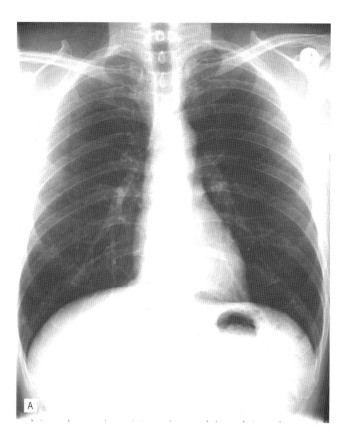

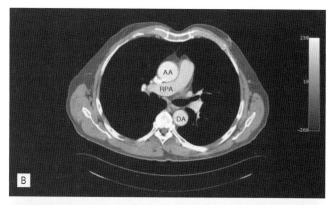

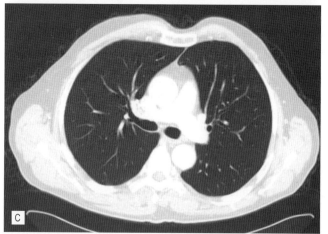

Figure 14.3 (A–C) Normal chest images. (A) Chest radiograph. The radiograph provides a quick and inexpensive overall view of the chest. The air-containing lungs are black because of little attenuation of the X-ray beam. The central pulmonary arteries and heart are well defined by the surrounding lung. However, the chest wall soft-tissue structures are poorly seen because of similar attenuation of the beam, i.e. lack of contrast. The denser bones, e.g. clavicles and ribs, are white. The heart overlies and obscures the thoracic spine in this view. **(B** and **C)** Axial CT chest. In **(B)** the viewing settings are optimized (i.e. window and level) to show the soft tissues to best effect. AA, ascending thoracic aorta; DA, descending thoracic aorta; RPA, right pulmonary artery. **(C)** Same patient and same level. However, by changing the viewing settings the lungs are now seen in exquisite detail. Note the improved anatomical depiction and improved tissue contrast in the CT images. CT solves the problem of overlapping structures obscuring the anatomy. The mediastinal and chest wall structures are now well seen.

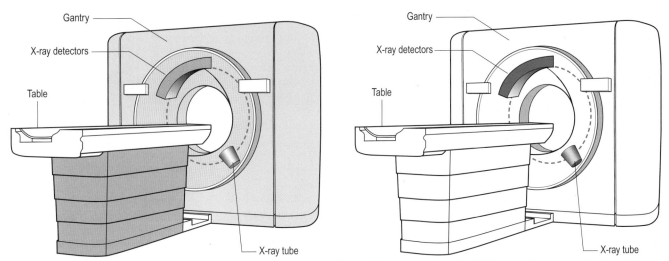

Figure 14.4 (A, B) CT scanner. (A) The table on which the patient lies and the gantry through which the patient passes during a CT scan. **(B)** The position of the X-ray tube and detectors within the gantry. The X-ray tube and detectors rotate around the patient. The X-rays pass through the patient and are collected by the detectors, which lie opposite. The detectors produce an electrical signal, which is fed into a computer to construct a cross-sectional image.

X-rays exit the body, reflecting the different tissue types that the X-ray beam has passed through. As Roentgen discovered, the X-rays will stimulate a fluorescent screen to produce light, which can be captured on specialized photographic film to produce an image of the body part. This is referred to as a radiograph or X-ray. Obtaining a good radiograph has many similarities to obtaining a good photograph. For example, if the subject moves, the photographic image will be blurred; if not enough light is available, the image will be dark. Similarly, if the radiograph is not exposed correctly, the image will be limited. This is particularly a problem with large patients. These issues are the same for all imaging studies.

Radiographs are relatively inexpensive, quick to perform and widely available. As a result, they continue to make up the bulk of imaging studies. Similar to the camera, radiographic images have moved away from film and are now mainly of digital format.

Image quality depends on the ability to discriminate between two adjacent objects, also called spatial resolution; with X-rays, this is very good. However, the ability to see a structure also depends on the difference in the attenuation of the X-ray beam between different tissues, i.e. tissue contrast. For example, bone, which attenuates most of the beam, is well outlined against adjacent soft tissue such as muscle, which does not attenuate the beam as much. Similarly, the lung parenchyma and cardiac silhouette is differentiated well from the surrounding air (Fig. 14.3A). However, differentiating soft tissue is a problem because of a similar attenuation of the beam; this means that the tissues all have a similar gray appearance, i.e. little or no contrast (Fig. 14.3A). This can be overcome to some extent by using contrast agents. Oral contrast with a barium solution, e.g. a barium enema, is used for evaluating the gastrointestinal tract. Intravenous and intra-arterial iodinated contrast agents for evaluating blood vessels and organs are used in arteriography and intravenous urograms.

Fluoroscopy uses continuous X-rays (in reduced doses) to allow real-time images. A device known as an image intensifier allows you to view the images on a TV screen. Although the radiation dose used to produce a particular image is much reduced compared with a standard radiograph, care must be taken not to prolong the procedure and cause unwanted exposure of the patient to high doses. Types of procedures using this technique include barium studies, arteriograms and internal fixation of fractures in the operating room.

Standard X-ray images produce a two-dimensional display of a three-dimensional structure; this means that there is an overlap of structures resulting in part of the anatomy being hidden. For example, on a frontal chest radiograph, the overlying heart obscures the spine (compare the chest radiograph in Fig. 14.3A with the chest CT in Fig. 14.3B and C). This can be alleviated somewhat by obtaining additional views such as a lateral view. However, the problem of overlapping structures has been overcome following the introduction of computerized axial tomography (CAT or CT scan) in the 1970s, made possible with the advent of the computer and the ability to capture and store data digitally.

COMPUTED TOMOGRAPHY

A computed tomography (CT) scan also utilizes X-rays to produce images but, instead of being stationary, the X-ray tube rotates around the patient (Fig. 14.4). Specialized detectors collect the emerging X-rays and produce an electrical signal that is fed into a computer; this information is then used to construct a cross-sectional image (Fig. 14.3B). The initial CT technique took several hours to acquire the data and several days for the computer to reconstruct the images. Modern scanners are very fast and can image the entire abdomen and pelvis in seconds. Multislice CT scanners are now replacing single-slice technology and, as the name indicates, multiple slices can be produced per rotation of the X-ray tube. This has the advantage of covering more territory and shortening scan times. This technology can produce very thin axial slices allowing the production of isotropic data sets, i.e. it has the ability to acquire a volume of data that can be viewed in any plane without distorting the image. Until this innovation, CT scans were generally limited to an axial display;

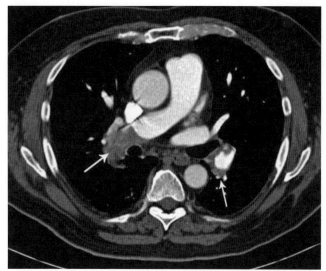

Figure 14.5 Acute chest pain. CT is now being used increasingly for evaluating acute chest pain. Here is an example of an acute pulmonary embolus. This 72-year-old male presented with bilateral leg pain and swelling, chest pain and shortness of breath. The lower limb ultrasound (not shown) demonstrated bilateral deep vein thrombosis. The CT (above) was obtained following intravenous contrast. Note that the contrast in the right pulmonary artery shows an abrupt cut-off, and low attenuating gray material (representing the embolus) is seen in the proximal right lower lobe pulmonary artery (right arrow). Compare with normal chest CT in Figure 14.3. This represents a large pulmonary embolus. A smaller embolus is seen on the left side (left arrow). CT plays a major role in evaluating chest disease. The scan takes a few seconds, making it an ideal modality for emergency situations such as this.

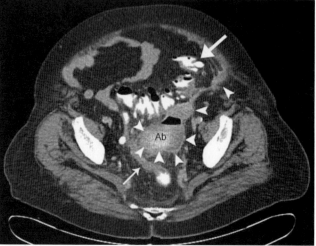

Figure 14.6 Abdominal pain. This can be difficult to evaluate on clinical grounds alone in the elderly as illustrated in this case of diverticulitis and diverticular abscess. This is a CT scan of the pelvis of a 70-year-old woman with minimal abdominal pain. Acute intra-abdominal processes can be a diagnostic dilemma in the elderly as symptoms and signs may be minimal or absent, as in this case. CT is very helpful in this situation. The CT demonstrates diverticular disease involving the barium-filled sigmoid colon (large arrow). The arrowheads show the track of the perforation leading to the abscess in the pelvis (Ab). The rectum is seen to the right and posterior to the abscess (small arrow). The abscess was drained surgically along with resection of the sigmoid colon. Note how the intra-abdominal and subcutaneous fat acts as a natural contrast, allowing separation and good delineation of adjacent soft tissues; this is one of the few advantages of being overweight.

now images can routinely be displayed in any plane giving multiplanar (MPR) and three-dimensional reconstruction capabilities. This allows more information to be gleaned from the study and improves diagnostic accuracy (Figs 14.5 and 14.6), particularly with complicated pathology such as complex fractures (see Fig. 14.7).

CT scanning is used to image all parts of the body. The speed of the examination makes this a particularly attractive investigation for older patients who may find it difficult to lie still for long periods of time. It also makes it the preferred method for examining very sick and injured patients when time is of the essence (Figs 14.5 and 14.6). The relatively large size of the gantry (the part of the machine that the patient passes through) (see Fig. 14.4) has almost eliminated the problem of claustrophobia. As with standard X-rays, CT demonstrates superb lung and bone detail (Figs 14.3C and 14.7). Fluids, such as ascites and cystic structures are well defined as are calcifications and acute and subacute hemorrhage (see Fig. 14.12A–C). Fat, particularly in the abdomen, is a natural contrast agent and is useful in defining adjacent organs and inflammation (see Fig. 14.6); however, CT still requires additional contrast agents to improve visualization. Oral contrast, usually in the form of dilute barium, aids visualization of the bowel (see Fig. 14.6), and intravenous contrast is used to optimize the evaluation of veins and arteries and the vascularity of organs. The addition of intravenous contrast material also allows further uses of CT, for example pulmonary embolism is now routinely evaluated by this method (see Fig. 14.5). The speed of the new multislice scanners allows the beating heart and

coronary arteries to be evaluated. The ability of CT to demonstrate an artery is now as good as the more invasive procedure of diagnostic arteriography and, in complex anatomical situations, may be better. As a result, many arterial lesions, such as aneurysm, dissection and stenosis, are diagnosed and evaluated with CT (Fig. 14.8), and the more invasive diagnostic arteriogram is now mainly used for therapy (e.g. treatment of a narrowed artery and aortic aneurysm with specially designed stents, which can be placed percutaneously via adjacent non-diseased vessels).

ULTRASOUND

Ultrasound has been used since the 1950s to produce medical images using sound waves. The frequency of the wave used to produce the images is in the range of 1–20 MHz. It is called ultrasound because this frequency is above the human audible range of 2–20 kHz. The probe or transducer used during the examination is responsible for both producing the sound and collecting the sound waves reflected from the patient's organs and tissues. The received sound is converted to an electrical signal and, from this, an image is developed by a computer and displayed in real time on a TV monitor. In addition, by using the Doppler effect, the returning sound waves can be used to evaluate blood flow. It is excellent for imaging soft tissues and has a long list of uses, including imaging of the major abdominal and pelvic organs. Superficial structures are particularly well seen, for example, the thyroid, superficial tendons, muscles, veins and arteries (see Figs 14.14C and 14.15E and F).

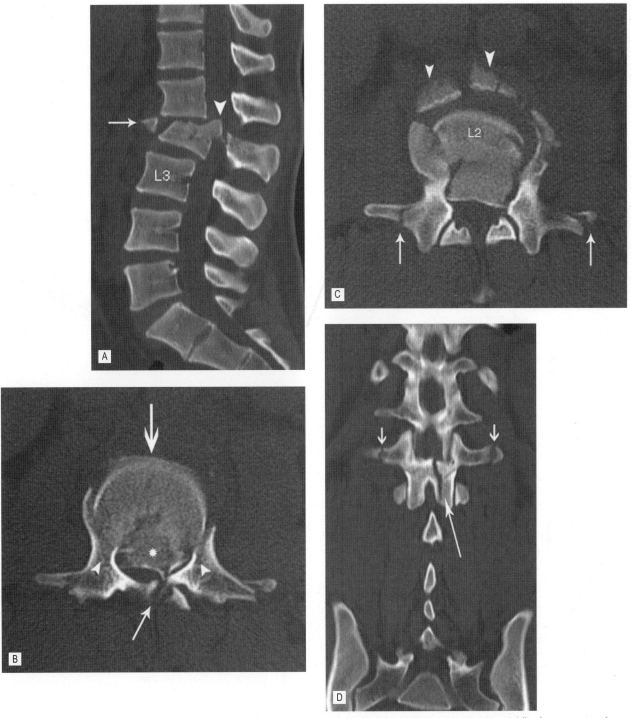

Figure 14.7 (A–D) Severe burst fracture with dislocation at L2. CT with multiplanar (MPR) reconstruction vividly demonstrates the components of this complex fracture, which resulted following a motor vehicle accident. **(A)** The sagittal MPR shows posterior displacement of the body of L2. There is a large, central, superior retro-pulsed fragment. An anterior and superior fragment has been avulsed. **(B)** The axial image at the level of the retro-pulsed fragment (*) demonstrates severe narrowing of the spinal canal. The vertebral body has been driven between the pedicles with fractures at the junction of the vertebral body and pedicles. **(C)** Just caudal to **(B)** shows the avulsed anterior fragments (arrow head) and fractures through both transverse processes (arrows). **(D)** There is widening of the interpedicle distance and a sagittal fracture through the lamina best seen on this coronal MPR. The fracture is unstable with disruption of all three columns. The patient had a significant neurological deficit and was treated with spinal decompression and instrument fixation.

The combination of real-time, multiplanar and vascular imaging makes ultrasound an excellent tool for imaging the heart. The lack of ionizing radiation and substantiated adverse effects have made it a popular imaging technique in all age groups. The relatively inexpensive equipment costs and portability have added to this. It is an excellent tool for guiding percutaneous needle biopsies, especially superficially located lesions such as breast and thyroid masses. There are some negative aspects of ultrasound. Unlike all other imaging

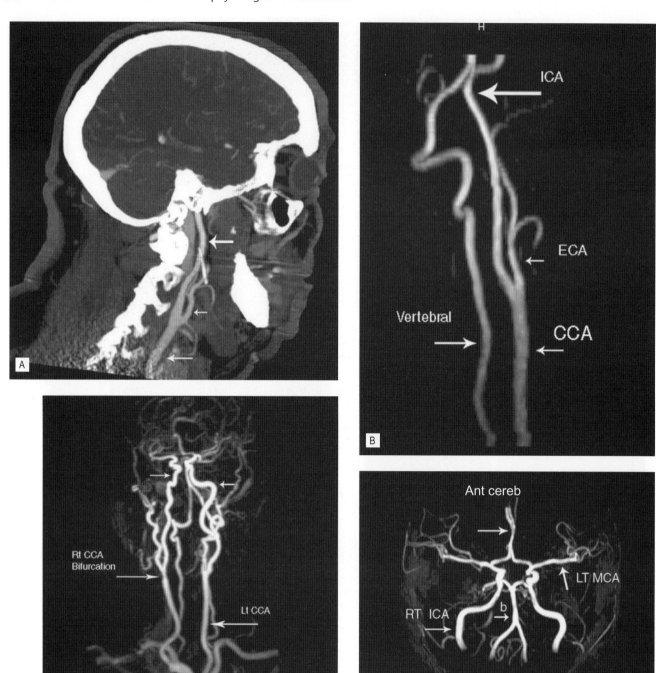

Figure 14.8 (A–D) Non-invasive vascular imaging. Examples of noninvasive imaging of the carotid arteries and intracranial arteries using CT (CTA) and MR (MRA). **(A)** CTA following intravenous contrast shows a sagittal MPR image of the common carotid artery (CCA; lower arrow) and the cervical portion of the internal carotid artery (ICA; upper arrow) and external carotid artery (ECA; middle arrow). **(B)** 2D time of flight MR image of the cervical carotid artery and its branches. This sequence does not use intravenous contrast. **(C)** 3D MRA following intravenous gadolinium allows a larger area to be evaluated. Here the aortic arch (Arch) and the three great vessels and both carotid arteries are seen. The cervical and intracranial (upper arrows) portions of both ICAs are seen. Note the narrowing at the right CCA bifurcation. **(D)** 3D time of flight MRA showing the intracranial vessels and central circle of Willis. Ant cereb, anterior cerebral arteries; b, basilar artery; LT MCA, left middle cerebral artery; RT ICA, right internal carotid artery. Atherosclerosis is a common problem in the elderly and can cause severe narrowing of the carotid artery particularly at the CCA bifurcation. This is a common cause of stroke and is a treatable condition. In the past this was diagnosed with angiography, an invasive procedure. The cervical portions of the carotid arteries are usually evaluated with ultrasound first. However, both CT and MR allow evaluation of the whole carotid system including the aortic arch and intracranial vessels. Noninvasive imaging of other vessels in the body is now routine, and the individual circumstances will determine which of the three modalities is used.

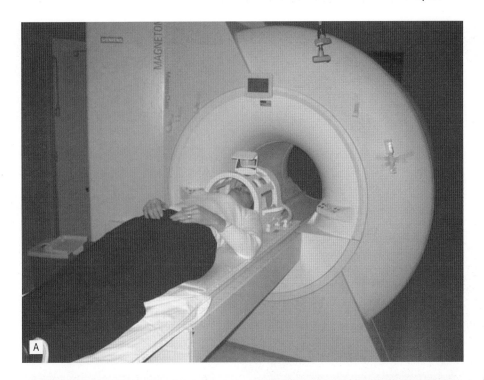

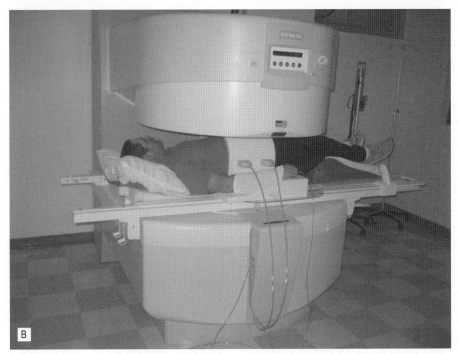

Figure 14.9 (A, B) Examples of MRI machines. (A) This patient is getting ready for a head scan in this closed, high field strength MRI scanner. The cage around the head contains the radiofrequency (RF) coils. Note that the bore of the magnet is fairly long and not that wide. This can be a problem for large patients and patients who suffer from claustrophobia. Elderly patients may become disorientated in this enclosure. New wide-bore MRI scanners help alleviate this problem. **(B)** Example of an open MR scanner. These scanners may not be capable of all the imaging sequences and can take longer to acquire the images but image quality is good and they are usually well tolerated by patients who suffer from claustrophobia. The large belt around the patients abdomen is an RF coil.

methods, it relies heavily on the expertise of the sonographer/sonologist to produce diagnostic images. Sound is reflected by bone and air, limiting evaluation of the chest, abdominal organs, which may be hidden by overlying gas-filled loops of bowel, and the brain, which is surrounded by the protective cranium.

MAGNETIC RESONANCE IMAGING

The phenomenon of magnetic resonance was discovered in the 1930s and initially used to determine the composition of chemical compounds. In the 1970s, it was realized that the same techniques could be used in medical imaging

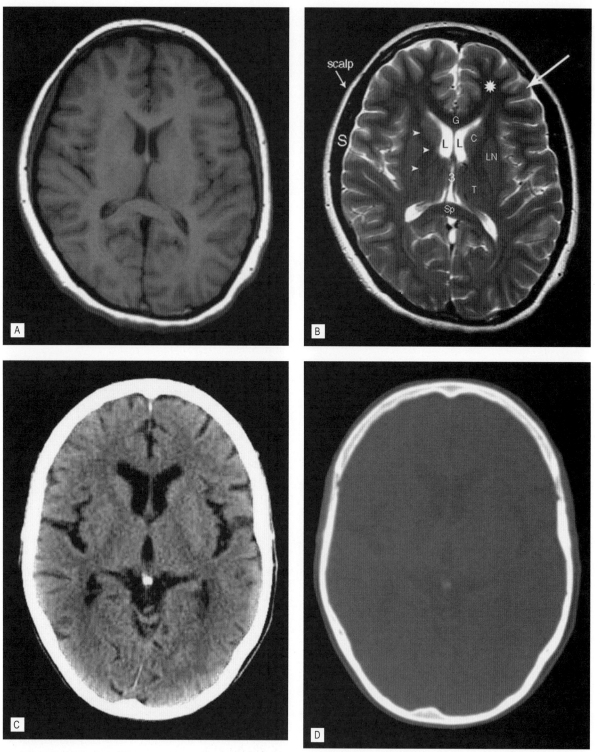

Figure 14.10 (A–D) Normal MRI and CT brain. (A) T1-weighted spin echo (SE) image (T1WI) and **(B)** T2-weighted turbo spin echo (TSE) image (T2WI). **(C)** CT optimized for viewing soft tissues. **(D)** Same CT optimized for viewing bone. All obtained without intravenous contrast at the level of the lateral (L) and third (3) ventricle. The T1 and T2 images are the basic sequences used in MRI, but there are several other sequences that are used which display certain pathologies to greater effect. CT, however, has only one sequence but by altering the level of attenuated tissues displayed the bony skull is seen to better effect. This is demonstrated in **(D)**, which shows the same CT scan with the view settings (level and window) optimized to demonstrate bone. Note the improved tissue contrast with MR allowing improved definition of the gray matter in the cerebral cortex (arrow) versus the white matter in the adjacent left frontal lobe (*). CSF in the third, lateral ventricles and sulci on the T2WI is bright and dark on the T1WI and CT. Note the skull is bright on CT, indicating increased attenuation of the X-ray beam. Calcium in the pineal gland is also bright (image **C**). The bright area surrounding the brain on the two MRI images, however, is subcutaneous fat in the scalp. Cortical bone does not produce a signal and the signal void (black area) between the scalp and the brain is the skull (S). G, genu and Sp, splenium of the corpus callosum; C, head of the caudate nucleus; L, lentiform nucleus; T, thalamus; arrow heads, internal capsule.

and, by the 1980s, magnetic resonance imaging (MRI) units were in clinical use. Magnetic resonance uses radio waves and a strong magnetic field to produce the image; as with ultrasound, it does not use ionizing radiation. The technique relies on the fact that some atomic nuclei have magnetic properties that act like microscopic magnets when placed in a strong magnetic field. The human body has an abundance of these in the form of the hydrogen ion that makes up water. These align with the direction of the bore of the magnet when the patient lies in the MRI machine (Fig. 14.9). If these nuclei are stimulated by a radio wave at a specific frequency, known as the resonant frequency, they gain energy and move into a transverse plane, perpendicular to the main magnetic field. This results in a radio wave being emitted by the rotated nuclei, which allows their position to be recognized. The radio waves are emitted and received by a device called a radio frequency (RF) coil, analogous to the ultrasound transducer that transmits and receives the sound waves. The coils are placed close to the patient. The head coil, used to image the brain, looks like a cylindrical cage that surrounds the patient's head (Fig. 14.9A). As with ultrasound, the received signal, in this case radio waves, creates an electrical signal, which is fed into a computer to produce an image (Fig. 14.10A, B).

The high tissue contrast (i.e. the difference in signal between tissue types) afforded by magnetic resonance is responsible for the excellent depiction of soft tissue anatomy. There are two main types of pulse sequences used in MRI, which produce images of the same area but with a different contrast; these are known as T1- and T2-weighted images. This is achieved by varying the time when the RF pulse is emitted and when the returning RF wave is received. Fluid gives a low signal on T1 images and a bright signal on T2 images, whereas fat gives a high signal on T1 and T2 images (when using the faster T2 turbo spin echo [TSE] sequence). Unique to MRI is the ability to selectively remove or null particular tissues from the image. For example, fat, which is bright and may obscure pathology, can be removed by a technique called fat saturation or 'fat sat' for short (see Figs 14.13E and 14.15D). This is an extremely useful technique, which also makes it possible to confirm that a structure is fat-containing (e.g. a lipoma) by obtaining images before and after fat saturation.

MRI is also routinely used to evaluate blood vessels (see Fig. 14.8). These images can be generated without the use of intravenous contrast agents although contrast-enhanced studies are also used to acquire additional information. The latest and faster MRI sequences allow routine evaluation of the beating heart and are a valuable tool in complementing cardiac ultrasound and cardiac nuclear medicine studies. Magnetic resonance spectroscopy has the ability to evaluate the chemical composition of tissue and has shown promise in the diagnosis of cerebral tumors. MRI is also used to evaluate brain function, the so-called functional MRI.

NUCLEAR MEDICINE

There are some fundamental differences between nuclear medicine and the other imaging modalities. Whereas the other modalities rely mainly on a change in anatomy caused by a pathological process, nuclear medicine is able to show images of changes in function or physiology as a result of pathological change. The energy source in nuclear medicine is a radionuclide that emits ionizing radiation in the form of gamma rays, which come from the same part of the electromagnetic spectrum as X-rays. The radionuclides are tagged with a biological compound that is used by a living tissue; this combination is called a radiopharmaceutical. Unlike the other forms of imaging, the radiopharmaceutical is placed inside the patient, usually by an intravenous route, and taken up by the organ/cells or pathological process of interest. During decay of the radionuclide, gamma rays are emitted and pass out of the body and are collected by a gamma camera to produce an image. The most common radionuclide used is technetium 99 m, and a common study is a bone scan in which the technetium is labeled with diphosphonate (Tc-MDP) (Fig. 14.11A, B). This is quickly taken up by bone, particularly in areas of bone remodeling, for example fracture repair and most bone metastases. The camera is positioned over the area of interest and images obtained in a two-dimensional plane (the planar image) (Fig. 14.11C). As in CT, images can also be obtained by rotating the camera slowly around the patient to obtain a cross-section or tomogram. This is referred to as SPECT (single photon emission tomography), and is used in, for example, SPECT bone imaging and thallium SPECT imaging of the heart.

The ability of nuclear medicine to show cellular function can be demonstrated by positron emission tomography or PET. In this technique, the radionuclide fluorine-18, in combination with glucose [18-flourodeoxyglucose (FDG)], is readily incorporated into cells allowing the utilization of glucose to be imaged; this is proving to be an extremely useful way to diagnose and monitor disease. For instance, it has been shown that FDG accumulates in most tumors to a greater amount than in normal tissue, allowing recognition of the tumor (Fig. 14.11D). It is used to diagnose, stage and evaluate the treatment response of several tumors. This list is growing and includes lung, colon, breast, head and neck cancer, lymphoma and melanoma. Positron-emitting radionuclides also produce gamma rays but require a specially designed camera for imaging. With small lesions or complex anatomical areas, PET may not provide enough anatomical detail to accurately depict the exact site of the lesion. By performing a CT scan at the same time as the PET scan (PET/CT) and fusing the images, anatomical localization of the lesion is improved, and the two modalities used together have proved to be complementary, resulting in a more accurate diagnosis.

SCREENING, INTRAVENOUS CONTRAST AND SAFETY

SCREENING

Using imaging to screen for disease, particularly cancer, has been a desirable goal for many years; however, the development of an effective screening test has been elusive. Screening mammography is an exception. A review of eight randomized controlled trials demonstrated a 20% reduction in breast cancer mortality when women aged 40–74 years of age were invited for screening; this represents a significant reduction in mortality (Smith et al., 2004). The National Cancer Institute, the American Cancer Society and the American College of Radiology recommend annual mammography screening for all women

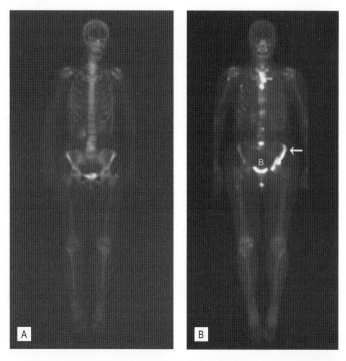

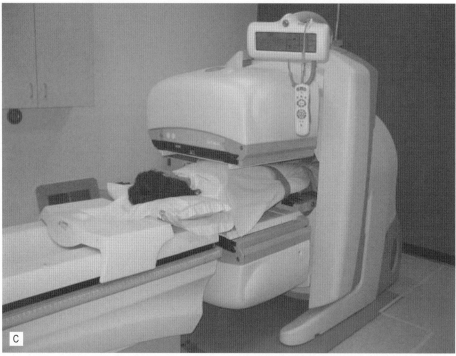

Figure 14.11 (A–C) Nuclear medicine whole body bone scan. (A) Normal bone scan. This anterior view was obtained 4 h after the intravenous injection of the radionuclide – Tc99^m MDP. The images show expected bone uptake in a 60-year-old female. The scan is routinely delayed to allow clearance of the radionuclide from the blood and soft tissues which would interfere with bone visualization. Note the symmetry of uptake. Increased activity at the shoulder and iliac wings in the pelvis is normal. Activity in the lower neck is due to normal thyroid cartilage activity. The tracer is cleared through the kidneys hence expected increased activity in the bladder and kidneys. Increased activity at L4/5 is due to degenerative disk and facet joint disease. **(B) Bone metastases.** Anterior view of a 65-year-old woman with metastatic bone disease from breast carcinoma. Increased activity is seen in the spine, left ilium (white arrow), sternum, the proximal right humerus and femur. The bone scan is used to diagnose the presence, extent and response of disease to treatment. **(C) Nuclear medicine gamma camera.** There are two gamma cameras (dual head), one above and one below the patient. This allows anterior and posterior images to be collected simultaneously, speeding up the examination. The cameras can be rotated around the patient to allow oblique and lateral projections.

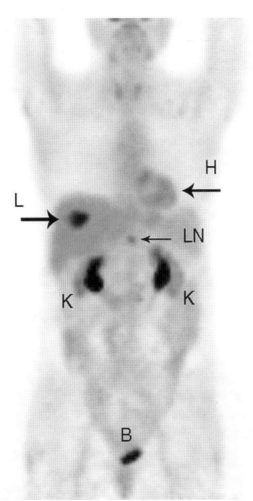

Figure 14.11 (D) Positron emission tomography (PET). Example of a PET scan with fluorodeoxyglucose (FDG). It was obtained to stage the colon cancer in this 60-year-old woman. Note the round area of increased activity in the liver (L arrow) from a single metastasis. This confirmed the CT findings. Increased activity in a small upper abdominal lymph node (LN) is also consistent with metastatic disease. This was not suspected on CT which relies on lymph node enlargement to make the diagnosis. FDG is excreted via the kidneys, hence the normal activity in the kidneys (K) and bladder (B). Normal activity is also seen in the heart (H).

over 40 years of age. All mammography facilities in the United States of America are regulated under the federal Mammography Quality Standards Act (MQSA). Despite these advances, it must be remembered that no perfect test has been found; breast cancer still remains the second most common cancer in women after lung cancer. The sensitivity and specificity of mammography screening is 83–95% and 90–98% respectively. Sensitivity is especially reduced in women with dense breasts. Breast self-examination and clinical examination remain essential for diagnosis.

The National Lung Screening Trial (NLST) has shown that low dose CT screening decreases the mortality from lung cancer and guidelines for its use are being developed. CT colonography is a new technique, which uses MPR and three-dimensional reconstruction to noninvasively view the colon, and is being evaluated as a possible screening tool for colorectal cancer. For these and other trials, including the effectiveness of imaging guided therapies such as RF

> **Box 14.1**   *Risk factors for iodinated contrast-induced nephropathy*
>
> - Age >60
> - History of renal disease, including:
>   - Dialysis
>   - Renal transplant
>   - Single kidney
>   - Renal surgery
>   - Acute renal injury
>   - Renal cancer
> - Hypertension
> - Diabetes
> - Gout

tumor ablation, refer to the American College of Radiology Imaging Network website (www.acrin.org) and the National Comprehensive Cancer network (www.nccn.org).

ISSUES RELATED TO INTRAVENOUS CONTRAST

Intravenous contrast agents are widely used and considered safe. However, adverse reactions can occur. For the most part these are minor reactions that do not require treatment, including hives, nausea and facial swelling. More moderate reactions that require observation and/or treatment include hypotension, bronchospasm and bradycardia. Rarely, the reaction may be life-threatening, requiring immediate treatment and usually hospitalization. With, present day, nonionic low osmolar iodinated contrast media (LOCM), used with X-ray and CT, the incidence of a severe reaction is 1–2 per 10000 examinations. Gadolinium chelates, which are used as intravenous contrast agents for MRI, are very well tolerated and have a much lower incidence of adverse reactions; severe reactions are extremely rare. Patients who have previously reacted to contrast are more likely to do so again. Current practice is to pretreat these patients with corticosteroids at least 6h prior to injection. An antihistamine, such as 50mg of diphenhydramine, is also used and given 1hour before the contrast injection. This may prevent or minimize a minor or moderate contrast reaction but has not been shown to prevent a major life-threatening event.

Iodinated contrast-induced nephropathy is a risk, particularly in patients with pre-existing renal failure (Box 14.1). It is usually transient, with renal function returning to the baseline within 10 days. Adequate hydration prior to the examination is important. In patients with poor renal function or repeated severe contrast reactions, it is recommended that the study be undertaken without contrast or by using a different imaging modality.

According to the ACR manual on contrast media, version 8 (see Bibliography), gadolinium does not cause renal toxicity. Also patients with end-stage renal disease requiring regular dialysis can be given iodinated contrast agents. However, recent reports have indicated that a new and rare disease, nephrogenic systemic fibrosis (NSF), may occur in patients with moderate to end-stage renal disease and acute renal injury following the administration of a gadolinium-based contrast agent. If you have patients with renal failure, particularly end-stage disease, who may require MRI, it

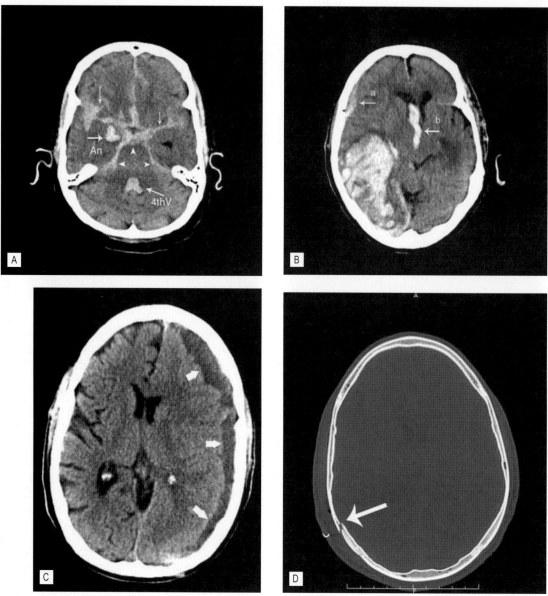

Figure 14.12 (A–D) Brain imaging. MRI and CT are used to image the brain. Both have their strengths and weaknesses. Generally speaking, MRI is the modality of choice. However, when speed is of the essence, such as in an emergency situation or with patients unable to lie still, CT is preferred. CT is used in patients unable to undergo MRI such as those who suffer from claustrophobia. In the acute setting, CT is usually the initial choice because of its availability, fast examination times and ability to identify acute intracranial blood, skull and facial fractures **(A–D)**. **(A) Subarachnoid hemorrhage** in a 75-year-old female who presented with an acute severe headache behind the right eye. Acute blood is seen in the basal cisterns (arrow heads), Sylvian fissure (arrows) and 4th ventricle (4th V). Acute blood appears white on CT and is easily differentiated from the darker brain parenchyma. This was caused by a rupture of a right posterior communicating artery aneurysm (An). The 15 mm triangular white area to the right of the circle of Willis represents blood around and thrombus within the aneurysm. Treatment was surgical clipping. In the right candidate, such aneurysms can be treated by placing small metal coils into the aneurysm and sealing them off; this is achieved by threading small catheters up to the brain via arteries in the groin and using fluoroscopy to guide the placement. **(B) Intracerebral hemorrhage** in a 90-year-old patient who presented with acute collapse. There is a large cerebral hematoma with considerable mass affect on the adjacent brain. Blood has ruptured into the lateral and 3rd ventricle (arrow b) and there is a small subdural component (arrow a). Elderly hypertensives are at particular risk for intracerebral hemorrhage. **(C) Chronic subdural hematoma.** The small arrows show a rim of chronic hematoma between the brain and the inner table of the skull. In contrast with acute blood, chronic subdural blood appears gray or dark on CT. Note the mass effect on the adjacent brain with loss of the sulci (compare opposite side) and shift of midline structures to the right. Subdural hematomas result from tearing of cortical bridging veins following head trauma. With an obvious episode of trauma and alteration of mental status, the diagnosis is straightforward. However, the episode of trauma may be minor, particularly in patients on anticoagulants. In the elderly, subtle changes of behavior may be difficult to define and the patient may not remember the traumatic event, making clinical diagnosis difficult. Not surprisingly, most chronic subdurals occur in the elderly. Symptoms are headache followed by deteriorating neurological function. Treatment is surgical drainage. **(D) Skull fractures.** Easily appreciated on CT, as shown by the arrow.

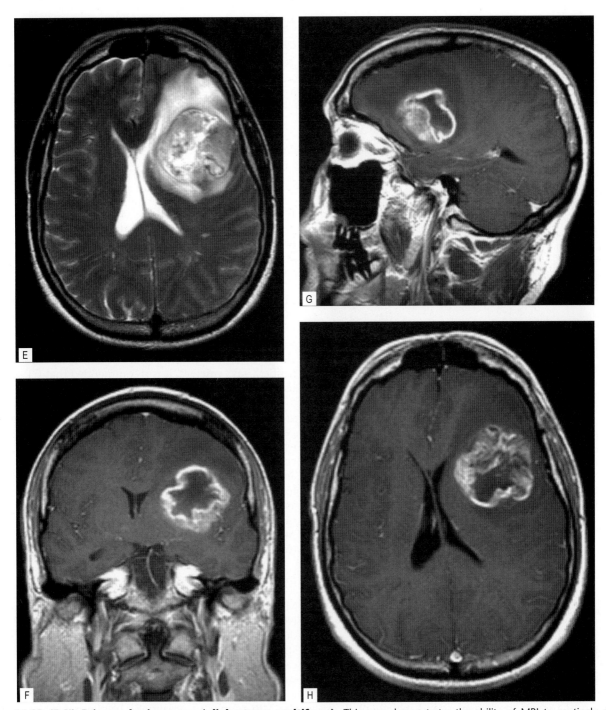

Figure 14.12 (E–H) Primary brain tumor (gliobastoma multiform). This case demonstrates the ability of MRI to routinely display pathology in multiple planes and the superior soft tissue depiction. The brain tumor in the left frontal region is well defined on these sagittal, coronal and transverse images **(E–H)**. The T1-weighted images **(G** and **H)** were obtained following intravenous gadolinium and show bright areas of enhancement in the periphery of the lesion. The bright area in the T2-weighted image **(E)** surrounding the tumor indicates associated edema. **(H)** The central part of the tumor is fluid-containing, dark on T1 **(C)** and bright on T2 **(E)**, and probably indicates cystic change or central necrosis. Mass effect on the adjacent structures is well appreciated.

is suggested that you also contact your MRI center for their current guidelines before ordering the test. Also for current American College of Radiology guidelines refer to the current ACR manual on contrast media (see Bibliography).

Patients using metformin to treat diabetes are at risk of developing lactic acidosis if the blood level of metformin is high. Metformin is excreted via the kidneys.

Therefore, the development of renal failure following intravascular iodinated contrast in patients taking metformin is of added concern. Current recommendations, with some modifications, are to stop metformin before administration of intravenous contrast and recommence after 48 hours, once it is established that renal function has not been affected.

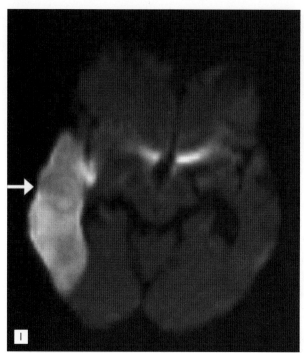

Figure 14.12 (I) Stroke. This is a clinical diagnosis. CT and MR are both used in patient evaluation. Although CT is usually used initially it may appear normal in the first few hours. Traditionally, its value is the assessment of stroke mimics, such as tumor and any associated hemorrhage. More recently, CT and MR have been used to assess perfusion of the brain and level of arterial vascular obstruction or stenosis with noninvasive vascular imaging (see Fig. 14.8). This figure is an example of diffusion-weighted MR (DWI) and acute brain infarct. This 85-year-old woman presented with acute onset of confusion, left-sided weakness and visual field defect. MRI is capable of measuring the motion of water through brain tissue. With acute infarction diffusion becomes restricted in those areas affected. This represents the bright area in the right temporal lobe (arrow). This is in the vascular territory supplied by the inferior division of the right middle cerebral artery. The change can be seen within minutes of the event and has revolutionized stroke diagnosis.

Table 14.1 **Typical radiation doses**	
Dose (mSV)	
Natural background	3.0/year
Chest X-ray (marrow)	0.1
Mammogram (breast)	0.7
Nuclear medicine	2.0–10.0
CT scan: head	2.0
CT scan: abdomen	10.0

A WORD ABOUT RADIATION EFFECTS

X-rays used in radiography, fluoroscopy and CT, and gamma rays used in nuclear medicine, have enough energy to cause ionization of atoms within the body. This form of energy or radiation is called ionizing radiation, and it can result in damage to DNA and the induction of tumors, both benign and malignant. Bone marrow, gastrointestinal tract, mammary glands, gonads and lymphatic tissue are most susceptible, and children are more susceptible than adults. The latency period for solid tumors is 25+ years, whereas for leukemia it is 5–7 years. While the higher the exposure, the greater the likelihood of getting cancer, there is no demonstrable threshold at which this can occur. In contrast, a single high dose can cause immediate cell death and may cause cataracts, skin burns and hair loss.

Imaging studies are only one source of ionizing radiation. Everyone is exposed to natural background radiation, which, in the US, is approximately 3 mSv/year. Table 14.1 lists some typical radiation doses. It is unknown exactly what the cancer risk is from diagnostic studies. It is assumed that there is a potential risk; however, the risk may be zero or very small. This is especially so with a chest X-ray where the dose is small and estimated to be equivalent to 10 days of background radiation. These factors must be weighed against the risk to the patient's health if the study is not performed.

From Table 14.1, it is clear that the examination resulting in the most patient exposure is a CT scan, which is of particular concern in children. If a patient needs a CT scan in order to improve their health and there is no other way of obtaining the information, then the choice is easy. However, until a clearer picture of the exact risks of diagnostic X-rays emerges, it is recommended that CT scans be used prudently.

Using the argument that the greater the dose, the greater the risk, strategies to reduce patient exposure are part of modern radiological practice. These include using exposures as low as reasonably achievable (ALARA), modern CT scanners that reduce radiation dose by using automatic exposure control, new image reconstruction techniques and trained personnel. Alternative studies such as MRI or ultrasound, which do not use ionizing radiation, are an option and for recommendations refer to the American College of Radiology Appropriateness Criteria (www.acr.org/ac).

MRI SAFETY

MRI uses no ionizing radiation and is a safe procedure. No long-term biological effects from MRI have been described. However there are some caveats. MRI uses a strong static magnetic field and ferromagnetic objects can become airborne projectiles. These include stainless-steel surgical instruments, ferrous oxygen tanks and car keys, and, therefore, such items are not allowed into the MRI room. Ferromagnetic implants may move with potential catastrophic consequences; certain cerebral aneurysm clips, especially the older type, are in this category. Newer magnetic resonance-safe clips are of no concern. If it is not possible to determine the type of clip used prior to the scan, the procedure is not undertaken. Implantable devices are assessed on a case-by-case basis. Generally, cardiac valve replacements, annuloplasty rings, arterial stents and joint replacements are safe. However, these devices may cause image artefacts, which may limit the usefulness of the study. Other contraindications include cochlear implants and most cardiac pacemakers. However, and more importantly, the Revo™ and second generation Advisa™ (Medtronic, 710 Medtronic Parkway Minneapolis MN 55432) MRI SureScan™ pacing systems are designed to allow

Table 14.2 Advantages and disadvantages of the various imaging modalities

	X-ray	CT	Nuclear Medicine	MRI	Ultrasound
Ionizing radiation	Yes, but the dose is usually small	Yes; has the highest doses	Yes	No	No
Scan time	Fast	Fast	May need delayed images	30–60 min	10–30 min
Cross-sectional, multiplanar and three-dimensional images	No	Yes, but current technology requires additional time	Yes; shows function-limited anatomical detail	Yes; routine and no extra time for reconstruction	Yes; three-dimensional is new but likely to be used more
Mobility/bedside imaging	Yes	No	No	No	Yes
Cost	Inexpensive	Expensive	PET scanners are expensive	Most expensive	Relatively inexpensive
Claustrophobia	No	Uncommon	Rarely	Yes; 1–4%	No
Large patients	No weight limit; image quality reduced	Weight limit; image quality reduced	Generally no weight limit; image quality reduced	Weight limit; also, if patient too wide they will not fit in the magnet bore	Images for deep structures limited; superficial images OK
Strengths	Still the most widely used imaging modality; fast and inexpensive; lungs and bones well seen; good overall view of anatomy	Fast; maximum amount of information in a short time frame; excellent in emergencies, e.g. acute hemorrhage, intra-abdominal air, complicated fractures; lung, bone and vessels well seen	Unsurpassed functional imaging; excellent for diffuse bone metastases; PET good for diagnosis and treatment of cancer; thallium and sestamibi used in diagnosis of IHD	Best for soft tissue and bone marrow; imaging of choice for brain, spine and musculoskeletal; nonionizing; list of uses increasing	Fast, mobile, real time and nonionizing; first line in many situations especially superficial structures; used for abdomen, pelvis, heart, carotids and limb DVT

DVT, deep vein thrombosis; IHD, ischemic heart disease; PET, positron emission tomography

implanted patients the ability to undergo an MRI scan under the specified MRI conditions for use. Expect similar devices in the near future from other manufacturers.

Metallic foreign bodies within the orbit are a contraindication and, if concern exists, a radiograph of the orbits is obtained prior to the study.

The magnetic field gradients used to produce a magnetic resonance image produce their own set of potential problems. These gradients can stimulate peripheral nerves but, at the Food and Drug Administration (FDA) limit for gradient field strength, this is not a practical problem. The loud knocking noises heard while in the scanner are produced by the changing field gradients. The noise has the potential to induce hearing loss and earplugs or noise-abating headphones must be worn.

Because of the potential for the RF pulse to heat the body, the FDA has recommended RF exposure limits. Care must also be taken to prevent burns that may develop from electrical currents in materials that are capable of producing a conductive loop, such as electrocardiogram (EKG) leads. Technical staff receive specific and continuous safety training, and rigorous patient screening, including a detailed safety form, is completed prior to any study. Removable metallic objects including jewelry, car keys and hairpins, are not permitted in the MRI room; credit cards should also be excluded as they will become damaged.

Only MRI-safe equipment is allowed in the suite and the patient is closely monitored during the scan.

WHICH IMAGING STUDY TO CHOOSE?

All of the imaging modalities have their strengths and weaknesses and none is perfect (Table 14.2). It is important to decide which test will answer the clinical problem with least risk and cost to the patient. New research and the march of technology mean that this will always be a moving target; what is the best test today may be old hat tomorrow. However, one of the most useful pieces of information for the imaging facility and interpreting radiologist is the clinical history. This information is critical in order to answer the clinical question and tailor the examination to ensure that the appropriate images are acquired.

In general, MRI with its superb tissue contrast and ability to image bone marrow with routine multiplanar imaging and nonionizing radiation is the method of choice for most brain, spine and musculoskeletal lesions (see Figs 14.12E–I, 14.13C–E, G–J, 14.14A–G, 14.15A–D and 14.16A–C). It also has an increasing role to play in the evaluation of the abdomen and pelvis. Noninvasive imaging of the biliary and pancreatic ducts, so-called MRCP, is now a routine investigation, replacing older more invasive studies.

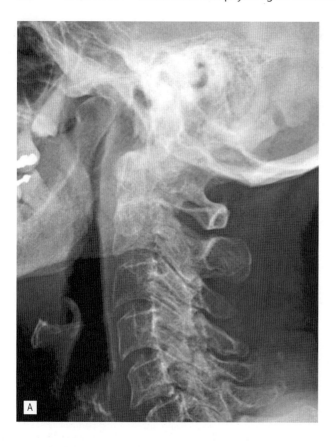

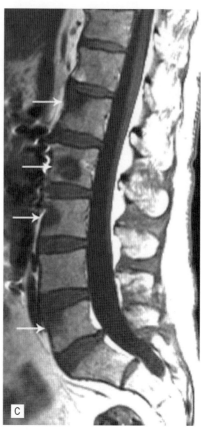

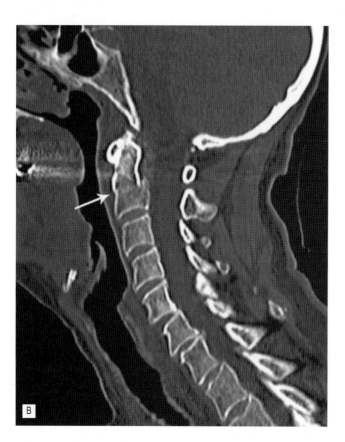

Figure 14.13 (A–C) Neck and back pain. Neck and back pain are common clinical problems. The following four cases show how CT and MR can be used to evaluate spine pain. **(A)** and **(B) Cervical spine injury in the elderly.** Lateral radiograph and sagittal, multiplanar reconstructed computed tomogram (MPR/CT) of a 78-year-old woman with neck pain following a minor fall. **(A)** The radiograph shows mild swelling of the prevertebral soft tissues at C2 of concern for a bony injury but none definitely detected. **(B)** The CT clearly demonstrates an undisplaced fracture through the base of the odontoid. This case serves to illustrate several common clinical situations. Firstly, both falls and neck pain are common in the elderly. Cervical spine fractures are also common in the elderly and odontoid fractures are disproportionately represented. Secondly, fractures of the cervical spine often occur following minor trauma and may, initially, not be suspected. Osteopenic bones add to the difficulty of diagnosis. MPR/CT overcome many of the limitations of plain radiographs and can be useful when plain films do not fit the clinical picture or further detail is required of a known fracture (see Fig. 14.7A–D). Suspected cord injury is best evaluated with MRI. **(C) Vertebral metastasis.** Sagittal T1-weighted image of the lumbar spine in a 57-year-old patient with back pain and lung cancer. The changes are typical for metastatic vertebral disease. Multiple oval areas of low signal (arrows) are seen replacing the bone marrow at multiple levels. The spine is the most common site of skeletal metastases, which are seen most frequently with breast, lung and prostate cancer. Whereas whole body nuclear medicine bone scanning is the preferred method for accessing total skeletal involvement (Fig. 14.11B), MR is the preferred method for evaluating the spine. Because of its superior imaging of bone marrow it can identify metastatic disease, to the spine, earlier than other techniques. In addition it is able to evaluate other causes of back pain and possible causes of neurological deficits including cord compression.

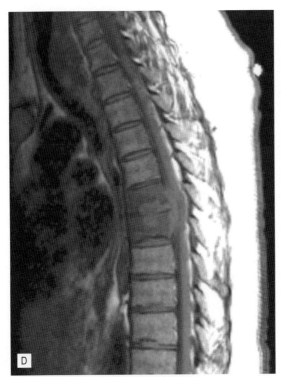
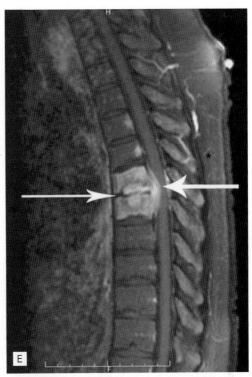

Figure 14.13 (D–E) Diskitis. This is an infection of the intervertebral disk, which usually occurs via blood borne bacteria which implant in the vertebral endplate and spread to the disk. It typically presents with focal back pain and tenderness. Elderly diabetics and the immunocompromised are particularly susceptible. MRI with excellent soft tissue and bone marrow detail has proven an accurate way to diagnose and monitor response following antibiotic treatment. **(D)** Sagittal T1-weighted image without intravenous gadolinium. **(E)** Sagittal T1 image following intravenous contrast. In this image, the bright fat signal has been removed (bright fat in **D** is now gray* in **E**) by a technique called fat saturation and allows dramatic appreciation of the increased enhancement (the bright area) across the disk and adjacent endplate (arrows) indicating infection. Note also involvement of the adjacent epidural space and compression of the spinal cord.

Ultrasound is often used as the initial modality for evaluating the abdomen, especially the gall bladder and bile ducts. Ultrasound is a good place to start when evaluating renal masses and possible renal obstruction as a cause for renal failure. It is the method of choice for initially evaluating uterine and ovarian masses. It allows excellent detail of superficial structures and is a reasonable place to start with superficial masses, for example thyroid masses. Joint and tendon pathology is usually evaluated with MRI but nonosseous problems, e.g. the rotator cuff, biceps and Achilles tendon tears, are well evaluated with ultrasound (see Figs 14.14C and 14.15E, F). For patients who are unable to undergo MRI, ultrasound or CT may be helpful.

In the case of trauma and emergency situations, X-ray and CT are the modalities of choice; they are readily available and quick to perform. Modern CT is very fast, with a typical brain scan taking only a few seconds. CT is very accurate at demonstrating acute intracerebral hemorrhage (see Fig. 14.12A–C). Acute chest and abdominal problems are routinely evaluated with CT (see Figs 14.5 and 14.6). With stroke, CT is currently used in an initial evaluation; however, CT has a limited ability to diagnose this important condition in the first few critical hours when treatment options need to be decided. Its role is mainly in excluding intracranial hemorrhage and stroke mimics such as tumors (see Fig. 14.12A–C). This situation is changing, and new sequences such as perfusion CT and MRI can evaluate areas in the brain with no perfusion, or limited perfusion, that are at risk for further infarct and

which may benefit from intervention with intravenous or intra-arterial thrombolysis using tissue plasminogen activator (tPA). MRI is able to diagnose stroke within minutes of the event. A sequence called diffusion imaging has revolutionized the diagnosis of this acute problem (see Fig. 14.12I) and is likely to play a major role along with perfusion imaging in acute stroke management.

Fractures are best evaluated by X-ray imaging. However, in the elderly, in whom bone density is reduced, undisplaced fractures may not be apparent (see Fig. 14.13A, B). Limited mobility, as in patients with spine and complex fractures, may reduce the usefulness of standard radiographs (see Fig. 14.16). MRI, with its ability to display bone marrow edema, has proved useful in evaluating the presence of acute compression fractures, metastatic disease of the spine and suspected fractures, especially hip fractures, not detected on initial radiographs (see Figs 14.13C, F–J and 14.16A, B). CT, with its multiplanar three-dimensional capabilities and superb bone detail, is well suited for the evaluation of complex and difficult-to-diagnose fractures (see Figs 14.7, 14.12D, 14.13A, B and 14.16D, E).

Nuclear medicine bone scans are also used in this situation; however, in the elderly, it may take a few days for the nuclear medicine scan to become positive. For diffuse bone metastases, whole body nuclear bone scanning is best, whereas spine metastases are evaluated well with MRI (see Figs 14.11B and 14.13C). Nuclear medicine still has a major role to play in the diagnosis of pulmonary embolus despite the move to CT.

(cont'd p. 102)

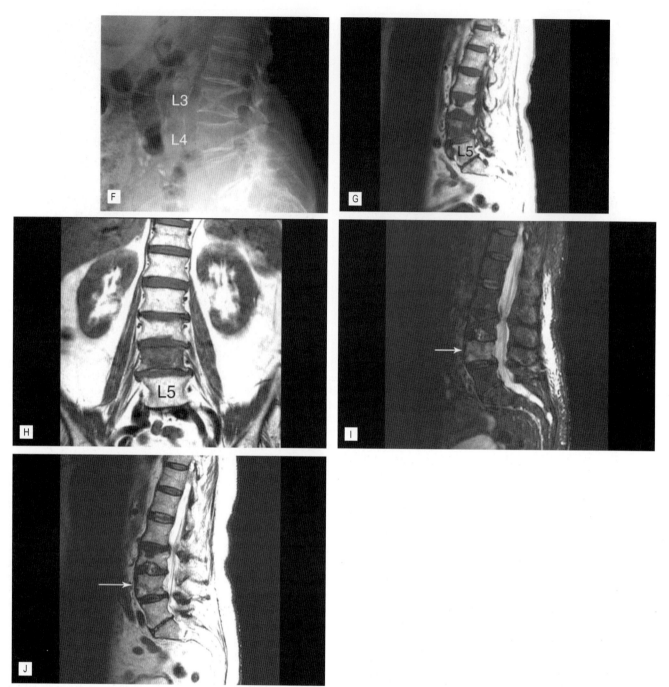

Figure 14.13 (F–J) Vertebral compression fractures. Vertebral fractures are a common cause of back pain in the elderly. This 70-year-old sustained a lumbar compression fracture following a fall. The case illustrates how MR is used to determine if the fracture on X-ray is recent or old and diagnose occult fractures. The radiograph **(F)** shows a fracture at L3. MRI also shows the fracture. However, on the sagittal and coronal T1 images **(G** and **H)** the vertebra is bright, the same as all the other vertebrae with the exception of L4 which is dark. L4, however, is bright on the STIR (short tau inversion recovery) or fluid-sensitive image **(I)**. What does this mean? The radiograph certainly shows a fracture at L3. However, it is an old fracture that has healed. This is confirmed on the MR where the signal of this vertebra is normal. L4 represents the acute fracture as seen by the bone marrow edema – dark on T1, bright on STIR. The fracture has not resulted in any loss of height of the vertebra, making it hard to pinpoint on the radiograph. A sagittal T2-weighted image **(J)** shows the fracture line. This serves to illustrate a frequent problem. In older individuals, compression fractures, usually related to osteoporosis, are common. The radiograph is able to show the fracture, providing there is compression of the vertebra or a fracture line. However, unless a recent study is available for comparison, it is not able to tell if this is new or old, and, as in this case, it can underdiagnose injury. The MR by demonstrating the bone marrow edema is able to show that an acute fracture has occurred and that it occurred at L4, not L3 as suggested on the radiograph. It is important to know which vertebra is involved prior to treatment and MR is frequently used to sort out this common conundrum.

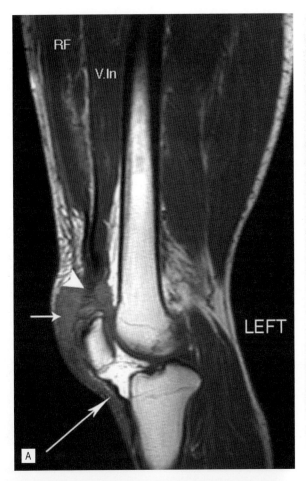

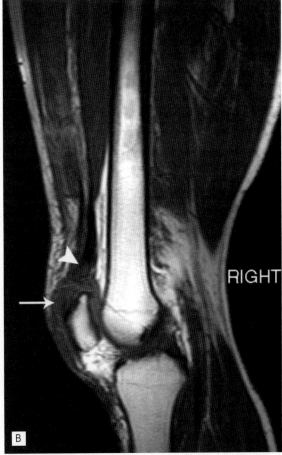

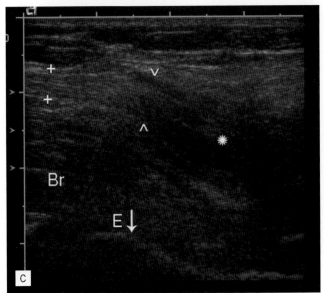

Figure 14.14 (A–C) Superficial soft tissues. MRI is very useful for evaluating superficial soft tissue pathology, particularly complex and acute problems. Lesions with calcium require X-ray. Ultrasound can be used for small or focal lesions. Radio-opaque foreign bodies need X-ray, whereas non-radio-opaque foreign bodies can be evaluated with ultrasound. (**A** and **B**) **Acute bilateral quadriceps rupture.** This 59-year-old male was unable to extend his knees after a fall. The sagittal T1-weighted image of both knees shows rupture of both quadriceps tendons at the attachment to the patella (arrow head). Loss of the normal dark signal of the tendon is seen. There is an associated hematoma on both sides (arrow), left > right. (V.In, vastus intermedius, RF, rectus femoris muscle). Note the crumpled patellar tendon and slight distal patellar displacement on the left side (long arrow). Quadriceps rupture is more common above the age of 40 and considered to be secondary to tendon degeneration. Bilateral rupture is unusual, however. MRI allows excellent depiction of this problem. The tendons were surgically reattached. **(C) Ultrasound of biceps tendon rupture**. This 71-year-old woman presented with anterior elbow and upper forearm pain and swelling following a fall. She tried to catch herself by grabbing the table with her hand while the elbow was flexed. This is a sagittal ultrasound of the lower end of the biceps tendon as it starts to dive towards its insertion onto the radial tuberosity, just below the elbow. The tendon is torn from the tuberosity. The normal linear fibers of the tendon (+ +) are interrupted and irregular (between the two arrows > <). The distal tendon is bulbous, representing degenerated torn tendon, fibrous tissue and surrounding edema (*). These findings were confirmed at surgery during reattachment of the tendon to the tuberosity. Brachialis muscle deep to the biceps tendon (Br). Anterior bony margin of the elbow (label E).

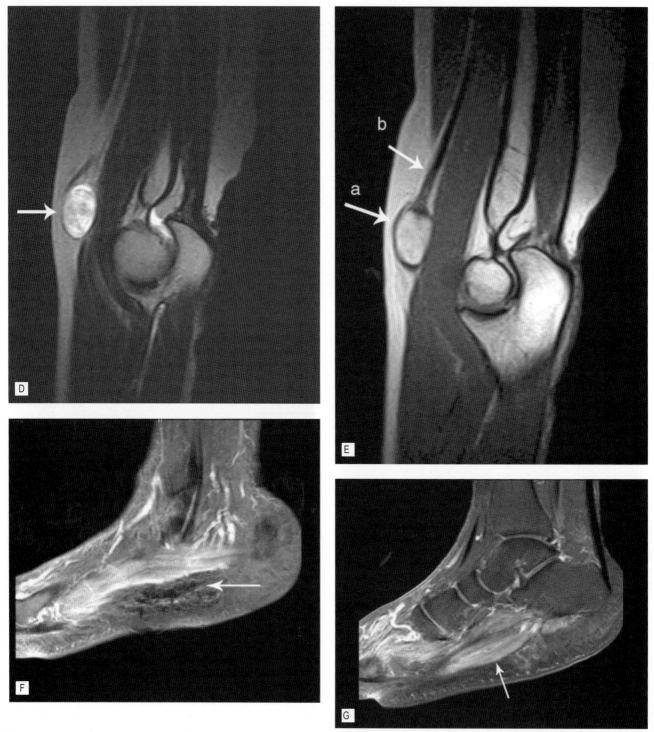

Figure 14.14 (D–G) (**D** and **E**) **Nerve sheath tumor**. This 56-year-old female presented with hand numbness, upper extremity pain and soft tissue mass anterior to the elbow. The nerve sheath tumor is exquisitely demonstrated by MR. The nerve in image (**E**) (arrow b) can be seen running into the tumor (arrow a). The MR findings are characteristic with the tumor bright on T2 (**D**) and enhancing with gadolinium on the T1 image (**E**). Findings confirmed at surgery. (**F** and **G**) **Foot infection: cellulitis and osteomyelitis**. A combination of radiographs and nuclear medicine has traditionally been used to evaluate osteomyelitis in the foot. MR with its excellent soft tissue and bone marrow depiction is able to show both soft tissue and bone infection. This case shows an MRI of a 54-year-old diabetic with diffuse foot swelling and infected non-healing plantar ulcer. (**F**) and (**G**) are sagittal views of the foot. They are T1-weighted images with fat saturation obtained after intravenous injection of gadolinium chelate. There is increased enhancement of the plantar soft tissues (bright area and vertical arrow) indicating infection. The bright tubular structures are veins. The black area or signal void is due to gas in adjacent devitalized tissue (horizontal arrow). These findings were confirmed at surgery.

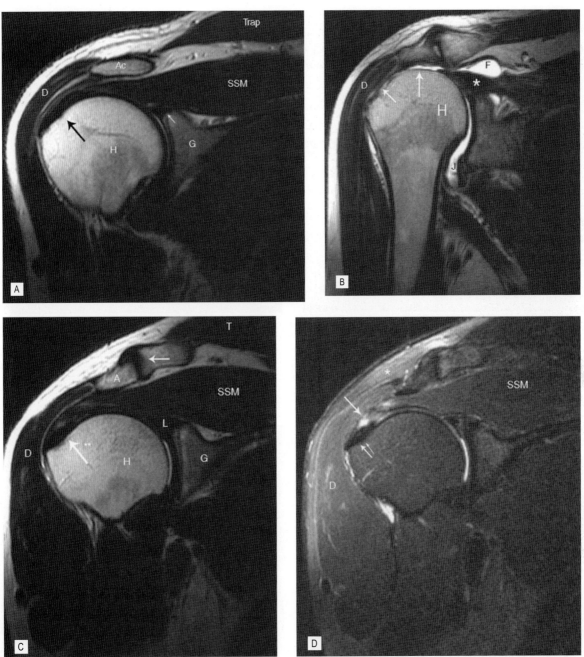

Figure 14.15 (A–D) Shoulder pain. Shoulder pain is a common symptom in the elderly often caused by tears of the rotator cuff. MRI with its superb soft tissue contrast and multiplanar abilities is well suited for imaging the rotator cuff. In patients unable to undergo MRI, ultrasound with its ability to image superficial soft tissue structures is an excellent technique for evaluating the rotator cuff. **(A) Normal right shoulder MRI.** This is a coronal view using a T2-weighted imaging sequence (T2WI). This view is part of a MR assessment of the rotator cuff, a common source of tendon tears. The supraspinatus muscle (SSM), part of the rotator cuff, is well seen. The muscle arises from the supraspinous fossa of the scapula. It passes under the acromion to insert anteriorly on the greater tuberosity (black arrow) of the humerus (H) shown above. The lateral margin of the deltoid (D) is well seen in this view, arising from the lateral and upper margin of the acromion (Ac). Superior labrum (small white arrow), trapezius muscle (Trap). **(B) Full thickness tear of the supraspinatus tendon.** Compare normal shoulder in **(A).** This coronal MRI, T2WI shows that this patient has sustained a large full thickness tear of the supraspinatus tendon. Note how the greater tuberosity and superior humeral head (arrows) are now bare. The tendon is retracted medially almost to the superior margin of the glenoid. (*) The humeral head is displaced superiorly and abuts the under surface of the acromion. Fluid is seen in the subacromial bursa (F) and in the glenohumeral joint (J). **(C and D) Partial tear of the supraspinatus tendon. (C)** is a coronal MRI, T2W1, showing mild increase in signal in the bursal or superior fibers of the tendon (white arrow and two stars). Note the normal bright signal from the subcutaneous fat overlying the deltoid. Acromioclavicular joint (small white arrow), glenoid (G), labrum (L), trapezius muscle (T). **(D)** Same area using an additional fat saturation sequence to remove the fat signal. Note how the subcutaneous fat is now gray. (*) Note also the bright signal in the tendon caused by the tear is better appreciated (single arrow). (Double arrow, normal dark signal from unaffected lateral margin of tendon.)

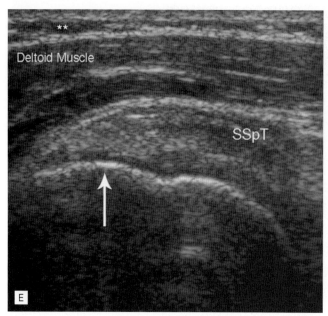

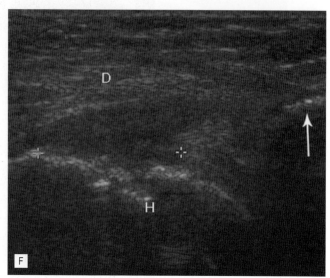

Figure 14.15 (E–F) **(E) Normal right shoulder ultrasound.** Compare this to the normal coronal MRI view of the shoulder with **(A)**. The supraspinatus tendon (SSpT) is well seen inserting into the greater tuberosity of the humerus (white arrow). (** Subcutaneous fat overlying the deltoid). **(F) Right shoulder ultrasound: full thickness tear.** Compare this to the MRI full thickness tear **(B)**. The horizontal echogenic fibers of the tendon are separated by a distance of 1.7 cm (++). The space is filled with hypoechoic material representing fluid and granulation tissue. Acromion (arrow), deltoid muscle (D), greater tuberosity and head of humerus (H).

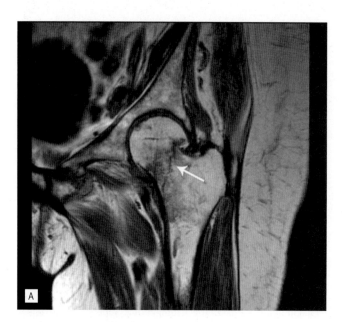

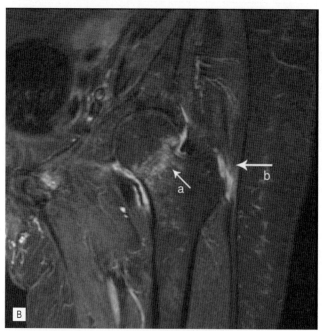

Figure 14.16 (A–B) Hip pain. This 76-year-old woman experienced left hip pain following a fall. The hip radiograph was normal. **(A)** is a T1-weighted coronal image of the left hip. This shows the fracture line (arrow) and gray areas in the adjacent bone marrow representing edema. **(B)** is a fluid-sensitive coronal image showing a linear bright area representing edema at the level of the fracture (arrow a). While the radiograph was negative, the MR was able to confirm the clinical suspicion of a fracture and allow treatment in a timely manner. Note the associated partial tear of the gluteus medius at its insertion (**B**, arrow b) illustrating MRI's ability to show other causes of hip pain following trauma such as adjacent muscle strain or tears and pelvic fractures.

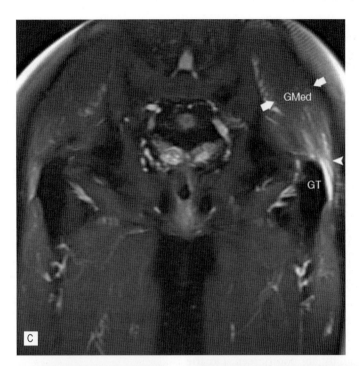

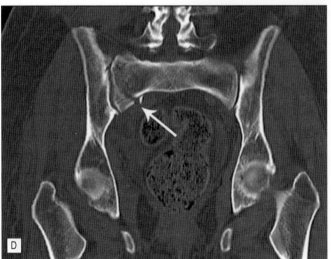

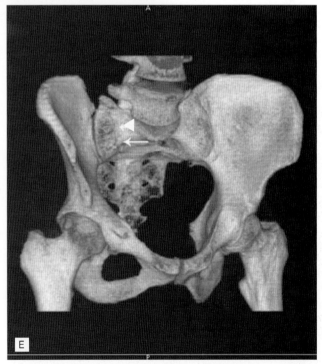

Figure 14.16 (C–E) (C) Tear of the gluteus medius muscle. This is a coronal fluid-sensitive MRI (STIR) scan of the pelvis and both hips in a 76-year-old women with left trochanteric pain. This demonstrates a full thickness tear of the lateral fibers of the gluteus medius muscle (GMed, between arrows) at its insertion onto the greater trochanter (GT) of the left femur (arrow head). So-called trochanteric pain syndrome is more common in middle-aged and elderly women. This has often been ascribed to trochanteric bursitis. However, with the advent of MRI it is now felt that this syndrome is more likely due to tendinopathy of the gluteus minimus and medius muscles, which both insert into the greater trochanter, and the bursitis is a secondary effect. The changes are analogous to tears of the rotator cuff of the shoulder. (**D** and **E**) **Hip pain**. This 56-year-old female experienced right hip and pelvic pain following a fall. The radiographs were normal. (**D**) is a coronal reconstructed CT image showing a fracture of the right sacrum (arrow). (**E**) is a 3D volume-rendered image elegantly demonstrating the fracture (arrows). The right hip was normal.

Acute cholecystitis, bile leaks, intestinal bleeding and infection are other diagnoses that can be made with nuclear medicine. FDG PET, as outlined above, has a major and increasing role to play in cancer imaging (Fig. 14.11D). It also has a role in the diagnosis of brain disorders including Alzheimer's disease, Parkinson's disease and seizures. In the future, it will also likely be used in the evaluation of myocardial perfusion.

Diagnostic vascular imaging is now mainly performed noninvasively using ultrasound, CT and MRI. Long and deep vessels, e.g. the thoracic and abdominal aorta and entire lower limb arterial supply, are best seen with magnetic resonance arteriography (MRA) and computed tomography arteriography (CTA) (see Fig. 14.8). Ultrasound with Doppler is very effective for short superficial vessels and is excellent for evaluating carotid artery stenosis in the neck. It is also the best test for deep vein thrombosis in the upper and lower limb.

Infection of the foot, especially with diabetes, is a common problem. The foot is first evaluated with X-ray imaging. This provides a lot of basic information including the presence of arthritis and neuropathic changes. However, plain film changes of osteomyelitis are a late finding and soft-tissue infection and viability are poorly seen. On the contrary, MRI has proven very useful in evaluating foot and spine infection (Figs 14.13D, E and 14.14F, G). For more information/updates go to the ACR website and navigate to Appropriateness Criteria (see Bibliography).

CONCLUSION

Medical imaging has come a long way in the past 100 years. The improvements have mirrored developments in technology. This has brought faster imaging times, improved anatomical detail and, more recently, molecular imaging. As a result, medical imaging is an important and integral part of modern medical practice. Future developments promise to build on these capabilities and help provide insight into the cause of disease, improved diagnosis, earlier detection, and improved and targeted treatment regimens. With constant change in the capabilities of the various modalities, new knowledge of disease processes and each patient's unique set of problems, it is not possible to be dogmatic on which modality is best suited for a given situation. However, an understanding of the strengths and weaknesses of the current imaging modalities will be of benefit when deciding the appropriate study for addressing the patient's particular clinical problem.

Finally, despite all of the spectacular progress over the past 100 years, medical imaging remains but one tool in the clinical armamentarium and is still no substitute for a good clinical history and physical examination.

Acknowledgments

I would like to thank the technical staff from the Radiology Department, Lancaster General Hospital and MRI Group, Lancaster, Pennsylvania. With special thanks to Chris Weir, Mark Housman, Idriz Dizdarevic, Dean Hollenbacher, Kory Mollica, Kevin Barnhar, Doug Peterson, Corinne Daubenhauser. Also to Jerry Kornfield for computer and graphics advice.

NOTE

Left and right sides are defined from the perspective of the radiologist looking at the patient from the foot of the bed. The patient's right side is opposite the radiologist's left. This is why in Figure 14.12C the shift is to the patient's right although in the image it is to the left.

REFERENCE

Smith RA, Duffy SW, Gabe R et al 2004 The randomized trials of breast cancer screening: what have we learned? Radiol Clin North Am 42:793–806

BIBLIOGRAPHY

American College of Radiology Imaging Network. www.acrin.org.
Grainger & Allison's Diagnostic Radiology: A Textbook of Medical Imaging, 5th edn. This is a good general radiology text.
Magnetic Resonance Imaging Special Issue. Journal of Orthopedic and Sports Physical Therapy 41(11) 2011.
Radiologic Clinics of North America. www.theclinics.com. Excellent up-to-date monographs published bimonthly.
Radiological Society of North America (RSNA). http://rsna.org. Membership is necessary to gain access to all the resources but there are lots of free articles and information. Click on 'Patient information'. There is lots of information here, including the 'Radiology in motion' section with short, funny, video clips on various imaging modalities.
The American College of Radiology. www.acr.org. Again, membership is required for full access but there is a lot of free information. For evidence-based guidelines on the most appropriate way to image patients, go to 'Quality and Patient Safety'. From the pop-up menu choose 'Appropriateness Criteria'. www.acr.org/Quality-Safety/Appropriateness-Criteria. Also in this section is the Manual on Contrast Media and MR Safety: www.acr.org/Quality-Safety/Resources/Contrast-Manual.
The National Comprehensive Cancer network. www.nccn.org.

Musculoskeletal disorders

Chapter 15

Posture

TIMOTHY L. KAUFFMAN • MICHELLE A. BOLTON

CHAPTER CONTENTS

INTRODUCTION

Posture is the alignment of body parts in relationship to one another at any given moment. Posture involves complex interactions between bones, joints, connective tissue, skeletal muscles and the nervous system, both central and peripheral. The complexity of these interactions is compounded when one considers the near infinitesimal variety of human balance, motor control and movement in relation to gravity. Furthermore, with the passage of time, each organism undergoes change resulting from microtrauma, frank injuries and the effects of disease on the neuromusculoskeletal system which result in the common and unique variations of aging posture.

Posture is commonly assessed using a grid or plumb line, with the patient in a static standing position; however, within the aging population, this becomes more difficult because of the age-associated increase in postural sway. This can be seen in the two photos in Figure 15.1 of a 98-year-old man taken only moments apart. The postural control mechanisms produce minor shifts in weight in order to avoid fatigue, excessive tissue compression and venous stasis. Hence, a photographic assessment of posture represents a fixed instant of a postural set. Thus, posture is actually a relative condition requiring full body integration and both static and dynamic balance control, as shown in Figure 15.2.

Multiple factors are involved in common age-related postural changes. These factors may be pathological, degenerative or traumatic, or may result from primary musculoskeletal changes, primary neurological changes or a combination of diminutions in the neuromusculoskeletal system.

Degenerative joint disease is a common age-related pathology involving bony and joint surface changes (see Chapters 19 and 24). The osteophytes that result from arthritis may prevent normal joint motion, cause pain and possibly encroach on nerves with a subsequent radiculopathy that includes muscle weakness and imbalance. Postural adjustments may be the result of attempts to unload weight from an osteophyte in order to reduce pain or to accommodate a radiculopathy.

AXIAL AND APPENDICULAR SKELETAL CHANGES

The common age-associated postural changes in the axial skeleton and their clinical implications are enumerated in Table 15.1 and may be seen in Figures 15.3 and 15.4. The idiosyncratic effects of 20 years of aging can be seen by comparing the images of the 78-year-old man in Figures 15.3B and 15.4B with the photographs in Figures 15.1 and 15.5, which were taken when the man was 98 years old. In the lateral view, note the large increases in trunk kyphosis and hip flexion. By comparing images of the posterior view at different ages (Fig. 15.4B and Fig. 15.5), the kyphoscoliosis with upper extremity extension, increased hip and knee flexion and loss of muscle mass in all four extremities and trunk are evident. A different individual, aged 93 years and shown in Figure 15.3C, also demonstrates extension of the upper extremities. The 98-year-old man's postural set (Figs 15.1 and 15.5) may be affected by his complaints of right hip pain, and decreased sensation and strength in the lower extremities. He lives in assisted living and uses a wheeled walker for most ambulation.

It is important to note that not all of these changes should be classified as being faulty or abnormal. Some of the adjustments may be normal compensatory changes resulting from other neuromusculoskeletal alterations in the spine, extremities or central control mechanisms (Barrey et al., 2011). For example, the head-forward position, especially when there is an increased extension of the upper cervical spine, may be the result of the body's attempts to counter a dorsal kyphosis caused by wedged thoracic vertebrae.

The effect of osteoporosis in the vertebrae on posture and vice versa is profound, with an abundance of recognized and silent fractures and probable microfractures (see Chapters 18 and 60). Katzman et al. (2012) found hyperkyphosis, an exaggerated anterior concavity

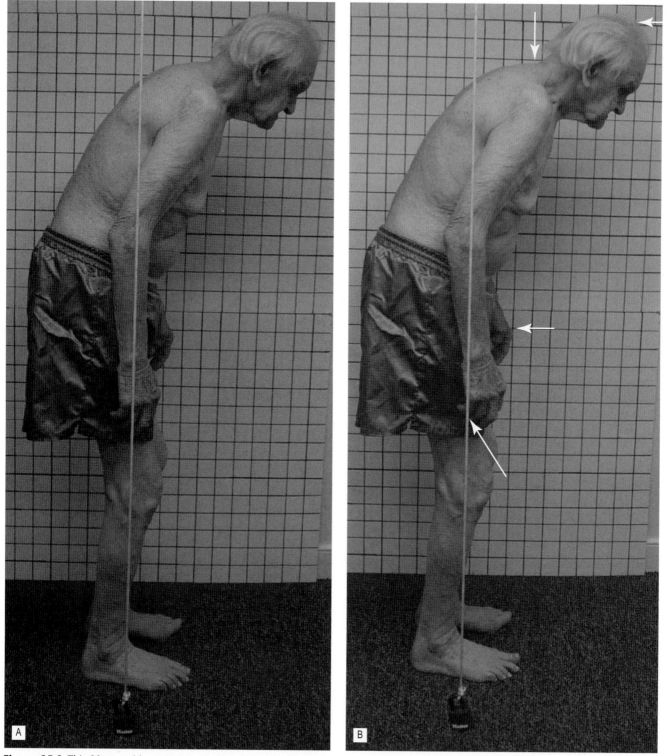

Figure 15.1 This 98-year-old man's posture shows a subtle shift of the hands forward, trunk and head more erect and right great toe extension. The photos were taken less than 1 second apart.

or 'dowager's hump' to be associated with older age, less body weight, lower spine bone mineral density and spine muscle density.

Spinal spondylosis is found in the vast majority of people by the age of 55. This may include deterioration of the spinal facet joints, loss of vertebral height, narrowing of the spinal canal or neural foramina, loss of intervertebral disc space, anterior lipping, formation of bony bridges and calcification of the periarticular connective tissue. Clinically, these changes may cause pain and

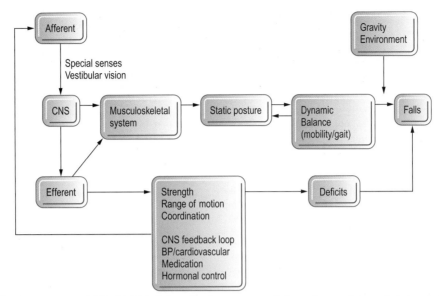

Figure 15.2 Factors affecting posture and falls. Multiple interactive forces govern static posture and dynamic balance. CNS, central nervous system; BP, blood pressure. *(From Kauffman T 1990 Impact of aging-related musculoskeletal and postural changes on falls. Top Geriatr Rehabil 5:34–43.)*

Table 15.1 Age-associated postural axial skeletal changes and their clinical implications

Axial Skeletal Changes	Clinical Implications
Head forward	Shifts center of mass forward; may increase dizziness because of a compromised basilar artery
Dorsal kyphosis	Reduces trunk motions for breathing and motor responses; encourages scapular protraction; may provoke shoulder pathologies
Flat lumbar spine	Reduces trunk/hip extension for gait strides
Occasional kyphosis of lumbar spine	Results from compression of vertebral bodies; not reversible
Increased lordosis (least common)	Results in tightness of trunk/hip extensors; weakened abdominals
Posterior pelvic tilt	Results from prolonged sitting; reduces trunk/hip extension for gait strides
Scoliosis	May alter balance, breathing and extremity motions

reduction in spinal motions, especially the subtle rotation motions involved in segmental rolling and the normal reciprocal pattern of the extremities in normal gait. The sit-to-stand motion may be more difficult because of the loss of coordinated spine flexion and extension.

In the appendicular skeleton, numerous combinations of changes occur as a result of a lifetime of wear and tear, habit, trauma and pathology in the neuromusculoskeletal system. These changes result in the unique postural features of aging individuals. The common age-associated extremity changes and clinical implications are enumerated in Table 15.2 and may be seen in Figures 15.3 and 15.4.

SOFT TISSUE

Postural changes caused by soft-tissue alterations may be a result of previous injuries that have lengthened or tightened tendons, ligaments and joint capsules. Collagen, a major component of skin, tendons, cartilage and connective tissue, may become increasingly stiff because of cross-linkage between fibers. Elastin is another major fibrous component of connective tissue found in skin, ligaments, blood vessels and lungs. With increasing age, elastin is supplanted by pseudoelastin, which is a partially degraded collagen or faulty elastin protein.

Additional soft-tissue changes that may lead to postural alterations can be found in the muscle. The muscle length may be increased or decreased. There is a loss of muscle fibers, which is likely to result in reduced strength. Type II muscle fibers are denervated and reinnervated as type I as aging progresses (Ditroilo et al., 2012), thus altering the fiber relationship, possibly influencing postural control responses and mechanisms. In addition, there is an increase in noncontractile tissue because of deposition of fat and collagen, causing the muscle to become increasingly stiff. Muscle tone may increase, decrease or vary because of changes in nervous system control. A more extensive discussion of these neuromuscular changes may be found in Chapters 2 and 5.

CLINICAL CONSIDERATIONS

Falls are significant problems for aging persons and may represent a failure of the neuromusculoskeletal posture

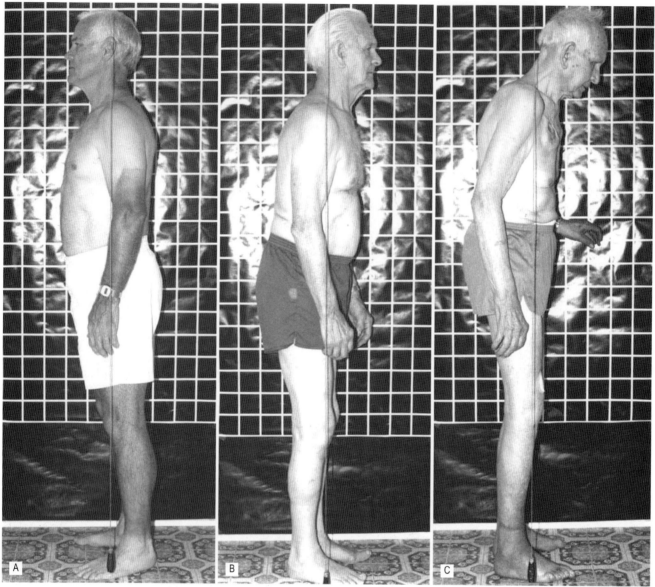

Figure 15.3 Lateral posture of **(A)** a 60-year-old man; **(B)** a 78-year-old man; and **(C)** a 93-year-old man.

control system. Centrally, the basal ganglia and cerebellum have important roles in modulating posture (see Chapter 5). Backward disequilibrium is associated with vascular lesions in the brain, normopressure hydrocephalus and hypertonia of extensor muscles (Manckoundia et al., 2008). Barbieri et al. (2010) reported that their older subjects perceived vertical posture as being posterior by 1°–2.5° compared to persons under 50 years. In response to postural perturbations, older persons used an increased active stiffness and damping (reduces oscillations) to control sway when compared to younger subjects and this may represent degradation in sensory and motor function (Cenciarini et al., 2010).

In the geriatric population, posture should be assessed not only in standing and sitting positions but also in bed, especially in a patient confined to bed because of injury or illness. It is particularly important to prevent pressure areas, and special care should be taken to avoid muscle imbalances resulting from prolonged positioning. Areas of concern are the triceps surae, hip and knee flexors, and hip abductors and adductors, especially after hip surgery. It is common for the patient to assume a supine but side-bent posture that may lead to muscle imbalance. The patient who side-bends toward the operative side will suffer a contralateral hip abductor lengthening and an ipsilateral hip abductor shortening. The converse is true for the patient who side-bends away from the operative side. These muscle imbalances will become significant during rehabilitation when the patient attempts to regain independent ambulation and may contribute to a Trendelenburg gait (see Chapter 16 for discussion of muscle lengthening and the concept of stretch-weakness changes).

Ryan and Fried (1997) found that kyphosis was associated with slower speeds of gait and stair climbing

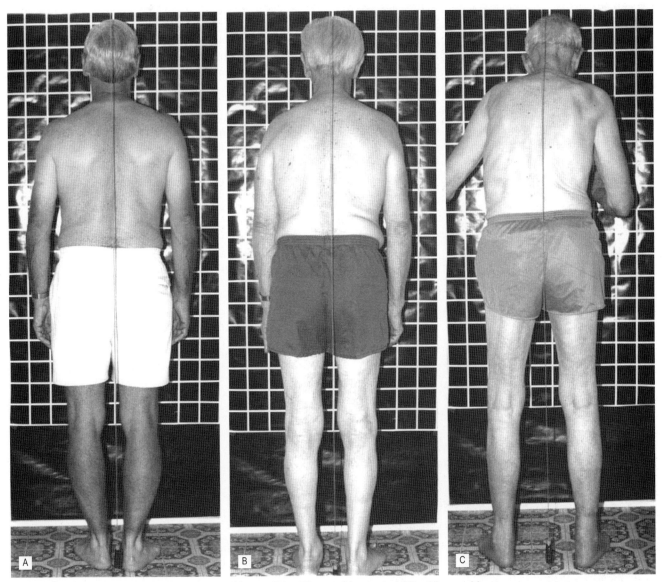

Figure 15.4 Posterior posture of **(A)** a 60-year-old man; **(B)** a 78-year-old man; and **(C)** a 93-year-old man.

and difficulties with reaching or heavy lifting in community dwellers between the ages of 59 and 89. Sinaki et al. (2005) reported that community dwelling females with osteoporotic-related kyphosis had reduced antero-posterior displacement and velocity and increased mediolateral displacement and velocity on a balance force platform when compared with slightly younger healthy control subjects. The kyphotic subjects also had greater balance abnormalities when measured on posturography.

Hyperkyphosis measured in the supine position in 1578 older community dwelling males and females was significantly associated in a stepwise manner with declining self-reported function for bending, walking, climbing and rising from a chair. Grip strength was also significantly associated with this postural change; the greater the kyphosis, the less strength (Kado et al., 2005). Slower speeds were reported by Katzman et al.

(2011) on the Timed Up and Go Test for persons with greater kyphotic angles.

Brown et al. (1995) demonstrated the important relationship between the strength of postural muscles in the lower extremities and functional tasks including walking, stair climbing and getting up from a chair. Weakness of calf muscles coupled with insufficient strength of the scapulothoracic stabilizers can contribute to increased kyphotic posture and loss of balance, especially when reaching forward with the upper extremities.

Menz et al. (2005) reported significant associations between the foot posture index and walking speed and balance impairments. Foot posture index, navicular drop and arch index are significantly associated with medial compartment knee osteoarthritis (Levinger et al., 2010). Clinical intervention should be undertaken in the case of postural changes if they cause pain, impair function or are likely to lead to future impairment. The typical

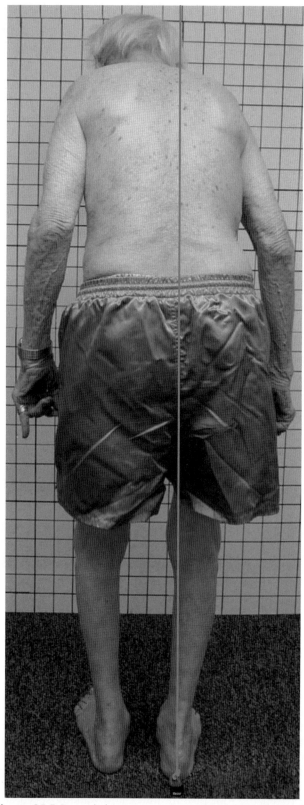

Figure 15.5 Postural changes are quite evident in this 98-year-old man when compared with his posture 20 years earlier (Fig. 15.4B). This degree of change is unique to this individual but is common in aging individuals. Note the kyphoscoliosis with extension of the upper extremities, increased hip and knee flexion and loss of muscle mass in all four extremities and trunk.

Table 15.2 Age-associated postural extremity changes and their clinical implications

Extremity Skeletal Changes	Clinical Implications
Scapular protraction or abduction	Alters normal scapulohumeral rhythm, leading to painful shoulder conditions
Tightness/contractures in elbow flexion, wrist ulnar deviation, finger flexion	Reduces reach and hand function
Hip flexion contractures (loss of hip extension to neutral or 0°)	Reduces stride length; may increase energy cost of mobility and may increase postural control requirements, especially if change is unilateral
Knee flexion contractures (loss of knee extension to neutral or 0°)	Reduces stride length and gait push-off; may increase energy cost of mobility and may increase postural control requirements, especially if change is unilateral
Varus/valgus changes at hip, knee, ankle	Reduces stride length and gait push-off; may increase energy cost of mobility and may increase postural control requirements especially if change is unilateral. Usually is a cause of pain because of mechanical deformation and strain on musculoskeletal tissues

Box 15.1 Clinical interventions for postural changes causing pain or dysfunction

1. Brace, support, immobilize, protect
2. Heat, cold, electrical stimulation
3. Therapeutic exercise to enhance functional muscle strength, tone, length, coordination, and balance between agonist and antagonist
4. Medications
5. Surgery

interventions listed in Box 15.1 are not listed in order of importance. One or all of the interventions may be appropriate, depending upon the clinical assessment and the individual patient's condition and prognosis.

CONCLUSION

It is crucial to note that common postural changes occur with increasing age but their characteristics are unique to each individual. Although not present in a young healthy adult, the new postural alignments are not necessarily faulty. As noted above, they may indicate normal compensation for degradation in the neuromusculoskeletal alignment or a loss of control of any of its component parts. Many of these changes have taken place slowly over decades and may not be ameliorated easily, if at all.

REFERENCES

Barbieri G, Gissot A, Perennou D 2010 Ageing of the postural vertical. Age (Dordr) 32:51–60

Barrey C, Roussouly P, Perrin G et al 2011 Sagittal balance disorders in severe degenerative spine. Can we identify the compensatory mechanisms? Eur Spine J 20(Suppl 5):626–633

Brown M, Sinacore D, Host H 1995 The relationship of strength to function in the older adult. J Gerontol A Biol Sci Med Sci 50:55–59

Cenciarini M, Loughlin P, Sparto P et al 2010 Stiffness and damping in posture control increase with age. IEEE Trans Biomed Eng 57:267–275

Ditroilo M, Cully L, Boreham C et al 2012 Assessment of musculo-articular and muscle stiffness in young and older men. Muscle Nerve 46:559–565

Kado D, Huang M, Barrett-Connor E et al 2005 Hyperkyphotic posture and poor physical functional ability in older community-dwelling men and women: the Rancho Bernardo Study. J Gerontol A Biol Sci Med Sci 60(5):633–637

Katzman W, Vittinghoff E, Kado D 2011 Age-related hyperkyphosis, independent of spinal osteoporosis, is associated with impaired mobility in older community-dwelling women. Osteroporos Int 22:85–90

Katzman W, Cawthon P, Hicks G et al 2012 Association of spinal muscle composition and prevalence of hyperkyphosis in healthy community-dwelling older men and women. J Gerontol A Biol Sci Med Sci 67:191–195

Levinger P, Menz H, Fotoohabadi M et al 2010 Foot posture in people with medial compartment knee osteoarthritis. J Foot Ankle Res 3:29

Manckoundia P, Mourey F, Perennou D, Pfitzenmeyer P 2008 Backward disequilibrium in elderly subjects. Clin Interv Aging 3:667–672

Menz H, Morris M, Lord S 2005 Foot and ankle characteristics associated with impaired balance and functional ability in older people. J Gerontol A Biol Sci Med Sci 60(12):1546–1552

Ryan S, Fried L 1997 The impact of kyphosis on daily functioning. J Am Geriatr Soc 45:1479–1486

Sinaki M, Brey R, Hughes C et al 2005 Balance disorder and increased risk of falls in osteoporosis and kyphosis: significance of kyphotic posture and muscle strength. Osteoporosis Int 16:1004–1010

Chapter 16

Muscle weakness and therapeutic exercise

TIMOTHY L. KAUFFMAN • KAREN KEMMIS

CHAPTER CONTENTS

INTRODUCTION

Muscle weakness has long been associated with aging and is a significant factor in morbidity and loss of function. However, skeletal muscle may be considered the largest organ in the body and has new-found hormonal actions (Doria et al., 2012; Ertek & Cicero, 2012), thus the role of muscle involves more than just providing strength. Muscle is involved with movement, which is crucial for joint nutrition as well as for cardiopulmonary health. Also, muscle is related to the circulatory system, as smooth muscle supports the walls of arteries and skeletal muscle is involved in the return of venous blood. Muscle is also involved in bone health and density. It provides impetus to the nervous system, as primary sensory fibers of the muscle spindle respond to muscle length changes. A principal source of body heat comes from muscle and, additionally, it provides a cushion of compressible tissue that helps to absorb impact in the event of trauma.

DEFINITIONS

Muscle is principally noted for its roles in strength and movement. Sarcopenia is the loss of skeletal muscle mass, strength and function, and is a component of the frailty syndrome (Frontera et al., 2012) and sarcopenia may be associated with a higher risk of death (Landi et al., 2013). Strength may be defined as the tension that is generated by contracting muscle and is best expressed as a force. Torque, a result of angular displacement, is the product of force and the perpendicular distance from the line of the force's action to the axis of rotation. Time is also a consideration for the tension that is generated and thus should be considered muscle power.

The generation of muscle tension is determined largely by the cross-sectional area of the muscle and the recruitment of motor units. Other biomechanical factors, such as muscle length and angle of displacement, and physiological factors, such as metabolism and muscle fiber type, also influence strength. Insufficient strength to perform a functional motor task should be considered weakness.

There are various types of muscle contractions. When there is no change in muscle length, a static contraction occurs, which is also referred to as isometric (same length). Dynamic contractions are a lengthening or shortening of a muscle, also called eccentric and concentric contractions respectively. Isotonic (same tone) contractions involve movement of a constant weight through a motion. Normally, raising a weight is a concentric contraction and lowering it is an eccentric contraction. When a mechanical device resists the tension generated by the contracting muscle, thereby controlling the speed of the limb's movement, an isokinetic (same speed) contraction occurs. Isokinetic devices are essential for assessing torque at various speeds, which is clinically important because of the age-related loss of fast-twitch type II muscle fibers (see Chapter 2). This loss is one of several factors that probably contribute to the increasing inability to recover from a stumble, which results in an increased risk of injury.

ASSESSMENT

Assessment of muscle strength can be performed using a manual muscle test (MMT). Although the MMT is an ordinal scale measurement, it is invaluable because it can be performed in every treatment setting. When using the MMT, it is crucial to specify the type of contraction being performed. The original MMT was designed to be an assessment of strength throughout the available range of motion (ROM), but it has been modified in many circumstances to a 'make' test, in which the patient performs an isometric contraction at a specific joint position. Modification of the MMT may be especially necessary for aging patients and others who have painful arcs or restrictions in motion (Kauffman, 1982). When measuring plantar flexor strength in the weight-bearing position on one leg, Jan et al. (2005) found that men and women between 61 and 80 years of age were able to heel raise a mean of 4.1 and 2.7 times respectively. Men and women aged between 21 and 40 years were able to perform 22.1 and 16.1 repetitions respectively. Clarity in documentation is enhanced when these specifics (type of test and position) are recorded.

In contrast, a 'break test' is used when the patient is asked to hold the joint in a specific position and the evaluator attempts to break the tension that is generated. This changes an isometric to an eccentric contraction and is likely to generate a greater force. It should be noted that in healthy muscle, the highest tension is generated with an eccentric contraction followed by an isometric contraction, and the least tension is generated with an isotonic contraction. This is an important consideration when measuring strength with a hand-held dynamometer because a 'make test' is different than a 'break test'. Caution should be used when measuring strength with the MMT in aging individuals because of the frequent necessity of modifying the test positions. In the aging patient, the test positions as enumerated in the standard manuals may have to be modified because of injury or disease. Also, a more functional position may be necessary because areas of weakness may be found only in certain positions of the joint's ROM. These areas of weakness may be the result of joint-surface irregularities or changes in periarticular connective tissue and muscle length.

Hand-held and isokinetic dynamometers are very useful for assessing strength. Caution must be used to avoid pain in and injury to swollen areas and ulcerated or atrophied skin; the verbal extolling that frequently accompanies this testing may have to be restrained. Also, a greater risk of injury because of age-related changes in periarticular connective tissue (see Chapters 4 and 61) should be considered when dynamometers are being used.

Another strength-assessment technique described in research but almost never in the clinic is the 1RM or 10RM technique. The 'RM' stands for repetition maximum: a 1RM test measures the maximal weight (dynamic and isotonic) that can be moved through the ROM once, and 10RM is the maximal weight that can be moved 10 times. Some guessing is involved in determining the starting test weight, which may be too heavy or too light, and weight adjustments must be made accordingly. These techniques are safe for older patients but caution must be used during testing to avoid injury. Manor et al. (2006) reported another method of assessing strength (and really power and endurance) by using elastic bands and recording the number of complete repetitions of the joint motion that can be achieved in 30 seconds. They found that the elastic band technique was significantly correlated with a 30-second test using dumb-bells and with maximal isokinetic torque.

Perhaps more important than a frank measurement of the force of a muscle contraction is a functional assessment of motor performance, such as the ability to ascend and descend a flight of steps or to raise a 1 kg (2 lb 3 oz) can of food onto the second shelf of a cupboard. Noting that a patient was able to ascend six steps before catching a toe or failing to elevate the lower extremity would be a functional parameter of muscle performance. Endurance is an important consideration, too, especially as it relates to functional outcomes. It is one factor in the 10RM test and is frequently measured with isokinetic devices. In activities of daily living, endurance is always a consideration; for example, carrying a full 1-gallon jug (3.6 kg [8 lb]) of water from the refrigerator to the kitchen table requires muscular strength and endurance.

STRENGTH TRAINING

Strength training research since the 1980s has shown that the potential to increase strength is maintained in older people (Kauffman, 1985). A task force from the Section on Geriatrics of the American Physical Therapy Association has developed 'Principles of Exercise Training in Aging Persons', as shown in Table 16.1. The benefits of strength training with isometric, isotonic and isokinetic routines have been shown. Simple calisthenics without the use of machines are efficacious. Hypertrophy occurs even in individuals aged 90 years and above, although hypertrophy itself is not necessarily a primary objective of care; however, as noted above, muscle mass does act as a shock absorber. Functional outcomes are related to strength and motor performance and should be the objective of rehabilitation.

Newman and associates (2006) reported that grip strength and isokinetic quadriceps strength were strongly related to mortality but that muscle size was not. Stenholm et al. (2012) reported similar findings. Exactly how strength and mortality are associated is unclear but these researchers suggested that the assessment of strength may measure other important aspects of the aging process. It is possible that sarcopenia and frailty, nutrition, disuse, inflammatory factors and hormonal factors related to strength, such as testosterone and insulin-like growth factor (IGF), may contribute to the strength–mortality association. For excellent reviews of the benefits of exercise on diseases, disability, performance and longevity see Warburton et al. (2006) and Kokkinos (2012).

Table 16.1	**Principles of exercise training in aging persons***
	Definition
Principle	
Overload[a]	Tissue must be exposed to increased load or strain to improve function.
	Overload applies to all aspects of the exercises prescription, including Frequency, Intensity, Time and Type (FITT principles).
	Overload should be applied during all forms of exercise, including aerobic capacity/endurance conditioning; or reconditioning balance, coordination and agility training; body mechanics and postural stabilization; flexibility exercises; gait and locomotion training; relaxation; and strength, power, and endurance training
Specificity	The beneficial effects of exercise are primarily specific to the body part involved in the exercise, the type of exercise and/or the skill or activity performed
Progression	An optimal level of exercise will provide the most favorable results. As the patient/client improves, intensity of a particular exercise should be reassessed and advanced to overload the stimuli and optimize results
Recuperation/recovery	Training should not be rushed. The body needs recovery time to avoid undue fatigue and/or injury
Use/disuse	Tissue will maintain or increase function with use and lose function with disuse
Components of the exercise prescription	
Frequency	How often an exercise is performed, typically stated in times per day or days per week
Intensity	How hard an exercise is performed, based on the individual's capacity
Time/Duration	How long an exercise is performed, typically in minutes or repetitions
Type/Mode	The particular exercise performed

[a]Definition from: American Physical Therapy Association. Guide to Physical Therapist Practice, 2nd edn. Phys Ther 2001;81:9–746.
*Adapted from Certified Exercise Experts for Aging Adults Educational Program of the Section on Geriatrics, American Physical Therapy Association, 2013.

MODIFYING STRENGTH TRAINING

When planning a strength training routine for geriatric patients, it is crucial to consider the need to modify the training regimen in order to accommodate pathology in the cardiopulmonary and cardiovascular systems as well as in the neuromusculoskeletal system. Guidelines for exercise in patients with heart disease are presented in Chapter 39. The aging individual is more susceptible to skin tears as well as injuries to muscles, joints and ligaments; however, injuries can be minimized with the use of individualized and sound exercise techniques (Dodd et al., 2004). Fatigue, poor physical work capacity and deconditioning are important considerations, especially in the frail elderly who have multiple diagnoses. The Valsalva maneuver must be avoided. Isometric exercises are safe, provided that the hold time is no more than 5–10 seconds, the standard isometric contraction. Blood pressure has been shown to be adversely affected by isometric contractions longer than 30 seconds in duration.

Aging patients who need an exercise program benefit from individualized instruction that is tailored to meet functional goals. Some individuals are fully cognitive and capable of engaging in standard strengthening and fitness exercises. Others do not have the same physical, cognitive or communicative abilities and, to be effective, the exercise program must be modified.

Monitoring response to exercise is requisite. This is achieved by observing and recording pulse rate, respiratory rate, perceived exertion and quality of movement. For example, asynchronous muscle contractions or obtaining full ROM for only the first 6 repetitions and not all 10 would be indicative of low quality of movement.

Blood pressure should be taken before, during and after exercise, especially in patients with known or suspected cardiovascular, cardiopulmonary or cerebrovascular disease. However, the repeated measurements with the use of a sphygmomanometer can become cumbersome in busy outpatient clinics and in home healthcare. A pulse oximeter is used to measure oxygen levels and may be helpful for establishing safe exercise parameters. Clinically, the talk test is beneficial. This is a simple safeguard that avoids overloading patients beyond capability by talking with them during the exercise routine. When overexercised, the patient will become dyspneic and be unable to talk in two- to three-word sentences.

Postexercise hypotension is a concern in patients who experience light-headedness or near-syncope, especially after endurance training. In these cases, further workup is necessary to rule out cardiac, cardiopulmonary or other potential causes of the problem. These symptoms may result from carotid sinus hypersensitivity when the pulse is taken at the carotid artery. Compression at the carotid sinus may send impulses to the vasomotor and cardioinhibitory centers in the medulla, resulting in hypotension (Ziegelstein, 2004).

TRAINING CONSIDERATIONS

To obtain optimal results, an exercise program for an aging adult should be prescribed based on the individual's abilities and goals. When prescribing each exercise, the therapist should consider each exercise principle and include all components of an exercise prescription. These principles and components apply to all types of exercises, including those to improve aerobic capacity/endurance, muscle performance or balance. Exercises should be monitored and adjusted as the individual progresses to achieve the most favorable outcome.

Exercise can be performed with weights, bands, balls and with body weight alone using isometric, isotonic and isokinetic contractions. The overload principle is necessary but care must be taken to avoid excessive overload. Some patients with cognitive or communicative difficulties may benefit from gestures or ROM exercises, including passive, active assistive, active and resistive exercises, as well as proprioceptive neuromuscular facilitation. Physical contact may assist not only in attaining a desired movement but also in establishing a trusting rapport between patient and care provider. Also, the benefit of sensory stimulation to muscle activation has been recognized, especially in work with individuals with neurological conditions.

Functional activities done repeatedly, such as sit-to-stand 10 times, will not only strengthen muscles but also enhance coordination, endurance and motor learning. Neural adaptations will occur in the motor cortex and in the spinal level that facilitates activation of individual muscles and coordinates groups of muscles. Practice is important for skill acquisition (see Chapter 5).

Some patients have pathologies, for example chronic obstructive pulmonary disease, or are too deconditioned to effectively undergo typical exercise routines such as closed chain activities, progressive resistive exercise and standard aerobic programs; however, they may benefit from a graded circuit routine using a combination of chair exercises and, if possible, ambulatory activities. Sample circuit exercises are provided in Box 16.1. The speed and number of repetitions of these simple exercises can be increased or decreased according to the patient's response to exercise. Walking exercises can also be added. Some individuals may only be able to exercise for 1 minute with this type of circuit routine, whereas others may be able to advance to 3–4 minutes. The talk test or perceived exertion are helpful for monitoring response to the activity. A rest of 1–5 minutes should be taken before repeating the routine. It is safe to start the routine again when the pulse rate has returned to the pre-exercise level. Exercise machines clearly have benefits for some patients. Weight-training units, bicycles, stair-steppers and rowing machines are all beneficial. As mentioned above, simple calisthenics and walking are mainstays in the exercise armamentarium for aging patients. Use of low weights at the ankles and wrists can increase the physical work carried out during simple walking exercises. Aquatic exercise is excellent for strengthening, conditioning and balance retraining, especially after joint replacement, back surgery or in those with painful arthritic joints (see Chapter 73).

SPECIAL CONSIDERATIONS POST STROKE

In a study performed by Mount et al. (2005), it was found that individuals older than 50 years of age who had had a stroke more than 6 months previously could make improvements by undertaking balance and functional activities. This case study consisted of four subjects who underwent a balance intervention twice a week for 8 weeks. Activities varied from a warm-up, including stretches and yoga-like poses, to dynamic gait and Theraball™ exercises. Each class lasted approximately 1 hour. All subjects were assessed using the Berg Balance Scale (BBS) and Performance Oriented Mobility Assessment (POMA), before and after intervention. All four subjects made gains in their functional balance as measured by these two assessment tools. This study illustrates that gains can be made after a traditional course of therapy. Further research is needed to determine the effect of this class in improving functional balance and decreasing the risk/incidence of falls.

Exercise clearly yields favorable effects on disease modification and recovery, and many of these result from systemic actions, including the brain. Archer (2011) presents an excellent review article about the benefits of exercise on executive function, cognition, Alzheimer's disease and brain activities like neuronal arborization and vascular angiogenesis. Aerobic-type exercises showed favorable benefits on brain-derived neurotrophic factor, IGF-1 and neurogenesis. Exercise three or more times weekly has been shown to delay the onset of dementia and to demonstrate benefits in physical performance and cognition (Larson et al., 2006).

WHEN STRENGTH TRAINING IS NOT EFFECTIVE

When an aging patient is undergoing a strength-training routine but there is no marked improvement in strength, a number of factors may be involved in reducing the patient's potential to improve muscular performance. First, adequate nutrition is critical. Sufficient

> **Box 16.1 Sample circuit exercises for the severely deconditioned or chairbound patient**
>
> 1. Check pre-exercise pulse, respiratory rate or pulse oximetry.
> 2. Raise both arms over head 10 times.
> 3. Straighten each knee 10 times (alternate sides).
> 4. Abduct both arms 10 times.
> 5. Flex each hip 10 times.
> 6. Boxing motions of the upper extremities.
> 7. Seated walk in place with reciprocal contralateral upper and lower extremity flexion.
> 8. Repeat above routine, OK to increase speed or expand to additional exercises, if possible, such as wheelchair push-ups; elbow flexion/extension; sit-to-stand; shoulder shrugs; gluteal squeezes; deep inspiration and forced exhalation; resistive exercise with or without elastic tubing; walking. Length of exercise should vary based on the patient's ability and limitations. These more exertional exercises are best performed after the easier warm-up exercises in 2 to 5.
> 9. Check post-exercise pulse, respiration rate or pulse oximetry.
> 10. Rest until heart rate returns to approximately pre-exercise rate, then repeat the routine, if appropriate.

calorie and protein intake is necessary if any exercise routine is to be performed. However, malnutrition is common among the elderly; frequently, ill health precedes it. Decreased physical activity may also contribute to malnutrition, and bereavement, depression, dementia and living alone are all factors that can result in a decreased appetite. Changes in the gastrointestinal tract (see Chapter 8) and medications may also diminish food and fluid intake. Vitamin D deficiency is a factor in osteoporosis that can contribute to back pain and subsequent weakness.

Second, dehydration is an important consideration when conducting exercises with patients, especially in the home-health setting. Adequate hydration is a concern not only during hot humid months but also during cold dry periods. Dehydration can alter mental status and thus decrease receptiveness to exercise. Lightheadedness, syncope and orthostatic hypotension may also present as findings in the dehydrated elderly patient.

The use of statins for hypercholesterolemia may cause muscle complaints such as weakness, myalgia, myositis and even rhabdomyolysis, which can be fatal. These complaints may occur in 10–20% of patients using statins and if suspected a 6-week drug holiday may be helpful (Fernandez et al., 2011). Other factors that may limit muscle responses to exercise include poorly oxygenated blood resulting from chronic lung disease and faulty or reduced cardiac responses. Beta blockers and pacemakers often reduce the ability of the heart to respond to the increased demands from exercise, thereby circumscribing the effects of exercise (see Chapters 6, 7, 39 and 43).

BLOOD CHEMISTRY IMBALANCES

Iron deficiency anemia is not likely to occur in aging individuals with a sensible, balanced diet; however, it may be found in those with neoplasms and gastrointestinal bleeding. This may manifest as decreased hemoglobin or hematocrit levels in the blood chemistry, and the patient may present with fatigue and weakness.

Magnesium is a mineral that is important for normal muscle contraction, and a deficiency is commonly found with low serum levels of calcium, potassium and phosphate. Hypomagnesemia is associated with muscle excitability, hyperreflexia, tetany, seizures, ataxia, tremors and weakness (*Merck Manual of Geriatrics* 2011).

Faulty calcium regulation may also contribute to changes in muscle performance. Hypercalcemia is often associated with primary hyperparathyroidism but may also be found after immobilization in patients with Paget's disease or with malignancies with bone metastases. The elevated calcium levels depress nervous system responses and muscle actions become sluggish and weak (*Merck Manual of Geriatrics* 2011). Hypocalcemia is caused by low serum calcium or low extracellular fluid concentration of calcium ions. It is associated with hypoparathyroidism, renal disease and vitamin D deficiency (Anderson & Xu, 2005). This may increase the excitability of the neuronal membrane leading to spontaneous discharging and tetany contractions, possibly

manifesting as carpopedal spasm. Trousseau's sign is an evaluative procedure used to determine the presence of tetany from hypocalcemia by inducing carpopedal spasm 3–4 minutes after reducing blood flow to the hand with the use of a tourniquet or blood pressure cuff on the arm (Urbano, 2000). Carpopedal spasm is a condition usually found in confused, aging individuals. It manifests as hyperflexion at the wrist and the metacarpal phalangeal and proximal interphalangeal joints on the third to the fifth fingers (Fig. 16.1). The distal interphalangeal joints of these three fingers are commonly hyperextended as they come into contact with the palm. The thumb and the index finger are usually in opposition and pointing. This condition can lead to tissue maceration and ulceration of the palm and the hands.

Reversal of Trousseau's sign is simple but treatment of longstanding carpopedal spasm is frustrating and often not effective. The goal is to prevent further injury. ROM exercises, in or out of water, may be helpful. Use of padding, washcloths or finger spreaders may be tried. Splinting and electrical stimulation to the wrist and finger extensors may be considered.

Hypokalemic myopathy results from decreased serum potassium, which is often secondary to the chronic use of diuretics. Muscle weakness develops slowly over days to weeks and may be the result of hyperpolarization of nerves and muscles, or tetany (Chawal, 2011).

Hypophosphatemia is a low serum phosphate level. Phosphate is normally stored in bone as hydroxyapatite and contributes to energy metabolism and cell membrane function and regulation. Phosphate loss may lead to muscle weakness.

Hyponatremia is decreased serum sodium and excess water relative to the sodium. It is common in patients suffering from diarrhea, vomiting or suctioning. Use of diuretics may also contribute to this condition. Hyponatremia may present with fatigue, muscle cramps and depressed deep-tendon reflexes. Hypernatremia is an increased serum sodium; it may present with symptoms of weakness, lethargy and orthostatic hypotension (Chawal, 2011).

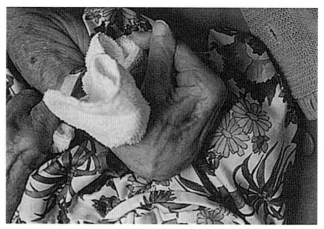

Figure 16.1 Carpopedal spasm manifests with hyperflexion at the wrist and at the metacarpal phalangeal and proximal joints of the third to fifth fingers.

HORMONAL IMBALANCES

Hyperthyroidism can cause acute myopathy in elderly patients (Anderson & Xu, 2005). It may also cause myokymia, which is a continuous quivering or undulating muscle movement. Proximal limb muscle weakness and muscle fatigue may be present.

Hypothyroidism may present with impaired energy metabolism within muscles and decreased contractile force (Anderson & Xu, 2005). Fatigue, muscle weakness and muscle cramps may be seen, resulting from impaired calcium uptake by the sarcoplasmic reticulum.

Prolonged use of corticosteroids in chemotherapy or in conditions such as myasthenia gravis or Cushing's disease may cause a corticosteroid myopathy. Muscle atrophy may be present and may involve most skeletal muscles, but weakness usually occurs first in the hip and quadriceps muscles. Mild aching in the muscles is not uncommon (*Merck Manual of Geriatrics* 2011).

ASTHENIA

Asthenia, is an ill-defined condition characterized by generalized weakness and usually involving mental and physical fatigue. The patient undergoing radiation therapy or chemotherapy may suffer from asthenia and thus may not tolerate the rigors of rehabilitation as defined by the Medicare system (twice-a-day treatments as inpatients in rehabilitation units or a minimum of three times a week in the home or outpatient setting). Other factors that may contribute to asthenia include anemia, malnutrition, infection, metabolic disorders and the use of medications such as methyldopa (Aldomet), Bactrim, Cardizem (Diltiazem), dexamethasone (Decadron), Donnatal, amitriptyline (Elavil), propranolol (Inderal), digoxin (Lanoxin), metoprolol (Lopressor), Novahistine, promethazine (Phenergan), Relafen (Nabumetone), co-careldopa (Sinemet) and alprazolam (Xanax). Asthenia is a factor in the rehabilitation of many frail patients (see Chapter 65).

STRETCH WEAKNESS

Stretch weakness is a theoretical construct for the clinical problem that results when a muscle remains in one position for a prolonged time (Kendall & McCreary, 1983). This is in contrast to the increased tension that is generated by brief quick stretches, such as those that occur with manual stretches or polymetrics. It is thought that weakness manifests as the muscle remains elongated beyond its neutral physiological resting length (Gossman et al., 1982). The exact physiology and morphology are not clearly known and the concept is not universally accepted; however, it remains a tenable theory.

Stretch weakness may be caused by a combination of factors including change in sarcomere length and number, length of noncontractile musculotendinous structures, muscle spindle bias, joint structure and ROM, neural input including excitability of spinal motoneuronal pools (Barry & Carson, 2004), habitual postures, gravity and pain. Often, a muscle imbalance between agonist and antagonist results. It is unclear how long it takes for these changes to occur in aging individuals but

it is most likely gradual over months and years unless paralysis or surgery is involved. Rassier et al. (1999) reported that, in laboratory animals (rabbits), significant increases in sarcomere numbers, which altered the shape of the length–tension curve, were found only 8 weeks after surgical release. In humans, applying the classical length–tension curve concept is difficult because of the changing joint movements and the line of action of the muscle. It is important to recognize that force–length properties can and will adapt to the functional requirements imposed on the muscle (Rassier et al., 1999).

The chronically shortened muscle will lose sarcomeres over time, which will decrease muscle resting length. The shortened muscle will have a leftward shift on the length–tension curve. On the other hand, the chronically lengthened, or elongated, muscle will have an increase in the number of sarcomeres. This will increase the resting length of muscle, and shift the length–tension curve to the right (Gossman et al., 1982). These shifts indicate that, in the shortened muscle, the tension generated is greater in the shortened range, and in the elongated muscle, tension is greater in the longer range, which may be beyond normal postural alignment.

Stretch weakness is commonly seen in postural malalignment and is often associated with arthritic and osteoporotic changes, as can be seen in Table 16.2. As noted by Gossman et al. (1982), the habitually or posturally elongated muscle may test stronger at its new lengthened position but weaker in its more normal resting or postural position.

THE RISK OF PROLONGED SITTING

An example of stretch weakness is seen in the patient who spends an excessive amount of time sitting in a chair, possibly even sleeping in a chair at night. This posture, involving hip, knee and trunk flexion, is likely to lead to increased resting-muscle length of the trunk extensors, knee vastus muscles and the hip extensors. Additionally, periarticular connective tissue may shorten anteriorly at the hip and posteriorly at the knee. Bony and cartilaginous changes may also occur at these joints and in the connective tissue. Full joint ROM is needed in order for proper nutrition to occur and, therefore, a person's inability to move through full ROM decreases joint nutrition.

Typically, a patient in this circumstance stands with hips and knees flexed, a position that has a higher energy cost than normal erect posture with a 0° extension at the hips and knees. When tested in the seated position for hip extension, strength on the MMT is likely to register in the good (4 out of 5) range. However, if the patient is placed prone, the standard test position, the stretch-weakened hip extensors are in a shortened position and are likely to grade in the fair (3 out of 5) range. The same may be found in knee extension with good strength in the midrange and fair strength at terminal extension. An extensor lag may be present. Some patients are capable of performing a locking isometric muscle contraction, which grades as good (4 out of 5) or even normal (5 out of 5), but dynamic contraction in the terminal range may reveal less than good strength.

Table 16.2	**Common areas of stretch weakness**	
Muscles Involved	**Contributing Factors and Manifestations**	**Related Conditions**
Scapular retractors or adductors	Prolonged sitting; dorsal kyphosis and head forward	Shoulder dysfunction, DJD, vertebral collapse, rib fracture
Gluteus maximus	Prolonged sitting; flat or kyphotic lumbar spine, loss of erect bipedal posture	Spinal DJD, vertebral collapse, hip DJD
Trunk extensors	Prolonged sitting; loss of erect posture, dorsal kyphosis	Faulty postural control, vertebral collapse
Knee extensors	Prolonged sitting; loss of erect posture, extensor lag at full knee extension	DJD
Gluteus medius	Hip fracture; trunk side-bent in bed, compensated or uncompensated gluteus medius limp	Scoliosis, leg-length shortening, hip DJD
Ankle dorsiflexors	Prolonged sitting or bedrest with feet resting in plantar flexion position; no heel strike or poor clearance of toes during swing phase of gait	Heel-cord shortening, gait/balance disturbance

THE RISK OF FLEXED POSTURE

A flexed posture frequently occurs in aging individuals, showing the characteristic thoracic kyphosis, forward head and hip/knee flexion. Individuals with the flexed posture generally display muscle imbalances of spine extensors, ankle plantar flexors and dorsiflexors. These muscles, along with the pectoralis major/minor and the hip flexors, are also involved in more severe cases of flexed posture. Change in strength and ROM can lead to further disturbances with gait such as decreased velocity, increased base of support and reduced stride length and cadence. Abnormal loading of these joints can also lead to articular degeneration (Balzini et al., 2003). Compression fractures of thoracic vertebrae also have a negative effect on respiratory capacity, as noted in Chapter 18. Also see Chapters 15, 60 and 72.

TREATMENT CONSIDERATIONS FOR STRETCH WEAKNESS

Treatment should be directed toward (i) improving muscle strength throughout the joint's ROM, especially working the stretch-weakened muscles in the functionally appropriate physiological range; (ii) creating greater physiological balance between agonists and antagonists; (iii) achieving closer to normal postural alignment, both resting and active; (iv) preventing further losses in strength and function; (v) improving balance and gait performance; and (vi) using neurophysiological techniques to enhance motor control. Resistance training itself will not only enhance strength but will also cause favorable neural adaptations with improvements in motor unit recruitment, coordination of synergistic muscles and less agonist–antagonist co-activation (Barry & Carson, 2004).

Emphasis should be placed on motor and postural control and active muscle actions of the agonist as well as on stretching of tightened antagonists and soft tissues. Caregivers and families must be taught about the dangers of prolonged sitting and immobility. Simple sit-to-stand and ROM exercises, especially in the antigravity muscles, are valuable.

In the above case of the prolonged sitting posture, terminal knee extension and the fully erect posture may be gained by working on static quad sets, static weight loading with weights at 0° of knee extension, extensor thrust exercises, bilateral and unilateral toe raises (plantar flexion) and gentle knee bends emphasizing return to full knee extension. Passive ROM may be needed to attain full extension; trunk extension strengthening exercises are also likely to be beneficial. These exercises should be considered not only for the additional ROM and strengthening that they produce but also for their proprioceptive and kinesthetic input into the postural control mechanism and their ability to teach the patient the necessary motion. By gaining good to normal (4 or 5 out of 5) strength in terminal hip and knee extension, a fully erect and energy-efficient posture may be attained; however, this is not always the case as the automatic postural control mechanism of this postural set may not be reprogrammable and one must consider that hip/trunk extension may aggravate spinal stenosis.

CONCLUSION

The loss of muscle strength and muscle tissue (sarcopenia) in aging individuals is an important but reversible condition that influences health, function and quality of life. Humane rehabilitative care requires paying attention to medical diagnoses, nutrition and blood chemistry as well as to the typical muscular evaluation. Recognizing the potential limitations of the muscular system when exercising, allows realistic treatment goals and outcomes to be established.

Amelioration is possible, especially when following the principles of exercise training as shown in Table 16.1, in some, albeit not all, cases.

REFERENCES

Anderson W, Xu L 2005 Endocrine myopathies. eMedicine from WEBMD. www.emedicine.com/neuro/topic125.htm

Archer T 2011 Physical exercise alleviates debilities of normal aging and Alzheimer's disease. Acta Neurol Scand 123:221–238

Balzini L, Vannucchi L, Benvenuti F et al 2003 Clinical characteristics of flexed posture in elderly women. J Am Geriatr Soc 51:1419–1426

Barry B, Carson R 2004 The consequences of resistance training for movement control in older adults. J Gerontol A Biol Sci Med Sci 59:730–754

Chawal J 2011 Stepwise approach to myopathy in systemic disease. Front Neurol 2:49

Dodd K, Taylor N, Bradley S 2004 Strength training for older people. In: Morris M, Schoo A (eds) Optimizing Exercise and Physical Activity in Older People. Butterworth–Heinemann, Edinburgh, pp. 125–157

Doria E, Buonocore D, Focarelli A et al 2012 Relationship between human aging muscle and oxidative system pathway. Oxid Med Cell Longev article number 830257.

Ertek S, Cicero A 2012 Impact of physical activity on inflammation: effects on cardiovascular disease risk and other inflammatory conditions. Arch Med Sci 8:794–804

Fernandez G, Spatz E, Jablecki C, Phillips P 2011 Statin myopathy: a common dilemma not reflected in clinical trials. Cleve Clin J Med 78:393–403

Frontera W, Zayas A, Rodriquez N 2012 Aging of human muscle: understanding sarcopenia at the single muscle cell level. Phys Med Rehabil Clin N Am 23:201–207

Gossman M, Sahrmann S, Rose S 1982 Review of length-associated changes in muscle. Phys Ther 62:1799–1808

Jan M, Chai H, Lin Y et al 2005 Effects of age and sex on the results of an ankle plantar-flexor manual muscle test. J Am Phys Ther Assoc 85:1078–1084

Kauffman T 1982 Association between hip extensor strength and stand-up ability in geriatric patients. Phys Occup Ther Geriatr 1(3):39–45

Kauffman T 1985 Strength training effect in young and aged women. Arch Phys Med Rehabil 66:223–226

Kendall F, McCreary E 1983 Muscles: Testing and Function, 3rd edn. Williams & Wilkins, Baltimore, MD

Kokkinos P 2012 Physical activity, health benefits and mortality risk. International Scholarly Research Network Cardiology. Article ID 718789.

Landi F, Cruz-Jentoft A, Liperoti R, Russo A 2013 Sarcopenia and mortality risk in frail older persons aged 80 years and older: results from the ilSIRENTE study. Age and Ageing 42:203–209

Larson E, Wang L, Brown J et al 2006 Exercise is associated with reduced risk for incident dementia among persons 65 years old and older. Ann Intern Med 144(2):73–81

Manor B, Topp R, Page P 2006 Validity and reliability of measurements of elbow flexion strength obtained from older adults using elastic bands. J Geriatr Phys Ther 29:16–19

The Merck Manual of Geriatrics (Beers MH, Berkow R, eds) 2011 3rd edn. [Online]. Merck & Co. Inc., Whitehouse Station, NJ. (Accessed at www.merckmanuals.com/professional/geriatrics.html December 2013)

Mount J, Bolton M, Cesari M et al 2005 Group balance skills class for people with chronic stroke: a case series. J Neurol Phys Ther 29(1):24–33

Newman A, Kupelian V, Visser M et al 2006 Strength, but not muscle mass, is associated with mortality in the Health, Aging and Body Composition Study cohort. J Gerontol A Biol Sci Med Sci 61:72–77

Rassier DE, MacIntosh BR, Herzog W 1999 Length dependence of active force production in skeletal muscle. J Appl Physiol 86:1445–1457

Stenholm S, Harkanen T, Saino P et al 2012 Long-term changes in handgrip strength in men and women accounting the effect of right censoring due to death. J Gerontol A Biol Sci Med Sci 67:1068–1074

Urbano F 2000 Signs of hypocalcemia: Chvostek's and Trousseau's signs. Hosp Physician 36:43–45

Warburton D, Nicol C, Bredin S 2006 Health benefits of physical activity: the evidence. Can Med Assoc J 174:801–809

Ziegelstein R 2004 Near-syncope after exercise. J Am Med Assoc 292:1221–1226

Chapter 17

Motor neuron pathologies: postpolio syndrome and ALS

MARILYN E. MILLER

CHAPTER CONTENTS

POSTPOLIO SYNDROME (PPS)

Postpolio syndrome (PPS) is defined as aging with polio-myelitis. Bottomley and Lewis (2008) state: 'Diseases of the neuromuscular system … are much more responsible for the decrements seen in aging than [are] the effects of normal aging'. Researchers estimate that 33–80% of polio survivors anywhere in the world will acquire PPS (Elrod et al., 2005; Ragonese et al., 2005). The higher the age of initial onset of polio, the lower the rate of PPS. PPS is reported to be the most prevalent progressive neuromuscular disease in North America (Elrod et al., 2005), with a significantly higher rate in women than in men (Ragonese et al., 2005). The more than one million PPS survivors in the United States of America, many of whom are in their later retirement years, find that their needs are increasing as they acquire other disabilities that accompany the natural changes of aging. To help these survivors avoid complications, rehabilitation professionals need to be sensitive to some of the special issues of PPS (Bartels & Omura, 2005).

The main clinical features of PPS are persistent new weakness, muscular fatigue, general fatigue and pain. The cause of PPS onset is unknown but contributing factors may be the aging motor neuron, muscle overuse and disuse, chronic physical stress and the impact of socioeconomic conditions (Ragonese et al., 2005; Trojan & Cashman, 2005). Pain is a persistent and common problem in persons with PPS, highlighting the need for effective and accessible pain treatments for this population (Stoelb et al., 2008). Attention to an overall healthy lifestyle and prompt identification and treatment of secondary conditions before they progress to greater impairment and/or disability are important to preserve function and maintain quality of life in PPS patients (Stuifbergen, 2005).

A systematic review of research to date indicates that conclusions cannot be drawn from the literature with regard to the functional course or prognostic factors in late-onset PPS; in fact, prognostic factors have not been identified (Stolwijk-Swuste et al., 2005). Weakness of muscle itself defines the functional consequences experienced by individuals with PPS. There is little evidence that the fatigue common in PPS is related to an increase in intrinsic fatigability of muscle fibers (Thomas & Zijdewind, 2006). Thus, this PPS fatigue must be accounted for by other sources, as yet unidentified, perhaps similar to the fatigue reported by multiple sclerosis patients and other diagnoses that involve spinal motor neuron death.

Researchers (Kalpakjian et al., 2005) have developed and validated an Index of Post-Polio Sequelae (IPPS), which offers clinicians a standardized scale to assess the severity of PPS. The IPPS measures the severity of commonly reported late effects problems. IPPS (Kalpakjian, 2004) assesses the degree of severity among 12 commonly reported problems, ranging from slight (1) to extreme (5). The 12 problems are: muscle weakness involved, muscle weakness uninvolved, muscle atrophy, joint pain, muscle pain, fatigue, sleep problems, breathing problems, swallowing problems, cold intolerance, contractures and carpal tunnel syndrome. PPS is usually slowly progressive, with no specific interventions identified. However, an interdisciplinary management program is useful in controlling PPS symptoms (Trojan & Cashman, 2005). Bartels and Omura (2005) have also recommended an interdisciplinary management program that may include (i) pharmacological interventions, limited to some anticholinergic agents, dopaminergic agents or amantadine; (ii) appropriate exercises, bracing and support; and (iii) the use of speech therapy and respiratory support when bulbar or respiratory symptoms are indicated. Persons with PPS may develop dysphagia, even though no swallowing problems were present in the initial onset of polio (Silbergleit et al., 1991). Brehm et al. (2006) recommend maintaining function in individuals with PPS, focusing on stabilizing or decreasing the energy demands of physical activities with exercise programs and/or improvements in assistive devices for walking.

Of particular interest to physical therapists are the PPS findings related to gait, a significant functional determinant of personal independence. A study by Horemans et al. (2005), which investigated the relationship between walking tests, walking activity in daily life and perceived mobility problems in a PPS population in The Netherlands, documented that PPS patients do not necessarily match their activity pattern to their perceived mobility problems. This study reported that PPS patients with the lowest test performance walked less in daily life. This same study also found no significant correlation between perceived mobility problems and walking activities. These researchers further reported that walking in daily life may be more demanding than walking under standardized conditions, an important finding to consider clinically and in future research. In their study of gait, Hebert and Liggins (2005) used a knee–ankle–foot orthosis (KAFO) to compare the locked-knee joint versus the automatic stance-control knee joint in a 61-year-old male subject with PPS. This case indicated that a stance-control KAFO appears to improve gait biomechanics and improve energy efficiency compared with a locked-knee KAFO.

The study by Brehm et al. (2006) compared the energy demands of walking in adults with PPS with those of matched healthy control subjects; this was achieved by assessing muscle strength and strength asymmetry. The findings indicated a significant difference between the groups for all walking parameters. Walking speed was 28% less while energy consumption and energy cost were higher in PPS subjects than in healthy subjects. Further, the walking parameter measures were more variable for the PPS subjects than the healthy subjects. Reduced walking efficiency was strongly associated with the degree of lower extremity muscle weakness, correlated with comfortable walking speed, and accounted for 59% of the variance. This study also reported that the energy cost of walking was associated with muscle strength asymmetry. The physical strain of performing submaximal activities in relation to the severity of the polio paresis appeared to be a determinant of the change of physical functioning over time. As noted, these researchers recommend maintaining function in individuals with PPS by stabilizing or decreasing the energy demands of physical activities. Tiffreau et al. (2010) report aquatic therapy has a positive impact on pain and muscle function. While submaximal aerobic training and low intensity muscular strengthening have shown positive effects on muscular strength and the cardiorespiratory system in persons affected by PPS, in persons reporting severe fatigue it is recommended to adapt the daily exercise routine to the individual specific case.

The almost complete eradication of polio in the industrialized nations has been an important achievement in world health policy. UNICEF formed the Global Polio Eradication Initiative in 1988 and has since made dramatic strides toward its goal (UNICEF, 2006). Rehabilitation professionals and counselors must be knowledgeable about PPS and its possible impact on employment. The physical symptoms can be severe enough to significantly alter work function, impose lifestyle changes and decrease quality of life (Elrod et al., 2005). Important barriers to work participation are encountered, particularly on the components of activity and environment, from the International Classification of Functioning, Disability and Health (ICF) model (Zeilig et al., 2012). The lessons learned now from PPS survivors may serve to improve care for future PPS survivors.

AMYOTROPHIC LATERAL SCLEROSIS (ALS)

Amyotrophic lateral sclerosis (ALS), which is also called motor neuron disease and in the US is sometimes referred to as Lou Gehrig's disease, results in neuron death in the brain and spinal cord. Dupuis and Loeffler (2009) report it is the most frequent adult onset motor neuron disorder. The AARP and ALS Association websites report there are about 30000 persons in the US living with ALS, with 5000 new cases identified annually. Early stages cause movement problems and fatigue, progressing to immobility, respiratory failure and death. More men than women are diagnosed, about 10% is familial, although most cases are random. Although research is ongoing, within the current status for persons with this terminal diagnosis much can be done to manage the physical and emotional symptoms to maintain or enhance quality of life. Smith (2000) reminds us that early diagnosis is not always desirable and that in ALS there is a question about the reliability of clinical diagnostic methods. Further, Smith (2000) states: 'until it is possible to alter the treatment outcome there is little to be gained by early detection'. ALS is fatal within 2–5 years, although approximately 10% of persons with ALS may live 8 years or more. The mind remains alert and in control of sight, hearing, smell, touch and taste. Bowel and bladder functions are not usually affected. The weakness in muscle groups will not be clinically apparent until a large proportion of motor units are lost.

Dadon-Nachum et al. (2011) report: 'This motor unit loss and associated muscle function which precedes the death of motor neurons may resemble the "die back" phenomena. Studies have indicated that in the early stages the nerve terminals and motor neuron junctions are partially degraded while the cell bodies in the spinal cord are mostly intact. If cell body degeneration is late compared with axonal degenerations, early intervention could potentially prevent loss of motor neurons.' Recent results in mouse models showed the key pathological event was the destruction of the neuromuscular junction (NMJ) rather than neuron death. These results suggest neuromuscular junction dismantlement is likely the result of chronic energy deficiency at the level of the whole organism. Krakora et al. (2012) state: 'The importance of NMJ has received relatively little attention in ALS, possibly because compensation mechanisms mask NMJ loss for prolonged periods. ... [R]esearch should focus on the potential for preserving NMJs in order to delay or prevent disease progression.' Related is the work of Gould and Oppenheim (2011) 'to examine the role of neurotrophic factor (NTF) and the intracellular cell death pathway in regulating the survival of spinal and lower motor neurons in the development, after injury and in response to disease'. Human stem cell replacement/gene replacement investigated by Hefferan et al. (2012) calls for 'a more clinically adequate treatment, strategies will likely require both spinal and supraspinal targets'. While Garbuzova-Davis et al. (2008) highlight the novel finding in ALS blood–brain barrier dysfunction: '[Future research may] focus on motor neuron terminals in order to delay or prevent the progressive degradation.'

Simmons (2005) calls for multidisciplinary clinics to support the patients and their caregivers for symptom management to optimize quality of life in the areas of respiration, nutrition, secretions, communication, pseudobulbar affects, therapy and exercise, spasticity and cramps, pain, depression and suicide, cognitive changes, advance directives, and care at end of life. Felgoise et al. (2010) reports psychological assessment of ALS has centered around depression, hopelessness and anxiety. Because psychological health impacts lifespan and quality of life Felgoise et al. (2010) call for broadly based mental health assessment and treatment using tools such as the Brief Symptom Inventory (BSI).

The impact on caregiver wellbeing cannot be underestimated. Boerner and Mock (2012) studied ALS patients and their caregivers for associations of two components of patient suffering – patient physical symptoms and mental distress – with caregiver wellbeing and found in regression analysis there were significant associations of patient distress with caregiver negative affect. Patient support was associated with greater caregiver positive affect, and patient symptoms and support were associated with greater likelihood of caregiver benefit-finding. Boerner and Mock (2012) call for support interventions for caregivers and ALS patients to identify and address challenges in support exchanges between caregivers and patients.

ALS rarely causes pain. ALS is not considered rare, as it is found in 7 out of 100 000 persons. Most diagnoses occur at between 40 and 70 years of age. There is not yet a cure, medicines relieve symptoms and perhaps prolong survival. Exercise is also considered to prolong function and survival. Kujala (2009) states 'there is accumulating evidence that in patients with chronic disease exercise therapy is effective in improving the prognostic risk factor profile and in certain diseases, delaying mortality'. Dalbello-Haas et al. (2008), as a result of systematic review of randomized and quasi-randomized studies of exercise in ALS using the ALS Functional Rating Scale (AFSRS), found a significant weighted mean improvement in the exercise group compared with the control group. However, no statistically significant differences in quality of life, fatigue or muscle strength were found. The studies reviewed were too small to determine to what extent strengthening exercises were beneficial or harmful (Dalbello-Haas et al., 2008). Several studies examined by McCrate and Kaspar (2008) were found to indicate that moderate exercise improves ALS patients' scores on functionality tests and ameliorates disease symptoms. They give 'possible explanations for these findings as exercise induced changes in motor neuron morphology, muscle-nerve interaction, glial activation, and altering levels of gene expression of anti-apoptotic proteins and neurotrophic factors in the active tissue'.

With regard to the outlook for treating spasticity in ALS patients, Ashworth et al. (2006) provided a systematic review of treatment of spasticity. In the single randomized study that met the inclusion criteria for review, they concluded 'individualized, moderate intensity, endurance type exercises for the trunk and limbs may help reduce spasticity in motor neuron disease'. Repetitive transcranial magnetic stimulation (rTMS) has also been examined in the treatment of ALS. To date there is insufficient evidence from systematic reviews of randomized trials to draw conclusions about the efficacy and safety of rTMS in the treatment of ALS.

Extensive lists of websites related to ALS can be found at the Medline Plus URL: www.nih.gov/medlineplus/amyotrophiclateralsclerosis.html.

REFERENCES

Ashworth NL, Satkunam LE, Deforge D 2006 Treatment for spasticity in amyotrophic lateral sclerosis/motorneuron disease. Cochrane Database Syst Rev(1):CD004156

Bartels MN, Omura A 2005 Aging in polio. Phys Med Rehabil Clin North Am 16(1):197–218

Boerner K, Mock SE 2012 Impact of patient suffering on caregiver well-being: the case of amyotrophic lateral sclerosis patients and their caregivers. Psychol Health Med 17(4):457–466

Bottomley J, Lewis C 2008 Geriatric Rehabilitation: A Clinical Approach, 3rd edn. Pearson/Prentice Hall, Harlow, p 67

Brehm MA, Nollet F, Harlaar J 2006 Energy demands of walking in persons with postpoliomyelitis syndrome: relationship with muscle strength and reproducibility. Arch Phys Med Rehabil 87(1):136–140

Dadon-Nachum M, Melamed E, Offen D 2011 The 'dying-back' phenomenon of motor neurons in ALS. J Mol Neurosci 43(3):470–477

Dalbello-Haas V, Florence JM, Krivickas LS 2008 Therapeutic exercise for people with amyotrophic lateral sclerosis or motor neuron disease. Cochrane Database Syst Rev 16(2):CD005229

Dupuis L, Loeffler JP 2009 Neuromuscular junction destruction during amyotrophic lateral sclerosis: insights from transgenic models. Curr Opin Pharmacol 9(3):342–346

Elrod LM, Jabben M, Oswald G et al 2005 Vocational implications of post-polio syndrome. Work 25(2):155–161

Felgoise SH, Chakraborty BH, Bond E et al 2010 Psychological morbidity in ALS: the importance of psychological assessment beyond depression. Amyotroph Lateral Scler 11(4):352–358

Garbuzova-Davis S, Saporta S, Sanberg PR 2008 Implications of the blood–brain barrier disruption in ALS. Amyotroph Lateral Scler 9(6):375–376

Gould TW, Oppenheim RW 2011. Motor neuron trophic factors: therapeutic use in ALS? Brain Res Rev 67(1–2):1–39, doi: 10.1016/j.brainresrev.2010.10.003. (Epub 2010)

Hebert JS, Liggins AB 2005 Gait evaluation of an automatic stance-control knee orthosis in a patient with postpoliomyelitis. Arch Phys Med Rehabil 86(8):1676–1680

Hefferan MP, Galik J, Kakinohana O et al 2012 Human neural stem cell replacement therapy for amyotrophic lateral sclerosis by spinal transplantation. PLoS One 7(8):e42614

Horemans HL, Bussmann JB, Beelen A et al 2005 Walking in postpoliomyelitis syndrome: the relationships between time-scored tests, walking in daily life and perceived mobility problems. J Rehabil Med 37(3):142–146

Kalpakjian CZ 2004 Participants, their health status and data about menopause. Post-Polio Health Int 20(1: Winter)

Kalpakjian CZ, Toussaint LL, Klipp DA et al 2005 Development and factor analysis of an index of post-polio sequelae. Disabil Rehabil 27(20):1225–1233

Krakora D, Macrander C, Suzuki M 2012 Neuromuscular junction protection for the potential treatment of amyotrophic lateral sclerosis. Neurol Res Int Epub August 7 doi: 10.1155/2012/379657

Kujala UM 2009 Evidence on the effects of exercise therapy in the treatment of chronic disease. Br J Sports Med 43(8):550–555

McCrate ME, Kaspar BK 2008 Physical activity and neuroprotection in amyotrophic lateral sclerosis. Neuromol Med 10(2):108–117

Ragonese P, Fierro B, Salemi G et al 2005 Prevalence and risk factors of post-polio syndrome in a cohort of polio survivors. J Neurol Sci 236(1–2):31–35

Silbergleit AK, Waring WP, Sullivan MJ et al 1991 Evaluation, treatment, and follow-up results of post polio patients with dysphagia. Otolaryngol Head Neck Surg 104(3):333–338

Simmons Z 2005 Management strategies for patients with amyotrophic lateral sclerosis from diagnosis through death. Neurologist 11(5):257–270

Smith RA 2000 Effects of the early diagnosis of amyotrophic lateral sclerosis on the patient: disadvantages. Amyotroph Lateral Scler Other Neuron Disord 1(suppl1):S75–S77

Stoelb BL, Carter GT, Abresch RT et al 2008 Pain in persons with post polio syndrome: frequency, intensity, and impact. Arch Phys Med Rehabil 89(10):1933–1940

Stolwijk-Swuste JM, Beelen A, Lankhorst GJ et al 2005 The course of functional status and muscle strength in patient with late-onset sequelae of poliomyelitis: a systematic review. Arch Phys Med Rehabil 86(8):1693–1701

Stuifbergen AK 2005 Secondary conditions and life satisfaction among polio survivors. Rehabil Nurs 30(5):173–179

Thomas CK, Zijdewind I 2006 Fatigue or muscles weakened by death of motoneurons. Muscle Nerve 33(1):21–41

Tiffreau V, Rapin A, Serafi R et al 2010 Post-polio syndrome and rehabilitation. Ann Phys Rehabil Med 53(1):42–50

Trojan DA, Cashman NR 2005 Post-poliomyelitis syndrome. Muscle Nerve 31(1):97–106

UNICEF 2006 Immunization plus. Available at: www.unicef.org/immuniztion/index_polio.html. Accessed April 2006

Zeilig G, Weingarten H, Shemesh Y et al 2012 Functional and environmental factors affecting work status in individuals with long-standing poliomyelitis. J Spinal Cord Med 35(1):22–27

Chapter 18

Osteoporosis and spine fractures

STEPHEN BRUNTON • BLAINE CARMICHAEL • DEBORAH GOLD • BARRY HULL •
TIMOTHY L. KAUFFMAN • BARBARA KOEHLER • ALEXANDRA PAPAIOANNOU •
RANDOLPH RASCH • HILMAR H.G. STRACKE • EERIC TRUUMEES

CHAPTER CONTENTS

INTRODUCTION

Osteoporosis, the most common bone disorder in humans, is a major concern for aging persons, with significant implications for morbidity and mortality. Osteoporosis is defined as a skeletal disorder with compromised bone strength as determined by bone density and bone quality. Specifically, bone mineral density (BMD) of 2.5 standard deviations or more below the young normal mean at the hip or spine is osteoporosis and osteopenia is 1–2.5 standard deviations. In the United States of America, the estimated cost of care in 2005 for osteoporotic related fractures was $17 billion (NOF, 2010). There are nearly 9 million osteoporotic-related fractures a year worldwide (WHO, 2007). There are multiple risk factors, some of which are amenable to lifestyle choices, as shown in Box 18.1.

Osteoporotic vertebral compression fractures (VCFs) represent a significant challenge to societies and health

---

Box 18.1 *Osteoporosis risk factors*

- Deficiency of estrogen, vitamin D and calcium
- Smoking
- Excessive alcohol intake
- Lack of exercise
- High caffeine, salt or aluminum (anti-acids) intake
- Cancer and chemotherapy
- Routine use of glucocorticoids
- Gastro-intestinal disorders
- Hyperparathyroidism
- Diabetes mellitus

Adapted from NOF, 2010 and US Department of Health and Human Services 2004 *Bone health and osteoporosis: a report of the Surgeon General. Available at: www.surgeongeneral.gov/library/bonehealth. Accessed 26 July 2005.*

---

delivery systems. Individuals with a VCF experience a decreased quality of life (QOL) and also show increases in digestive and respiratory morbidities, anxiety, depression and death (Papaioannou et al., 2002; Gold, 2003; Koehler et al., 2011; Edidin et al., 2013). Most importantly, these patients have as much as a five-fold increased risk of another fracture within 1 year of the initial fracture (Lindsay et al., 2001). Up to two-thirds of VCFs are undiagnosed and, even if diagnosed, many patients are treated only acutely; few are managed long term for the prevention of fractures (Papaioannou et al., 2003b,) Thus, this chapter on osteoporosis will focus on VCFs.

According to the National Osteoporosis Foundation (NOF, 2010), primary care physicians (PCPs) need to take a proactive role in assessing the risk for or presence of VCFs and in maintaining or improving general bone health. Many patients consider back pain a normal part of aging and do not discuss it with their physician. Further, the PCP needs to act as the central point of care for a patient with a VCF, working with a spine doctor, physical therapist, clinical social worker, pharmacist and dietician to provide optimal management. To optimize interventions aimed at maintaining function and minimizing disability, all health professionals working in this field should have an in-depth understanding of the patient's functioning and health status as well as a conceptual framework to guide communication among health professionals, clinical research and patient care. Addressing this need, the World Health Organization (WHO) has introduced the International Classification of Functioning, Disability and Health (ICF) (Gradinger et al., 2011; Koehler et al., 2011).

The International Classification of Functioning, Disability and Health (ICF) of the WHO is a conceptual framework and should be used for communication among health professionals, clinical researchers and those involved in patient care.

KEY POINTS AND RECOMMENDATIONS

Key points and recommendations concerning VCFs are summarized below:

- VCFs are common but often silent consequences of osteoporosis (strength of recommendation (SOR): A).
- The risk of death is increased several-fold during the year following a VCF (SOR: B).
- Calcium and vitamin D supplementation, antiresorptive and anabolic agents, and weight-bearing exercises are helpful in preventing secondary VCFs (SOR: A).
- The incidence of fractures can be reduced by 40–60% with pharmacological therapies (SOR: A).
- Magnetic resonance imaging of the spine is probably the single most useful test for evaluating a fracture (SOR: C).
- Vertebroplasty or kyphoplasty should be considered for patients in whom a progressive kyphotic deformity or intractable pain develops (SOR: A).

SOR: A = consistent and good quality evidence. SOR: B = inconsistent or limited quality evidence. SOR C: = consensus, usual practice, opinion, disease-oriented evidence.

PREVALENCE OF VCFs

Of the nearly 9 million fractures that occur each year worldwide, over 1.4 million are spinal fractures (WHO, 2007). One in two women and one in five men aged 50 years and older will have an osteoporosis-related fracture (NOF, 2010). The incidence of VCF increases progressively with age and the risk for males over 65 years of age is increased. VCF are about as common in Asian as for Caucasian women and less common for African-American women (Alexandru & So, 2012).

CLINICAL CONSEQUENCES OF VCFs

Active efforts to diagnose VCFs are critical because only about one-third of radiographically diagnosed VCFs cause symptoms (Black et al., 1996), often just moderate back pain. However, vertebral and other osteoporotic fractures produce cumulative and often irreversible damage (Papaioannou et al., 2002), fracture-related medical problems (Alexandru & So, 2012) and increased risk of death. For example, lung function is reduced significantly in patients with a thoracic or lumbar fracture: one thoracic compression fracture may cause a 9% loss of the forced vital capacity (FVC) (Leech et al., 1990). A four-fold higher prevalence of severe VCFs has been reported in patients with chronic obstructive pulmonary disease than in matched controls, as well as impaired lung function as measured by the percentage decrease in FVC (Papaioannou et al., 2003b).

Multiple VCFs cause height loss, thoracic hyperkyphosis, loss of lumbar lordosis and subsequent compression of the internal organs as the spine no longer holds the body upright (Yamaguchi et al., 2005; Katzman et al.,

---

Box 18.2 *Clinical consequences of VCFs*

- Protuberant abdomen
- Difficulty fitting clothes because of kyphosis, protuberant abdomen
- Back pain (acute and chronic)
- Height loss
- Reflux
- Early satiety
- Weight loss
- Reduced lung function
- Shortness of breath
- Impaired physical functioning
- Fear of fracture and falling
- Impaired activities of daily living (e.g. bathing, dressing)
- Depression
- Sleep disturbance
- Difficulty bending, lifting, descending stairs, cooking
- Increased length of fracture-related hospital stay by 2.0 days
- Increased mortality

From Papaioannou et al., 2001, 2002, 2003b; Yamaguchi, 2005.

2010). The rib cage presses on the pelvis, reducing the thoracic and abdominal space; with severe disease, this space may measure less than two finger widths. Box 18.2 provides some examples of the other effects of VCFs on a patient's life.

ASSESSMENT AND DIAGNOSIS

Symptomatic VCFs usually present as acute thoracic or lumbar back pain. Importantly, little correlation exists between the degree of vertebral body collapse and pain level. Evaluating the patient's risk, taking a history, conducting a physical examination and ordering radiological studies are essential parts of the assessment and diagnosis of a suspected VCF (Fig. 18.1).

Form 18.1 shows the standardized assessment and outcome measure using the ICF Core Set for osteoporosis (brief version) that is recommended by the WHO in a modified version for use in clinical practice (Koehler et al., 2011). Form 18.2 uses information from Case Study B to show possible changes between before and after the operation by using the ICF Core Set.

RISK FACTORS

Low Bone Mineral Density

BMD should be tested in women age 65 and men age 70 unless there are risk factors (see Box 18.1), in which case testing may be indicated earlier (NOF, 2010). BMD is a better predictor of osteoporotic fracture than cholesterol is for coronary heart disease or blood pressure is for stroke (Tosi et al., 2004). If a patient has a fracture, the PCP should determine if the patient has had a workup for or diagnosis of osteoporosis; in the absence of a previous diagnosis of osteoporosis, the patient should be tested. Many VCFs occur in women with normal or osteopenic BMD scores, suggesting the presence of contributing risk factors, which include long-term corticosteroid use.

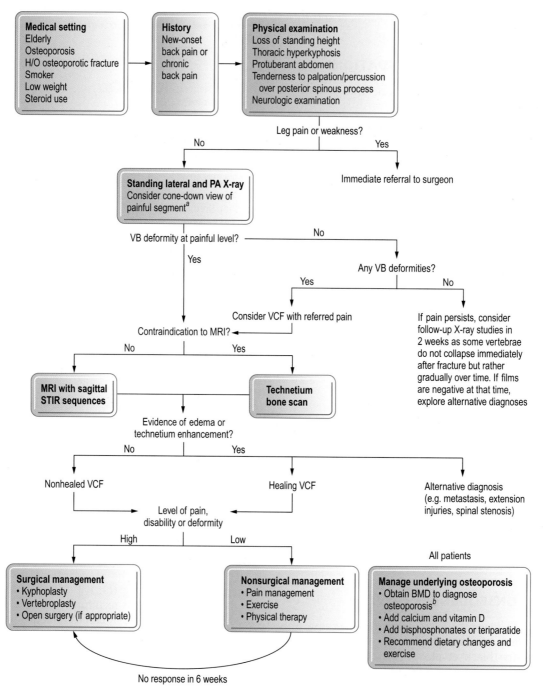

Figure 18.1 Management algorithm for acute painful VCFs. [a]Subtle T11–L1 fractures may be missed because they are at the lower end of a T spine and the top of an L spine film. Moreover, parallax obscures anatomical detail at the edges of an X-ray film. [b]If no osteoporosis, consider malignancy or other trauma as causes. H/O, history of; BMD, bone mineral density; MRI, magnetic resonance imaging; PA, posteroanterior; STIR, short tau inversion recovery; VB, vertebral body; VCF, vertebral compression fracture.

PATIENT HISTORY

Previous Fracture

A history of a VCF and other fractures, for example of the wrist, is also a strong predictor of a subsequent VCF (Lindsay et al., 2001).

DIAGNOSIS

Physical Examination

The physical examination should be performed with the patient standing so that signs of osteoporosis, for example kyphoscoliosis, are more apparent. The recommended

		Before					After				
		0	1	2	3	4	0	1	2	3	4
Body Functions = physiological functions of body systems (including psychological functions)											
b152	Emotional functions										
b280	Sensation of pain										
b710	Mobility of joint functions										
b730	Muscle power functions										
Body Structures = anatomical parts of the body such as organs, limbs and their components											
s750	Structure of lower extremity										
s760	Structure of trunk										
Activities and Participation = execution of a task or action by an individual and involvement in a life situation											
d430	Lifting and carrying objects										
d450	Walking										
d920	Recreation and leisure										
Environmental Factors = make up the physical, social and attitudinal environment in which people live and conduct their lives, +/–											
e110	Products or substances for personal consumption										
e355	Health professionals										
e580	Health services, systems and policies										
Additive problems											

(b), Body Functions; (s), Body Structures; (d), Activities and Participation; (e), Environmental Factors.
0 = NO problem (0–4%), 1 = MILD problem (5–24%), 2 = MODERATE problem (25–49%),
3 = SEVERE problem (50–95%), 4 = COMPLETE problem (96–100%). + Or – means (–) problems or
(+) resources influencing the health problem.
Adapted from Koehler, 2011.

Form 18.1 The ICF Core Set for osteoporosis brief version as a tool for assessment and outcome measure.

procedure is as follows. Beginning at the top and working down, depress the thumb on or over the spinous processes to examine the spine. Although VCFs can occur from the occiput to the sacrum, they most often occur in the midthoracic region and at the thoracolumbar junction (Tanigawa et al., 2012). Ask the patient to indicate the presence of pain; repeat the spine examination as necessary to pinpoint the actual pain location. Pain associated with spinal palpation may indicate a compression fracture. Often, there is an accentuation of the normal spinal contour at the level of injury with associated prominence of the spinous processes in the painful area. The presence of a spinal deformity by itself does not indicate the cause

or timing of the fracture. If there is no identifiable sharp pain, suspect other age-related spine problems. Have the patient flex and extend the spine; these movements often exacerbate pain resulting from VCFs. Moderate muscle spasm or splinting may occur as the antigravity muscles of the spine attempt to unload the pressure on the wedged anterior vertebral body. A postural record can be made with a flexible ruler (Katzman et al., 2010) and a screen for balance dysfunction should be performed. A neurological examination should also be performed. In rare cases, osteomyelitis mimics symptoms of a VCF.

Other findings associated with an increased risk of osteoporosis or spinal fracture are listed in Box 18.3.

		Before					After				
		0	1	2	3	4	0	1	2	3	4
Body Functions = physiological functions of body systems (including psychological functions)											
b152	Emotional functions										
b280	Sensation of pain										
b710	Mobility of joint functions										
b730	Muscle power functions										
Body Structures = anatomical parts of the body such as organs, limbs and their components											
s750	Structure of lower extremity										
s760	Structure of trunk										
Activities and Participation = execution of a task or action by an individual and involvement in a life situation											
d430	Lifting and carrying objects										
d450	Walking										
d920	Recreation and leisure										
Environmental Factors = make up the physical, social and attitudinal environment in which people live and conduct their lives, +/−											
e110	Products or substances for personal consumption				−				+		
e355	Health professionals				+			+			
e580	Health services, systems and policies				+			+			
Additive problems											

(b), Body Functions; (s), Body Structures; (d), Activities and Participation; (e), Environmental Factors.
0 = NO problem (0–4%), 1 = MILD problem (5–24%), 2 = MODERATE problem (25–49%),
3 = SEVERE problem (50–95%), 4 = COMPLETE problem (96–100%). + Or − means (−) problems or
(+) resources influencing the health problem.

Form 18.2 Case Study B using the ICF Core Set for osteoporosis brief version before and after the operation.

Box 18.3   Findings on physical examination suggestive of multiple osteoporotic vertebral body compression fractures

- Rib–pelvis distance: two finger-breadths between the inferior margin of the ribs and the superior surface of the pelvis in the midaxillary line
- Self-report of humped back
- Tooth count less than 20 teeth
- Wall–occiput distance: inability to touch occiput to the wall when standing with back and heels to the wall
- Weight less than 51 kg (women)

Radiology

During the physical examination, a radio-opaque marker may be applied to the skin next to the most painful region; this may, however, obscure evidence of neoplasm or endplate erosions suggestive of osteomyelitis. Standing posteroanterior and lateral radiographic studies may be ordered, with instructions to the radiologist that the objective is to rule out a VCF. A symptomatic VCF does not always show collapse on the initial radiograph and magnetic resonance imaging (MRI) may be needed.

Magnetic Resonance Imaging

If the source of pain remains undetermined, MRI may rule out a malignant tumor, identify the presence of a fracture and help identify appropriate treatment (see Chapter 14). A T1 sequence of an acute fracture will be darker than other vertebral bodies; a T2 sequence will be brighter. A short tau inversion recovery (STIR) sequence is ideal because it is very sensitive for osseous edema following a VCF. Routine imaging of the entire spine is probably not appropriate because of the expense. If the MRI does not reveal edema, the fracture has most likely healed and is not the cause of the pain. When an MRI is contraindicated, a technetium bone scan may be used.

PRIMARY CARE MANAGEMENT OF VCFs

For patients with an osteoporotic fracture, treatment should be aimed at recovery and prevention of a second fracture (Eisman et al., 2012). PCPs should seek to prevent or rehabilitate fractures with nonpharmacological and pharmacological therapies as well as with lifestyle changes and other practices that protect bone (Box 18.4). Management guidelines should focus on (i) decreasing pain; (ii) preserving or increasing function; (iii) preventing additional fractures; and (iv) restoring spine alignment, if possible (Table 18.1).

In the past, conventional treatment included bedrest, opioid analgesics and back bracing to reduce the pain. Unfortunately, prolonged bedrest can contribute to further bone loss, thereby increasing the risk of subsequent fractures. Mobility and balance retraining along with

---

> **Box 18.4 *Rehabilitation of chronic back pain in patients with VCFs***
>
> - Practice good body mechanics.
> - Avoid activities such as forward bending that increase compression on vertebrae.
> - Prescribe an appropriate therapeutic exercise program.
> - Strengthening exercises for the trunk, pelvis, thighs and lower extremities.
> - Emphasis should be on trunk extension and avoidance of trunk flexion and rotation.
> - Tai chi activities have been shown to be beneficial at increasing strength, balance and posture.
> - Gentle aerobic activity, including walking, even with the use of a wheeled walker with hand brakes, may improve mobility.
> - Exercises should be done for a minimum of 30 min at least three times weekly.
> - Use appropriate medications for pain control and bone enhancement.
> - Assess and treat as needed any psychosocial issues.
> - Use modalities for pain control and as adjuncts to exercises.
> - Utilize community support to supplement patient knowledge and understanding of disease.
>
> Consider complementary and alternative treatment approaches such as acupuncture, guided visualization, relaxation techniques or biofeedback.
>
> *Adapted from Katzman et al., 2010; NOF, 2010.*

Table 18.1 **Medical management of a VCF**

	Management
Who to screen Patient type	Women >65 years with no other risk; adult women with a previous history of fracture; women and men on corticosteroids >3 months
What to look for BMD finding	Within 1 SD of the mean: diagnosis normal; between 1 and 2.5 SD below the mean: diagnosis osteopenia; at least 2.5 SD below the mean: diagnosis osteoporosis[a]. The risk of fracture increases with age and with each SD below the mean. A minimum of 2 years may be needed to reliably measure a change in BMD, but a longer interval may be adequate for repeated screening to identify new cases of osteoporosis
Other prominent risk factors (also see Box 18.1)	Previous fracture, low body weight, persistent back pain
What to do All patients	Advocate 1200–1500 mg calcium with 800–1000 IU vitamin D daily and weight-bearing exercise; educate on importance of good exercise and calcium intake; prescribe and encourage compliance with a medication that increases BMD; refer to physical therapy if help is needed to promote an osteoporosis exercise program; identify any coexisting medical conditions that cause or contribute to bone loss (Cushing's syndrome, diabetes mellitus, inflammatory bowel syndrome, multiple myeloma, end-stage renal disease, chronic metabolic acidosis) by ordering initial lab workup that includes: complete blood count; spinal films; chemistry profile (calcium, total protein, albumin, LFTs, creatinine, electrolytes); 24-h urine calcium; vitamin D levels (25-hydroxy vitamin D, dihydroxyvitamin D-25 levels); thyroid-stimulating hormone; erythrocyte sedimentation rate; alkaline phosphatase; phosphorus
Acute treatment	Bedrest (prolonged bedrest can lead to further bone loss); analgesics (NSAIDs may inhibit repair of the bone fracture, whereas opioids may cause constipation); braces; pharmacological treatment of osteoporosis; for patients with persistent back pain, refer to a spine specialist for workup for vertebroplasty or kyphoplasty
Long-term management	Patient may require home care for an assessment of risk of falls at home; be aware that VCF may cause loss of physical functioning and depression in patients; be prepared for a consultation to assess social and physical functioning
Prevention strategies	Physical therapy: gait and back strengthening, education on proper lifting etc., appropriate use of walker or cane; patient education: smoking cessation, calcium and vitamin D supplements, medication, importance of BMD results, exercise; environmental assessment: lighting, carpeting, living on one floor vs multilevel

From Papaioannou et al., 2001; NOF, 2010; NICE, 2012.
BMD, bone mineral density; LFTs, liver function tests; NSAIDs, nonsteroidal anti-inflammatory drugs; SD, standard deviation; VCF, vertebral compression fracture
[a]Young adult mean.

strengthening, breathing and posture exercises were not prominent in conservative care. Opioid analgesics should be used cautiously as their central nervous system effects may increase the risk of falling.

NONPHARMACOLOGICAL PREVENTION STRATEGIES

Exercise

Weight-bearing, balance, aerobic and resistance exercises have been reported to maintain or increase BMD and promote mobility, agility, muscle strength and postural stability (Kemmler et al., 2012). Cheung and Giangregorio (2012) summarized that older persons engaging in strength training activity can enhance their BMD, and exercises to challenge balance may reduce the risk of falls and fractures. Gomez-Cabello et al., (2012) conducted a systematic review of the effects of training on bone mass in older male and female adults. They concluded that aerobic activities, such as walking, have less beneficial effect on BMD than strength training and multi-component training activities. An active lifestyle starting at a young age is encouraged (NOF, 2010). The benefits of bicycling are many but they do not appear to have beneficial effects on hip BMD.

Diet

Adequate daily intake of dietary or supplementary vitamin D and calcium is essential. There has been some recent concern that calcium supplements may be associated with a small increase for adverse cardiovascular events; however, this is not well established with impeccable research evidence. After careful scrutiny of the data, Heaney et al. (2012) advocate the continued use of the guidelines as set forth in Table 18.1.

Patient Education and Counseling

Because compliance with an exercise program or pharmacological regimen declines as early as 1 year after initiation (Papaioannou et al., 2003a), patient education is essential. Referral to a clinical social worker may be useful to identify premorbid anxiety and depression. The ICF Core Set is a tool for assessment and outcome measure by gaining the patient's perspective and also provides an educational aspect – see Table 18.1 (Gradinger et al., 2011; Koehler et al., 2011).

Physical Therapy

Physical therapy is essential to prevent deformity by strengthening antigravity muscles and promoting postural retraining. Breathing exercises encourage thoracic expansion, improve pulmonary function and reduce the risk of pulmonary compromise. A description of rehabilitation for spine fracture is provided in Chapter 24.

Bracing

To allow early physical therapy and control pain, use of a limited contact brace may be warranted. However, long-term bracing is discouraged. Compliance with bracing is low, especially with the rigid body jackets or the Knight–Taylor orthoses. Lightweight thoracolumbar braces (easier to put on and take off) may improve compliance. For lumbar fractures, a chairback brace is recommended, whereas cruciform anterior spinal hyperextension (CASH) or Jewett braces are appropriate for thoracic fractures. Lumbar corsets are not recommended as they place additional stress on fractures at the thoracolumbar junction (see Chapter 69). Braces may need to be adjusted for individual patients by an orthotist or therapist; customized braces can also be ordered from orthotic facilities.

Pharmacological Therapy

Pharmacological therapy is an important component of care for patients with osteoporosis. Other than the acute management of pain, the role of pharmacological therapy is to maintain or increase BMD and reduce the risk of future fractures. There are a number of available agents including estrogen, estrogen agonists/antagonists also known as Selective Estrogen Receptor Modulators (SERMs), parathyroid hormone and bisphosphonates, but there are some potential negative side-effects (NOF, 2010). Calcitonin, approved since the 1980s in the US, has recently had reports of increased risks of cancer and the efficacy for fracture reduction has not been clearly established. Thus, the European Medicines Agency and others recommend that calcitonin is not used for osteoporosis and fracture prevention (Overman et al., 2013). Strontium ranelate is used in Europe but not in the US at the time of this writing. Denosumab is the latest bone enhancing medication approved for use in the US. The choice of a specific drug is dependent on the patient's fracture risk, tolerance and the drug side-effects, but medications should always be used in combination with exercise, instruction in body mechanics, good posture, calcium and vitamin D.

SURGICAL MANAGEMENT OF VCFs

Kyphoplasty and vertebroplasty, two minimally invasive procedures, stabilize a VCF, reduce pain, increase spinal function and restore normal daily function. Open surgical treatment can address deformity but is reserved for cases of neurological deficit. In many cases, poor bone strength precludes the use of orthopedic screws or other open surgical treatment. Kyphoplasty and vertebroplasty are performed by orthopedists, neurosurgeons and interventional radiologists. Both procedures involve an incision site of less than 1 cm and can be performed on an inpatient or outpatient basis under local or general anesthesia. Kyphoplasty restores spinal alignment, theoretically reducing the risk of subsequent fractures.

There are some risks and controversy about these procedures, mainly cement leakage and increased risk of new fractures. Klazen et al. (2010) reported no significant increase in VCF 1 year after vertebroplasty when compared to nonsurgical care. A back exercise program after vertebroplasty demonstrated significantly better results at 1 and 2 years on the visual analog pain scale and on the Oswestry Disability Index (Chen et al., 2012). However, Kallmes et al. (2009) reported that there were no superior benefits in pain reduction or scores on the Roland Morris Disability Questionnaire when

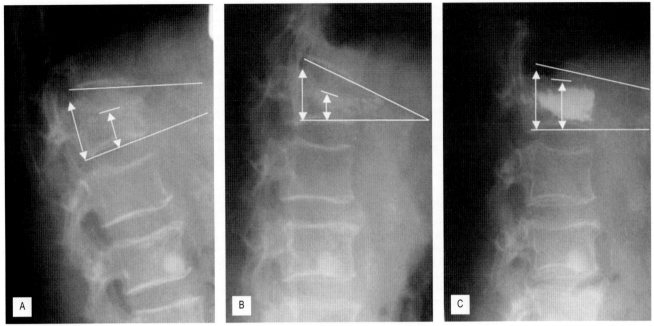

Figure 18.2 Kyphoplasty: effect on vertebral height and reduction of spinal deformity. **(A)** Immediately post fracture, kyphosis = 16°; **(B)** post fracture + 4 days, kyphosis = 25°; **(C)** post kyphoplasty, kyphosis = 10°. *(Reproduced with permission of Dr Isador Lieberman.)*

comparing persons who had vertebroplasy or simulated procedures without injection of bone cement.

KYPHOPLASTY: AN OVERVIEW

Kyphoplasty involves the stabilization of the fracture using bone cement (polymethylmethacrylate [PMMA]). The procedure is initiated by inserting a balloon tamp into the vertebral body under fluoroscopic guidance. The balloon is inflated, restoring vertebral height and moving the weight-bearing axis posteriorly to reduce spinal deformity (Fig. 18.2). The size of the void created by the balloon is determined, the balloon is removed and the void is filled with a precise amount of cement at low pressure to minimize extravasation. Pain reduction occurs in 60–97% of patients with rapid improvement in daily activity levels and QOL; benefits are sustained for at least 2 years (Lieberman et al., 2001). In one study only 8% of patients had a subsequent fracture within 2 years (Giannotti et al., 2012). Physical functioning shows significant improvement, with an increase from 12 to 47 in the physical functioning subscale score of the Short Form 36 (Lieberman et al., 2001), a survey assessing health status in eight different areas, including physical functioning, bodily pain and general mental health.

The extent of fracture deformity correction has been expressed variously in different studies as the angular correction (i.e. Cobb angle), the amount of correction or the degree to which the vertebral body returns to the expected height. Overall, a mean 50% of the lost height is restored. Acute or 'readily reducible' fractures are typically corrected to 90% of their prefracture height (Lieberman et al., 2001). Early referral of appropriate patients is important because the likelihood of

height restoration decreases with time after the injury. However, the age of the fracture is irrelevant if the fracture is painful and STIR-sequence MRI reveals edema at the culprit vertebrae. Procedure-related complication rates range from 0.2% to 0.7% and include extravasation, embolism and nerve root injury.

VERTEBROPLASTY: AN OVERVIEW

Initially used to treat symptomatic hemangiomas of the vertebral body, vertebroplasty is now used more frequently in the management of painful osteoporotic VCFs. Unlike kyphoplasty, a balloon tamp is not involved and so this procedure may not restore height or reduce spinal deformity. Bone cement is injected under fluoroscopic guidance into the vertebral body to stabilize the fracture in its current position. Pain relief is achieved but in one study 18% of the patients experienced new vertebral fractures and underwent additional vertebroplasties (Al-Ali et al., 2009). Unfortunately, the spinal deformity remains as the fracture is cemented in place. The failure and complication rates are low, but extravasation of the cement into veins, soft tissue and disc occurred in 33% of cases without any complications (Al-Ali et al., 2009). There is concern that bone cement leakage can cause nerve injury and embolism is possible.

Tanigawa et al. (2012) reported significant improvements in pulmonary function for vital capacity (VC) and FVC 1 month post vertebroplasty. This is important because the long-term effect of VCF is pulmonary compromise, which can be fatal. Following either procedure, it is important that calcium, vitamin D and other pharmacological and rehabilitative measures be implemented to prevent a secondary VCF.

CASE STUDY A

KYPHOPLASTY

A 69-year-old woman experiences excruciating and immediate back pain after slipping on ice. X-ray studies demonstrate marked collapse of the L2 vertebra. Nonoperative management with bracing, nasal miacalcin, opioids, relative rest and physical therapy fail to control pain. Patient is nonambulatory. MRI STIR sequences demonstrate intense uptake in the L2 vertebral body, whereas the T1 marrow signal is decreased. Subsequent radiographs demonstrate further collapse of the vertebra. Because of progressive deformity and intense pain, a kyphoplasty is performed, with balloons inserted into the L2 vertebral body under local anesthesia. Serial inflation of the balloons allows restoration of lost vertebral body height; the fracture is stabilized with PMMA. A postoperative computed tomography (CT) scan reveals excellent restoration of the vertebral morphology without cement leak. Long-term therapy with a bisphosphonate, vitamin D and calcium are also instituted.

CASE STUDY B

VERTEBROPLASTY

A 74-year-old woman with primary osteoporosis complains of 4 weeks of gradually increasing low back pain after having picked up a potted plant. Radiographs reveal a mild superior endplate fracture of L3. Initial management (brace, physical therapy and pain medications) fails to relieve pain. The patient's pacemaker precludes an MRI scan. A bone scan and CT scan demonstrate intensely increased uptake suggestive of an acute fracture without evidence of lytic lesion or canal compromise. To relieve intractable pain, a vertebroplasty is performed under local anesthesia. The patient notes immediate relief of her pain. Postoperative plain radiographs and a CT scan demonstrate an appropriate cement mantle with only mild intravascular leakage. Long-term therapy with a bisphosphonate, vitamin D and calcium are also instituted.

CONCLUSION

VCF is a relatively common consequence of osteoporosis. Back pain is the typical presenting symptom; patients older than 50 years with acute back pain should undergo a clinical workup for a VCF. Primary care clinicians have important roles as educators about bone health and as providers of pharmacological therapies. Additionally, they are critical in coordinating the multidisciplinary care of a patient with a VCF. Kyphoplasty and vertebroplasty stabilize a VCF, increase spinal function and restore normal daily function. They provide rapid pain improvement with a low complication rate. Restoration of the vertebral height is an added benefit of kyphoplasty. Standardized international and multidisciplinary assessment and outcome measures with the ICF Core Set of the WHO could be useful for daily practice as well as research and development (Gradinger et al., 2011; Koehler et al., 2011).

Acknowledgment

Modified with permission from Brunton S, Carmichael B, Gold D et al., 2005 Vertebral compression fractures in primary care: recommendations from a consensus panel. J Fam Pract 54:781–8. The publication's recommendations stemmed from a review of the literature and panel members' clinical experiences. Highlighted are the impact of VCFs on overall QOL, risk factors for VCFs and a discussion of management options for patients with VCFs.

REFERENCES

Al-Ali F, Barrow T, Luke K 2009 Vertebroplasty: what is important and what is not. AJNR Am J Neuroradiol 30:1835–1839

Alexandru D, So W 2012 Evaluation and management of vertebral compression fractures. Perm J 16:46–51

Black DM, Cummings SR, Karpf DB et al 1996 Randomised trial of effect of alendronate on risk of fracture in women with existing vertebral fractures. Fracture Intervention Trial Research Group. Lancet 348:1535–1541

Chen B, Zhong Y, Huang Y et al 2012 Systematic back muscle exercise after percutaneous vertebroplasty for spinal osteoporotic compression fracture patients: a randomized controlled trial. Clin Rehabil 26:483–492

Cheung A, Giangregorio L 2012 Mechanical stimuli and bone health: what is the evidence? Curr Opin Rheumatol 24:561–566

Edidin A, Ong K, Lau E et al 2013 Life expectancy following diagnosis of a vertebral compression fracture. Osteoporos Int 24:451–458

Eisman J, Bogoch E, Dell R et al 2012 Making the first fracture the last fracture: ASBMR task force on secondary fracture prevention. J Bone Miner Res 27:2039–2046

Giannotti S, Carmassi F, Bottai V et al 2012 Comparison of 50 vertebral compression fractures treated with surgical (kyphoplasty) or nonsurgical approach. Clin Cases Miner Bone Metab 9:184–186

Gold DT 2003 Osteoporosis and quality of life, psychosocial outcomes and interventions for individual patients. Clin Geriatr Med 19:271–280

Gomez-Cabello A, Gonzalez-Aguero A, Casajus JA et al 2012 Effects of training on bone mass in older adults a systemic review. Sports Med 42:301–325

Gradinger F, Koehler B, Khatami R et al 2011 Problems in functioning from the patient perspective using the International Classification of Functioning, Disability and Health (ICF) as a reference. J Sleep Res 20(1 Pt 2):171–182

Green A, Colon-Emeric C, Bastian L et al 2004 Does this woman have osteoporosis? JAMA 292:2890–2900

Heaney R, Kopecky S, Maki KC et al 2012 A review of calcium supplements and cardiovascular disease risk. Adv Nutr 2(6):763–771

Kallmes D, Comstock B, Heagerty P et al 2009 A randomized trial of vertebroplasty for osteoporotic spinal fractures. N Engl J Med 361:569–579

Katzman W, Wanek L, Shepherd J et al 2010 Age-related hyperkyphosis: its causes, consequences and management. J Ortho Sports Phys Ther 40:352–360

Kemmler W, Häberle L, von Stengel S 2013 Effects of exercise on fracture reduction in older adults a systematic review and meta-analysis. Osteoporos Int 24(7):1937–1950

Klazen C, Venman A, de Vries J et al 2010 Percutaneous vertebroplasty is not a risk factor for new osteoporotic compression fractures: results from VERTOS II. AJNR Am J Neuroradiol 31:1447–1450

Koehler B, Kirchberger I, Glaessel A et al 2011 Validation of the International Classification of Functioning, Disability and Health Comprehensive Core Set for Osteoporosis: the perspective of physical therapists. J Geriatric Phys Ther 34:117–130

Leech JA, Dulberg C, Kellie S et al 1990 Relationship of lung function to severity of osteoporosis in women. Am Rev Respir Dis 14:68–71

Lieberman IH, Dudeney S, Reinhardt MK et al 2001 Initial outcome and efficacy of 'kyphoplasty' in the treatment of painful osteoporotic vertebral compression fractures. Spine 26:1631–1638

Lindsay R, Silverman SL, Cooper C et al 2001 Risk of new vertebral fracture in the year following a fracture. JAMA 285:320–323

NICE (National Institute for Health and Care Excellence) 2012. Osteoporosis: assessing the risk of fragility fracture. NICE Clinical Guideline 146. NICE, UK. (Accessed at guidance.nice.org.uk/cg146 March 2014)

NOF (National Osteoporosis Foundation) 2010 Clinician's Guide to Prevention and Treatment of Osteoporosis. NOF, Washington DC

Overman R, Borse M, Gourlay M 2013 Salmon calcitonin use and associated cancer risk. Ann Pharmacother 47:1675–1684

Papaioannou A, Adachi JD, Parkinson W et al 2001 Lengthy hospitalization associated with vertebral fractures despite control for comorbid conditions. Osteoporos Int 12:870–874

Papaioannou A, Watts NB, Kendler DL et al 2002 Diagnosis and management of vertebral fractures in elderly adults. Am J Med 113:220–228

Papaioannou A, Adachi JD, Winegard K et al 2003a Efficacy of home-based exercise for improving quality of life among elderly women with symptomatic osteoporosis related vertebral fractures. Osteoporos Int 14:677–682

Papaioannou A, Parkinson W, Ferko N et al 2003b Prevalence of vertebral fractures among patients with chronic obstructive pulmonary disease in Canada. Osteoporos Int 14:913–917

Tanigawa N, Kariya S, Komemushi A et al 2012 Added value or percutaneous vertebroplasty: effects on respiratory function. AJR Am J Neuroradiol 198:W51–W54

Tosi LL, Bouxsein ML, Johnell O 2004 Commentary on the AAOS position statement: recommendations for enhancing the care for patients with fragility fractures. Techniques Orthopediques 19:121–125

WHO (World Health Organization) 2007 Scientific Group on the Assessment of Osteoporosis at Primary Health Care Level. WHO, Geneva

Yamaguchi T, Sugimoto T, Yamauchi M et al 2005 Multiple vertebral fractures are associated with refractory reflux esophagitis in postmenopausal women. J Bone Miner Metab 23:36–40

Chapter 19
Rheumatic conditions

JUNE E. HANKS • DAVID LEVINE

INTRODUCTION

Rheumatic disease, commonly known as arthritis, is a term used to describe a collection of diseases affecting the joints and soft tissues. Arthritis-related musculoskeletal disorders contribute significantly to disability globally (Vos et al., 2012) and in the United States of America (Hootman et al., 2006). Predictions indicate that by the year 2030, arthritis will affect one-quarter of the US population, with women being more often affected than men (Cheng et al., 2010). A diagnosis of arthritis may be established following careful attention to clinical manifestations, laboratory tests, radiographic and imaging studies, and responses to drug therapy. Although arthritis can affect anyone, certain types of arthritis are commonly associated with aging. Discussed below is the pathophysiology, medical management and recommended therapy for the following rheumatic conditions: osteoarthritis, rheumatoid arthritis, systemic lupus erythematosus, gout, pseudogout, polymyalgia rheumatica, bursitis and tendinitis.

OSTEOARTHRITIS

Osteoarthritis (OA), also called osteoarthrosis or degenerative joint disease, is the most common joint disorder and one of the leading causes of disability in the elderly. The condition involves cartilage degeneration, the remodeling of subchondral bone and overgrowth of bone at joint margins. Joint effusion and thickening of the synovium and capsule also may occur. OA affects women more than men, though both genders are affected with severity increasing with age (Deyle et al., 2012). The most affected joints are the weight-bearing synovial joints of the lower extremity, the spine and the carpometacarpal and distal interphalangeal joints of the hand (CDC, 2013a).

OA occurring without a predisposing condition is called 'primary OA', whereas 'secondary OA' results from a local or systemic factor such as trauma, developmental deformity, infection, or following cartilage damage due to another disease or another form of arthritis. The disease process of OA affects the entire joint, including the articular cartilage, synovium, subchondral bone and surrounding supportive connective tissues. The most marked changes in OA involve the articular cartilage. In an unaffected joint, the articular cartilage provides a smooth, almost frictionless weight-bearing joint surface which spreads and minimizes local loads. Repeated excessive loading of normal cartilage and subchondral bone, or normal loading of biologically deficient cartilage and subchondral bone, may lead to microcracks and uneven distribution of chondrocytes. The degenerating, thinning cartilage is less able to redistribute forces, leading to greater force transference to the subchondral bone (Egloff et al., 2012). The reaction is subchondral bone hardening and the formation of osteophytes (bone spurs) at joint margins. As the joint surface deteriorates, the joint capsule may become lax, leading to joint instability. OA is evidenced on radiographs by decreased joint space, osteophyte formation, subchondral sclerosis and subchondral trabecular fractures. Radiographic evidence of OA is present in the majority of older individuals, though not all individuals are symptomatic. Generally, however, a positive correlation exists between clinical and radiographic findings. Factors contributing to OA include aging, excess body weight, occupational or sport joint injury, and metabolic or endocrine disorders (Deyle et al., 2012).

Clinical characteristics include joint pain, stiffness, tenderness, instability and enlargement. Periarticular muscle atrophy and weakness occur, contributing to disability. Early in the disease course, pain is worsened by activity and relieved by rest. With disease progression, pain is often present even at rest and may lead to significant functional impairment. Articular cartilage is devoid of nerve endings, thus the pain associated with OA arises from innervated intraarticular and periarticular structures. In the spine, bony overgrowth may encroach on emerging nerve roots, causing pain. Stiffness, usually occurring in the mornings and following periods of rest, is relieved by movement. Motion limitation may be caused by irregular joint surface movement due to cartilage degeneration, muscle spasms due to pain, muscle weakness due to disuse and osteophyte formation. Crepitus, a clicking or crackling sound, may occur as the joint is moved. Joints may enlarge due to synovitis, joint effusion, connective tissue overgrowth, or osteophyte formation. Joint deformity may occur, as forces are inappropriately distributed between joint structures.

Inflammation is not a typical characteristic of OA, but may occur as the irritated synovium contributes to the activation of chondrocytes causing production of a wide range of inflammatory mediators that release cartilage-damaging products. The imbalance between chondrocyte synthesis and degradation stimulates further production of proinflammatory mediators and proteinases. The naturally occurring tissue inhibitors become overwhelmed and crystals may be deposited in the degenerating cartilage, sometimes breaking off into the joint and creating acute or chronic inflammation (Walker, 2004).

The aim of therapeutic intervention is to relieve symptoms, maintain and improve function, and limit the degree of functional impairment. Typical therapeutic interventions for OA include education, rest, pharmacologic agents, exercise, weight reduction and possibly surgery. Patients should be instructed in joint protection and energy conservation techniques to help prevent acute flare-ups and to help minimize joint stress and pain. Regularly administered pharmacologic agents include analgesics and nonsteroidal anti-inflammatory drugs (NSAIDs). Intraarticular corticosteroid injections may benefit acute joint inflammation.

Rehabilitation should include appropriate weight-bearing and non-weight-bearing exercise. The Ottawa Panel Evidence-Based Clinical Practice Guidelines recommends therapeutic exercise, particularly strengthening and general activity, with or without manual therapy, in managing pain and functional impairment of OA (Ottawa Panel, 2005), though manual therapy in addition to exercise may enhance pain relief (Jansen et al., 2011). Individualized programs should include strengthening, range of motion and cardiovascular fitness. To minimize stress on the joints, the design of the strengthening program should be one using low weight and high repetitions. Aquatic therapy, elliptical training and cycling are examples of therapeutic exercise that allow patients to place decreased stress through their affected joints while allowing for aerobic training (Ottawa Panel, 2005; Sinusas, 2012). Exercise in water is an excellent activity since buoyancy in water reduces the effect of gravity and the loading effect on joints. Resistive exercise producing increased joint pain during or following exercise probably indicates too much resistance is being used, stress is being placed at an inappropriate part of the range of motion, or the exercise is being incorrectly performed. Stretching exercises incorporating a low load, prolonged stretch, performed three or more times a day, will lead to more appropriate length–tension relationship for the muscles surrounding the affected joints and may lead to decreased stress in the intraarticular and periarticular joint structures. Home exercise programs must be carefully planned and monitored.

Heat may decrease pain and stiffness and cold may decrease pain and inflammation. Splints, braces and gait devices, such as crutches, a walker or rolling walker, may be helpful to decrease joint stress. If excess weight is present, weight loss may alleviate or even prevent the onset of symptoms, and should always be incorporated into the patient's therapeutic program.

Surgical interventions such as arthroscopy, arthroplasty and angulation osteotomy may provide symptomatic relief, improved motion and improved joint biomechanics. The most common major orthopedic procedure performed in the elderly is hip surgery, the indications being fracture or pain due to OA. A large percentage of hip and knee replacements are for OA. While elderly patients are at higher risk for complications than younger patients, most have a satisfactory outcome and significant relief of pain. Experimental surgical techniques to stimulate cartilage repair or transplant cartilage are generally not successful, though select patient populations with focal defects may benefit (Kreuz et al., 2009).

RHEUMATOID ARTHRITIS

Rheumatoid arthritis (RA), one of the most common of the rheumatic diseases, is a chronic, systemic, inflammatory, autoimmune disorder. Clinical features vary among individuals and within the same individual over the course of the disease. The hallmark feature of RA is chronic inflammation of the synovium, peripheral articular cartilage, and subchondral marrow spaces. In response to the inflammation, granulation tissue (pannus) forms leading to the erosion of articular cartilage. Early in the disease process, the synovitis may be clinically detected as warmth and swelling in joints. As the disease progresses, joint immobility and reduced vascularity of the synovium makes the degree of inflammation more difficult to detect. Inflammation in tendon sheaths may lead to tendon fray or rupture. The clinical manifestation of synovial inflammation is morning stiffness related to immobilization that lasts greater than 2 hours after rising. As a systemic connective tissue disease, RA may manifest systemic and extraarticular pathological changes that are the predominant feature of the disease process in some persons. Systemic and extraarticular manifestations include muscle fibrosis and atrophy, vasculitis, pericarditis, fatigue, weight loss, generalized stiffness, fever, anemia, pleural effusion, interstitial lung disease, keratoconjunctivitis, increased susceptibility to infection, and neurological compromise leading to sensory and/or motor loss. Subcutaneous, non-tender nodules may occur on the extensor surface of the forearm or other pressure areas. The effect of RA is broad, ranging from mild symptoms resulting in only occasional pain and discomfort, and only slight decrease in function, to severe symptoms with significant pain, decreased function and joint deformity.

The prevalence of RA increases with age, is 2–3 three times higher in women than men, and has a peak incidence in the sixth decade (CDC, 2013b). The onset of RA may be acute, but is usually insidious. The clinical course of RA is variable and unpredictable. Patients with RA who smoke, have diabetes, or are physically inactive tend to be at higher risk for developing comorbidities such as cardiovascular or respiratory disease (Verstappen & Symmons,

2011). In the initial stages, joint pain and stiffness are prevalent, especially in the mornings. With disease progression, motion becomes more limited and ankylosis may develop. Radiographic evidence of the disease becomes apparent over time. Treatment effectiveness may be difficult to determine due to spontaneous exacerbations and remissions. Testimonials of 'cures' with unproven remedies are common, as certain treatment approaches may have been initiated during the initial stages of a spontaneous remission.

The etiology of RA is unknown. Evidence exists for a genetic predisposition for the disease that may be triggered by bacteria or viruses. The pathogenesis of RA is better understood than the etiology. The characteristic chronic inflammatory process begins with synovitis, developing as microvascular endothelial cells become swollen and congested. As the disease advances, the synovium becomes progressively thickened and edematous, with projections of synovial tissue invading the joint cavity. Pannus, tumor-like thickened layers of granulation tissue, infiltrates the joints destroying periarticular bone and cartilage. Fibrotic ankylosis may eventually occur, with bony malalignment, visible deformities, muscle atrophy and subluxation of joints. In advanced RA, bony ankylosis and significant disability may occur.

A definitive diagnosis is based on a combination of clinical manifestations and laboratory findings, as there is no laboratory test specific for RA. Frequent laboratory findings in persons with RA include decreased red blood cell count, increased erythrocyte sedimentation rates (ESR) and positive rheumatoid factor (RF). A positive test of RF is not diagnostic, as RF is found in a small percentage of normal individuals and in persons with other autoimmune diseases. However, high concentration of RF is associated with greater long-term risk of RA (Nielsen et al., 2012).

Joint manifestations occur bilaterally, affecting principally the small joints of the hands and feet, ankles, knees, wrists, elbows and shoulders. Typically, the metacarpophalangeal and proximal interphalangeal joints of the hand are affected, with sparing of the distal interphalangeal joints. RA can affect the hip, knee, ankle and small joints of the foot. In axial involvement, the upper cervical spine is most affected. Tenosynovitis of the transverse ligament of the first cervical vertebra and disease of the cervical apophyseal joints may lead to instability and cord compression. A thorough neurological examination should be conducted to determine involvement. Most of the joints ultimately affected by RA will be involved during the first year of the disease.

Joint deformities result from synovitis, pannus formation, cartilage destruction and voluntary joint immobilization due to pain. The change in joint mechanics from cartilage degeneration and the erosive effect of chronic synovitis may lead to ligament laxity. The changed mechanics result in abnormal lines of pull from tendons, leading to joint deformity. Additionally, tenosynovitis may occur, causing an obstruction of tendon movement within the tendon sheath and/or tendon rupture. Nodular thickening may occur, leading to a 'locking' sensation or rupture of the tendon. Synovitis can lead to compression of nerves, particularly in the carpal tunnel and, less commonly, the tarsal tunnel. The ulnar nerve may be compressed at the elbow or in the hand.

Common deformities of the hand include radial deviation of the wrist, ulnar deviation at the metacarpophalangeal joints, and deformities in the fingers. Flexion deformity of the elbow and loss of shoulder motion is common. Due to the weight-bearing nature of the lower extremity, major disability can result, particularly in the toes and ankle. Cock-up deformities of the toes and subluxation of the metatarsal heads with concurrent migration of the metatarsophalangeal fat pad result in significant pain in walking.

Effective treatment of RA attempts to reduce the inflammation, provide pain relief, maintain and restore joint function, and decrease the development of joint deformity. Medications include NSAIDs, corticosteroids, slow-acting antirheumatic drugs, and disease-modifying antirheumatic drugs (DMARDs) (Singh & Cameron, 2012). Patients must balance activity and rest. Fatigue may be decreased with appropriate rest, which may include 8–10 hours of sleep at night and an afternoon nap. Energy should be conserved for daily activities. Prolonged bed rest has not proven to be beneficial. Therapeutic exercise cannot alter the course of the disease, but can help prevent deformity and loss of motion and muscle strength. Clinical practice guidelines developed by the Ottawa Panel emphasize shoulder, hand, knee and whole body functional strengthening at low intensities (Ottawa Panel, 2004a). Active and passive range of motion exercise, pain-free isometrics, proper positioning and posture should be performed regularly to achieve functional goals. Joint-stressing activities should be avoided. Aquatic therapy is an excellent medium for active individual or group structured exercise, though the water temperatures for patients with RA may need to be higher than usual. Splints and assistive devices should be used as needed to protect the joints. During active inflammatory periods, exercise should be performed carefully, with special care taken to protect the joints. Heavy resistive exercise should be avoided, as the joint compression that occurs with this exercise could increase pain and contribute to joint damage. Since the limitation of motion is due to distended joint capsules and not to adhesions, forceful stretching should be avoided. During times of remission, non- or low-impact aerobic conditioning such as swimming or stationary bicycling can be performed within the patient's tolerance. Gentle stretching can be performed. Relaxation exercises often help to decrease muscle tension and stress.

Clinical evidence exists for the inclusion of low-level laser therapy (Brosseau et al., 2005; Alves et al., 2011; Bálint et al., 2012), therapeutic ultrasound, thermotherapy and transcutaneous electrical stimulation in the management of RA (Ottawa Panel, 2004b). Surgical procedures may be performed with goals to reduce pain, improve function, and correct instability or deformity. Common surgical procedures include tenosynovectomy, tendon repair, synovectomy, arthrodesis and arthroplasty.

SYSTEMIC LUPUS ERYTHEMATOSUS

Systemic lupus erythematosus (SLE) is an autoimmune disease primarily affecting young women. The peak incidence of SLE occurs between the ages of 15 and 40, but the disease may affect both younger and older persons, with a female to male ratio of approximately 10:1. The disease course varies widely from a relatively benign to life-threatening illness (Robbins, 2001). Most deaths occur due to infection (Chen et al., 2008).

The etiology of SLE is unknown, but may involve immunologic, environmental, hormonal and genetic factors. The prime causative mechanism is thought to be autoimmunity in which tissues are damaged as antibodies are produced against many body tissues and tissue components such as blood vessels, red blood cells, lymphocytes and various organs. Antibodies directed against components of the cell nucleus, antinuclear antibodies (ANA), are found in most SLE patients.

Two ANA molecules, ANA-DNA and ANA-Sm, are unique to SLE and are used as diagnostic criteria. The diagnosis of SLE is based on clinical manifestations supported by laboratory tests. Clinical criteria to classify SLE include skin rash, renal dysfunction, blood disorders, arthritis, cardiopulmonary dysfunction, neurological/psychiatric problems and abnormal immunologic tests (Petri et al., 2012). Clinically apparent nephritis develops in many cases and biopsies may be used to assess the degree of kidney damage. Photosensitive skin disorders are common, especially acute inflammatory rash on the malar regions of the face, known as 'butterfly rash', or on the upper extremities or trunk. Subacute symmetrical and widespread lesions or chronic disc-shaped, scaly lesions may appear. Pleurisy, pericarditis, chronic interstitial lung inflammation, heart valve abnormalities, and thromboses are common with varying degrees of severity. Neurological and psychiatric manifestations include seizures and psychosis. Gastrointestinal manifestations include diffuse abdominal pain, nausea and vomiting, and anorexia. The arthritis associated with SLE may be symmetrical or nonsymmetrical and typically affects the small joints of the hands, wrists and knees. Typically, the arthritis is non-erosive, but deforming arthropathy, particularly of the hands, can develop as a consequence of recurrent inflammation.

While the short-term prognosis has improved in recent years, the long-term outlook for patients with SLE is generally poor, with complications resulting from either the disease itself or as a consequence of treatment. Late complications of SLE include end-stage renal disease, atherosclerosis, pulmonary emboli, venous syndromes, avascular necrosis, and neuropsychological dysfunction and bacteriacemia (Chen et al., 2008).

Treatment of SLE is determined by disease activity and severity. Drugs that suppress inflammation and interfere with immune system functioning are commonly prescribed. NSAIDs may be used to treat musculoskeletal complications. Skin lesions may be treated with corticosteroids and antimalarial agents. Corticosteroids are used in the treatment of systemic symptoms of SLE such as pericarditis, nephritis, vasculitis and CNS involvement. In some patients, cytotoxic drugs such as methotrexate, azathioprine and cyclophosphamide are prescribed. In the absence of lupus nephritis or neuropsychiatric lupus, the drug belimumab appears effective and well tolerated (Boyce & Fusco, 2012).

Patient education is paramount in the treatment of SLE. The patient must understand that periods of remission and exacerbation are typical. Many patients with SLE are photosensitive and must be reminded to avoid or reduce sun exposure when possible. Due to the increased risk of infection, emphasis should be placed on prompt evaluation for unexplained fever. The fatigue associated with SLE may be reduced through cardiovascular fitness and muscular strengthening interventions (Ayan & Martin, 2007; Yuen et al., 2011). Heat may be used to relieve joint pain and stiffness. Regular active exercise may prevent contractures.

GOUT

Gout is a metabolic disease characterized by the deposition of monosodium urate crystals in connective tissues, resulting in painful arthritis. The hyperuricemia associated with gout may result from a variety of factors, including a genetic defect in purine metabolism, leading to an overproduction and/or undersecretion of uric acid. Other associated factors include obesity, diet, lifestyle, renal dysfunction and hemoglobin levels. Diuretics can lead to an underexcretion of uric acid and may play a role in the pathogenesis of gout (Rakieh & Conaghan, 2011). Primary gout typically occurs in men, with peak incidence in the fifth decade, and commonly causes short-term disability. Gout may also occur in postmenopausal women, especially when diuretics are used. Secondary gout occurs primarily in the elderly and results from the hyperuricemia associated with diseases such as diabetes mellitus and hypertension. The mechanisms are not fully defined, but are likely due to diminished renal function, dehydration, decreased tissue perfusion, and the effect of certain drugs leading to uric acid overproduction or underexcretion. Gout is relatively common in organ transplant recipients due to the use of cyclosporine and reduced renal function, regardless of the organ transplanted.

The clinical course of gout typically follows four stages: asymptomatic, acute, intercritical and chronic. An asymptomatic period of urate crystal deposition in connective tissue often appears prior to the first episode of gouty arthritis. The initial episode of gout is typically sudden, often occurring during the night. The patient awakes with severe unexplained joint pain and swelling. The first metatarsophalangeal joint is commonly affected. The ankle, tarsal joints and knee may also be involved. Trauma, alcohol, drugs, or acute medical illness may precipitate acute attacks. The intercritical stage is characterized by symptom-free periods which may last from months to years. The presence of crystal deposition persists during these asymptomatic periods and aspiration of synovial fluid may confirm the diagnosis. The chronic stage of gout is characterized by tophi, large masses of urates within the subarticular bone or surrounding soft tissues. Less commonly, tophi form in the internal organs. Tophi deposits precipitate joint erosion and tendon rupture. The arthritic clinical manifestation of chronic gout may resemble RA, though gout is usually more asymmetrical and can involve any joint.

Not all persons with hyperuricemia will develop gout. The presence of monosodium urate crystals in synovial fluid is generally considered necessary to establish a definitive diagnosis. Even during asymptomatic periods, monosodium urate crystals may be demonstrated in synovial fluid aspirated from previously involved joints, as well as from joints that have never been involved. Serum uric acid levels are less helpful in definitive diagnosis, especially in the acute phase, but will eventually become elevated.

Treatment of gout is aimed at early intervention for acute attacks, reducing hyperuricemia, preventing recurrence, and preventing erosive joint damage and kidney complications. During acute attacks, NSAIDs, colchicines or corticosteroids may be used to relieve symptoms. Urate-lowering therapy may be used for long-term control (Doghramji et al., 2012). Included in the treatment regimen are bedrest, joint immobilization and local cold application to inflamed joints. Attack frequency may be decreased by certain dietary and lifestyle changes. Recommended dietary modification includes the avoidance of alcohol and a restriction of purine-rich foods, such as liver, kidneys, shellfish, salmon, peas, beans and spinach. Weight loss and the avoidance of repetitive trauma are helpful prophylactic measures that may allow one to avoid drug therapy during intercritical periods. Infected or ulcerated tophi may require excision.

Practical considerations include the use of a bed cradle to keep bed covers off inflamed joints, the intake of plenty of fluids to prevent the formation of kidney stones, prompt treatment of acute attacks, and rapid attention to the side-effects of drug therapies. Assistive devices may also be used to decrease stress on inflamed joints.

PSEUDOGOUT

Pseudogout (PG), a chronic recurrent arthritis similar to gout, results from calcium pyrophosphate dihydrate (CPPD) crystal deposition in articular and periarticular structures. The presence of CPPD crystals in joint tissue is common in the elderly, and there is only a weak correlation with joint pain. The risk of CPPD-associated disease increases with age, but occurs half as commonly as gout, with a near-equal occurrence in men and women. The pattern of joint involvement is symmetrical, though possibly more advanced on one side. Acute PG is characterized by self-limiting attacks of acute joint pain and swelling. Any synovial joint may be affected, but the knee is the most common. The pain associated with PG is less severe than with gout. Calcification from CPPD crystal deposits will characteristically be demonstrated on well-exposed radiographs of the knees and wrists. Acute attacks may be provoked by surgery, trauma, or severe illness. Joint inflammation and destruction may occur simultaneously or independently, thus resembling other rheumatic diseases. Definitive diagnosis is made through the demonstration of CPPD crystals. Acute attacks are managed through joint aspiration to relieve pressure, injection of steroids, administration of analgesics and NSAIDs, as well as the use of oral or intravenous colchicines.

Persons with PG may experience multiple joint involvement, with low-grade inflammation lasting for weeks or months. The morning stiffness, fatigue, synovial thickening and flexion contractures associated with PG may lead to a misdiagnosis of RA. The pattern of joint degeneration in PG is distinctive from OA, in that symmetrical involvement is most typical. Rehabilitation of persons with PG should focus on joint protection during acute attacks, maintenance of range of motion and energy conservation practices.

POLYMYALGIA RHEUMATICA

Polymyalgia rheumatica (PMR) is a common systemic inflammatory disorder in the elderly and is characterized by the gradual development of persistent pain, weakness and stiffness in proximal muscles, in combination with fever, weight loss and high ESR. More common in women than men, PMR occurs mostly in those over 50 years of age, with peak incidence between 60 and 75 years of age (Charlton, 2008). Symptoms are usually symmetric and onset may be abrupt. Stiffness is typically worse in the morning. Tenderness and stiffness is most common in the muscles of the shoulder, pelvic girdles and neck, but may be present in the knees, wrists and hands. Differential diagnosis of PMR from hypothyroidism, malignancies, RA, SLE and infectious diseases, is critical. Giant cell arteritis (GCA), also known as temporal arteritis, is a systemic inflammatory disorder affecting large and medium-sized blood vessels. The pain presentation may be similar to that in PMR and the conditions may coexist in some persons. The vasculitis associated with GCA may lead to severe occlusive disease and result in stroke and blindness (Weyand et al., 2012). Symptoms include headache, visual disturbance, scalp tenderness and abnormalities in the temporal arteries.

The diagnosis of PMR is based on clinical manifestation supported by laboratory tests such as high ESR and C-reactive protein. Results of muscle enzyme tests and biopsies and plain film radiographs do not contribute to differential diagnosis. PMR responds dramatically to prednisone therapy; thus, the response is used in diagnosis as well as treatment. The lowest dose of prednisone to control symptoms is optimal, and long-term side-effects such as osteoporosis, diabetes, hypertension and gastrointestinal problems should be monitored and treated. The disease is typically self-limiting, lasting 2–7 years. Patients should be warned of the signs and symptoms of GCA. Later in the course of the disease, stretching and strengthening exercises may be helpful. Modalities such as ice and electrical stimulation may be used to decrease pain. The use of assistive devices may decrease the risk of falls.

BURSITIS

A bursa is a small sac with a synovial-like membrane containing a fluid that is indistinguishable from synovial fluid. Located in areas of potential friction, bursae are commonly located between bones and ligaments, skin, or muscles. An example is the ischial bursa that lies between the ischial tuberosity and the gluteus maximus. Bursitis is defined as inflammation of the bursa, and may occur in the superficial bursae of the shoulder, greater trochanter, knee or elbow or in deeper bursae of the ischial tuberosity, iliopsoas, and popliteal areas. As a response to the stimulus of inflammation, the lining membrane may produce excess fluid, causing distension of the bursa.

Bursitis may be caused by an acute trauma, such as a direct blow to the area, for example when trochanteric bursitis develops as a result of a fall on the greater trochanter. Chronic trauma may be causative, as is seen with overuse syndromes such as olecranon bursitis resulting from leaning on the elbow for extended time periods. Septic bursitis may occur secondary to the entry of bacteria from a puncture wound or fissuring of the bursal sac, as may occur with other disease processes such as RA, gout, tuberculosis and syphilis. The bursal fluid may be aspirated and cultured to determine if infection is present.

Clinical characteristics may include joint distension (effusion), pain, redness, increased temperature and loss of function at the involved joint. Pain is usually worsened by activity at the involved joint and relieved by rest; however, pain may continue to be present at rest but with a lesser severity. The pain is typically described as a deep aching discomfort. Both active range of motion (AROM) and passive range of motion (PROM) are usually normal, with increased pain at the end of the range in the direction of stress to the bursa (e.g. elbow flexion with olecranon bursitis). Range of motion may be limited due to pain if the condition is very acute or the bursa becomes pinched during the movement, as with shoulder flexion or abduction causing the subacromial bursa to be pinched under the acromion process. Resistive testing is usually negative, as the bursa is a non-contractile tissue, but discomfort may be caused from the contraction of neighboring muscles encroaching on the swollen bursa. Palpation directly over the area is typically painful.

Therapeutic interventions for acute bursitis include protecting and resting the area, icing, anti-inflammatory medications, and iontophoresis or phonophoresis using betamethasone or dexamethasone. Relieving the cause of the bursitis by altering postures or modifying environmental factors is helpful. An example is padding wheelchair armrests or wearing protective elbow pads to reduce trauma to the olecranon bursa. Another example is discontinuing work performed overhead, a position that may further aggravate an inflamed subdeltoid bursa. Oral NSAIDs or local corticosteroid injections may be beneficial in reducing the inflammation and pain. As the acute inflammation subsides, pain-free AROM is encouraged to help to increase metabolism in the area and decrease swelling. In cases of chronic bursitis, determining the cause of the problem becomes the most important factor in successful treatment. A patient with chronic trochanteric bursitis may benefit from stretching of a tight iliotibial band. Surgical intervention is uncommon and depends on the extent of the disease process. Surgery usually has the goal of creating more area for structures to move, such as an acromioplasty or removal of osteophytes from the undersurface of the acromion process and acromioclavicular joint.

TENDINITIS

Tendinitis is defined as inflammation of a tendon; tenosynovitis is defined as inflammation of a tendon and tendon sheath. The tendon may become inflamed in many areas and due to several mechanisms. Inflammation may occur within the tendon itself, at the area where the tendon fuses with the muscle (musculotendinous junction) or where the tendon attaches to bone (tenoperiosteal junction). Determining the exact location of the lesion is extremely important, as successful treatment needs to be directed at the exact lesion site. Tenosynovitis may occur from overuse, unaccustomed activity, or puncture wounds. In the absence of a precipitating trauma, the presence of tenosynovitis may indicate a systemic inflammatory process.

A common cause of tendinitis is anatomical or biomechanical constraint to the tendon, such as supraspinatus tendon impingement by the coracoacromial arch. Other common mechanisms include microtrauma due to repeated overload, such as the flexor tendons of the hand undergoing repeated contractions in a keyboard operator, and macrotrauma to a tendon. Calcific tendinitis occurs when calcium deposits form in the tendon, resulting in decreased blood supply to the tendon. Commonly affected tendons are the Achilles, rotator cuff, bicipital, patellar, common extensor group of the wrist and the posterior tibial. In the geriatric population, pain from Achilles or posterior tibial tendinitis must be differentiated from pain of vascular origin, such as thrombosis or thrombophlebitis. Calf deep vein thrombosis may be identified by the clinical Homan's sign test or by Doppler ultrasonography.

Clinical characteristics of tendonitis include pain, edema, redness, increased temperature and loss of function at the involved joint. Symptoms are typically worsened by use of the involved tendon, especially with eccentric loading of the tendon, as when going down stairs with patellar tendinitis. Use of the tendon in a range of motion where it is likely to be impinged (painful arc) also will reproduce the patient's pain. An example is the painful arc produced by overhead abduction with supraspinatus tendinitis. Though commonly relieved by rest, pain may be present even at rest, if acute. Active motion may be painful with muscle contraction of associated tendons. Passive motion may be painful, especially those motions resulting in full elongation of the tendon, such as full shoulder extension, elbow extension, and pronation with bicipital tendinitis. Resistive testing is the key clinical diagnostic test, with the tendon being strong and painful upon resistance. Palpation directly over the tendon is typically painful. In the case of a partial tear of the tendon, the resisted motion will characteristically present as weak and painful.

Typical therapeutic interventions for acute tendinitis include protection and rest of the area, ice and anti-inflammatory medications. Also essential is relieving any possible causes of the tendinitis by altering or modifying work and/or environmental factors that may be contributing to the problem, such as an office worker with extensor carpi ulnaris tendinitis who may further aggravate the condition by continuing to type. Corticosteroid injection into the tendon or tendon sheath may be beneficial in acute cases, but is not indicated for chronic lesions (Jacobs, 2009).

As the acute inflammation subsides, painfree active motion is encouraged to help provide nutrition to the area and decrease swelling. In cases of chronic tendinitis, determining the cause of the problem becomes the most important factor in successful treatment. If a patient has a chronic supraspinatus tendinitis, the cause, such as weak shoulder external rotators or a bone spur on the inferior side of the acromion, needs to be identified. Chronic tendinitis is usually the result of poor blood flow to the injured area combined with a continued stress that does not allow for adequate maturation of the healing tissue. Transverse friction massage may be used in chronic tendinitis to increase the mobility of the scar and stimulate healing of the scar tissue with normal fiber alignment. Surgical intervention is only performed when conservative measures have not improved the condition. These procedures usually have the goal of creating more area for structures to move, such as an acromioplasty or removal of osteophytes from the undersurface of the acromion process and acromioclavicular joint in impingement syndrome.

CONCLUSION

Considering the increasing prevalence of rheumatic conditions especially in the aging population, therapists should be aware of signs and symptoms, current research, medical management and therapeutic interventions. One should note that there are more than 100 types of arthritis and many persons live with chronic joint symptoms, but have not yet been diagnosed with the disease. The clinician should engage in prevention and self-management education, make appropriate referrals to other healthcare providers, and advocate for access to advances in medical care, surgery and physical rehabilitation.

REFERENCES

Alves AC, de Carvalho PD, Parente M et al 2013 Low level laser therapy in different stages of rheumatoid arthritis: a histological study. Lasers Med Sci 28(2):529–536

Ayan C, Martin V 2007 Systemic lupus erythematosus and exercise. Lupus 16:5–9

Bálint G, Barabas K, Zeitler Z et al 2011 Ex vivo soft-laser treatment inhibits the synovial expression of vimentin and α-enolase, potential autoantigens in rheumatoid arthritis. Phys Ther 91(5):665–674

Boyce EG, Fusco BE 2012 Belimumab: review of use in systemic lupus erythematosus. Clin Ther 34:1006–1022

Brosseau L, Welch V, Wells GA et al 2005 Low level laser therapy (Classes I, II and III) for treating rheumatoid arthritis. Cochrane Database Syst Rev 2005(4):CD002049, doi: http://dx.doi.org/10.1002/14651858.CD002049.pub2

CDC (Centers for Disease Control and Prevention) 2013a Osteoarthritis. [Online] Available at: www.cdc.gov/arthritis/basics/osteoarthritis.htm. Accessed January 2013

CDC (Centers for Disease Control and Prevention) 2013b Rheumatoid arthritis. [Online] Available at: www.cdc.gov/arthritis/basics/rheumatoid.htm. Accessed January 2013

Charlton R 2008 Polymyalgia rheumatica and its links with giant cell arteritis. Clin Med 8:498–501

Chen MJ, Tseng HM, Huang YL et al 2008 Long-term outcome and short-term survival of patients with systemic lupus erythematosus after bacteraemia episodes: 6-yr follow-up. Rheumatology (Oxford) 47:1352–1357

Cheng YJ, Hootman JM, Murphy LB et al 2010 Prevalence of doctor-diagnosed arthritis and arthritis-attributable activity limitation – United States, 2007–2009. MMWR Morbid Mortal Wkly Rep 59(39):1261–1265

Deyle GD, Gill NW, Allison SC et al 2012 Knee OA: which patients are unlikely to benefit from manual PT and exercise? J Fam Pract 61:E1–E8

Doghramji PP, Mandell BF, Pop RS 2012 Casebook consults: improving outcomes in gout (multimedia activity). Am J Med 125:S1

Egloff C, Hugle T, Valderrabano V 2012 Biomechanics and pathomechanisms of osteoarthritis. Swiss Med Wkly 142:w13583, doi: http://dx.doi.org/10.4414/smw.2012.13583

Hootman J, Bolen J, Helmick C et al 2006 Prevalence of doctor-diagnosed arthritis and arthritis-attributable activity limitation – United States, 2003–2005. MMWR Morbid Mortal Wkly Rep 55:1089–1092

Jacobs JW 2009 How to perform local soft-tissue glucocorticoid injections. Best Pract Res Clin Rheumatol 23:193–219

Jansen MJ, Viechtbauer W, Lenssen AF 2011 Strength training alone, exercise therapy alone, and exercise therapy with passive manual mobilisation each reduce pain and disability in people with knee osteoarthritis: a systematic review. J Physiother 57:11–20

Kreuz PC, Muller S, Osssendorf C et al 2009 Treatment of focal degenerative cartilage defects with polymer-based autologous chondrocyte grafts: four-year clinical results. Arthritis Res Ther 11:R33

Nielsen SF, Bojesen SE, Schnohr P et al 2012 Elevated rheumatoid factor and long term risk of rheumatoid arthritis: a prospective cohort study. BMJ 345:e5244

Ottawa Panel 2004a Ottawa Panel Evidence-based Clinical Practice Guidelines for therapeutic exercises in the management of rheumatoid arthritis in adults. Phys Ther 84:934–972

Ottawa Panel 2004b Ottawa Panel Evidence-based Clinical Practice Guidelines for electrotherapy and thermotherapy interventions in management of rheumatoid arthritis in adults. Phys Ther 84:1016–1043

Ottawa Panel 2005 Ottawa Panel Evidence-based Clinical Practice Guidelines for therapeutic exercises and manual therapy in the management of osteoarthritis. Phys Ther 85:907–971

Petri M, Orbai A, Alarcon GS et al 2012 Derivation and validation of the Systemic Lupus International Collaborating Clinics classification criteria for systemic lupus erythematosus. Arthr Rheum 64:2677–2688

Rakieh C, Conaghan PG 2011 Diagnosis and treatment of gout in primary care. Practitioner 255:17–20

Robbins L (ed) 2001 Clinical Care in the Rheumatic Diseases, 2nd edn. American College of Rheumatology, Atlanta, GA

Singh JA, Cameron DR 2012 Summary of AHRQ's comparative effectiveness review of drug therapy for rheumatoid arthritis (RA) in adults – an update 2012. J Manag Care Pharm 18(4 Supp C):S1–S18

Sinusas K 2012 Osteoarthritis: diagnosis and treatment. Am Fam Phys 85:49–56

Verstappen SM, Symmons DP 2011 What is the outcome of RA in 2011 and can we predict it? Best Pract Res Clin Rheumatol 25:485–496

Vos T, Flaxman AD, Naghavi M et al 2012 Years lived with disability (YLDs) for 1160 sequelae of 289 diseases and injuries 1990—2010: a systematic analysis for the Global Burden of Disease Study 2010. Lancet 380:2163–2196

Walker JM, Helewa A 2004 Physical Rehabilitation in Arthritis, 2nd edn. Saunders, St Louis, MO, p 67

Weyand CM, Liao YJ, Goronzy JJ 2012 The immunopathology of giant cell arteritis: diagnostic and therapeutic implications. J Neuroophthalmol 32:259–265

Yuen YK, Holthaus K, Kamen DL et al 2011 Using Wii Fit to reduce fatigue among African American women with systemic lupus erythematosus: a pilot study. Lupus 20:1293–1299

Chapter 20

The shoulder

EDMUND M. KOSMAHL

CHAPTER CONTENTS

INTRODUCTION

Shoulder pain and dysfunction are common problems for seniors. The prevalence of musculoskeletal shoulder complaints ranges from 14.3% to 32.0% (Satish et al., 2001; Chaaya et al., 2012), with 21% reporting bilateral symptoms. Shoulder disorders are associated with substantial functional limitation, because functional limitation is correlated with pain during active shoulder motion (Ozaras et al., 2009). Important activities such as feeding, dressing and personal hygiene can be compromised. Pain and shoulder mobility restrictions are significantly associated with long-term decreases in quality of life measures (Nesvold et al., 2011).

Because shoulder impairment and pain can produce functional limitation, tests and measures of pain, impairment and functional limitation should be incorporated in the examination of the aging shoulder. Visual analog scales are valid and reliable measures of pain (Bergh et al., 2000). The Shoulder Pain and Disability Index (Bicer & Ankarali, 2010) and the Disabilities of the Arm, Shoulder and Hand Outcome Questionnaire (Slobogean et al., 2010) are measures of shoulder function for which validity and reliability have been established. The purpose of this chapter is to review rehabilitation concepts for the following shoulder problems that may cause pain and dysfunction in seniors: (1) degenerative rotator cuff; (2) fracture of the proximal humerus; (3) arthroplasty; and (4) shoulder pain with hemiplegia.

DEGENERATIVE ROTATOR CUFF

The rotator cuff is comprised of the musculotendinous insertions of the supraspinatus, infraspinatus, teres minor and subscapularis muscles. These structures are important for nearly all shoulder functions, especially activities that require overhead arm function. Rotator cuff pathology is the most common affliction of the adult shoulder (Akpinar et al., 2003).

Advancing age is the factor most highly correlated with degenerative tendinopathy of the rotator cuff (Feng et al.,

2003). A lifetime of activity can lead to degeneration of the rotator cuff in association with osteoarthritis of the glenohumeral and acromioclavicular joints. Degeneration can cause partial- or full-thickness tears in the cuff.

Degeneration of the rotator cuff can be associated with subacromial impingement syndrome. The mobility of the thoracic spine and scapulae is decreased in patients with subacromial impingement syndrome (Seitz et al., 2012). Theoretically, subacromial impingement can be induced by excessive thoracic kyphosis and protracted scapulae (Lewis et al., 2005; Kalra et al., 2010). These postural misalignments place the glenoid and acromion in a downward and forward position. This position may encourage subacromial impingement when the arm is elevated (Fig. 20.1; see Chapter 15 Posture). When range of motion (ROM) limitations and postural malalignments are present, interventions should include exercises to increase mobility and establish a more upright posture.

Exercises for degenerative rotator cuff should be designed to avoid worsening a subacute inflammatory

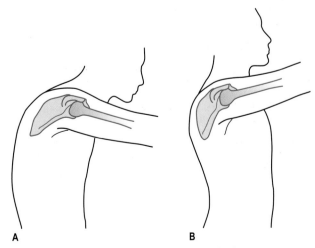

A   B

Figure 20.1 Excessive thoracic kyphosis **(A)** leads to impingement in the subacromial space during elevation of the arm. Upright posture **(B)** allows arm elevation without impingement.

Table 20.1 **Interventions for degenerative rotator cuff**	
Impairment	Intervention
Pain and inflammation	Rest, modalities (cold, nonthermal ultrasound, electrical stimulation)
Excessive thoracic kyphosis and limited mobility	Thoracic spine extension exercises
Protracted scapulae and limited mobility	Scapular retraction exercises
Decreased shoulder ROM	Passive and assisted ROM exercises (assistance from noninvolved upper extremity, overhead pulley, wand)
Decreased strength of shoulder musculature	Isometrics, side-lying isotonics for internal and external rotators, assisted eccentric lowering of arm from overhead
Decreased function	Gradual introduction: touch top of head, back of neck, low back – adapt activities of daily living to functional capabilities

ROM, range of motion

process. The therapist should incorporate exercises to avoid positions that cause subacromial impingement and pain. Table 20.1 summarizes rehabilitation interventions for degenerative rotator cuff without tear.

When tear of the degenerative rotator cuff exists, the history and presentation are typical. The patient usually does not report trauma. A common scenario involves the sudden inability to raise the arm overhead during a functional activity. Pain may or may not be reported. The patient cannot hold the arm in the 90° abducted position (failure of the drop-arm test). Because of the poor condition of the degenerative tissues, operative repair for tears of the rotator cuff is less often considered for older persons. Surgical repair produces less satisfactory outcomes in persons older than 65 years (American Academy of Orthopaedic Surgeons, 2011a). The metaphor of 'trying to anastomose cooked spaghetti' may be helpful to conceptualize the rationale for nonoperative management of degenerative rotator cuff tear.

The success of nonoperative management for rotator cuff tear is associated with the initial amount of ROM and strength (Tanaka et al., 2010). For this reason, it is unreasonable to expect full functional return for the patient with degenerative rotator cuff tear who cannot actively raise the arm above the head at initial evaluation. Management should be aimed at decreasing inflammation and pain (when present), maintaining full passive ROM, and maximizing strength and functional ability. The interventions summarized in Table 20.1 are appropriate for the patient with degenerative rotator cuff tear. Because the restoration of full, active, overhead mobility is less likely for these patients, assisted ROM exercises often must be continued indefinitely. This is important to prevent additional pathology, such as adhesive capsulitis.

FRACTURE OF THE PROXIMAL HUMERUS

Seventy-five percent of proximal humerus fractures occur in older persons (Chu et al., 2004), and of these, 75% occur in women. Low bone mass, falls and frailty are risk factors. Ninety-two percent of proximal humerus fractures are the direct result of a fall. These realities suggest that screening and intervention for fall risk, frailty and bone health are worthwhile preventive measures, and should be part of a comprehensive rehabilitation program after proximal humeral fracture.

Most fractures at the proximal humerus are nondisplaced or minimally displaced and can be managed nonoperatively (Bell et al., 2011). Management involves a period of sling immobilization followed by early ROM exercises. The sling is worn when not exercising. There is no clear consensus regarding the length of time for immobilization prior to initiating exercises. Starting exercise earlier can reduce pain and improve shoulder activity (Bruder et al., 2011). Although initial formation of bone callus takes about 3 weeks, there is evidence that mobilization at 1 week instead of 3 weeks alleviates short-term pain without compromising long-term outcome (Handoll & Ollivere, 2010). One should expect loss of function of the joint capsule and muscles about the shoulder during the period of immobilization. This is a function of fibrous adhesions that may develop in response to bleeding in the capsule.

The exercise program should begin with active-assistive motion within pain tolerance (Hodgson et al., 2003). It is unwise to apply passive stretching until there is radiographic evidence of fracture union (usually about 6 weeks). Resistance exercises should be avoided during this period. Isometric exercises may be considered from the time of injury provided there is no risk of displacement of the fracture fragments by muscular contraction. This is a concern whenever the fracture involves the greater or lesser tuberosities. Sub-maximal isometric exercise may be appropriate to encourage muscle contractility without risking displacement of fracture fragments. An outline of general exercise interventions for nonoperative proximal humeral fracture appears in Table 20.2.

About 15% of fractures of the proximal humerus involve displacement of fragments that is greater than 1 cm or angulation of fragments that is more than 45°. The four important fracture fragments are: (1) humeral head; (2) greater tuberosity; (3) lesser tuberosity; (4) humeral shaft. These fractures usually require operative reduction and internal fixation (ORIF) to allow fracture healing and return of function. More serious fractures can interrupt the blood supply to the humeral head. This interruption can lead to necrosis, which may require hemiarthroplasty.

Rehabilitation following ORIF varies depending on the classification of the injury (see Table 20.3) and stability of fixation. Close communication with the surgeon can facilitate proper progression of the rehabilitation program without risking a delay in healing or re-injury. Some older patients may not be candidates for ORIF because they cannot reasonably be expected to tolerate (or survive) anesthesia. In other cases, osteoporosis may reduce bone stock to the point where hardware fixation cannot be achieved. Complete restoration of function may be an

Table 20.2 Exercise interventions for proximal humeral fracture (non-operative)

Problem	Exercise	Timeline
Maintain or improve ROM	Assisted ROM (wand, wall climbing, pendulum)	7–14 days, or radiographic evidence of callous (usually 3 weeks)
	Passive ROM, stretching (overhead pulley)	Radiographic evidence of union, usually 6 weeks
Maintain or improve strength	Submaximal isometrics	No risk of fragment displacement, usually immediately
	Full active ROM against gravity	Radiographic evidence of union, usually 6 weeks
	External resistance isotonics	Ability to perform full active ROM against gravity, radiographic evidence of union, usually 6 weeks
Maximize function	Touch top of head, back of neck, low back	Assisted – radiographic evidence of callous, usually 3 weeks Unassisted – radiographic evidence of union, usually 6 weeks

ROM, range of motion

Table 20.3 Neer classification for proximal humeral fractures

Category	Description
I One-part	Non- or minimally displaced
II Two-part	One part displaced >1 cm or angulated >45°
III Three-part	Two parts displaced and/or angulated from each other, and from remaining part
IV Four-part	Four parts displaced and/or angulated from each other
V Fracture-dislocation	Displacement of humeral head from joint space with fracture

Adapted from Neer CS II. Displaced proximal humeral fractures: I. Classification and evaluation. J Bone Joint Surg 1970;52A:1077.

unrealistic goal for these patients. In the past decade, locking plate technology has been used to achieve stable fixation of fractures in spite of weakened osteoporotic bone (Cornell & Omri Ayalon, 2011). Every attempt should be made to maximize functional outcomes (e.g. dressing and grooming).

SHOULDER ARTHROPLASTY

Shoulder arthroplasty options include total shoulder arthroplasty (TSA), stemmed hemiarthroplasty, resurfacing arthroplasty and reverse TSA (American Academy of Orthopaedic Surgeons, 2011b). Table 20.4 contains details about these surgical procedures.

Hemiarthroplasty is often the procedure of choice for older persons who have suffered three- or four-part fractures, especially if there has been substantial damage to the articular surface of the humerus, or when there is substantial osteoporosis. The primary indication for TSA is severe, chronic and progressive pain related to arthritis of the glenohumeral joint. Reverse total shoulder arthroplasty is favored when rotator cuff deficiency coexists with the indication for arthroplasty.

Important considerations during rehabilitation after arthroplasty include the condition of soft tissues, whether soft tissues were repaired, preoperative function, and the surgical approach (Wilcox et al., 2005). Rehabilitation protocols are generally divided into phases, and progression is dependent on soft tissue healing times and achievement of clinical criteria. Rehabilitation principles after TSA or hemiarthroplasty are similar, and are summarized in Table 20.5.

Because outcomes after TSA or hemiarthroplasty for persons with concomitant rotator cuff deficiency have been suboptimal, reverse total shoulder arthroplasty (RTSA) has become popular for these patients (Boudreau et al., 2007). Rotator cuff deficiency modifies shoulder biomechanics, causing the TSA humeral head component to migrate superiorly during elevation, leading to dysfunction and component loosening. The RTSA prosthesis uses a convex glenoid component and a concave humeral component. The center of rotation is moved inferior and medial, which improves the mechanical advantage of the deltoid muscle. This is thought to improve the ability of the deltoid to elevate the arm without causing superior migration of the humeral component. Following RTSA, patients with rotator cuff deficiency regain from 100° to 138° of active elevation, which is more than after TSA.

Principles of rehabilitation and precautions for RTSA are different than for TSA or hemiarthroplasty, because there is a potential for less stability with the RTSA prosthesis design. RTSAs dislocate more frequently than conventional TSAs. If dislocation occurs after RTSA, it happens in a position of internal rotation, adduction and extension, which is different from TSA or hemiarthroplasty (external rotation and abduction). Therefore, reaching behind the back is avoided.

Because the RTSA shoulder is typically rotator cuff deficient, deltoid and scapular muscle function becomes important for stability and function. If teres minor function is absent, the expectation for return of active external rotation function diminishes. The rehabilitation program must emphasize these muscles, and functional expectations must be tempered by the status of the rotator cuff. Generally, most patients should be able to regain 105° of active elevation (Boudreau et al., 2007). Rehabilitation after RTSA is divided into phases that are guided by soft tissue healing and progression criteria (see Table 20.6 for details).

As one can appreciate from the preceding information, there are a myriad of surgical variables that may influence the course of postoperative rehabilitation. The

Table 20.4	**Shoulder arthroplasty surgical procedures**		
Procedure	**Surgery Details**	**Indications**	**Other**
Total shoulder arthroplasty	Humeral component: metal stem and ball, may be cemented. Glenoid component: plastic cup, usually cemented	Osteoarthritis with intact rotator cuff	Better pain relief than hemiarthroplasty
Stemmed hemiarthroplasty	Humeral component only: metal stem and ball, may be cemented	Arthritis or severe fracture involving only the humerus (glenoid cartilage intact). Severely weakened glenoid bone. Arthritis with severe rotator cuff tendon tear	Less pain relief than total shoulder arthroplasty
Resurfacing arthroplasty	Humeral component only: cap prosthesis resurfaces humerus (no stem)	Glenoid cartilage intact. No humeral fracture. Preserve humeral bone	Reduced risk of component wear and loosening. Easier to convert to total shoulder arthroplasty in future
Reverse total shoulder arthroplasty	Humeral component: plastic cup on metal stem. Glenoid component: metal ball	Cuff tear arthropathy (arthritis with complete tear of rotator cuff, inability to elevate arm above 90°). Revision of failed total shoulder arthropathy	Reversal of components moves center of rotation giving deltoid a better mechanical advantage to elevate arm

Adapted from Shoulder joint replacement. American Academy of Orthopaedic Surgeons. Available at: http://orthoinfo.aaos.org/topic.cfm?topic=A00094. Accessed July 2012.

Table 20.5	**Rehabilitation principles for total shoulder arthroplasty and hemiarthroplasty**	

Phase I: Immediate Postoperative (lasts 4–6 weeks postop)

Goals	Precautions	Interventions
Soft tissue healing. Restore passive range (shoulder). Restore active range (distal joints). Control pain, inflammation	No active range, stretching or lifting. Avoid hyperextension, extremes of rotation	Sling 3–4 weeks. Passive elevation (scapular plane). IR to chest, ER 30°. Active motion (distal joints). Cryotherapy. Scapular isometrics. Pendulums

Criteria for progression

Tolerates exercise program
PROM: 90° PROM elevation, 45° ER in plane of scapula, 70° IR in plane of scapula

Phase II: Early Strengthening (not before 4 weeks postop)

Goals	Precautions	Interventions
Avoid overstressing healing soft tissues. Full passive range. Restore active range. Control pain, inflammation. Dynamic shoulder stability	No lifting. Avoid hyperextension. Establish proper mechanics before instituting active exercises against gravity	Sling when sleeping. Active motion in pain-free range. Submaximal isometrics (pain-free). Cryotherapy. Scapular and distal strengthening (resistance)

Criteria for progression

Tolerates exercise program
PROM 140° flexion, 120° abduction, 60° ER and 70° IR in plane of scapula
100° active elevation against gravity with proper mechanics

Phase III: Moderate Strengthening (not before 6 weeks postop)

Goals	Precautions	Interventions
Restore strength, power and endurance. Optimize neuromuscular control. Return to function	No heavy (>3 kg), sudden, jerky lifting, pushing, pulling	Wean from sling. Strengthening (resistance) all muscle groups

Criteria for progression

Tolerates exercise program
120° active elevation against gravity with proper mechanics

(continued)

Table 20.5 (Continued)

Phase IV: Advanced Strengthening (not before 12 weeks postop)

Goals	Precautions	Interventions
Restore strength, power, and endurance Return to function	Avoid stress to anterior capsule	Progress strengthening program Moderately challenging functional and recreational activities Home program

Criteria for discharge

Non-painful AROM

Maximum expected function, strength, power and endurance

Adapted from Wilcox R III, Arslanian LE, Millett PJ. Rehabilitation following total shoulder arthroplasty. J Orthop Sports Phys Ther 2005;35(12):821–36.
AROM, active range of motion

Table 20.6 Rehabilitation principles for reverse total shoulder arthroplasty

Phase I: Immediate Postoperative (6 weeks postop)

Goals	Precautions	Interventions
Joint protection Soft tissue healing Partial passive range (shoulder) Restore active range (distal joints) Control pain, inflammation Function with assistance	No internal rotation/adduction/extension No active range, stretching or lifting	Sling 3–4 weeks Passive elevation (scapular plane), ER 30° Active motion (distal joints) Cryotherapy Submaximal, pain-free isometrics (scapular day 1, deltoid day 21) Pendulums

Criteria for progression

Tolerates exercise program

Able to activate deltoid and scapular muscles in plane of scapula

Phase II: Active Range and Early Strengthening (6–12 weeks postop)

Goals	Precautions	Interventions
Avoid overstressing healing soft tissues Partial passive and active range Control pain, inflammation Dynamic shoulder stability	No lifting > 0.5 kg Avoid hyperextension Establish proper mechanics before instituting active exercises against gravity	Active motion in pain-free range Submaximal, pain-free isometrics (external and internal rotation) Cryotherapy Gentle deltoid, scapular and distal strengthening (resistance)

Criteria for progression

Tolerates exercise program

Isotonic activation of deltoid and scapular muscles

Phase III: Moderate Strengthening (12 weeks postop)

Goals	Precautions	Interventions
Improve strength Return to function	No heavy (>2.7 kg), sudden, jerky lifting, pushing, pulling	Gentle strengthening (resistance) all muscle groups

Criteria for progression

Tolerates exercise program

Motion and strength progress with proper mechanics

Phase IV: Home Program (16 weeks postop)

Goals	Precautions	Interventions
Restore strength Return to function (light household and recreational activities)	Avoid stress to posterior capsule	Progress strengthening program Moderately challenging functional and recreational activities Home program

Criteria for discharge

Non-painful AROM

Elevation 80°–120°, external rotation 30°

Adapted from Boudreau et al. Rehabilitation following reverse total shoulder arthroplasty. J Orthop Sports Phys Ther 2007;37(12):734–43.
AROM, active range of motion

therapist must communicate carefully with the surgeon to ensure an adequate understanding of the particulars of each case. Realizing a successful functional outcome following shoulder arthroplasty requires a well-coordinated and consistent effort by patient, surgeon and therapist. The patient may consider the outcome successful if pain has been reduced enough to allow an uninterrupted night of sleep. Significant functional loss preoperatively, especially as related to coexisting degenerative rotator cuff disease, may necessarily limit expectations for functional outcomes.

SHOULDER PAIN WITH HEMIPLEGIA

In the preface to his book, Cailliet (1980) stated: 'The hemiplegic patient can improve his ambulation, communication, balance, and self-care through treatment, but in the overall picture of functional return, the shoulder remains an enigma.' Unfortunately, the intervening years have added little in the way of understanding the causes and effective interventions for the patient with shoulder pain and hemiplegia.

Reports about the incidence of this problem vary from 5% to 84% (Turner-Stokes & Jackson, 2002; Ratnasabapathy et al., 2003; Klit et al., 2011). Operational definitions used for patient selection may account for these differences. For example, 'pain', 'tenderness', 'mild shoulder discomfort' and 'adhesive capsulitis' are all terms that have been used to identify patients with hemiplegia and shoulder pain.

The causes of shoulder pain with hemiplegia are poorly understood. A combination of factors may be at fault (Gilmore et al., 2004). Unfortunately, there is little empirical evidence to support or refute causality for any of these associated factors. Still, it appears that there are statistically significant relationships between shoulder pain with hemiplegia and the following associated factors: loss of ROM, especially external rotation or scapular upward rotation during movement, poor return of function, biceps or supraspinatus tendinopathy, glenohumeral subluxation and complex regional pain syndrome (Aras et al., 2004; Pong et al., 2012; Hardwick & Lang, 2011). It is important to note that a statistically significant relationship does not imply causality. Whether therapeutic interventions aimed at decreasing these suggested causes will reduce the incidence of shoulder pain with hemiplegia remains to be proven.

In the absence of a clear understanding about the causes of shoulder pain with hemiplegia, interventions should be directed by clinical observations. Evaluation and re-evaluation of signs, symptoms and responses to interventions must continually be used to reformulate the intervention plan. Patients should be evaluated for signs of musculoskeletal impairments (capsulitis, rotator cuff degeneration and tears, tendinitis, bursitis etc.). Interventions for these impairments should be similar to intervention regimens for patients without hemiplegia who exhibit musculoskeletal shoulder impairments. Preventing the loss of external rotation ROM as a result of capsulitis appears to be a particularly important therapeutic goal. The intelligent use of exercise and modalities should have a beneficial effect on musculoskeletal causes of shoulder pain with hemiplegia.

Glenohumeral subluxation as an etiology for shoulder pain with hemiplegia is a multidimensional problem. Theoretically, inferior subluxation places abnormal stresses on periarticular structures and leads to pain. The tension created by inferior subluxation can lead to ischemia, which is thought to cause inflammation and pain. One approach suggests various types of slings to reduce the glenohumeral subluxation. Although a sling can accomplish reduction, it may delay return of voluntary muscular control. Because flaccidity is a suspected cause of shoulder pain with hemiplegia, the anticipated gains afforded by reduction of the subluxation may be derailed by a delay in return of voluntary muscular control. Some slings are designed to reduce the subluxation while simultaneously allowing functional use of the extremity (Harvey et al., 2009). These are preferable to slings that prevent voluntary use.

Another approach to the glenohumeral subluxation problem focuses on return of voluntary muscular control. The muscles that upwardly rotate the scapula (trapezius and serratus anterior) and elevate the humeral head (supraspinatus and deltoid) are the targets of this approach. The scapular muscles are important for maintaining a vertical position of the glenoid fossa. The humeral elevators can maintain the humeral head in the glenoid fossa as long as the fossa is not rotated downwards. The requisite synergy between these muscle groups dictates that if any of these muscles are dysfunctional (flaccid or spastic), subluxation is likely to occur. Therapeutic interventions for this problem include exercise, electromyographic biofeedback and functional electric stimulation. Interventions should be designed to restore normal voluntary control of these muscles.

Renzenbrink and IJzerman (2004) have shown that percutaneous electrical stimulation can produce statistically significant improvement in pain, subluxation, pain-free range of external rotation and Fugl-Myer Motor Test scores at 18 weeks post intervention. They used indwelling electrodes in the supraspinatus, upper trapezius, and posterior and middle deltoid to deliver biphasic, balanced pulses (20 mA, 12 Hz, 10–200 μs, 10 s on/10 s off) 6 hours daily for 6 weeks. By contrast, Yelnik et al. (2003) demonstrated the effectiveness of botulinum toxin injection in spastic subscapular muscles to reduce shoulder pain and increase ROM. The success of these apparently dichotomous approaches underscores the need to carefully evaluate the signs and symptoms for each person as recovery progresses. Clearly, patients with flaccid paralysis must be cared for differently than patients with spastic paralysis.

Another issue to consider is that of poor positioning and handling of the affected upper extremity. Although not established empirically, many feel that poor handling produces trauma and causes pain. This is thought to be more of a problem for patients with flaccid paralysis. Until proven otherwise, prudence dictates that caregivers should use the utmost of care when positioning and handling the affected upper extremity. The affected upper extremity should be positioned so the scapula is protracted, the glenohumeral joint slightly flexed and abducted, and wrist and fingers slightly extended (Turner-Stokes & Jackson, 2002). Pillows, lapboards and slings may be incorporated into positioning interventions. Caregivers should not use the affected upper extremity when assisting for transfer or ambulation. The rapid restoration of voluntary motor control should be high on the list of therapeutic goals for the patient with flaccid paralysis.

Shoulder pain with hemiplegia is poorly understood. Possible interventions are variable because of the lack of understanding about causes. Patients with hemiplegia and shoulder pain should be evaluated for presence of all of the suspected possible causes. Intervention should be directed at reducing possible causes that can be identified on a case-by-case basis.

REFERENCES

Akpinar S, Ozkoc G, Cesur N 2003 Anatomy, biomechanics, and physiopathology of the rotator cuff. Acta Orthop Traumatol Turc 37(Suppl 1):4–12

American Academy of Orthopaedic Surgeons 2011a Rotator cuff tears. [Online] Available at: http://orthoinfo.aaos.org/topic.cfm?topic=a00064. Accessed October 2012

American Academy of Orthopaedic Surgeons 2011b Shoulder joint replacement. [Online] Available at: http://orthoinfo.aaos.org/topic.cfm?topic=A00094. Accessed July 2012

Aras MD, Gokkaya NK, Comert D et al 2004 Shoulder pain in hemiplegia: results from a national rehabilitation hospital in Turkey. Am J Phys Med Rehabil 83(9):713–719

Bell J, Leung B, Spratt K et al 2011 Trends and variation in incidence, surgical treatment, and repeat surgery of proximal humeral fractures in the elderly. J Bone Joint Surg Am 93:121–131

Bergh I, Sjostrom B, Oden A et al 2000 An application of pain rating scales in geriatric patients. Aging (Milano) 12(5):380–387

Bicer A, Ankarali H 2010 Shoulder pain and disability index: a validation study in Turkish women. Singapore Med J 51(11):865–870

Boudreau S, Boudreau E, Higgins LD, Wilcox RB, 2007 Rehabilitation following reverse total shoulder arthroplasty. J Orthop Sports Phys Ther 37(12):734–743

Bruder A, Taylor NF, Dodd KJ 2011 Exercise reduces impairment and improves activity in people after some upper limb fractures: a systematic review. J Physiother 57(2):71–82

Cailliet R 1980 The Shoulder in Hemiplegia. FA Davis, Philadelphia, PA

Chaaya M, Slim ZN, Habib RR 2012 High burden of rheumatic diseases in Lebanon: a COPCORD study. Int J Rheum Dis 15(2):136–143

Chu S, Kelsey J, Keegan T 2004 Risk factors for proximal humerus fracture. Am J Epidemiol 160:360–367

Cornell C, Omri Ayalon O 2011 Evidence for success with locking plates for fragility fractures. HSS J 7:164–169

Feng S, Guo S, Nobuhara K et al 2003 Prognostic indicators for outcome following rotator cuff tear repair. J Orthop Surg (Hong Kong) 11(2):110–116

Gilmore PE, Spaulding SJ, Vandervoort AA 2004 Hemiplegic shoulder pain: implications for occupational therapy treatment. Can J Occup Ther 71(1):36–46

Handoll HH, Ollivere BJ 2010 Interventions for treating proximal humeral fractures in adults. Cochrane Database Syst Rev 2010(12) CD000434

Hardwick DD, Lang CE 2011 Scapula and humeral movement patterns and their relationship with pain: a preliminary investigation. Int J Ther Rehabil 18(4):210–220

Harvey R, Macko R, Stein J et al (eds) 2009 Stroke Recovery and Rehabilitation Demos Medical Publishing, New York

Hodgson S, Mawson S, Stanley D 2003 Rehabilitation after two-part fractures of the neck of the humerus. J Bone Joint Surg Br 85B(3):419–422

Kalra N, Seitz A, Boardman III N et al 2010 Effect of posture on acromiohumeral distance with arm elevation in subjects with and without rotator cuff disease using ultrasonography. J Orthop Sports Phys Ther 40:633–640

Klit H, Finnerup NB, Overvad K et al 2011 Pain following stroke: a population-based follow-up study. PLOS ONE 6(11):1–9

Lewis J, Wright C, Green A 2005 Subacromial impingement syndrome: the effect of changing posture on shoulder range of movement. J Orthop Sports Phys Ther 35:72–87

Nesvold IL, Reinertsen KV, Fosså SD et al 2011 The relation between arm/shoulder problems and quality of life in breast cancer survivors: a cross-sectional and longitudinal study. J Cancer Surviv 5(1):62–72

Ozaras N, Cidem M, Demir S et al 2009 Shoulder pain and functional consequences: does it differ when it is at dominant side or not? J Back Musculoskelet Rehabil 22(4):223–225

Pong YP, Wang LY, Huang YC et al 2012 Sonography and physical findings in stroke patients with hemiplegic shoulders: a longitudinal study. J Rehabil Med 44(7):553–557

Ratnasabapathy Y, Broad J, Baskett J et al 2003 Shoulder pain in people with a stroke: a population-based study. Clin Rehabil 17(3):304–311

Renzenbrink GJ, IJzerman MJ 2004 Percutaneous neuromuscular electrical stimulation (P-NMES) for treating shoulder pain in chronic hemiplegia. Effects on shoulder pain and quality of life. Clin Rehabil 18(4):359–365

Satish S, Postigo LG, Ray LA et al 2001 Chronic rheumatologic symptoms in a tri-ethnic sample of men and women aged 75 and older. J Gerontol A Biol Sci Med Sci 56(8):M471–M476

Seitz AL, McClure PW, Finucane S et al 2012 The scapular assistance test results in changes in scapular position and subacromial space but not rotator cuff strength in subacromial impingement. J Orthop Sports Phys Ther 42:400–412

Slobogean GP, Noonan VK, O'Brien PJ 2010 The reliability and validity of the Disabilities of Arm, Shoulder, and Hand, EuroQol-5D, Health Utilities Index, and Short Form-6D outcome instruments in patients with proximal humeral fractures. J Shoulder Elbow Surg 19(3):342–348

Tanaka M, Itoi E, Sato K 2010 Factors related to successful outcome of conservative treatment for rotator cuff tears. Upsala J Med Sci 115:193–200

Turner-Stokes L, Jackson D 2002 Shoulder pain after stroke: a review of the evidence base to inform the development of an integrated care pathway. Clin Rehabil 16:276–298

Wilcox III R, Arslanian LE, Millett PJ 2005 Rehabilitation following total shoulder arthroplasty. J Orthop Sports Phys Ther 35(12):821–836

Yelnik AP, Colle FM, Bonan IV 2003 Treatment of pain and limited movement of the shoulder in hemiplegic patients with botulinum toxin A in the subscapular muscle. Eur Neurol 50(2):91–93

Chapter 21
Total hip arthroplasty

MARK A. BRIMER

INTRODUCTION

The total hip arthroplasty (THA) is an orthopedic procedure that is performed 280000 times annually in the United States of America (Cram et al., 2012). THA is one of the most common surgical procedures performed in the US and worldwide (Lohmander et al., 2006). The presence of severe and continuing pain and disability and the inability to perform one's job or participate in social and leisure activities generally make the decision to undergo the surgery easier for the patient and surgeon. THA is generally considered a safe procedure with major complication rates of approximately 3% for a primary procedure and 8% for revision procedures (Khatod et al., 2008). Overall, because of an aging society, it is anticipated an increasing number of elderly people will be undergoing total joint arthroplasty (Reininga et al., 2012).

INDICATIONS FOR THA

The primary indications for a total hip replacement are:

- severe osteoarthritis
- rheumatoid arthritis
- avascular necrosis
- traumatic arthritis
- hip fractures
- benign and malignant bone tumors
- arthritis associated with Paget's disease
- ankylosing spondylitis
- juvenile rheumatoid arthritis.

There are relatively few contraindications to the THA procedure other than active local or systemic infection and other medical conditions (e.g. diabetes mellitus, peripheral vascular disease) that increase the risk of perioperative complications or death (Barrett et al., 2005). Hemiarthroplasty, or partial reconstruction of the hip, is performed when the acetabular cartilage is intact and joint pathology is limited to the femoral side of the joint (Dalury, 2005).

Previously, obesity had been considered a contraindication to surgery because of a reported high mechanical failure rate in heavier patients. The prospect of long-term reduction in pain and disability for heavier patients may, however, offset the risk associated with potential mechanical failure (Phillips et al., 2003).

Data indicate that 62% of all THA procedures performed in the US are performed in women, with two-thirds of those procedures being performed in persons older than 65 years of age. The highest age-specific rate of THA in men is between the ages of 65 and 74 years. For women, the highest age-specific rate is between 75 and 84 years.

If the patient desires to undergo bilateral hip replacement sequentially, it is recommended that he or she wait at least 6 weeks between operations to avoid increased risk of complications from the presence of an occult venous thrombus from the first procedure. Otherwise, the bilateral procedure poses no increase in frequency of postoperative complications.

Historically, aseptic loosening of implanted components was identified as a major problem with THA. This problem was especially prevalent in younger and more active patients and in those who had undergone revision surgery. In the past two decades, however, the number of complications involving mechanical loosening has declined significantly. The incidence of mechanical loosening has decreased, as a result of improved fixation techniques, to the point where more than 90% of all total joints are never revised.

THE SURGICAL APPROACHES FOR THA

The primary surgical approaches used for THA are the anterolateral and the posterior approaches. The choice of surgical approach often depends upon the surgical training of the physician. Many of the difficulties associated with using the anterolateral approach are related to the anterior third of the gluteus medius muscle, which partially obstructs the insertion of the stem of the component into the femur. This has become a more critical element with the introduction of cementless technology. The anterolateral approach does, however, provide excellent exposure of the acetabulum, which is why some

Table 21.1 THA gait training and ROM guidelines

	Arthroplasty			
	Conventional (Cemented THA)	Bipolar Osteonics Ingrowth	Porous Coated	Trochanteric Osteotomy[a]
Mobilize (out of bed)	POD 1–2	POD 2	POD 2	POD 2–5
Ambulation, WB	PWB to WB as tolerated at discharge	(Porous coated stem, bipolar head) PWB 40–50 lb	PWB 40–50 lb	PWB
ROM of hip flexion	Same criteria for all: POD 2, up to 30°; POD 4–6, up to 60°; POD 6–10, up to 90°			
Precautions	Applies to all: avoid dislocation forces at hip, which are a combination of hip flexion, adduction and internal rotation; no hip flexion greater than 90°			
				No resisted abduction of hip; initially walk with a slightly abducted gait

From K. Lawrence, Orthopedic Team Supervisor of Physical Therapy Department, Medical College of Virginia, Richmond, VA, with permission.
POD, postoperative day; WB, weight-bearing; PWB, partial weight-bearing; ROM, range of motion
[a]No active abduction.

surgeons prefer that approach. Additionally, some data indicate patients receiving the anterior approach for THA tend to recover more quickly and have improved early outcomes, with dislocation rates at less than 1% (Moskal et al., 2013).

Regardless of the approach taken, difficulties are occasionally encountered. When using the posterior approach, there is a tendency to place the femoral component in less than normal anteversion, thereby leading to less postoperative external rotation because of the presence of an intact anterior capsule. A patient who undergoes the anterolateral approach commonly demonstrates less internal rotation postoperatively and a weaker hip abductor that is associated with surgical interference with the function of the abductor muscle.

There have been reports about the effectiveness of the minimally invasive approach to THA. The minimally invasive approach for hip arthroplasty was designed to transect less muscle and tendon. Therefore, it was expected to reduce hospital length of stay, pain levels, promote a quicker recovery and yield an improved cosmetic appearance (Berger, 2004). Total blood loss utilizing the minimally invasive procedure has been determined to be less than with conventional arthroplasty (Higuchi et al., 2003). Studies indicate the use of this procedure has not been found to increase the rate of postoperative dislocation (Siguier et al., 2004).

THE CEMENT AND CEMENTLESS TECHNIQUES

There are two available surgical mechanisms that can be used to properly secure the acetabular and femoral stem components. The cement technique adheres one or both of the replacement components to the surface of the bone with the use of polymethylmethacrylate bone cement. The cementless technique relies upon bone growth into porous or onto roughened surfaces for fixation.

The choice of which component to use with a particular patient may be based upon the individual's level of strenuous physical activity, age, health and wellbeing, and bone density. Surgical revision of both component types,

as evaluated by the use of modern techniques, has been reported to be less than 5% for the cemented femoral component over a 10-year period. The number of uncemented acetabular components requiring revision in a 7-year follow-up is approximately 2%.

Of primary concern in the cementless implants is the importance of the precise mechanism of load transfer to the bone. If the fit in the proximal femur is too loose and the distal end is too tight, then the proximal part of the component will be stress-shielded which could cause increased porosity or bone loss. If the proximal segment is well fitted but the distal end underfills the medullary cavity, then the patient may exhibit distal toggling while under load, which causes persistent thigh pain.

REHABILITATION

Preoperative care is beneficial for some individual patients but research has yet to support this in controlled studies and thus is best determined by the surgeon and the patient.

INPATIENT POSTOPERATIVE REHABILITATION CONSIDERATIONS

The primary concern following THA is to have the patient begin to walk. Patients with uncomplicated THAs are generally encouraged to ambulate, beginning on postoperative day 1 (Wright, 2004). Although ambulation may be brief in duration, the role of the therapist is to encourage mobility, self-care and proper weight-bearing and gait, and to teach the patient how to get into and out of bed in the proper manner. (See Table 21.1 for THA gait training and ROM guidelines.)

In the initial stages, most orthopedic surgeons recommend that the patient does not exceed 90° of hip flexion after surgery. Especially if the posterior approach has been used, it is important to instruct the patient to avoid internal rotation and adduction of the hip. Any of these motions, singularly or in combination, may produce a dislocation of the replacement. The complication of hip dislocation is more likely to occur in a patient who

Box 21.1   *THA postoperative concerns*

Therapists are advised to individualize these programs by adding or subtracting exercises depending on the patient's postoperative condition. Additional preoperative instructions to the patient may address the following immediate postoperative concerns:

1. Most THA procedures require the presence of an abduction pillow or wedge placed between the legs when the patient is in bed or in a wheelchair.
2. Patients are cautioned not to exceed 90° of flexion of the operative hip.
3. Passive or forcible movement of the hip that causes pain is contraindicated.
4. Internal rotation and adduction are contraindicated.
5. The patient is encouraged to perform active ankle exercises (rhythmic active dorsal and plantar flexion) frequently during the first few days postoperatively to prevent thrombophlebitis.
6. No weight-bearing or standing should take place unless under the direct supervision of the physical therapist.
7. Transfers and log-rolling should be performed away from the operative side, with the leg supported by a staff member.

From Echternach J 1990 Physical Therapy of the Hip. Churchill Livingstone, New York, with permission.

Box 21.2   *Homecare instructions for THA patients*

First 6 weeks postoperatively:

DO NOT

- Sit in low chairs or sofas
- Cross your legs
- Force your operated leg to flex (bend) or rotate at the hip
- Sit down on the floor of a bath tub
- Lean forward or raise your knee higher than your hip
- Discard the walking assistive device until instructed to do so
- Drive until permitted
- Force hip abduction, external rotation or extension if your doctor has performed an anterolateral surgical approach

DO

- Use help for putting on shoes and stockings
- Use your compression stockings
- Exercise as instructed
- Sleep on your back
- Place a pillow between your knees when sitting or sleeping
- Use caution when sitting and reaching towards the floor or towards the phone/table on the operative side. These motions encourage hip flexion and adduction, which are motions to be protected on the operative side
- Use caution getting into and out of bed and on and off a toilet seat. Avoid hip adduction, internal rotation and flexion approach beyond 90° if your doctor has performed a posterolateral approach

presents with a neurological disorder or is mentally confused. A common mechanism to prevent dislocation is the use of an abduction pillow. Abduction pillows are, as a general rule, used for a 1-month period (Box 21.1).

The hospital rehabilitation department that is preparing the patient for home or skilled-nursing placement should address the environment in which the patient will be placed. For example, a patient returning home should be thoroughly informed about the proper use of an elevated toilet seat, the possibility of encountering steps or stairs and how to deal with carpeted surfaces and the surfaces encountered outside the home. It is particularly important that a patient understands the proper positions for sleeping and what types of chairs are considered too low for comfortable and safe seating. A patient who plans return visits to the physician in the office must be instructed on how to properly enter, sit in, and exit from a car to avoid excessive hip flexion.

Activities of daily living should be discussed with the patient and immediate caregivers. Because a large majority of THA procedures are performed in the geriatric population, special consideration should be given to visual, balance and endurance losses that may have occurred. Patients have long been encouraged to use safe ambulation procedures until outpatient rehabilitation gait training needs can be addressed (Jagmin, 1998).

OUTPATIENT AND HOME-HEALTHCARE REHABILITATION CONSIDERATIONS

In the outpatient or home-healthcare environment, the focus is on restoring normal activities of daily living and safe walking techniques (Box 21.2). In the

initial stages (0–6 weeks), the patient should be advised to follow all dislocation precautions. These include the avoidance of excessive hip flexion and, in the case of the posterior approach, adduction and internal rotation. The patient should continue the use of elevated chairs and toilet seats until cleared by the surgeon to do otherwise.

In the 6 weeks following surgery, rehabilitation should focus on hip abduction (presuming no contraindications exist) and mild hip flexor and extensor strengthening. The patient may progress to standing with full weight-bearing, as permitted by the surgeon. A patient who has undergone the cementless technique may be required to maintain limited weight-bearing until sufficient new bone growth can be seen by the physician on X-ray. Falls risk assessment should be part of the continuous re-examination process during rehabilitation.

DESIRED REHABILITATION OUTCOMES FOR THE THA PATIENT

Most patients who undergo THA require limited outpatient physical therapy once a normal gait pattern can be resumed. The use of home programs as well as general conditioning exercises allows the patient to resume normal activities quickly. Gait may progress from using a walker to using a cane and then to using no assistive

Question	Score
1. **Please describe any pain in your hip:**	
A. No pain	44
B. Slight pain or occasional pain	40
C. Mild, no effect on ordinary activity, pain after unusual activity, uses aspirin or similar medication	30
D. Moderate pain that requires pain medicine stronger than aspirin/similar medications. I'm active but have had to make modifications and/or give up some activities because of pain	20
E. Marked or severe pain that limits activity and requires pain medicine frequently	10
F. Totally disabled – wheelchair or bed ridden	0
2. **Amount and type of support used:**	
A. None	11
B. Cane for long walks	7
C. Cane all the time	5
D. 2 canes	2
E. 1 crutch	3
F. 2 crutches or walker	0
G. Unable to walk	0
3. **Limp. This should be judged at the end of a long walk using the type of support chosen in question 2.**	
A. None	11
B. Slight	8
C. Moderate	5
D. Severe	0
4. **Distance that you can walk. This should be judged with the aid of a support if you use one.**	
A. Unlimited	11
B. 5–6 blocks	8
C. 1–4 blocks	5
D. In the house only	2
E. Unable to walk	0
5. **Climbing stairs:**	
A. Normally	4
B. Need a banister or cane or crutch	2
C. Must put both feet on each step/severe trouble climbing stairs	1
D. Unable to climb stairs	5
6. **Shoes and socks:**	
A. Can put on socks and tie a shoe easily	4
B. Can put on socks and tie a shoe with difficulty	2
C. Cannot put on socks and shoes	0
7. **Sitting:**	
A. Comfortable in any chair	5
B. Comfortable only in high chair, or can sit comfortably for only 0.5 hour	3
C. Cannot sit for 0.5 hour because of pain	0

From Mahomed N et al., 2001 The Harris Hip Score: comparison of patient self-report with surgeon assessment. J Arthroplasty 16:575–580, with permission from Elsevier.

Form 21.1 Self-administered hip-rating questionnaire

devices, as tolerated by the patient. Differences in leg length should be assessed and a shoe insert recommended if gait abnormalities persist. Once component stability has been obtained and dislocation potential has lessened, many surgeons encourage their patients to gain additional range of motion (ROM) in the hip. Patients are generally encouraged to resume, in moderation, physical activities such as golf, tennis, bicycle riding and walking.

The Self-Administered Hip-Rating Questionnaire shown in Form 21.1 has been used to assess patients' perspectives on outcomes after THA. As can be seen in

Figure 21.1, most benefits were obtained in 6 months, and some favorable changes took place after 6 months. The greatest functional improvements occurred in stair climbing, wearing normal shoes, and performing housework well.

CONCLUSION

When rehabilitating a patient who has received a THA, it is important to understand the specific procedures and to implement properly the specific guidelines for mobility,

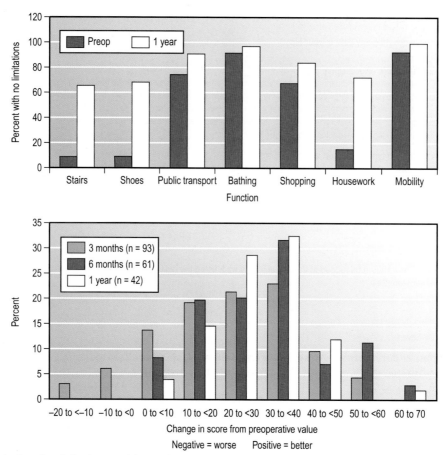

Figure 21.1 Change in function following total hip arthroplasty. Top graph shows changes in activities of daily living. Bottom graph shows changes in functional scores at 3, 6 and 12 months postoperatively. *(From Johanson NA, Charlson ME, Szatrowski TP et al., 1992A self-administered hip-rating questionnaire for the assessment of outcome after total hip replacement. J Bone Joint Surg Am 74:587–97, with permission from Elsevier.)*

weight-bearing, and ROM. Normal recovery timelines and progressions must be followed, with special attention to physician recommendations. Favorable functional outcomes are expected in 6–12 months.

REFERENCES

Barrett J, Losina E, Baron JA et al 2005 Survival following total hip replacement. J Bone Joint Surg Am 87:1965–1971

Berger RA 2004 Mini-incision total hip replacement using an anterolateral approach: technique and results. Orthop Clin North Am 35:143–151

Cram P, Lu X, Callaghan JJ et al 2012 Long term trends in hip arthroplasty utilization and volume. J Arthroplasty 27(2):278–285e2

Dalury DF 2005 The technique of cemented total hip replacement. Orthopedics 28:s853–856

Higuchi F, Gotoh M, Yamaguchi N et al 2003 Minimally invasive uncemented total hip arthroplasty through an anterolateral approach with a shorter skin incision. J Orthop Sci 6:812–817

Jagmin MG 1998 Postoperative mental status in elderly hip surgery patients. Orthop Nurs 17:32–42

Khatod M, Inacio M, Paxton EW 2008 Knee replacement epidemiology, outcomes, and trends in Southern California: 17,080 replacements from 1995 through 2004. Acta Orthop 79(6):812–819

Lohmander L, Engesaeter LB, Herberts P et al 2006 Standardized incidence rates of total hip replacement for primary hip osteoarthritis in the 5 Nordic countries: similarities and differences. Acta Orthop 77(5):733–740

Moskal J, Capps SG, Scanelli JA 2013 Anterior muscle sparing approach for total hip arthroplasty. World J Orthop 4(1):12–18

Phillips CB, Barrett JA, Losina E et al 2003 Incidence rates of dislocation, pulmonary embolism, and deep infection during the first six months after elective total hip replacement. J Bone Joint Surg Am 85:20–26

Reininga IH, Stevens M, Wagenmakers R et al 2012 Minimally invasive total hip and knee arthroplast-implications for the elderly patient. Clin Geriatric Med 28(3):447–458

Siguier T, Siguier M, Brumpt B 2004 Mini-incision anterior approach does not increase dislocation rate: a study of 1037 total hip replacements. Clin Orthop Rel Res 426:164–173

Wright JM 2004 Mini-incision for total hip arthroplasty: a prospective, controlled investigation with 5-year follow-up evaluation. J Arthroplasty 5:538–545

Chapter 22
Total knee arthroplasty

MARK A. BRIMER

INTRODUCTION

Total knee replacement (TKR), also referred to as total knee arthroplasty (TKA), is one of the most common surgical procedures performed for patients with severe arthritis of the knee (Mahomed et al., 2005). Between 1991 and 2010, annual primary TKA increased 161% from 93 230 to 243 802 and revision TKA volume increased 109% from 9650 to 19 871 (Cram et al., 2012). Although there are over 150 brand name implants currently on the market, along with custom prostheses (Bush et al., 2006), they may be divided into three categories: the linked prosthesis, the resurfacing implant and the conforming implant.

THE THREE CATEGORIES OF IMPLANTS

In the *linked prosthesis,* the femoral and tibial components are physically fastened together at the time of manufacture or at some point during the surgical procedure. The linked prosthesis may be fully constrained, thereby permitting only flexion and extension, or it may permit flexion, extension and limited axial rotation. Used primarily in the 1970s, the linked prosthesis is no longer commonly used because of the loosening of components that occurs when stresses are applied to the tibial side of the joint. These prostheses may, however, be appropriate for patients who have markedly unstable knees or after failure of one or more previous arthroplasties.

A *resurfacing implant* has a flat polyethylene tibial surface that articulates with the metallic femoral condylar component. A resurfacing implant requires proper balancing of the collateral and cruciate ligaments and, therefore, is not indicated in a case in which either the cruciate or the collateral ligament is absent or deficient. Because a large number of patients with advanced arthritis have a missing or attenuated cruciate ligament and compromised soft-tissue balancing, which is necessary for the procedure to succeed, resurfacing implants are not the primary choice of many surgeons.

A *conforming implant* consists of a metallic femoral condylar component and a polyethylene tibial component. Designed to resist some of the translatory and shear stresses, they have a long record of use: 95% of all TKR procedures (Heck et al., 1998). The design of the conforming implant requires surgical sacrifice of the anterior cruciate ligament and, in some cases, depending upon the design of the particular implant, of the posterior cruciate ligament as well. The posterior cruciate is almost always removed in cases in which the patient presents a fixed varus or valgus contracture of 15–20° and the associated fixed flexion deformity.

FIXATION OF THE IMPLANT

The typical surgical approach has for many years been a conventional one. Recently, computer-navigated TKA has been investigated. Kim et al. (2012) reported no difference in clinical function, alignment or survivorship of the components that underwent computer-navigated versus conventional TKA. Regardless of approach, surgical fixation of all of the knee components is accomplished through one of two methods. The first involves the use of polymethylmethacrylate bone cement; one or both of the components is cemented to the bone surface. In the second method, the implants are inserted and one or both of the components are attached in a cementless manner. Although cemented knee components are still utilized, the preferred mechanism for attachment is cementless. Some of the problems that have been identified with the use of cemented components include the following:

1. The polymethylmethacrylate bone cement is known to become brittle. If the cement fragments in the joint, it can become trapped between components, which results in excessive component wear.
2. As the polymethylmethacrylate hardens, it is known to become thermotoxic to adjacent bony cells. It has also been known to decrease leukotaxis (attract leukocytes) and thereby increase the risk of infection at the implant site.
3. The use of bone cement is known to make surgical revision more difficult.

The cementless technique relies upon bone growth into porous or roughened surfaces for firm fixation. Proper and precise surgical placement of cementless components is essential if firm component attachment is to be obtained. Studies indicate that bone will not grow across gaps greater than 1–2 mm.

The choice of component may be based upon the patient's level of strenuous physical activity, age, health and wellbeing, and bone density. The primary contraindication to the use of a cementless component is severe osteoporosis. Loosening of the tibial tray is cited as the most common cause of failure in TKA but the mechanism remains unclear (Gebert de Uhlenbrock et al., 2012). Unicompartmental knee arthroplasty has been associated with consistently worse survival rates then TKA in worldwide arthroplasty registers (Baker et al., 2012).

Monitoring for potential infection is particularly important in TKA because a large amount of foreign material has been implanted in a superficial joint. Although a TKA is a relatively safe orthopedic procedure, wound-healing difficulties can occasionally be seen, including problems such as marginal wound necrosis, skin sloughing, sinus tract formation and hematoma formation (Norton et al., 1998). The presence of any of these complications may adversely affect the outcome. This is especially true with regard to range of motion (ROM) in cases in which therapy must be stopped until the problem can be resolved. The use of the minimally invasive TKR may reduce the potential for postoperative complications (Bonutti et al., 2004). However, more recent studies do not consistently report advantages of the minimally invasive approach for elderly patients (Liebensteiner et al., 2012; Reininga et al., 2012).

REHABILITATION

Preoperative care is beneficial for some individual patients but research has yet to support this in controlled studies and thus is best determined by the surgeon and the patient.

INPATIENT POSTOPERATIVE REHABILITATION CONSIDERATIONS

The primary concern after a TKA is to see that the patient begins to walk (Katz et al., 2004). A patient with an uncomplicated TKA is generally encouraged to walk on postoperative day 1, even if ambulation time is brief. The role of the therapist is to encourage mobility, self-care, proper weight-bearing and gait, and getting into and out of bed in the proper manner (Kane et al., 2005). Quadriceps femoris muscle strength is an important determinant of physical function, therefore improving quadriceps weakness is an important goal for orthopedic surgeons and rehabilitation specialists (Saleh et al., 2010).

During the first few days after surgery, many surgeons ask their patients to use a continuous passive motion (CPM) device to maximize ROM results. These devices are used in conjunction with physical therapy exercises and ROM and gait training sessions two or three times

a day. Patients are often encouraged to remain in the CPM device unless attending a physical therapy session or resting.

When a hospital rehabilitation department is preparing a patient to go home or to a skilled-nursing facility, staff members should consider the environment into which the patient is being discharged. For example, a patient returning home should be thoroughly trained in how to negotiate steps and flights of stairs, carpeted surfaces and surfaces that might be encountered outside the home. It is particularly important that the patient understand the proper positioning of the knee during sleep in order to prevent unwanted contractures.

Performance of the activities of daily living should be discussed with the patient and the immediate caregivers. Because a large majority of TKA procedures are performed in members of the geriatric population, special attention should be paid to any impairment in vision, balance, or endurance that may have occurred. A falls risk assessment should be performed and documented. Patients should be encouraged to monitor the integrity of the wound site on a daily basis and to use safe ambulation procedures until outpatient gait training needs can be addressed.

OUTPATIENT AND HOME HEALTHCARE REHABILITATION CONSIDERATIONS

In the outpatient or home healthcare rehabilitation environment the focus is on restoring the ability to perform normal activities of daily living, ROM of the knee and teaching safe ambulation. In the initial stages (0–4 weeks) it is vital to maximize ROM. Functional ROM is considered to be between 110° and 120° of flexion and full extension. Patients should be actively involved in home programs that focus upon the prevention of flexion or extension contractures of the knee. Neuromuscular electrical stimulation (NMES) can facilitate the recovery of quadriceps muscle strength after TKA, but the optimal intensity (dosage) of NMES on strength after TKA has yet to be determined (Stevens-Lapsley et al., 2012).

In the period between 0 and 4 weeks after surgery, rehabilitation should focus upon strength gains in the quadriceps, hamstring, hip flexor and hip extensor muscles. The patient may be allowed to progress to walking with full weight-bearing, as indicated by the physician. A patient who has undergone the cementless technique may be weight-bearing as tolerated immediately after surgery, or may be required to maintain limited weight-bearing for a period of 4–6 weeks or until sufficient new bone growth can be seen on an X-ray.

DESIRED REHABILITATION OUTCOMES FOR THE TKA PATIENT

Patients who undergo TKA commonly require extensive outpatient physical therapy for a period of approximately 6 weeks in order to maximize ROM. Swelling may persist for several months until sufficient collateral circulation can develop. The use of home ROM programs as well as general conditioning exercises

Table 22.1 Knee Society clinical rating system

Patient Category

A. Unilateral or bilateral (opposite knee successfully replaced)
B. Unilateral, other knee symptomatic
C. Multiple arthritis or medical infirmity

Pain	Points	Function	Points
None	50	Walking	
Mild or occasional	45	Unlimited	50
Stairs only	40	>10 blocks	40
Walking and stairs	30	5–10 blocks	30
Moderate		<5 blocks	20
Occasional	20	Housebound	10
Continual	10	Unable	0
Severe	0	Stairs	
Range of motion	25	Normal up and down	50
(5° = 1 point)		Normal up; down with rail	40
Stability (maximum movement in any position)		Up and down with rail	30
		Up with rail; unable down	15
Anteroposterior		Unable	0
<5 mm	10	Subtotal	
5–10 mm	5	Deduction (minus)	
10 mm	0	Cane	5
Mediolateral		Two canes	10
<5°	15	Crutches or walker	20
6–9°	10	Total deductions	
10–14°	5	Function score	
15°	0		
Subtotal			
Deductions (minus)			
Flexion contracture			
5–10°	2		
10–15°	5		
16–20°	10		
>20°	15		
Extension lag			
<10°	5		
10–20°	10		
>20°	15		
Alignment			
5–10°	0		
0–4° (3 points each degree)	15		
11–15° (3 points each degree)	15		
Other	20		
Total deductions			
Knee score (if total is a minus number, score is 0)			

From Insall JN, Dorr LD, Scott RD et al., 1989 Rationale of the knee society clinical rating system. Clin Orthop 248:13–14.

allows the patient to resume normal activities quickly. Strenuous exercise is to be avoided until approved of by the physician. A knee evaluation scale is shown in Table 22.1; it may be helpful in documenting postsurgical outcomes.

The patient may progress from using a walker to using a cane and then to ambulating with no assistive devices, as tolerated by the individual. Differences in leg length should be assessed and a shoe insert recommended if gait abnormalities persist. After several months, patients are often encouraged to resume, in moderation, physical activities such as golf, tennis, bicycle riding and walking (Lingard et al., 2004).

CONCLUSION

TKA is a surgical procedure commonly used in cases of advanced knee arthritis. Implants can be divided into three categories: linked prostheses, resurfacing implants and conforming implants. The components of the knee replacement may be surgically fixed with bone cement, or a cementless technique can be used. Rehabilitation is similar after the use of both of these methods, but a patient who has had the cementless procedure may be limited in weight-bearing for 4–6 weeks. Following discharge from the inpatient setting, continued rehabilitation should advance functional activities, restore normal ROM (110–120° of flexion and full extension are desirable), and ensure safe walking. Normal physical activities can be resumed several mouths after the operation.

REFERENCES

Baker PN, Petheram T, Avery PJ et al 2012 Revision for unexplained pain following unicompartmental and total knee replacement. J Bone Joint Surg Am 94(17):e1261–e1267

Bonutti PM, Mont MA, McMahon M et al 2004 Minimally invasive total knee arthroplasty. J Bone Joint Surg Am 86:26–32

Bush JL, Wilson JB, Vail TP 2006 Management of bone loss in revision total knee arthroplasty. Clin Orthop Rel Res 452:186–192

Cram P, Lu X, Kates SL et al 2012 Total knee arthroplasty volume, utilization, and outcomes among Medicare beneficiaries, 1991–2010. JAMA 308(12):1227–1236

Gebert de Uhlenbrock A, Puschel V, Puschel K et al 2012 Influence of time in-situ and implant type on fixation strength of cemented tibial trays – a post mortem retrieval analysis. Clin Biomech 27(9):929–935

Heck DA, Melfi CA, Mamlin LA et al 1998 Revision rates after knee replacement in the United States. Med Care 26:661–669

Kane RL, Saleh KJ, Wilt TJ et al 2005 The functional outcomes of total knee arthroplasty. J Bone Joint Surg 87:1719–1724

Katz JN, Barrett J, Mahomed NN et al 2004 Association between hospital and surgeon procedure volume and the outcomes of total knee replacement. J Bone Joint Surg Am 86:1909–1916

Kim YH, Park JW, Kim JS 2012 Computer-navigated versus conventional total knee arthroplasty a prospective randomized trial. J Bone Joint Surg 94(22):2017–2024

Liebensteiner MC, Krismer M, Koller A et al 2012 Does minimally invasive total knee arthroplasty improve isokinetic torque? Clin Orthop Rel Res 470(11):3233–3239

Lingard EA, Katz JN, Wright EA et al 2004 Predicting the outcomes of total knee arthroplasty. J Bone Joint Surg Am 86:2179–2186

Mahomed NN, Barrett J, Katz JN et al 2005 Epidemiology of total knee replacement in the United States Medicare population. J Bone Joint Surg 87:1222–1228

Norton EC, Garfinkel SA, McQuay LJ et al 1998 The effect of hospital volume on the in-patient complication rate in knee replacement patients. Health Serv Res 33:1191–1210

Reininga IH, Stevens M, Wagenmakers R et al 2012 Minimally invasive total hip and knee arthroplasty – implications for the elderly patient. Clin Geriatr Med 28(3):447–458

Saleh KJ, Lee LW, Gandhi R et al 2010 Quadriceps strength in relation to total knee arthroplasty outcomes. Instr Course Lect 59:119–130 Southern Illinois University, Springfield, Illinois, USA

Stevens-Lapsley JE, Balter JE, Wolfe P et al 2012 Relationship between intensity of quadriceps muscle neuromuscular electrical stimulation and strength recovery after total knee arthroplasty. Phys Ther 92(9):1187–1196

Chapter 23
The aging bony thorax

STEVEN PHEASANT

INTRODUCTION

The bony thorax has the primary function of protecting the organs of circulation and respiration. Some protection is also given to the liver and stomach. Secondarily, the bony thorax contributes to the mechanics of breathing through the attachment of the muscles of respiration to the ribs. These elements are shown in Figure 23.1. Lastly, the bony thorax serves as the foundation from which the shoulder complex functions, therefore influencing the efficiency of the upper extremity (Edmondston et al., 2012).

The thorax is composed of 12 thoracic vertebrae posteriorly, the sternum anteriorly and 12 pairs of ribs, which encircle the thorax. The first seven pairs of ribs are true ribs, with joints that attach the thoracic vertebrae to the sternum. The lower five pairs are considered false ribs since they do not attach directly to the sternum. Rib pairs 8, 9 and 10 attach to the sternum by way of their costal cartilage attachments to the seventh pair of ribs. Rib pairs 11 and 12 do not have attachments anteriorly to the sternum and are referred to as floating ribs. These bony relationships are shown in Figures 23.2 and 23.3.

The sternum is composed of three parts – the manubrium, the body and the xiphoid process – that are connected by fibrocartilage. The manubrium is the most superior and has notches for the clavicles. The body is a thin flexible bone and is the part used for closed cardiac compression. The xiphoid process is attached to the distal part of the body (Jenkins, 2009).

Each rib has a small head at the posterior end that presents upper and lower facets divided by a crest. Each facet articulates with the adjacent vertebral body. The next part of the rib, the tubercle, articulates with the transverse process of the corresponding vertebra. The shaft of the rib curves gently from the neck to a rather sharp bend called the angle of the rib. Successive ribs are separated by an intercostal space which is occupied by the intercostal muscles. The inferior border of each rib contains a costal groove in which the costal nerves and blood vessels run (Jenkins, 2009).

KINESIOLOGY

MECHANICS OF THE RIBS

There are two basic kinds of rib movements. The pump-handle type is noted at the upper ribs, where movement is limited by joint articulations anteriorly and posteriorly. When the upper ribs move upward, because of the costosternal joints, the sternum follows by moving forward and gliding upward. This thoracic movement increases the anteroposterior diameter and depth of the thorax.

The lower ribs move outward and upward during inspiration. This movement increases the transverse diameter of the thoracic cage. The movement is similar to a bucket-handle movement and is given this name. These two movements (pump-handle and bucket-handle) increase the volume of the thorax, which contributes to the negative pressure responsible for air exchange during inhalation (Frownfelter & Dean, 2006; Jenkins, 2009).

The excursion of the ribs during both quiet and deep breathing has been observed to decrease with advancing age. The reduction in movement has been noted to particularly involve the excursion of the upper ribs during deep breathing, affecting the pump-handle mechanism, and a reduction in the lower rib during quiet breathing, affecting the bucket-handle mechanism. The reduction in rib excursion suggests a compromise of inspiratory capacity as a consequence of an aging thorax (Kaneko & Horie, 2012).

MUSCLES OF THE THORAX

The primary muscle of respiration is the large dome-shaped diaphragm, which separates the thoracic and abdominal cavities. It has two halves, each of which has attachments anteriorly to the sternum at the posterior aspect of the xiphoid process.

Laterally, the diaphragm arises from the inner surfaces of the lower ribs and the lower six costal cartilages. Posteriorly, the diaphragm attaches to the vertebral bodies of the upper three lumbar vertebral bodies as well as the fascial coverings of the psoas major and quadratus lumborum. From

157

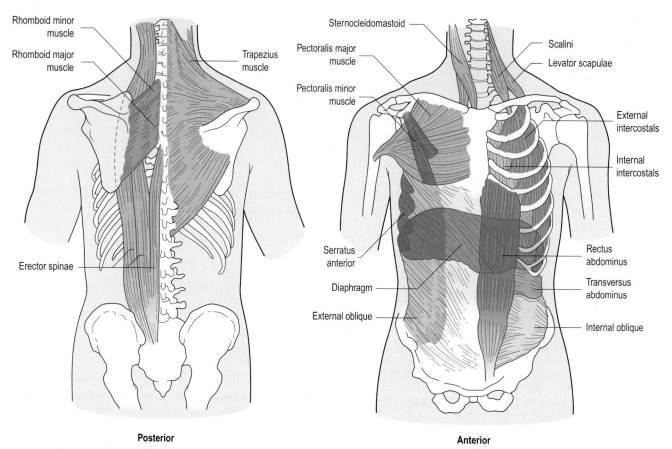

Figure 23.1 Muscles of ventilation, posterior and anterior views. *(From Starr JA 1995 Pulmonary system. In: Sgarlat-Myers R (ed), Saunders Manual of Physical Therapy Practice. WB Saunders, Philadelphia, PA,* p. 259, *with permission.)*

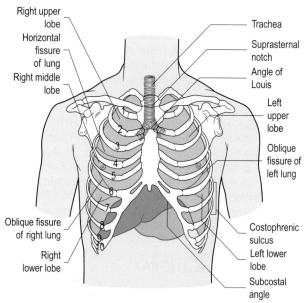

Figure 23.2 The bones of the thorax, anterior view. *(From Starr JA 1995 Pulmonary system. In: Sgarlat-Myers R (ed), Saunders Manual of Physical Therapy Practice. WB Saunders, Philadelphia, PA,* p. 254, *with permission.)*

these vast origins, the diaphragm spans the abdomen to insert into a central tendon at the pinnacle of the dome. The diaphragm descends as it contracts, increasing the vertical dimension of the thoracic cavity contributing to the

negative pressure responsible for air exchange during inhalation (Frownfelter & Dean, 2006; Neumann, 2010).

The intercostal muscles also play a role in inhalation, are comprised of three layers of muscle and occupy the spaces between adjacent ribs. The most superficial layer is made up of the external intercostals, which have a fiber direction that traverses in an inferior and medial direction in a course similar to that of the external abdominal oblique muscle. The external intercostal muscles consist of 11 pairs corresponding with each intercostal space and attaching the inferior border of the superior rib to the superior border of the inferior rib. The intermediate layer is comprised of the internal intercostals, which have fiber orientations that resemble the internal abdominal oblique muscles traveling in an inferior and lateral fashion and also consists of 11 pairs. The deepest layer of the intercostal muscles is the intercostal intimi. Although less defined, their fiber direction is similar to that of the internal intercostals. These 11 external and 11 internal intercostals, along with the erector spinae, rectus abdominus, internal oblique abdominals and transverse abdominals, also contribute to respiration.

The external intercostals and portions of the internal intercostals have been reported to contribute to pump- and bucket-handle elevation of the ribs, therefore contributing to increasing both the anterior/posterior and lateral dimensions of the thorax during quiet inhalation, further reducing the negative intrathoracic pressure and aiding the flow of air into the lungs (Frownfelter & Dean, 2006; Neumann, 2010).

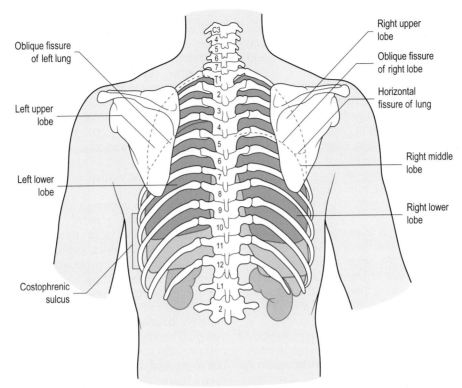

Figure 23.3 The bones of the thorax, posterior view. *(From Starr JA 1995 Pulmonary system. In: Sgarlat-Myers R (ed), Saunders Manual of Physical Therapy Practice. WB Saunders, Philadelphia, PA, p. 254, with permission.)*

POSTURAL STRESSES ON THE THORACIC SPINE

The thoracic spine possesses a naturally occurring kyphosis. The kyphosis is, in part, due to the wedge shape of the thoracic vertebral bodies (taller dorsally and shorter ventrally). Both the magnitude of the thoracic kyphosis and the resultant postural stresses imposed on the vertebral bodies increase substantially with a forward-thrust head posture. Increased postural stresses render the thoracic vertebral bodies vulnerable to compression fractures, particularly in those who are osteoporotic. Compression fractures in the thoracic spine can lead to increased vertebral wedging, greater postural stresses and a progressive thoracic kyphosis that further compounds the impairment (Katzman et al., 2010). The incidence of thoracic compression fractures in those over 70 years of age is 19%, of which 30% will suffer multiple fractures due in large part to the above mentioned biomechanical factor (Waterloo et al., 2012). Information regarding vertebral compression fracture management and rehabilitation can be found in Chapters 24 and 25.

PATHOLOGIES INVOLVING THE BONY THORAX

OBSTRUCTIVE LUNG DISEASES

Obstructive lung diseases cause an overinflated state in the lungs. The thoracic cage tends to assume the inspiratory position and the diaphragm becomes low and flat. The anteroposterior (AP) and transverse diameters of the chest are increased, and the ribs and sternum are always in

a state of partial or complete expansion. In this population, the abdominal musculature assists expiration by forcing the diaphragm back to its resting position. This increased abdominal activity and the resultant trunk flexion movement may, in part, be responsible for the four-fold increase in vertebral compression fractures observed in those with chronic obstructive pulmonary disease (COPD) (Brunton et al., 2005; Frownfelter & Dean, 2006).

RESTRICTIVE LUNG DISEASES

In restrictive lung diseases, the lungs are prevented from fully expanding because of restrictions in the lung tissue, pleurae, muscles, ribs or sternum. The AP and transverse diameters of the chest should increase with inspiration, but do not increase to normal levels in these conditions. Interstitial fibrosis, sarcoidosis and pneumoconiosis are examples of disease processes that decrease elasticity (or compliance) of the lung tissue.

Tumors or abnormalities in the pleural tissue, such as pleurisy, pleuritis and pleural effusion, cause compression of the lungs. Any condition that elevates the diaphragm and prevents full excursion of this muscle diminishes the ability of the chest to expand. Examples of such conditions are ascities, obesity and abdominal tumors of any kind (Watchie, 2010).

Numerous musculoskeletal conditions cause disturbed respiratory mechanics. The autoimmune (collagen) diseases can affect any joint in the body, including the costochondral and costovertebral joints. Additionally, these are systemic diseases and thus can also involve the pleural or lung tissue as well. Rheumatoid arthritis, systemic lupus erythematosus and scleroderma are examples. Other less severe forms of autoimmune disease such as fibromyalgia and dermatomyositis may affect the musculature and can cause pain and restriction of the myofascial structures and thereby limit chest expansion.

Costochondritis is another common condition affecting the chest wall. The inflammation of the costochondral junction is often seen in individuals over 40 years of age and can be caused by coughing, strenuous exercise or physical activities that stress the upper extremities. Costochondritis is a self-limiting condition but can be a source of chest pain that may be mistaken for myocardial infarction. It can also be confused with the less common 'Teitze syndrome' that tends to be seen in a younger population (Proulx et al., 2009).

Orthopedic conditions such as kyphosis, scoliosis and kyphoscoliosis, affect primarily the vertebral segments and costovertebral articulations. Even with mild changes of spine alignment, the mechanics of the ribs and sternum are altered. In severe cases, the lung tissue, heart and major vessels may be compromised by the deformity and altered mechanics.

Scheuermann's disease is characterized by hyperkyphosis of the thoracic spine and, though typically seen in adolescents, may not present until adulthood. Scheuermann's disease is defined by three successive thoracic vertebrae demonstrating anterior wedging of >5° with management determined by the magnitude of the deformity. Long-term follow-up of individuals with thoracic deformity due to Scheuermann's disease have a propensity for increased thoracic pain, decreased extension range of motion (ROM) of the thoracic spine and decreased strength of the thoracic spinal extensors. Individuals with a thoracic kyphosis exceeding 100° have also been shown to have reduced forced vital capacity due to compromised respiratory mechanics (Wood et al., 2012).

Ankylosing spondylitis can be considered in the autoimmune and orthopedic categories. It is considered separately here because of the severe consequences it can have on the thorax. In this condition, there is gradual fusion of spinal zygapophyseal joints, starting usually in the sacroiliac joints. As more and more of the spine becomes involved, X-rays demonstrate a bamboo-like image (bamboo spine). There is a calcification of the spinal segments as well as of the costovertebral joint, which causes severe restriction of chest expansion (Braveman, 2008).

Paget's disease is a chronic condition that results in abnormal bone degradation and regrowth. The resultant bone has inferior structural properties and often results in bony deformity. Although the effects are not unique to the spine, the thoracic spine can certainly be involved, and the disease should be considered as a possible source of pathology in the aging spine (Lane, 2009).

Trauma, accidental or surgical, can cause muscle splinting which may restrict chest expansion or relaxation. After thoracic and cardiovascular surgery there is a tendency for the patient to breathe in a shallow, rapid and guarded manner, usually not using the diaphragm but, rather, accessory muscles such as the scalenes and sternocleidomastoids. Even after healing, the posture of such patients has often changed and shows an increase in thoracic kyphosis, a marked forward-thrust head, protraction of the shoulder girdles and an adducted and internally rotated position of the shoulders. The acquired posture compromises not only spinal and respiratory function but function of the upper extremities as well.

Another type of trauma to the thorax that is not often considered is injury that occurs in a motor vehicle accident. If the person is using a seat belt/shoulder strap type of restraint at the time of the accident, the shoulder strap may cause damage to the thoracic fascial structures, muscles, or sternum and ribs, as well as fractures. However, soft-tissue and joint injuries are often overlooked even though they may contribute to painful postural and respiratory dysfunction.

Compression fractures in the thoracic spine are commonplace in the geriatric population. The increased mechanical stresses that result from the forward-thrust head, rounded shoulder, kyphotic posture that frequently follows a thoracic compression fracture, predispose the individual to further pain, reduced spinal motion and compromised respiratory function (Waterloo et al., 2012) (see Chapters 24 and 25). A 9% reduction in forced vital capacity has been reported as a consequence of thoracic vertebral compression fractures. Additionally, multiple compression fractures may lead not only to increasing pain but to a protruding abdomen, thereby reducing abdominal cavity space. This could subsequently create difficulty with digestion. The deformity due to multiple compression fractures may also allow the floating ribs to rest upon the iliac crests, leading to another potential source of pain (Brunton et al., 2005).

When muscular, fascial, spinal, rib, or sternal components are the cause of restriction of lung capacity, the patient may benefit from physical therapy that can improve mechanics and lower the pain factor, thus improving quality of life in spite of the underlying disease process.

ASSESSMENT

History is very important. Understanding the underlying disease process or mechanism of trauma can help in defining the problem list and the goals for a particular patient. Histories of the present illness as well as of past medical and surgical problems are vital to proper examination and treatment. Laboratory and radiographic data, medication lists, particularly pulmonary and cardiac drugs, and psychosocial information should be gathered.

Examination can be broken down into components, starting with general appearance (Box 23.1). This consists of assessing level of consciousness, which can indicate adequacy of oxygenation of brain tissues. Body type is evaluated as normal, obese, or cachectic. An obese person has higher energy demands, even for simple activities. General appearance can also indicate whether the person is deconditioned. Also, some respiratory conditions are caused by excessive weight which can cause restriction of the diaphragm. The cachectic patient may have had weight loss associated with a carcinoma, or eating may take too much energy, so caloric intake becomes insufficient.

In evaluating posture, the therapist should note any spinal malalignment or unusual postures. The extremities are observed for nicotine stains (which indicate a history

Box 23.1 Steps in clinical assessment of patients with breathing dysfunction

1. General appearance
   Level of consciousness
   Body type: obese, cachectic
2. Posture
3. Skin and color
   Face
   Fingers
4. Vital signs
5. Respiratory pattern
   Rate
   Rhythm
   Accessory muscles
6. Chest wall movement
   Axilla
   Xiphoid tip
   Lower costal border
   Quiet and maximal inhalation and exhalation
7. Range of motion
   Neck
   Upper extremity
   Trunk
   Lower extremity
8. Auscultation
9. Strength
   Trunk posture
10. Functional abilities
    Activities of daily living
    Gait
11. Palpation
    Skin
    Fascia
    Muscles
12. Joint mobility
    Costosternal
    Costovertebral
    Spinal
13. Psychosocial factors
    Patient's goals
    Family's goals

of heavy smoking), clubbing of the fingers or toes (a sign of cardiopulmonary or small bowel disease), swollen joints, tremors and edema. Any of these parameters may indicate respiratory system impairment.

The color of the skin and face should be noted. A patient might show evidence of a bluish tinge to the mucous membranes or nail beds, indicating severe arterial oxygen desaturation (Frownfelter & Dean, 2006).

Posture should be noted initially, especially sitting and standing patterns. In a patient with COPD usually there is a forward-thrust head, increased kyphosis in the thoracic area, and abduction and protraction of the shoulder girdles. If there is less than a two finger space between the iliac crests and the lower ribs, osteoporosis should be suspected and further appropriate workup and care should be considered (Brunton et al., 2005). There may be elevation of the shoulder girdles as well, if the accessory muscles of breathing are the primary respiratory muscles. With spinal curvature, there are changes in posture from the sagittal and frontal views. When trauma is the

mechanism of dysfunction, any or all of the above can be seen, as well as changes related to joint dysfunction and muscle involvement.

Reliance on accessory muscles for respiration may result in hypertrophy and strain leading to possible ROM restrictions and pain. Bracing postures or slightly forward bent postures may also be assumed to assist with respiration in those in respiratory distress. Although the postures may be assumed to assist respiration, the postures themselves may be a source of pain due to the mechanical strain that may accompany them.

The depth of inspiration and whether expiration is passive (as is normally expected at rest) or forced should also be observed. Vital signs, including blood pressure, heart rate and rhythm, and respiratory rate and rhythm should be noted. It may be pertinent to assess these at rest and with exertion. Pulmonary function volumes and diseases are described in Chapters 7 and 45. Pulmonary function might have to be assessed by means of spirometry. Respiratory patterns include not only rate and rhythm but also identification of the particular muscles used for respiration (Watchie, 2010).

Chest wall excursion can be recorded taking circumferential measurements with a tape measure at the floor of the axillae, at the tip of the xiphoid and at the lower costal border at the midaxillary line of the 10th rib. These measurements should be taken during quiet breathing for inspiration and expiration, as well as with maximum inspiration and forced expiration. These landmarks (or others of the therapist's choice) should be consistent and reproducible.

Auscultation, or listening to the breath sounds, is another important aspect of assessment. When possible, the patient should sit forward for this part of the examination. The anterior and middle lobes can best be auscultated at the front of the patient, whereas the posterior lobes are best heard at the patient's back. The patient should breathe in and out through an open mouth. A comparison of breath sounds in each segment of each lung should assess the intensity, pitch and quality.

There is a system of nomenclature and it is helpful to use these standard terms. Quality is defined as absent, decreased, normal, or bronchial. If abnormal sounds are heard, they can be further described as crackles, rales, wheezes, or rhonchi. During vocalization, sounds can be normal, increased, or decreased. All the above can help to define the area of the chest and lungs involved in the pathology. One can also hear rubs from the pleura or from the pericardium. (See Figure 23.4 for auscultation sites.)

ROM assessment, formal or functional, should include the head, neck, upper extremities, lower extremities and trunk. Emphasis on specific areas may change depending on the pathology. However, as the neck, upper back and shoulder girdles are consistently involved to a large degree, these areas must be accurately assessed on an ongoing basis. Flexibility is an important parameter to consider, especially that of the anterior chest muscles. The pectoralis major and minor, sternocleidomastoid and scalenes may all be shortened or overused. Unless a normal length can be regained in these muscles, normalization of posture cannot occur.

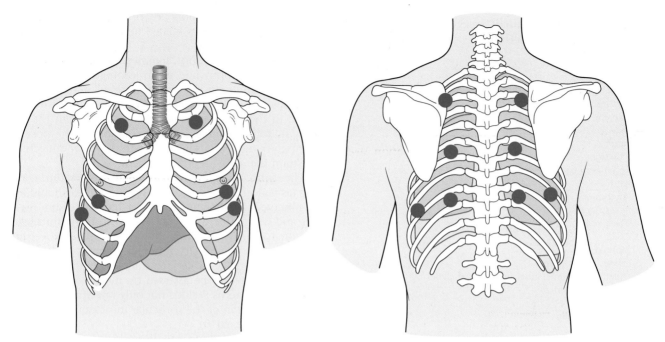

Figure 23.4 Anterior, lateral and posterior auscultation sites. *(From Starr JA 1995 Pulmonary system. In: Sgarlat-Myers R (ed), Saunders Manual of Physical Therapy Practice. WB Saunders, Philadelphia, PA, p. 270, with permission.)*

Strength may also be specifically or functionally tested. In most cases, testing of functional strength is all that is necessary. However, when working on postural correction, it may be important to test specifically the trapezius, rhomboids and rotator cuff muscles as well as neck and back extensors. Coordination among muscle groups should be examined.

It is extremely important to note functional abilities, as it is these activities that most concern outcome measures. Basics such as bed mobility, transfers, feeding, bathing and toileting may be possible but higher-level activities such as housekeeping, food preparation and shopping may be limited. Whatever the functional limitation, it is important to note them in measurable ways. Gait pattern, balance, endurance and need of assistive devices should be evaluated. The ability to traverse a specific distance in a measured time clarifies functional mobility. For example, Brown et al. (2010) reported a walking endurance of 200 m as a distance to be used as a baseline goal for ambulating in the community. Similarly, a walking velocity of 30 m/min has been reported as a minimum to allow safe street crossing. Both are measures that are particularly important for community dwelling individuals (Andrews et al., 2010).

On palpation, skin, fascia and each layer should be pliable and extensible, and each layer should be separated from adjacent layers. With the absence of any of these qualities, movement at any or all layers or planes may be restricted and painful, thus creating guarding or spasm, which may prevent normal joint kinematics and mobility.

Joint mobility can be restricted by surgical, traumatic, or soft-tissue conditions. The costosternal and costovertebral joints may be involved, which limits general mobility of the ribs in their upward and downward movements. The sternum can also be prevented from gliding by soft-tissue restriction or dysfunction of the sternoclavicular joints and costoclavicular joints on one or both sides. To a lesser extent but still important are the spinal joints of the cervical and thoracic areas. The scapulothoracic joints may also affect the mobility of the ribs, and certainly affect posture.

The joints can be assessed by passive mobility testing involving A-P, P-A springs at the costosternal, costovertebral, cervical and thoracic segments. Monitoring the excursion of each rib anteriorly and/or laterally during inspiration and expiration may reveal any dysfunction. At the first rib, a distal spring at the midpoint of the supraclavicular space and A-P and P-A springs can be used to assess mobility. Glides of the scapula in all planes detect disturbances of the scapulothoracic joints. Particular care should be exercised when assessing passive joint mobility of the vertebral and costal structures in patients with osteoporosis.

Psychological factors can affect a patient's condition, goals, treatment plan and outcome measurements. The patient's family situation, the availability of a caregiver and the type of dwelling should be recorded. The patient's and the family's reactions to the disease process may affect the pathology and the outcome, so it is important to allow the patient to discuss problems and concerns. It is to be hoped that the patient's and family's goals are congruent with those of the medical providers.

INTERVENTION

Optimal breathing is performed by the diaphragm, with distal excursion on inspiration and return to baseline or elevation on expiration, normal or forced. This results in expansion of the lower chest and abdomen on inspiration and retraction in these areas on expiration. The person should be encouraged to inhale through the nose (to filter, warm and moisturize the air) and to exhale through pursed lips to ensure the emptying of the alveoli (Watchie, 2010).

Diaphragmatic, pursed lipped and timed breathing exercises have each demonstrated favorable outcomes in regards to distance covered during a 6-minute walk test in a population of individuals with COPD. Ventilation feedback training, however, was determined to be less effective than exercise training in the same population (Holland et al., 2012).

Lateral costal expansion can also be promoted as this requires rib movement in a bucket-handle fashion and may improve mobility. Use of tactile stimulation over the diaphragm or the lateral costal margins can facilitate the proper function. Resistance may also be performed by using weights on the diaphragm area or by resisting chest expansion with elastic exercise bands or tubing. When a specific area of the lungs is not expanding, segmental breathing exercises may be useful. Again, tactile stimulation may provide the sensory input that will promote increased expansion at the area (Watchie, 2010).

In conjunction with proper breathing techniques, postural correction exercises can assist with more efficient breathing patterns. However, in the case of chronic cardiopulmonary diseases, the aforementioned postural adaptations may have occurred to assist air exchange, and if so, correction of these postures can be detrimental to the patient's overall condition. Each case must be considered on an individual basis.

In order to improve posture, several factors must be considered. Some muscles will have shortened, whereas others will have been overstretched and weakened. Joints may have lost passive mobility in one or several planes. Body awareness and proprioception may be impaired, so high patient motivation and a long-time commitment to exercise and body awareness are necessary. ROM, strengthening and flexibility exercises are vital for postural changes, functional improvements and general wellbeing. All areas of the body should be considered, but practicality stresses exercises for the most severely involved areas. When pulmonary disease is present, the ability of the muscles to extract oxygen can be enhanced by strengthening exercises. This improved extraction of oxygen allows the patient better efficiency and endurance during routine activities (Ortega et al., 2002).

Strengthening exercises may include any or all of the following: active ROM, progressive resistive exercises with gradually increasing weight and repetition, and use of exercise equipment, such as a bicycle ergometer, treadmill, rowing machine, or ski machine. Proprioceptive neuromuscular facilitation exercises and closed-chain activities or functional activities with increasing time and difficulty can enhance strength and fitness.

For patients with musculoskeletal conditions in the thoracic or rib area, physical therapy modalities including heat, cold, ultrasound and electric stimulation may be indicated (see Chapters 66 and 67).

If during the evaluation, restriction of skin, fascia, or muscle is identified, manual techniques may be used to regain tissue extensibility. Treatment techniques are identified by many different names, but the goals of all such techniques are the same – to improve the extensibility of tissues and to allow one layer to move separately from adjacent layers.

Mobilization of the joints may be necessary in order to recover full ROM, full flexibility and correct posture. The first rib as well as the costosternal and costovertebral joints can be mobilized by A-P, P-A spring and distal glide mobilizations in grades I–IV, depending on the patient's condition and tolerance. Mobilization techniques used on the ribs can encourage elevation or depression.

CONCLUSION

The bony thorax is often overlooked in caring for an aging patient unless there is frank pathology. In addition to overt pathologies of the thorax, insidious age-related declines contribute to changes in structure and function that necessitate thorough assessment. Breathing, posture, mobility, and strengthening exercises are important rehabilitation interventions.

REFERENCES

Andrews A, Chinworth S, Bourassa M et al 2010 Update on distance and velocity requirements for community ambulation. J Geriatr Phys Ther 33(3):128–134
Braveman SE 2008 Ankylosing spondylitis. In: Frontera WR (ed) Essentials of Physical Medicine and Rehabilitation: Musculoskeletal Disorders, Pain, and Rehabilitation, 2nd edn. Saunders Elsevier, Philadelphia, PA
Brown CJ, Bradberry C, Howze SG et al 2010 Defining community ambulation from the perspective of the older adult. J Geriatr Phys Ther 33(2):56–63
Brunton S, Carmichael B, Gold D et al 2005 Vertebral compression fractures in primary care. Supplement to J Fam Pract. [Online] 54(9):781–8. (Accessed at www.jfponline.com January 2013)
Edmondston S, Ferguson A, Ippersiel P et al 2012 Clinical and radiological investigation of thoracic spine extension motion during bilateral arm elevation. J Orthop Sports Phys Ther 42(10):861–869
Frownfelter D, Dean E 2006 Principles and Practice of Cardiopulmonary Physical Therapy, 4th edn. Mosby Elsevier, St Louis, MO
Holland AE, Hill CJ, Jones AY et al 2012 Breathing exercise for chronic obstructive pulmonary disease: review. Cochrane Database Syst Rev 10:CD008250, doi: http://dx.doi.org/10.1002/14651858.CD008250.pub2
Jenkins D 2009 Hollinshead Functional Anatomy of the Limbs and Back, 9th edn. Saunders, St Louis, MO
Kaneko H, Horie J 2012 Breathing movements of the chest and abdominal wall in healthy subjects. Respiratory Care 57(9):1442–1451
Katzman WB, Wanek L, Shepherd JA et al 2010 Age-related hyperkyphosis: its causes, consequences, and management. J Orthop Sports Phys Ther 40(6):352–360
Lane N 2009 Paget's disease of bone, 8th edn. In: Firestein GS (ed) Kelley's Textbook of Rheumatology, vol. 2. Saunders Elsevier, Philadelphia, PA, pp. 1593–1595
Neumann DA 2010 Kinesiology of the Musculoskeletal System, Foundations for Rehabilitation, 2nd edn. Mosby Elsevier, St Louis, MO
Ortega F, Toral J, Cejudo P et al 2002 Comparison of effects of strength and endurance training in patients with chronic obstructive pulmonary disease. Am J Respir Crit Care Med 166(5):669–674
Proulx AM, Zryd TW 2009 Costochondritis: diagnosis and treatment. Am Fam Physician 80(6):617–620
Watchie J 2010 Cardiopulmonary Physical Therapy, 2nd edn. WB Saunders, Philadelphia, PA
Waterloo S, Ahmed L, Center J et al 2012 Prevalence of vertebral fractures in young women and men in the population-based Trømso study. BMC Musculoskelet Disord 13(3) Epub 17 January 2012. doi: http://dx.doi.org/10.1186/1471-2474-13-3, PMCID: PMC3273434
Wood KB, Melikian R, Villamil F 2012 Adult Scheuermann kyphosis: evaluation, management, and new developments. J Am Acad Orthop Surg 20(2):113–121

Chapter 24
The geriatric spine

TIMOTHY L. KAUFFMAN • RICHARD HAYDT

CHAPTER CONTENTS

INTRODUCTION

The aging process can be 'a pain in the neck' or a 'pain in the back', literally as well as figuratively. Early in the 20th century, Schmorl and Junghann (1932) reported that 90% of males over the age of 50 and 90% of females over the age of 60 have radiographic evidence of spinal degeneration.

In regards to the lumbar spine, by the age of 45 or 50 approximately 75% of men and 60% of women have lumbar disc degeneration at grades 1–4. By age 65 the incidence increases to over 90% and 80% respectively, with increased frequency of grade 3–4 degeneration. In addition to degeneration of the lumbar discs, degeneration and spondylosis of the facet or zygapophyseal joints are common (Badley, 1987). In the cervical spine it is common for elderly individuals to experience neck symptoms, with the majority of them related to cervical spondylosis or degenerative disease of the cervical spine (Modic et al., 1989).

Spine conditions commonly occur as a result of degeneration of the intervertebral discs, with loss of the water content within the disc and subsequent disc collapse. The resultant increased loads on spinal osseous elements such as facet joints, uncovertebral joints and vertebral bodies can lead to osteophyte formation on these structures. Degenerative disc bulging, osteophyte formation and ligamentum flavum hypertrophy can encroach upon the nerve roots in the intervertebral foramen or on the spinal cord in the central canal. Lee et al. (2012) reported that the cumulative incidence of cervical and lumbar spine degeneration in the US population ranged from 12.7% to 51.5% during a recent 5- to 25-year period.

CERVICAL SPINE

COMMON CLINICAL SYNDROMES

Cervicalgia

Cervicalgia – defined as neck pain – tends to be located posteriorly in the area of the paraspinous muscles. It can easily be aggravated by driving, computer use and physical inactivity. Patients often complain of occipital headaches as well as interscapular pain. Symptoms are exacerbated by neck motion and by fully abducting the arms. The symptoms are relieved by various therapeutic modalities, including hot packs, ultrasound, electrical stimulation, traction and manual techniques such as joint and soft tissue mobilization. Immobilization with a cervical orthosis along with neck-strengthening exercises may be helpful. It should be noted, however, that older patients have difficulty wearing a soft collar because it tends to be too large and uncomfortable. Rigid supports should be used rarely.

Radiculopathy

Radiculopathy – defined as pain in a specific nerve root distribution – can result from herniation of a disc or from constriction, where the nerve root exits the spinal foramina due to the presence of osteophytes. Lower motor neuron signs and symptoms may result. Clinically, it is characterized by pain and paresthesia both proximally and distally along the involved nerve root dermatomes. It is not uncommon to find overlapping symptoms in multiple dermatomes. Additionally, weakness can be present in corresponding myotomes with C5–6 and C6–7 interspaces most commonly involved (Rana, 2011).

Myelopathy

Myelopathy – often missed but more commonly found in patients over 55 years of age. Radiographs show the typical osteophytes and narrowing of disc spaces. Compression of the spinal cord is likely if the spinal canal diameter is less than 10mm. Typical neurological findings include lower motor neuron and reflex changes at the level of the lesion and upper motor neuron involvement below the level of the lesion. Spastic gait or other gait abnormalities are the most common clinical concern due to spinal cord compression (Beers et al., 2011). The myelopathy tends to have an insidious onset and develops gradually over a long period of time.

HISTORY, PHYSICAL EXAMINATION AND IMAGING

During history-taking and physical examination it is important to differentiate between cervical spine radiculopathy and cervical myelopathy. It is extremely important to specify the type of pain and its anatomical distribution (Rana, 2011). Complaints of deep aching pain and a burning sensation specifically bilaterally or in both upper and lower extremities are suggestive of spinal cord involvement. Many patients lose hand dexterity.

Most patients present with decreased neck range of motion (ROM) and paraspinous muscle spasm. There may be tenderness directly over the spinous process. Radicular pain is typically exacerbated by moving the neck or shoulders and it is common for pain to radiate either within a specific nerve distribution down the arm, into the scapular region or proximately into the occiput. A clinical prediction rule (CPR) can aid the clinician in diagnosing cervical radiculopathy (Wainner et al., 2003). Predictor variables are: (1) cervical spine rotation toward the involved side <60°; (2) positive upper limb tension test; (3) positive cervical spine distraction test (symptom relief); and (4) a positive Spurling test. The presence of three or more predictor variables indicates a moderate shift in probability that a patient will test positive for cervical spine radiculopathy using needle electromyography. In cases of cervical myelopathy, both upper and lower neurological examination should be performed. Imaging modalities are extremely useful in differentiating various types of cervical disease. Probably the most useful test is computerized tomography (CT) with intrathecal contrast which provides excellent differential between bone and soft tissue lesions and can accurately demonstrate canal size and foraminal narrowing. Magnetic resonance imaging (MRI) is useful as a noninvasive way of evaluating the spinal cord, soft tissues and neural structures (Rana, 2011). Plain radiographs can demonstrate bony changes and obvious foraminal narrowing, but tend to be more generalized (see Chapter 14).

DIFFERENTIAL DIAGNOSIS

In generating a differential diagnosis when working with an older individual, other diseases should be considered (Rana, 2011). Cancerous conditions that can refer pain to the neck region include metastatic lesions, leukemia, cervical spine bone or spinal cord tumors, lung cancer, Pancoast tumor, esophageal cancer and thyroid cancer. Neoplasms, the most common being metastatic tumors from carcinoma of the breast, prostate, kidney or thyroid, should be sought. Pain resulting from metastatic disease tends to be more intense at night and is often unremitting. Viscerogenic conditions such as angina, myocardial infarction or aortic aneurysm should be ruled out. Additionally, the pulmonary conditions such as a pneumothorax, pneumonia and tracheobronchial irritation should be ruled out as well (Goodman & Snyder, 2013).

Sepsis of the skeleton occurs infrequently in the cervical spine but is commonly seen in the lumbosacral spine and can occur following urogenital procedures. In those over the age of 65, sepsis of skin, soft tissue and bone accounts for 4.4% of all patients hospitalized for sepsis (Martin et al., 2006). Other inflammatory diseases can also lead to myelopathy; they include rheumatoid arthritis, ankylosing spondylitis, Reiter's syndrome and diffuse idiopathic skeletal hypertrophy (DISH). However, most patients with such diseases present with other joint symptoms before the cervical spine becomes involved (Rana, 2011).

Cervical disc disease must be differentiated from primary shoulder disorders (Rana, 2011). Rotator cuff tendonitis, subacromial bursitis and acromioclavicular joint problems can present with shoulder pain that radiates into the paraspinous muscle area. It is possible for a patient to have both primary shoulder disease and degenerative disc disease of the cervical spine. Selective injections, particularly into the subacromial space or the glenohumeral joint, can be helpful in differential diagnosis. Polymyalgia rheumatica should also be considered when an older patient presents specifically with significant proximal pain and stiffness in the morning. This can develop into an acute emergency if the patient develops temporal arteritis and visual difficulties. A patient who presents with these symptoms should be referred to a physician immediately for evaluation and treatment.

Other neurological findings that may be confused with cervical radiculopathies include compressive neuropathies such as entrapment of the suprascapular nerve, with pain in the upper scapular region and atrophy of the rotator cuff musculature. Median and ulnar nerve compression and thoracic outlet syndrome also present with shoulder pain, along with paresthesia or weakness. Differentiation can be determined by nerve conduction studies or electromyelograms (see Chapters 32 and 33).

The bilateral vertebral arteries pass through the foramen transversarium and join to form the basilar artery and supply the circle of Willis. Age-related degenerative changes in the cervical spine may compromise this circulation, especially when the neck is extended, and are a possible cause of dizziness or balance complaints (Kesson & Atkins, 2005).

TREATMENT

The majority of cervical symptoms in the geriatric patient can be treated by means of physical therapy and careful monitoring. Surgery is indicated primarily in a patient with myelopathy, progressive compression of the spinal cord or significant nerve root encroachment that causes pain and progressive weakness in a specific nerve distribution. In a study involving patients over 55 years of age, 3 weeks of mechanical traction and exercise showed improvement of neck pain (Raney et al., 2009). Escortell et al. (2008) studied 90 patients with subacute or chronic neck pain, with 47 patients randomly allocated for manual therapy and 43 for transcutaneous electrical stimulation. Both manual therapy and transcutaneous electrical stimulation were found to reduce neck pain, although there were no differences between the groups. Manual techniques, such as mobilization and stretching, are often helpful but the vertebrobasilar system must be cleared. Clinically, cervical spondylosis, and especially vertebral artery compromise, may limit cervical spine ROM exercises, mobilization, manipulation and the use of the Hallpike maneuver. Cervical manipulation should be used with extreme caution because of the documented risk of encroachment on the vertebral arteries and the possibility of stroke (Carlesso et al., 2010).

If the symptoms of cervical myelopathy or radiculopathy do not respond to conservative measures an anterior cervical discectomy and fusion (ACDF) procedure is commonly performed. Good to excellent results have been obtained in 88–94% of patients undergoing the ACDF procedure. Total disc replacement (arthroplasty) surgery has been recently developed and performed, with studies showing comparable or even better results (Smith et al., 2012). In a systematic meta-analysis, Fouyas et al. (2002) reported evidence that cervical spine surgery for spondylotic radiculopathy or myelopathy did not provide greater benefits than were derived from conservative therapy at 1 or 2 years.

THORACIC SPINE

DISORDERS OF THE THORACIC SPINE

The most common disorder of the thoracic spine in geriatric patients results from osteoporosis. Nearly 44 million Americans have osteoporosis and 50% of women and 20% of men over the age of 50 will incur a fracture due to osteoporosis (NOF, 2010). As bone mass decreases in elderly individuals, the vertebral bodies are at particular risk for compression fractures. A patient with multiple compression fractures in the thoracic spine can develop a severe kyphotic deformity ('dowager's hump'). Minimal trauma or none at all may create fragility fractures in the geriatric population with low bone mineral density (see Chapters 18 and 60). In a new fracture there is significant tenderness, with palpation of the spinous process and paraspinous muscle spasm. The neurological examination generally remains intact.

Compression fractures must be differentiated as old from new, and from malignancies. Plain radiographs are not the 'gold standard' (see Chapter 14, Figure 14.13). It is not uncommon for a patient with multiple myeloma or metastatic disease to present with a compression fracture (Rana, 2011). A bone scan, which may demonstrate lesions in other skeletal areas, is useful in differentiating a malignancy from a compression fracture resulting from osteoporosis.

Other thoracic spinal abnormalities include infections and degenerative disc disease. DISH is commonly found in the thoracic spine, presenting as stiffness and local pain. Other visceral problems can present as acute thoracic back pain in older patients, particularly ruptured aortic aneurysms, angina, myocardial infarctions, mediastinal tumors, breast cancer, lung infections, acute pneumonia, pneumothorax, peptic ulcer disease, kidney disease, pancreatic disease and acute cholecystitis (Goodman & Snyder, 2013). A careful physical examination and laboratory and diagnostic studies can differentiate viscerogenic from spinal disorders.

TREATMENT OF COMPRESSION FRACTURES

Treatment of compression fractures involves analgesics and brief bedrest followed by gradual mobilization and weight-bearing with assistive devices, if required. Caution must be exercised because the biomechanics (long lever arm) of lifting a walker can actually provoke increased thoracic pain. A wheeled walker reduces biomechanical strain. Prolonged bedrest leads to further osteopenia caused by disuse and to other complications, including pneumonia and urinary incontinence. If analgesics are incapable of resolving these symptoms or if polypharmacy is a concern, a transcutaneous electrical nerve stimulation (TENS) unit may be helpful in relieving pain. External immobilization such as Jewett or other hyperextension braces are often of little use for these patients because they can be extremely uncomfortable and often cause chest compression and resultant difficulties in lung expansion and breathing. If necessary, a simple extended corset can be used for support. The Spinomed lightweight moldable brace has been shown to improve trunk strength, improve forced expiratory volume and decrease kyphosis, pain and postural sway (Pfeifer et al., 2004). Within a period of 1–2 weeks, once the symptoms have resolved, extension exercises may be useful in preventing further kyphotic deformity.

If pain persists for longer than 2–3 months, surgical intervention with kyphoplasty or vertebroplasty may be beneficial (see Chapter 18); however, efficacy is not clearly established (Kallmes et al., 2009). Chen et al. (2011) reported that a post-vertebroplasty back exercise program resulted in more favorable daily function at 2 years compared to non-exercise grouped patients. New studies investigating combined interventions of surgery with exercise, posture and body mechanics are needed. Vitamin D deficiency, a risk factor for osteoporotic fractures, and hyperkyphosis contribute to weakness and mobility dysfunction and are amenable to intervention (Katzman et al., 2010; Boucher, 2012).

LUMBAR SPINE

DISORDERS OF THE LUMBOSACRAL SPINE

Clinically, the aging spine presents with a loss of height and mobility. Degenerative changes in discs and spondylosis of the zygopophyseal joints are common, with changes starting as early as the second decade of life and progressing with age (Siemionow et al., 2011). It is estimated that, by the age of 45, approximately 75% of males and 60% of females have some lumbar disc degeneration at grades 1–4. The amount increases to over 90% and 80%, respectively, by the age of 65, with increased frequency of grade 3–4 degeneration (Badley, 1987). The changes include loss of the water content, which diminishes from nearly 90% at birth to 65–71% at 75 years. Reductions also occur in the proteoglycans and number and structure of collagens (Kesson & Atkins, 2005), thereby diminishing the pliability of the intervertebral disc leading to disc collapse and protrusion. As discs collapse, instability in the adjacent vertebrae develops, often causing mechanical low back problems. In addition, significant arthritic change can lead to stenosis of the central spinal canal or the intervertebral foramina of the nerve roots.

Patients with spinal stenosis tend to have a classic presentation. Typically, there is pain in the lower back or pain radiating down both legs, usually after walking for a brief time. Symptoms are relieved with sitting or flexion of the spine but recur when walking is resumed. These symptoms of neurogenic claudication are similar to the experience of lower limb claudication resulting from vascular compromise. However, with vascular claudication, symptoms of lower extremity (LE) pain are induced by physical activity, when blood flow demand of the muscles is inadequate, and relieved by rest when muscular blood flow demand decreases. Unlike neurogenic claudication, vascular claudication is not influenced by spine postures. Clinicians often use a bicycle test to differentiate between neurogenic and vascular claudication. With neurogenic claudication LE symptoms are typically present when cycling with the spine in extension and relieved with the spine in flexion. With vascular claudication LE symptoms are not influenced by posture and are relieved with rest from cycling activity. Fritz et al. (1997a) used a two-stage treadmill to differentiate between vascular and neurogenic claudication. Treadmill walking on a 15° incline (flexed spine posture) allowed for increased tolerance compared to level treadmill walking (extended spine posture). Recovery time was more prolonged with neurogenic claudication. Physical examination of a patient with spinal stenosis often demonstrates symptoms after hyperextension of the spine which leads to narrowing of the spinal canal in the lumbosacral region resulting in cord compression. The symptoms may also be aggravated by stenosis of the vertebral foramina, which often leads to radicular symptoms in addition to the claudication.

Treatment of spinal stenosis in severe cases is almost always surgical; however, age-related comorbidities may limit this option. Often, multiple vertebrae require decompression and fusion is accompanied by spinal instrumentation to provide rigidity and stability of the spine until the vertebrae have fused. The results of decompressive spinal surgery for stenosis tend to indicate better outcomes than conservative treatment (Pearson et al., 2012), but long-term effects of surgery are variable; thus conservative care like manual therapy and strengthening exercises may offer alternatives (May & Comer, 2013).

Less invasive surgical procedures are being performed to maintain the dimensions of the spinal canal and intervertebral foramen. An interspinous process distraction spacer is surgically placed to prevent spinal canal narrowing, intervertebral foramen narrowing and compression of the spinal neural elements. These devices allow motion but limit segmental spine extension. Nandakumar et al. (2010) reported the Xstop device was effective in decompression of the stenosed segment after 2 years. These less invasive techniques are particularly adventitious in the elderly population with numerous comorbidities.

In mild cases, nonsteroidal anti-inflammatories and, occasionally, epidural steroid blocks may be helpful in relieving the patient's symptoms. In addition to history and physical examination, the diagnosis of spinal stenosis can easily be made with the use of computerized tomography, with or without intrathecal contrast. Lumbosacral supports and corsets are often uncomfortable and provide little if any relief of symptoms. Abdominal exercises and stretching provide the most relief to a patient suffering from mechanical low back pain. Occasionally, massage, hot packs and ultrasound are also useful in resolving symptoms. Reduced weight-bearing walking in an aquatic program or harness suspension on land have been shown to reduce symptoms and improve exercise tolerance (Fritz et al., 1997b). It is important to remember many patients with spinal stenosis have osteoporosis as well as concomitant degenerative changes, thus, a therapeutic exercise program should be individualized. This program should include postural retraining and overall strengthening and conditioning, with stenosis favoring flexion and osteoporosis extension (see Chapter 60).

HISTORY AND DIFFERENTIAL DIAGNOSIS

A review of systems for a viscerogenic origin of low back pain is imperative. Disorders of the cardiovascular, gastrointestinal, renal, urologic and gynecologic systems often cause low back pain (Goodman & Snyder, 2013). Therefore, the medical history is very important because back pain can result from pathologies in specific structures such as the aorta (especially aneurysm), kidney, bowel, uterus or prostate (Kesson & Atkins, 2005; Goodman & Snyder, 2013). When a patient experiences acute low back pain without trauma, silent compression fracture, infection or neoplasm must be considered. Radiographic studies and laboratory tests should differentiate the abnormalities.

Unexplained weight loss and pain without cause may raise a suspicion of cancer. Multiple myeloma, a neoplastic disorder involving immature plasma cells in bone marrow often produces back or rib pain. Non-Hodgkin's lymphoma may also involve bone (Beers et al., 2011). Metastatic bone disease from primary breast or prostate cancers is frequently found in the lumbar spine and may present in a variety of ways. Metastasis from colon cancer is less common but can occur (Lurie et al., 2000). Neoplastic bone pain is usually a boring pain that often wakes the patient at night; rest does not relieve the pain. These symptoms are significant in a patient with a history of cancer (Kesson & Atkins, 2005). Weakness and fatigue may also be reported.

Osteomyelitis, discitis and other spinal infections must be ruled out, especially because radiographic evidence of degenerative changes is common in the aging spine (see Chapter 14). Lurie and associates (2000) presented the case of an 80-year-old man with arthritic changes in the spine and hips, including severe spinal stenosis. Treatment with rest and medications, including codeine, was ineffective. The patient had a decompressive laminectomy without relief of symptoms. After further workup and sound clinical reasoning, the patient was started on intravenous antibiotics for a spine infection, which rendered a gradual improvement. It should be noted that spinal infections mimic back pain and radicular complaints but they do not always present with typical features of infection. Fortunately, spinal infections are not common, accounting for about 0.01% of cases in primary care (Lurie et al., 2000).

OSTEOMALACIA

Osteomalacia means 'soft bones' and involves the failure of newly formed or remodeling bone to mineralize, resulting in an excess of unmineralized bone matrix (osteoid). Osteomalacia refers to the adult form of this condition; rickets is the same disease process but targets the epiphysis in the growing skeleton. Osteomalacia results from inadequate or delayed mineralization of mature cortical and spongy bone; this occurs because of the loss, altered intake or altered metabolism of 1,25-dihydroxyvitamin D3 (vitamin D3) and phosphate (Beers et al., 2011).

The gross histopathological and radiological abnormalities of osteomalacia are the common result of a number of different diseases. In general, osteomalacia is considered to be commonly caused by altered metabolism of vitamin D3 or phosphate or both, a condition for which the elderly population is at particular risk. Recent advances in the understanding of the biochemistry of vitamin D3 metabolism have provided new insight into this condition. In developed countries, elderly individuals, particularly the housebound or institutionalized, are vulnerable to osteomalacia.

Vitamin D3 deficiency may be caused by an inadequate intake of vitamin D3, minimal or no exposure to ultraviolet radiation or by defective intestinal absorption of vitamin D3, as is observed in malabsorption syndromes such as jejunoileal bypass or celiac disease. Also, there may be an age-related diminished response of the intestine to vitamin D3. In normal individuals, the main source of vitamin D3 is dermal synthesis. There is an age-related decrease in the dermal synthesis of 7-dehydrocholesterol, the precursor of vitamin D3. A deficiency can occur if there is a defect in vitamin D3 metabolism. Most diseases are not caused by simple vitamin D3 deficiency but involve abnormal production or regulation of its synthesis in the liver or kidneys.

Renal disorders are the main cause of difficulty in metabolizing phosphate. When phosphate depletion is a causative factor for osteomalacia, the serum phosphorus is markedly depressed. In osteomalacic patients, it is common to find very low plasma phosphate levels. Alimentary phosphate deficiency is additionally aggravated by vitamin D3 deficiency. Vitamin D3 promotes jejunal phosphate absorption and renal phosphate reabsorption (Beers et al., 2011).

Patients may have vague generalized bone pain, multiple fractures, thoracic kyphosis and loss of height because of multiple vertebral compression fractures, and deformity of the lower limbs because of the malunion or bowing associated with pseudofractures. Osteomalacia can affect bone turnover to the extent that fractures occur in situations that otherwise might constitute only a minimal to moderate impact stress. Lumbar scoliosis may develop because of the altered biconcave shape of affected vertebral bodies. The patient may complain of generalized dull aching bone pain and muscle weakness, particularly in the proximal muscle groups in the lower extremities (referred to as pelvic girdle myopathy)

and back. This diffuse skeletal pain is typically exacerbated by physical activity and tenderness may be elicited by palpation. Muscle weakness is a common accompaniment to prolonged vitamin D3 deficiency. A waddling gait manifests with this condition and generalized muscle atrophy may be evident. Falls risk is increased (Boucher, 2012) and functional activities such as climbing stairs and ambulation may become difficult.

The stereotypical presentation of osteomalacia can be cured or improved with appropriate therapy for the specific underlying abnormality. Although there may be different underlying causes of this skeletal disorder, most signs and symptoms resolve with supplementation of vitamin D3, which aims to restore plasma calcium and phosphate levels to normal. Concurrent with appropriate pharmacological therapy, physical management strategies should include postural and strengthening exercises and gait retraining in order to attain maximal functional status. There are no apparent contraindications, but sound judgment should be used and proper precautions taken when treating a patient who has osteomalacia with ultrasound, electrical stimulation, heat or cold, or when loading the bone with weight-bearing and resistive exercises.

PAGET'S DISEASE

Paget's disease, also known as osteitis deformans, is a common bone disorder among the elderly; it rarely affects people below the age of 40. Approximately 60% of those affected are male. Paget's disease, a chronic asymmetrical focal bone disease featuring increased osteoclastic bone resorption and aberrant secondary osteoblastic bone formation, is the second most common metabolic bone disorder after osteoporosis (Goodman & Snyder, 2013).

The overall structure of the bone demonstrates a mosaic pattern in which packets of bone are laid down subsequent to a phase of osteoclastic bone resorption. The bone that becomes enclosed in individual packets consists of true woven bone as well as lamellar bone. There is marked net bone formation, which is essentially normal. Bone biopsy remains important for the differentiation between malignancy and the Pagetic bone (Beers et al., 2011).

Unlike osteomalacia, radiographs and bone scans are definitive in revealing an active disease process in Paget's disease. The typically focal nature of Paget's disease and the extent of spread in individual bones makes the bone scan useful in differentiating Paget's disease from other bone diseases, including metastatic carcinoma. A bone scan demonstrates an increased uptake of isotopes at diseased sites, reflecting the activity of bone formation.

Specific patterns of radiographic changes are featured, including radiolucent areas of patchy arrangement that indicate increased bone resorption, as well as evidence of regional bone formation processes represented by cortical and cancellous thickening and sclerosis, and uneven widths of affected bones. Patchy areas of resorption typical of Paget's disease are referred to as osteoporosis circumscripta. In the pelvis, there may be evidence of sclerosis along the iliopectineal line. In the vertebrae, cortical thickening and expansion are characteristic but this appearance may be difficult to distinguish from osteoblastic metastasis, which occurs without cortical thickening. In Pagetic bone, neoplastic changes occur in less than 1% of cases but osteosarcoma is associated with Paget's disease in the elderly. In addition, fibrosarcoma and chondrosarcoma may occur (Beers et al., 2011).

CLINICAL PRESENTATION

Approximately 90% of individuals affected by Paget's disease are asymptomatic. Diagnosis is usually made by reports of bone pain or deformity, radiography or detection of elevated serum alkaline phosphatase levels upon routine biochemical testing. The most common complaints reported are pain, skeletal deformity and changes in skin temperature. Other clinical manifestations include diminished mobility and unsteady gait; in more severe cases of Paget's disease, pathological fractures may manifest. The major clinical features are outlined in Table 24.1.

Bone pain is often nocturnal and is thought to be the result of increased pressure on the periosteum or associated hyperemia. Other causes of pain may be nerve root compression or nerve entrapment if the diseased bone involves neural foramina. The deep-rooted pain of Paget's disease is often unresponsive to simple analgesics and is more likely to be experienced when at rest than during movement. The efficacy of physical modalities in treating Pagetic pain is unclear and is best applied on an individual basis. Mixed sensorineural and conductive hearing loss is a common clinical manifestation of Paget's disease. Auditory nerve compression occurs when

Paget's disease involves the petrous temporal bone, and encroachment on the internal auditory meatus may cause compression of cranial nerve VIII, leading to hearing loss. Conduction deafness may result from otosclerosis or indirect involvement of the cochlea or ossicles and is also a common finding in patients with Paget's disease. Because of abnormal bone remodeling processes inherent in the progression of Paget's disease, bone architecture becomes distorted in patients in the advanced stages of disease. Mobility becomes difficult because weight-bearing exacerbates the development of deformities, and pathological fractures occur most commonly in the long weight-bearing bones of the lower extremities (in the femoral neck and the subtrochanteric and tibial regions). An increase in skull size, lateral bowing of the long bones (especially the tibia, femur and humerus) and dorsal kyphosis are typical deformities in the Paget's patient.

CONCLUSION

Common disorders of the aging spine are the result of osteoporosis and degenerative changes. However, the cause of the patient's complaints must be investigated with appropriate laboratory and radiographic studies because other bone disorders, metastatic disease and visceral problems may present as spine pain.

In most cases, it is extremely important that elderly patients with any kind of spinal disorder be mobilized as quickly as possible to prevent further disuse, including muscle weakness, deep vein thrombosis and pneumonia. Attempts should be made to provide appropriate assistive devices so that patients can be ambulatory as soon as possible, and rehabilitation interventions must be individualized.

Table 24.1	**Major clinical features of advanced Paget's disease**
Bones	**Clinical Features**
Skull	Headaches, deafness, expanded skull size, cranial palsies
Facial bones	Deformity, dental problems
Vertebrae	Nerve root compression, cord compression
Long bones	Deformity, e.g. bowing of tibia (anterior) or femur (lateral)
	Secondary osteoarthritis
	Incremental fissure fractures
	Excessive operative bleeding
General	Bone pain
	Malaise
	Immobility
	Deformity
	Bone sarcoma
	Heat over affected bones
	High-output cardiac failure

From Anderson DC, Richardson PC 1992 Paget's disease of bone. In: Brocklehurst JC, Tallis RC, Fillit UM (eds) Textbook of Geriatrics and Gerontology. Churchill Livingstone, New York, pp. 783–791, with permission.

REFERENCES

Badley E 1987 Epidemiological aspects of the ageing spine. In: Hulkins D, Nelson M (eds) The Ageing Spine. Manchester University Press, Manchester, pp. 1–18

Beers M, Berkow R et al (eds) 2011 Merck Manual of Geriatrics, 3rd edn. Merck & Co., Inc., Whitehouse Station, NJ. www.freebooks-4doctors.com

Boucher B 2012 The problems of vitamin deficiency in older people. Aging Dis 3:313–329

Carlesso LC, MacDermid JC, Santaguida LP 2010 Standardization of adverse event terminology and reporting in orthopaedic physical therapy: application to the cervical spine. J Orthop Sports Phys Ther 40:455–463

Chen B, Zhong Y, Huang Y et al 2011 Systemic back muscular exercise after percutaneous vertebroplasty for spinal osteoporetic compression fracture patients: a randomized controlled trial. Clin Rehabil 26(6):483–492

Escortell ME, Lebrijo PG, Perez MY et al 2008 Randomized clinical trial for primary care patients with neck pain: manual therapy versus electrical stimulation. Spanish Med Soc Primary Care Fam Commun 40(7):337–343

Fouyas IP, Stratham PF, Sandercock PA 2002 Cochrane review on the role of surgery in cervical spondylotic radiculomyelopathy. Spine 27(7):736–747

Fritz J, Ernhard R, Delitto A et al 1997a Preliminary results of the use of a two stage treadmill test as a diagnostic tool in the differential diagnosis of lumbar spinal stenosis. J Spinal Disord 10:410–416

Fritz J, Erhard R, Vignovic M 1997b A nonsurgical treatment approach for patients with lumbar spinal stenosis. Phys Ther 77:962–973

Goodman C, Snyder TE 2013 Differential diagnosis for physical therapists: screening for referral. Saunders Elsevier, Philadelphia, PA, pp. 547,558.

Kallmes DF, Comstock BA, Heagerty PJ et al 2009 A randomized trial of vertebroplasty for osteoporotic spinal fractures. N Engl J Med 361:569–579

Katzman W, Wanek L, Shepherd JA et al 2010 Age related hyperkyphosis: its causes, consequences and management. J Orthop Sports Phys Ther 40(6):352–360

Kesson M, Atkins E 2005 Orthopaedic Medicine: A Practical Approach. Elsevier, Oxford, pp. 267–352, 515–576

Lee M, Dettori JR, Standaert CJ et al 2012 The natural history of degeneration of the lumbar and cervical spines. Spine 37:pS18–pS30

Lurie J, Gerber P, Sox H 2000 A pain in the back. N Engl J Med 343:723–726

Martin G, Mannino D, Moss M 2006 The effect of age on the development and outcome of adult sepsis. Crit Care Med 34:15–21

May S, Cromer C 2013 Is surgery more effective than non-surgical treatment for spinal stenosis and which non-surgical treatment is more effective? A systematic review. Physiother 99:12–20

Modic MT, Ross J, Masaryk T 1989 Imaging of degenerative disease of the cervical spine. Clin Orthop Relat Res 239:109–120

Nandakumar A, Clark NA, Peehal JP et al 2010 The increase in dural sac area is maintained at 2 years after X-stop implantation for the treatment of spinal stenosis with no significant alteration in lumbar spine range of movement. Spine 10(9):762–768

NOF (National Osteoporosis Foundation) 2010 Clinician's Guide to Treatment and Prevention of Osteroporosis. NOF, Washington, DC

Pearson A, Lurie J, Tosteson T et al 2012 Who should have surgery for spinal stenosis? Spine 37:1791–1802

Pfeifer D, Begerow B, Minnie H 2004 Effects of a new spinal orthosis on posture, trunk strength, and quality of life in women with postmenopausal osteoporosis: a randomized trial. Am J Phys Med Rehabil 83:177–186

Rana S 2011 Diagnosis and management of cervical spondylosis. In: Gellman H (ed) Orthopedic Surgery. Medscape Reference

Raney NH, Peterson EJ, Smith TA et al 2009 Development of a clinical prediction rule to identify patients with neck pain likely to benefit from cervical traction and exercise. Euro Spine J 18(3):382–391

Schmorl G, Junghann S 1932 Die gesunde und Kranke Wirtel Saule im Rontgenbild. Georg Thieme, Leipzig

Siemionow K, Masuda K, Anderson G et al 2011 The effects of age, sex ethnicity and spinal level on the rate of intervertebral disc degeneration: a review of 1712 intervertebral discs. Spine (Phila PA 1976) 36(17):1333–1339

Smith JS, Helgeson MD, Albert TJ 2012 The argument for anterior cervical discectomy and fusion over total disc replacement. Semin Spine Surgery 24:2–7

Wainner RS, Fritz JM, Irrgang JJ et al 2003 Reliability and diagnostic accuracy of the clinical examination and patient self report measures for cervical radiculopathy. Spine 28:52–62

Chapter 25

Orthopedic trauma

P. CHRISTOPHER METZGER • MARK LOMBARDI

CHAPTER CONTENTS

INTRODUCTION

As the average age expectancy approaches 80 years in the United States of America, musculoskeletal injuries can be expected to increase in number. This statement takes on significant ramifications when coupled with the knowledge that an estimated 78 million 'baby boomers' are either in their seventh decade or rapidly approaching it. The baby boomer population consists of anyone born between 1946 and 1964 according to the US Census Bureau. Today, more than ever, many geriatric patients lead very active and productive lives. Unfortunately, such a lifestyle can be dramatically affected by an inadvertent slip or fall that may produce an orthopedic injury. As these injuries become more prevalent they can be expected to have a profound effect on both society and its already stressed healthcare system. This chapter focuses on the rehabilitation of such orthopedic injuries in the geriatric population.

Rehabilitation may be defined as the restoration of normal form and function after an injury or an illness (Dirckx, 2001). What is meant by 'normal form and function' varies from individual to individual. The desired goal for the injured patient is to return them to their preinjury activities, knowing that this may not always be possible.

Fractures of the proximal femur are a common and increasing cause of hospitalization. In 2004 there were more than 320 000 hospital admissions necessitated by hip fractures in the US. It is projected that there will be more than 500 000 hip fractures by 2040 (CDC, 2010). At a cost of approximately $27 000 per patient one can see the staggering economic burden produced by such injuries. Roughly 4% of all deaths from injury in the US are caused by hip fractures (Bergen et al., 2008). In the geriatric population hip fractures are usually associated with low energy trauma. Death may occur when there is exacerbation of medical comorbidities (e.g. diabetes mellitus, coronary artery disease, chronic obstructive pulmonary disease etc.) caused by the resulting immobility or postoperative complications. Only 25% of these patients will make a full recovery, 30% will require nursing home care and 50% will require the use of a cane or walker. Within approximately 12 months, 30% of these patients will die (Moran & Wenn, 2005). Data from Europe indicate that hip fractures pose the same problems (Lippuner et al., 2005). Such statistics point out the need for expert and efficient musculoskeletal care.

The goal of fracture care in this age group is early mobilization and the eventual restoration of function. Prolonged periods of immobility increase the risk of deep vein thrombosis (DVT), pulmonary embolism, pressure ulcers, pneumonia and joint contractures. Surgical intervention, when necessary, is best performed within 48 hours after injury if the patient has been deemed medically stable. The patient, family, orthopedic surgeon and all those who provide ancillary services must understand that often there is a decrease in the healing potential of a geriatric patient. (See Chapter 60, Fracture Considerations.)

BASIC PRINCIPLES FOR REHABILITATION

The goals of rehabilitation are to: (1) control and reduce inflammation, (2) restore motion, (3) develop motor control and coordination, (4) regain strength and (5) restore function. The rehabilitation process in pelvic or lower extremity injuries is begun by mobilizing the patient. This consists of getting the individual out of bed into a chair and is followed by ambulation with external support (cane, crutches or walker). At the same time, joint mobility and flexibility must be restored. This is accomplished with active, active-assisted and passive range of motion (ROM) exercises. As both mobility and ROM are regained, emphasis must be placed on reacquiring strength, joint stability, motor control, proprioception and coordination.

It is desirable to start mobilization as soon as the patient's medical condition permits. Learning to ambulate with either crutches or a walker in a partial weight-bearing fashion is a challenge for most. The amount of energy required to perform limited weight-bearing is

30–50% greater than that required for normal ambulation (Hsu et al., 2008). This added demand can be particularly taxing for the elderly individual, especially if there is a decreased cardiopulmonary reserve.

In upper extremity injuries, patient mobilization is usually not as difficult to attain. The only necessary instructions may be to keep the arm elevated and to educate the patient on how to get in and out of bed and chairs without putting pressure on the injured extremity. In general, the more severe injuries, those with upper and lower extremity involvement, pose a greater obstacle to mobilization. In such instances initial attention may have to focus on simple transfers from bed to chair because ambulation may not be possible. The use of adaptive equipment, such as forearm supports on assistive devices, may prove to be necessary. The geriatric patient may already have some pre-existing impairment of mobility that has to be taken into consideration. The goal of rehabilitation is to get the patient back to their preinjury status if at all possible.

MOTION

One of the therapist's responsibilities is to instruct and assist the patient in the restoration of ROM after injury. At all times, the physician should communicate with the therapist regarding any precautions or restrictions. Such communication should take place on a regular basis and must always be documented.

MOTOR CONTROL AND COORDINATION

Motor control is necessary before any active exercises can begin or progress. Sometimes electrical stimulation is needed to activate muscles that demonstrate atrophy, muscle inhibition or painful muscle guarding (Hopkins & Ingersoll, 2000). Coordination is crucial to motor control. It involves smooth and accurate movement of the joints in the kinetic chain. The timing and sequencing of movements of ipsilateral and contralateral joints requires neural control and musculoskeletal integrity. For example, a humeral fracture that disrupts the coordinated movement of the involved arm also reduces the contralateral arm swing during normal reciprocal gait. Proper breathing, decreased muscular guarding and reduced abnormal flexor and adductor tone in either the upper or lower extremities facilitates improved muscle activity and coordination.

STRENGTHENING

When some degree of comfortable motion and muscle control are attained, strengthening can be started. Increased strength often results in increased motion. It has been shown that age is no barrier to regaining or even increasing strength. (See Chapter 61, Contractures and Stiffness.)

An effective method of strengthening is progressive resistive exercise (PRE). Initial efforts with strengthening may begin with isometric training. Isometric strength training may provide increased joint stability, promoting improved joint motion, as ROM increases. As the patient's strength increases, the therapist may elect to progress strengthening through techniques that exercise each muscle group with enough resistance to allow 20–30 repetitions. It is recommended that the therapist break the patient's sets/reps into more manageable bouts of exercise to prevent fatigue that often can lead to poor performance or injury. Once 30 repetitions can be achieved, the resistance is increased and the progression of repetitions from 20 to 30 is repeated. Another method involves the patient completing three sets of 10–15 repetitions, decreasing the resistance with each set, or three sets using the same resistance but decreasing the number of repetitions (from 20 to 15 to 10).

ADAPTATION

At some point during rehabilitation it may become evident that there will be some permanent functional limitation or disability. Changes in anatomy and consequently in function, resulting from the injury, may force changes in the patient's movement patterns thus affecting their lifestyle. In order to adapt to these changes different training techniques or equipment may be needed. These needs may be apparent early in the rehabilitation period if, for instance, there has been a major amputation. In other cases, it may become evident later in the course of rehabilitation that permanent loss of joint motion or strength is inevitable and that compensation during work or play is required. Loss of joint motion during the rehabilitation period should be communicated with the physician on an ongoing basis in an attempt to minimize the degree or severity of loss.

The ability to restore some form of useful activity in the involved extremity is one of the primary goals of rehabilitation, although it may not always be attainable. It may be that the patient will need to adjust to a more sedentary lifestyle or pursue activities that are less physically demanding. Learning to accept these limitations is part of regaining a meaningful life.

TREATMENT OF OSTEOPOROSIS

Osteoporosis is a metabolic bone disease characterized by decreased bone mass and bone quality. Changes in bone mineral density (BMD) and quality increases the patient's risk of fragility fractures. Osteoporosis is a 'silent' condition that is generally asymptomatic until a fracture occurs (Sinaki, 2003). It is defined by a BMD that is 2.5 or more standard deviations below that of normal young adults (WHO, 2003). In the US it has been estimated that 4–6 million women and 1–2 million men greater than 50 years of age have osteoporosis. In 2005 the cost for treating osteoporotic fractures in the US was $17 billion and is expected to increase by 50% by 2025 (Lim et al., 2009). It can therefore be seen that early detection and treatment of osteoporosis would play an essential role in decreasing healthcare costs. (See Chapter 18, Osteoporosis and Spine Fractures.)

There have been promising results in the treatment of osteoporosis and osteopenia through calcium supplementation, adequate vitamin D intake and the use of biphosphonates, estrogen and progesterone (Hormone

Replacement Therapy – HRT) (Martin, 2012), calcitonin, teriparatide and testosterone. Pharmacological intervention is not without risk and the therapist should work with the patient, physician and nutritionist to insure that the patient is monitored and progressed appropriately (Martin, 2012). If possible, regular physical activity, including weight-bearing and resistive exercise, may also be helpful if introduced and advanced appropriately following recommended guidelines to safe exercise in patients with osteoporosis/osteopenia (Martin, 2012).

REHABILITATION AFTER SPECIFIC INJURIES

FRACTURES OF THE PROXIMAL HUMERUS

Fractures of the proximal humerus are the third most commonly encountered fractures in the geriatric population, with only hip and distal radius fractures seen occurring more often. The frequent occurrence of this fracture in the elderly population certainly suggests an association with osteoporosis and impaired balance. A fall onto an outstretched hand (FOOSH) is the most common mechanism of injury for these fractures. Fortunately approximately 85% of these fractures are either nondisplaced or minimally displaced (Flynn, 2011). These fractures can be treated by sling and swathe immobilization for 10–14 days followed by gentle ROM exercises. Elbow flexion and extension as well as forearm pronation and supination can be started during this period of immobilization. Prior to initiating the exercise program for the shoulder, clinical continuity (the fracture moves as a single unit) must be present.

If there is stability at the fracture site, passive and active assisted ROM is started early. This consists of pendulum exercises and supine external glenohumeral rotation with a stick. About 3–4 weeks after the fracture has occurred, active-assisted forward elevation, pulley exercise, extension and isometrics can be added (Withrow et al., 2010). After this first phase has been complete, active and early resistive exercises become important. Therabands are often used to strengthen the shoulder rotators and deltoid muscle. A program that emphasizes further stretching and strengthening is appropriate 3 months after fracture.

It is important in the early stages of fracture healing for the patient to avoid using the affected arm when getting into and out of bed or a chair. Such actions can displace the fracture even when there has been stable internal fixation. Displacement is more likely to occur in the patient with multiple injuries or limited cognitive capabilities. Throughout the entire rehabilitation program, the therapist should be working with and assessing functional mobility of the cervical spine, scapula, elbow, wrist and hand. Most patients with fractures of the proximal humerus do obtain satisfactory results; however, it must be understood that usually there is some resultant loss of motion and strength. Complications include malunion, delayed union, nonunion, loss of motion, stiffness and post-traumatic arthritis.

Open treatment may prove to be necessary when a displaced fracture cannot be reduced. Treatment options consist of either a closed reduction with percutaneous pinning, an open reduction with internal fixation using a precontoured locking plate or hemi-arthroplasty when the articular surface is non-reconstructable.

The results of open reduction with internal fixation for proximal humerus fractures demonstrate good surgical outcomes when correct surgical technique is employed. Brunner et al. (2009) reported that the most common postoperative complication was screw perforation into the glenohumeral joint. Primary hemiarthroplasty is usually successful in eliminating pain; however, in many instances only moderate function and poor strength levels were achieved. It is felt that the reduction in function is due to lack of rotator cuff integrity (Gronhagen et al., 2007).

FRACTURES OF THE DISTAL RADIUS

Distal radial fractures account for approximately 20% of all fractures and therefore are the most common fractures seen in the upper extremity. Such fractures usually occur following a FOOSH and are seen quite often in the geriatric population, particularly women with osteoporosis (Flynn, 2011). A Colles' fracture involves the distal radial metaphysis and demonstrates dorsal angulation and displacement. Often there may be comminution and intraarticular extension of the fracture. A Smith's fracture demonstrates volar angulation of the distal radius with resultant instability.

Treatment options for these fractures include simple cast immobilization, closed reduction with cast application, closed reduction with external fixation and open reduction with internal fixation. The trend today is toward open reduction and internal fixation using a volar fixed-angled locking plate for displaced intraarticular fractures. The usual indications are radial shortening of more than 3 mm, dorsal tilt greater than 10° or intraarticular displacement of more than 2 mm (American Academy of Orthopedic Surgeons, 2011). The possible complications that may result from this particular type of fracture include delayed union, nonunion, malunion, median nerve compression, tendon damage, post-traumatic arthritis and loss of motion.

Restoration of motion and strength, which leads to improved function, is of vital importance in the rehabilitation of these fractures. Early rehabilitation includes management of pain and edema, digital ROM and care of the surgical site (Smith et al., 2004). After appropriate consultation with the attending physician, ROM and strengthening exercises for areas of the upper extremities that are not immobilized should be initiated immediately, if possible, to prevent residual stiffness in the shoulder, elbow and hand. Once immobilization is no longer necessary, active-assisted and active exercises are encouraged in all six directions – flexion, extension, radial and ulnar deviation, pronation and supination. Modalities such as hydrotherapy, electrical stimulation, heat, cold, or ultrasound may be helpful. Depending on the status of fracture healing and the amount of stiffness, the therapist may incorporate specific mobilization techniques to increase the ROM. The initiation of muscle control and coordination may be difficult when motion is painful. In addition to addressing the inflammatory process, which causes pain and swelling, the therapist should attend to head, neck and trunk posture, which may contribute to the patient's discomfort and limitation of movement. As ROM in the wrist increases, strengthening exercises using motion against resistance should be included in the treatment plan. The final goal should be to restore ROM and strength of the injured wrist to preinjury levels. Unfortunately this is not always possible and some degree of impairment may remain as a result of the fact that normal architecture could be restored secondary to the severity of the injury (Smith et al., 2004).

When rehabilitating a patient who has undergone an open reduction with internal fixation using a volar plate, attention must be directed accordingly to prevent a contracture of the pronator quadratus, which could cause a limitation of forearm rotation.

INTERTROCHANTERIC FRACTURES

An intertrochanteric fracture occurs along the line that is located between the greater and lesser trochanters. These fractures are seen most commonly in the elderly and are usually the result of a fall. The goal of care for this particular type of fracture should be to restore the patient to his or her preinjury status as quickly as possible. The potential benefits of operative intervention include rapid mobilization, ease of nursing care, shorter hospitalization, decreased mortality and restoration of function.

Stable intertrochanteric fractures are still best treated with a sliding screw (Flynn, 2011). The treatment of the unstable intertrochanteric fracture remains somewhat controversial but often requires the use of a cephalomedullary nail. The surgery should be performed within the first 48 hours if at all possible. The success of the surgical procedure largely depends upon: (1) bone quality, (2) fracture pattern, (3) accuracy of the reduction and (4) the adequacy of internal fixation.

The major goal of rehabilitation after an intertrochanteric fracture is to enable the patient to walk, especially if they were ambulatory prior to the injury. Mobilization of the patient should be initiated almost immediately after completion of the surgical procedure. ROM exercises are encouraged as soon as the initial pain subsides and the patient can safely cooperate with the physical therapist. ROM in all directions is advised, to prevent flexion and adduction contractures that can make ambulation more difficult. Getting the patient to a level where they can control the involved limb is essential to permit adequate mobility in bed, preventing and/or lessening the occurrence of pressure ulcers, to allow for independent transfers into and out of bed and to promote the initiation of weight-bearing and restoration of gait (Kagaya & Shimada, 2007). Balance and coordination instructions are given concurrently with all phases of rehabilitation.

Usually the patient should get out of bed and transfer to a chair on the day following surgery. With intertrochanteric fractures, partial weight-bearing may often be necessary. The weight-bearing status is determined by the accuracy and stability of the reduction achieved at the time of surgery, bone quality, premorbid status and mental alertness. The patient who is not strong enough to manage partial weight-bearing or not coherent enough to understand the therapist's instructions may be limited to a wheelchair and/or pre-gait activities, such as sit to stand and static stance with weight shift until they are stronger or until the fracture has healed sufficiently to permit full weight-bearing. Early assisted swing (slide) phase of gait of the involved leg may be helpful in facilitating proper weight-bearing and restoration of functional gait in the future. This is achieved with the patient standing in parallel bars or with a walker, and simply sliding the foot of the involved leg forward and backward or lifting the involved leg over a lower obstacle (cane, cup or cone) that is placed on the floor in front of the patient.

Strengthening the hip abductors gradually reduces the Trendelenburg gait pattern commonly seen following a hip fracture. PREs are used, starting with abduction while standing or the use of a sliding board while supine. As strength increases, the patient is instructed to perform the exercises while lying on the contralateral side, thus abducting against gravity. Coexisting musculoskeletal and cardiovascular conditions may necessitate modification of these positions. Once 20–30 repetitions can be performed, progressive resistance is added. Strengthening the hip flexors, extensors, rotators and adductors is also important to insure restoration of muscle strength, flexibility and endurance to allow progression of gait.

After the fracture heals and rehabilitation is complete, occasional decreased mobility may be the end result. Patient adaptation may involve having to accept the permanent use of a cane or walker to aid in balance, reduce Trendelenburg characteristics associated with weak abductors seen in gait, and to increase patient confidence, safety and mobility. The patient with an intertrochanteric fracture should be expected to transfer and ambulate independently before being discharged home. If this is not possible, placement in an assisted living facility or a nursing home may be necessary.

FEMORAL NECK FRACTURES

Femoral neck fractures occur most commonly in the eighth decade of life as a result of bone that is weakened by either osteoporosis or osteomalacia. The most common mechanisms of injury are either a fall that causes a direct blow to the greater trochanter or forced lateral rotation of the lower extremity (Bucholz et al., 2009). If the fracture is displaced, often the arterial supply to the proximal end of the femur is disrupted, thus creating an environment favorable to the development of either a nonunion or avascular necrosis.

Elderly patients with nondisplaced or valgus impacted fractures can be treated with percutaneous pin fixation using cannulated screws (Flynn, 2011). The displaced fracture is best treated with hemiarthroplasty using a cemented stem. Today a trend is developing that suggests perhaps total hip arthroplasty is favorable over simple hemiarthroplasty for the highly functional elderly patient (Flynn, 2011).

If a posterior approach is used when either a hemiarthroplasty or total hip arthroplasty is performed, caution must be used for the first several weeks in order to prevent hip dislocation (see Chapter 21, Total Hip Arthroplasty). A dislocation may occur with a combination of excessive hip flexion, adduction and internal rotation. The avoidance of this position in the early postoperative period is imperative. Safety measures must also be taken when patients are putting on their stockings and shoes, recumbent in bed, sitting upright or rising from a chair or recliner. In cases in which the stability of the prosthesis is in question, an abduction pillow is extremely helpful. The patient should also be instructed to sit in a lean-back chair so that the hip is flexed no more than 90°. In most cases, when a prosthesis is inserted, a graduated weight-bearing program is indicated.

Recent studies suggest that the therapist work in concert with the medical team to address changes in affect identified in patients having sustained a femoral neck fracture (Olofsson et al., 2005).

SUPRACONDYLAR FRACTURES OF THE FEMUR

The supracondylar region of the distal femur is often weakened by osteoporosis and thus even low energy forces can create complex fracture patterns. The resulting fractures are often comminuted, displaced and intraarticular, making management quite difficult. Years ago treatment consisted of traction and cast bracing, which unfortunately often resulted in a loss of joint motion. Today internal fixation techniques (intramedullary nailing or plate fixation) have been developed that allow for an anatomical reconstruction of the distal femur, more rigid internal fixation and earlier patient mobilization, thus allowing for improved ROM and function. Indications for nonoperative treatment include nondisplaced fractures, fractures occurring in patients who are not candidates for surgery, and fractures in patients who do not ambulate.

If rigid internal fixation has been achieved at the time of surgery, the use of a continuous passive motion machine may often prove to be quite helpful. This encourages increased motion, less postoperative swelling and reduces the incidence of quadriceps adhesions. For the first 6 weeks partial weight-bearing with a walker is allowed only if stable fixation is present. At the 6-week point, weight-bearing can be increased to tolerance providing there is radiographic evidence of healing. Full weight-bearing with external support is often not possible until the 12th week. In instances in which stable fixation has not been achieved supplemental support with a cast brace may prove to be necessary.

The same principles that govern motor control, coordination, strengthening and adaptation in fractures of the proximal femur apply to fractures of the distal femur. In addition, attention to distal lower extremity pain, weakness and decreased ROM will be required. The therapist should be aware of and proactive in the management of any patient having weight-bearing restrictions and decreased mobility issues as a result of lower extremity fracture and surgery with regard to an increased incidence of DVT or pulmonary emboli (PE). While Homan's Sign is but one tool that the therapist has at their disposal to assess for DVT, they need to be aware that the test has a low sensitivity (<50%) and be familiar with other methods of patient assessment and monitoring (Riddle & Wells, 2004).

FRACTURES OF THE TIBIAL PLATEAU

Fractures of the tibial plateau (Fig. 25.1) involve the proximal tibial articular surface. Fracture patterns vary greatly. Sometimes associated soft tissue damage may be quite significant. In the elderly, often a low energy mechanism of injury produces such a fracture. The goals of treatment should be the attainment of an accurate reduction and if at all possible the institution of early ROM exercises. Delayed weight-bearing often is necessary to prevent the fracture site from collapsing.

For nondisplaced fractures of the proximal tibia that are stable to both varus and valgus stresses nonoperative treatment is appropriate. Such treatment may also prove necessary in the nonambulatory or medically unstable individual. Initially a hinged knee brace, locked in full extension, is applied. Approximately 2 weeks after injury, should the individual's clinical condition permit, the brace is adjusted to allow early gentle ROM exercises. Weight-bearing must be delayed for 6–12 weeks, depending upon the amount of comminution and the rate of radiographic healing.

When radiographs indicate an articular step-off of 2 mm or more, surgical intervention is often carried out. The goal of surgery is to restore bony anatomy, achieve bone and soft tissue healing without complications, and to provide adequate fixation allowing early joint motion. Early joint ROM is initiated as early as is felt appropriate to minimize postoperative stiffness. Often, supplemental bone grafting may very well be necessary in the face of a significant metaphyseal defect. As with nondisplaced fractures, weight-bearing may very well be delayed for 6–12 weeks.

Complications of tibial plateau fractures include nonunion, delayed union, malunion, post-traumatic arthritis, DVT, postoperative infection and loss of motion. Rehabilitation should emphasize pain control, restoration of ROM and strength, and a return to preinjury status. Again, with all traumatic lower extremity fractures that result in impaired mobility and limited weight-bearing, the therapist needs to be acutely aware of the signs/symptoms of DVT and/or PE.

COMPRESSION FRACTURES OF THE SPINE

As with other fractures in the elderly, osteoporosis plays a major role in compression fractures of the vertebral body. Vertebral compression fractures are the most common osteoporotic fractures and their incidence is expected to increase as the baby boomer population ages. These fractures are seen more commonly in women than in men and although often resulting from a fall on the buttocks, may occur spontaneously through movement and be the initial sign that the patient is osteoporotic (Sinaki, 2003).

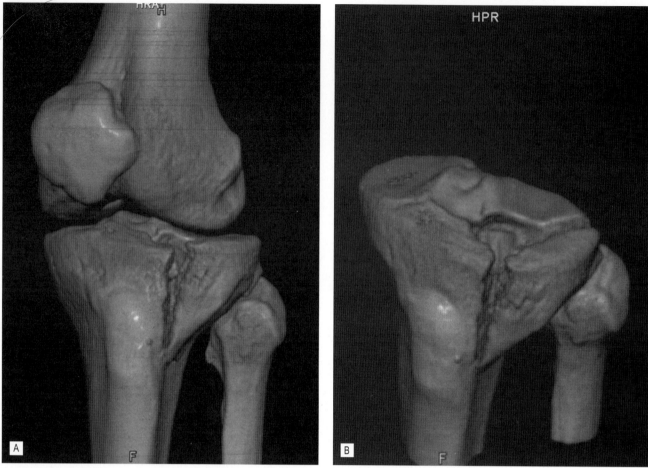

Figure 25.1 (A) Computerized tomography demonstrating the split component of a lateral tibial plateau fracture. **(B)** The same study showing significant depression of the lateral tibial plateau.

Initial nonsurgical treatment consists of appropriate activity modification, the taking of a mild analgesic and bracing. Once the pain begins to subside, the patient is encouraged to start moving. (See Chapters 18 and 60.) Physical therapy should concentrate on increasing the patient's knowledge of safety, posture, transfers, the performance of daily living activities and ambulation. Care is taken so as to avoid forceful flexion as this often duplicates the mechanism of injury. Gentle extension and exercises of the trunk are useful in attaining patient mobility. Postural exercise should include activities of the shoulder and scapulae to ensure overall strengthening and spinal stability (Martin, 2012). Occasional wearing of either a lumbar or thoracolumbar support may be helpful.

Surgical treatment may be indicated in the patient with a neurological deficit resulting from an exaggerated kyphotic deformity. Treatment options include vertebroplasty or kyphoplasty, and open surgery.

CONCLUSION

The aging of the baby boomer population coupled with an expected increase in life expectancy will most certainly result in an increase in the number of musculoskeletal injuries in the geriatric population. Excellent and efficient orthopedic care will become more important with the passage of time. Such care will hopefully enable patients to attain the highest possible level of function, satisfaction, comfort and quality of life.

REFERENCES

American Academy of Orthopedic Surgeons 2011. www.aaos.org

Bergen G, Chen L, Warner M et al 2008 Injury in the United States: 2007 Chartbook. National Center for Health Statistics, Hyattsville, MD

Brunner F, Sommer C, Bohrs C et al 2009 Open reduction and internal fixation of proximal humerus fractures using a proximal humeral locked plate: a prospective multicenter analysis. J Orthop Trauma 23(3):163–172

Bucholz RW, Heckman JD, Court-Brown CM et al 2009 Rockwood and Green's Fractures in Adults, 2 vols. Lippincott, Williams & Wilkins, Philadelphia, PA

CDC (Centers for Disease Control and Prevention) 2010 Older adult falls data and statistics. www.cdc.gov/homeandrecreationalsafety/Falls/data.html

Dirckx JH (ed) 2001 Stedman's Concise Medical Dictionary for the Health Profession, 4th edn. Lippincott, Williams & Wilkins, Philadelphia, PA

Flynn J 2011 Orthopedic Knowledge Update 10. American Academy of Orthopedic Surgeons, Rosemont, IL

Gronhagen CM, Abbaszaden H, Revay SA et al 2007 Medium term results after primary hemi-arthroplasty for comminuted proximal humerus fractures: a study of 46 patients followed up for an average of 4.4 years. J Shoulder Elbow Surg 16(6):766–773

Hopkins JT, Ingersoll CD 2000 Arthrogenic muscle inhibition: a limiting factor in joint rehabilitation. J Sport Rehabil 9(2):135–159

Hsu J, Michael J, Fisk J 2008 AAOS Atlas of Orthoses and Assisted Devices, 4th edn. Mosby/Elsevier, Philadelphia PA

Kagaya H, Shimada Y 2007 Treatment and rehabilitation after hip fracture in the elderly. Crit Rev Phys Rehabil Med 19(2):97–113

Lim LS, Horksene LJ, Sherin KA 2009 CPM prevention practice committee: screening for osteoporosis in the adult US population: ACPM position statement on preventative practice. AM Prev Med 36(4):366–375

Lippuner K, Hauselmann HJ, Szucs TD 2005 A model on osteoporosis impact in Switzerland 2000–2020. Osteoporosis Int 16(6):659–671

Martin M 2012 Working with Osteoporosis and Osteopenia: Part A. MelioGuide. MedBridge Education. www.medbridge.com

Moran CG, Wenn RT 2005 Early mortality after hip fracture: is delay before surgery important? J Bone Joint Surg 87(3):483–489

Olofsson B, Lundstrom M, Borssen B et al 2005 Delerium is associated with poor rehabilitation outcome in elderly patients treated for femoral neck fractures. Scand J Caring Sci 19(2):119–127

Riddle D, Wells P 2004 Diagnosis of lower-extremity deep vein thrombosis in outpatients. Phys Ther 84:729–735

Sinaki M 2003 Critical appraisal of physical rehabilitation measures after osteoporotic vertebral fracture. Osteoporos Int 14:773–779

Smith D, Brou K, Henry M 2004 Early active rehabilitation for operatively stabilized distal radius fractures. J Hand Ther 17:43–49

WHO (World Health Organization) 2003 Prevention and management of osteoporosis. WHO, Geneva, Technical Report Series No. 921

Withrow P, Stoecker J, Stevens K et al 2010 Non-operative management of a patient with a two-part minimally displaced proximal humerus fracture: a case report. Physiother Theory Pract 26(2):120–133

Neuromuscular and neurological disorders

UNIT CONTENTS

Chapter 26

Neurological trauma

DENNIS W. KLIMA

CHAPTER CONTENTS

INTRODUCTION

A key component of geriatric rehabilitation includes the management of older patients who have sustained neurological trauma to the brain or spinal cord. Therapists must consider the impact of these injuries, along with adjacent neural changes that occur during the aging process. Management of older patients with both spinal cord (SCI) and traumatic brain injuries (TBI) requires the integration of musculoskeletal, neuromuscular and cognitive interventions to enable them to effectively progress towards established goals.

A thorough history must first be obtained from the patient or family to ascertain the previous level of function. A systems review will further corroborate any changes in physical status, affect and cognition that have occurred following the sustained injury. Selected tests and measures typically combine traditional examination activities along with instruments specifically geared towards patients with TBI or SCI. A summative evaluation will then be formulated, along with an appropriate rehabilitation diagnosis and prognosis. With both patient populations of individuals who have sustained a TBI or SCI, the rehabilitation diagnosis is influenced by a multitude of mitigating factors such as age-related changes in organ systems, as well as injury complications such as heterotopic ossificans and autonomic nervous system dysfunction.

The International Classification of Function, Disability and Health model (ICF) illustrates how both TBI and SCI affect an older patient's ability to perform functional tasks and participate in community-related activities and employment (Fig. 26.1) (Salter et al., 2011). Strategic functional mobility interventions are implemented to address all established goals within the body structure/function, activity and participation domains. Outcomes may be measured through a variety of instruments, including the Functional Independence Measure, or FIM, which has shown appropriate psychometric support for patients with both SCI and TBI (Corrigan et al., 1997).

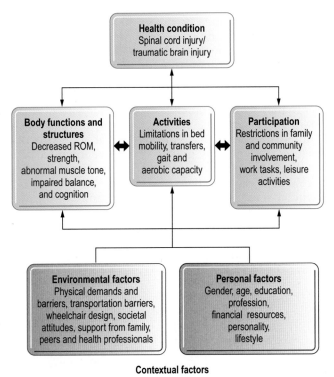

Figure 26.1 International Classification of Functioning, Disability and Health: spinal cord injury and traumatic brain injury. ROM, range of motion.

TRAUMATIC BRAIN INJURY

Over one million people sustain a TBI each year in the United States of America; moreover, TBI injuries account for one-third of all injury-related deaths (Faul et al., 2010; Brain Injury Association of America, 2012). The leading cause of TBI for those aged 65 or older is a fall-related episode, and current hospitalization rates continue to increase for individuals over the age of 80 who sustain head injuries (Bhullar et al., 2010). TBI is the principal cause of seizure disorders worldwide, and the World Health Organization adapted criteria for head injury surveillance in 1993.

Head injury sequelae can be devastating for a geriatric client and affect nearly every component of the quality of life, including self-care, employment and leisure activities. Poor recovery outcomes may warrant institutional placement if caregiving demands exceed available resources in the home environment. Fall prevention strategies for older clients are essential in preventing head injury. Geriatric individuals generally sustain falls secondary to either intrinsic or extrinsic causes. For example, intrinsic causes include sensory changes or vestibular pathology that impede effective balance modulation. Environmental barriers and obstacles resulting in trips and slips are included in the extrinsic category. Appropriate balance measures such as the Berg Balance Scale (Berg et al., 1992) or Timed Up and Go Test (Posiadlo & Richardson, 1991) can assist in identifying those clients most at risk for falling.

Head injuries may be characterized as either open or closed; open head injuries involve open penetration to the skull. The initial site of impact following a traumatic insult to the brain is known as the coup injury. A rebound effect often occurs in the cranium following the initial impact and causes a contre-coup injury (Fig. 26.2). Patients may also sustain additional complications because of skull fractures or hematomas. Skull fractures vary from relatively nonthreatening simple linear fractures to those with extensive comminuting fragments that require cranioplasty procedures (Fig. 26.3). Additionally, patients can incur complications such as internal organ damage or both spinal and extremity fractures. Patients may undergo extensive intensive care monitoring because of uncontrolled intracranial pressure or resultant seizure activity.

Initial trauma assessments are performed using the Glasgow Coma Scale (GCS). Composed of three divisions, this instrument assesses three areas of function in individuals following head injury: motor performance, eye opening and verbal response (Table 26.1) (Teasdale & Jennett, 1974). Scores from 13 to 15 designate mild injury; from 9 to 12, moderate injury; and from 3 to 8, severe TBI. The rehabilitation team members should be aware of the initial GCS score and subsequent complications at the time of injury so that any examination or intervention activities can be adjusted. Patients' prognostic functional recovery can be predicted by the initial FIM score, duration of post-traumatic amnesia and initial GCS score (Sandhaug et al., 2010).

Interventions for the geriatric client with a TBI include integrated strategies for both cognitive and neuromuscular impairments. Following recovery from a head injury, patients may be classified according to behavior associated with the Rancho Los Amigos Levels

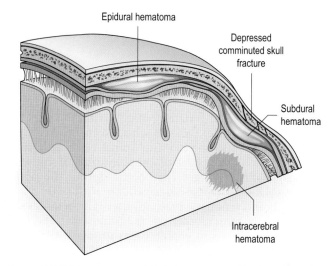

Figure 26.3 Hematoma and skull fracture complications following traumatic brain injury. (*Reprinted with permission from Klima D 2006 Clients with traumatic brain injury. In: Umphred D, Carlson C (eds) Neurorehabilitation for the Physical Therapist Assistant. Slack, Thorofare, NJ. Illustration by Tim Phelps, CMI.*)

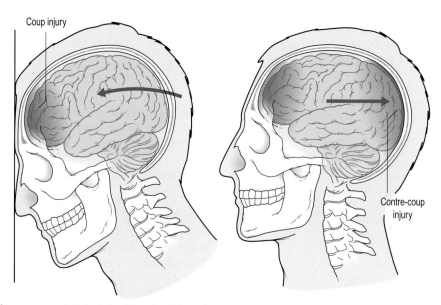

Figure 26.2 Coup and contre-coup injuries following traumatic brain injury. (*Reprinted with permission from Klima D 2006 Clients with traumatic brain injury. In: Umphred D, Carlson C (eds) Neurorehabilitation for the Physical Therapist Assistant. Slack, Thorofare, NJ. Illustration by Tim Phelps, CMI.*)

Table 26.1	**Glasgow Coma Scale**	
	Response	**Score**
Eyes open	Spontaneously	4
	To verbal command	3
	To pain	2
	No response	1
Best motor response		
To verbal stimulus	Obeys command	6
To painful stimulus	Localizes pain	5
	Flexion–withdrawal	4
	Flexion–abnormal (decorticate rigidity)	3
	Extension (decerebrate rigidity)	2
	No response	1
Best verbal response	Oriented and converses	5
	Disoriented and converses	4
	Inappropriate words	3
	Incomprehensible sounds	2
	No response	1
Total		3–15

Table 26.2	**Rancho Los Amigos levels of cognitive function**
I	No Response
II	Generalized response
III	Localized response
IV	Confused–agitated
V	Confused–inappropriate
VI	Confused–appropriate
VII	Automatic–appropriate
VIII	Purposeful–appropriate

of Cognitive Function. Consisting of eight stages, this classification scheme illustrates progressive improvement from minimally responsive behavior to near full cognitive recovery (Table 26.2). This tool has been widely used to track such outcomes as patients' functional recovery and hospital length of stay (Fakhry et al., 2004).

LEVELS I–III: COMA EMERGENCE

The initial stages depict coma emergent behavior. Patients may progress from initially exhibiting no response to demonstrating a variety of localized responses such as a hand squeeze or facial grimace. The rehabilitation team members may elect to track progress through a standardized coma emergence rating form such as the JFK Coma Recovery Scale–Revised (Schnakers et al., 2009). Neurobehavioral assessments can aid in delineating between diagnostic criteria for minimally conscious and vegetative state conditions. Patients reaching maximum scores on these instruments may then have more advanced goals and intervention plans established. Patients emerging from minimally responsive states are progressively mobilized through tilt-table or standing-frame activities. Patients are started on a sitting schedule to gradually increase sitting time. A variety of sensory stimulation activities are utilized throughout functional tasks. Geriatric clients must be monitored carefully for vital sign fluctuations given premorbid medical conditions and adverse effects of bedrest acquired from extended intensive care unit (ICU) monitoring.

LEVEL IV: THE AGITATED CLIENT

Level IV depicts the agitated patient who cannot process the multitude of sensory experiences within the immediate environment. Individuals in this stage tend to exhibit disconcerted, agitated behavior, which often escalates to bursts of hostility. Therapists must adjust treatment activities by scheduling shorter treatment sessions or holding sessions in quiet areas to avoid sensory overload. Therapists should also model calm behavior and allow agitated patients to feel that they have control over the immediate situation. Treatment sessions are structured accordingly to avoid or minimize painful or fearful activities. The Agitated Behavior Scale is an instrument that documents levels of agitation among patients with TBI (Bogner et al., 2000).

LEVELS V–VIII: PROGRESSIVE COGNITIVE RECOVERY

In levels V–VIII, cognitive recovery progresses from behavior that is confused and inappropriate to eventual appropriate and purposeful behavior. Unfortunately, older clients who sustain more severe injuries and complications may not achieve full recovery. In addition, both cognitive and neuromuscular recovery may not occur in tandem. The ultimate challenge in geriatric head trauma rehabilitation focuses on integrating both cognitive and functional training strategies to effectively guide the patient towards maximal functional independence. The cognitive dimension of therapeutic interventions adds a level of complexity that necessitates specialized skills to facilitate psychomotor skill attainment and community re-entry.

Cognitive impairment following a TBI may be substantial. Patients demonstrate slower processing and require increased time to optimize task performance. A diminished attention span may also be apparent and patients require ongoing redirection to the designated task. Learning of functional skills occurs at a diminished rate and suitable time allotment and cue sequences must be constructed within a treatment session to optimize skill acquisition. Memory deficits may continue to be problematic. In addition, rehabilitation clinicians must be reminded that the issue of impaired judgment is still prominent in the final stages of the Rancho continuum. Patients at higher functional levels of mobility may still be unable to problem-solve in the event of an emergency situation.

Cognitive and functional interventions are merged in a variety of ways. For example, dual task activities are created to assess the patient's problem-solving ability during functional tasks. Patients can be challenged to react in the event of an emergency situation. In addition, elements of memory can be incorporated by observing and reinforcing safety strategies taught during previous sessions. Patients may continue to have difficulty with advanced gait and balance activities such as tandem stance (Walker & Pickett, 2007), sensory reweighting tasks (Pickett et al., 2007) and running (Williams et al., 2012). At discharge, appropriate family training and instructions should be given to those family members who are caregivers for the older adult patient recovering from a TBI.

It is estimated that 200 000 individuals are currently living in the US with activity and participation limitations sustained from SCI, with over 12 000 new cases sustained each year (Bernhard et al., 2005). This includes those individuals who are aged 65 years or older. Major causes of SCI worldwide include motor vehicle accidents, acts of violence and recreational activities. In addition, atypical causes globally in developing countries include falls from trees, injuries on construction sites and spinal injuries sustained while carrying heavy loads on the head (Lee et al., 2013). Injuries to the cervical spine often result in tetraplegia (also known as quadriplegia), with resultant impairments to all four extremities, the trunk and the pelvic organs. The term paraplegia indicates resultant lower extremity paralysis from a designated lesion occurring below the cervical spine and is associated with varying levels of trunk involvement in accordance with the lesion level. Functional outcomes parallel specific levels of function and benchmark muscles spared following an injury (Table 26.3). Geriatric clients may have similar causes of spinal cord pathology because of neoplasms or spinal stenosis conditions.

A comprehensive examination should be performed to address all resultant impairments (body structure/function), activity limitations and disabilities (participation) in the geriatric patient with SCI. Examination strategies are often aligned with major components of the American Spinal Injury Association (ASIA) examination instrument (Fig. 26.4), including key muscles indicative of important myotome levels. Residual muscle function and sensory integrity is linked to the ASIA Impairment Scale (Table 26.4) to discern complete or incomplete involvement (ASIA, 2000; Teeter et al., 2012). A thorough musculoskeletal assessment is performed to determine the presence or absence of available intact musculature and the extent to which key muscle groups will be able to assist in functional activities. Detailed range of motion (ROM) is examined to recognize pertinent joint integrity restrictions. Sensory testing should be completed to identify those dermatomal fields that are intact, impaired or absent. Finally, a full mobility examination identifies the patient's ability to perform important functional activities such as transfers, pressure relief, wheelchair propulsion and bed mobility tasks. Aerobic capacity is assessed through vital sign responses,

Table 26.3 Key muscles used to determine neurological classification of spinal cord injury (ASIA)

Level	Muscle Groups Associated with Spinal Level
C5	Elbow flexors (biceps brachii)
C6	Wrist extensors (extensor carpi radialis longus and brevis)
C7	Elbow extensors (triceps)
C8	Finger flexors (flexor digitorum profundus)
T1	Small finger abductors (abductor digiti minimi)
L2	Hip flexors (iliopsoas)
L3	Knee extensors (quadriceps)
L4	Ankle dorsiflexors (tibialis anterior)
L5	Long toe extensors (extensor hallucis longus)
S1	Ankle plantar flexors (gastrocnemius/soleus)

Sensory levels are utilized to determine C1–4, T2–L1 and S2–5 neurological levels.

pulse oximetry and tolerance to all activities performed; in addition, examination of the patient's respiratory function should include an assessment of the patient's breathing pattern, ventilatory muscle strength and overall cough quality.

FUNCTIONAL TRAINING

Of paramount importance to older individuals suffering from a SCI is the transition to wheelchair mobility. Following medical stabilization, patients in rehabilitation learn wheelchair propulsion techniques according to the level of damage to their spinal cord and residual muscle function. For example, patients with lesions below the C6 level learn to manually propel a wheelchair; however, higher lesions may necessitate the need for electric wheelchair operation. Endurance and strength impairments may prohibit the geriatric client from successfully navigating the home and community environments, and goals may need to be adjusted.

Older adults with an SCI present a major challenge to rehabilitation clinicians. Often, patients are slower to achieve their target functional outcomes because of pre-existing comorbidities; in addition, contextual and personal factors may be more challenging for older adults with a SCI (Franceschini et al., 2011). For example, patients with injuries at or below the C7 level should achieve independence in all bed mobility activities; however, the older client with insufficient upper extremity strength may be slower to achieve established outcomes. The use of bedrails and other adaptive equipment will assist patients in effectively transitioning from the supine position to sitting. Certain geriatric patients with respiratory pathology will be unable to assume or tolerate the prone position, thus requiring adaptations to therapeutic exercise programs and bed mobility maneuvers.

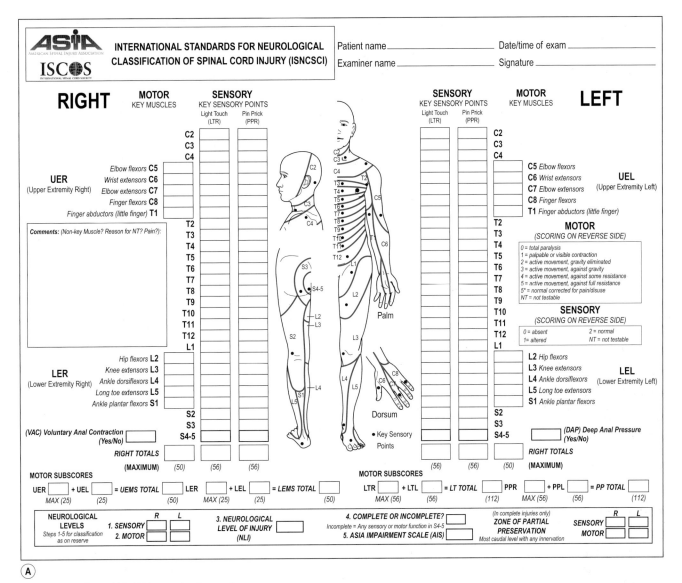

Figure 26.4 (**A** and **B**) ASIA examination tool.

Two major priorities for the geriatric client with an SCI include pressure relief and continued strengthening exercise programs. Older adults are more susceptible to pressure ulcers following an SCI and ongoing pressure relief mechanisms should be emphasized (Chen et al., 2005). For individuals with injuries above the C7 level, pressure relief will involve hooking the upper extremity onto the handgrip and incorporating a side-to-side lean. More dependent patients must utilize other modified positional leaning strategies or tilt maneuvers within the power chair. Patients with injuries at or below the C7 level will incorporate a full or modified push-up. Pressure relief strategies should be performed several times hourly to avoid pressure ulcer development.

Therapeutic exercise interventions for older adults with an SCI include both stretching and strengthening activities. Key muscle groups, such as the finger flexors in tetraplegia and trunk extensors in paraplegia, should remain tight. Hamstring flexibility, however, should be

optimized to facilitate transfers and dressing activities. Shoulder girdle strength is maximized in rehabilitation to accomplish the task of ongoing wheelchair propulsion, given that the upper extremities may be striking the handrim as many as 3500 times per day (Boninger et al., 2000). Major shoulder muscles are involved with both the push and recovery phases of wheelchair propulsion among individuals with both paraplegia and tetraplegia (Table 26.5) (Mulroy et al., 2004). Unfortunately, repetitive trauma to the shoulder joint or pain syndromes can significantly hinder wheelchair propulsion in geriatric clients with longstanding injuries. Upper extremity therapeutic exercise programs have been effective in reducing the incidence of shoulder pain among individuals with SCI (Nash, 2005).

In geriatric patients, the issue of ambulation following SCI is multifaceted. Patients must have the requisite strength, endurance and control to don and doff braces, arise to standing and ambulate with the appropriate gait

Muscle Function Grading

0 = total paralysis

1 = palpable or visible contraction

2 = active movement, full range of motion (ROM) with gravity eliminated

3 = active movement, full ROM against gravity

4 = active movement, full ROM against gravity and moderate resistance in a muscle specific position

5 = (normal) active movement, full ROM against gravity and full resistance in a functional muscle position expected from an otherwise unimpaired person

5* = (normal) active movement, full ROM against gravity and sufficient resistance to be considered normal if identified inhibiting factors (i.e. pain, disuse) were not present

NT = not testable (i.e. due to immobilization, severe pain such that the patient cannot be graded, amputation of limb, or contracture of > 50% of the normal range of motion)

Sensory Grading

0 = Absent

1 = Altered, either decreased/impaired sensation or hypersensitivity

2 = Normal

NT = Not testable

Non Key Muscle Functions (optional)

May be used to assign a motor level to differentiate AIS B vs. C

Movement	Root level
Shoulder: Flexion, extension, abduction, adduction, internal and external rotation **Elbow:** Supination	C5
Elbow: Pronation **Wrist:** Flexion	C6
Finger: Flexion at proximal joint, extension, **Thumb:** Flexion, extension and abduction in plane of thumb	C7
Finger: Flexion at MCP joint **Thumb:** Opposition, adduction and abduction perpendicular to palm	C8
Finger: Abduction of the index finger	T1
Hip: Adduction	L2
Hip: External rotation	L3
Hip: Extension, abduction, internal rotation **Knee:** Flexion **Ankle:** Inversion and eversion **Toe:** MP and IP extension	L4
Hallux and Toe: DIP and PIP flexion and abduction	L5
Hallux: Adduction	S1

ASIA Impairment Scale (AIS)

A = Complete. No sensory or motor function is preserved in the sacral segments S4–5.

B = Sensory Incomplete. Sensory but not motor function is preserved below the neurological level and includes the sacral segments S4–5 (light touch or pin prick at S4–5 or deep anal pressure) AND no motor function is preserved more than three levels below the motor level on either side of the body.

C = Motor Incomplete. Motor function is preserved below the neurological level**, and more than half of key muscle functions below the neurological level of injury (NLI) have a muscle grade less than 3 (Grades 0–2).

D = Motor Incomplete. Motor function is preserved below the neurological level**, and at least half (half or more) of key muscle functions below the NLI have a muscle grade ≥ 3.

E = Normal. If sensation and motor function as tested with the ISNCSCI are graded as normal in all segments, and the patient had prior deficits, then the AIS grade is E. Someone without an initial SCI does not receive an AIS grade.

** For an individual to receive a grade of C or D, i.e. motor incomplete status, they must have either (1) voluntary anal sphincter contraction or (2) sacral sensory sparing <u>with</u> sparing of motor function more than three levels below the motor level for that side of the body. The International Standards at this time allows even non-key muscle function more than 3 levels below the motor level to be used in determining motor incomplete status (AIS B vs. C).

NOTE: When assessing the extent of motor sparing below the level for distinguishing between AIS B and C, the *motor level* on each side is used; whereas to differentiate between AIS C and D (based on proportion of key muscle functions with strength grade 3 or greater) *the neurological level of injury* is used.

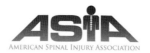

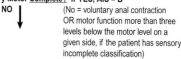

AMERICAN SPINAL INJURY ASSOCIATION

INTERNATIONAL STANDARDS FOR NEUROLOGICAL CLASSIFICATION OF SPINAL CORD INJURY

INTERNATIONAL SPINAL CORD SOCIETY

Steps in Classification

The following order is recommended for determining the classification of individuals with SCI.

1. Determine sensory levels for right and left sides.
The sensory level is the most caudal, intact dermatome for both pin prick and light touch sensation.

2. Determine motor levels for right and left sides.
Defined by the lowest key muscle function that has a grade of at least 3 (on supine testing), providing the key muscle functions represented by segments above that level are judged to be intact (graded as a 5).
Note: in regions where there is no myotome to test, the motor level is presumed to be the same as the sensory level, if testable motor function above that level is also normal.

3. Determine the neurological level of injury (NLI)
This refers to the most caudal segment of the cord with intact sensation and antigravity (3 or more) muscle function strength, provided that there is normal (intact) sensory and motor function rostrally respectively.
The NLI is the most cephalad of the sensory and motor levels determined in steps 1 and 2.

4. Determine whether the injury is Complete or Incomplete.
(i.e. absence or presence of sacral sparing)
*If voluntary anal contraction - **No** AND all S4–5 sensory scores = **0** AND deep anal pressure = **No**, then injury is **Complete**. Otherwise, injury is **Incomplete**.*

5. Determine ASIA Impairment Scale (AIS) Grade:

Is injury <u>Complete</u>?   If YES, AIS = **A** and can record
NO ↓   ZPP (lowest dermatome or myotome on each side with some preservation)

Is injury Motor <u>Complete</u>?   If YES, AIS = **B**
NO ↓   (No = voluntary anal contraction OR motor function more than three levels below the motor level on a given side, if the patient has sensory incomplete classification)

Are <u>at least</u> half (half or more) of the key muscles below the <u>neurological</u> level of injury graded 3 or better?

NO ↓   YES ↓

AIS = C   AIS = D

If sensation and motor function is normal in all segments, AIS = E
Note: AIS E is used in follow-up testing when an individual with a documented SCI has recovered normal function. If at initial testing no deficits are found, the individual is neurologically intact; the ASIA Impairment Scale does not apply.

Ⓑ

Figure 26.4 (Continued)

Table 26.4 ASIA Impairment Scale

A = Complete. No sensory or motor function is preserved in the sacral segments S4–S5

B = Sensory Incomplete. Sensory but not motor function is preserved below the neurological level and includes the sacral segments S4–S5 (light touch, pin-prick at S4–S5, or DAP), AND no motor function is preserved more than three levels below the motor level on either side of the body

C = Motor Incomplete. Motor function is preserved below the NLI and more than half of key muscle functions below the single NLI have a muscle grade < 3 (Grades 0–2)

D = Motor Incomplete. Motor function is preserved below the NLI and at least half (half or more) of key muscle functions below the NLI have a muscle grade > 3

E = Normal. If sensation and motor function as tested with the ISNCSCI are graded as normal in all segments, and the patient had prior deficits, then the ASIA grade is E. Someone without an initial SCI does not receive an ASIA grade

ASIA, American Spinal Injury Association; DAP, deep anal pressure; NLI, neurological level of injury; ISNCSCI, International Standards for Neurological Classification of Spinal Cord Injury (see Fig. 26.4).

Table 26.5 **Shoulder muscle activation pattern in SCI during wheelchair propulsion**	
Push Phase (Following Initial Contact)	**Recovery Phase (Return to Handrim)**
Anterior deltoid	Middle deltoid
Pectoralis major	Posterior deltoid
Supraspinatus	Supraspinatus
Subscapularis (tetraplegia)	Subscapularis (paraplegia)
Infraspinatus	Middle trapezius
Serratus anterior	Triceps brachii
Biceps brachii	

devices. Older patients may lack sufficient requirements in any one of these areas. Patients with injuries between levels L3 and L5 will as a minimum require an ankle–foot orthosis and upper extremity assistive device for ambulation. Higher lesions require more extensive bracing. In a study of 41 patients with SCI who were aged 50 or older, patients who achieved ambulation were those with lower classifications (ASIA C and D) on follow-up after their injury (Alander et al., 1997). Current interventions with body weight support treadmill training and robot-assisted devices should be used in conjunction with, rather than in place of, overground and task-oriented locomotor training to facilitate stepping and ambulation among select older individuals with SCI (Dobkin & Duncan, 2012).

COMMON MANAGEMENT ISSUES FOR CLIENTS WITH TBI AND SCI

Upper motor neuron damage may result in extensive resultant spasticity among geriatric clients, and tone management becomes an essential priority. The Modified Ashworth Scale (Bohannon & Smith, 1987) is utilized to grade hypertonic muscle groups and should be especially employed when implementing specific interventions to problematic muscle groups. Serial casting and splinting techniques are used to manage more severe spasticity, although therapists must use caution with older clients who have diabetes or compromised skin integrity. Medical management of hypertonicity may include the use of such centrally acting antispasmodics as lioresol (Baclofen), diazepam (Valium), or medications that act directly on muscle tissue itself such as dantrolene sodium (Dantrium).

Rehabilitation team members should be attentive to heterotopic ossificans, also known as myositis ossificans, following a TBI or SCI. Caused by ectopic bone formation, this condition can potentially result in significant joint ROM restrictions and pain. Therapists must acknowledge all abnormal joint end-feels when performing therapeutic exercise activities. Commonly affected joints include the hips, knees, shoulders and elbows. Diphosphates are used pharmacologically to inhibit the abnormal calcium metabolic process. Milder forms of heterotopic ossificans will not impose major functional limitations, although joints progressing to ankylosis will impede effective mobility activities such as transfers.

Management of both medical and autonomic complications of central nervous system trauma is a priority for all rehabilitation professionals. These conditions may become medical emergencies. For example, patients with spinal cord lesions above the T6 level may experience episodes of autonomic dysreflexia. Patients often experience such symptoms as a pounding headache, chills and profuse sweating in response to a noxious stimulus. Events triggering an episode of autonomic dysreflexia include restrictive clothing, a kinked catheter line and fecal impaction. Therapists should attempt to both recognize and eliminate the noxious stimulus if possible. Furthermore, the patient should be brought to a sitting position to alleviate dangerously elevated blood pressure.

Patients with both TBI and SCI should be monitored for episodes of orthostatic hypotension. Lower extremity paralysis and periods of prolonged bedrest are common predisposing factors. Geriatric patients are particularly at risk and should receive preventative graduated pressure stockings as indicated. Patients will require gradual postural changes when adjusting to the vertical position through use of a reclining wheelchair seating system and tilt-table activities. Ongoing skin inspections should occur for early detection of adverse swelling or deep vein thrombosis.

Neurological trauma sustained during injuries frequently includes trauma to the peripheral nervous system. Peripheral nerve damage can especially occur following a fall episode. For example, axillary nerve injury is a complication of humeral fractures, and sacral plexus damage and pelvic fractures often accompany high velocity injuries such as motor vehicle accidents. Additionally, brachial plexopathies can also arise from traumatic origins. Therapists must be vigilant during patient examinations to identify additional peripheral nerve damage not detected initially following medical management of the injuries sustained.

CONCLUSION

Comprehensive management of the geriatric client with neurological trauma requires strategic implementation of interventions designed to improve functional mobility limitations while, at the same time, integrating the older patient's premorbid condition and limitations imposed by age-related changes in organ systems. Appropriate outcome measures are utilized to both track and prognosticate the patient's status in the continuum of recovery. Common complications in SCI and TBI, such as heterotrophic ossificans and hypertonicity, must be recognized and treatment activities altered accordingly. Effective management will integrate and augment current evidence-based activities in the plan of care, as well as recognize the unique needs of the geriatric client who has sustained trauma to the brain or spinal cord.

REFERENCES

Alander D, Parker J, Stauffer E 1997 Intermediate-term outcome of cervical spinal cord-injured patients older than 50 years of age. Spine 22(11):1189–1192

ASIA (American Spinal Injury Association) 2000 International Standards for Neurological and Functional Classification of Spinal Cord Injury. American Spinal Injury Association, Chicago, IL

Berg K, Wood-Dauphine SL, Williams JI et al 1992 Measuring balance in the elderly: validation of an instrument. Can J Public Health 83:S9–11

Bernhard M, Gries A, Kremer P et al 2005 Spinal cord injury (SCI) – prehospital management. Resuscitation 66(2):127–139

Bhullar IS, Roberts EE, Brown L et al 2010 The effect of age on blunt traumatic brain-injured patients. Am Surg 76(9):966–968

Bogner JA, Corrigan JD, Bode RK et al 2000 Rating scale analysis of the Agitated Behavior Scale. J Head Trauma Rehabil 15(1):656–669

Bohannon RW, Smith MB 1987 Interrater reliability of a modified Ashworth scale of muscle spasticity. Phys Ther 67:53–54

Boninger ML, Baldwin M, Cooper RA et al 2000 Manual wheelchair pushrim mechanics and axle position. Arch Phys Med Rehabil 81:608–613

Brain Injury Association of America 2012. www.biausa.org/Pages/cdc_report.html

Chen Y, Devivo MJ, Jackson AB 2005 Pressure ulcer prevalence in people with spinal cord injury: age-period-duration effects. Arch Phys Med Rehabil 86(6):1208–1213

Corrigan JD, Smith-Knapp K, Granger CV 1997 Validity of the Functional Independence Measure for persons with traumatic brain injury. Arch Phys Med Rehabil 78:828–834

Dobkin BH, Duncan PW 2012 Should body weight-supported treadmill training and robotic-assistive steppers for locomotor training trot back to the starting gait? Neurorehabil Neural Repair 26(4):308–317

Fakhry SM, Trask AL, Waller MA, (Neurotrama Task Force) 2004 Management of brain injured patients by an evidence-based medicine protocol improves outcomes and decreases hospital charges. J Trauma 56(3):492–500

Faul M, Xu L, Wald MM et al 2010 Traumatic Brain Injury in the United States: Emergency Department Visits, Hospitalizations, and Deaths. Centers for Disease Control and Prevention, National Center for Injury Prevention and Control, Atlanta, GA

Franceschini M, Cerrel Bazo H, Lauretani F et al 2011 Age influences rehabilitative outcomes in patients with spinal cord injury (SCI). Aging Clin Exp Res 23(3):202–208

Lee BB, Cripps RA, Fitzharris M et al 2013 The global map for traumatic spinal cord injury epidemiology: update 2011, global incidence rate. Spinal Cord:1–7, doi:10.1038/sc.2012.158

Mulroy BJ, Farrokhi S, Newsam CJ et al 2004 Effects of spinal cord injury level on the activity of shoulder muscles during wheelchair propulsion: an electromyographic study. Arch Phys Med Rehabil 85:925–934

Nash MS 2005 Exercise as a health-promoting activity following spinal cord injury. J Neurol Phys Ther 29:87–103

Pickett TC, Radfar-Baublitz LS, McDonald SD et al 2007 Objectively assessing balance deficits after TBI: role of computerized posturography. J Rehabil Res Dev 44(7):983–990

Posiadlo D, Richardson S 1991 The Timed 'Up and Go': a test of basic functional mobility for frail elderly persons. J Am Geriatr Soc 39:142–147

Salter K, McClure JA, Foley NC et al 2011 Community integration following TBI: an examination of community integration measures within the ICF framework. Brain Inj 25(12):1147–1154

Sandhaug M, Andelic N, Vatne A et al 2010 Functional level during sub-acute rehabilitation after traumatic brain injury: course and predictors of outcome. Brain Inj 24(5):740–747

Schnakers C, Vanhaudenhuyse A, Giacino J et al 2009 Diagnostic accuracy of the vegetative and minimally conscious state: clinical consensus versus standardized neurobehavioral assessment. BMC Neurol 9:35, doi: 10.1186/1471-2377-9-35

Teasdale G, Jennett B 1974 Assessment of coma and impaired consciousness: a practical scale. Lancet 2:81–84

Teeter L, Gassaway J, Taylor S et al 2012 Relationship of physical therapy inpatient rehabilitation interventions and patient characteristics to outcomes following spinal cord injury: the SCIRehab project. J Spinal Cord Med 35(6):503–526

Walker WC, Pickett TC 2007 Motor impairment after severe traumatic brain injury: a longitudinal multicentre study. J Rehabil Res Dev 44(7):975–982

Williams G, Schnache AG, Morris ME 2012 Self-selected walking speed predicts ability to run following traumatic brain injury. J Head Trauma Rehabil 28(5):379–385

Chapter 27

Rehabilitation after stroke

MAUREEN ROMANOW PASCAL • SUSAN BARKER

CHAPTER CONTENTS

INTRODUCTION

A cerebrovascular accident (CVA), commonly referred to as a stroke, is the interruption of blood flow to brain tissue. The brain tissue that has been deprived of oxygen is damaged or dies. According to the World Health Organization (WHO), the standard definition of stroke is 'A focal (or at times global) neurological impairment of sudden onset, and lasting more than 24 hours (or leading to death), and of presumed vascular origin' (WHO, 2006). Strokes can be ischemic or hemorrhagic. Ischemic stroke is the most common type, accounting for 88% of CVAs. Ischemic strokes can be thrombotic or embolic. Thrombotic CVA is caused by a thrombus that develops in an artery supplying part of the brain. Embolic CVA is caused by blood clots that form outside the brain and travel through the bloodstream to the brain (WHO, 2006). Hemorrhagic CVA is the result of arterial bleeding into brain tissue or near the surface of the brain. It is usually the result of trauma, vascular abnormality, or hypertension. Hemorrhagic CVA can be either intracerebral or subarachnoid. Intracerebral hemorrhage is the result of bleeding into brain tissue. Subarachnoid hemorrhage is the result of bleeding into the space between the arachnoid layer and the pia mater.

Worldwide, stroke is the leading cause of disability in developed countries. It is estimated there are approximately 12.6 million individuals living with stroke throughout the world. Of these, about 8.9 million live in low- to middle-income countries (Hachinski et al., 2010). Countries in Africa and Northern Asia have the highest concentrations of people living with disability, or disability-adjusted life years (DALYs), for both men and women (Mendis et al., 2011) (Figs 27.1 and 27.2). Stroke is the second leading cause of death, with more than 85% of these deaths occurring in low- and middle-income countries combined, compared to high-income countries (WHO, 2011) (see Fig. 27.3). While mortality due to stroke is expected to decline in developed countries, the burden of disability is expected to increase. This indicates a increasing need for quality stroke rehabilitation, but more importantly, global efforts to reduce the prevalence of stroke.

RISK FACTORS

Some risk factors for stroke are non-modifiable. These include age, gender, race, family history and history of prior stroke or heart attack. CVA risk doubles for every decade beyond age 55. CVA is more common in men than women, and African-Americans and Hispanics are at greater risk for CVA than Caucasians. A person's risk of CVA is increased if an immediate family member has had a CVA (Goodman & Fuller, 2009).

Among the modifiable risk factors for CVA, hypertension is most important, since about 30% of adults in most countries have hypertension (Mackay & Mensah, 2004). Hypertension accounts for up to 54% of all strokes (Lawes et al., 2008). Patients with atrial fibrillation have five times greater risk of stroke, but treatment with anticoagulants can reduce that risk by two-thirds. Physical inactivity increases stroke risk, and even light physical activity can decrease that risk. Other modifiable risk factors include cigarette smoking or other tobacco use, a diet low in fruits and vegetables, heavy alcohol consumption, being overweight or obese, hypercholesterolemia and the combination of smoking and oral contraceptive use (Kwiatkowski et al., 1999; WHO, 2006).

SIGNS AND SYMPTOMS

Signs and symptoms of a possible CVA include weakness or altered sensation of the face, arm, and/or leg, headache, vision changes (field cuts, blurriness), confusion, dizziness and alterations in speech (Sullivan et al., 2004; WHO, 2006). Development of these signs or symptoms indicates the individual should receive immediate medical attention. Other symptoms may include headache, dizziness or vertigo, seizure or difficulty swallowing. If these symptoms are combined with weakness or sensory changes, it is likely the individual is having a stroke. If the stroke is ischemic, blood supply may be restored

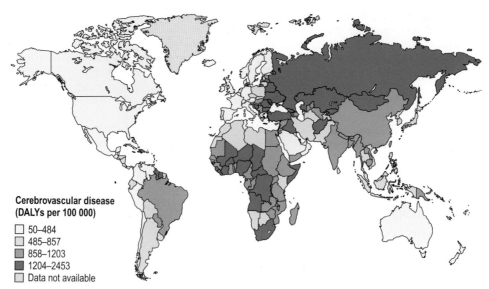

Figure 27.1 World map showing the burden of cerebrovascular disease in males (DALYs, age standardized, per 100 000). *(Reproduced from Mendis et al., 2011, Fig. 21, p. 13, with permission from the World Health Organization. © WHO, 2011.)*

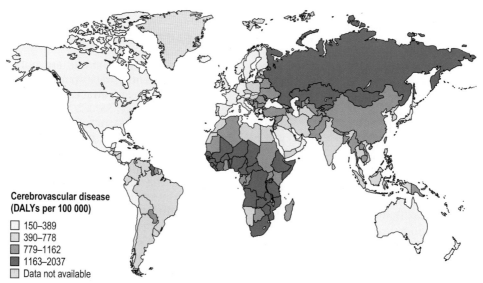

Figure 27.2 World map showing the burden of cerebrovascular disease in females (DALYs, age standardized, per 100 000). *(Reproduced from Mendis et al., 2011, Fig. 21, p.13, with permission from the World Health Organization. © WHO, 2011.)*

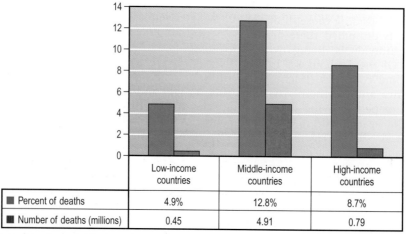

	Low-income countries	Middle-income countries	High-income countries
Percent of deaths	4.9%	12.8%	8.7%
Number of deaths (millions)	0.45	4.91	0.79

Figure 27.3 Stroke-related death and country income.

through a thrombolytic agent such as tissue plasmino-gen activator; however, this treatment has only been demonstrated to improve outcomes if administered within the first 3 hours of the event (Clark et al., 1999; Kwiatkowski et al., 1999).

DIAGNOSIS

According to the World Health Organization's STEPS Stroke Manual, 'stroke is a clinical diagnosis, and is not based on radiological findings'. However, in most developed countries, definitive diagnosis of stroke is often made based on results of a computed tomography (CT) or magnetic resonance imaging (MRI) scan. CT is used more commonly than MRI, as CT is generally more available and less expensive than MRI (Calautti & Jean-Claude, 2003). Both CT and MRI can provide information about areas of infarction or hemorrhage (Kidwell et al., 2004). Diffusion-weighed MRI has been shown to be superior in the diagnosis of acute ischemic stroke, which is an important factor in the decision about the use of thrombolytic medication (Etgen et al., 2004). However, since CT can exclude the diagnosis of hemorrhagic stroke, can be performed more quickly than MRI and is more readily available, it remains the more common imaging modality (Edlow, 2011). In addition to CT and MRI, echocardiography and ultrasound may be used to identify the location of the blood clot responsible for an ischemic event (Gunaratne, 2012).

PROGNOSIS

Impaired motor function after a stroke may lead to long-term disability. Early return of motor function is a good prognostic indicator of future functional improvement. Regaining voluntary shoulder and finger movements within 7 days of a stroke is associated with a good return of arm function (Nijland et al., 2010). Return of leg strength within 1 week is a good predictor of return to independent walking (Stinear, 2010). In a study conducted in The Netherlands, Kwakkel et al. found that, at 5 weeks post stroke, physical therapists and occupational therapists are able to accurately predict a patient's walking ability and manual dexterity at 6 months post stroke (Kwakkel et al., 2000).

Imaging modalities may be used to determine prognosis after stroke. Functional MRI (fMRI) and transcranial magnetic stimulation (TMS) both show potential for more widespread use as prognostic tools. fMRI can be used to evaluate the cortical activation patterns used to perform a functional movement. The pattern used by a patient after a stroke is well-correlated with level of recovery and outcomes (Carey et al., 2002; Ward et al., 2003; Ward & Cohen, 2004; Stinear, 2010). Patients who demonstrate activation maps similar to controls (i.e. they activate the left cortex for right-sided movements) have fewer residual impairments. Patients who demonstrate activation of the primary motor cortex ipsilateral to the lesion, plus bilateral activation of supplementary areas, generally have greater impairments and a poorer outcome (Ward & Cohen, 2004). Due to the limited availability and costs associated with performing fMRI it is not currently in wide use.

TMS is an imaging modality that shows some potential for prognosis in the future. TMS can be used to stimulate the primary motor cortex and elicit a motor response peripherally. The presence or lack of evoked potentials in the targeted muscles provides information about the integrity of the corticomotor pathway. Similarly to fMRI, the test looks at the patient's ability to use the cortex on the side of the brain most affected by the stroke (ipsilesional) to control the contralateral extremities. As with fMRI, the ability to use the ipsilesional cortex to elicit motor function is associated with improved functional outcomes. Both fMRI and TMS are used for testing upper extremity more than lower extremity function (Stinear, 2010).

Severity of stroke can play a role in prognosis. Patients who sustain a severe middle cerebral artery stroke tend to have a poor prognosis for functional use of the affected upper extremity. The chance of recovery declines if it takes longer for the patient to make functional gains, or to regain active hand motion (Kwakkel et al., 2000).

There are many other factors that will affect a patient's outcome after stroke, including the presence of comorbidities such as hypertension, diabetes mellitus and overweight and obesity. The presence of cognitive or perceptual limitations may limit understanding of directions, negatively affecting a patient's motivation or insight into the deficits of the stroke. None of these factors precludes a good outcome, but they may increase the time it takes a patient to demonstrate functional improvement during rehabilitation.

One specific problem that tends to lengthen the time for rehabilitation is pusher syndrome, a disorder related to a stroke that affects the right or left posterolateral thalamus. In pusher syndrome, or contraversive pushing, the patient shifts excessive weight onto the weaker side, resulting in difficulty maintaining upright sitting or standing. The patient has an impaired perception of vertical, does not attempt to correct the faulty posture and resists correction by another individual. Intervention for pusher syndrome includes using a landmark or visual cue to help the patient identify vertical in the environment. Pusher syndrome rarely lasts more than 6 months post stroke, so although rehabilitation takes longer, the long-term outcome tends not to be greatly affected (Karnath & Broetz, 2003).

One comorbidity that can affect the outcome is metabolic syndrome (see Chapter 46). Metabolic syndrome increases the risk of diabetes mellitus, heart disease and stroke. A patient with metabolic syndrome has at least one of the following factors: large waist circumference, high triglycerides, low HDL cholesterol, insulin resistance and/or hypertension (National Heart, Lung, and Blood Institute, 2011). In one recent study by Mi et al., Chinese individuals with metabolic syndrome, and specifically those with central obesity, were found to be at higher risk for having another stroke within a year of the first stroke (Mi et al., 2012). This finding has implications for patient education about healthy lifestyles, both before and after a stroke.

One other factor that greatly affects prognosis is whether or not the patient will be given the opportunity to participate in a quality rehabilitation program. WHO and the World Stroke Organization both recommend rehabilitation services at a center that specializes in the treatment of stroke (WHO, 2006; Hachinski et al., 2010). The interventions that may be used to promote recovery are discussed below.

INTERVENTION

Several impairments and functional limitations may occur after a stroke. Hemiparesis involving the upper or lower extremity, or both, is one of the most common impairments that may need to be addressed by occupational therapists and physical therapists. Patients may also experience sensory loss or altered sensation in the area of the body affected by the stroke. Other common impairments include decreased balance, sensory, visual and perceptual deficits, impaired cognition, impaired communication, decreased coordination, increased tone and spasticity and decreased motor control. Functional limitations often include decreased functional mobility in bed, transfers, gait and activities of daily living (ADLs), especially those that are usually bimanual, e.g. dressing and bathing. The large spectrum of possible impairments in body structure or function, activity limitations and participation restrictions is the reason a team approach that includes physical and occupational therapists, speech-language pathologists, physicians, nurses and other health professions is crucial to the rehabilitation approach.

The paresis following a stroke appears related to several structural and physiological changes that occur after a stroke, including a decrease in the number of muscle fibers, change in the types of muscle fibers and muscle recruitment patterns, and decreases in peripheral nerve conduction velocity. The functional result is a decrease in ability to produce adequate muscle force (Patten et al., 2004).

Improving physical function plays an important role in quality of life after a stroke. Duncan et al. have researched quality of life in people with stroke and have found that decreased physical abilities have the greatest effect on quality of life after stroke. Loss of hand function is reported as the most disabling (Duncan et al., 2003).

One of the most commonly used treatment interventions for post-stroke rehabilitation is the Bobath approach, or neurodevelopmental treatment. This approach focuses on encouraging, or facilitating, normal movement and inhibiting abnormal movement patterns. Strengths of the Bobath approach are that many of the treatment techniques are designed to encourage increased functional mobility, and treatments are often performed in functional positions. Many experienced therapists who use the Bobath method apply motor learning principles and perform techniques during functional activities (Lennon & Ashburn, 2000). Another strength of this approach is that it can be performed with minimal equipment, making it a good choice for therapists who have limited resources for rehabilitation. The Bobath approach has evolved to focus less on the reacquisition of normal movement and more on the use of problem-solving strategies during functional tasks, focusing on encouraging postural control

(Huseyinsinoglu et al., 2012). Despite its wide use, there is currently no evidence that the Bobath approach is more effective than other methods used in stroke rehabilitation. Conversely, there is also no evidence that it is an ineffective approach (Paci, 2003). Due to the training involved, and the variety of techniques that may be employed in the Bobath method, researchers have found it difficult to perform controlled studies of this method.

Other common methods used in stroke intervention include proprioceptive neuromuscular facilitation, and intervention approaches developed by Brunnstrom, Rood, Johnstone and Ayres (O'Sullivan & Schmitz, 2007). Like the Bobath method, the effectiveness or ineffectiveness of these strategies has not been supported by controlled research studies (Van Peppen et al., 2004). Similar to the Bobath approach, these interventions can be performed with little equipment.

It is now well acknowledged that stroke rehabilitation must be designed to maximize the neuroplasticity that can occur as the nervous system attempts to recover. One important factor in promoting neuroplasticity and recovery is making the rehabilitation activities salient, specific and functional. The activities need to have enough intensity and repetition to promote learning (Kleim & Jones, 2008). The task-oriented approach is based on the concept that learning is goal-oriented (Gordon, 2000). While the task-oriented approach does not preclude hands-on activity, it does imply that the patient participates in some exploration of the task, including trial-and-error. One specific method based on the task-oriented approach is the Motor Relearning Programme. A Norwegian study demonstrated that this method can be effective in improving motor function and performance in ADLs in patients with acute stroke (Langhammer & Stanghalle, 2000).

Because the paresis that results from stroke is related to functional limitations, strength training is an intervention that may be appropriate in post-stroke rehabilitation (Canning et al., 2004; Morris et al., 2004; Patten et al., 2004; Forrester et al., 2008). Several studies have demonstrated functional improvements in patients who participated in both strength training and task-oriented functional training (Morris et al., 2004; Patten et al., 2006; Jørgensen et al., 2010). There does not seem to be a link between strength training and increased spasticity (Patten et al., 2004).

Modalities that are frequently used in stroke rehabilitation include functional electrical stimulation (FES) and neuromuscular electrical stimulation (NMES). A recent innovation in the use of FES for the lower extremity is a neuroprosthesis, a device worn by the patient in place of an ankle–foot orthosis or hand splint. The device incorporates FES to promote proper timing of stimulation of muscles during a functional activity. In the lower extremity it is designed to stimulate the ankle dorsiflexors during the swing phase of gait to help reduce or eliminate foot drop. Some lower extremity neuroprostheses can also stimulate ankle plantarflexors at the end of stance to improve push-off (Mesci et al., 2009; Embrey et al., 2010). Currently there is limited evidence to support the use of FES to increase lower extremity strength (Ferrante et al., 2008), and NMES to increase upper extremity strength (Van Peppen et al., 2004). There is strong evidence to support the use of NMES to both decrease inferior subluxation of the glenohumeral joint, and to increase shoulder external rotation passive range of motion (Van Peppen et al., 2004).

Some of the newer interventions that have been developed for rehabilitation of patients with stroke target specific impairments or functional limitations. One of these is constrained-induced therapy (CIT), which is also known as constraint-induced movement therapy and forced use. This intervention targets the hemiparetic upper extremity. A constraining device such as a sling or mitt is applied to the stronger upper extremity to promote increased use of the affected arm (Mark & Taub, 2002). The current protocol requires 'massed practice with the more affected arm on functional activities, shaping tasks in the training exercises, and restraint of the less-affected arm for a target of 90% of waking hours' (Mark & Taub, 2002). The protocol has been most successful with patients who have some ability to extend the affected wrist and fingers. It has been less successful in patients with little active movement, although improvement is still possible (Mark & Taub, 2002; Lin et al., 2010). Wolf et al. demonstrated CIT can promote recovery of hand function in patients who are 1 year post stroke (Wolf et al., 2006).

An intervention that specifically targets walking ability is body-weight supported treadmill training (BWS-TT). In this intervention, a portion of the patient's weight is suspended using a sling attached to an overhead harness. The patient is then assisted in performing gait training on a treadmill. Results from several randomized controlled trials indicate that BWS-TT can help to increase endurance for walking and improve gait speed (Hesse, 2004; Peurala et al., 2005; Lindquist et al., 2007; Tilson et al., 2010). Current evidence does not support using this method to improve walking ability or postural control, except with a specialized split-belt treadmill (Van Peppen et al., 2004; Reisman et al., 2007). In contrast, gait training on a treadmill without body weight support has been shown to improve walking ability (McCain & Smith, 2007; Luft et al., 2008).

Some interventions that are currently being studied use advanced technology to help reduce impairments and functional limitations after a stroke. These include the use of robotic training to improve gait and upper extremity motor control (Lum et al., 2002; Stein et al., 2004; Riener et al., 2005; Frick & Alberts, 2006) and virtual reality (Merians et al., 2002; Weiss et al., 2003; Deutsch et al., 2004). Some interventions, such as mirror therapy (Sütbeyaz et al., 2007; Yavuzer et al., 2008) and aquatic therapy (Noh et al., 2008; Chon et al., 2009), require less technology and have recent research supporting their use. As research in these areas continues, they will likely prove to be valuable adjuncts to current physical therapy practice.

CONCLUSION

Stroke is a global problem that can result in a multitude of impairments and functional limitations. Improvement of healthcare and public awareness of the importance of reducing risk factors may help to decrease the incidence and severity of this condition, and decrease the global burden of this non-communicable disease. There are currently many types of physical therapy interventions used to improve the functional abilities of patients after a stroke. More randomized, controlled clinical research is needed in this area to help therapists make informed decisions about which interventions are most appropriate for the patients with whom they work.

References

Calautti C, Jean-Claude B 2003 Functional recovery after stroke in adults. Stroke 34:1553–1575

Canning CG, Ada L, Adams R et al 2004 Loss of strength contributes more to physical disability after a stroke than loss of dexterity. Clin Rehabil 18:300–308

Carey JR, Kimberley TJ, Lewis SM et al 2002 Analysis of fMRI and finger tracking training in subject with chronic stroke. Brain 125:773–778

Chon SC, Oh DW, Shim JH 2009 Watsu approach for improving spasticity and ambulatory function in hemiparetic patients with stroke. Physiother Res Intern 14(2):128–134

Clark WM, Wissman S, Albers GW et al 1999 Recombinant tissue-type plasminogen activator (alteplase) for ischemic stroke 3 to 5 hours after symptom onset. JAMA 282(21):2019–2026

Deutsch JE, Merians AS, Adamovich S et al 2004 Development and application of virtual reality technology to improve hand use and gait of individuals post stroke. Restor Neurol Neurosci 22:371–386

Duncan PW, Bode RK, Min Lai S et al 2003 Rasch analysis of a new stroke-specific outcome scale: the Stroke Impact Scale. Arch Phys Med Rehabil 84(7):950–963

Edlow JA 2011 Evidence-based guideline: the role of diffusion and perfusion MRI for the diagnosis of acute ischemic stroke: report of the therapeutics and technology subcommittee of the American Academy of Neurology. Neurology 76:2036–2038

Embrey DG, Holtz SL, Alon G et al 2010 Functional electrical stimulation to dorsiflexors and plantar flexors during gait to improve walking in adults with chronic hemiplegia. Arch Phys Med Rehabil 91:687–696

Etgen T, Grafin von Einsiedel H, Rottinger M et al 2004 Detection of acute brainstem infarction by using DWI/MRI. Eur Neurol 3(52):145–150

Ferrante S, Pedrocchi A, Ferrigno G et al 2008 Cycling induced by functional electrical stimulation improves the muscular strength and the motor control of individuals with post-acute stroke. Eur J Phys Rehabil Med 44:159–167

Forrester LW, Wheaton LA, Luft AR 2008 Exercise-mediated locomotor recovery and lower-limb neuroplasticity after stroke. J Rehabil Res Devel 45(2):205–220

Frick EM, Alberts JL 2006 Combined use of repetitive task practice and an assistive robotic device in a patient with subacute stroke. Phys Ther 86(10):1378–1386

Goodman CC, Fuller K 2009 Pathology: Implications for the Physical Therapist, 3rd edn. WB Saunders, St Louis, MO

Gordon J 2000 Assumptions underlying physical therapy intervention: theoretical and historical perspectives. In: Carr J, Shepherd R, Gaithersburg MD (eds) Movement science: foundations for physical therapy in rehabilitation. Aspen Publishers Inc., New York

Gunaratne PS 2012 Stroke Care. S Godage & Brothers (Pvt) Ltd, Colombo, Sri Lanka

Hachinski V, Donnan GA, Gorelick PB et al 2010 Stroke: working toward a prioritized world agenda. Int J Stroke 5(4):238–256

Hesse S 2004 Recovery of gait and other motor functions after stroke: novel physical and pharmacological treatment strategies. Restor Neurol Neurosci 22:359–369

Huseyinsinoglu BE, Ozdincler AR, Krespi Y 2012 Bobath concept versus constraint–induced movement therapy to improve arm functional recovery in stroke patients: a randomized controlled trial. Clin Rehabil 26(8):705–715

Jørgensen JR, Bech-Pedersen DT, Zeeman P et al 2010 Effect of intensive outpatient physical training on gait performance and cardiovascular health in people with hemiparesis after stroke. Phys Ther 90:527–537

Karnath H-O, Broetz D 2003 Understanding and treating 'pusher syndrome'. Phys Ther 83:1119–1125

Kidwell CS, Chalela JA, Saver JL et al 2004 Comparison of MRI and CT for detection of acute intracerebral hemorrhage. JAMA 292(15):1823–1830

Kleim JA, Jones TA 2008 Principles of experience-dependent neural plasticity: implications for rehabilitation after brain damage. J Speech Lang Hearing Res 51:S225–S239

Kwakkel G, van Dijk GM, Wagenaar RC 2000 Accuracy of physical and occupational therapists' early predictions of recovery after severe middle cerebral artery stroke. Clin Rehabil 14:28–41

Kwiatkowski TG, Libman RB, Frankel M et al 1999 Effects of tissue plasminogen activator for acute ischemic stroke at one year. N Engl J Med 340:1781–1787

Langhammer B, Stanghalle JK 2000 Bobath or motor relearning programme? A comparison of two different approaches of physiotherapy in stroke rehabilitation: a randomized controlled study. Clin Rehabil 14:361–369

Lawes CMM, Vander Hoorn S, Rodgers A 2008 Global burden of blood-pressure-related disease, 2001. Lancet 371:1513–1516

Lennon S, Ashburn A 2000 The Bobath concept in stroke rehabilitation: a focus group study of the experienced physiotherapist's perspective. Disabil Rehabil 22(15):665–674

Lin K-C, Chung H-Y, Wu C-Y et al 2010 Constraint-induced therapy versus control intervention in patients with stroke: a functional magnetic resonance imaging study. Am J Phys Med Rehabil 89:177–185

Lindquist ARR, Prado CL, Barros RML et al 2007 Gait training combining partial body-weight support, a treadmill, and functional electrical stimulation: effects on poststroke gait. Phys Ther 87:1144–1154

Luft AR, Macko RF, Forrester LW et al 2008 Treadmill exercise activates subcortical neural networks and improves walking after stroke. Stroke 39:3341–3350

Lum PS, Burgur CG, Shor PC et al 2002 Robot-assisted movement training compared with conventional therapy techniques for the rehabilitation of upper-limb motor function after stroke. Arch Phys Med Rehabil 83(7):952–959

McCain KJ, Smith PS 2007 Locomotor treadmill training with body-weight support prior to over-ground gait: promoting symmetrical gait in a subject with acute stroke. Top Stroke Rehabil 14(5):18–27

Mackay J, Mensah G 2004 Atlas of heart disease and stroke. WHO Press, Geneva, Switzerland

Mark VW, Taub E 2002 Constraint-induced movement therapy for chronic stroke hemiparesis and other disabilities. Restor Neurol Neurosci 22:317–336

Mendis S, Puska P, Norrving B et al (eds) 2011 Global Atlas on Cardiovascular Disease Prevention and Control. World Health Organization, Geneva

Merians AS, Jack D, Boian R et al 2002 Virtual reality-augmented rehabilitation for patients following stroke. Phys Ther 82:898–915

Mesci N, Ozdemir F, Kabayel DD et al 2009 The effects of neuromuscular electrical stimulation on clinical improvement in hemiplegic lower extremity rehabilitation in chronic stroke: a single-blind, randomized, controlled trial. Disabil Rehabil 31(24):2047–2054

Mi D, Zhang L, Wang C et al 2012 Impact of metabolic syndrome on the prognosis of ischemic stroke secondary to intracranial atherosclerosis in Chinese patients. PLoS ONE 7(12):1–5, doi: 10.1371/journal.pone.0051421 (accessed 28 February 2013)

Morris SL, Dodd KJ, Morris ME 2004 Outcomes of progressive resistance strength training following stroke: a systematic review. Clin Rehabil 18:27–39

National Heart, Lung, and Blood Institute 2011 What is metabolic syndrome? Available at: www.nhlbi.nih.gov/health/health-topics/topics/ms/. Accessed February 2013

Nijland RH, van Wegen EE, Harmeling-van der Wel BC et al 2010 Presence of finger extension and shoulder abduction with 72 hours after stroke predicts functional recovery: early prediction of functional outcome after stroke: the EPOS cohort study. Stroke 41:745–750

Noh DK, Lim J-Y, Shin H-I et al 2008 The effect of aquatic therapy on postural balance and muscle strength in stroke survivors – a randomized controlled pilot trial. Clin Rehabil 22:966–976

O'Sullivan SB, Schmitz TJ 2007 Stroke. In: Physical Rehabilitation, 5th edn. FA Davis Company, Philadelphia, PA

Paci M 2003 Physiotherapy based on the Bobath concept for adults with post-stroke hemiplegia: a review of effectiveness studies. J Rehabil Med 35:2–7

Patten C, Lexell J, Brown HE 2004 Weakness and strength training in persons with poststroke hemiplegia: rationale, method and efficacy. J Rehabil Res Dev 41(3A):293–312

Patten C, Dozono J, Schmidt SG et al 2006 Combined functional task practice and dynamic high intensity resistance training promotes recovery of upper extremity motor function in post-stroke hemiparesis: a case study. J Neurol Phys Ther 30(3):99–115

Peurala SH, Tarkka IM, Pitkänen K et al 2005 The effectiveness of body weight-supported gait training and floor walking in patients with chronic stroke. Arch Phys Med Rehabil 86:1557–1564

Reisman DS, Wityk R, Silver K et al 2007 Locomotor adaptation on a split-belt treadmill can improve walking symmetry post-stroke. Brain 130:1861–1872

Riener R, Net T, Colombo G 2005 Robot-aided neurorehabilitation of the upper extremities. Med Biol Eng Comput 43:2–10

Stein J, Krebs HI, Frontera WR et al 2004 Comparison of two techniques of robot-aided upper limb exercise training. Am J Phys Med Rehabil 83(9):720–728

Stinear C 2010 Prediction of motor recovery after stroke. Lancet Neurol 9:1228–1232

Sullivan KJ, Hershberg J, Howard R et al 2004 Neurological differential diagnosis for physical therapy. J Neurol Phys Ther 28(4):162–168

Sütbeyaz S, Yavuzer G, Sezer N et al 2007 Mirror therapy enhances lower-extremity motor recovery and motor functioning after stroke: a randomized controlled trial. Arch Phys Med Rehabil 88:555–559

Tilson JK, Sullivan KJ, Cen SY et al 2010 Meaningful gait speed improvement during the first 60 days post stroke: minimal clinically important difference. Phys Ther 90(2):196–208

Van Peppen RPS, Kwakkel G, Wood-Dauphinee S et al 2004 The impact of physical therapy on functional outcomes after stroke: what's the evidence? Clin Rehabil 18:833–862

Ward NS, Brown MM, Thompson AJ et al 2003 Neural correlates of outcome after stroke: a cross-sectional fMRI study. Brain 126:1430–1448

Ward NS, Cohen LG 2004 Mechanisms underlying recovery of motor function after stroke. Arch Neurol 61(12):1844–1848

Weiss PL, Naveh Y, Katz N 2003 Design and testing of a virtual environment to train stroke patients with unilateral spatial neglect to cross a street safely. Occup Ther Int 10(1):39–55

WHO (World Health Organization) 2006 WHO STEPS Stroke Manual: The WHO STEPwise approach to stroke surveillance. World Health Organization, Geneva

WHO (World Health Organization) Media Centre 2011 The 10 leading causes of death by broad income group, 2008. World Health Organization, Geneva. Available at: www.who.int/mediacentre/factsheets/fs310/en. Accessed February 2013

Wolf SL, Winstein CJ, Miller JP et al 2006 Effect of constraint-induced movement therapy on upper extremity function 3 to 9 months after stroke. JAMA 296(17):2095–2104

Yavuzer G, Selles R, Sezer N et al 2008 Mirror therapy improves hand function in subacute stroke: a randomized controlled trial. Arch Phys Med Rehabil 89:393–398

Chapter 28
Neurocognitive disorders

JAMES SIBERSKI

CHAPTER CONTENTS

INTRODUCTION

Dementia affected 36 million people around the world in 2010; in 2030 that number will rise to 65 million (Hughes, 2011) and will continue to increase unless interventions are developed. With regard to Alzheimer's disease (AD) alone, unpaid caregivers provide 210 billion dollars' worth of care, and total reimbursement payments for healthcare for all of the dementias are projected to be $1.1 trillion in 2050 (in 2012 dollars) (Alzheimer's Association, 2012). It can be said that the dementia crisis is upon us.

When discussing the rehabilitation of individuals diagnosed as being demented one needs to define what was or is dementia. In 2013, the American Psychiatric Association published their updated Diagnostic and Statistical Manual, DSM 5, which will effectively eliminate the term dementia. It will be replaced with the term 'neurocognitive disorder' (NCD). The DSM 5 will also split the NCD category into three broad syndromes: Delirium, Minor NCD and Major NCD.

The proposed revision for a Delirium is:

A. *Disturbance in attention (i.e. reduced ability to direct, focus, sustain, and shift attention) and orientation to the environment.*
B. *The disturbance develops over a short period of time (usually hours to a few days) and represents an acute change from baseline that is not solely attributable to another neurocognitive disorder, and tends to fluctuate in severity during the course of a day.*
C. *A change in an additional cognitive domain, such as memory deficit, disorientation, or language disturbance, or perceptual disturbance, that is not better accounted for by a pre-existing, established, or evolving other neurocognitive disorder.*
D. *The disturbances in Criteria A and C must not be occurring in the context of a severely reduced level of arousal such as coma.*

The proposed revision for a Minor Neurocognitive Disorder is:

A. *Evidence of modest cognitive decline from a previous level of performance in one or more of the domains outlined above based on:*
   1. *Concerns of the individual, a knowledgeable informant, or the clinician that there has been a modest decline in cognitive function; and 2. A decline in neurocognitive performance, typically involving test performance in the range of 1 and 2 standard deviations below appropriate norms (i.e. between the 3rd and 16th percentile) on formal testing or equivalent clinical evaluation.*
B. *The cognitive deficits are insufficient to interfere with independence (i.e. instrumental activities of daily living [more complex tasks such as paying bills or managing medications] are preserved), but greater effort, compensatory strategies, or accommodation may be required to maintain independence.*
C. *The cognitive deficits do not occur exclusively in the context of a Delirium.*
D. *The cognitive deficits are not primarily attributable to another mental disorder (e.g. Major Depressive Disorder, Schizophrenia).*

The proposed revision for a Major Neurocognitive Disorder is:

A. *Evidence of substantial cognitive decline from a previous level of performance in one or more of the domains outlined above based on:*
   1. *Concerns of the individual, a knowledgeable informant, or the clinician that there has been a substantial decline in cognitive function; 2. A decline in neurocognitive performance, typically involving test performance in the range of 2 or more standard deviations below appropriate norms (i.e. below the 3rd percentile) on formal testing or equivalent clinical evaluation.*
B. *The cognitive deficits are sufficient to interfere with independence (i.e. requiring assistance at a minimum with*

instrumental activities of daily living [more complex tasks such as paying bills or managing medications]).
C. *The cognitive deficits do not occur exclusively in the context of a Delirium.*
D. *The cognitive deficits are not primarily attributable to another mental disorder (e.g. Major Depressive Disorder, Schizophrenia).*

Once the clinician makes the diagnosis of Minor NCD or Major NCD, the clinician must then utilize the proposed criteria for the etiological subtypes of Minor and Major NCD, which are listed below:

Neurocognitive Disorder Due to Alzheimer's Disease
Frontotemporal Neurocognitive Disorder
Neurocognitive Disorder with Lewy Bodies
Vascular Neurocognitive Disorder
Neurocognitive Disorder Due to Traumatic Brain Injury
Substance/Medication-Induced Neurocognitive Disorder
Neurocognitive Disorder Due to HIV Infection
Neurocognitive Disorder Due to Prion Disease
Neurocognitive Disorder Due to Parkinson's Disease
Neurocognitive Disorder Due to Huntington's Disease
Neurocognitive Disorder Due to Another Medical Condition
Major or Mild Neurocognitive Disorder Due to Multiple Etiologies
Unspecified Neurocognitive Disorder.

(DSM 5, 2012)

There have been positive and negative views expressed from many quarters concerning the DSM 5 proposed changes. Suffice it to say that change is always difficult, costly and confusing to both professionals and patients. Professionals will need to become familiar with DSM 5 NCD in order to explain these changes to their patients.

Adding to the confusion, the Alzheimer's Association and the National Institute on Aging (NIA), for the first time in over 27 years, have changed the staging of AD. As a result of recent research, it is now understood that AD progresses on a spectrum with three stages. In the preclinical stage, where the brain changes, there are no symptoms, as it starts years, if not decades, before the early symptoms of AD become apparent. An upcoming section of this chapter on lifestyle rehabilitation will elaborate. The middle stage, mild cognitive impairment (MCI), is a term not used in DSM 5, which may initially confuse professionals and surely baffle patients. The final stage, AD, is marked by symptoms of cognitive decline or dementia. The Alzheimer's Association and NIA staging employs the term dementia while DSM 5 does not, perhaps creating a bit more confusion (Siberski, 2012).

NEUROCOGNITIVE DISORDERS AND ASSESSMENT

A rehabilitation program should begin with a competent assessment, with the primary goal being an accurate and early diagnosis. It must first be determined if there is a NCD or if the issue is a normal age-related change or perhaps even a delirium as the management strategies differ from those that would be utilized in a NCD. Once a NCD is diagnosed, the cause of the minor/major NCD must be

determined in order to start the rehabilitation course. In a cortical NCD, such as Alzheimer's dementia, the patient's executive function could be normal, especially in the early phases of the disease. In a frontal–subcortical NCD, such as NCD due to Lewy bodies, executive function would be impaired. This information is important to the treatment and rehabilitation strategies a therapist would utilize (Mendez & Cummings, 2003). The diagnostic workup should include the following components:

comprehensive history to look at cognitive and functional difficulties;
physical and neurological exam (including lab work and brain imaging) to rule out treatable causes of NCD;
medication review to see if medication(s) could be causing the problem;
mental status exam to rule in/out depression or other mental illnesses which can mimic the symptoms of AD;
cognitive and neuropsychological tests to ascertain cognitive function, which can include a neuropsychologist administering a battery of tests, computerized testing or a Mini Mental Status Exam (MMSE) used by many clinicians, or a Montreal Cognitive Assessment (MOCA).
(Cobert, 2012; Mendez & Cummings, 2003; Weiss et al., 2012)

Newer instruments, such as the Montreal Cognitive Assessment (Fig. 28.1), a screening tool developed to assist clinicians in detecting MCI, which the MMSE is unable to screen for, are gaining credibility because of improvements in sensitivity and decreasing susceptibility to cultural and educational biases. The MOCA offers the advantage of testing multiple cognitive domains with an easy scoring system and is free for clinical use (www.mocatest.org). The MOCA probes all four lobes of the brain. The MOCA is available in many different languages and comes with instructions and scoring (Galvin & Sadowsky, 2012).

REHABILITATION AND NEUROCOGNITIVE DISORDERS

A working definition of cognitive rehabilitation is 'Cognitive rehabilitation (CR) aims to enable people with cognitive impairments to achieve their optimum level of wellbeing by helping to reduce the functional disability resulting from damage to the brain' (Clare, 2012).

Contributions can be made by various clinicians, e.g. physical therapist, occupational therapist and nurses, by providing interventions at any phase of the cognitive decline in order to enhance patient participation in activities of daily living (ADLs) and communication to minimize caregiver burnout. The key strategy is to build on the patient's intact skills, to explore new possibilities for communication and to create a sense of safety and enjoyment that includes modified ADL tasks for the patient. The clearest means of communication is to relate in ways that allow the person to feel emotionally safe and to build from an emotional tone that is perceived by the patient as being nurturing and positive.

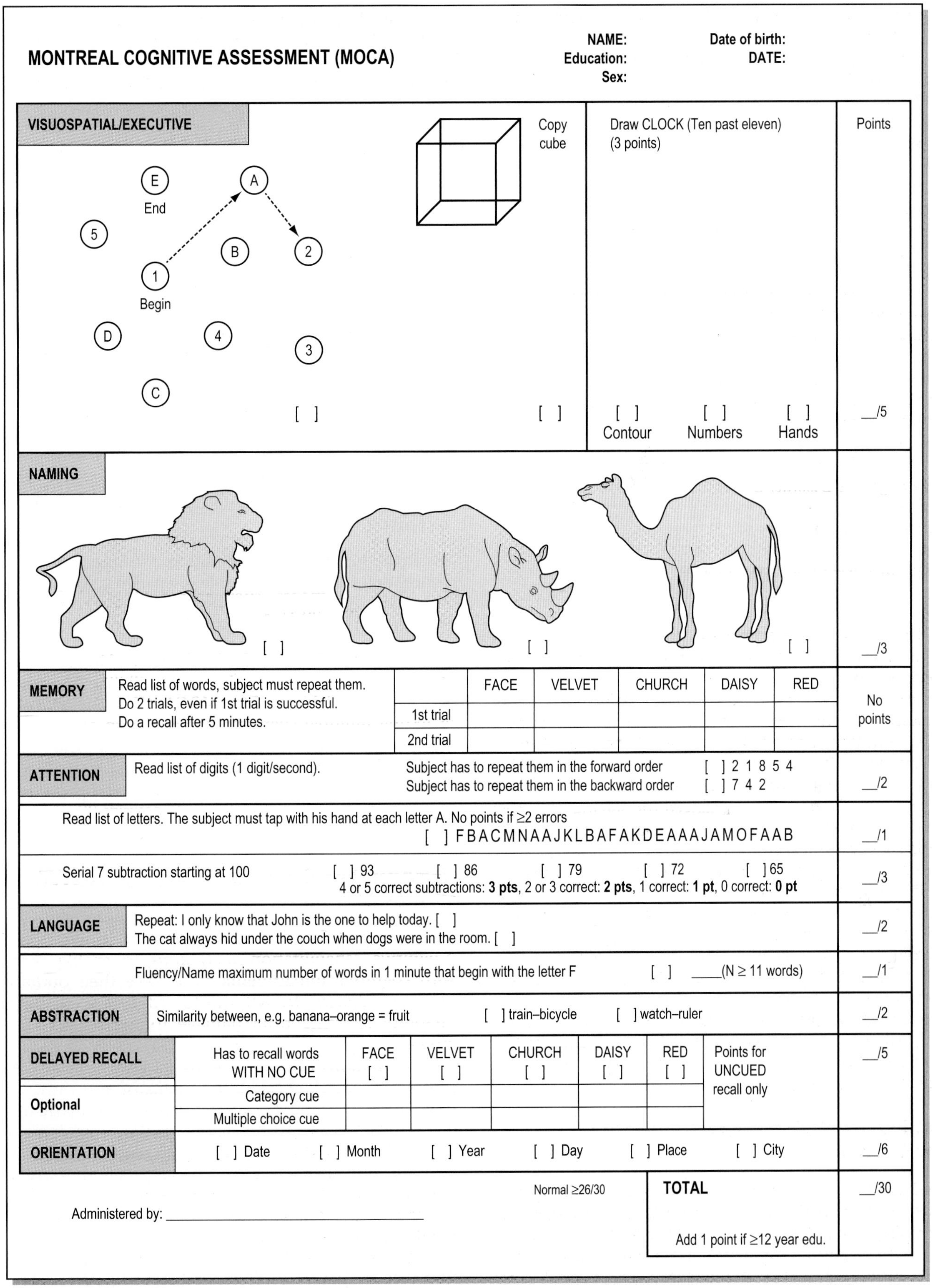

MONTREAL COGNITIVE ASSESSMENT (MOCA)

NAME:
Education:
Sex:

Date of birth:
DATE:

VISUOSPATIAL/EXECUTIVE		Points

Copy cube

[ ]

Draw CLOCK (Ten past eleven)
(3 points)

[ ]   [ ]   [ ]
Contour   Numbers   Hands

___/5

NAMING

[ ]   [ ]   [ ]

___/3

MEMORY	Read list of words, subject must repeat them. Do 2 trials, even if 1st trial is successful. Do a recall after 5 minutes.		FACE	VELVET	CHURCH	DAISY	RED	No points
		1st trial						
		2nd trial						

ATTENTION	Read list of digits (1 digit/second).	Subject has to repeat them in the forward order [ ] 2 1 8 5 4	___/2
		Subject has to repeat them in the backward order [ ] 7 4 2	

Read list of letters. The subject must tap with his hand at each letter A. No points if ≥2 errors
[ ] FBACMNAAJKLBAFAKDEAAAJAMOFAAB

___/1

Serial 7 subtraction starting at 100   [ ] 93   [ ] 86   [ ] 79   [ ] 72   [ ] 65
4 or 5 correct subtractions: **3 pts**, 2 or 3 correct: **2 pts**, 1 correct: **1 pt**, 0 correct: **0 pt**

___/3

LANGUAGE	Repeat: I only know that John is the one to help today. [ ]	___/2
	The cat always hid under the couch when dogs were in the room. [ ]	

Fluency/Name maximum number of words in 1 minute that begin with the letter F   [ ]   ____(N ≥ 11 words)

___/1

ABSTRACTION	Similarity between, e.g. banana–orange = fruit [ ] train–bicycle [ ] watch–ruler	___/2

DELAYED RECALL	Has to recall words WITH NO CUE	FACE [ ]	VELVET [ ]	CHURCH [ ]	DAISY [ ]	RED [ ]	Points for UNCUED recall only	___/5
Optional	Category cue							
	Multiple choice cue							

ORIENTATION	[ ] Date [ ] Month [ ] Year [ ] Day [ ] Place [ ] City	___/6

Normal ≥26/30

TOTAL

Add 1 point if ≥12 year edu.

___/30

Administered by: _____

Figure 28.1 Montreal Cognitive Assessment (MOCA) *(www.mocatest.org/).*

Empowering the patient during interactions with care-givers and family means that individuality and a sense of safety and self-determination are the most important outcomes for each interaction. For staff and family, this means that there is a need to become aware of what works for the patient and what the patient can emotionally sense if the intention of the caregiver is to support their confidence and self-esteem.

The therapeutic interventions that are required for a person with an NCD necessitate that the therapist be trained beyond the entry level. When a therapist or assistant is interested in working with older individuals with cognitive impairment, advanced training in kinesthetic contact, communication, procedural learning, neurological rehabilitation and handling skills is necessary. Emphasis on mastering neurological rehabilitation techniques to empower the patient through functional training and kinesthetic cueing is critical. The therapist works closely with caregivers to enhance the effectiveness of daily tasks that are important to the patient. Patients should always be seen for treatment in their own environment, if possible, and any new therapists should be introduced by someone who has a history of months of nurturing contact with the patient (Willingham et al., 1997; Van Wynn, 2001; Holtzer et al., 2004).

REHABILITATING LIFESTYLE

The modification of risk factors has been cited as a cornerstone for NCD prevention until medication can be developed that will prevent or stop the progression of NCD. In order to accomplish this, individuals will have to rehabilitate their lifestyles. Evidence suggests that lifestyle factors for cardiovascular disease are contributors to the development of NCDs, particularly AD and NCD due to vascular disease. Lifestyle rehabilitation that addresses issues such as obesity, high cholesterol, diabetes, high blood pressure and smoking could be effective in preventing or postponing the development of NCD (Desai, 2010). Dr Gary Small, the director of the UCLA longevity center, in his book *The Alzheimer's Prevention Program*, noted that the three most important words in AD prevention are timing, timing, timing. In the book, Dr Small states:

A particular brain-protective treatment that is effective at one point in time can be less effective if we wait too long to use it. In fact some therapies may even be harmful if the timing is slightly off. The most effective point in time for using a certain treatment may be years, even decades, before any symptoms of mental decline are noticeable.

By rehabilitating a patient's lifestyle to include dietary changes such as eating fruits and vegetables for a 4-year period reduces the risk of NCD by 44%. Patients who engage in complex mental activity and/or learn new things in midlife reduce the risk of NCD by 48%. Depending on when a patient initiates the lifestyle changes he/she could add up to 4 years of symptom-free life (Small & Vorgan, 2011: 17). To rehabilitate one's lifestyle the patient needs the information discussed above. The rehabilitation therapist may have many opportunities to convey this information to patients, medical doctors during scheduled checkups, physical therapists, occupational therapists, nurses etc. while providing therapy during midlife encounters and to all rehabilitation therapists during workshops and conferences.

SUPPORTING QUALITY OF LIFE

The interventions necessary to support a good quality of life for each patient fall into the categories of treating excess disability, reducing patient stress and creating a supportive environment. The family generally needs referral to a family support group or to formal counseling so that they can work through their emotional reactions (i.e. grief and anger). Counseling is often helpful in answering questions from grandchildren who may not have been present to see the gradual decline but who are then introduced to a person who looks like their grandparent but who does not even recognize them. Children are often fine at accepting the limited abilities of a relative if they are given the right tools and support, enabling them to be comfortable and feel safe in the situation.

NEUROPLASTICITY, NEUROGENESIS, SYNAPTOGENESIS

In terms of NCD and rehabilitation, it is important to recognize that the brain is capable of change at any age. This is called neuroplasticity. Although the shrinking, older brain may have less capacity to change, the capacity is still present. The cognitive, sensory and motor activities must be strenuously and continually challenged in order to accomplish this change. Neurogenesis is the neural plasticity occurring when the individual creates new neurons (Cozolino, 2008; Desai, 2010). The possibility exists that therapeutic stimulation of neurogenesis could have a positive impact on brain repair in later life, including the diseased brain (Desai, 2010). Synaptogenesis is the formation of synapses between neurons in the nervous system and it continues throughout the lifespan. Enrichment increases synaptogenesis by as much as 150–200% in animal studies. Human studies have now shown that enrichment can increase neurogenesis in the adult hippocampus (Levi et al., 2003). Challenging activities, new learning and exercising can mend the brain. Evidence indicates that learning and other challenging activities triggers the brain to grow (Cozolino, 2008). Neuroplasticity, neurogenesis and synaptogenesis will be utilized by rehabilitation therapists when they are employing their rehabilitation techniques.

REHABILITATION INTERVENTIONS

It is always incumbent on the rehabilitation therapist to do due diligence by investigating the rehabilitation techniques, therapies and interventions in terms of best practice. The next step is to develop a cognitive rehabilitation treatment plan starting with:

- Diagnosis – this is the type of NCD being treated.
- Assessment/evaluation – this is identifying and developing strengths and needs. Strengths are used to address needs and needs are prioritized.

- Long-term and short-term goals – these are patient's goals, not therapist's goals. The patient/family should have appropriate input.
- Interventions, approaches, therapies – these are what the therapist uses to assist the patient in attaining goals.
- Evaluation of effectiveness – this is whether the goal was achieved and a new goal is established. If the goal was not achieved, monitor the progress to determine if the goal should be continued or replaced with a new goal (Clare, 2012).

THERAPIES AND APPROACHES

Currently, there are four medications therapeutically used to treat NCDs. These medications can slow the progression of the NCD, especially in AD. Aricept was recently found to be effective in treating NCDs due to Lewy bodies (Mori et al., 2012). Three of the four drugs, Aricept, Exelon and Razadyne, are cholinesterase inhibitors. It has been suggested that these drugs can have a positive impact on activities of daily living, improve behavior (Hughes, 2011) and help with cognition (Mendez & Cummings, 2003). According to the NIA website, Namenda, the fourth drug:

. . . is used to treat the symptoms of Alzheimer's disease. Memantine (Namenda) is in a class of medications called NMDA receptor antagonists. It works by decreasing abnormal activity in the brain. Memantine can help people with Alzheimer's disease to think more clearly and perform daily activities more easily, but it is not a cure and does not stop the progression of the disease (www.nia.nih.gov/).

It is approved for late-stage NCD due to AD and, as a rule, is prescribed with one of the cholinesterase inhibitors. When the medical practitioner orders one of these drugs for a patient with NCD it should aid in the patient's rehabilitation by slowing the progression of the NCD.

Regardless of an NCD diagnosis, all patients exhibiting memory problems should have their sensory systems evaluated. Sensory memory, the shortest of all types of memory, may depend on the patient's ability to hear. If sensory systems are not functioning appropriately they will have a negative impact on memory and rehabilitation expectations. Vision assessment, hearing tests etc. should be utilized. If on evaluation deficiencies are noted, attempts should be initiated to repair or improve function.

Therapists can also attempt to engage the remaining episodic memory, a type of long-term memory enabling the individual to remember events and experiences of personal significance. The objective is to build on the remaining episodic memory and encourage the learning of important new information or the relearning of previously known information.

Another approach is to work with the procedural memory, which is the memory of performing skills and tasks. Explicit memory is conscious recollection, while implicit memory is unconscious. Implicit or procedural memory is generally stronger than explicit. The intention is to restore the ability to perform selected activities of daily living. It

has been demonstrated that with practice, patients can learn new skills.

Therapists can also implement behavioral and environmental modifications for those patients who are disinhibited with NCD due to frontal temporal disorder. Due to their inability to inhibit their behavior, these patients can present with many dysfunctional issues causing difficulties for themselves and distressing family and staff (Davis, 2005).

SLEEP

The rehabilitation therapist needs to assess sleeping patterns and insure that the patient is getting quality sleep. Sleep deprivation has been associated with poor memory, attention and concentration. It is when an individual is sleeping that their memory is consolidated (Cozolino, 2008: 214). Memory consolidation is a process by which new and unstable memory traces after being acquired are reconfigured into more permanent forms of long-term storage. Rehabilitation therapists need to assess sleep and should they discover an issue, attempt to correct it in order to improve cognitive functioning. There is evidence that sleep has an effect on modulating synaptic plasticity in the brain and that lack of sleep in the older person inhibits neurogenesis. The older patient can present with many sleep disorders such as apnea and restless leg syndrome (Desai, 2010).

COMPUTERIZED COGNITIVE TRAINING PROGRAMS

Currently, there is much development in progress to explore computer-based cognitive training programs. Companies such as Cognifit and Posit Science have developed graduated cognitive exercises to enhance brain plasticity. Programs developed by these and other companies have shown benefit in enhancing cognitive abilities (Desai, 2010). Cognitive training may improve cognition in patients after coronary artery bypass grafting (CABG). Older adults who undergo CABG experience postoperative cognitive decline but it has been demonstrated that cognitive training improved their memory and attention. The findings suggest that this training can be a useful rehabilitation tool (Bherer, 2012). Another study indicated that an Integrated Cognitive Stimulation and Training Program (ICSTP) utilizing computer-based programs, blended with paper and pencil exercises, generally had positive effects on cognitive and memory functioning scores compared to a matched control group in individuals aged 65 years and above. These effects were sustained with no additional treatment after 8 weeks. Statistically significant improvements of scores on the Dementia Rating Scale occurred for mildly and moderately impaired treatment participants (Bucher & Siberski, 2009). Computer-based cognitive training programs are improving, and rehabilitation therapists need to explore the range of possibilities that these programs can provide for patients with NCDs.

VALIDATION THERAPY, REALITY ORIENTATION THERAPY, REMINISCENCE THERAPY AND REMOTIVATION THERAPY

Rehabilitation therapists must not ignore the psychosocial group therapies designed to maintain verbal ability and prevent excess disability, i.e. disability caused by disuse. If the patient's verbal, group, social etc. skills are allowed to atrophy, we fail to enable people with cognitive impairments to achieve their optimum level of wellbeing. The goal is to reduce the functional disability resulting from damage to the brain. Several therapies have a role in maintaining wellbeing. When utilized by staff in long-term care facilities, validation therapy increased positive feelings and decreased negative feelings (Davis, 2005). It also reduces stress on patients since their feelings will not be invalidated. Validation therapy accomplishes this by validating the truth of the feelings and by not addressing the truth of the facts. Reality orientation assists the patient with time, place and person issues. Some studies have shown a reduction in negative behavior and an increase in self-control. Reminiscence therapy uses the relatively spared long-term memory with patients who have a NCD. In the groups, peers can help, encourage and support other group members for experiencing altruism. Patients' verbal ability is reinforced and social skills are facilitated (Davis, 2005). Remotivation is a simple group therapy (five basic steps) of an objective nature in which topics such as flowers, cooking, fishing etc. are used in an effort to reach the unwounded areas (strengths) of the patient's personality to encourage them to think about reality in relation to themselves. Remotivation therapy can be used with NCD patients, particularly AD. It also helps to prevent excess disability, focuses on abilities and not weaknesses, supports desired behavior and inspires communication on both the verbal and nonverbal levels. Validation therapy, reality orientation therapy, reminiscence therapy and remotivation therapy can all accommodate the more cognitively impaired patient. However, validation therapy is best for those who are the most impaired and reality orientation is more beneficial for those who are moderately impaired and for those patients who respond well to cognitive enhancing drugs. Reminiscence therapy is effective for the higher to lower functioning patients since it utilizes long-term memories which are preserved until late in most NCDs. While remotivation therapy is appropriate for moderate to higher functioning patients, it is appropriate for a wide variety of diverse populations.

EXERCISE AND COGNITIVE IMPAIRMENT

Exercise delivers more oxygen to the brain improving brain health and plasticity of the frontal lobes and exercise has been shown to add neurons to the hippocampus (Cozolino, 2008). Rehabilitation of patients should include an exercise component. Regular exercise is important to aging successfully and protects the brain in the older population. More research is needed with controlled studies to better understand the relationship between aging and dementia (Desai, 2010). However, clinically it may be seen that patients with social disengagement and little or no appropriate stimulation are often withdrawn, confused, physically aggressive and depressed. Almost 20%, and possibly as many as 86%, of patients with dementia are depressed (Teri & Wagner, 1992); however, with social and physical activity (walking 15–20 min daily), behavior and cognition may be more appropriate (Merck Manual, 2000). Depression is a treatable condition that is common in demented patients; this is important because physical performance is more likely to decline in depressed individuals (Chow & MacLean, 2001). As advocated by Crooks and Geldmacher (2004), physical therapy is indicated to curtail loss in physical performance.

Teri et al. (2003) conducted a randomized controlled study of 153 community-dwelling patients with a diagnosis of AD. Their intervention was caregiver training for behavior management and exercise assistance and encouragement. At 3 months, the exercise group, who carried out 60 min/week of aerobic, strength, balance and flexibility activities, scored significantly better on physical performance and depression tests when compared with control subjects who received routine medical care. At 2 years, they again significantly outscored the routine-care group on physical performance scores and showed a decrease of 19–50% in the rate of institutionalization for behavioral problems.

As the world ages, the findings of three papers merit further consideration and investigation. Exercising for three or more times a week (Larson et al., 2006) and programs in which women walked for at least 1.5 hours a week (Weuve et al., 2004) were significantly associated with better physical performance, cognition and delayed onset of NCD. Men who walked less than 0.25 miles daily showed a 1.8-fold excess risk for dementia compared with those who walked more than 2 miles daily (Abbott et al., 2004).

ANTICHOLINERGIC MEDICATIONS

The rehabilitation of patients with NCD will require a medication review by a medical professional competent in prescribing for the needs of the older patient. There are many anticholinergic medications that can have a negative impact on the cognitive abilities of NCD patients. These drugs treat vertigo, migraine, Parkinson's disease, depression, diarrhea, allergies, urinary incontinence, sleep issues, psychosis and other conditions. Common anticholinergic side-effects include dry mouth, constipation, headache, mental changes and dizziness. Anticholinergic CNS side-effects include sedation, decreased concentration, forgetfulness, falls, confusion and delirium. Anticholinergic medications can exacerbate memory impairment resulting in increased memory deficits, confusion and disorientation, agitation, hallucinations and delirium (Kemper et al., 2007) in patients with mild and major NCD. In the United States of America the general population's use of anticholinergic medications is very high and 74% of elderly nursing home residents with dementia take anticholinergic medications (Chatterjee et al., 2010). The rehabilitation therapist needs to assess the NCD patient for anticholinergic medication use whether it be prescribed medication or over-the-counter medication such as Tylenol PM, Benadryl or others. Cholinesterase inhibitors (Aricept, Exelon, Razadyne) which are used to treat NCDs, especially in the case of AD, may counter the effect of anticholinergic drugs.

CASE STUDY

HISTORY (ABBREVIATED)

Jack, a 77-year-old successful businessman, has a spouse and several children who are all concerned about his memory, which has been poor for some time and is getting worse. He has a history of strokes, diabetes, depression and he cries very easily. He does not hear well and sleeps poorly. In the past, when he was diagnosed with AD, he had been taking Aricept and Namenda, but not at present. He spends his day sitting in a chair and dozing. He still maintains an office but is less interested. At the time treatment was initiated, he would drink his morning coffee, eat breakfast and required help with dressing and with other ADLs.

ACTIONS TAKEN

A comprehensive assessment (following Fig. 28.1) revealed a major NCD due to vascular issues as well as a depression. On the computerized cognitive evaluation Jack scored 2 standard deviations below the norm in several cognitive domains. He also scored 1 standard deviation above the norm for verbal abilities and close to normal on one or two other cognitive areas. His depression was assessed and was rated as severe. Of the several stokes which were noted, one of the two recent strokes was in the frontal region of the brain.

TREATMENT PLAN AND RESULTS

All medical issues were addressed and the required adjustments were made. Both the family and Jack were given the results of the evaluation and were educated as to what NCD due to vascular issues is and what to expect. The treatment was also discussed and the medication changes were introduced. The antidepressant was initially minimally increased and then raised again with good results. Jack began to dress himself, tidy up, was eager to go fishing and with the exception of crying, appeared less depressed and less apathetic. Jack had always been an emotional person with a tendency to choke up but not overtly weep. The thought was that the crying was

not related to depression but due to the damage from strokes, particularly damage to the frontal lobe which prevented inhibiting the crying behavior. Jack eventually enrolled in a memory care program conducted by a graduate student, which met for 1 hour on 2 days each week for a period of 6 weeks. A combination of graded computerized cognitive exercises, paper and pencil exercise and socialization were provided. Although Jack claimed that he disliked games, puzzles and computers, he thrived. He never cried during the program and there was even a reduction in crying in general. Jack stated that he enjoyed the program and at one point, announced to the group 'it is the fastest hour of the day'. Jack often became upset when he had problems remembering things, such as the date, his daily to-do list etc. When a dry-erase white board was mounted outside of the bathroom (reality orientation) he began to check it on a daily basis, became oriented and less upset. He was also fitted for and now wears two hearing aids, which have addressed the auditory issues. Currently, Jack has maintained a level of independence that was not anticipated as achievable by him or by his family. His quality of life has improved. Although it is neither perfect nor at the level he prefers, it is better than he initially feared it would be.

The goals for this treatment plan were that Jack will:

agree to take medications 100% of the time to control medical and psychiatric conditions in order to improve his quality of life (*achieved and will continue to monitor*);
participate in a cognitive rehabilitation program two times each week to prevent the premature loss of cognitive skills (excess disability) and to enhance his independence (*achieved and will need to find another placement after completion of program*);
have his hearing assessed and if necessary, wear hearing aid(s) (*achieved*);
check the white board daily to determine what his schedule is and what it is that he needs to do to stay on track (*partially achieved*).

Therefore, this drug combination should be avoided as it will be detrimental in the rehabilitation effort of the NCD patient (Brauser, 2011) if any degree of rehabilitation is anticipated.

CONCLUSION

Cognitive rehabilitation for patients with NCD is currently possible. It will only improve as additional baby boomers age and demand better cognitive care. Since the number of baby boomers will ultimately overwhelm the medical and rehabilitative communities with both their sheer numbers and with the projected rise in NCD due to AD and other causes, lifestyle rehabilitation needs to be pursued aggressively. More research will be required to refine techniques and interventions. Recognizing that cognitive impairments can be caused by temporary conditions that can be reversed is vital. When the NCD deficits are progressive, the stage to which it has progressed affects the intervention. Since the involvement of family and caregivers is crucial, educating them must be a priority. Every change that enhances the treatment of the patient, facilitates their participation in self-care and improves the quality of life is of great value. The rehabilitation therapist who works with cognitively impaired

patients can appreciate their contributions as not only rewarding but will discover, like Jack in the Case Study, that it results in the fastest hour of the day.

REFERENCES

Abbott R, White L, Ross G et al 2004 Walking and dementia in physically capable elderly men. J Am Med Assoc 292:1447–1453

Alzheimer's Association 2012 Alzheimer's disease facts and figures. Alzheimer's & Dementia 8:2

Bherer L 2012 Cognitive training after CABG found beneficial in elderly population. J Behav Med 35:557–568

Brauser D 2011 Meds prescribed for Alzheimer's may cancel each other out. Medscape 7 November. Available at: www.medscape.com/viewarticle/753019. Accessed November 2013

Bucher M, Siberski J 2009 Preserving cognition through an integrated cognitive stimulation and training program. Am J Alzheimer's Dis Other Dement 24(3):234–245

Chatterjee S, Mehta S, Sherer JT et al 2010 Prevalence and predictors of anticholinergic medication use in elderly nursing home residents with dementia. Drugs Aging 27(12):987–997

Chow TW, MacLean CH 2001 Quality indicators for dementia in vulnerable community-dwelling and hospitalized elders. Ann Intern Med 135:668–676

Clare L 2012 Cognitive rehabilitation and people with dementia. In: Stone JH, Blouin M (eds) International Encyclopedia of Rehabilitation. Center for International Rehabilitation Research Information and Exchange (CIRRIE), Buffalo, NY

Cobert J 2012 Tarascon Adult Psychiatrica. Jones & Bartlett, Sudbury, MA

Cozolino L 2008 The Healthy Aging Brain. WW Norton, New York

Crooks EA, Geldmacher DS 2004 Interdisciplinary approaches to Alzheimer's disease management. Clin Geriatr Med 20:121–139

Davis LA 2005 Educating individuals with dementia. Top Geriatric Rehabil 21(4):304–314

Desai AK 2010 Healthy Brain Aging: Evidence Based Methods to Preserve Brain Function and Prevent Dementia. Clin Geriatr Med 26(1):xi–xii

Diagnostic and Statistical Manual of Mental Disorders, 5th edn. (DSM 5) 2013 American Psychiatric Association, Arlington, VA

Galvin JE, Sadowsky CH 2012 Practical guidelines for the recognition and diagnosis of dementia. J Am Board Fam Med 25(3):367–382

Holtzer R, Stern Y, Rakitin BC 2004 Age related differences in executive control of working memory. Mem Cognit 8:1333–1345

Hughes JC 2011 Alzheimer's and other dementias. Oxford University Press, New York

Kemper RF, Steiner V, Hicks B et al 2007 Anticholinergic medications use among older adults with memory problems. J Gerontol Nurs 33(1):21–31

Larson E, Wang L, Bowen J et al 2006 Exercise is associated with reduced risk for incident dementia among persons 65 years of age and older. Ann Intern Med 144(2):73–81

Levi O, Jongen-Relo A, Feldon J et al 2003 ApoE4 impairs hippocampal plasticity isoform-specifically and blocks the environmental stimulation of synaptogenesis and memory. Neurobiol Dis 13:273–282

Mendez MF, Cummings JL 2003 Dementia: A Clinical Approach. Butterworth–Heinemann, Philadelphia, PA

Merck Manual 2000. In: Beers M, Berkow R et al (eds) The Merck Manual of Geriatrics, 3rd edn. Merck & Co., Inc., Whitehouse Station, NJ, pp. 357–377

Mori E, Ikeda M, Kosaka K et al 2012 Donepezil for dementia with Lewy bodies: a randomized, placebo-controlled trial. Ann Neurology 72(1):41–52

Siberski J 2012 Dementia and DSM 5: changes, cost, and confusion. Aging Well 5(6):12–16

Small G, Vorgan G 2011 Alzheimer's Prevention Program. Workman Publishers, New York

Teri L, Wagner A 1992 Alzheimer's disease and depression. J Consult Clin Psychol 60:379–391

Teri L, Gibbons L, McCurry S et al 2003 Exercise plus behavioral management in patients with Alzheimer disease. JAMA 290:2015–2022

Van Wynn EA 2001 A key to successful aging: learning-style patterns of older adults. J Gerontol Nurs 9:6–15

Weiss D, Morgan MJ, Kinnealey M 2012 A Practitioner's Guide to Clinical Occupational Therapy. Austin, TX, Pro-ed

Weuve J, Kang J, Manson J et al 2004 Physical activity, including walking, and cognitive function in older women. JAMA 292:1454–1461

Willingham DB, Peterson EW, Manning C et al 1997 Patients with Alzheimer's disease who cannot perform some motor skills show normal learning of other motor skills. Neuropsychology 11(2):262–271

Chapter 29

Multiple sclerosis

DIANE MADRAS

CHAPTER CONTENTS

INTRODUCTION

As the life expectancy of the general population increases, so does the life expectancy of the population of older adults with disabilities. Life expectancy in those with multiple sclerosis (MS) is relatively normal, although some studies report lifespan may be reduced by 6–14 years (Stern, 2005). Therefore, aging with MS presents unique challenges for the physical therapist and the patient alike. Issues for people aging with MS pertain to minimizing disability and morbidity, and promoting functional independence and maximizing quality of life (Cruise & Lee, 2005).

Although there are data relating to all of the sequelae of MS, much of the early research on this disease involved younger subjects. Research is now beginning to examine the effects of aging on populations with MS. Many of the physiological changes of aging are similar to the effects of MS. The similarities include muscle atrophy, decreased cardiopulmonary reserve, impaired temperature regulation and depression (Stern, 2005).

This chapter will highlight the signs and symptoms associated with MS and identify issues that should be addressed in the rehabilitation of the aging patient who presents with MS.

OVERVIEW/EPIDEMIOLOGY

MS, the most common disabling neurological disease in young adults (Goodman & Snyder, 2000), is most commonly diagnosed between 20 and 40 years of age. Although the cause remains unknown, several predisposing factors have been identified. Childhood forms were recently identified (Pugliatti et al., 2006; Govender et al., 2010; Absoud et al., 2011). Women are affected twice as often as men, and a family history of MS increases the risk by 10-fold. MS may be the result of a genetic predisposition or may be triggered by a virus or environmental factor. Environmental factors (Conradi et al., 2011) may affect the onset of symptoms since MS is five times more prevalent in the colder climates of North America and Europe than in tropical areas (Goodman & Snyder, 2000).

NATURAL HISTORY/CLASSIFICATION

MS is classified as a progressive autoimmune disease characterized by chronic central nervous system (CNS) inflammation, demyelination and axonal damage. Demyelination leads to scarring (gliosis), which develops into plaques. The plaques (lesions) are distributed throughout the white matter of the CNS, leading to a wide array of brain and spinal cord syndromes (Goodman & Snyder, 2000; Stern, 2005). The plaques slow or block neuronal transmission resulting in motor and sensory disturbances and other symptoms such as fatigue, depression and pain. Clinically, patients can present with weakness, ataxia, visual disturbances, numbness, paresthesias, heat intolerance, fatigue, depression, pain, bowel and urinary dysfunction. Symptoms are variable, making the course of MS highly unpredictable. The progression of MS is related to several factors, including the neurological status 2 years post onset, and the frequency and severity of exacerbations and remissions. Disease-modifying drugs decrease the frequency and severity of exacerbations with variable success (Tremlett et al., 2010).

Approximately 85% of patients experience an abrupt onset of symptoms. Disease classification is based on the clinical course of signs and symptoms as the patient is followed over time. Approximately 80–85% of patients are initially diagnosed with relapsing–remitting MS, characterized by acute episodes of worsening symptoms (referred to as either relapses or exacerbations) with complete or incomplete recovery of function. Relapsing–remitting MS (the most common form) is characterized by symptoms that develop over a period of a few hours to a few days, followed by complete or incomplete recovery and a stable course known as 'remission' between relapses.

Table 29.1	**Classification of MS based on clinical course**
Relapsing remitting	Fluctuating course; sudden onset of new symptoms or reappearance of previous symptoms followed by complete or incomplete recovery. Slow accumulation of disability
Secondary progressive	Absence of remission with more rapid progression of symptoms and accumulating disability; develops from relapsing–remitting course
Primary progressive	Slow progression of symptoms from onset of disease with no remission of symptoms, and steady accumulation of disability
Clinically isolated syndrome	MRI evidence and a single episode of MS exacerbation followed by very slow or little accumulation of disability

Almost 50% of patients with relapsing–remitting MS eventually develop secondary progressive MS (SP-MS), characterized by gradual neurological deterioration with or without superimposed acute relapses. Approximately 10% of patients over 40 years of age diagnosed with MS experience continued disease progression from the outset with only minor fluctuations in function and are classified as primary progressive (PP-MS).

Progressive-relapsing MS, a rare form of the disease, is characterized by gradual neurological deterioration from the onset of symptoms and subsequent superimposed relapses (Stern, 2005). A relatively new classification of MS has been established, known as clinically isolated syndrome (CIS), where an individual with findings on magnetic resonance imaging (MRI) suggestive of MS experiences a single episode followed by a benign disease course (Nielsen et al., 2007; Mastorodemos et al., 2010). Table 29.1 summarizes each of the major subtypes of MS.

DIAGNOSIS/MEDICAL MANAGEMENT

DIAGNOSIS

The prevalence of MS is increasing worldwide, as diagnostic criteria become more refined and MRI technology improves (Albertyn et al., 2010; Chen et al., 2010; Cheng et al., 2010). The diagnosis of MS is usually made based on a variety of information sources such as a thorough medical history, physical, neurological and laboratory examination and, potentially, imaging studies. Usually the patient presents to a medical professional reporting one or more symptoms occurring intermittently over time. Suspicion of MS increases when abnormalities noted on physical examination and MRI with gadolinium are disseminated in space and time. Although the diagnostic criteria are still under debate, the use of the Poser and revised McDonald criteria are improving the accuracy of diagnosing CIS and MS worldwide (Polman et al., 2011). MS lesions visible on MRI are thought to identify white matter lesions and demonstrate the breakdown in the blood–brain barrier occurring during acute MS activity (when a symptom is present for less than 6 weeks). The physiological process of normal aging (Schuster et al., 2011) can also produce hyper-intense

foci in the subcortical region on MRI, therefore the older adult with MS presents a challenge for differentiating between new disease activity, normal aging and a stroke. Imaging of both the brain and spinal cord can assist in the differential diagnosis of MS or other neurological disease processes (Bot et al., 2012). Patients with MS are classified on the Expanded Disability Status Scale published by Kurtzke in 1983.

MS MANAGEMENT

The availability of disease-modifying drugs has increased since 1993, with nine therapeutic agents currently available. Presently, there are two oral medications – Aubagio (teriflunomide) and Gilenya (fingolimod) – and four subcutaneous injectable medications – Betaseron (interferon beta-1b), Copaxone (glatiramer acetate), Extavia (interferon beta-1b) and Rebif (interferon beta-1a). One intramuscular injectable medication – Avonex (interferon beta-1a) – and two delivered by infusion – Novantrone (Mitoxantrone) and Tysabri (Natalizumab) – are also available (National Multiple Sclerosis Society, 2012).

EXACERBATION MANAGEMENT

Minimizing duration and severity of an exacerbation (or flare) is the goal of medical management of patients with MS during an exacerbation. The primary medications administered during acute episodes are Solu-Medrol (methylprednisolone), Decadron (dexamethasone), or ACTH (adrenocorticotropic hormone). Corticosteroids may become problematic in an older individual since potential side-effects include immunosuppression and increased osteoporosis from lack of activity (National Multiple Sclerosis Society, 2012).

AGING WITH AND CLINICAL FEATURES OF MS

Many clinical manifestations are shared by aging and MS, such as ophthalmic changes, cognitive dysfunction, bowel and bladder dysfunction, sensory changes, balance dysfunction and sexual dysfunction, all of which can contribute to decreased quality of life.

The physiological changes that occur during the process of aging present additional challenges for MS patients, caregivers and practitioners. Although many traditional physical therapy approaches are effective in the management of the ailments associated with aging, elderly patients with MS require special consideration. One consideration in older adults is their susceptibility to adverse drug side effects because of decreased physiological reserve impacting liver and kidney function. Table 29.2 outlines the various manifestations associated with aging with MS and issues that require special consideration (Stern, 2005).

One of the hallmarks of MS is fatigue. Individuals with MS frequently have limitations in activities of daily living (ADLs), employment, social relationships, self-care and activities that require physical effort. The greatest challenge for clinicians and patients alike is determining what is 'normal fatigue' or what is 'pathological' fatigue, associated with the disease state. Regardless of the cause, fatigue can

Table 29.2 Clinical manifestations and special considerations in the older adult with MS

Clinical Feature	Description	Impact of Aging	Treatment Considerations
Ophthalmological symptoms	Affects 80% of patients. Leads to decreased ADLs and employment. Most common: optic neuritis, internuclear ophthalmoplegia and nystagmus. Symptoms: blurred vision, scotoma, impaired color vision and contrast sensitivity, pain with eye movement	In older population: presbyopia, cataracts, macular degeneration and glaucoma compound visual disturbances. Leads to further isolation and decreased self-care	Environmental adaptations include outlining doorways and stairs. Reduce glare and use magnifiers. Diplopia: eye patching or glasses with prism lenses
Fatigue	One of the most debilitating symptoms, occurring in over two-thirds of patients. Includes decreased energy; malaise; motor weakness during sustained activity; and difficulty concentrating. Interferes with work, family and social life	Look for secondary causes, e.g. infection; cancer; anemia; hypothyroidism; rheumatological conditions; diseases of the cardiovascular, pulmonary, renal or hepatic systems. Other factors include depression, pain, deconditioning or exposure to heated environment	Medication side-effects also contribute: TCAs; benzodiazepines; anticonvulsants; beta blockers; interferons; anti-spasticity medications. Intervention includes energy conservation and aerobic exercise. Medication: caution with older adults, e.g. use of stimulants, i.e. amantadine, associated with risk of cardiac side-effects
Heat intolerance	Frequently associated with increase in severity of symptoms. Excessive heat is caused by weather, over exercising or fever	Elderly vulnerable to hyperthermia because of loss of homeostatic temperature regulation, decreased ANS function, decreased sweat gland function, loss of subcutaneous fat	Outside activity should be performed in early morning; use air-conditioning in home and car; wear light clothes or cooling vest; avoid saunas, hot tubs. Ideal pool temperature 85°F (29.4°C)
Depression	Most common mood disorder; caused by a neuroanatomical or neurochemical changes. Incidence three times greater than the general population	Often overlooked because of symptoms of fatigue, decreased activity level and decreased concentration. Depression rating scales have limited utility in the MS population	Use of antidepressants also helpful in pain management. There are depressive side-effects from other medications including anxiolytics; beta blockers; methyldopa; clonidine; reserpine; steroids. There is a 7.5 times greater risk of suicide: duration and severity of disease not factors but major depression, living alone and alcohol abuse are
Cognitive dysfunction	Mild cognitive dysfunction; 5–10% have severe condition. Deficits include decreased short-term memory, reasoning, verbal fluency, abstract reasoning and speed of information processing. Intellectual functions intact	In aging, slowing of frontal lobe processes leads to decreased learning rate. Aging MS patient at greater risk for cognitive impairment	Medications may also be a factor, for example anticholinergics, antispasmodics, opioids, benzodiazepines, TCAs. Use lists, calendars and journals to assist with memory deficits
Sensory disturbance	Most common initial symptom: affects > 50% of patients. Includes paresthesia; numbness; loss of proprioception; neuropathic pain; acute pain because of inflammation; chronic pain from increased muscle tone or musculoskeletal changes	Seen with longer duration of disease, therefore common in older patients. Aging associated with musculoskeletal degeneration; may aggravate symptoms. With aging patient, rule out other etiology of pain, i.e. cervical spondylosis: look for neck and reticular pain; muscle atrophy; decreased deep tendon reflexes	MS patients often under-treated for pain. Pain treated with opioid analgesics, and NSAIDs, antiseizure medications, antidepressants and antispecificity agents. Intrathecal baclofen pump may be beneficial for intractable pain and spasming. Assess posture and wheelchair seating. Use appropriate assistive devices to decrease strain and overuse of muscles if inefficient gait is observed. Assess skin integrity with sensory loss
Cerebellar symptoms	Seen in one-third of patients. Disabling tremors affect any muscle group. Increases fatigue because of increased energy consumption	Aging also affects balance in general population: cerebellar symptoms may further increase fall risk	No effective medications. Review fall precautions. Home assessment may be helpful to increase safety

Table 29.2 (Continued)			
Clinical Feature	Description	Impact of Aging	Treatment Considerations
Motor loss and spasticity	Present in > 60% of patients; results from corticospinal involvement. Lower extremities involved more than upper extremities. Energy requirement increases for activity with spasticity	Weakness associated with aging because of lower motor neuron denervation and atrophy. Rule out secondary causes in aging patient with spasticity: infections, skin breakdown, spinal stenosis with myelopathy	Oral medications for spasticity must be monitored closely. Baclofen: lower initial dose and slower titration decreases risk of sedation and confusion. Benzodiazepines: increased half-life and higher association with agitation and disequilibrium
Bladder dysfunction	Affects 96% with > 10 years history; detrusor hyperreflexia is most common. Urinary tract dysfunction can lead to bladder or renal stones and frequent UTI	Anatomical and physiological changes because of aging can cause urinary frequency, hesitancy, retention and nocturia. Incontinence can be caused by delirium, atrophic vaginitis, enlarged prostate, constipation	Elderly sensitive to urological side-effects of medications used to treat MS. Take into consideration level of disability; manual dexterity; other medical problems; provide social support for decisions regarding intermittent catheterization versus indwelling catheter
Bowel disturbance	Constipation most common because of pelvic floor spasticity, decreased gastrocolic reflex, decreased hydration, medication, immobility, weak abdominal muscles	Slowed motility of gastrointestinal tract seen in older adult	Medications (anti-cholinergics, TCAs, antihypertensives, iron, calcium, opioids) may exacerbate constipation in elderly; regular bowel program may be necessary; rehabilitation to increase mobility may also be beneficial

ADLs, activities of daily living; ANS, autonomic nervous system; NSAIDs, nonsteroidal anti-inflammatory drugs; TCA, tricyclic antidepressants; UTI, urinary tract infection

limit function up to 60% of the time. Acute fatigue is present for less than 6 weeks while chronic fatigue is present for longer than 6 weeks. Intrinsic (MS-related) fatigue can be made worse by heat and is often one of the first symptoms of MS, often preceding a relapse. The pathophysiology of fatigue is complex and can be associated with dysregulation of the immune system and CNS changes such as neuroendocrine or neurotransmission processing. Fatigue may be considered a secondary complication of MS because of sleep disturbance resulting from nocturnal muscle spasm, incontinence, pain, decreased physical activity and deconditioning, or medication side-effects. Depression and inactivity also appear to be related to fatigue (MacAlastair & Krupp, 2005).

Fatigue is closely associated with heat intolerance. The symptoms of MS are made worse by heat. Weather, exercise or overexertion can magnify symptoms. Aging patients with MS are more vulnerable to the effects of heat as normal aging decreases sweat gland and temperature regulatory function (Stern, 2005).

Depression in an aging individual with MS can be related to neuroanatomical, neurochemical changes, or to the effects of dealing with potential long-term disability. Depression is one of the most common mood disorders seen with MS and the incidence of depression is three times greater in patients with MS than the general population. The suicide risk is 7.5 times higher in patients with MS, although the suicide rate is not associated with the duration or severity of MS but rather to alcohol abuse and living alone (Stern, 2005).

Other behavioral changes and cognitive dysfunction seen in MS include emotional lability and euphoria. The basis of the behavioral responses related to CNS involvement or resulting from psychological stress triggered by limitations and disabilities is unclear (Stern, 2005).

Sensory and visual changes, lower extremity weakness, spasticity, cerebellar and corticospinal involvement, heat intolerance and fatigue are often seen in combination in MS. These signs and symptoms can be important features in a debilitating spiral that leads to medical complications such as osteoporosis and cardiac disease. The medical conditions and sequelae associated with MS align with numerous Preferred Practice Patterns (American Physical Therapy Association, 2003). Further descriptions of specific Practice Patterns and their use are discussed under Physical Therapy Examination below.

The ability to maintain one's balance requires the integration of multiple sensory and motor systems. Impaired vision, loss of proprioception and vestibular impairment result in a decrease in information regarding postural control in any given environment. Motor control, controlled in the cerebellum, vestibulospinal inputs and corticospinal signals are also essential in maintaining balance. Spasticity and lower extremity weakness contribute to balance and gait cycle changes in patients with MS. This, in turn, can lead to increased energy consumption, contributing to fatigue and limitations in mobility. Increased fatigue and limited mobility can lead to depression, which in turn can lead to a decrease in physical activity, resulting in lowered aerobic capacity, creating a vicious cycle of decreasing activity, depression, leading to increased risk of cardiac disease (MacAlastair & Krupp, 2005; Stern, 2005).

Of note, swallowing disorders can affect up to 20% of patients with MS (Stern, 2005). Increasing age can contribute to the development of esophageal reflux and hiatal hernia, which can negatively impact nutritional intake in elderly patients with MS.

Sexual disturbance in patients with advanced age and MS may be primary (MS caused) or secondary. Primary sexual dysfunction results from CNS lesions that cause decreased genital sensation, orgasmic response, erectile function in men and vaginal lubrication in women. Secondary dysfunction is a result of other symptoms of MS, such as spasticity, bowel and bladder dysfunction (Stern, 2005).

As people age and decrease activity, loss of bone density is a common risk, especially in the spine and femoral neck. In people aging with MS, the use of corticosteroids can contribute to the development of osteoporosis which, when coupled with decreased balance, increases the risk of injury from falling. This fact is particularly troubling when treating a patient with MS, since a fall in a patient with poor bone density can lead to catastrophic events (Stern, 2005).

QUALITY OF LIFE

Quality of life is important in the intervention of a patient aging with MS, since the unpredictable nature of the progressive disability can pose a challenge to the healthcare practitioner and patient alike. The medical needs of the aging patient with MS are different from the general population. Issues threatening quality of life include: (1) fear of further loss of mobility and independence; (2) becoming a burden to family and caregivers, physically, financially or psychologically; (3) nursing home placement, since the timing of placement is earlier in patients with MS. Typically, decisions related to long-term care occur when people are in their late 70s; however, for patients with MS decisions arrive sooner, nearer to age 55 years (Finlayson, 2004). For the effective management of MS throughout the life of the patient, the outcome of any intervention needs to include a quality of life assessment.

FUNCTIONAL SCALES

Three scales are commonly used to quantify function in the individual with MS. The Kurtzke Expanded Disability Status Scale (EDSS) quantifies disability in the MS population (Kurtzke, 1983), according to signs and symptoms observed during a neurological examination. The Multiple Sclerosis Functional Composite measure consists of a 25-foot walk, nine-hole peg test and paced auditory serial addition test (Fischer et al., 1999). The MS Quality of Life Inventory (MSQLI) assesses 10 scales that are generic and MS-specific (DiLorenzo et al., 2003). The scales have also been useful in studies on the effects of rehabilitation and exercise.

PHYSICAL THERAPY EXAMINATION

Examination of a patient with MS should consist of a history, systems review and physical examination. The physical examination should address cardiopulmonary function and endurance, sensory and motor status, posture, balance and coordination, gait and ambulatory status, wheelchair

---

Box 29.1   *Standardized test and measures frequently used in examination of MS patients*

FATIGUE
- Fatigue Severity Scale

BALANCE
- Berg Functional Balance Scale
- Tinetti Performance-Oriented Mobility Assessment
- Forward reach
- Dynamic posturography
- Dizziness Handicap Inventory
- ABC fall scale
- Best test
- 30 second chair rise
- Sit to stand test

GAIT
- Gait Abnormality Rating Scale (GARS)
- Dynamic Gait Index
- 2-minute walk test
- 10-gait speed

---

seating and mobility. The history/patient interview will help determine and prioritize which tests and measures to carry out. It is essential to prioritize what the examination should include and how much can be accomplished in the first session since endurance can be limited in the individual with MS, especially those of advanced age. Obtaining baseline measures of strength, balance, endurance, gait, transfers and community mobility are essential not only for the current episode of care but also for future episodes. Pulmonary function should be assessed, even if only simple measures such as forced vital capacity are possible. Since the course of MS is unique to the individual and unpredictable, both the practitioner and patient need an accurate clinical picture of the patient's status before rehabilitation begins, to reflect back on at a later time of re-evaluation. This information may be useful in identifying relapses or remissions, quantifying progressive worsening in physical mobility and measuring response to medical interventions. Box 29.1 lists some appropriate tests and measures that are frequently used in the examination of patients with MS. As with the examination of any patient, the selection of appropriate tests should reflect the individual's needs. Judicious use of any measurement must bear in mind the physical, emotional and functional components of each patient.

A comprehensive source of examination measures and intervention strategies is the Guide to Physical Therapist Practice (American Physical Therapy Association, 2003). This guide describes physical therapist practice, defines the role of physical therapists in numerous settings and delineates tests, measures and interventions that are utilized in physical therapist practice. The Guide aligns MS into five Preferred Physical Therapist Practice Patterns and lists an array of current options for the management of patients presenting with a diagnosis of MS.

PHYSICAL THERAPY INTERVENTION

Rehabilitation of the older adult with MS should be tailored to the specific needs of the individual. In general, intervention should be designed to maximize the patient's mobility; educate the patient and caregiver regarding maintenance or improvement of aerobic capacity and endurance without increasing fatigue; and enable the patient to remain independent. All of the patient's impairments should be addressed with the goal of improving function and minimizing disability. In addition, all concurrent medical conditions, which frequently accompany MS in the aging patient, need to be considered. As well as the neurological impairments seen in MS, the degenerative musculoskeletal and cardiopulmonary changes of aging need to be identified and managed during the course of care.

Modifications may need to be made throughout the episode of care, for example performing balance retraining activities on a compliant foam may be more difficult for the aging patient with severe degenerative joint disease (DJD) in both knees and ankles, and aerobic training activities should be more closely monitored with the elderly patient with MS who has a pacemaker. Home exercise programs should be reviewed more carefully, written clearly and possibly enlarged for optimal comprehension and adherence. A review of the home program should occur on a regular basis, ruling out any possible activities that may be worsened by pain or shortness of breath.

Since the fear of falling and imbalance are significant concerns in the general older population, prevention of falls and fall risk modifiers should be included in the rehabilitation of most patients aging with MS. Box 29.2 provides a list of modifiable intrinsic and extrinsic factors that can be addressed to reduce fall risk.

Rehabilitation has played a major role in addressing the deficits and improving function in patients with MS. Exercise is considered the first line of intervention in the treatment of fatigue. Exercise not only counteracts deconditioning from inactivity but also has the positive benefits of increasing self-esteem, improving mood, combating social isolation and decreasing the risk of cardiovascular disease (MacAlastair & Krupp, 2005) and mental deterioration (White & Castellano, 2008). There have been numerous studies supporting traditional therapeutic activities and aerobic exercise as a plausible means of increasing endurance, functional activity and quality of life in the adult aging with MS. Various physical therapy regimens ranging from sensorimotor adaptation (Rasovna et al., 2005), individualized programs for therapeutic activities, resistance activities, balance and gait training (Romberg et al., 2005) and aerobic exercise on a stationary bike (Romberg et al., 2004; Kileff & Ashburn, 2005) have had significant positive effects in the MS population at all ages. Outcomes from these studies include increased endurance, ability to walk further, decreased fatigue, decreased depression, decreased disability and maybe improved quality of life (Romberg et al., 2004, 2005; Kileff & Ashburn, 2005; Rasovna et al., 2005).

Although there are numerous positive outcomes observed, special attention should be paid when implementing rehabilitation in the older adult with MS. The aging patient with MS may need increased recovery times following exercise. There is also a reduction in training capacity in patients with neuromuscular diseases (Stuerenberg & Kunze, 1999). Rigid rules associated with Medicare, i.e. the need for patients to receive physical therapy for 3 hours per day, may negatively affect the progress of an older adult with MS because overexercising may compound the challenges of fatigue. Exercise prescription should be tailored to each patient carefully; education should include instruction in how to monitor activities and fatigue in an appropriate way. Monitoring fatigue, endurance and aerobic capacity during physical activities and home exercise regimens stresses the importance of the balance between maintaining physical activity and energy conservation techniques. The Borg Perceived Level of Exertion Scale can assist the patient in assessing their tolerance to exercise (see Chapter 39, Exercise Considerations for Aging Adults).

Gait disturbance is usually caused by weakness, ataxia, sensory loss and spasticity. Achieving independence with mobility can be accomplished with a variety of assistive devices and gait training (Stern, 2005). The age of the patient, as well as other demographic and environmental factors and medical conditions, will determine which assistive device is most appropriate. Concerns in the population aging with MS include energy conservation. Seating, baskets and hand brakes may be helpful accessories for a rolling walker. Built-up or molded hand grips are useful for the aging patient with arthritic changes in the hand and wrist to prevent secondary dysfunction such as carpal tunnel syndrome. Ankle–foot orthoses can increase knee stability and toe clearance and enable the patient to walk more efficiently. Caution is required when selecting an orthosis since a heavy device will increase energy demands during ambulation and be counterproductive. New functional electrical stimulatory devices are available to assist with ambulation and hand function (Bioness, Valencia, CA). Because of weight issues, hip–knee–ankle orthoses are generally avoided (Stern, 2005).

Box 29.2   Risk factors for falls in older adults

Intrinsic factors	Extrinsic factors*
Women >men	Poor lighting
>80 years	Clothing too long
Incontinence	Footwear
Medical conditions	Stairs
Medication use	Curbs
Low or high physical	Ramps
activity level/exercise*	Ice, snow
Sensory: vision, proprioception, vestibular*	Wet surfaces
Weakness: hips, knees, ankles*	Obstacles, clutter
Decreased range of motion*	
Balance and gait deficits*	
Insight regarding safety, and actual deficits and risk-taking*	

*Items that are modifiable factors.

CONCLUSION

Aging with the chronic, progressive and unpredictable nature of MS is challenging. The clinical consequences of the older adult with MS are far-reaching, affecting literally every aspect of life. It is important to monitor the effects of this disease as well as the medical conditions associated with the aging process, e.g. cancer, stroke, diabetes, arthritis and cardiac disease. Management of the signs and symptoms of MS requires a team effort involving multiple healthcare professionals, the patient and their caregivers, and social supports. Many of the symptoms of MS can be addressed through education on the subjects of energy conservation, provision of appropriate exercise regimens and appropriate compensatory strategies and adaptive equipment. Because fatigue, depression, sleep disturbance and deconditioning are interrelated, an appropriate exercise program is critically important to the rehabilitation of the older adult with MS.

REFERENCES

Absoud M, Cummins C, Chong WK et al 2011 Paediatric UK demyelinating disease longitudinal study (PUDDLS). BMC Pediatr 11:68

Albertyn C, O'Dowd S, McHugh J et al 2010 Compliance with McDonald criteria and red flag recognition in a general neurology practice in Ireland. Mult Scler 16(6):678–684

American Physical Therapy Association 2003 The Guide to Physical Therapist Practice, 2nd edn. APTA, Alexandria, VA

Bot JC, Barkhof F, Lycklamà NG et al 2012 Differentiation of multiple sclerosis from other inflammatory disorders and cerebrovascular disease: value of spinal MR imaging. Radiology 223:46–56

Chen S-Y, Lo C-P, Hsu W-L et al 2010 Modifications to the McDonald MRI dissemination in space criteria for use in Asians with classic multiple sclerosis: the Taiwanese experience. Mult Scler 16(10):1213–1219

Cheng X-J, Cheng Q, Xu L-Z et al 2010 Evaluation of multiple sclerosis diagnostic criteria in Suzhou, China: risk of under-diagnosis in a low prevalence area. Acta Neurol Scand 121:24

Conradi S, Malzahn U, Schröter F et al 2011 Environmental factors in early childhood are associated with multiple sclerosis: a case-control study. BMC Neurol 11:123

Cruise CM, Lee MHM 2005 Delivery of rehabilitation services to people aging with a disability. Phys Med Rehabil Clin North Am 16:267–284

DiLorenzo T, Halper J, Picone MA 2003 Reliability and validity of multiple sclerosis quality of life inventory in older individuals. Disability Rehabil 25:891–897

Finlayson M 2004 Concerns about the future among older adults with multiple sclerosis. Am J Occup Ther 58:54–63

Fischer JS, Rudick RA, Cutter GR et al 1999 The multiple sclerosis functional composite measure (MSFC): an integrated approach to MS clinical outcome assessment. National MS Society Clinical Outcomes Assessment Task Force. Mult Scler 5:244–250

Goodman CC, Snyder TEK 2000 Differential Diagnosis in Physical Therapy, 4th edn. WB Saunders, Philadelphia, PA, pp 402–403

Govender R, Wieselthaler NA, Ndondo A et al 2010 Acquired demyelinating disorders of childhood in the Western Cape, South Africa. J Child Neurol 25(1):48–56

Kileff J, Ashburn A 2005 A pilot study of the effect of aerobic exercise on people with moderate disability multiple sclerosis. Clin Rehabil 19:165–169

Kurtzke JF 1983 Rating neurologic impairment in multiple sclerosis: an expanded disability status scale (EDSS). Neurology 33:1444–1452

MacAlastair WS, Krupp LB 2005 Multiple sclerosis-related fatigue. Phys Med Rehabil Clin North Am 16:483–502

Mastorodemos V, Nikolakaki H, Tzagournissakis M et al 2010 Benign multiple sclerosis in Crete. Mult Scler 16(6):701–706

National Multiple Sclerosis Society 2012 Therapies to stop MS. Available at: www.nationalmssociety.org/research/stop/index.aspx. Accessed December 2012

Nielsen JM, Moraal B, Polman CH et al 2007 Classification of patients with a clinically isolated syndrome based on signs and symptoms is supported by magnetic resonance imaging results. Mult Scler 13(6):717–721

Polman CH, Reingold SC, Edan G et al 2011 Diagnostic criteria for multiple sclerosis: 2010 revisions to the MacDonald criteria. Ann Neurol 69:292–302

Pugliatti M, Riise T, Sotgiu MA et al 2006 Evidence of early childhood as the susceptibility period in multiple sclerosis: space-time cluster analysis in a Sardinian population. Am J Epidemiol 164(4):326–333

Rasovna K, Krasensky J, Havrdova E et al 2005 Is it possible to actively and purposely make use of plasticity and adaptability in the neurorehabilitation treatment of multiple sclerosis patients? A pilot project. Clin Rehabil 19:170–181

Romberg A, Virtanen A, Aunola S et al 2004 Exercise capacity, disability and leisure activity of subjects with multiple sclerosis. Mult Scler 10:212–218

Romberg A, Virtanen A, Ruutianen J 2005 Long-term exercise improves functional impairment but not quality of life in multiple sclerosis. J Neurol 252:839–845

Schuster L, Essig M, Schröder J 2011 Normales Altern und seine Bildgebungskorrelate [Normal aging and imaging correlations] [German]. Radiologe 51(4):266–272

Stern M 2005 Aging with multiple sclerosis. Phys Med Rehabil Clin North Am 16:219–234

Stuerenberg HJ, Kunze K 1999 Age effects on serum amino acids in endurance exercise at the aerobic/anaerobic threshold in patients with neuromuscular diseases. Arch Gerontol Geriatrics 28:183–190

Tremlett H, Zhao Y, Rieckmann P et al 2010 New perspectives in the natural history of multiple sclerosis. Neurology 74(24):2004–2015

White LJ, Castellano V 2008 Exercise and brain health – implications for multiple sclerosis: Part 1: neuronal growth factors. Sports Med 38(2):91–100

Chapter 30

Parkinson's disease

MICHAEL L. MORAN

CHAPTER CONTENTS

INTRODUCTION

Parkinson's disease (PD), also known as paralysis agitans, is a progressive neurodegenerative disease that affects approximately 1% of those over the age of 60 years. With the aging of the population, this number is expected to increase. For example, PD affects approximately one million people in the United States of America. Globally, the number of individuals with PD was estimated at 4 million in 2005, and is expected to reach 9 million by 2030 (Georgy et al., 2012). Men and women are equally affected.

PD results from a loss of pigmented neurons in the substantia nigra which leads to a reduction in the production of the neurotransmitter dopamine. The resulting movement disorders are characterized by tremor, rigidity, bradykinesia and postural instability. Diagnosis is usually made by observation of signs and symptoms and may be facilitated by positron emission tomography (PET) scans as well as single photon emission computer tomography (SPECT) (Winogrodzka et al., 2005). Magnetic resonance imaging (MRI) and computerized tomography (CT) can be useful in differentiating PD from other disorders. A clinical presentation that mimics but is different from PD is called Parkinson's syndrome or parkinsonism.

Parkinsonism is a frequent cause of functional impairment in the elderly. The diagnosis is based on an evaluation of four signs: resting tremor, akinesia, rigidity and postural abnormalities. Parkinsonism may be caused by PD and can be a part of the clinical presentation of other neurodegenerative diseases (Bhalsing et al., 2013).

SIGNS AND SYMPTOMS

The signs and symptoms of PD vary, depending on the stage of the disease. The early stage may include tremor (often unilateral) and a sense of fatigue. The middle stage usually includes tremors, varying degrees of rigidity, bradykinesia, postural changes, instability and the patient may begin to require assistance from caregivers. The final stage of PD includes extensive motor disorders, requiring that the patient be assisted in performing activities of daily living (ADLs) and moving. Cognitive changes (depression, dementia) commonly accompany PD (Johnson & Galvin, 2011).

Tremors are present at rest and usually disappear as a patient attempts to move and during sleep. The term given to the commonly observed repetitive finger movements is 'pill-rolling'. Clinically, it has been observed that PD patients move slowly, and with inconsistent acceleration, and this bradykinesia is often noticeable when the patient progresses from the early stages of the disease. A complete lack of movement (akinesia) may occur. PD patients can 'freeze' in a certain position (including standing) and then spontaneously begin to move again. Rigidity has been linked to the development of contractures, fixed kyphosis and loss of pelvic mobility. Postural instability most likely reflects central nervous system pathology as well as the musculoskeletal changes mentioned above.

INTERVENTIONS

The management of PD usually combines nonpharmacological and pharmacological treatments. The former should include a multidisciplinary approach involving various therapies (physical, occupational and speech) emphasizing the patient's independence and training of the caregiver. Musculoskeletal changes associated with aging should not be confused with the changes typically seen in PD: a forward-thrust head, increased thoracic kyphosis, posterior pelvic tilt and a slow, shuffling gait. Instead, a PD patient should be objectively evaluated using an appropriate device such as the Unified Parkinson's Disease Rating Scale (Goetz et al., 2008; Table 30.1). The clinical assessment can be video recorded, which allows changes in movement disorders to be more easily tracked. Also, research has shown that various tools, such as the Timed Up and Go Test and the Dynamic Gait Index, have acceptable measurement error and test–retest reliability. Tools such as these can help clinicians determine whether a change in a patient with PD is a true change (Huang et al., 2011).

Table 30.1 **Unified Parkinson's disease rating scale (modified Hoehn and Yahr staging)**

Stage 0	No signs of disease
Stage 1	Unilateral disease
Stage 1.5	Unilateral plus axial involvement
Stage 2	Bilateral disease, without impairment of balance
Stage 2.5	Mild bilateral disease, with recovery on pull test
Stage 3	Mild to moderate bilateral disease; some postural instability; physically independent
Stage 4	Severe disability; still able to walk or stand unassisted
Stage 5	Wheelchair bound or bedridden unless aided

Source: www.ncbi.nlm.nih.gov/books/NBK27684.

NONPHARMACOLOGICAL MANAGEMENT

Therapeutic intervention should begin as early in the disease state as possible. Avoiding soft tissue contracture, loss of joint range of motion, reduction in vital capacity, depression and dependence on others enhances the quality of life of the PD patient. It is important to include caregivers and others significant to the patient in goal-setting and planning interventions.

Intervention should be goal-oriented (i.e. preventing loss of function is the desired outcome) and individually tailored, based on the stage the patient is in. Relaxation exercises may be useful to reduce rigidity and there is some support for the idea that strengthening exercises may help to prevent falling. However, patient adherence to exercise programs is an important issue (Pickering et al., 2013). Stretching and active range of motion (ROM) exercises are vital, and the patient should be provided with a home program to facilitate improvement in functional postural alignment. Breathing and endurance exercises can help to maintain vital and aerobic capacities. They are important, as PD patients have a high incidence of pulmonary complications such as pneumonia. Balance, transfer and gait activities (including weight shifting) are also recommended.

Balance training should include repetitive training of compensatory steps (Jobges et al., 2004), and practice at varied speeds as well as self-induced and external displacements. Self-induced displacements are necessary to help the patient in tasks such as leaning, reaching and dressing. Displacements of an external origin may be expected if a patient is walking in crowds or attempting to negotiate uneven or unfamiliar terrain. External displacements may be simulated by the use of gradual resistance via rhythmic stabilization. Neurofeedback (Rossi-Izquierdo et al., 2013) and tai chi (Tsang, 2013) have been shown to improve balance in patients with PD.

Transfer training should focus on those activities reasonably expected of the patient. At a minimum, bed mobility and transfers, and chair and commode transfers should be considered. Limitations in active trunk and pelvic rotation may impair a PD patient's mobility in bed. Satin sheets or a bed cradle may reduce resistance to movement from friction. An electric mattress warmer may ease mobility by reducing the need for and thus the weight of covers. If the PD patient cannot be taught to perform a transfer independently, accommodations should he considered. Examples include bed rails or a trapeze, a lift chair and a commode with arms.

Specific training may enhance a PD patient's ability to perform some transfers such as sit to stand. Evidence indicates that strategies designed to facilitate tibialis anterior activation may improve sit to stand performance (Bishop et al., 2005). Mak and Hui-Chan (2008) reported that cued task-specific training was better than exercise in improving sit to stand in patients with PD. More recently, Mak et al. (2011) noted that limb support and ill-timed peak forward center of mass velocity, rather than dynamic stability, play dominant roles in determining successful sit to stand performance in patients with PD.

Gait training should focus on musculoskeletal limitations that can be quantified. PD patients tend to have limitations in ankle dorsiflexion, knee flexion/extension, stride length, hip extension and hip rotations. Joint mobilization and soft-tissue stretching can be effective to increase ROM and improve gait. It is important to include trunk mobility (rotation) and upper extremity ROM (large, reciprocal arm swings) in a comprehensive gait training program for PD patients. Ebersbach et al. (2010) reported that high amplitude movements were an effective technique to improve motor performance in patients with PD.

Rhythm or music may facilitate movement, but the use of assistive devices such as canes and walkers is not always appropriate for PD patients. At times, the use of an assistive device increases a festinating gait or aggravates problems with balance or coordination. Care should be taken to avoid excessive musculoskeletal stress and falls. Conditions such as osteoporosis may predispose a patient to injury.

For PD patients, a primary problem is difficulty in motor planning. Complex tasks such as transferring out of bed and walking to the bathroom have to be broken down into simple components (Bakker et al., 2004). It is important for patients and caregivers to remember that verbal and physical cuing (and other forms of assistance) should be oriented toward completion of a number of simple tasks in order to accomplish the overall goals of maintaining function and mobility. It has been noted that stress, fatigue, anxiety, or need to hurry imposed by the caregiver may exacerbate the freezing associated with PD. Further, Schenkman et al. (2011) stated that functional loss occurs at different points in the disease process, depending on the task under consideration.

When examining and planning interventions for a PD patient, common age-related changes must be considered. For instance, older individuals are more sensitive to glare and benefit from contrasting colors when determining depth. These facts are especially evident when working in some environments during activities such as gait training on steps. Further, some signs and symptoms of PD have been confused with changes associated with aging. PD patients may present with a reduced or lost sense of smell, handwriting that is difficult or impossible to read, and changes in sleep patterns.

Specific nonpharmacological interventions include biofeedback, proprioceptive neuromuscular facilitation, Feldenkrais and the Alexander Technique (Stallibrass,

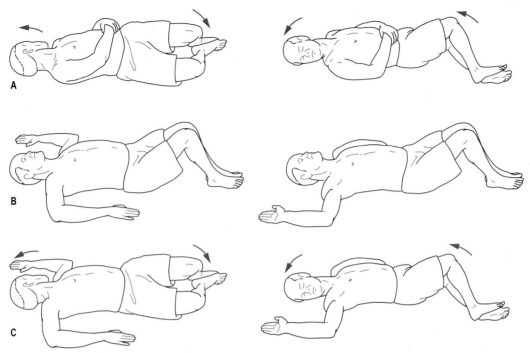

Figure 30.1 A sequence of exercises that can be used in the supine position to increase the range of motion of the neck and trunk. Any combination of motions can be used. **(A)** Head is slowly rotated side-to-side within the available range of motion while lower extremities are rotated side-to-side in the opposite direction. **(B)** Upper extremities are positioned with 45° of shoulder abduction with 90° of elbow flexion. One shoulder is externally rotated; the opposite shoulder is internally rotated. From this initial position, the shoulders are slowly rotated back and forth from an internally to an externally rotated position. **(C)** In an advanced exercise, the head, shoulders and lower extremities are simultaneously rotated from one position to the other. *(From Turnbull GI 1992 Physical Therapy Management of Parkinson's Disease. Churchill Livingstone, New York, with permission.)*

2002). In addition, treadmill training, spinal flexibility training, Qigong and tango dancing appear to be of some benefit for people with PD (Morris et al., 2010). Technology can also play a role in helping patients with PD: Ledger et al. (2008) reported that auditory cueing devices can improve walking speed, stride length and freezing.

Stretching, active ROM and strengthening exercises should emphasize safety: patients should be placed in a fully supported position initially and progressed to unsupported positions. In addition, spinal mobility must be oriented toward complete full normal rotation, including elongation of trunk musculature. A loss of pelvic motion occurs and can be addressed by means of lateral and anterior/posterior tilts; for instance, the functional task of standing from a seated position can incorporate anterior pelvic tilts. Mobility in bed, such as rolling over, can include trunk rotation. To improve postural (i.e. balance) responses, a variety of balance activities has been recommended (Hirsch et al., 2003). It is noted, however, that a variety of tasks should be practiced, as skills tend to be task-specific (de Lima-Pardini et al., 2012). Examples of some of the mobility skills are shown in Figures 30.1, 30.2 and 30.3.

The patient with PD may experience frustration because of a loss of independence in performing normal activities. That frustration may lead to social withdrawal as symptoms worsen. Social withdrawal can be related to facial involvement – the 'mask' face typical of patients with PD, which includes prolonged eyelid closure, slurred speech and drooling. Drooling may be reduced by

correcting forward head posture and using speech therapy to address tongue and swallowing dysfunctions. Speech therapy may also assist in improving voice volume and inspiratory muscle strength (Simberg et al., 2012). Sucking ice chips 20–30 minutes before a meal may help swallowing and decrease coughing and choking. See Chapter 54 for additional information about dysphagia.

PHARMACOLOGICAL MANAGEMENT

Pharmacological management of PD includes dopamine replacement (Sinemet, a combination of carbidopa and levodopa), dopaminergic drugs that act at the postsynaptic site such as pergolide (Permax) and bromocriptine (Parlodel), anticholinergic drugs like trihexyphenidyl (Artane), and neuroprotective medications (drugs that help prevent further dopaminergic cell death) including selegiline (Eldepryl). A drug that can be used to test for suspected PD is amantadine (Symmetrel), as it is believed to have dopaminergic and anticholinergic properties.

Medications used for PD have a great number of side-effects that can hamper rehabilitation. Nausea, vomiting, confusion, lightheadedness, hypotension and dyskinesia are only a few clinical signs that may be evident. Some clinical problems may be medication-related; Sinemet and Parlodel can cause hallucinations, vivid dreams, leg cramps and daytime drowsiness. In addition, levodopa is associated with the 'on–off' syndrome in which the PD patient demonstrates periods of time when motor control is intact (on) or not (off). As dosages increase, a wearing

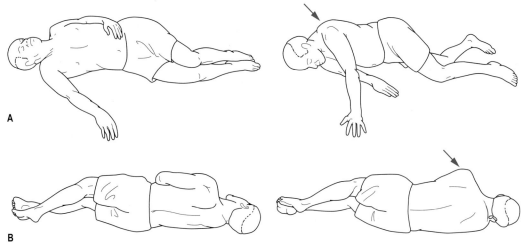

Figure 30.2 In a side-lying position, the thorax is slowly rotated forwards and backwards relative to the pelvis while the upper extremity is protracted and retracted relative to the thorax. *(From Turnbull GI 1992 Physical Therapy Management of Parkinson's Disease. Churchill Livingstone, New York, with permission.)*

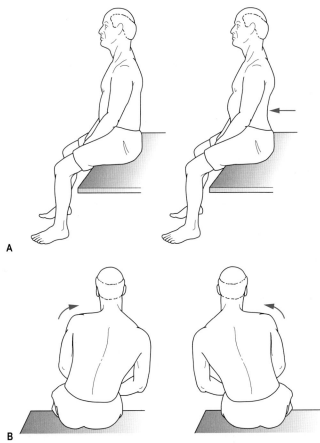

Figure 30.3 Pelvic exercises in the sitting position. **(A)** The pelvis is anteriorly and posteriorly tilted while the shoulders remain at midline. **(B)** The pelvis is laterally tilted (by lumbar lateral flexion) while the shoulders remain at midline. *(From Turnbull GI 1992 Physical Therapy Management of Parkinson's Disease. Churchill Livingstone, New York, with permission.)*

off effect may be noted; this is a deterioration of motor performance as the time nears for the next dose of medication. Because of these limitations of levodopa, some physicians delay using it, preferring to start with drugs such as selegiline. Generally, as the disease progresses, finding the right dose of medication becomes difficult and patients may be over- or under-medicated (Lindahl & MacMahon, 2011).

SURGICAL TREATMENT

Surgical treatments are varied, as are the long-reported outcomes (Ansari et al., 2002). Specific techniques have included basal ganglia stereotactic surgery, thalamotomy, a surgical lesion of the thalamus (which is reported to reduce tremor), chronic thalamic stimulation and pallidotomy, a surgical lesion of the globus pallidus (which is reported to alleviate bradykinesia more than tremor). Patients apparently demonstrate reduced dyskinesia associated with anti-Parkinson medications following thalamotomy and pallidotomy. Fetal tissue transplant procedures have been done in some countries but are banned in others. Strategies for using stem cells to benefit patients with PD have been reported in the literature (Gibson et al., 2012). Deep brain stimulation is a technique used to treat some of the symptoms of PD. Williams et al. (2010) reported that surgery can improve quality of life and motor function, and reduce the need for medication to control symptoms.

COGNITIVE AND SOCIAL ISSUES

Cognitive deficits that have been associated with PD are dementia and depression (mood disorders) (Heisters & Bains, 2012). These deficits are demonstrated by changes in cognitive abilities such as memory impairments, spatial abilities, word finding and dealing with new or complex tasks. Cognitive deficits should be considered when planning a treatment program for PD patients, as modifications may be required to accommodate specific patient limitations. Varying the style of interaction and reducing the pace of communication may be helpful. Therapists should use caution when deciding that a PD patient is being uncooperative or stubborn, as cognitive deficits may not have been adequately addressed. Possibly, cognitive changes from an earlier injury such as a cerebrovascular accident may already exist. It is important to educate caregivers regarding a patient's cognitive deficits and find strategies to reduce frustration for both.

CONCLUSION

PD is a neurodegenerative disease that results from a loss of pigmented neurons in the substantia nigra and leads to movement disorders characterized by tremors, rigidity, bradykinesia and postural instability. Therapeutic interventions should begin in the early stages of the disease in order to enhance mobility and quality of life. Pharmacological intervention is a mainstay in the treatment of PD, but therapists must be cognizant that the potential side-effects of medicines and the on–off syndrome may hamper rehabilitation. Surgical interventions continue to be developed.

REFERENCES

Ansari SA, Nachanakian A, Biary NM 2002 Current surgical treatment of Parkinson's disease. Saudi Med J 23(11):1319–1323

Bakker M, Munneke M, Keus SHJ et al 2004 Postural instability and falls in patients with Parkinson's disease. Ned Tijdschr Fysiother 114(3):63–66

Bhalsing K, Suresh K, Muthane UB et al 2013 Prevalence and profile of restless legs syndrome in Parkinson's disease and other neurodegenerative disorders: a case control study. Parkinsonism Relat Disord 19(4):426–430

Bishop M, Brunt D, Pathare N et al 2005 Changes in distal muscle timing may contribute to slowness during sit to stand in parkinsons disease. Clin Biomech 20(1):112–117

De Lima-Pardini AC, Papegaaij S, Cohen RG et al 2012 The interaction of postural and voluntary strategies for stability in Parkinson's disease. J Neurophysiol 108(5):1244–1252

Ebersbach GE, Ebersbach A, Edler D et al 2010 Comparing exercise in Parkinson's disease – the Berlin LSVT BIG study. Mov Disord 25(12):1902–1908

Georgy E, Barnsley S, Chellappa R 2012 Effect of physical exercise – movement strategies programme on mobility, falls, and quality of life in Parkinson's disease. Int J Ther Rehabil 19(2):88–96

Gibson SA, Gao GD, McDonagh K et al 2012 Progress on stem cell research towards the treatment of Parkinson's disease. Stem Cell Res Ther 3(2):11

Goetz CG, Tillet BC, Shaftman SR et al 2008 Movement disorder society sponsored revision of the unified Parkinson's disease rating scale (MDS-UPDRS): scale presentation and clinimetric results. Mov Disord 23(15):2129–2170

Heisters D, Bains J 2012 Side effects of treatment for Parkinson's disease. Nurs Residential Care 14(5):230–233

Hirsch MA, Toole T, Maitland CG et al 2003 The effects of balance training and high-intensity resistance training on persons with idiopathic Parkinson's disease. Arch Phys Med Rehabil 84(8):1109–1117

Huang S, Hsieh C, Wu R et al 2011 Minimal detectable change of the Timed Up and Go Test and the Dynamic Gait Index in people with Parkinson disease. Phys Ther 91(1):114–121

Jobges M, Heuschkel G, Pretzel C et al 2004 Repetitive training of compensatory steps: a therapeutic approach for postural instability in Parkinson's disease. J Neurol Neurosurg Psychiatry 75(12):1682–1687

Johnson DK, Galvin JE 2011 Longitudinal changes in cognition in Parkinson's disease with and without dementia. Dement Geriatr Cogn Disord 31(2):98–108

Ledger S, Galvin R, Lynch D et al 2008 A randomized controlled trial evaluating the effect of an individual auditory cueing device on freezing and gait speed in people with Parkinson's disease. BMC Neurol 8:46

Lindahl AJ, MacMahon D 2011 Parkinson's: treating the symptoms. Br J Nursing 20(14):852–857

Mak MK, Hui-Chan CW 2008 Cued task specific training is better than exercise in improving sit to stand in patients with Parkinson's disease: a random controlled trial. Mov Disord 23:501–509

Mak MK, Yang F, Pai Y 2011 Limb collapse, rather than instability, causes failure in sit to stand performance among patients with Parkinson disease. Phys Ther 91(3):381–391

Morris ME, Martin CL, Schenkman ML 2010 Striding out with Parkinson disease: evidence based physical therapy for gait disorders. Phys Ther 90(2):280–288

Pickering RM, Fitton C, Ballinger C et al 2013 Self reported adherence to a home based exercise program among people with Parkinson's disease. Parkinsonism Relat Res 19(1):66–71

Rossi-Izquierdo M, Ernst A, Soto-Varela S et al 2013 Vibrotactile neurofeedback balance training in patients with Parkinson's disease: reducing the number of falls. Gait Posture 37(2):195–200

Schenkman M, Ellis T, Christiansen C et al 2011 Profile of functional limitations and task performance among people with early and middle stage Parkinson disease. Phys Ther 91(9):1339–1354

Simberg S, Rae J, Kallvik E et al 2012 Effects of speech therapy on voice and speech in Parkinson's after a 15 day rehabilitation course: a pilot study. Int J Ther Rehabil 19(5):273–286

Stallibrass C 2002 Randomized controlled trial of the Alexander Technique for idiopathic Parkinson's disease. Clin Rehabil 16(7): 695–708

Tsang WW 2013 Tai chi training is effective in reducing balance impairments in patients with Parkinson's disease. J Physiother 59(1):55

Williams A, Gill S, Thelekat V et al 2010 Deep brain stimulation plus best medical therapy versus best medical therapy alone for advanced Parkinson's disease (PD SURG trial): a randomized, open-label trial. Lancet Neurol 9(6):581–591

Winogrodzka A, Wagenaar RC, Booij J et al 2005 Rigidity and bradykinesia reduce interlimb coordination in Parkinsonian gait. Arch Phys Med Rehabil 86(2):183–189

Chapter 31

Tremor and other involuntary movement

WENDY ROMNEY • MICHELLE E. WORMLEY • MICHELLE M. LUSARDI

CHAPTER CONTENTS

INTRODUCTION

Many of the neuromuscular diseases common with aging have signs and symptoms that include extraneous or involuntary movement. Some have little impact on functional ability whereas others can significantly compromise an older adult's ability to safely or efficiently accomplish functional tasks. In order to select the most appropriate measures of impairment and function, and to develop a plan of care that will enhance safety and function, rehabilitation professionals need to differentiate between the possible causes, characteristics and management of the various involuntary movements and dyskinesias encountered when working with older adults. In this chapter, we define the most common types of dyskinesia, present a classification of movement dysfunction and review the evidence for examination and functional interventions in individuals who exhibit involuntary movement.

DEFINITION OF TERMS

DYSKINESIA

The term dyskinesia is used when extraneous or unintended motion is routinely observed during postural and/or functional tasks. Tremor is the most common form of dyskinesia. Other forms of dyskinesia include: dystonia, clonus, choreoathetosis and ballism. Dyskinesia occurs at various levels within the central nervous system (CNS). Dystonia (fixed abnormal postures) and clonus (recurrent hyperactive deep-tendon responses to sudden changes in muscle length) are common in diseases affecting the pyramidal (voluntary) motor systems. Tremors at rest, writhing choreoathetosis and ballism suggest impairment in the extrapyramidal system at the level of the basal ganglia. Tremors that increase in severity with movement often indicate cerebellar dysfunction. Fasciculation, often mistaken for tremor, occurs as a result of an adverse drug reaction or denervation.

TREMOR

Tremor, the most prevalent involuntary movement, is characterized by a rhythmic oscillation around a fixed axis, often congruent with the axis of motion of the affected joint or joints (Alty & Kempster, 2011). The frequency (period) and waveform (timing, sequence of muscle activity) of a particular type of tremor is remarkably consistent over time, although the amplitude of the tremor may vary with internal factors (e.g. fatigue, anxiety, stress, emotions) or external factors (e.g. ambient temperature, alcohol or other substance use, environmental conditions or demands) (Bhidayasiri, 2005).

Tremor appears to be the result of alternating contraction of muscles on either side of a joint. The underlying CNS mechanisms of tremor are not clearly understood; there are several interactive factors that may contribute to the motor expression of tremor: the oscillating tendencies of the mechanical systems of joints and muscles; short- and long-loop spinal cord and brainstem reflexes; closed-loop feedback systems of higher motor centers, including the cerebellum.

Identifying when a tremor occurs (activation) is one strategy for classification: tremor may occur only during movement (action tremor), only when at rest (resting tremor), when trying to maintain a relatively fixed posture (postural tremor), or under all of these conditions. Other strategies for identifying tremor involve observing anatomical location, frequency and amplitude. Most tremors increase with higher levels of stress, anxiety or fatigue and decrease or disappear during periods of sleep (Daroff et al., 2012).

FASCICULATION

Fasciculation is spontaneous discharge from whole or partial motor units, that may be mistaken for tremor (Daroff et al., 2012). On careful observation, fasciculations present as random twitching rather than the rhythmic oscillating contraction seen in tremor. Fasciculation can occur in motor neuron diseases like amyotrophic lateral sclerosis or primary lateral sclerosis. Fasciculation may also be seen as a result of anticholinergic drugs and stimulants (e.g. excessive caffeine), electrolyte imbalance or sodium deficiency, muscle denervation, nerve root irritation (herniated intervertebral disc or spondylosis). Fasciculation can sometimes be observed in periods of extreme stress or fatigue, or following excessive strenuous exercise.

MYOCLONUS

Myoclonus (clonus) is sudden, brief involuntary movement caused by muscular contractions (positive myoclonus) or inhibitions (negative myoclonus). Due to its rhythmic involuntary nature, it can resemble tremor (Weiner & Lang, 2005). Myoclonus occurs under three circumstances:

1. as the expression of the hyperactive spinal cord-level stretch (deep tendon) reflex related to pathology of the pyramidal system (e.g. stroke, cerebral palsy, multiple sclerosis or spinal cord injury) or, in some instances, occurring in 'normal' individuals who are very anxious, stressed or fatigued;
2. during a partial or generalized seizure as a result of abnormal electrical activity of motor areas of the cerebral cortex;
3. less commonly, as a component of a familial, idiopathic or physiologically induced movement disorder (Blumenfeld, 2010).

Myoclonus associated with hyperactive stretch reflexes can be transient (lasting for several beats) or sustained over a period of time (mimicking tremor). It can be 'triggered' by rapid elongation of affected muscles, as in deep-tendon reflex testing; rapid passive range of motion (commonly examined at the ankle with a quick stretch of the gastrocsoleus by dorsiflexion); or during position change. The peripheral mechanism of myoclonus is the same as that of the stretch reflex: annulospiral 'endings' around intrafusal fibers within the muscle spindle are stimulated by elongation of muscle tissue. Information about change in length is carried to the CNS via 1a afferent neurons in peripheral nerves. These 1a neurons synapse directly with alpha-motor neurons in the anterior horn of the spinal cord or motor cranial nerve nuclei. If stimulated sufficiently, alpha-motor neurons trigger the activation of the motor units of the elongated extrafusal muscle. The resulting contraction elongates the antagonistic muscles on the other side of the joint, triggering the stretch reflex. Deep tendon reflexes are classified as follows: 0 (absent), 1+ (hypoactive), 2+ (normal), 3+ (hyperactive response without clonus) and 4+ (hyperactive response with myoclonus) (Paz & West, 2008). Many individuals with myoclonus associated with pyramidal system dysfunction also exhibit a positive Babinski response when the lateral plantar surface of the foot is stimulated (an upward-pointing hallux with fanning of the second to the third toes).

Myoclonus observed during seizures may involve a single limb segment (in a partial seizure of the opposite motor cortex) or rhythmic jerking of multiple limbs (in a generalized tonic–clonic seizure of the entire cortex). The combination of altered consciousness and myoclonus differentiates the involuntary movement of seizures from tremor. An electroencephalogram (EEG) recorded during either partial or generalized seizure demonstrates abnormal electrical activity of the motor cortex, whereas EEG patterns in those with tremor are less likely to be grossly abnormal (Raethjen et al., 2007; Muthuraman et al., 2008; Shibasaki, 2012).

Hiccups and 'sleep starts' (nocturnal myoclonus) are examples of physiologically triggered myoclonus. Movement-triggered myoclonus has been reported during recovery from severe cerebral hypoxia or ischemia following myocardial infarction or near drowning. Myoclonus may occur as a component of uremic or hepatic encephalopathy and with degenerative disorders, as in Alzheimer's disease. Occasionally, myoclonus may be caused by drug toxicity (e.g. penicillin, tricyclic antidepressant, levodopa) (Rowland & Pedley, 2010).

TICS

Tics are brief and intermittent movements (motor tics) or sounds (phonic tics) that can resemble myoclonus and tremor as well as the dance-like involuntary movement of chorea (Daroff et al., 2012). Tics can be classified as 'simple', involving brief irregular muscle twitching of an isolated body segment, as in the case of repetitive eye blinking, throat clearing, or shoulder shrugging. Tics can also present as 'complex', for example in the case of coordinated, patterned movements involving several muscles, as in arm gesturing, skipping while walking, and whistling or stuttering (Rowland & Pedley, 2010; Daroff et al., 2012). Those experiencing tics will describe a sense of increasing muscle tension that can only be relieved when the stereotypical movement occurs. Tics differ from other types of involuntary movement in that they are somewhat under voluntary control and can be suppressed for a length of time. Idiopathic tics often occur for short periods of time, sometimes in childhood, and may be associated with anxiety or other psychological stress factors. Tics differ from other dyskinetic movement disorders as they may be evident during all stages of sleep, although they may subside with sleep. Tics associated with Tourette's syndrome may persist over the lifespan and include vocalizations (barking, grunting, echolalia and repetitive swearing) as well as stereotypical facial or extremity movement.

DYSTONIA

Dystonia is a movement disorder characterized by a sustained positioning or a very slowly changing abnormal synergistic movement (Alarcon et al., 2004). It can affect one or more body segments, often observed as tonic abnormal posturing in individuals with longstanding damage to the pyramidal motor system (e.g. severe equinovarus after significant stroke or other acquired brain injury, or spastic cerebral palsy). Dystonic positions are described as abnormal; they cannot be accurately mimicked or recreated volitionally. Individuals with dystonia associated with pyramidal system dysfunction may also exhibit myoclonus and hypertonicity.

Some dystonias are idiopathic and may be familial (e.g. spastic torticollis). Others occur only during one specific motor activity (e.g. writer's cramp or laryngeal dystonia during public speaking). Facial hemispasm is an intermittent focal dystonia related to compression or irritation of the seventh cranial nerve. If idiopathic torsion dystonia develops in later life, it most commonly affects axial, facial or upper extremity muscles and may challenge feeding, communication and other activities of daily living (ADLs). Most idiopathic dystonias are nonprogressive.

Secondary dystonias may be associated with damage to the putamen nucleus of the basal ganglia resulting from a tumor, ischemia or infarct, or head injury. Dystonia may be one of the signs of progressive degenerative diseases such as supranuclear palsy, Huntington's disease, Wilson's disease or Parkinson's disease. Dystonic postures may emerge in the end-stages of Alzheimer's disease.

Medications used to manage dystonia and spasticity must be closely monitored owing to adverse side-effects. Medications include: benzatropine mesylate (Cogentin), diazepam (Valium), dantrolene (Dantrium), haloperidol (Haldol), baclofen (Lioresal, Clofen), tizanidine hydrochloride (Zanaflex), carbamazepine (Tegretol) and Gabapentin (Neurontin) (Ciccone, 2007; Gladson, 2010). Severe focal dystonia may be temporarily treated with injection of botulinum toxin.

CHOREA

Chorea is a less common dyskinesia consisting of the random and rapid involuntary contractions of muscle groups, mostly of the extremities or face (Rowland & Pedley, 2010). Proximal and/or distal muscle groups of the extremities may be affected. Typically, muscles of the axial skeleton are not involved; therefore, postural control is not significantly compromised.

Chorea occurs when there is damage to the corpus striatum (basal ganglia), especially the caudate nucleus and putamen; however, the exact localization and pathophysiology of chorea is uncertain (Patestas & Gartner, 2006). Some choreas are hereditary (e.g. Huntington's disease), whereas others are a consequence of another physiological disease or trauma (Blumenfled, 2010). Choreic movement also occurs with tardive dyskinesia, a complication of the long-term use of certain neuroleptic drugs (e.g. in the management of schizophrenia) or dopamine toxicity (e.g. in the management of Parkinson's disease) (Caligiuri et al., 2000).

The quality of choreiform movement is often described as graceful or dance-like. Individuals learn to blend their involuntary movement with a purposeful movement in an attempt to mask or minimize the unwanted movement (e.g. a choreic movement of the arm over the head might be turned into smoothing of the hair). People with chorea will often have difficulty sustaining contractions (e.g. 'milk-maid's handshake' – the patient contracts and relaxes when asked to maintain a constant, firm grip during a handshake). As with tremor, choreiform movements

become more obvious in periods of stress and may disappear during sleep. Pseudochorea has been reported in individuals with impairment of proprioception resulting from multiple sclerosis and other diseases of the dorsal columns.

ATHETOSIS

Athetosis is a continuous, slow, involuntary, writhing movement. Athetosis is mostly observed in muscles of the extremities (distal to proximal) but it can also involve muscles of the face, neck and postural muscles of the trunk. It may be associated with dystonic postures, chorea or spasticity. Athetoid movements that are brief may be associated with chorea (choreoathetosis). Writhing movements that are sustained, may be associated with dystonia (athetotic dystonia). Individuals with athetosis have difficulty sustaining positions at rest and during volitional movement. Athetosis affects the efficacy of postural control when sitting and standing, as well as during both transitional and skilled movements necessary for mobility and activities of daily living. Athetosis is slower and less jerky than chorea and unable to be sustained, as with dystonia.

Athetosis occurs when there has been damage to the corpus striatum (caudate and putamen) in the basal ganglia, most often in children with perinatal ischemia and hypoxia or severe bilirubin toxicity. In the past, athetosis was referred to as the basal ganglia form of cerebral palsy. Currently, the term dyskinetic cerebral palsy is preferred and the use of athetosis is recommended only to indicate a particular type of movement independent of etiology. Although the severity of athetosis does not change with maturity, function may become more challenging in aging individuals with athetosis because of typical age-related changes and increased incidence of musculoskeletal and neuromuscular pathologies that are common later in life. Pseudoathetosis may occur in adulthood due to severe distal sensory loss (Spitz et al., 2006).

BALLISMUS OR BALLISM

Ballismus is a rarely occurring movement disorder that presents as wild and forceful flinging movements of one or more of the extremities that are rapid and nonpatterned (Arminoff, 2008; Klein, 2005). Trunk and facial muscles are usually spared and bulbar functions (e.g. speaking, swallowing, breathing) are not impaired. Ballismus is usually unilateral (hemiballismus) and movements are much more stereotypical and disruptive than those seen in chorea. It may be suggested that ballism and chorea represent a continuum rather than distinct entities (Daroff et al., 2012). Ballismus differs from other dyskinesias in that these involuntary motions do not tend to decrease in frequency or amplitude during periods of sleep.

Ballismus is thought to occur when there has been damage or disruption to the subthalamic nuclei in the diencephalon. Alteration of neural output from the subthalamus apparently 'releases' the activity of the globus pallidus nuclei, which unleashes stereotypical synergistic movement of the limb girdle and extremity. It occurs most often as the result of a 'lacunar' stroke of the lenticulostriate branches of the middle cerebral artery, which damages the subthalamus deep in one cerebral hemisphere.

Haloperidol (Haldol) is often used to control unwanted and disruptive motion during the acute and early rehabilitation phases of care, and to promote more effective sleeping. Fortunately, hemiballistic movement tends to diminish in both amplitude and frequency in the weeks following a stroke; however, more subtle choreoathetotic movements may persist (Blumenfled, 2010).

ASTERIXIS

Asterixis, also referred to as negative myoclonus, occurs as a brief and recurrent loss of sustained muscle contractions in postural muscles of the extremities and trunk (Rubboli & Tassinari, 2006; Rowland & Pedley, 2010). Asterixis is observed during neurological examination when the person being assessed exhibits 'flapping' of the hands when asked to hold their arms horizontally with wrists extended against gravity. Asterixis may occur in individuals with toxic metabolic encephalopathy as a result of hepatic, renal or pulmonary disorders. It has also been reported as a consequence of drug toxicity, during anticonvulsant therapies and when there is a lesion interrupting interconnections between the brainstem and thalamus.

AKATHISIA (RESTLESS LEG SYNDROME)

Akathisia, often called restless leg syndrome, is a distressing subjective sense of tension and discomfort of the limbs that is often associated with agitation and a need to move around, but that is not always relieved by movement (Weiner & Lang, 2005). Restless leg syndrome occurs in 10–35% of people over the age of 65 (Milligan & Chesson, 2002). Those with the clinical diagnosis of akathisia report difficulty sitting or lying still and a powerful urge to move. They may pace or rock in place and often complain of difficulty sleeping. Akathisia can be idiopathic or can be an extrapyramidal side-effect of antipsychotic medication. It may be the presenting symptom in someone who is developing tardive dyskinesia (see Drug-induced Movement Disorders below). The FDA has approved three drugs for the management of restless leg syndrome, including pramipexol (Mirapex), ropinirole (Requip) and gabapentin enacrabil (Neurontin Horizan) (Milligan & Chesson, 2002).

CLASSIFICATION AND DIFFERENTIAL DIAGNOSIS OF TREMORS

Neurologists and therapists use a variety of subjective and observed characteristics when examining the movement dysfunction of individuals who experience tremor (Bhidayasiri, 2005; Alty & Kempster, 2011; Crawford & Zimmerman, 2011). These factors include: when the tremors occur, the frequency and amplitude, the body segments affected by the tremor, whether there is a family history, their responsiveness to medications and their association with additional CNS signs and symptoms (Table 31.1).

Table 31.1	Comparison of classification strategies for tremor			
Type of Tremor	**Frequency (cps)[a]**	**Behavior**	**Characteristics**	**Response to Medication**
Normal physiological	7–12	At rest	Not observable without instrumentation	Increases with sympathetic activity
Enhanced physiological	7–11	Action	Low amplitude, visible bilaterally with outstretched arms, increases with anxiety, stress	Increases with certain medications and metabolic conditions; uncommonly treated
Essential	8–10	Postural, action	Symmetric, involves hands and wrists (handwriting large and tremulous), lower extremities, head or voice; may improve with alcohol, prevalence increases with advanced age	Decreases with beta blockers, primidone, thalamic DBS
Parkinsonian tremor	4–5	Rest	Asymmetric, involves distal extremities (handwriting small and illegible), decreased with voluntary movement; other signs include bradykinesia, postural instability and rigidity	Decreases with anticholinergics, amantadine, MAO inhibitors, catechol-O-methyltransferase inhibitors and levodopa, dopamine agonists, thalamic DBS
Intention/ cerebellar	3–5	Action, postural	Ispilateral involvement to lesion, amplitude increases with intention. Other signs: abnormal finger to nose, ataxia, abnormal heel to shin test, hypotonia	Decreases with dansetron, isoniazid, physostigmine, carbamazepine, clonazepam, thalamic DBS
Psychogenic	4–10	Rest, postural or action	Abrupt onset, spontaneous remission, extinction with distraction, involves both arms, head and lower extremities, absence of other neurological signs, associated with stressful life event	May be referred to psychiatry services for identification and management of illness

Sources: Alty and Kempster, 2011; Bhidayasiri, 2005; Daroff et al., 2012; Deuschl et al., 1998; Klein, 2005.
[a]Frequency range: low 0–4, middle 4–7, high 7–12 cps (cycles per second).
Monoamine oxidase (inhibitor), MAO

Because the frequency (period) of most tremors is remarkably stable within and across individuals, one classification strategy focuses on the frequency of the tremor as it typically occurs. This requires electromyographic (EMG) recording or use of a sensitive accelerometer; tremor frequency cannot be reliably assessed by observation alone. Amplitude of tremor is more variable, both within and among individuals (e.g. becoming more pronounced under stressful conditions or with fatigue), and therefore is not a useful indicator of severity of tremor.

A more common way to classify tremor is based on when the tremor is observed. A resting tremor occurs in an otherwise relaxed or inactive body part. Resting tremors are commonly observed in individuals with Parkinson's disease (e.g. 'pill-rolling' tremor of the hands), as described in Chapter 30, and may also be seen in those with normal pressure hydrocephalus, heavy metal poisoning and neurosyphilis, or as a side-effect of the use of neuroleptic medications. A postural tremor occurs when a body part (limb or trunk) is maintained in a sustained, often antigravity, position. Postural tremor is frequently a component of essential tremor and may also be observed in Parkinson's disease, hereditary motor and sensory neuropathy (Charcot–Marie–Tooth disease) and spastic torticollis. An action tremor (kinetic tremor) occurs during volitional movement. In those with essential tremor, the amplitude of an action tremor remains stable throughout the excursion or performance of the movement. Action tremors that worsen (increase in amplitude) during the trajectory of the movement, especially as the movement goal is approached, are referred to as intention tremors. Intention tremors are clinically evaluated using 'finger-to-nose' or 'heel-to-shin' movement tasks. Intention tremors are classic signs of cerebellar dysfunction.

Neurologists often evaluate the response to medication as a means of confirming or clarifying the diagnosis of a movement disorder.

The amplitude of resting tremors often decreases when anticholinergic medications are administered. The amplitude of essential tremors (whether action or postural) tends to diminish with consumption of alcohol or administration of beta blockers. Cerebellar intention tremors are unresponsive to pharmacological intervention and intensify with alcohol consumption (Rowland & Pedley, 2010; Alty & Kempster, 2011; Crawford & Zimmerman, 2011).

PHYSIOLOGICAL TREMOR

Physiological tremor is a normal phenomenon that is usually so mild that it cannot be easily observed at rest (Whitney et al., 2003). A fine physiological tremor of 11–13 cycles per second (cps) can be detected in healthy individuals on EMG; this is usually not observable without instrumentation. Because this minimal amplitude physiological tremor is normal in all muscles of the body, it is observed during movement and while holding antigravity positions. Factors that contribute to physiological tremor include the resonant properties of musculoskeletal structures; synchronization of agonist/antagonist motor neuron activity coupled by afferent neurons from the muscle spindle; and the cardioballistic force of the heartbeat. Physiological tremor affects all muscles of the body simultaneously whereas most pathological tremors tend

to affect selected body segments. Physiological tremor may become 'enhanced' with any mechanism that triggers sympathetic nervous system activity (beta-adrenergic activity and catecholamine release), including stress, anxiety, fright, sleep deprivation, alcohol ingestion, certain classes of cardiac medication, CNS stimulants, exercise and fatigue. The amplitude of physiological tremor also increases in hypoglycemia, thyrotoxicosis, alcohol and sedative withdrawal, carbon monoxide exposure and heavy metal poisoning. Toxic levels of certain medications (lithium, bronchodilators, tricyclic antidepressants) may also lead to tremor. Physiological tremor typically becomes more difficult to detect with advancing age.

ESSENTIAL TREMOR

Essential tremor can be observed as a postural and/or action tremor, commonly affecting neck and axial muscles, expressed as a nodding rotation of the head or an oscillating flexion/extension movement of the trunk (Sullivan et al., 2004). It may be apparent during upper extremity tasks that require holding a fixed proximal position. Involvement of the muscles of the larynx and pharynx may compromise phonation and swallowing. As an action tremor, essential tremor may interfere with the efficiency of fine motor tasks such as writing, grooming or bringing food on utensils toward the mouth. A recent meta-analysis has indicated the prevalence of essential tremor to be between 0.01% and 20.5% of the population. The prevalence in individuals aged 65 years or older is 4.6% and may be as high as 21.7% in those 95 or older (Louis & Ferreira, 2010).

Essential tremor, although considered benign because it is not associated with progressive neuropathology, is generally bilateral and can significantly interfere with functional activities in older adults. There is often a temporary decrease in symptoms (for approximately 30 minutes) after ingestion of alcohol (Mostile & Jankovic, 2010). Propranolol and other beta-blocker medications are prescribed for long-term management when essential tremor interferes with function, except when contraindicated by other concurrent conditions (e.g. congestive heart failure, atrioventricular (AV) heart block, asthma, insulin-dependent diabetes). Primidone (Mysoline), an anticonvulsant, may also be prescribed. Sedatives, tranquilizers and anticholinergics have little impact on essential tremor.

Thalamic deep brain stimulation (DBS), a procedure that uses implanted pulse generators in the subthalamic nucleus or globus pallidus, has been performed in individuals with essential tremor. Reports have indicated a reduction in contralateral tremor by as much as 75% in up to 90% of the cases (Pahwa et al., 2006). This procedure is only considered in healthy patients who are cognitively intact and when the tremor is resistant to medications. Side-effects are rare but may include neurological implications such as an intracranial hematoma, headaches, dyspraxia and word-finding difficulties (Daroff et al., 2012).

RESTING TREMOR

Resting tremor is a tremor at rest that disappears with volitional movement. Resting tremor is one of the most common symptoms of Parkinson's disease and may also be seen in other neurological conditions such as normal pressure hydrocephalus, progressive supranuclear palsy and the cumulative encephalopathy in those with repetitive head injury (Krauss & Jankovic, 2002; Jankovic & Tolosa, 2007). It most often involves oscillating supination/pronation of the forearm or lumbrical flexion/extension of the thumb and fingers (e.g. 'pill-rolling' tremor). Parkinsonian resting tremor has a relatively low period/frequency when compared with other types of tremor. Although the underlying mechanism is unclear, it may be the result of compromised nigral–striatal function. Anticholinergic medications (e.g. trihexyphenidyl/Artane, benzatropine/Cogentin) are more effective in reducing resting tremor than dopamine agonists or levodopa. Surgical ablation of the contralateral ventral lateral (VL) nucleus of the thalamus has been used to reduce the amplitude of severe resting tremor.

INTENTION TREMOR

An intention tremor is a tremor that becomes obvious and often exaggerated as the need for precise movement increases (also known as rubral, cerebellar or 'course' tremor) (O'Suilleabhain & Dewey, 2004; Weiner & Lang, 2005). With intention tremor, there is oscillation of increasing amplitude during voluntary movement, especially as the movement draws to its conclusion. Intention tremor is one of the symptoms of cerebellar dysfunction, especially if there has been damage to the superior cerebellar peduncle because of diffuse axonal injury, multiple sclerosis or infarction/ischemia in the midbrain and upper pons. Because damage to these structures compromises the ongoing 'feedback' necessary for 'error control', intention tremor is most apparent when fine-skilled motor tasks are attempted. In addition, intention tremor has been observed in alcohol, barbiturate or sedative intoxication and with high serum levels of some anticonvulsants (e.g. phenytoin/Dilantin and carbamazepine/Tegretol).

Intention tremor affects proximal and distal musculature of the extremities. In very severe cases, there may be observable postural tremor in addition to the classic disruption of goal-oriented volitional movement. Individuals with intention tremor may also exhibit other symptoms of cerebellar dysfunction including nystagmus, hypotonia, dysmetria, movement decomposition and gait ataxia. For reasons not well understood, the amplitude of cerebellar intention tremor often decreases when the eyes are closed.

NEUROPATHIC TREMOR

Occasionally, tremor has also been observed in individuals with significant peripheral neuropathy; however, the presentation of neuropathic tremor is much less stereotypical than essential, resting and intention tremors (Daroff et al., 2012). It is not well understood how and why tremor occurs in individuals with neuropathy.

Neuropathic tremor occurs in some, but not all, individuals with longstanding diabetes, end-stage renal disease, chronic alcoholism, hereditary sensory–motor neuropathy (Charcot–Marie–Tooth disease) and infectious neuropathies such as acute Guillain–Barré syndrome. These tremors may present as action and resting tremors

based on whether it is of demyelinating or inherited origin. Management of these tremors can be challenging because many of the medications that are successful in controlling extraneous movement are not as effective in the presence of peripheral neuropathy (Puschmann & Wszolek, 2011). These disorders need to be diagnosed in a timely manner as they can be treated with immuunosuppressive therapies, such as corticosteroids, intravenous immunoglobulin (IVIG), cyclophosphamide or plasma exchange.

POST-TRAUMATIC TREMOR

Individuals of any age who have sustained a severe acquired brain injury may develop a tremor within a month or years after the actual trauma and can have a mixed presentation. The tremor most commonly manifests itself 1–4 weeks after the traumatic event, and it is similar to essential tremor (Krauss & Jankovic, 2002; O'Suilleabhain & Dewey, 2004). A delayed-onset post-traumatic tremor, evolving 12–18 months post injury, has also been reported. Delayed-onset post-traumatic tremor often persists for several years or longer. It is not possible to identify a specific lesion eliciting the tremor by magnetic resonance imaging (MRI) or computed tomography (CT) scanning. This type of tremor is not particularly responsive to the medications used to control essential tremor. Often, the magnitude of this post-traumatic tremor decreases over time; however, it may remain problematic for some individuals.

ORTHOSTATIC TREMOR

In very rare circumstances, an older adult may experience a tremor in their lower extremities only during unsupported standing or during preparation for assuming a standing position. If the tremor is severe, it can interfere with transitional movement (e.g. sit-to-stand) and with postural control (Whitney et al., 2003). Orthostatic tremor is usually perceived by the individual as difficulty with stability (unsteadiness) while standing, when not supported by an assistive device or other external support, and is frequently associated with an increased fear of falling. Orthostatic tremor has a higher frequency/faster period (14–18 cps) than most other tremors, although its amplitude tends to be small. Orthostatic tremor does not respond to alcohol or propranolol, as seen in essential tremor, but does respond to clonazepam. Levodopa and gabapentin have also been recently used to treat orthostatic tremor and beneficial results have been noted (Daroff et al., 2012). Orthostatic tremor can significantly affect quality of life and limit functional ability.

METABOLIC TREMOR

Metabolic tremor is characterized by a recent-onset postural tremor. Hyperthyroidism is the most common cause of metabolic tremor and presents as a high frequency tremor of the upper extremities that is similar to an enhanced physiological tremor as seen with anxiety or stressful triggers. Additional systemic signs accompany the tremor, such as excessive sweating or weight loss, which will differentiate it from an essential tremor. Other metabolic causes include renal failure, hypoglycemia and liver disease (Alty & Kempster, 2011).

PSYCHOGENIC TREMOR

Psychogenic tremor is a psychiatric condition that appears as involuntary movement, differing in characteristics and consistency from action, intention or resting tremors (Alty & Kempster, 2011). Within an individual, psychogenic tremor may migrate from one area of the body to another. Onset is typically abrupt and may occur after a stressful life event; most other types of tremor are insidious. The frequency and amplitude of psychogenic tremor are inconsistent and variable over time. In most other types of tremor, the amplitude tends to increase when individuals are given competitive, anxiety-producing cognitive tasks (e.g. beginning at 100 and serially subtracting 7); in psychogenic tremor, the amplitude tends to decrease (or completely disappear) when attention is focused elsewhere.

HOLMES' TREMOR

Holmes' tremor is an uncommon tremor caused by damage to the cerebellar connections to the thalamus and brainstem (Seidel et al., 2009). Holmes' tremor was previously referred to as rubral tremor, midbrain tremor, thalamic tremor and Benedikt's syndrome. This tremor is a postural tremor of the proximal limbs characterized by slow frequency and large oscillations. It can be present at rest, during postural control (sitting) and may increase with movement. Multiple sclerosis and brain injury are common causes for Holmes' tremor (Alty & Kempster, 2011).

CLASSIFICATION AND DIFFERENTIAL DIAGNOSIS OF DYSKINETIC CONDITIONS

The other types of dyskinetic conditions that are encountered in geriatric rehabilitation are most often associated with a long-term disorder with which the individual has aged; however, some medication-related movement disorders are newly diagnosed.

HUNTINGTON'S CHOREA

Huntington's chorea is an autosomal dominant hereditary progressive disorder involving degeneration of the corpus striatum (Rowland & Pedley, 2010; Daroff et al., 2012). The gene for Huntington's is located on the short arm of chromosome 4. The three characteristic signs of Huntington's chorea are movement disorder (chorea), dementia and personality disorder. The first signs and symptoms of the disease appear in midlife (35–40 years) as restlessness, emotional lability, neurosis or personality disorders. Over time, cognitive impairment becomes more apparent and choreiform involuntary movement develops, often impairing judgment, locomotion and mobility, speech production and swallowing. As the severity of symptoms increases, functional status deteriorates. Dystonia and rigidity may develop late in the disease process.

On CT or MRI there is marked bilateral degeneration of the caudate nucleus, enlargement of the anterior horn of the lateral ventricles and cerebral atrophy. Treatment of Huntington's disease is symptomatic; choreiform movement can sometimes be managed with dopamine-blocking agents such as haloperidol, reserpine or tetrabenazine. Individuals with Huntington's disease may have to cope with their increasingly debilitating impairments for 10–25 years, until the disease takes their life.

WILSON'S DISEASE (HEPATOLENTICULAR DEGENERATION)

Wilson's disease (WD) is a rare autosomal recessive hereditary disorder of copper metabolism, with a mutation on chromosome 13 (Rowland & Pedley, 2010; Daroff et al., 2012). Many patients present in childhood with signs of liver disease and failure associated with the accumulation of copper. Although initial symptoms typically appear in adolescence and early adulthood, presentation may first occur as late as 60 years of age. If undetected early in life, Wilson's disease can be fatal.

Nearly half of patients with WD present with CNS signs and symptoms (Daroff et al., 2012). Neurological symptoms of poorly managed WD include resting or postural tremor, chorea of the extremities, dystonia, pseudobulbar palsy and cognitive dysfunction. The abnormal liver function associated with WD eventually leads to chronic cirrhosis. Traditionally, the acute management of the disease began with penicillamine, but more recent treatment strategies include the use of trientine and zinc (removes excess copper) or ammonium tetrathiomolybdate (to block copper absorption), which are less toxic but still being researched. Orthotopic liver transplantation has been found to correct the underlying pathology in those individuals in severe hepatic failure without the presence of neurological symptoms (Daroff et al., 2012).

PAROXYSMAL KINESIGENIC DYSKINESIA

Paroxysmal kinesigenic dyskinesia (PKD or paroxysmal kinesigenic epilepsy), formerly known as paroxysmal choreoathetosis, presents as jerking and writhing movements of the limb and trunk when an individual is unexpectedly startled or disturbed (Daroff et al., 2012). The movements may be unilateral or bilateral lasting about 1 minute and can occur up to 100 times daily. Paroxysmal dyskinesia initiates in childhood, however this condition persists later in life. PKD is responsive to anticonvulsant medication such as carbamazepine and phenytoin.

PAROXYSMAL NONKINESIGENIC DYSKINESIA

Paroxysmal nonkinesigenic dyskinesia (PNKD), formerly known as familial choreoathetosis, is a rare autosomal dominant hereditary movement disorder that is relatively benign, with onset in childhood or early teens (Rowland & Pedley, 2010). In this condition, the individual experiences intermittent 'attacks' or spells of dystonia, chorea, athetosis, ballismus or a combination of movements that are associated with periods of physical exertion or ingestion of alcohol or caffeine. The 'attack' frequency can range from several episodes per month to several episodes per day, and last between 10 minutes to several hours (Daroff et al., 2012). This condition may lessen with age.

SENILE CHOREA

Senile (or essential) chorea is a late-appearing idiopathic movement disorder that evolves in the absence of psychotropic or dopamine therapy, Huntington's chorea, dementia or familial movement disorders (Daroff et al., 2012). Also known as oral–facial–lingual dyskinesia, senile chorea primarily affects the muscles of the mouth, tongue and jaw. It is important to differentiate the abnormal involuntary movements of senile chorea from the similar facial movements that occur in tardive dyskinesia and the lip and jaw movements commonly observed in older individuals who have lost all of their teeth and are no longer able to wear dentures. Antidopaminergic drugs are the most effective when monitored carefully to assess for the development of tardive dyskinesia.

TOURETTE'S SYNDROME

Tourette's syndrome is a genetically determined chronic neuropsychiatric disorder that is characterized by multiple motor and vocal tics (Hallett, 2003; Daroff et al., 2012). Symptoms may occur initially in childhood or adolescence and persist into adulthood and later life. Initially, many individuals with Tourette's are misdiagnosed with a psychiatric illness.

Initial motor tics typically involve the face and eyes, and may eventually include vocalizations (repetitive grunts, barks, throat clearing, cursing, echolalia). Repetitive motor tics of the extremities can resemble chorea. Although Tourette's is documented as an autosomal dominant trait, other hypotheses are: it is considered to be a disorder of the basal ganglia that involves excessive levels of the transmitter dopamine; a limbic system disorder involving dysfunction of the central endogenous opioid system; and reports of Tourette's following head trauma, toxic and metabolic encephalopathies, and Huntington's disease are more likely to be coincidental than causal.

Tourette's can cause considerable social, vocational and functional impairment and may also be associated with obsessive–compulsive behavior, attentional and executive dysfunction, sleep disorders and aggressive behavior (Hankey & Wiardlaw, 2008). Lifelong pharmacological intervention including dopamine-blocking agents, clonidine, haloperidol or pimozide can assist with community reintegration without compromising life expectancy.

DRUG-INDUCED MOVEMENT DISORDERS

Extrapyramidal dysfunction also occurs as the undesirable side-effect of antipsychotic drugs and other medications (Caligiuri et al., 2000; Lee et al., 2005; Morgan & Sethi, 2005). Because drug metabolism and excretion mechanisms become less efficient with aging, older adults are more susceptible to drug toxicity and adverse drug reactions; the medications that older adults are prescribed may

remain physiologically active for longer periods of time, especially if dosage is not adjusted for age and body composition (Ciccone, 2007; Gladson, 2010). Classes of medications associated with extrapyramidal side-effects are outlined in Table 31.2.

Antipsychotic medications have recently been classified as either 'traditional' or newer 'atypical' antipsychotics according to their efficacy and side-effects. Traditional antipsychotics are associated with more side-effects, including an increased incidence of extrapyramidal side-effects, as compared to the atypical medications. The psychotropic medications most likely to cause extrapyramidal dysfunction include haloperidol (Haldol) and fluphenazine (Prolixin). Tricyclic antidepressants may have similar effects in some individuals. Akathisia is often the initial indicator of iatrogenic extrapyramidal dysfunction and, over time, many susceptible individuals develop a condition that mimics Parkinson's disease, including hypokinesia, rigidity, stooped and flexed upright posture, shuffling gait and balance impairment.

An acute dyskinetic reaction can occur within days of initiation of therapy with antipsychotic medications, tricylic antidepressants, phenytoin, carbamazepine, propranolol and certain calcium-channel blockers. Although this is more common in young adults, it can occur in older adults as well. The relatively sudden onset of choreiform movement of the face, head and neck, or limbs can be frightening but typically resolves as the offending medication is withdrawn (Ciccone, 2007; Gladson, 2010).

Tardive dyskinesia is the most severe form of medication-related extrapyramidal movement dysfunction, typically developing 3–12 months into the use of dopamine antagonists (Paulson, 2005). Individuals who develop tardive dyskinesia demonstrate involuntary rhythmic choreoathetoid movements of the face, mouth and tongue (e.g. repeated tongue thrusts, lip smacking, sucking, grimacing, blinking). Some may also experience chorea of the extremities and dystonia (e.g. torticollis, occulogyric crisis, opisthotonos). These extrapyramidal signs may develop slowly and progressively worsen until the precipitating medication is reduced in dosage or discontinued; sometimes, symptoms of tardive dyskinesia persist even after the medication is discontinued. If the medication that triggers tardive dyskinesia cannot be discontinued, mild extrapyramidal symptoms can be managed with anti-Parkinson's medication, benzodiazepines, or calcium-channel blockers. Severe cases of tardive dyskinesia may need to be managed with dopamine-blocking agents, which themselves carry the risk of orthostatic hypotension. The use of newer, atypical antipsychotics has been associated with a lower risk of tardive dyskinesia, even in high-risk patients (Ciccone, 2007).

Certain other medications also carry a risk of extrapyramidal side-effects. It is not uncommon for individuals taking levodopa for the long-term management of Parkinson's disease to develop choreic movements of the face, tongue and (less commonly) lower extremities (Elble, 2002). The severity of symptoms is dosage-related, fluctuating with the levels of circulating L-dopa. Although more frequent administration of smaller doses may reduce the chorea, the disabling bradykinesia and gait disturbance typical of Parkinson's may intensify.

Table 31.2	Medications associated with extrapyramidal side-effects	
Type of Medication	Symptoms	Examples
Antipsychotic/ neuroleptic	Akathisia, pseudo-Parkinson's chorea, tardive dyskinesia, acute dyskinetic reaction	*Traditional antipsychotics:* chlorpromazine, triflupromaxine, fluphenazine, perphenazine, trifluoperazine, promazine, mesoridazine, thiothizene, haloperidol, loxapine, molindone *Atypical antipsychotics:* aripiprazole, clozapine, olanzapine, quetiapine, risperidone, ziprasidone
Antidepressants	Chorea, athetosis, akathisia Tremor, myoclonus, pseudo-Parkinson's chorea	Tricyclic antidepressants, mono-oxide inhibitors Lithium carbonate, amoxapine
Stimulants	Postural tremor, chorea	Amphetamines, methadone, methylphenidate, fenfluramine, caffeine, cocaine
CNS depressants/ sedatives	Physiological intention tremor, chorea, dystonia	Alcohol, diazepam
Anticonvulsants	Intention tremor, chorea, asterixis	Phenytoin, valproic acid, carbamazepine, phenobarbital, clonazepam
Anti-Parkinson's medications	Akathisia, chorea, dystonia	Amantadine, bromocriptine, levodopa
Other types of medication	Tremor	Bronchodilators (theophylline, doxapram), hypoglycemics, corticosteroids
	Chorea, tremor	Gastrointestinal medications (cimetidine, terfenadine)
	Chorea, dystonia, tremor	Antiarrhythmic medications (propranolol, tocainide)
	Tardive dyskinesia	Antiemetic medications (prochlorperazine, thiethylperazine, promethazine)
	Intention tremor, ataxia	Cyclosporin A
	Chorea	Estrogen/oral contraceptives, sleeping medications

Chorea is an infrequent side-effect of anticonvulsant medications such as phenytoin and carbamazepine. If chorea develops, the triggering medication should be withdrawn, even if blood levels are within the therapeutic range. The onset of choreiform movement is one of the many signs of lithium toxicity. Certain CNS stimulants (e.g. amphetamines, methylphenidate) may also induce oral–facial choreiform movement.

USE OF THE ICF MODEL FOR EXAMINATION AND INTERVENTIONS FOR INDIVIDUALS WITH TREMOR AND DYSKINESIA

The International Classification of Functioning, Disability and Health (ICF) model, discussed in Chapter 5, is a classification of health and health-related domains that guide the interdisciplinary team on decisions for examination and treatment (World Health Organization, 2001). Although rehabilitation professionals working in geriatric health-care settings are likely to encounter older individuals who have aged with a concurrent movement disorder (e.g. dyskinetic cerebral palsy) or have developed dyskinesia associated with a pathology that is more prevalent in later life (e.g. dystonia after stroke, Parkinson's disease), the evidence in the clinical research literature regarding the impact of nonpharmacological and nonsurgical interventions on tremor and other dyskinesias is incomplete. The final section of this chapter aims to provide a guideline for assessing and developing a treatment plan for individuals with tremor based on the ICF model.

EXAMINATION

Examination of an older adult with a movement disorder should include a thorough chart review and history. Specific questions regarding onset period may guide the rehabilitation professional to complete a more extensive neurological examination or indicate the need for referral to another healthcare provider. Precipitating and relieving factors that trigger or reduce symptoms of tremor can assist with classifying the dyskinetic movement. Underlying medical history, including comorbidities, surgical history, a systems review and medication history, may determine specific characteristics of movement disorders. An accurate list of both current medications and chronic use of medications assist with determining the source of tremor. Medications with potential side-effects can be found in Table 31.2. Past exposure to dopamine receptor-blocking agents (levodopa, antipsychotics/neuroleptics) could elicit a movement disorder even if the medication has been discontinued.

A brief review of cardiopulmonary, musculoskeletal, neuromuscular, communication, cognition and language systems will assist with gathering information regarding the patient's ability to function or determine the need for referral to an additional healthcare provider. A family history concentrating on dyskinetic movement disorders and other

Table 31.3 **Examination of patients with movement disorders, guided by the ICF model**		
Body Structures and Function	**Activitie**	**Participation**
Tremor location	Balance	Employment
Symmetry	Self-reported	status
Frequency	measures	
Fast	Standardized	Community
Slow	assessments	activities
Amplitude		
Fine	Functional mobility	Household
Course	Bed mobility	responsibilities
Activation	Transfers	
Rest	Gait	Quality of Life
Posture	(i) Qualitative	Measurement
Action	(ii)	Scales
Coordination testing	Quantitative	
(cerebellar)	Stairs	
Visual screening (CNS)	ADLs	
DTR (CNS	IADLs	
dysfunction)		
Sensation		
Strength		
Posture		
Cognition		

Central nervous system, CNS; deep tendon reflex, DTR; activities of daily living, ADL; instrumental activities of daily living, IADL

neurological conditions is of interest when considering congenital sources of movement disorders (Alty & Kempster, 2011). Social history is also significant and includes an inquiry regarding the individual's vocation and avocation, living environment, diet, drug and alcohol use. Recent life changing events that increase anxiety, stress, or fatigue may be the source of a new onset tremor or may exacerbate a pre-existing tremor. The individual's social history along with the home environment will provide information regarding prior level of function and assist with determining the patient's expectations for rehabilitation in order to guide goal-setting. A summative examination strategy using the ICF model is outlined in Table 31.3.

INTERVENTION

When designing a treatment plan for an older individual with a movement disorder, it is important to keep in mind where he or she is in the rehabilitation process in order to address activity limitations or participation restrictions. The phases of the rehabilitation process may include rehabilitation, compensatory training and/or preventative measures. Identification of the appropriate phase will assist with devising a treatment plan that may assist with returning the individual to his/her prior level of function, modify functional mobility activities in order to compensate for the existing movement disorder, or prevent avoidable issues surrounding safety and skin integrity.

REHABILITATIVE PHASE

The rehabilitative phase may include educating the individual or family members about the movement disorder, providing possible referral sources to involve other members of the rehabilitation team, offering recommendations to address social concerns surrounding the movement disorder, and identifying interventions that may improve or maintain function. The most compelling evidence in the field of movement disorders focuses on exercise aimed at preserving or improving cardiovascular fitness, strength and flexibility; enhancing the functional status of individuals coping with movement disorders by reducing the risk of deconditioning and physical compromise associated with inactivity and a sedentary lifestyle (Bilodeau et al., 2000; Reuter & Engelhardt, 2002; Bilney et al., 2003; Robichaud et al., 2005; Zesiewicz et al., 2005; Keogh et al., 2010; O'Connor & Kini, 2011).

COMPENSATORY PHASE

The compensatory phase may include the use of adaptive equipment or assistive devices to maintain or possibly improve function. Training with assistive devices and/or adaptive equipment may address limitations in mobility, locomotion and activities of daily living in individuals with various types of tremor, dystonia, chorea or athetosis (American Physical Therapy Association, 2003). A maintenance home exercise program focusing on strengthening, flexibility and cardiovascular fitness may be prescribed. The evidence regarding the usefulness of cuff weights during functional activities such as feeding (theoretically providing more intense proprioceptive information to the cerebellum) in individuals with intention tremor is conflicting (McGruder et al., 2003; Meshack & Norman, 2002).

PREVENTATIVE PHASE

The goal of the preventative phase is to maintain the individual's safety, the safety of others and to prevent skin breakdown and other musculoskeletal deformities. The use of resting or tone-inhibiting splints and positioning may be helpful in slowing secondary musculoskeletal complications (such as severe contracture) in individuals with dystonia (Lusardi & Bowers, 2012). Periodic reassessment and adjustment of fitness/wellness activities is especially important for those with progressive CNS disorders. A neurological reassessment is important to identify changes in disease progression that may warrant referral to a primary care physician or neurologist. In addition, pathologies that result in movement disorders often increase the daily physiological (caloric) demand, while at the same time compromising swallowing, coughing and other bulbar functions (Ahmed et al., 2008; Delikanaki-Skaribas et al., 2009). Referrals to registered dieticians and speech-language pathologists may be indicated and is an important component of the effective interdisciplinary approach to caring for individuals with movement disorders.

CONCLUSION

To be most effective in the care of older adults with tremor and other dyskinesias, physical therapists and other rehabilitation professionals must be familiar with the various movement dysfunctions, the etiology and progression of the underlying pathological process and their medical (pharmacological and/or surgical) management. It is especially important to recognize extrapyramidal symptoms of adverse drug reactions and toxicity in older adults. Although rehabilitation interventions may not directly reduce the severity of tremor or other involuntary movement, functional assessment and training play an important role and have a powerful impact on quality of life, as well as in preventing secondary impairments of the musculoskeletal and cardiovascular systems that may occur as a consequence of inactivity.

References

Ahmed NN, Sherman SJ, VanWyck D 2008 Frailty in Parkinson's disease and its clinical implications. Parkinsonism Relat Disord 14:334–337

Alarcon F, Zijlmans JC, Duenas G et al 2004 Post-stroke movement disorders: report of 56 patients. J Neurol Neurosurg Psychiatry 75:1568–1574

Alty JE, Kempster PA 2011 A practical guide to the differential diagnosis of tremor. Postgrad Med J 87:623–629

American Physical Therapy Association 2003 Guide to Physical Therapy Practice, 2nd edn (revised) [Online]. Alexandria, VA: APTA. Available at: http://guidetoptpractice.apta.org/. Accessed November 2012

Arminoff M 2008 Neurology and General Medicine, 4th edn. Churchill Livingstone, Philadelphia, PA

Bhidayasiri R 2005 Differential diagnosis of common tremor syndromes. Postgrad Med J 81:756–762

Bilney B, Morris ME, Perry A 2003 Effectiveness of physiotherapy, occupational therapy, and speech pathology for people with Huntington's disease: a systematic review. Neurorehabil Neural Repair 17:12–24

Bilodeau M, Keen DA, Sweeney PJ et al 2000 Strength training can improve steadiness in persons with essential tremor. Muscle Nerve 23:771–778

Blumenfeld J 2010 Neuroanatomy Through Clinical Cases, 2nd edn. Sinauer Associates, Inc., Sunderland, MA

Caligiuri MR, Jeste DV, Lacro JP 2000 Antipsychotic-induced movement disorders in the elderly: epidemiology and treatment recommendations. Drugs Aging 17:363–384

Ciccone CD 2007 Pharmacology in Rehabilitation, 4th edn. FA Davis, Philadelphia, PA

Crawford P, Zimmerman EE 2011 Differentiation and diagnosis of tremor. Am Fam Physician 83:697–702

Daroff R, Fenichel J, Jankovic J et al 2012 Bradley's Neurology in Clinical Practice, 6th edn. Saunders, Philadelphia, PA

Delikanaki-Skaribas E, Trail M, Wong WW et al 2009 Daily energy expenditure, physical activity, and weight loss in Parkinson's disease patients. Mov Disord 24:667–671

Deuschl G, Bain P, Brin M, AHS 1998 Consensus statement of the Movement Disorder Society on tremor. Mov Disord 13:2–23

Elble RJ 2002 Tremor and dopamine agonists. Neurology 58:S57–S62

Gladson B 2010 Pharmacology for Rehabilitation Professionals. WB Saunders, Philadelphia, PA

Hallett M 2003 Movement Disorders: Handbook of Clinical Neurophysiology. Elsevier, Philadelphia, PA

Hankey G, Wiardlaw JM 2008 Clinical Neurology. Demos Medical Publishing, London

Jankovic J, Tolosa E 2007 Parkinson's Disease and Movement Disorders, 5th edn. Lippincott Williams & Wilkins, Philadelphia, PA

Keogh JW, Morrison S, Barrett R 2010 Strength and coordination training are both effective in reducing the postural tremor amplitude of older adults. J Aging Phys Act 18:43–60

Klein C 2005 Movement disorders: classifications. J Inherit Metab Dis 28:425–439

Krauss JK, Jankovic J 2002 Head injury and posttraumatic movement disorders. Neurosurgery 50:927–939 discussion 939–40

Lee PE, Sykora K, Gill SS et al 2005 Antipsychotic medications and drug-induced movement disorders other than parkinsonism: a population-based cohort study in older adults. J Am Geriatr Soc 53:1374–1379

Louis ED, Ferreira JJ 2010 How common is the most common adult movement disorder? Update on the worldwide prevalence of essential tremor. Mov Disord 25:534–541

Lusardi MM, Bowers DM 2012 Orthotic decision making in neurological and neuromuscular disease. In: Lusardi MM, Jorge M, Neilson CC (eds) Orthotics and Prosthetics in Rehabilitation, 3rd edn. Elsevier Saunders, St Louis, MO

McGruder J, Cors D, Tiernan AM et al 2003 Weighted wrist cuffs for tremor reduction during eating in adults with static brain lesions. Am J Occup Ther 57:507–516

Meshack RP, Norman KE 2002 A randomized controlled trial of the effects of weights on amplitude and frequency of postural hand tremor in people with Parkinson's disease. Clin Rehabil 16:481–492

Milligan SA, Chesson AL 2002 Restless legs syndrome in the older adult: diagnosis and management. Drugs Aging 19:741–751

Morgan JC, Sethi KD 2005 Drug-induced tremors. Lancet Neurol 4:866–876

Mostile G, Jankovic J 2010 Alcohol in essential tremor and other movement disorders. Mov Disord 25:2274–2284

Muthuraman M, Raethjen J, Hellriegel H et al 2008 Imaging coherent sources of tremor related EEG activity in patients with Parkinson's disease. Conf Proc IEEE Eng Med Biol Soc:4716–4719

O'Connor RJ, Kini MU 2011 Non-pharmacological and non-surgical interventions for tremor: a systematic review. Parkinsonism Relat Disord 17:509–515

O'Suilleabhain P, Dewey Jr RB 2004 Movement disorders after head injury: diagnosis and management. J Head Trauma Rehabil 19:305–313

Pahwa R, Factor SA, Lyons KE et al 2006 Practice Parameter: Treatment of Parkinson disease with motor fluctuations and dyskinesia (an evidence-based review): report of the Quality Standards Subcommittee of the American Academy of Neurology. Neurology 66:983–995

Patestas MA, Gartner LP 2006 A Textbook of Neuroanatomy. Blackwell, Malden, MA

Paulson GW 2005 Historical comments on tardive dyskinesia: a neurologist's perspective. J Clin Psychiatry 66:260–264

Paz J, West M 2008 Acute Care Handbook for Physical Therapists, 3rd edn. Saunders Elsevier, St Louis, MO

Puschmann A, Wszolek ZK 2011 Diagnosis and treatment of common forms of tremor. Semin Neurol 31:65–77

Raethjen J, Govindan RB, Kopper F et al 2007 Cortical involvement in the generation of essential tremor. J Neurophysiol 97:3219–3228

Reuter I, Engelhardt M 2002 Exercise training and Parkinson's disease: placebo or essential treatment? Phys Sportsmed 30:43–50

Robichaud JA, Pfann KD, Vaillancourt DE et al 2005 Force control and disease severity in Parkinson's disease. Mov Disord 20:441–450

Rowland L, Pedley T 2010 Merritt's Neurology, 12th edn. Lippincott Williams & Wilkins, Philadelphia, PA

Rubboli G, Tassinari CA 2006 Negative myoclonus: an overview of its clinical features, pathophysiological mechanisms, and management. Neurophysiol Clin 36:337–343

Seidel S, Kasprian G, Leutmezer F et al 2009 Disruption of nigrostriatal and cerebellothalamic pathways in dopamine responsive Holmes' tremor. J Neurol Neurosurg Psychiatry 80:921–923

Shibasaki H 2012 Cortical activities associated with voluntary movements and involuntary movements. Clin Neurophysiol 123:229–243

Spitz M, Costa Machado AA, Carvalho Rdo C et al 2006 Pseudoathetosis: report of three patients. Mov Disord 21:1520–1522

Sullivan KL, Hauser RA, Zesiewicz TA 2004 Essential tremor. Epidemiology, diagnosis, and treatment. Neurologist 10:250–258

Weiner W, Lang K 2005 Behavioral Neurology of Movement Disorders (Advances in Neurology), 2nd edn. Lippincott Williams & Wilkins, Philadelphia, PA

Whitney S, Wrisley DM, Musolino MC et al 2003 Orthostatic tremor: two persons in a balance disorder practice. J Neurol Phys Ther 27:46–53

World Health Organization (WHO) 2001 International Classification of Functioning, Disability and Health (ICF). WHO, Geneva. Available at: www.who.int/classifications/icf/en. Accessed December 2012

Zesiewicz TA, Elble R, Louis ED et al 2005 Practice parameter: therapies for essential tremor: report of the Quality Standards Subcommittee of the American Academy of Neurology. Neurology 64:2008–2020

Chapter 32

Generalized peripheral neuropathy

ANITA CRAIG • JAMES K. RICHARDSON

INTRODUCTION

Peripheral nerve disorders are common in the elderly and have significant impact on their function and quality of life. It is also important to recognize the impact of underlying peripheral neuropathy (PN) when rehabilitating the elderly for other conditions. Approximately 10% of Americans over the age of 60 have PN as a result of diabetes and another 10% have PN due to other causes, with a prevalence of PN of about 20% in the older American population (Richardson & Ashton-Miller, 1996). The prevalence of PN in the elderly requiring rehabilitation is undoubtedly much higher. This chapter will address recognition and treatment strategies to successfully rehabilitate elderly patients with functionally significant generalized PN.

CAUSES OF PERIPHERAL NEUROPATHY IN THE ELDERLY

PN can be caused by a number of conditions that are especially common in the older population. Certainly the most common cause is diabetic PN (George & Twomey, 1986), but other etiologies such as alcoholism, renal disease, thyroid disease and neoplasm are commonly encountered (Box 32.1). In patients referred for

---

Box 32.1   *Common causes of PN in older adults*

- Alcohol abuse
- Diabetes mellitus
- Chronic obstructive pulmonary disease (COPD)
- Monoclonal gammopathy (benign or malignant)
- Neoplasm
- Medications and chemotherapeutic agents
- Renal disease
- Thyroid disease
- Vitamin B_{12} deficiency

---

subspecialty evaluation of PN, an underlying cause cannot be determined in 10–23% of cases (Wolfe & Barohn, 1998) and idiopathic PN is more common in older populations, even when comparing those younger than 80 to those greater than 80 years old (Verghese et al., 2001).

A number of pharmaceutical agents can cause neuropathies. Many agents used in the treatment of cancer can induce severe neuropathies and those neuropathies can be a treatment-limiting side-effect. General chemotherapy-induced adverse effects are more common in the elderly; however, in the limited studies that have evaluated common therapeutic agents, pacitaxel and cisplatin-based chemotherapy, elderly patients do not have a greater risk for developing PN, nor do they demonstrate greater severity of PN. However, given the greater number of elderly patients undergoing cancer treatment, chemotherapy-induced PN is an important entity, occurring in up to 30–40% of patients undergoing chemotherapy. Onset of PN may be acute or subacute, and may present days to months after initiation of treatment. Sometimes signs and symptoms appear or progress for up to 2 months after cessation of the agent, the so called 'coasting phenomenon' (Guitiérrez-Guitiérrez et al., 2010). Reduction in dose, slower infusion rates, or longer periods between doses may bring improvement, however sometimes cessation of treatment is required. Often symptoms of PN will improve, but in some cases recovery can be incomplete. A number of other non-chemotherapeutic drugs can cause PN. Because the elderly tend to be on multiple pharmaceuticals it is important to scrutinize the medication list of any elderly patient presenting with signs of PN (Box 32.2).

RECOGNIZING A GENERALIZED PERIPHERAL NEUROPATHY

PNs can be characterized by the type of nerve fibers affected, whether they affect the nerve axon or the myelin, and the pattern of distribution of the affected nerves. The majority of PNs are diffuse and symmetrical in distribution; however, many vasculitic disorders present with asymmetrical or multifocal neuropathies (Craig & Richardson, 2003). Neuropathies affecting somatic or autonomic small fibers can be difficult to diagnose as they can present with profound neuropathic pain but have relatively normal physical and electrodiagnostic examinations (Hoitsma et al., 2004).

Neuropathic processes generally affect the nerve in a length-dependent manner, with longer nerves being more susceptible. Because lower extremities are longer than upper extremities and because sensory nerves are longer than motor nerves (as a result of the former's intraspinal dendritic processes), distal lower extremity sensory function is the first and most severely affected in diffuse PN, followed by distal lower extremity motor function, distal upper extremity sensory function, and lastly distal upper extremity motor function. In addition, nerves that are more vulnerable to compressive neuropathies, such as the median and peroneal (fibular) nerves, are more susceptible to injury in those already compromised by PN.

Patients' historical presentations can be quite variable, due to individual insight into their PN symptoms, as well as rapidity and acuity of onset. Many patients are acutely aware of their numbness and pain, whereas others note only vague sensory abnormalities such as a sensation of walking on pillows or simply that they have to be more careful with activities involving balance. When pain or numbness is apparent to the patient, it is generally noted to be most profound in the forefoot and lessen proximally. In the upper extremities, if symptoms are present they too will follow in a distal to proximal gradient. Often, however, upper extremity symptoms will manifest as difficulty performing fine motor tasks such as buttoning or picking up small objects without using visual feedback. Loss of motor strength is often not present, but in more severe disease foot drop or loss of hand dexterity may develop. Balance problems are often present, with insidious need to touch something when walking on uneven surfaces or in low lighting, as well as difficulty climbing stairs without the use of a railing. In predominantly small fiber neuropathies severe pain can be a prominent feature. Autonomic symptoms may be present, including increased or decreased sweating, dry eyes, erectile dysfunction, gastroparesis and skin temperature changes. Cardiovascular involvement limits activity tolerance and increases risk of sudden death and myocardial ischemia (Boulton et al., 2005). Clinically significant orthostatic hypotension is of particular concern in older patients given the association between postural hypotension and falls.

On physical examination, there is a loss of sensory function in a distal-to-proximal gradient. Multiple sensory modalities should be assessed. Vibratory sensation is particularly sensitive for large fiber neuropathies. This is best evaluated with a 128 Hz tuning fork maximally struck and placed at the base of the great toe, the malleolus, and the tibial tuberosity. Accuracy of the test may be improved by first familiarizing the patient with the vibratory stimulus at the clavicle. The number of seconds that the patient can perceive the vibration at each location is recorded. In PN the number of seconds that the vibration is felt increases proximally. If the patient is able to perceive the vibration for greater than 10 seconds at the great toe, PN is absent; if the sensation is present for less than 10 seconds at the malleolus, PN is likely to be present. Proprioception is also a good assessment of large fiber sensory function. This is tested by assessing the patient's ability to perceive 8–10 small (1 cm) movements at the great toe. The inability to identify correctly at least 8–10 movements has been correlated with decreased ankle inversion/eversion proprioception (Vanden Bosch et al., 1995). Light touch using a 10-guage monofilament and pinprick will also reveal sensory loss in a distal to proximal gradient. In a patient with a purely small fiber neuropathy pinprick sensation may be decreased with relatively spared vibratory sensation.

Muscle stretch reflexes are affected, with Achilles tendon reflexes almost uniformly lost in PN, and the patellar and internal hamstring reflexes to a lesser degree. The Achilles reflexes can be obtained either with direct percussion or by the planter strike technique, which may be more reliably obtained in the older population (O'Keefe et al., 1994). Absence of Achilles tendon reflex, with or without facilitation, the inability to perceive at least 8–10 great toe movements, and the loss of vibratory sensation within 8 seconds are predictive of electrodiagnostically significant PN in older populations (Richardson, 2002).

Deficits of motor function can be seen in a distal to proximal gradient as well. Early motor strength loss may be recognized by easy fatigability; therefore, detection of subtle weakness may be improved by testing a muscle with multiple resistance maneuvers (McComas et al., 1995). The intrinsic musculature of the foot is commonly atrophied in PN, which cause changes in the architecture of the foot, with extension of the metatarsophalangeal joints in extension and interphalangeal joints in flexion (hammer toes). Toes move minimally or only in a stiff gross manner. In more advanced PN the anterior compartment, and to a lesser degree the posterior compartment, leg muscles weaken and atrophy. When PN has progressed to this point usually the intrinsic muscles of the hand become involved. Gross motor function is also affected. Patients may have a positive Romberg's sign, wherein the patient is stable standing with feet together when eyes are open, but unstable with eyes closed.

Table 32.1 **Clinical findings in functionally significant peripheral neuropathy**	
Test or Condition	**PN Functionally Significant**
Vibratory sensation with 128 Hz tuning fork	Obvious gradient Perceived at malleolus <5–6 seconds
Foot deformity and callouses	Present
Achilles reflex	Absent
Position sense at the great toe	<8 out of 10 correct responses
Unipedal stance	<5 seconds on each of three attempts

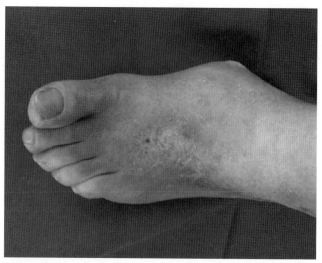

Figure 32.1 Foot deformity caused by Charcot arthropathy. *(From Brodsky JW 2007 The diabetic foot. In: Coughlin MJ et al. Surgery of the Foot and Ankle, 8th edn. Mosby/Elsevier, Philadelphia, PA, with permission from Elsevier.)*

This suggests a deficit in somatosensory input and an excessive reliance upon vision for balance. A positive Romberg sign suggests a relatively severe PN; however, many patients with functionally significant PN demonstrate a negative Romberg's sign. A more sensitive test of balance impairment due to PN is the assessment of unipedal stance time. If the patient can balance on one foot for 10 seconds or more (the best of three tries on the foot of their choice), functionally significant PN is not likely to be present. If the patient can balance on one foot for only 3–4 seconds or less, then the PN is functionally significant. It should be noted that the unipedal stance test is not used to identify PN, but rather to determine the extent of loss of balance caused by the PN once it has been identified by the other elements of the clinical examination (Hurvitz et al., 2000). Table 32.1 lists clinical characteristics of a patient with functionally significant PN.

Patients with PN may also demonstrate changes in the skin and architecture of the foot. Skin lesions or breakdown can be seen in an insensate foot with a predilection for the heel and metatarsal heads (see Chapter 49). The presence of PN is associated with an 8–18-fold greater risk of foot ulceration and a 2–15-fold greater risk of amputation (Paola & Faglia, 2006). Foot deformity caused by intrinsic muscle atrophy, as mentioned previously, increases the risk of ulceration by creating areas of excessive pressure. In severe PN, particularly associated with diabetes, Charcot arthropathy may develop. This condition is characterized by pathologic fracture, joint destruction and severe deformity, predominantly affecting the forefoot (Fig. 32.1). This condition results from autonomic dysfunction causing increased blood flow to the foot with resulting bone resorption and osteopenia. Initial presentation can mimic cellulitis or deep venous thrombosis, with a hot, swollen foot. Bone scan can be positive early in the course of this process, before radiographic evidence of fracture and dislocation. Early recognition and immobilization in a total contact cast or boot is important to reduce deformity (Vinik et al., 2008).

Few other diseases mimic PN. Lumbar stenosis, which like PN is common in the older population, can present in a similar fashion, with gradual numbness and weakness in the distal lower extremities. Lumbar stenosis, however, presents with increased pain with standing and walking, and improvement with sitting or lying down. There is usually some accompanying back pain as well. PN differs in that it is present at all times, or even worse at night. On physical examination, the patient usually does not show the symmetrical gradient of sensory loss that is seen in the PN patient. If there is motor involvement, the stenosis patient usually demonstrates asymmetrical weakness, also involving proximal gluteal as well as the distal musculature. In contrast, the patient with PN has symmetrical weakness that is always more severe distally and improves proximally. Another process that can be confused with PN is cervical myelopathy. Patients with this condition may present with balance difficulties, gait ataxia and falls, similar to the PN patients. Generally this can be readily differentiated by lack of overt sensory loss in the lower extremities as well as upper motor signs such as hyper-reflexia and clonus.

FUNCTIONAL IMPACT OF PERIPHERAL NEUROPATHY

PN has significant impact on the functioning of the older patient in rehabilitation. Studies have demonstrated that patients with isolated PN are about 20 times more likely to fall than patients without PN (Richardson et al., 1992; Richardson & Hurvitz, 1995). The subjects in these studies had PN but no other functionally relevant diagnoses and all were community ambulators without assistive devices. The impact of PN is undoubtedly equal or greater in rehabilitation patients with concomitant diagnoses and worse baseline functioning.

Patients with PN have been shown to have impaired ankle proprioception (Vanden Bosch et al., 1995) as well as decreased ability to maintain unipedal stance (Richardson et al., 1996) regardless of preparation time. Ankle inversion/eversion proprioceptive thresholds in subjects with PN were about 1.5°, compared to 0.3° in matched controls. At the ankle 1.5° of motion is enough to allow the body's center of mass to travel to the edge of the patient's base of support during unipedal stance before being perceived. This suggests that even under calm and deliberate settings those with PN will have difficulty performing tasks requiring unipedal stance, such as climbing stairs or dressing.

The inability of the elderly patient with PN to rapidly develop ankle strength (torque) contributes to gait dysfunction, inability to maintain unipedal stance and recover from postural challenges even when clinically normal strength is present. In testing of ability to recover from lateral lean, subjects with PN were unable to rapidly develop the torque around the ankle necessary to recover (Guitiérrez et al., 2001). Patients with PN are therefore doubly penalized when their center of mass is perturbed as it takes greater displacement before loss of balance is perceived and they are unable to quickly generate the corrective muscular torque to compensate, regardless of intact gross strength.

It is clinically observed that PN patients rarely fall in optimal environments, i.e. environments that the patient is familiar with, have good lighting, and are smooth and level. Irregular surfaces are often a cause of falls; they were found to underlie nearly 80% of falls in a prospective study of 20 older PN subjects (DeMott et al., 2007). In addition, older PN subjects demonstrate greater step time variability and step width–step length variability and greater decrease in step length and speed than control subjects when adapting to challenging environments (Richardson et al., 2004). These alterations in gait on irregular surfaces have implications for endurance as the altered gait pattern is less efficient. Additionally this has implications on community mobility where the maintenance of speed on irregular surfaces may be critical, for example when crossing a street.

In the older rehabilitation patient, PN is rarely isolated as in the research subjects described above; therefore, PN exacerbates the clinically obvious impairments already present. For example, if a patient with PN has hemiparesis or an above-knee amputation as the primary rehabilitation diagnosis then the patient's ability to use the 'good' lower extremity is also impaired. If the PN is not recognized, unrealistic expectation or caregiver confusion over difficulty with progression to certain goals may develop. Patients with ataxia from cerebellar or vestibular dysfunction or disruption of vision or the visual–spatial system will be even further compromised by underlying PN. The early recognition of PN in such patients allows for the formulation of reasonable goals and an early start to the learning process that enables patients to compensate for PN.

TREATMENT AND MANAGEMENT OF PERIPHERAL NEUROPATHY

When PN is identified or clinically suspected, should it be further investigated? The answer to this depends on the circumstances. Many causes of PN are quite common in the older population, for example diabetes, renal disease, critical care illness, peripheral vascular occlusive disease and alcoholism. The identification of PN in a patient with any of these disorders does not necessarily require further investigation, particularly if the symptom onset is gradual. If, however, the patient does not have any risk factors or if the onset of the PN is rapidly progressive, more investigation is warranted. PN can be the initial presenting sign of many treatable systemic diseases. Likewise if the patient is on any medications or chemotherapeutic agents that are known to cause PN, that agent needs to be identified and possibly discontinued or changed. In general PN predominantly affecting the nerve axons are associated with metabolic disorders or toxins, and those that affect the myelin are associated with immune processes that may sometimes be related to malignancy. Making the distinction on clinical grounds is challenging; clues to a demyelinating PN are early loss of reflexes with relative preservation of muscle mass, whereas clues to an axonal PN are maintenance of proximal reflexes and relatively greater muscle atrophy distally. Neuropathies that present with asymmetrical involvement should raise suspicion for autoimmune or vasculitic disorders.

Education is the most important intervention in terms of reducing the functional impact of PN. The patient and the patient's family must understand the nature of the disorder – that the patient has lost a special sense in the distal lower (and sometimes upper) extremities. They must further understand that, as a result of this lost special sense, the patient's balance is impaired and compensatory techniques will be necessary to avoid an increased risk of falls.

Visual input must be maximized to compensate for the impaired somatosensory input from the lower extremities. Reduced visual acuity and depth perception, and loss of visual field have been shown to increase the risk of falls (Lord et al., 2010) and this is likely to have even greater impact on patients already compromised by PN. The elderly often either wear no glasses or have outdated prescriptions. Vision should be tested and, if impaired, referral to the appropriate health professional is indicated. It is important to note, however, that dramatic changes in spectacle prescription can also at least temporarily increase risk of falls by causing obstacles to appear further or closer than the person is accustomed to. The use of multifocal lenses may increase the risk of falls as the lower lenses blur the lower visual field which is at a critical distance to perceived floor level objects that may present trip hazards. Patients who use multifocal glasses are more likely to fall outside their home and when walking up or down stairs (Lord et al., 2002). The use of single-lens glasses may be preferable, particularly for patients who engage in regular outside activities. Equally important is teaching the patient the importance of proper lighting, particularly at night. The patient must be encouraged to avoid the temptation not to put on their glasses and to leave the lights off so as not to disturb other household members during nocturnal trips to the bathroom.

Proper shoe wear is very important for patients with PN. Shoes that are best for balance have a wide base of support and thin soles. Thick crepe soles or the heavily cushioned soles of athletic wear should be avoided. If significant foot deformity exists, custom orthotics, possibly along with extra-depth shoes to accommodate the foot deformity should be prescribed. Sometimes a patient with poor balance finds plastic ankle–foot orthoses that are custom molded to be beneficial; however, care must be taken when fitting them to avoid the initiation of a foot wound. Patients with PN and caregivers should be educated on the importance of regular skin inspection of

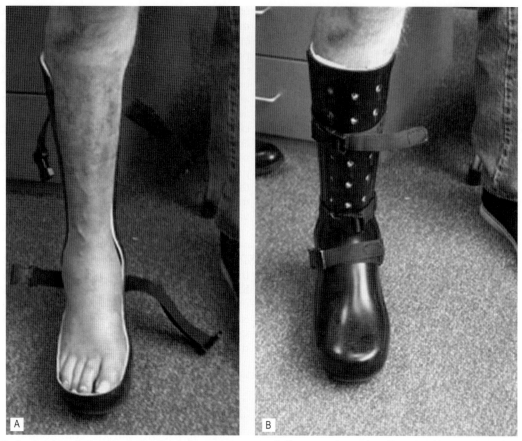

Figure 32.2 Bivalve total contact ankle foot orthosis for management of Charcot arthropathy. *(From Brodsky JW 2007 The diabetic foot. In: Coughlin MJ et al. Surgery of the Foot and Ankle, 8th edn. Mosby/Elsevier, Philadelphia, PA, with permission from Elsevier.)*

insensate feet. It is important to keep feet well moisturized and callouses and nail care diligently managed, possibly by podiatry or a diabetic foot care clinic. Patients with evidence of Charcot neuroarthropathy may require full contact casting or a boot for immobilization and a period of nonweightbearing in the acute stage (Fig. 32.2).

A patient with balance impairment due to PN can benefit from the use of a support when walking. The use of a cane for stabilization in PN has been studied (Ashton-Miller et al., 1996). Subjects were asked to transfer onto an unsteady surface that tilted during mid-transfer and maintain 3 seconds of unipedal balance. Under such conditions the PN subjects failed to maintain their balance without a cane about 50% of the time but succeeded with a cane about 96% of the time. It has been further demonstrated that, to obtain maximal benefit from a cane in preventing a fall, patients must be able to support approximately 25% of their body weight with the cane. The patient should be instructed to place the cane down with each contralateral footstep to assist in preventing falls away from the cane as well at towards it. Patients and family are often reluctant to accept the use of a cane. Acceptance and compliance may be greater if they are told that the cane is a substitute, like glasses or a hearing aid, for a special sense that has been lost and is a way to prevent falls, not a sign of infirmity. The patient may also comply better if the cane is used as needed and not all the time. A patient can usually be free of the cane when the lighting is good and the walking surface is firm, flat and familiar.

Other interventions can also be helpful in improving gait parameters and reducing the risk of falls, particularly on irregular surfaces. These include the use of ankle orthoses (AO) with medial and lateral supports and the use of a firm vertical support. All three interventions have been demonstrated to improve the step-width variability which suggests improved medial/lateral stability, and decreased step-width range (Richardson et al., 2004). The use of an AO and vertical wall also improved step-time variability, which has been prospectively associated with falls (Hausdorff et al., 2001). The mechanism of improvement in gait parameters with AO does not appear to be related to improvement in proprioceptive thresholds or unipedal stance time (Son et al., 2010) but may be related to stiffening of the ankle. Only the cane intervention was associated with decreased walking speed. Advantages of use of an AO over cane include the availability of both upper extremities and better walking speed; the disadvantage of an AO is the possibility of skin breakdown (Fig. 32.3).

There is clearly a role for exercise in the setting of neuropathy. Given the overwhelming evidence demonstrating the health and life-extending benefits of walking in older people with diabetes mellitus (Sluik et al., 2012), the goal of exercise is to maintain postural stability during gait on smooth and irregular surfaces. Recent work provides some clues as to the goals of an exercise prescription in this patient population. Data from 43 older subjects, about two-thirds of them with varying degrees of diabetic neuropathy, indicate that one-legged balance

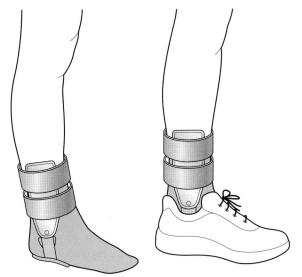

Figure 32.3 Ankle orthoses with medial and lateral support can improve gait parameters and balance with ambulation. *(Reproduced from Richardson JK, Thies S, De Mott T et al. 2004 Interventions improve gait regularity in patients with peripheral neuropathy while walking on an irregular surface under low light. J Am Geriatr Soc 52(4):510–515 with permission from Wiley.)*

(an important marker of frailty and fall risk) is governed by the ratio of laboratory-based measures of frontal plane hip strength to ankle proprioceptive threshold rather than age (Allet et al., 2012a). Importantly, hip adductor strength was as important as the more-emphasized hip abductor strength. If these findings are extrapolated to the dynamic scenario that occurs while walking and arresting a perturbation, then frontal plane hip rate of strength generation is critical, as suggested by Johnson et al. (2004). Therefore frontal plane hip strengthening, with an emphasis on the adductor musculature, is reasonable and the greater the severity of neuropathy the more aggressively hip rate of strength development should be emphasized. For patients with greater than grade 4 ankle dorsiflexion and inversion/eversion strength, strengthening of these groups is also of potential benefit, with the inversion group appearing to be the most important for navigation on irregular surfaces. (Allet et al., 2012b)

Pain, particularly nocturnal pain, can be a significant problem for the patient with PN. Neuropathic pain can be dull, tooth ache-like or cramping in large fiber neuropathy, or burning with hypersensitivity, as seen in small fiber neuropathy. Other sources of foot pain should be ruled out, such as lumbar radiculopathy, vascular claudication, plantar fasciitis, or Morton's neuroma. Treatment can be challenging and side-effects may be a significant limiting factor, particularly in the elderly. Topical agents have the advantage of having no systemic side-effects but application may be difficult for the patient. A trial of topical capsaicin is indicated if the patient has the intellectual ability and manual dexterity to apply it properly. It must be applied 3–4 times a day and may make the symptoms worse initially, but avoids the side-effects of oral agents. If the affected area is discrete a transdermal lidocaine patch can be used. Other options include a low dosage of one of the tricyclic antidepressants, such as nortryptiline or amytriptyline prior to bed. Serious potential side-effects include orthostatic hypotension, and possible cardiac arrhythmias, and are contraindicated in patients with prolonged QT interval, recent myocardial infarction, or conduction block. Patients over 40 should have a screening electrocardiogram prior to initiating any of this class of agents (Dworkin et al., 2003). Gabapentin at doses up to 3600 mg/day can be very effective in reducing pain, but side-effects such as somnolence and dizziness may exacerbate balance and gait problem, particularly upon initiating this agent, and should therefore be titrated slowly. Pregabalin and duloxetine are currently the only two drugs approved by the FDA to treat painful diabetic neuropathy. Pregabalin has similar side-effects to gabapentin and duloxetine may cause significant gastrointestinal upset. Second line agents include lamotrigine, carbamazepine, other selective serotonin uptake inhibitors, and clonidine. Opioids should be used very judiciously due to concerns for cognitive side-effects, particularly, in the elderly, physiologic dependency and addiction. Transcutaneous electrical nerve stimulation (TENS) can be helpful and, like capsaicin, it has the advantage of producing no systemic side-effects.

CONCLUSION

Approximately 20% of older Americans have PN, which is likely to have an impact on rehabilitation. Sensory impairment is usually more prominent than motor impairment and distal lower extremities are affected more than distal upper extremities. These changes usually impair balance control and this often leads to falls. Generalized PN usually compounds existing clinical impairments. The patient and the patient's family must be educated about the loss and advised of the potential risk for further injury and how to mitigate the risks. The use of assistive devices for mobility, therapeutic exercises for functional activities and medication or TENS for pain control is encouraged.

REFERENCES

Allet LA, Kim H, Ashton-Miller JA et al 2012a Frontal plane hip and ankle sensorimotor function, not age, predicts unipedal stance time. Muscle Nerve 45(4):578–585

Allet LA, Kim H, Ashton-Miller JA 2012b Which lower limb sensory and motor functions are required for functional gait on uneven surfaces in older persons with diabetic neuropathy? PMR 4(10):726–733

Ashton-Miller JA, Yeh MW, Richardson JK et al 1996 A cane lowers the risk of patients with peripheral neuropathy losing their balance: results from a challenging unipedal balance test. Arch Phys Med Rehabil 77:446–452

Boulton AJM, Vinik AI, Arezzo JC 2005 Diabetic neuropathies: a statement by the American Diabetes Association. Diabetes Care 28(4):956–962

Craig ASW, Richardson JK 2003 Acquired peripheral neuropathy. Phys Med Rehabil Clin North Am 14:365–386

DeMott TK, Richardson JK, Thies SB et al 2007 Falls and gait characteristics among older persons with peripheral neuropathy. Am J Phys Med Rehabil 86:125–132

Dworkin RH, Backonja M, Rowbotham MC et al 2003 Advances in neuropathic pain: diagnosis, mechanisms, and treatment recommendations. Arch Neurol 60:1524–1534

George J, Twomey JA 1986 Causes of polyneuropathy in the eldery. Age Ageing 15:247–249

Guitiérrez EM, Helber MD, Dealva D et al 2001 Mild diabetic neuropathy affects ankle motor function. Clin Biomech 16:522–528

Guitiérrez-Guitiérrez G, Sereno M, Miralles A et al 2010 Chemotherapy-induced peripheral neuropathy: clinical features diagnosis, prevention and treatment strategies. Clin Transl Oncol 12:81–91

Hausdorff JM, Rios DA, Edleberg HK 2001 Gait variability and fall risk in community-living older adults: a 1-year prospective study. Arch Phys Med Rehabil 82:1050–1056

Hoitsma E, Reulen JPH, de Baets M 2004 Small fiber neuropathy: a common and important clinical disorder. J Neurol Sci 227:119–130

Hurvitz EA, Richardson JK, Werner RA et al 2000 Unipedal stance testing as an indicator of fall risk among older outpatients. Arch Phys Med Rehabil 81(5):587–591

Johnson ME, Mille ML, Martinez KM et al 2004 Age-related changes in hip abductor and adductor joint torques. Arch Phys Med Rehabil 85:593–597

Lord SR, Dayhew J, Howland A 2002 Multifocal glasses impair edge-contrast sensitivity and depth perception and increase the risk of falls in older people. J Am Geriatr Soc 50(11):1760–1766

Lord SR, Smith ST, Menant JC 2010 Vision and falls in older people: risk factors and intervention strategies. Clin Geriatr Med 26:569–581

McComas AJ, Miller RG, Gandevia SC 1995 Fatigue brought on by malfunction of the central and peripheral nervous systems. Adv Exp Med Biol 384:495–512

O'Keefe ST, Smith T, Valancio R et al 1994 A comparison of two techniques for ankle jerk assessment in elderly subjects. Lancet 344:1619–1620

Paola LD, Faglia E 2006 Treatment of diabetic foot ulcer: an overview. Strategies for clinical approach. Curr Diabetes Rev 2:431–447

Richardson JK 2002 The clinical identification of peripheral neuropathy among older persons. Arch Phys Med Rehabil 83:1553–1558

Richardson JK, Ashton-Miller JA 1996 Peripheral nerve dysfunction and falls in the elderly. Postgrad Med 99:161–172

Richardson JK, Ching C, Hurvitz EA 1992 The relationship between electromyographically documented peripheral neuropathy and falls. J Am Geriatr Soc 40:1008–1012

Richardson JK, Ashton-Miller JA, Lee SG et al 1996 Moderate peripheral neuropathy impairs weight transfer and unipedal balance in the elderly. Arch Phys Med Rehabil 77:1152–1156

Richardson JK, Hurvitz EA 1995 Peripheral neuropathy: a true risk factor for falls. J Gerontol Ser A Biol Sci Med Sci 50A:211–215

Richardson JK, Thies SB, DeMott TK et al 2004 Interventions improve gait regularity in patients with peripheral neuropathy while walking on an irregular surface under low light. J Am Geriatr Soc 52:510–515

Sluik D, Buijsse B, Muckelbauer R et al 2012 Physical activity and mortality in individuals with diabetes mellitus: a prospective study and meta-analysis. Arch Intern Med 172(17):1285–1295

Son J, Ashton-Miller JA, Richardson JK 2010 Do ankle orthoses improve ankle proprioceptive thresholds or unipedal balance in older persons with peripheral neuropathy? Am J Phys Med Rehabil 89:369–375

Vanden Bosch CG, Gilsing M, Lee SG et al 1995 Effect of peripheral neuropathy on ankle inversion and eversion detection thresholds. Arch Phys Med Rehabil 76:850–856

Verghese J, Bieri PL, Gellido C et al 2001 Peripheral neuropathy in young-old and old-old patients. Muscle Nerve 24:1476–1481

Vinik AI, Strotmeyer ES, Nakave AA et al 2008 Diabetic neuropathy in older adults. Clin Geriatr Med 24(8):407–435

Wolfe GI, Barohn RJ 1998 Cryptogenic sensory and sensorimotor polyneuropathies. Semin Neurol 118:105–111

Chapter 33

Localized peripheral neuropathies

ANITA CRAIG • JAMES K. RICHARDSON

Chapter Contents

INTRODUCTION

Localized peripheral neuropathies are even more common than generalized neuropathies and the two often coexist. Because a diffusely diseased peripheral nervous system is less able to recover from a mechanical insult than a healthy one, it is a clinical rule that a patient with generalized peripheral neuropathy is at an increased risk for specific discrete neuropathies. Localized neuropathies can also be a sequelae of a number of traumatic and iatrogenic injuries, which may or may not be immediately apparent upon initial evaluation and treatment of the injured patient. In addition, mechanical insults are particularly common in the rehabilitation setting as patients learn alternative strategies for self-care and mobility. Such strategies often involve stressing intact musculoskeletal regions to compensate for regions that are impaired, which increases the risk of nerve trauma in the intact regions. Early recognition, prevention and, when necessary, treatment of these specific neuropathies are critical for the prevention of further impairment and disability in older patients.

This chapter will be organized around typical (and nonspecific) symptoms and complaints. The potentially responsible focal neuropathy will be identified for each symptom. The details of clinical presentation and approach to each potentially responsible focal neuropathy will also be discussed.

NUMB HAND

Hand numbness and pain are extremely common complaints. Usually, one of the three nerves that serve the hand distally – the median, radial or ulnar nerves – is at fault. Hand numbness is also a possible presentation of a more proximal process such as a radiculopathy or plexopathy.

MEDIAN NERVE COMPRESSION

Median mononeuropathy at the wrist (CTS) demonstrates a bimodal age distribution, with peaks at ages 50–54 years and 75–84 years (Bland & Rudolfer, 2003). While older individuals tend to have more severe muscle loss and electrophysiologic changes than younger patients, there is no difference in the subjective symptoms reported (Blumenthal et al., 2006). This raises the concern that older patients are underreporting their symptoms. Although classic median nerve compression at the wrist (CTS) involves the second and third digits the patient often senses that the 'whole hand is numb'. Usually the sensation in the thenar eminence will be spared as it is innervated by the palmar cutaneous branch which comes off proximal to the carpal tunnel and is thus spared. Pinprick sensitivity should be determined by first pricking a noninvolved area and then comparing the sensitivity between sides. Ask, 'If this (the normal side) is 100 percent, how much is this (the affected side)?' It is important not to ask the patient to indicate whether the sensation is sharp or dull because the sharp sensation is often maintained, even in the presence of a clinically significant localized or generalized neuropathy. An additional clue is the presence of Tinel's sign, tingling that radiates from the percussed median nerve at the site of entrapment. The site of entrapment is more distal than is often perceived, approximately 1–2 cm beyond the distal wrist crease (Fig. 33.1). Phalen's sign, in which the wrists are held in flexed positions for 30–60 seconds by pushing the dorsa of the hands together in front of the chest (Fig. 33.2) is often used in examination; however, it is overly sensitive because pain of a nature other than that caused by CTS is often elicited. A particularly misleading 'positive' Phalen's test occurs when the hands turn numb because of the stretching of compressed ulnar nerves across the flexed elbows rather than because of median nerve compression at the wrist. Attention should also be paid to the muscles in the hand that are served by the median nerve, those of the thenar eminence. An obvious difference in bulk and strength suggests significant axonal damage to the median nerve and a prolonged, often incomplete, recovery, even with surgical decompression. It is important to test the strength of the patient's thumb abductors by the examiner opposing them with their own.

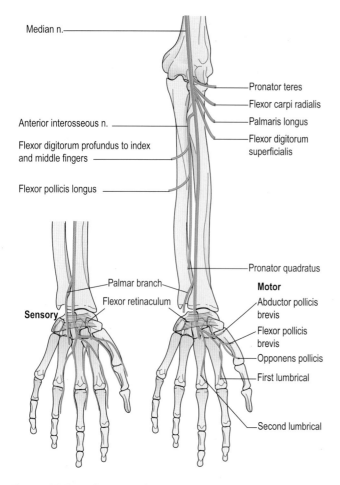

Figure 33.1 Median nerve branches and relationship to the transverse carpal ligament. *(Reproduced with permission from Pectoral girdle and upper limb: overview and surface anatomy. In: Standring S et al. (eds), Gray's Anatomy, 40th edn. Churchill Livingstone Elsevier, Edinburgh; 2008, p. 478.)*

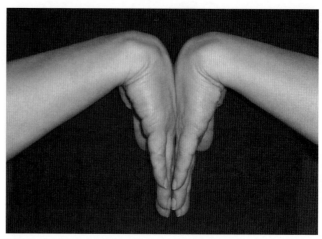

Figure 33.2 Phalen's maneuver for median nerve compression. *(Reproduced with permission from Craig AC, Richardson JK. Rehabilitation of patients with peripheral neuropathies. In: Physical Medicine and Rehabilitation, 4th edn. Saunders Elsevier, Philadelphia, PA; 2010.)*

Treatment

Treatment requires decreasing the pressure within the carpal tunnel. The pressure in the canal is increased in positions of hyperflexion or hyperextension. Avoidance of wrist extension and gripping is particularly difficult for those who use assistive devices such as walkers and canes. The temporary use of forearm platforms rather than hand grips on assistive devices lessens the pressure on the median nerve without compromising mobility and safety. The use of a splint, which prevents flexion and extension, particularly at night when a patient's tendency is to sleep with the wrist flexed or extended, is recommended. Wrist splints are readily available in the community, however they frequently hold the wrist in greater than 30° of extension and may aggravate symptoms. The optimal extension angle is 0–5° and thus the brace may need to be modified, which can be easily done by bending the metal dorsal plate to a more appropriate angle. A patient who routinely uses a sliding board is also at risk. Using splints during transfers may allow continued function without repetitively compressing the median nerve. Local steroid injections may offer relief for those who do not respond to conservative measures. Injections have been shown to

be superior to surgical decompression at 3 months, with significant clinical improvement in both nocturnal and diurnal symptoms and functional impairment. Two injections are usually required, administered 2 weeks apart (Ly-Pen et al., 2005). Injections can be very effective and associated with both improvements in symptoms and in electrophysiologic parameters (Aygul et al., 2005). Surgical decompression may be indicated with severe or rapidly progressive muscle loss, in the presence of a compressive mass, or after failure of conservative measures.

ULNAR NERVE COMPRESSION

The second most common cause of hand numbness is ulnar nerve compression. This occurs most commonly at the elbow. Decreased pinprick response in the ulnar distribution (the fourth and fifth digits), hand-intrinsic muscle wasting and a positive Tinel's sign over the ulnar nerve at the elbow are common findings. When it is severe, hand-intrinsic wasting leads to a characteristic hand position of hyperextension at the metacarpophalangeal joints and flexion at the interphalangeal joints. The interossei of the patient's hands should be tested against the interossei of the examiner's hands so that a true estimation of strength is possible. This is similar to the testing of the thumb abductors in CTS.

Cause and Treatment

The cause of an ulnar neuropathy in an older patient is usually compression at the elbow within the groove between the olecranon and the medial epicondyle, or the stretching of the nerve from a prolonged hyperflexed elbow position (Fig. 33.3) (Kincaid, 1983). The latter often occurs while a patient sleeps on one side holding the hand against the neck and chest. Compression commonly occurs in wheelchair users as forearms and elbows rest on wheelchair arms. Men are more likely to develop ulnar mononeuropathies at the elbow (UME) and older age is associated with greater risk, as is a present or prior history of smoking (Richardson et al., 2009). This suggests that external compression may be more of a significant

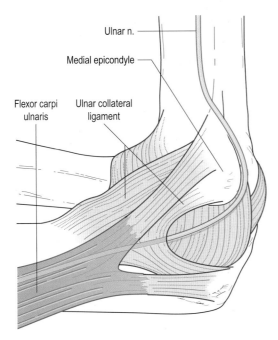

Figure 33.3 The vulnerability of the ulnar nerve to compressive or traction forces is illustrated. *(Reproduced with permission from McGann SA, Flores RH, Nashel DJ. Entrapment neuropathies and compartment syndromes. In: Hochberg MC et al. (eds), Rheumatology. Mosby/Elsevier, Philadelphia, PA; 2010, p. 785.)*

factor in the development of UME in women than in men. Treatment is best accomplished by protecting the elbow with an elastic pad, such as those often used by athletes. The pad can be maintained posteriorly during the day to prevent compression and anteriorly during sleep to prevent hyperflexion. If these measures are not successful, ulnar transposition surgery can be performed to remove the nerve from its usual position over a bony prominence. There are no randomly controlled studies comparing outcomes of conservative versus surgically treated UME. The general practice is to reserve surgical treatment for patients with severe, rapidly progressive neurologic deficit or who have failed conservative treatment (Caliandro et al., 2012). Compression of the ulnar nerve at the wrist is far less common but may occur with direct compression over the wrist and hypothenar eminence. This can be caused by the use of an assistive device, such as a walker or cane, or with wheelchair propulsion.

RADIAL NERVE INVOLVEMENT

One of the pitfalls in the treatment of CTS is the development of a radial sensory neuropathy of the distal forearm. In this situation, the splint compresses the superficial radial nerve over the distal and radial aspects of the forearm. The only clinical consequence is sensory loss as there is no radial motor function in the hand-intrinsic musculature. The numbness that was initially attributed to CTS persists in the second and third digits of the hand despite the splint. At this point, however, the numbness involves the dorsum of the hand rather than the palmar aspect, but the patient may not recognize or report this subtle change. Decreased pinprick and light-touch

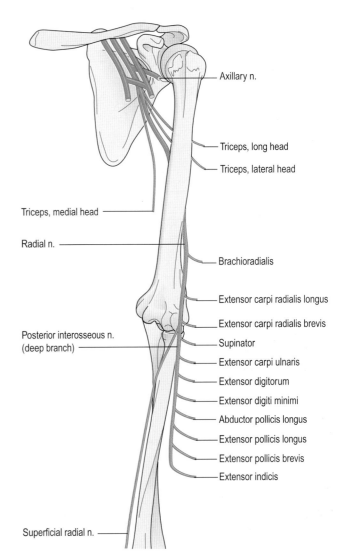

Figure 33.4 The radial nerve and its relationship to the humerus. *(Reproduced with permission from Pectoral girdle and upper limb: overview and surface anatomy. In: Standring S et al. (eds), Gray's Anatomy, 40th edn. Churchill Livingstone Elsevier, Edinburgh; 2008, p. 782.)*

sensation in the radial nerve distribution is noted on examination and, usually, a Tinel's sign can be noted with gentle percussion over the superficial radial nerve in the distal forearm. The CTS signs may coexist or may have resolved. Treatment should consist of discontinuing (if the CTS is resolved) or modifying the splint to relieve the compression of the nerve.

The radial nerve can also be affected proximally. This occurs most commonly following a humeral fracture after a fall by an osteoporotic patient but it can also occur after a prolonged compression of the posterolateral humerus (Fig. 33.4). When the radial nerve is injured proximally, the hand numbness in the radial distribution is accompanied by weakness of the brachioradialis muscle and the wrist and digit extensors (Fuller, 2003). At times, the nerve is not injured acutely at the time of fracture but becomes compressed by bony callus as the fracture heals. This pattern of injury would be most evident to the patient's rehabilitation team. Dynamic orthotics can

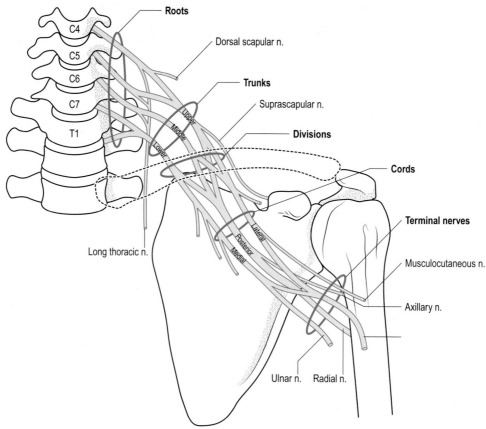

Figure 33.5 The lower trunk of the brachial plexus supplies the hand-intrinsic musculature and supplies sensation to the medial (ulnar) aspect of the forearm and hand; the upper trunk supplies the shoulder musculature and elbow flexors, giving sensation to the lateral aspect of the forearm and hand. *(Reproduced with permission from Wilbourn AJ. Brachial plexus lesions. In: Dyck PJ, Thomas PC (eds), Peripheral Neuropathy, 4th edn. Saunders Elsevier, Philadelphia, PA; 2005, p. 1340.)*

substitute for some of the extensor functions of the digits until the return of neurological function.

BRACHIAL PLEXOPATHY

Another cause of hand numbness that is seen in the older population is an injury to the brachial plexus (Fig. 33.5). Common causes include trauma, tumors and remote effects from radiation, most commonly to the chest and axilla during treatment for breast or lung cancer. Motor vehicle accidents typically affect the upper trunk; the patient's head is laterally flexed and the shoulders depressed. Such patients experience weakness in the humeral rotators and abductors and the elbow flexors, with numbness involving the lateral aspect of the arm and the first and second digits of the hand more than the fifth. Trauma after surgery usually results from the upper extremity being abducted and externally rotated, which leads to excessive stretching of the lower trunk of the plexus. This results in weakness of the hand-intrinsic musculature and numbness in the fourth and fifth digits.

Tumors – metastatic, recurrent or primary – can cause plexopathy. The two most common tumors to affect the plexus are those of the lung and breast. Classically, these tumors cause shoulder pain and a predominantly lower trunk plexopathy with numbness along the medial aspect of the forearm and hand weakness. Except for Pancoast's

syndrome, a carcinoma involving the apex of the lung, it is rare for the brachial plexopathy to be the first manifestation of the tumor. Finally, exposure of the upper chest or shoulder to radiation, for example in lymphoma and breast or lung cancer, can lead to plexopathy. Plexopathy does not occur in every patient who has received radiation therapy, but the likelihood increases with higher doses. Symptoms and signs of plexopathy can occur anywhere from a few months to several years after the completion of radiation therapy. Although it has been suggested that pain and lower trunk involvement are more commonly caused by recurrence of the tumor and upper trunk involvement by radiation effects, it is not possible to distinguish the two based on clinical grounds and a more extensive investigation is indicated. An acute brachial neuritis (Parsonage–Turner syndrome) can occur which may be preceded by an antecedent infection, surgery, or other stress to the immune system. The upper trunk is preferentially affected; however, isolated nerve involvement can occur (Stewart, 2000).

Regardless of cause, brachial plexopathies that are primarily demyelinating in nature can improve rapidly and leave a fully functional limb. Plexopathies that are associated with significant axon loss typically improve slowly and the patient is usually left with some residual weakness and sensory loss. Atrophy is an important clinical clue to significant axon loss; electrodiagnostic studies can determine much more precisely the degree and distribution of axon loss, thus assisting the rehabilitation clinician with prognosis.

CERVICAL RADICULOPATHY

Radiculopathy can be a cause of hand numbness in the older patient (Fuller, 2003). Although C7 is the level most commonly affected by acute disc herniations, C5 and C6 are the levels most commonly affected by chronic degenerative changes, and are therefore the most commonly affected in the older population.

With a cervical radiculopathy at this level the patient experiences numbness over the lateral aspect of the forearm and the first and second digits. Weakness occurs predominantly in the humeral rotators and elbow flexors. In a C7 radiculopathy the third digit feels numb and the elbow extensors and shoulder depressors are weak. With lower cervical radiculopathies (C8 and T1) the fourth and fifth digits are numb and weakness is most prominent in the hand-intrinsic musculature. Atrophy, weakness and decreased reflexes in the proper distribution are clues to the presence of a radiculopathy. In addition, if compression of the nerve roots by simultaneously extending, laterally flexing and rotating the head to the symptomatic side increases upper extremity symptoms and pain (Spurling's sign), radiculopathy is likely. Extension of the neck should be undertaken cautiously in the older patient with vascular or degenerative disease. The addition of axial compression of the head to the above maneuvers, as is often advocated in the Spurling's test, should be avoided in the older patient undergoing rehabilitation. Electrodiagnostic studies should be obtained to assist with specific diagnoses, prognostication and treatment.

Radiculopathies and plexopathies have functional ramifications. Upper plexopathies and high cervical radiculopathies lead to shoulder weakness; this weakness, in turn, predisposes the patient to rotator cuff tendinopathies and impingement. This is particularly true if the extremity is used regularly or is overused, for example during ambulation with a cane or walker. If possible, the extremity should not be used to assist with mobility skills. If this is not possible, the use of a platform rather than a standard cane or walker may be helpful, as these allow the shoulder to bear weight with less internal rotation. C7 radiculopathies cause weakness of shoulder depressors and elbow extensors. As a result, the extremity is much less effective during transfers. It can still assist with ambulation but less effectively and the patient may benefit from a shortening of the cane so that the elbow can lock when the cane is placed on the ground. Lower trunk plexopathies and C8/T1 radiculopathies result in hand and finger weakness. Assistive devices can still be used effectively but compensation for the weakened grip may have to be made. Activities of daily living (ADLs) that require fine motor function become very difficult and adaptive techniques are usually necessary.

STENOSIS AND MYELOPATHY

It should be noted that the same cervical degenerative processes that cause upper extremity radiculopathies in older patients can cause cervical stenosis and resultant myelopathy (Malcolm, 2002); this is particularly true following a fall or motor vehicle accident when the spinal cord is 'shaken' against a narrowed irregular cervical spinal canal. Such patients have weak atrophied upper extremities and minimally atrophied, often spastic, lower extremities; these changes are sometimes associated with bowel or bladder dysfunction. Muscle stretch reflexes give the best clinical clues. Depressed reflexes in the upper extremities associated with hyperactive reflexes and extensor plantar (Babinski) responses in the lower extremities suggest a cervical myelopathy. If this syndrome is suspected, then appropriate imaging studies and neurosurgical consultation are indicated.

FOOT-DROP

Foot-drop, or dorsiflexor weakness, is a common observation or complaint in the older population. Both upper motor neuron dysfunction leading to equinovarus posturing and lower motor neuron dysfunction can cause functionally significant foot-drop. This section focuses on the latter. The common areas of peripheral nerve compression that lead to foot-drop are demonstrated in Figure 33.6.

COMMON PERONEAL NEUROPATHY

The most frequent cause of foot-drop is a common peroneal neuropathy at the fibular head. Older patients in rehabilitation have many risk factors for such a lesion. Common peroneal neuropathy typically occurs in patients with prolonged hospitalization, weight loss, knee replacement surgery, plaster casts and fractures of the fibular head or neck (Fuller, 2003). Severe ankle sprains can cause peroneal nerve injury from traction injury due to tearing of the vasa nervorum (Stewart, 2008). Weakness occurs in the ankle dorsiflexors and evertors. Numbness and decreased sensation are present along the anterolateral calf and dorsum of the foot. At times, Tinel's sign can be found over the peroneal nerve just inferior and posterior to the fibular head. Significant wasting of the musculature of the anterior and lateral compartments suggests significant axon loss and a prolonged or incomplete recovery. Treatment includes protecting the peroneal nerve from further mechanical trauma. Weight gain in cachectic patients and careful positioning in bed to prevent knee hyperflexion and pressure over the area are helpful. As the patient becomes ambulatory, it is imperative that the ankle–foot orthosis prescribed to compensate for the foot-drop does not exacerbate the injury by putting pressure on the peroneal nerve adjacent to the fibular head.

DEEP PERONEAL NEUROPATHY

Less commonly, foot-drop can be caused by a deep peroneal neuropathy. The common peroneal nerve divides into the superficial and deep branches just distal to the fibular head. The deep branch provides innervation of the anterior compartment muscles, which are the ankle dorsiflexors and toe extensors, plus sensation to a small space between the dorsal aspects of the first and second toes. Lesions to the deep peroneal nerve are commonly

1 month and a history of any kind of cancer. Worsening pain at night is almost universal in patients with a malignant cause of back pain, but it also occurs commonly in benign causes of back pain. As a result, the absence of night pain is reassuring and suggests that the source of pain is not malignant, but the presence of night pain is less diagnostically helpful.

L5 radiculopathy can be differentiated clinically from a lesion at the fibular head by a variety of clinical findings. A patient with an L5 radiculopathy usually has the following: weakness in the hip abductors and knee flexors; loss of an internal hamstring reflex on the affected side; a positive straight-leg raising sign (straight-leg raising causes pain or dysesthesia in the anterolateral calf and dorsum of the foot); and absence of Tinel's sign at the fibular head. If the cause of the radiculopathy is not known, appropriate imaging studies should be performed. If the cause is benign, electrodiagnostic studies can provide prognostic information. As the patient begins to ambulate, it is important to use an orthosis to accommodate the foot-drop and also to support the weakened gluteal musculature by using a cane in the opposite hand. This helps to avoid a trochanteric bursitis on the affected side and difficulty during the swing phase of gait on the contralateral side.

SCIATIC NEUROPATHY

The sciatic nerve is made up of both the tibial division and peroneal division; however, sciatic neuropathy frequently presents predominantly with foot-drop due to preferential injury to the peroneal division. The reason for this is that the peroneal division of the sciatic nerve lies in a more lateral and superficial position as it travels through the buttock and proximal posterior thigh and is thus more vulnerable to external forces. Additionally, the peroneal division is more vulnerable to traction injury as it is tethered both proximally as it exits the pelvis and distally at the fibular head. Although in such instances foot-drop, or dorsiflexion weakness, is the predominant finding, close examination usually suggests that there is some degree of tibial division involvement as demonstrated by a decreased ankle muscle stretch reflex or plantar flexor weakness or both. In addition, sensation commonly decreases in both the peroneal and tibial distributions. Risk factors for sciatic neuropathies in older patients include hip surgery, repeated intramuscular injections in the hip, cachexia, malpositioning (hips flexed for too long in the lithotomy position, lying supine on an operating-room table) and a history of trauma to the hip or pelvis. Avoiding pressure over the posterior thigh and buttock is important to allow healing. Ankle–foot orthotics are important functionally but must be carefully fitted to prevent the development of a more distal peroneal neuropathy at the fibular head or a foot wound.

LUMBOSACRAL PLEXOPATHY

Several disorders that are common among older patients can affect the lumbosacral plexus which, in turn, can cause foot-drop. These include radiation exposure, proximal diabetic neuropathy and retroperitoneal disorders

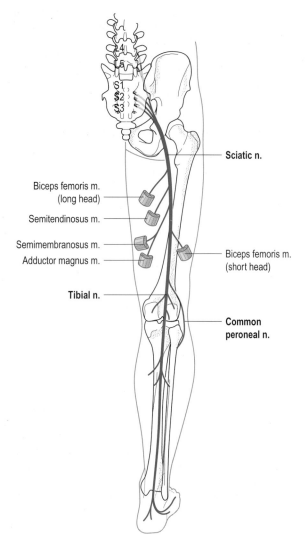

Figure 33.6 The common sites of compression or trauma that lead to foot-drop include the lumbar roots, sciatic nerve near the sciatic notch, and common peroneal nerve at the fibular head. *(Reproduced with permission from Katirji B, Wilbourn AJ. Mononeuropathies of the lower limb. In: Dyck PJ, Thomas PC (eds), Peripheral Neuropathy, 4th edn. Saunders Elsevier, Philadelphia, PA; 2005, p. 1494.)*

caused by anterior compartment syndromes that result from high pressure within the anterior compartment caused by tissue trauma, tibial fracture or hemorrhage. Compartment syndromes are usually handled surgically in the acute care setting. The deep peroneal nerve is not influenced by external compression forces or positioning.

L5 RADICULOPATHY

Another cause of foot-drop is a low lumbar (usually L5) radiculopathy. This can develop as the result of an acute disc herniation, which is uncommon in older populations, or more gradually as the result of degenerative changes. Such patients usually have a long history of low back pain with or without leg pain. It should be kept in mind that tumor can be a cause of back pain and radiculopathy, especially in patients over 50. Clinical clues that suggest a malignant cause of back pain and radiculopathy include an age greater than 50, insidious onset, pain for more than such as hematomas, aortic aneurysms, malignancies and abscesses. Radiation plexopathy does not occur in the lumbar region as frequently as it does in the cervical region. When it does occur, symptoms develop a few months to several years after the radiation therapy and are associated with relatively painless weakness. Proximal diabetic neuropathy typically causes symptoms in the thigh and hip although more distal involvement is possible and will be discussed in a later section (see under Diabetic neuropathy). Retroperitoneal hematomas can occur in any anticoagulated patient; the resultant neurological compromise is usually related to hemorrhage into the psoas muscle. Usually, the thigh muscles are more affected than the distal muscles. Several tumors that are common among older populations occur in the retroperitoneal area and lead to plexopathy. These include lymphoma and carcinomas of the prostate, bladder, kidney, cervix and colon. In 15% of cases, the initial manifestation of retroperitoneal tumors is lumbosacral plexopathy. Sensory and motor symptoms develop, as does pain.

All of these diagnoses have serious ramifications. If foot-drop develops and there are also proximal signs or symptoms suggestive of a plexopathy (weakness of the knee extensors, hip flexors and abductors and numbness proximal to the knee), proper diagnostic studies should be carried out as soon as possible. This typically involves investigation of the area with magnetic resonance imaging (MRI) or computed tomography (CT), and electrodiagnostic studies.

HIP AND THIGH NUMBNESS OR WEAKNESS

Numbness or weakness of the hip or thigh is a common problem in the older patient involved in rehabilitation. If there is no numbness and the complaints are bilateral, a muscular cause such as disuse or a metabolic myopathy is the likely underlying cause. This section focuses on patients who have associated numbness or unilateral symptoms.

MERALGIA PARESTHETICA

One of the most benign and common causes of thigh numbness is entrapment of the lateral femoral cutaneous nerve, often referred to as meralgia paresthetica (Fuller, 2003). This nerve is purely sensory and is vulnerable to compression as it exits the pelvis medial to the anterior superior iliac spine under the inguinal ligament. The nerve then travels distally, supplying sensory innervation to the anterior and lateral thigh. The nerve can be injured during a number of surgical procedures such as inguinal hernia repair, renal transplant, hip surgery and iliac crest bone graft harvesting (Shapiro & Preston, 2009). Entrapment can occur because of belts or restraints and commonly occurs because of thoracolumbosacral orthoses (TLSOs). Anxiety often develops in patients with TLSOs when meralgia paresthetica develops, as well as in their families and healthcare providers, as there is a natural concern that spinal instability is developing along with progressive neurological compromise. Patients can be reassured if the numbness is just over the anterior and lateral aspects of the thigh, and the knee muscle

stretch reflex and quadriceps muscle bulk are maintained. Further confirmatory evidence is sometimes available if Tinel's sign is found when the skin just medial and inferior to the anterior superior iliac spine is percussed. If the diagnosis is clear, no further studies are needed; although electrodiagnostic evaluation can rule out other diagnoses, it is surprisingly ineffective in confirming the presence of meralgia paresthetica and is generally not indicated.

The natural history of meralgia paresthetica is spontaneous resolution. If present, tightness of the rectus femoris and iliotibial band muscle tendon complexes should be corrected and this correction can help to hasten improvement. Avoiding external compression medial to the anterior superior iliac spine will prevent the prolongation of the syndrome. Judicious use of medications for neuropathic pain, such as gabapentin, can bring symptomatic relief. If symptoms become severe or longlasting, injection with local anesthetics and corticosteroids may be helpful; surgical treatment is also efficacious.

UPPER LUMBAR RADICULOPATHY

Thigh numbness and weakness resulting from an upper lumbar radiculopathy are more common among older than younger patients. One of the reasons is that as patients age, the L4/L5 and L5/S1 discs degenerate, decreasing movement at these interspaces. As motion and stress increase in the upper lumbar segments, disc displacement, injury and degenerative changes become more likely. An upper level (L2, L3 or L4) radiculopathy may result. The patient experiences unilateral knee weakness and numbness of the anterior and medial thigh. On examination, there is evidence of muscle wasting, which can be subtle and is best found by looking for side-to-side differences in vastus medialis oblique. Other findings include decreased sensation over the anterior and medial thigh and a reverse straight-leg raising sign. This occurs when the patient experiences dysesthetic pain into the anterior thigh while lying prone and having the thigh passively extended by the examiner at the same time as maintaining knee flexion at about 90°. Imaging studies are indicated in older patients to rule out malignant causes of radiculopathy. If the patient does not improve, electrodiagnostic studies are indicated to provide information concerning the location and severity of the lesion.

RETROPERITONEAL AND FEMORAL NEUROPATHY

Thigh numbness and weakness can result from any of the retroperitoneal processes described in the section on foot-drop. As is true for foot-drop, a careful examination usually demonstrates abnormalities of reflex, sensation or strength in the gluteals or leg muscles and in the thigh, which leads the examiner to suspect a plexopathy. In anticoagulated patients, however, an isolated femoral neuropathy can develop because of a hematoma in the iliacus muscle. The femoral nerve can also be injured during hip procedures, especially ones involving an anterior or anterolateral approach, and in procedures employing the lithotomy position (Warner et al., 2000). For comfort the patient keeps the lower extremity flexed at the hip.

Loss of patellar reflex and knee extension strength on the affected side is usually present while distal strength is preserved; sensory loss may be less remarkable and occurs over the anterior or lateral thigh and medial knee and leg.

GLUTEAL WEAKNESS

Weakness of the gluteal musculature can be subtle and difficult to identify. The superior gluteal nerve innervates the gluteus medius and minimus muscles and the tensor fascia lata. These muscles control hip abduction and external rotation of the hip, which, as mentioned in Chapter 32, is important for balance, particularly when compensating for peripheral neuropathy. The inferior gluteal nerve supplies the gluteus maximus. Injuries of these nerves usually are the result of iatrogenic cause. Up to 75% of patients will demonstrate electrophysiologic changes in these muscles after hip replacement surgery (Abitol et al., 1990). Clinical identification of these lesions can be masked by postoperative pain and weakness, and a clinically significant injury may only be suspected when gait difficulties persist long after the expected surgical healing and rehabilitation time. The persistence of gluteal weakness may be suspected when the patient has a persistent Trendelenburg gait, with pelvic tilt toward the strong side during gait and unipedal stance on the weak side in spite of adequate rehabilitation (Fig. 33.7). If such weakness is noted, particularly accompanied by deep gluteal pain, in a patient who has not had any medical or surgical intervention in the area, this should raise suspicion for an internal compressive lesion such as pelvic mass from colorectal cancer or iliac artery aneurysm (LaBan et al., 1982).

DIABETIC NEUROPATHY

Proximal diabetic neuropathy (also known by other terms including diabetic amyotrophy, diabetic polyradiculopathy, diabetic radiculoplexopathy) is included in this section as the major clinical manifestation often involves the thigh. However, it should be recognized that proximal diabetic neuropathy may involve multiple roots or multiple lesions at the level of the lumbosacral plexus. Commonly, the patient experiences the abrupt or subacute onset of pain in the hip and thigh. Lower extremity weakness soon develops and has a predilection for the anterior thigh musculature. The pain usually diminishes as the weakness develops, and the weakness is often accompanied by dramatic weight loss. Often, the pain and weight loss lead to a search for neoplasm. Most patients have evidence of a generalized polyneuropathy at the onset of the proximal diabetic neuropathy. Similarly, most patients are known to have diabetes when proximal diabetic neuropathy develops but it can be the presenting manifestation of diabetes (Polydefkis et al., 2003). Symptoms are usually bilateral but often so asymmetric that the less affected side is not functionally impaired.

Although there is no clear way to influence the recovery of the nerves from the presumed metabolic or vascular insult associated with proximal diabetic neuropathy, it makes good clinical sense to maximize the patient's neuromuscular anabolism by optimizing glycemic control

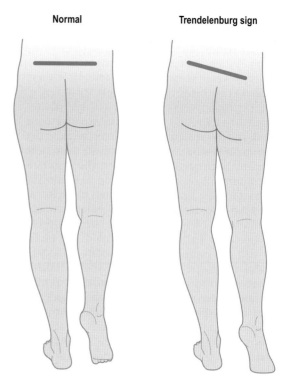

Figure 33.7 Trendelenburg sign suggests weakness of abductors of the hip. The pelvis tilts toward the strong side (right) with unipedal stance on the weak side. *(Reproduced with permission from Fredericson M, Chew K. Trochanteric bursitis. In: Frontera WR, Silver JK, Rizzo TD Jr (eds), Essentials of Physical Medicine and Rehabilitation, 2nd edn. Saunders Elsevier, Philadelphia, PA; 2008 p. 305.)*

and instituting a graded therapeutic exercise regimen. Joint protection with orthotics, particularly to stabilize the knee, is often indicated. Careful education of patient and family to prevent falls is critical, as the majority of these patients have peripheral neuropathy as well as marked proximal weakness. Pain control can be difficult. Tricyclic antidepressants (preferably with low anticholinergic side-effects), anticonvulsants, capsaicin and transcutaneous electrical nerve stimulation (TENS) units may be helpful. Pain lessens after the first few weeks or months and strength returns slowly over a period of 6–18 months. A full recovery occurs in slightly less than 50% of patients, but most have sufficient recovery to develop functional mobility skills. When the patient walks again it is important to avoid superimposed compression neuropathies as described above; the median, ulnar and peroneal nerves are at particular risk.

CONCLUSION

Localized peripheral neuropathies are common complaints; they manifest as numbness, weakness and radicular pain. The common causes of these clinical problems have been discussed for upper and lower extremities. Accurate diagnosis is crucial for prognosis and effective treatment, which is aimed at reducing compression or entrapment; educating the patient and family; teaching the proper use of protective equipment, orthotics or assistive devices; preventing further injury; controlling pain; and restoring or optimizing function.

REFERENCES

Abitol JJ, Gendron D, Laurin CA et al 1990 Gluteal nerve damage following total hip arthroplasty: a prospective analysis. J Arthroplasty 5:319–322

Aygul R, Ulvi H, Karatay S et al 2005 Determination of sensitive electrophysiologic parameters at follow-up of different steroid treatments of carpal tunnel syndrome. J Clin Neurophysiol 22:222–230

Bland JDP, Rudolfer SM 2003 Clinical surveillance of carpal tunnel syndrome in two areas of the United Kingdom. J Neurol Neurosurg Psychiatry 74:1674–1679

Blumenthal S, Herskovitz S, Verghese J 2006 Carpal tunnel syndrome in older adults. Muscle & Nerve 34:78–83

Caliandro P, La Torre G, Padua R et al 2012 Treatment for ulnar neuropathy at the elbow. Cochrane Database of Systematic Reviews 7:1–27

Fuller G 2003 Focal peripheral neuropathies. J Neurol Neurosurg Psychiatry 74(Suppl 2):II20–II24

Kincaid JC 1983 Minimonograph No. 31: The Electrodiagnosis of Ulnar Neuropathy at the Elbow. American Association of Electrodiagnostic Medicine, Rochester, MN

LaBan MM, Meerschaert JR, Taylor RS 1982 Electromyographic evidence of inferior gluteal nerve compromise: an early representation of recurrent colorectal carcinoma. Arch Phys Med Rehabil 63(1):33–35

Ly-Pen D, Andreu JL, de Blas G et al 2005 Surgical decompression versus local steroid injection in carpal tunnel syndrome. Arthritis Rheumatol 52(2):612–619

Malcolm G 2002 Surgical disorders of the cervical spine: presentation and management of common disorders. J Neurol Neurosurg Psychiatry 73:34–41

Polydefkis M, Griffin JW, McArthur J et al 2003 New insights into diabetic polyneuropathy. JAMA 290:1371–1376

Richardson JK, Ho S, Wolfe J et al 2009 The nature of the relationship between smoking and ulnar neuropathy at the elbow. Am J Phys Med Rehabil 88:711–718

Shapiro BE, Preston DC 2009 Entrapment and compression neuropathies. Med Clin North Am 93:285–315

Stewart JD 2000 Brachial plexus In: Focal Peripheral Neuropathies. Lippincott Williams & Wilkins, Philadelphia, PA, p. 117–155

Stewart JD 2008 Foot drop: where, why and what to do? Pract Neurol 8:158–169

Warner MA, Warner DO, Harper M et al 2000 Lower extremity neuropathies associated with lithotomy position. Anesthesiology 5:319–322

Neoplasms

UNIT CONTENTS

Chapter 34

Neoplasms of the brain

STEPHEN A. GUDAS

CHAPTER CONTENTS

INCIDENCE

Primary tumors of the central nervous system have an annual incidence rate of between 4.8 and 20 per 100 000 population; on average, this results in 23 100 new cases and 14 080 deaths annually in the United States of America (Siegel et al., 2013). Between 2000 and 2002, the rates were similar in Canada and Israel for men, and for both genders in New Zealand, Spain and the UK. Deaths in women were less frequent in Canada (2.76%), Israel (3.26%) and Japan (0.72%) (Cancer Mondial, 2012).

The actual age incidence is bimodal, with an early peak in infancy and childhood and another more sustained peak in the fifth to eighth decades. In adults, primary brain cancer is the thirteenth most frequent of all cancers. Because brain tumors affect the organ of intellect, humanity and function, they evoke powerful emotional and psychosocial sentiments. Contemporary neurooncology emphasizes some of the more hopeful clinical features of these tumors. Approximately 50% of patients with primary brain tumors are now successfully treated, many with an excellent long-term prognosis (Thapar & Laws, 1995). Older patients may be treated suboptimally, as comorbidity and age discrimination may influence the treatment choices (Basso et al., 2003; Brandes & Monfardini, 2003; McNamara, 2012).

Some very unique therapeutic considerations govern the diagnosis and management of tumors in the central nervous system, where the distinction between benign and malignant histology is not an absolute concept. A benign tumor of the brain will be just as lethal if it recurs and is surgically ineradicable as one that is similarly located but frankly malignant in histology. The brain lacks a defined lymphatic drainage system; this, in conjunction with the fact that brain neoplasms rarely, if ever, metastasize outside the central nervous system, gives these tumors special significance (Thapar & Laws, 1995). Tumors can be locally progressive and invasive, compressing nearby structures. Cerebral edema, especially in metastatic lesions, complicates the clinical picture and may be responsible, in part, for the symptomatology that is observed.

The exact pathophysiology and etiological features of most brain tumors remain obscure, despite the fact that, in small discrete groups of subpatients, a genetic predilection to brain tumor development has been identified. There is an increased incidence in patients with neurofibromatosis; familiar clustering has been observed (Blatt et al., 1986; Brandes & Monfardini, 2003). However, the fact that as many as 7% of patients with primary brain tumors have a blood relative with a history of a brain tumor is intriguing and demands further study (Thapar & Laws, 1995). Although there is currently scant evidence supporting a viral etiology of brain tumors, the concept cannot be completely ignored, considering the relationship between cerebral lymphomas and the Epstein–Barr virus (O'Neil & Illig, 1989).

Results of studies implicating environmental carcinogens in brain tumor etiology and development have been conflicting. There are some questionable positive statistical associations between brain tumor occurrence and working in the rubber, petrochemical and farming industries. Much work remains to be done regarding the etiology and pathogenesis of brain tumors. Tumors of the spinal cord and pituitary gland are excluded in this chapter; they are much less common than primary or secondary brain tumors, although they are just as important clinically for those elderly individuals who develop them.

CLINICAL RELEVANCE

Brain tumors are classified on the basis of both cellular origin and histological grade. Tumor location, independent of tumor pathology, may be a critical factor governing therapy and prognosis (Taphoom et al., 2005). Although neurons themselves have an extreme tissue density in the central nervous system, they have no reproductive capabilities and, therefore, are rarely the cause of tumors. Glial cells, on the other hand, have tremendous replicative ability and are the most common cell of origin of central nervous system tumors and account for more than half of all primary brain tumors. Tumors may also arise from the meninges, choroid plexus, blood vessels and primitive embryonal cells. Primary lymphomas of the brain, once uncommon and accounting for only 1–2% of brain tumors, have seen an appreciable rise in incidence in the last two decades, partly because they tend to occur in patients with acquired immunodeficiency syndrome (AIDS), transplant recipients and those who are immunocompromised (Roth et al., 2012).

The astrocytomas, graded from I to IV depending on their differentiation and degree of malignancy, are the most common tumors seen by healthcare practitioners. The glioblastoma multiforme is a grade IV astrocytoma, characterized by cellular atypia, high mitotic activity, florid endothelial proliferation and necrosis. These tumors are the classic type that can kill a patient in less than 6 months. They most often occur in patients between 45 and 65 years of age, which is somewhat later than lower grade gliomas (Thapar & Laws, 1995). Oligodendrogliomas comprise 30% of brain tumors and are characterized by a somewhat earlier age of occurrence, slow growth, calcification and indolent course; however, they are still seen in the elderly population. Meningiomas make up approximately 20% of brain tumors, have a 3:1 female–male ratio, occur more commonly in elderly individuals and carry a good prognosis with surgical removal. Regardless of tumor type, tumor recurrence after surgical removal is common and the tumors typically recur with a higher grade pathology, rendering difficult treatment decisions.

The brain has a surprisingly good tolerance for the compressive and infiltrative effects of an expanding cranial lesion but, in time, all tumors produce symptoms via several mechanisms: increased intracranial pressure, compression or destruction of brain tissue or cranial nerves and local electrochemical instability, which results in seizures (Thapar & Laws, 1995). Headache occurs in 30% of patients at diagnosis, and 70% will have headache during the course of the disease. Papilledema, increased intraoptic pressure, occurs in 50–70% of patients and is often detected early. Seizures are the presenting symptom in about one-third of patients and will occur in 50–70% of patients during the disease course.

Tumors in subcortical areas tend to be less epileptogenic. Altered mental status occurs in about 15–20% of cases; this is more commonly caused by tumors of the frontal lobe. Focal neurological signs are characterized by gradual and progressive loss of neurological function – this is especially important when the frontoparietal lobe is involved; hemiparesis and loss of sensation are of interest to rehabilitation clinicians. Tumors of the temporal lobe often cause seizure activity whereas tumors of the occipital lobe, uncommon in comparison to other brain areas, cause homonymous hemianopsia. Tumors of the cerebellum cause headaches, vertigo, ataxia, akinesia, and nausea and vomiting, all symptoms that can profoundly affect function. Many tumors cause considerable brain edema and this increased swelling may result in false localizing signs.

Computed axial tomography (CAT) scans and magnetic resonance imaging (MRI) have revolutionized the diagnosis of brain tumors. The former will detect 90% or more of tumors whereas the latter provides much greater anatomical detail and resolution in multiple planes, and is particularly useful in visualizing the skull base, brainstem and posterior cranial fossa. Cerebral angiography is rarely indicated, perhaps only when excessive vascularity is anticipated in surgery; however, outlining the blood supply of a brain tumor preoperatively can be of help to the surgeon in the planning approach and technique, especially in areas affording limited accessibility.

Metastatic complications of cancer are an escalating clinical problem, with brain metastases occurring in 20% of patients with cancer. Lung and breast tumors are the most common primary tumors, followed by renal cell carcinoma and melanoma (Talouret et al., 2012). Although usually occurring late in the clinical course of a malignancy, brain metastases are being seen earlier in some cancers, particularly lung carcinoma, where it is not uncommon to present with brain metastases as the first symptom of cancer. Tumors are more common in the frontal and parietal lobes because of the extensive vascular territory of the middle cerebral artery. Multiple metastatic lesions, many of them subclinical, are present in over one-half of cases. Solitary brain lesions may present a diagnostic problem in the face of an unknown primary tumor; histological confirmation may be necessary. Unlike primary brain tumors, the evolution of symptoms in brain metastases is rapid, often measured in days to weeks. This may be partially a result of cerebral edema, which is disproportionate when compared with edema caused by primary brain tumors. The symptoms caused by brain metastases are, in other ways, similar to those caused by a primary lesion.

THERAPEUTIC INTERVENTION

Advancing age alone remains a strong and independent negative prognostic factor in glioblastoma. Although there appears to be an increase in aggressiveness of treatment provided to the elderly, the gain for the oldest group is modest at best (Gulati et al., 2012). The treatment of malignant brain tumors is guided by the principle that it is worthwhile to prolong the lifespan of patients, as most of this remaining time is qualitatively good. However, one is cautioned against thinking that glioblastoma therapy is standardized and reduced in the elderly (Nghiemphu & Cloughesy, 2012). Fortunately, serious functional loss tends to occur late in the course of brain tumors. For virtually all types of brain tumors, surgical resection is the most important form of initial therapy. Surgery establishes the tissue diagnosis, quickly relieves intracranial pressure and the mass effect, and achieves the oncological cytoreduction that will facilitate later adjuvant or first-line chemotherapy (Basso et al., 2003; Gulati et al., 2012). Collectively, many advances in neurosurgical techniques, including lasers, intraoperative ultrasound and computer-based stereotaxic resection procedures, have afforded new dimensions to neurosurgical approaches and strategies. Even if not curative, tumor resection is a reasonable goal provided that a neurological deficit is not imposed. Although surgical treatment of high-grade gliomas causes low mortality and acceptable morbidity in patients older than 60, it is less beneficial in patients aged greater than 80 or with poor preoperative functioning (Kongland et al., 2013). Corticosteroids are a mainstay because they relieve cerebral edema, believed to be responsible for much of the symptomatology that is observed. Corticosteroids can sometimes produce dramatic improvements in clinical function and neurological status. The clinician treating a patient on prolonged corticosteroids should be aware of the increased risk of osteoporotic fracture.

Radiation therapy is a proven effective method of treatment for most brain tumors. The elderly may exhibit a poor clinical course and lower tolerance to radiation therapy; therefore, prospective randomized studies should be performed to define the best option for efficacy in light of the toxicity and effect on quality of life (Chinot, 2003; Tanaka et al., 2005). Older and younger individuals do not differ significantly in their response to radiation therapy; therefore, age alone should not be a consideration in decision-making. At the very least, a short-term survival advantage is obtained from radiation therapy and so it is often used in conjunction with surgery in tumor treatment. Recently, Barker et al. (2012) found that radiotherapy and concomitant temozolomide (TMZ) increased the 2-year overall survival rate from 14% to 41%. Effects of radiation therapy can be divided into acute and chronic; the acute brain syndromes seen as a result of edema and irritation of the brain microvasculature are self-limiting and respond well to steroid administration. Long-term chronic effects are fortunately uncommon and they include brain necrosis, endocrine disturbances and neurooncogenesis. The newer techniques of interstitial brachytherapy and stereotaxic radiotherapy employ different radiation physics compared with conventional external beam radiation; they are designed to deliver a highly concentrated, discrete and well-controlled dose of radiation directly to the tumor, sparing uninvolved brain tissue in the process. As the availability of these procedures has increased, so have the favorable clinical results that are reported.

Although chemotherapy has not made major breakthroughs in brain tumor treatment, some brain tumors in children have responded well. Chemotherapy can provide modest increases in survival for some patients but the gains may be overshadowed by other variables, such as age, performance status and neurological deficit. Immunotherapy has some clinical appeal, as brain tumors cause a marked reduction in immunocompetence. The potential use of biological response modifiers is being explored.

REHABILITATION

In terms of rehabilitation, clinical problems frequently arise that are amenable to therapeutic intervention. Any patient with a hemiparesis or other motor syndrome secondary to the tumor or its treatment will respond to therapeutic strategies structured to return and enhance motor function. All neurophysiological approaches are appropriate and may be tried sequentially or concomitantly. The efficacy of many of the standard exercise and facilitative approaches is empirical, and the choice of treatment is sometimes by trial and error. Postural and balance control exercises may be necessary, even in the absence of frank hemiparesis. For balance and coordination problems, location of the tumor may be a factor; rehabilitation may

be more efficacious with cerebellopontine angle tumors than with posterior fossa tumors (Karakaya et al., 2000). Pain management and proper breathing exercises are useful in many patients. Because so many patients exhibit symptoms attributable to brain edema, relief of this complication with corticosteroids will assist the healthcare practitioner in bringing improved clinical function to the patient.

Wheelchair prescription and management, evaluation for assistive devices and teaching skills used in activities of daily living (ADLs) and related activities are tantamount to a good functional outcome. The various therapeutic disciplines should combine their efforts in a team approach, each field contributing its own expertise. Nutrition intake should be monitored to prevent malnourishment, dehydration or excessive weight gain. To this end, patients should be evaluated for dysphagia, as dehydration and aspiration pneumonia can result from swallowing difficulties (Wesling et al., 2003). Nursing must attend to skin, bowel and bladder integrity, as well as infection control. Social interaction with other patients may be crucial to success. Family involvement and teaching are also integral; psychosocial support and intervention are very helpful, especially when the family is confronted with an individual who has altered mental status and severe motor/sensory deficit. Formal rehabilitation in an inpatient rehabilitation center setting is sometimes indicated, and the rehabilitation professional should be available to assist in this transition when it occurs. Patients may make functional gains during and after inpatient rehabilitation, but the gain in quality of life may not be significant until 1 month or more post discharge (Huang et al., 2001). Also, quality of life may not correlate well with functional outcome in rehabilitation.

In summary, the treatment of primary and metastatic tumors of the central nervous system offers unique and challenging clinical opportunities for the healthcare practitioner. Because the clinical course may be prolonged and sometimes indolent, the rehabilitation staff should be on hand to provide the services necessary to bring patients to their highest level of function. Newer and more exciting treatment techniques, particularly in the delivery of radiation therapy, will result in increased survival in selected patients and longer periods when the healthcare professional will be needed to respond to the clinical syndromes and rehabilitative problems that ensue.

REFERENCES

Barker CA, Change M, Chou JF et al 2012 Radiotherapy and concomitant temozolomide may improve survival of elderly patients with glioblastoma. J Neurosurg 109(2):391–397
Basso V, Monfardini S, Brandes AA 2003 Recommendations for the management of malignant gliomas in the elderly. Expert Rev Anticancer Ther 3(5):643–654
Blatt J, Jaffe R, Deutsch M et al 1986 Neurofibromatosis and childhood cancers. Cancer 57:1225–1228
Brandes AA, Monfardini S 2003 The treatment of elderly patients with high grade gliomas. Semin Oncol 30(6 Suppl 19):58–62
Cancer Mondial 2012 International Agency for Research for Cancer, World Health Organization. Available at: www-dep.iarc.fr/. Accessed March 2013.
Chinot OL 2003 Should radiotherapy be standard therapy for brain tumors in the elderly? Considerations. Semin Oncol 30(6 Suppl 19):68–71

Gulati S, Jakola AS, Johannesen TB 2012 Survival and treatment patterns of glioblastoma in the elderly: a population based study. World Neurosurg 78(5):518–526

Huang ME, Warlella JE, Kreutzer JS 2001 Functional outcomes and quality of life in patients with brain tumors: a preliminary report. Arch Phys Med Rehabil 82(11):1540–1546

Jemal A, Murray T, Ward E et al 2005 Cancer statistics 2005. Cancer J Clin 55(1):10–30

Karakaya M, Kose N, Otman S et al 2000 Investigation and comparison of the effects of rehabilitation on balance and coordination problems in patients with posterior fossa and cerebellopontine angle tumors. J Neurosurg Sci 44(4):220–225

Kongland A, Helseth R, Lund-Johansen M et al 2013 Surgery of high grade gliomas in the elderly. Acta Neurol Scand 128(3):185–193

McNamara S 2012 Treatment of primary brain tumors in adults. Nurs Stand 27(14):42–47

Nghiemphu PL, Cloughesy T 2012 Glioblastoma therapy in the elderly: one age does not fit all. Lancet Oncol 13(9):85–88

O'Neil BP, Illig JJ 1989 Primary central nervous system lymphoma. Mayo Clin Proc 64:1005–1009

Roth P, Martus P, Kiewe P et al 2012 Outcome of elderly patients with primary CNS lymphoma in the G-PVNSC-SG-1 trial. Neurology 79(9):890–896

Siegel RS, Nashanham M, Amedin J 2013 Cancer Statistics 2013 CA. Cancer J Clin 63(1):11–30

Talouret F, Chinot O, Metellus P et al 2012 Recent trends in epidemiology of brain metastases: an overview. Anticancer Res 32(ll):4655–4662

Tanaka M, Ino Y, Nagawaka K et al 2005 High dose conformal radiotherapy for supratentorial malignant glioma: an historical comparison. Lancet Oncol 6(12):953–960

Taphoom MJ, Stopp R, Coens C et al 2005 Health-related quality of life in patients with glioblastoma: a randomized controlled clinical trial. Lancet Oncol 6(12):937–944

Thapar K, Laws E 1995 Tumors of the central nervous system. In: Murphy GP, Lawrence W, Lenmhard RE (eds) American Cancer Society Textbook of Clinical Oncology, 2nd edn. American Cancer Society, Atlanta, GA, pp. 378–411

Wesling M, Brady S, Jensen M et al 2003 Dysphagia outcomes in patients with brain tumors undergoing inpatient rehabilitation. Dysphagia 18(3):203–210

Chapter 35

Neoplasms of the breast

STEPHEN A. GUDAS

CHAPTER CONTENTS

INCIDENCE

Breast carcinoma remains one of the most challenging diseases for healthcare practitioners and their patients. The disease's extensive metastatic capability, combined with intriguing responses to treatment, make breast cancer a compelling enigma for all involved in oncology. Until just a few years ago, breast cancer was the number one cause of cancer death in women in the United States of America and it is now surpassed only by cancer of the lung. Similarly, breast cancer is one of the leading causes of cancer-related deaths in many other countries (see Box 35.1). It was estimated that 234 580 new breast cancer cases would be seen and 40 030 people would die of the disease in the US in 2013 (Siegel et al., 2013). Currently the incidence is 122.3 per 100 000. Breast cancer death rates had been stable for over 50 years but have just recently begun to decrease, and this trend continues. Risk-adjusted incidence rates for breast cancer are lower than conventional incidence rates (Merrill & Sloan, 2012). Individuals with breast cancer are now living for considerably longer periods of time, and survivorship has increased appreciably. Screening for breast cancer in the elderly is also important (Walter & Covinski, 2001). The recognition that breast cancer is a treatable disease has set the stage for numerous clinical trials utilizing various forms of treatment; however, there are sometimes barriers to participation in clinical trials for older patients with breast carcinoma (Trimble et al., 1994; Kemeny et al., 2000). These barriers can range from comorbidities in the patient to investigator bias.

The median survival of patients with metastatic breast cancer is longer than 5 years, a considerable improvement from the past (Henderson, 1995; Franceschi & LaVecchia, 2001; Malik et al., 2013). As many as 10% of those who have metastatic disease will live for more than a decade. During this long interval, symptoms arise that may lead to functional disability. Thus, many geriatric patients with breast cancer will have problems related to both the disease process and its treatment.

Breast cancer in the geriatric patient does not differ greatly from that in younger individuals (Balducci & Yates, 2000; Diab et al., 2000). However, older patients have smaller cancers, more infiltrating lobular types, fewer ductal carcinomas in situ, and tumors are more frequently estrogen-positive (Malik et al., 2013). Also, knowledge of breast cancer in those older than 75 is reduced in terms of understanding symptoms and personal risk (Fentimen, 2013). It is common for clinicians to encounter patients with longstanding indolent disease. Considering treatment, women aged 70 or more who are enrolled in clinical trials are similar to their younger counterparts with regard to response rates, time interval to disease progression, survival and effects of chemotherapy (Christman et al., 1992; Dees et al., 2001). Many elderly patients with breast cancer suffer from intercurrent diseases that not only significantly reduce their life expectancy but also increase their operative risk. However, despite a high percentage of deaths from concomitant diseases, long-term survival of the elderly breast cancer patient is possible and comparable to the general population with breast cancer. Admittedly, there is a paucity of data from randomized trials on the risks and benefits of the newer and increasingly effective treatments in the older cancer patient (Jones et al., 2012).

Box 35.1 *The leading causes of cancer deaths in the United States of America, 2013*

MEN

1. Lung carcinoma
2. Prostate carcinoma
3. Colon and rectal carcinoma

WOMEN

1. Lung carcinoma
2. Breast carcinoma
3. Colon and rectal carcinoma

Other leading causes of cancer death include carcinoma of the pancreas, stomach and esophagus in men, and carcinoma of the ovaries, pancreas and stomach in women.

From Siegel et al., 2013.

CLINICAL RELEVANCE

The clinical relevance of breast cancer to the rehabilitation professional is engendered across the disease process: from detection to primary treatment, through a long period of metastatic disease, should it occur, and culminating in terminal patient care. Many forms of breast cancer are now treated with simple lumpectomy, segmental mastectomy or axillary node dissection. These procedures have not replaced the modified radical mastectomy, which is still necessary in many patients (Fisher et al., 2002). In a modified radical procedure, the breast and the axillary lymphatics are removed but the pectoralis major and minor are preserved. The patient is often discharged from hospital with surgical drains still in place, to be removed at the first clinical visit the following week. Although aggressive manipulation of the shoulder may not be indicated during the first few days, a temporary loss of abduction and forward flexion may be commonly observed.

The percentage of elderly patients undergoing immediate or delayed reconstruction is less than the percentage of younger individuals; however, more elderly patients are opting for breast reconstruction when it is feasible (Francheschi & LaVecchia, 2001). When possible, breast-conserving therapy rather than mastectomy should be offered to the older patient (Fentimen, 2013). Age alone should not be a factor in decision-making; the functional abilities and overall health of the elderly patient should take more importance. More extensive disease, such as a neglected or aggressive tumor that becomes attached to the chest wall or muscles, will naturally require a more extensive surgical approach to result in a definitive cure (Zidak et al., 2012).

The functional disabilities seen following mastectomy or breast-conserving procedures are usually temporary and respond favorably to physical therapy intervention. Elderly patients who do not gain their full range of motion within 6–8 weeks following surgery are not likely to do so (Lauridsen et al., 2005). The reasons for this observation are not entirely clear; a sedentary patient combined with an overly cautious therapist may be contributory factors. The window of opportunity to avoid functional decreases in range and function is not a large one, and an aggressive approach may be warranted (Springer et al., 2010).

Edema of the ipsilateral arm occurs in a significant percentage of cases. The incidence of this complication has declined considerably over the past few decades, largely because of early detection, improved radiation therapy and more limited surgical techniques and, most importantly, early and comprehensive management to effect control. In some cases, edema is severe and neglected, resulting in a grossly enlarged upper extremity with resultant loss of range and function. This is usually preventable with active rehabilitation interventions.

Few cancers can match carcinoma of the breast in terms of metastatic patterns; the disease spreads both lymphatically and hematogenously and the latter process can actually occur well before the primary cancer is detected and initial treatment begun. The skeleton is the most common site of bloodborne spread. Lesions favor the axial skeleton because of Batson's vertebral plexus of veins; the pelvis, spine, ribs, upper femora, upper humeri and scapulae are most frequently involved. Lesions are most often lytic, but blastic-predominating and mixed patterns may occur. Large lytic lesions in the long bones

carry the greatest risk of pathological fracture. The proximal femur is the area of most concern. In bony metastatic disease, pain usually heralds positive radiographs. Occasionally, however, pain may be severe in the absence of both radiographic evidence of the disease and scan positivity.

Differential diagnosis is extremely important. A patient who has no specific cause of pain, especially back or pelvic pain; a history of cancer; is awakened at night; gets no relief with rest; and is not responding/presenting like the typical back or shoulder pain patient should receive further workup. If radiography is negative, a bone scan or MRI may be integral in detecting metastatic bone disease.

Occasionally, axillary metastases and local recurrence in the chest wall produce troubling edema and complex wound care problems. More common are metastases to other organs, following or concomitant to bone metastases. The liver, pleura, lungs, central nervous system and intra-abdominal area can all be involved, with each area producing its particular array of symptoms. Liver metastases cause fatigue, early coffee or strong food intolerance, anorexia, metabolic disturbances and weakness – all rehabilitative problems. Pleural effusions are painful, debilitating and require frequent thoracentesis. Chest tubes may be in place, which limit mobility and function. Lung metastases are of several types. Parenchymal rounded lesions eventually coalesce but do not affect pulmonary function or cause symptoms until a critical amount of lung tissue is compromised. On the other hand, lymphangitic metastases, where the tumor is within the lymphatics of the lung, cause an early and distressing pulmonary syndrome of cough, dyspnea and intense sputum production. Metastases to the brain cause symptoms and signs that are comparable to primary brain tumors. Older individuals may not be diagnosed as readily because of concomitant illnesses and comorbidity.

Metastatic breast carcinoma, the second leading cause of epidural spinal cord compression after lung cancer, is a medical emergency. Sudden or subacute onset of sensory disturbances and motor weakness of the lower extremities in a metastatic breast cancer patient with known spinal disease warrants prompt attention. The pattern and degree of weakness may fluctuate and often the neurological condition improves with treatment, which is less likely in traumatic spinal injury. This presents a dynamic and sometimes frequently changing clinical picture to the healthcare practitioner. Metastases of any type will debilitate the patient. Pain may be one of the major limiting factors in any rehabilitative effort and, therefore, adequate pain control is tantamount to successful rehabilitative intervention. Older patients undergoing chemotherapy will need to be monitored for neutropenic infections, anemia and management of mucositis (Carrera et al., 2005).

It is clear that breast cancer is a complex disease process, resulting in a multiplicity of rehabilitation issues that are important for the clinician. Because patients are living longer with treatable metastatic disease, these issues will continue to pose unique and challenging problems to the clinicians who diagnose and treat them.

THERAPEUTIC INTERVENTION

The therapeutic treatment of and rehabilitative intervention in the elderly patient with breast cancer needs to be comprehensive and ongoing throughout the disease process. Preoperative physical therapy screening in a sound clinical practice is important, as the information imparted can do much to allay fears and establish a good clinical rapport with the patient. In an elderly patient, the common existence of premorbid functional loss of range of motion in the shoulder, on the operated side, underscores the value of preoperative intervention when possible. If a preoperative visit is not carried out, a physical therapy visit on the day after surgery is desirable. After a modified radical mastectomy or a lumpectomy with axillary node dissection, glenohumeral flexion and abduction should be limited to 90° until the surgical drains have been removed (Chen & Chen, 1999). Because the hospital stay of all patients having this procedure is short, early and consistent intervention assures optimal functional and physical return. The actual timing of exercise after surgery has been studied by several authors and results suggest that the incidence of seroma formation is not increased by waiting a few days after breast surgery before beginning exercises (Schultz et al., 1997; Nay et al., 1999; Shamley et al., 2005).

A scoliotic curvature is common in elderly women and should be a consideration when treating the elderly patient post mastectomy. This curve may be present before surgery; when the curve results from surgery and the weight imbalance that follows, positioning, trunk range of motion and strengthening exercises, and chest wall and breathing exercises may offset any problems.

Various exercises are utilized to regain shoulder range and function; no single program has proved to be superior to another in terms of functional results. Most regimens call for a gradual stretch of the pectoralis major muscle; pulley exercises and wall climbing are often used (Box et al., 2002; Morimoto et al., 2003). External rotation emphasis, slowly bringing the clasped hands behind the head, is another standard approach. Recall that many geriatric patients may already have a functional loss in external rotation before surgery. Complex lymphedema therapy, which involves bandaging, exercises and specialized massage, can be of immense benefit to patients with lymphedema (Moseley et al., 2005). Early monitoring for lymphedema is essential. The fitting of elastic compression garments has become a large part of the care of these individuals. The success of sequential pneumatic intermittent compression devices to decrease or control lymphedema is variable, even among younger patients. More important, perhaps, has been the acceptance of complex lymphedema therapy into mainstream postoperative care. The program is multidimensional and includes manual lymph drainage techniques followed by specific exercise, meticulous skin care and wrapping with elastic material of specific pressure. Complex lymphedema therapy has gained favor in clinical practice as an approach to lymphedema management, and certified lymphedema therapists should be consulted when swelling is an issue (Hwang et al., 1999;

Marcus et al., 2012). Lymphedema prevention through patient and family education is paramount.

Older breast cancer patients tend to have more bony and soft tissue disease than their younger counterparts and sometimes an indolent clinical course may be seen where bony metastases predominate (Ratner, 1980). However, even in older women with extensive bony disease, the lesions may be largely asymptomatic. Pain is made worse by activity, particularly weight-bearing. If a patient experiences a pathological fracture and is treated surgically or has the procedure performed prophylactically, aggressive rehabilitative therapy is warranted when the patient can tolerate it. Internal fixation of the femur facilitates nursing care, potentiates ambulatory ability and makes transportation of the patient easier. Ease of transportation is important in facilitating limb positioning during radiation therapy treatment. Early mobilization with cautious weight-bearing needs to be instituted and graduated exercises need to be performed for a maximum functional outcome to be expected. Strength and range of motion can be restored and the complications of a bed-ridden patient can be avoided.

Orthotic devices to relieve weight-bearing may be tried but extensive bracing should be avoided in the moribund patient, unless used for pain control. Thoracolumbar stabilization with an orthotic device may be required if the spine is heavily involved with tumor and has become unstable. Patients with liver metastases have poor exercise tolerance and this must be respected, while weighing up the difficulties that accompany the immobile patient. Pleural effusions and lung metastases will respond to chest physical therapy intervention. Epidural spinal cord compression is approached assertively, with all rehabilitation techniques pertinent to traumatic spinal cord injury being applicable. The changing weakness patterns, as well as the fairly frequent and sometimes dramatic motor return that is seen, merit intense rehabilitative efforts. The importance of supportive and palliative care for terminally ill geriatric breast cancer patients is integral to total patient care and is most appreciated by those patients who need it. Lastly, the current development of surveillance models for the rehabilitation of women with breast cancer is paramount, in keeping with integrative medicine and the total patient care concept (Gudas, 2012).

Breast cancer rehabilitation in the elderly patient begins with diagnosis, continues through the early post-surgical phase and is both reactive and active. As metastases spread and cause specific symptoms and disabilities, rehabilitation plays a major role in preventing immobility. Palliative and comfort care round out the intervention and, with patients living for an appreciably longer time, the period of rehabilitative care may span decades. Breast cancer in the elderly is a treatable disease and rehabilitation is an integral part of this treatment.

REFERENCES

Balducci L, Yates J 2000 General guidelines for the management of older patients with cancer. Oncology 14:221–227

Box RC, Reul-Hirshe HM, Bullock-Saxton JE et al 2002 Shoulder movement after cancer surgery: results of a randomized controlled study of postoperative physiotherapy. Breast Cancer Res Treat 75(1):35–50

Carrera I, Balducci L, Extermann M 2005 Cancer in the older person. Cancer Treat Rev 31(5):380–402

Chen SC, Chen MF 1999 Timing of shoulder exercise after modified radical mastectomy – a prospective study. Changgeng Yi Xue Zu Zhi 22(1):37–43

Christman K, Muss HB, Case LD et al 1992 Chemotherapy of metastatic breast cancer in the elderly. The Piedmont Oncology Association experience. J Am Med Assoc 268:57–62

Dees EC, OReilly S, Goodman SN et al 2001 A prospective pharmacologic evaluation of adjuvant chemotherapy in women with breast cancer. Cancer Invest 18:521–529

Diab SG, Elled RN, Clark GM 2000 Tumor characteristics and clinical outcome in elderly women with breast cancer. J Natl Cancer Inst 92:550–556

Fentimen IS 2013 Management of operable breast cancer in older women. J R Soc Med 106(1):13–18

Fisher B, Bryant J, Dignam J et al 2002 Tamoxifen, radiation therapy or both for prevention of ipsilateral breast tumor recurrence after lumpectomy in women with invasive breast cancer one centimeter or less in size. J Clin Oncol 20:4141–4149

Francheschi S, LaVecchia C 2001 Cancer epidemiology in the elderly. Crit Rev Oncol Hematol 39(3):219–226

Gudas S 2012 Report on the status of cancer rehabilitation: reexamination of the findings of the 1990 task force on medical rehabilitation research's panel on cancer rehabilitation. Rehab Oncol 30(3):15–20

Henderson IC 1995 Breast cancer. In: Murphy GP, Lawrence WL, Lenmhard RE (eds) American Cancer Society Textbook on Clinical Oncology, 2nd edn. American Cancer Society, Atlanta, GA, pp. 198–220

Hwang JH, Kwon JY, Lee KW et al 1999 Changes in lymphatic function after complex physical therapy for lymphedema. Lymphology 32:15–21

Jones EL, Leak A, Muss HB 2012 Adjuvant therapy of breast cancer in women 70 years of age and older: tough decisions, high stakes. Oncology 26(9):793–801

Kemeny M, Muss HB, Kornblith AB et al 2000 Barriers to participation of older women with breast cancer in clinical trials. Proc Soc Clin Oncol 19:602a

Lauridsen MC, Christiansen P, Hessor I 2005 The effect of physiotherapy on shoulder function in patients surgically treated for breast cancer: a randomized study. Acta Oncologica 44(5):423–424

Malik MK, Tartter PT, Belfer R et al 2013 Undertreated breast cancer in the elderly. J Cancer Epidemiol Epub 10 January 2013, doi: 10.1155/2013/893104

Marcus AL, Gaalied AB, Ayed FB et al 2012 Lymphedema of the arm after surgery for breast cancer: new physiotherapy. Clin Exp Obstet Gynecol 39(4):438–488

Merrill RM, Sloan A 2012 Risk adjusted female breast cancer incidence in the US. Cancer Epidemiol 36(2):137–140

Morimoto T, Tamura A, Ichihaia T et al 2003 Evaluation of a new rehabilitation program for postoperative patients with breast cancer. Nurs Health Sci 5(4):275–282

Moseley AL, Piller NB, Carati CJ 2005 The effect of gentle arm exercise and deep breathing on secondary arm lymphedema. Lymphology 38(3):136–145

Nay M, Lee TS, Kay SW et al 1999 Early rehabilitation program in postmastectomy patients: a prospective clinical trial. Yonsei Med J 40(1):1–8

Ratner LH 1980 Management of cancer in the elderly. Mount Sinai J Med 47:224–231

Schultz I, Bauholm M, Rondal S 1997 Delayed shoulder exercise in reducing seroma frequency after modified radical mastectomy: a prospective randomized study. Ann Surg Oncol 4(4):293–297

Shamley DR, Barker K, Simonite V et al 2005 Delayed vs. immediate exercise following surgery for breast cancer: a systematic review. Breast Cancer Res Treat 90(3):262–271

Siegel RS, Naishadham M, Jernal A 2013 Cancer statistics 2013. CA Cancer J Clin 63(1):11–30

Springer BA, Levy E, McGarvey C et al 2010 Pre-operative assessment enables early diagnosis and recovery of shoulder function in patients with breast cancer. Breast Cancer Res Treat 120(1):135–147

Trimble EL, Carter CL, Cain D et al 1994 Representation of older patients in cancer treatment trials. Cancer 74:2208–2214

Walter LC, Covinski KE 2001 Cancer screening in elderly persons. A framework for individualized decision-making. J Am Med Assoc 285:2750–2756

Zidak M, Lidak D, Cupurdija K et al 2012 Immediate breast reconstruction in relation to a woman's age. Coll Antropol 36(3):835–839

Chapter 36
Gastric and colon neoplasms

STEPHEN A. GUDAS

INCIDENCE

GASTRIC CANCER

Until 1940, gastric carcinoma had the highest mortality rate of all cancers; gastric cancer was the leading cause of cancer death. Despite the fact that the treatment and overall survival rate for gastric cancer patients in the United States of America has not changed appreciably in the past 50 years, the number of stomach cancer deaths has decreased considerably during this same period (Biondi et al., 2012). In other areas of the world, stomach cancer remains the most common form of cancer. In 2010, the age-standardized rate for stomach cancer deaths in Mexico in men was 5.27 per 100 000. In 2007, similar data from Venezuela showed a rate of 8.37 per 100 000 for men and 5.33 per 100 000 for women. In the UK the respective figures for 2010 are 10.48 and 3.61 per 100 000 (Cancer Mondial, 2013).

Ongoing studies are attempting to delineate the purported dietary factors that are believed to play a major role in the geographical differences in the incidence of stomach cancer. The role of *Helicobacter pylori* remains to be fully elucidated and described (Hunt, 2004). It was estimated that in 2013 there would 21 600 new cases of stomach cancer in the US and approximately 12 000 deaths (Siegel et al., 2013). Stomach cancer is now the third most commonly diagnosed gastrointestinal neoplasm, after colorectal cancer and pancreatic cancer. There is a slight male preponderance and the incidence is greater in older men, peaking between 50 and 70 years of age (Siegel et al., 2013).

Atrophic gastritis seems to be more common in countries that have a high incidence of gastric cancer, an association only partly explained by the natural progression of a dysplasia or inflammatory process to frank cancer. Similarly, there is a slight increase in the risk of gastric cancer in individuals who have undergone a partial gastric resection for peptic ulcer disease. The stimulus for this pathological chain of events has not been clearly defined. Although nitrosamines can produce carcinoma of the stomach in animal experiments, the synthesis of these compounds is blocked by normal stomach acid; however, this may explain the increased incidence of gastric carcinoma in individuals with pernicious anemia and the accompanying achlorhydria.

COLON CANCER

In the US, colon cancer is the third leading cause of cancer death for both men and women, with approximately 102 480 new cases per year and 50 830 deaths (Siegel et al., 2013). This is surpassed only by lung cancer and breast cancer in women, and lung cancer and prostate cancer in men. The average age at diagnosis is between 60 and 70 years (Bader, 1986). In patients with both gastric cancer and colon cancer, two-thirds of cases occur in individuals over the age of 65 (Enzinger & Mayer, 2004). The average survival rate for colorectal cancer is about 50%, and that figure has increased only slightly; older patients have an overall poorer survival (Patel et al., 2013).

There are several known predisposing conditions for colon cancer, the most common of which are ulcerative colitis and familial polyposis. In ulcerative colitis, length of disease is as important a factor as severity of symptoms in the progression of the disease to malignant transformation. If there is a strong predisposition to the development of colon cancer, a partial colectomy with preservation of sphincter function is possible and has been a rather remarkable clinical advance in recent years for the prevention of colon cancer. All patients with familial polyposis will eventually have malignant degeneration of one or more polyps. In the future, with major breakthroughs in the molecular biology of colon adenocarcinoma, medical genetics may be able to define a population of additional individuals with premalignant colon phenotypes to which model systems of genetics and screening can be applied, allowing polyps that are believed to presage colon cancer to be found and treated at an earlier stage.

CLINICAL RELEVANCE

GASTRIC CANCER

Gastric cancer most often arises from the distal portions of the lesser curvature of the stomach. However, there seems to be an increasing trend towards a more proximal origin.

In the US, by the time that gastric cancer has been diagnosed and the patient comes to surgery, the tumor has commonly already penetrated the muscular layers of the gastric wall and can frequently be seen on the outer serosal surface of the stomach (Donati & Nano, 2003; Dicken et al., 2005). The tumor frequently involves anatomical structures that are in close proximity to the stomach, with involvement of the pancreas and the transverse mesocolon being most frequent. In addition, gastric cancer spreads via the peritoneal surface of the abdominal cavity, making survival less certain if ascites or peritoneal tumor implants are present. In almost two-thirds of patients, gastric cancer will already have spread to the abdominal lymphatics when the patient is surgically explored; sentinel lymph nodes are usually involved and are therefore sampled (Donati & Nano, 2003). The gastric area is richly supplied lymphatically and this, along with an intricate mixture of vessels and nervous tissue, results in the rapid spread of the tumor and surgery that is risky and fraught with difficulty. Once regional lymphatics on the greater and lesser curvatures are involved, spread to the lymphatics along the hepatic and splenic vessels occurs and survival is much less certain.

Hematogenous dissemination of gastric cancer occurs late in the course of the disease; dissemination is most often to the liver via the portal vein but other distant sites may be involved. Spread may be asymptomatic; 25% of patients at autopsy show lung metastases, but they are not commonly detected clinically prior to death.

Clinically, gastric carcinoma presents most often with vague epigastric discomfort, postprandial pain or early satiety in eating. Because these somewhat nonspecific symptoms may be attributed to simple gastritis or dietary indiscretion, the elderly especially may delay seeking medical attention. Anemia, weakness and weight loss may all occur, alerting the patient to a more serious source of the discomfort. The physical examination of the elderly patient with gastric cancer may often be unrevealing, except when advanced disease is present (Sial & Catalano, 2001). A palpable tumor in the upper abdomen is not a common presentation but, when it does occur, it is usually a poor prognostic sign. A thorough workup is indicated in any elderly individual who exhibits persistent symptomatology. This is needed to evaluate the patient's risk and optimize surgical, chemotherapeutic and palliative outcomes (Sial & Catalano, 2001). An upper gastrointestinal endoscopy accompanied by biopsy of the suspected lesion will provide the diagnosis in over 95% of cases. Endoscopic ultrasound evaluation is a relatively new technique that shows some promise in that it enables the clinician to visualize all the walls of the stomach (Dicken et al., 2005).

COLON CANCER

Colon cancer spreads through the bowel wall, and the tumor–node–metastases (TNM) classification system has begun to replace the Duke's ABC terminology (related to size and depth of bowel invasion). In classic colon or rectal carcinoma, spread occurs sequentially from the bowel to pericolonic nodes or the rectal mesentery and its

nodes, to more regional nodes and eventually to venous channels. Because of the portal venous system, metastases most often occur in the liver, and much has been written concerning the various techniques and approaches to treat metastatic hepatic disease. The lungs and bone may also be involved, usually late in the course of the illness. Interestingly, direct extension of a rectal or low colonic tumor into the sacral area and eventual involvement of the lumbosacral plexus sometimes occurs, causing varying syndromes of plexopathy or nerve compression. In addition to the carcinoembryonic antigen (CEA) that is commonly followed in these patients, there are other potential tumor markers in the marrow that may be determinants of metastatic proclivity to certain distant sites. Following selected patients for detection and observation of metastatic expression is good clinical practice in the geriatric population.

Diagnosis of colon cancer is difficult despite the more widespread use of the digital exam and sigmoidoscopy, and the use of complete colonoscopy for high-risk patients. Circumferential or 'apple-core' lesions of the lower colon are usually the cause of changes in bowel habits, where almost complete obstruction may lead to a paradoxical diarrhea. More proximal lesions may cause weakness because of anemia from slow blood loss. Melena, blood in the stool, is a frequent and sometimes presenting sign of colon cancer. Frank obstruction is most common in the left colon, where the pain may be colicky. In rectal cancer, the pain may be gnawing and constant, the melena is bright red and tenesmus may occur. Liver metastases may compromise hepatic function, causing the patient to become weak and moribund. Other sites of metastases produce symptomatology that is specific to their location and occasionally function. Aging is associated with alterations in clinical and pathologic characteristics and decreased survival (Patel et al., 2013).

THERAPEUTIC INTERVENTION

GASTRIC CANCER

In gastric carcinoma, surgery is the only effective method of treatment where cure is the goal, and this approach is utilized for palliation as well. Survival rates remain low except in those with early carcinoma, which is not frequently diagnosed. The mortality rate from surgery is the same for fit elderly patients and younger patients (Kemeny, 2004). Biondi et al. (2012) found that 5-year cancer-specific survival did not show any significant differences when younger and older patients were compared. And although there may be no differences in short-term outcome after surgery, the hospital stay might be longer and the major complications rate higher in the elderly (Kimes et al., 2012). All patients are carefully screened and newer noninvasive diagnostic imaging has done much to assist in selectively identifying curable patients as opposed to those who require a palliative procedure. Unfortunately, only 40% of patients can be considered potentially curable. Distal, proximal or total gastrectomy may be performed, with various methods and pouches used to restore or assure continuity of the alimentary tract. Resection of adjacent organs may be required, making cure less likely. Careful abdominal exploration at the time of surgery is necessary not only to avoid unnecessary radical procedures but also to confirm the histological diagnosis. For the 60% of patients who are not curable but potentially operable, some type of palliative resection is usually done to relieve symptoms and prolong survival.

Because the common reason for palliation is anatomical unresectability, radiation therapy is often employed where surgery has failed. Postsurgical external beam radiation therapy may be used to relieve obstruction or control bleeding. Although some surgeons are trying intraoperative radiation therapy, trials are pending or in progress and the results are inconclusive. Many chemotherapeutic trials of various preparations have taken place over the years, with most regimens including 5-fluorouracil (Enzinger & Mayer, 2004).

The patient with gastric cancer usually needs rehabilitation post surgery, including assistance in mobilization and ambulation to avoid complications and to get the alimentary tract functioning again. Barring serious complications, older patients should be mobilized out of bed gently but definitely on the first postoperative day. Mild exercise programs are also helpful in restoring muscle strength and functional mobility.

After recovery from gastrectomy, long-term sequelae are more important than short-term ones. The former includes the 'dumping syndrome', where gastric transit is greatly accelerated; this can result, for example, from the loss of pyloric function controlling food entry into the duodenum. This can usually be controlled by diet and the more frequent employment of gastric reservoirs during surgery. Anemia and accompanying weakness may occur if there is impairment of iron absorption or loss of intrinsic factor when large portions of the stomach are surgically resected.

COLON CANCER

Colon cancer also is primarily treated surgically, with the creation of a temporary or permanent colostomy if the distal colon or rectum is resected (Gingold, 1981). More proximal tumors may allow end-to-end colonic anastomosis, a less radical procedure. During the surgical procedure the entire lesion is removed, analysis of the depth of invasion through the colonic wall is performed and lymphatic drainage is analyzed (Sobrero & Guglielmi, 2004). Intraoperative ultrasonography allows observation of the adjacent and noncontiguous abdominal organs. When utilizing less extensive procedures for low rectal cancer, where a low anterior resection is common, a major limiting factor is the lack of adequate preoperative staging techniques. The inability to define microscopic lymphatic spread contributes to the failure rate of surgical intervention. Sphincter preservation approaches, especially desirable in the elderly, should not result in sacrifice of curative surgical principles. Elderly surgical patients seem to tolerate the surgery reasonably well and chronological age alone is not a deterrent to surgery (Sobrero & Guglielmi, 2004). However, elderly patients may present with a slightly higher incidence of comorbidities, which may affect the incidence rates of postoperative complications (Gross et al., 2012).

The creation of a temporary or permanent colostomy or ileostomy engenders loss of voluntary control of bowel function. Ostomy rehabilitation has become a specialty in its own right, and enterostomal therapists and wound care specialists are called upon to manage postcolostomy care and instruction. The diversification of collecting devices, skin adhesives and related appliances has been remarkable over the past few decades. A regular elimination schedule, skin protection and odor control are a few of the many issues addressed in the postoperative care of these patients. Like gastric cancer patients, the postoperative colon cancer patient needs gentle but persuasive out-of-bed mobilization and exercises as required. Liver metastases are common and the healthcare worker involved with these patients should be alert to the decreased exercise tolerance, generalized weakness and cachexia that can occur. Even patients with widespread metastases from colon cancer can benefit from a therapeutic program that emphasizes exercise, ambulation and pain control.

There have been many clinical trials of radiation therapy and chemotherapy in the treatment of colon cancer. Most recently, it has been shown that concurrent or subsequent radiation therapy and chemotherapy affords a survival advantage and more trials are under way (Wasil & Lichtman, 2005). Evidence suggests that chemotherapy has similar relative effectiveness and safety for patients over 65 versus younger patients in stage III colon cancer (Hung & Mullins, 2013). An interdisciplinary team approach is the best method for supporting and rehabilitating the patient. It is of interest that less than 10% of gastric and colon cancer cases are unresectable at surgery and more than 50% of patients will be alive and free of disease 5 years after treatment (Renouf et al., 2013). These results are encouraging and continue to improve.

REFERENCES

Bader JF 1986 Colorectal cancer in patients older than 75 years of age. Dis Colon Rectum 29:728–734

Biondi M, Cananzi FC, Persiani R et al 2012 The road to curative surgery in gastric cancer treatment: a different path in the elderly? J Am Coll Surg 215:858–867

Cancer Mondial 2013 International Agency for Cancer Research. Available at: www.dep.iarc.fr/. Accessed March 2013

Dicken BJ, Bigam DL, Cass C et al 2005 Gastric adenocarcinoma: review and considerations for future directions. Ann Surg 241(1):27–39

Donati D, Nano M 2003 The role of lymphadenectomy in gastric cancer in elderly patients. Minerva Chir 58:281–289

Enzinger PC, Mayer RJ 2004 Gastrointestinal cancer in older patients. Semin Oncol 31(2):206–219

Gingold BS 1981 Local treatment for carcinoma of the rectum in the elderly. J Am Geriatr Soc 29:10–16

Gross G, Pindi A, Marentano S et al 2012 Major postoperative complications and survival of colon cancer elderly patients. BMC Surg Suppl S20:12

Hung A, Mullins CD 2013 Relative effectiveness and safety of chemotherapy in elderly and non elderly patients with stage III colon cancer: a systemic review. Oncologist 18(1):59–63

Hunt RH 2004 Will eradication of Helicobacter pylori infection influence the risk of gastric cancer? Am J Med 117(Suppl 15A):865–915

Kemeny NM 2004 Surgery in older patients. Semin Oncol 31(20): 175–184

Kimes EJ, Seu KW, Yoon KY 2012 Laparoscopy assisted distal gastrectomy for early gastric cancer in the elderly. J Gastric Cancer 12(4): 232–236

Patel SS, Nelson R, Sanchez S et al 2013 Elderly patients with colon cancer have unique tumor characteristics and poor survival. Cancer 119(4):739–747

Renouf DJ, Woods R, Speer C et al 2013 Improvements in 5 year outcomes of stage II/III rectal cancer relative to colon cancer. Am J Clin 36(6):558–564

Sial SH, Catalano MF 2001 Gastrointestinal tract cancer in the elderly. Gastroenterol Clin North Am 30(2):565–590

Siegel RS, Nashanham M, Amedin J 2013 Cancer statistics 2013. CA Cancer J Clin 63(1):11–30

Sobrero A, Guglielmi A 2004 Current controversies in the adjuvant therapy of colon cancer. Ann Oncol 15(Suppl 14):39–41

Wasil T, Lichtman SM 2005 Treatment of elderly cancer patients with chemotherapy. Cancer Invest 23(60):537–547

Chapter 37

Neoplasms of the skin

STEPHEN A. GUDAS

CHAPTER CONTENTS

INCIDENCE AND CLINICAL RELEVANCE

Skin cancer is one of the most common forms of cancer in humans and kills an estimated 12 650 individuals annually (Siegel et al., 2013). In total, 53% of skin cancer-related deaths occur in those over the age of 65 (Syrigos et al., 2005). The worldwide variation in the number of cases of melanoma (one type of skin cancer) and the subsequent deaths per year for both sexes is presented in Table 37.1 (Globocan, 2008).

Skin cancer tends to be a disease of the middle-aged and elderly (Stevenson & Ahmed, 2005), and age alone should not be an obstruction to seeking optimal treatment. The most common forms of skin cancer are basal cell carcinoma (BCC), squamous cell carcinoma (SCC) and malignant melanoma. Other rarer types occur and the skin can also be the site of metastatic tumors. Sarcomas of the skin can occur and are characterized by clinical heterogeneity. Cutaneous angiosarcoma, myxofibrosarcoma and leimyosarcoma arise predominantly in elderly patients (Mentzel, 2011).

When working with patients, all practitioners should be ever-vigilant for any skin changes that may warrant further evaluation. Careful inspection of the skin of any body part under examination should be part of a complete physical therapy evaluation. Figure 37.1 depicts the differences between common skin moles and skin cancers. Uncertainty in skin cancer risk perceptions is more common in the elderly (Buster et al., 2012). Also, when skin lesions present in the elderly, one needs to examine the presentation, contributing factors and associated systemic disorders (Na et al., 2012). BCC, the most common of the skin cancers, occurs primarily on sun-exposed skin surfaces (those areas of skin exposed to ultraviolet light). Although historically this disease affected more men than women, there is currently only a slight male preponderance. It is commonly a disease of older individuals; however, it is becoming more common in younger people, with some cases being diagnosed in only the third decade of life. Increased sun exposure, as culturally defined, and depletion of the protective ozone layer in the atmosphere, believed to be a result of increased air pollution, are both believed to play a role in the etiology of this disease. Those who work outdoors or who participate in extensive outdoor recreation are at most risk; cumulative exposure to ultraviolet light over time is the strong unifying factor. Ionizing radiation can also be implicated as causative; the resultant BCC occurs after a long latency period and is usually in the area of previous irradiation. The immune system may play an, as yet, undefined role but this is less well appreciated compared with SCC.

BCCs are locally destructive but rarely, if ever, metastasize (Friedman et al., 1995). Metastases usually occur in long-standing head and neck BCCs. The tumor follows the path of least resistance and so muscle, cartilage and bone are invaded late in the course of the illness. The primary lesion may vary in size and appearance but is most often of the nodular-ulcerative variety. The margin of the lesion typically demonstrates a pearly, raised or rolled border, with reactive telangiectasis and central necrosis. The head and neck are the most common locations.

SCC of the skin is a tumor of the keratinizing cells of the epidermis and its behavior is like SCC arising elsewhere in the body. It is the second most common skin cancer and the risk of occurrence increases dramatically with age (McNaughton et al., 2005). For SCC, the

Table 37.1 **Worldwide variation in the number of cases of skin melanoma and subsequent deaths**				
	Cases		Deaths	
	Men	Women	Men	Women
World	101 807	25 860	97 820	20 512
North America	37 959	5941	30 141	3351
North Africa	271	152	280	156
South America	3645	1503	3642	1153
Eastern Asia	3245	1755	2642	1347
Northern Europe	9088	2034	10 031	1566
Australia/ New Zealand	6624	825	4818	399

From the Globocan, 2008 database. www-dep.iarc.fr/GLOBOCAN_frame. htm.

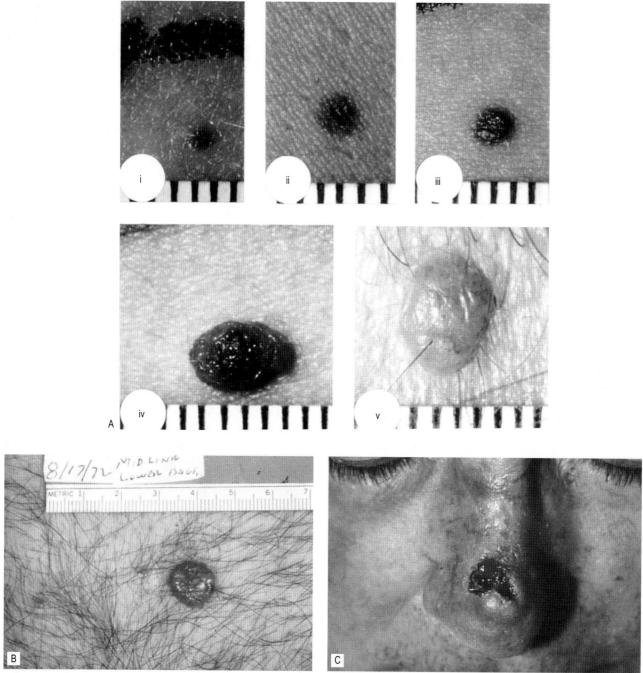

Figure 37.1 The differences between common skin moles and skin cancers. **(A)** Natural history of commonly acquired nevi (National Cancer Institute). Ordinary moles begin as uniformly tan or brown macules, 1–2 mm in diameter (i), expand to a larger macule (ii), progress to a pigmented papule that may be minimally (iii) or obviously (iv) elevated above the surface of the skin, and terminate as a pink or flesh-colored papule (v). These lesions are junctional (i, ii), compound (iii, iv) and dermal (v) nevi respectively. Note their smooth borders and clear demarcation from the surrounding skin. **(B)** Basal cell carcinoma. Small, reddish/brownish papule, often with telangiectatic blood vessels. May appear translucent and, when it is, is described as being 'pearly' in color. May have a central depression with rolled borders. **(C)** Squamous cell carcinoma (National Cancer Institute). Tends to arise from premalignant lesions and actinic keratoses; surface is usually scaly and often ulcerates (as shown here).

mean age at diagnosis is 68.1 and 72.7 years for men and women, respectively, with very few cases occurring before the age of 40. The factors that initiate or promote the development of SCC are the same as those for BCC; both are sun-exposure related and light-skinned poorly tanning individuals are at most risk. Other predisposing factors are exposure to ionizing radiation and chemical

carcinogens, both usually incurred in the workplace. The list of chemical carcinogens is extensive and is growing.

Unlike BCC, SCC has a propensity to metastasize to regional lymph nodes and distant sites. The metastatic potential of SCC is determined by tumor size, location, extent of cellular differentiation, whether mucocutaneous

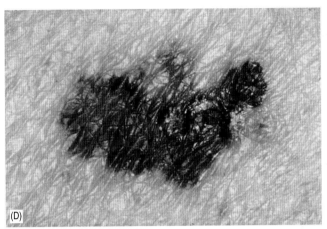

Figure 37.1 (D) Melanoma: color (Skin Cancer Foundation). A melanoma with coloring of different shades of brown, black or tan. Part of the ABCDs for the detection of melanoma.

or purely cutaneous and a host of other factors. SCC tumors may present in a variety of ways, from a nonhealing ulcer to a plaque-like lesion that is raised and erythematous. SCC typically lacks the pearly raised border and telangiectasia of BCC.

Malignant melanoma develops from the malignant transformation of the melanocyte, a cell of neural-crest origin that produces melanin pigment (Testori et al., 2004). It is surprising that the disease is not more common, considering that most individuals have numerous pigmented moles or other lesions. Melanoma accounts for about 3% of all cancers and is increasing in incidence, mainly as a result of increased sun exposure (Swetter et al., 2004). In the last few years, the survival rate has increased from 60% to 84%; this is not only because of newer and more intense methods of detection but also because of improved treatments. Melanoma may appear as a change in an existing mole, with rapid growth, bleeding or a change in color (Korner et al., 2013). However, the lesion can also arise de novo.

Four patterns of melanoma are seen: superficial spreading melanoma, nodular melanoma, lentigo melanoma and acral lentigo melanoma. The last two varieties occur almost exclusively in the elderly and carry a better prognosis because they tend to stay in situ longer (Stevenson & Ahmed, 2005). The nodular type has the worst prognosis because of the great depth of invasion, which may be unapparent at quick visual inspection. Pathological staging of melanoma is based on the microscopic assessment of thickness and level of invasion, the latter expressed as Clarke's level I–IV.

Melanoma does not kill by local extension of disease, but rather by distant metastases. No other human tumor approaches the metastatic potential and virulence of an aggressive melanoma (Testori et al., 2004). Virtually any organ in the body can be invaded but the regional lymph nodes are often involved first. Distant sites that can be invaded are the brain, lung and bone. Prognostic factors are multiple and variable, and depend on the stage of the disease at diagnosis. Tumor thickness is the most important and dominant variable; other factors include site, sex,

age of the patient, ulceration, number of nodes involved and length of disease. Older patients may not seek treatment and diagnosis early compared with younger individuals with pigmented tumors (Testori et al., 2004). Melanomas can metastasize years after the primary lesion has been successfully treated, a fact not often appreciated among healthcare workers.

THERAPEUTIC INTERVENTION

BCC and SCC are treated primarily by either surgery or radiotherapy. Curettage and electrodessication are commonly used for small tumors, with total surgical excision saved for larger lesions. The Mohs micrographic technique, a method employed for SCC and BCC, allows maximum conservation of normal tissues. Wide surgical margins are necessary; the fact that BCC and SCC can spread deeply into the tissue must be respected and recognized in surgical treatment procedures. Alternative removal methods include lasers, cryosurgery and radiation therapy, the last being a paradoxical method of treatment as it can also induce the development of cancer. Radiation therapy is best used for small lesions or in patients who cannot or will not tolerate a surgical procedure.

Both SCC and BCC can be treated with these methods but the propensity for SCC to metastasize must be considered. All therapies are designed to result in total tumor removal, the primary goal in treating these cancers. Recurrence rates are high in certain areas and in certain histological variants; this may call for more extensive surgery or an alternate technique. Many older individuals can be freed from tumors with the techniques described above. Follow-up visits are essential to promptly diagnose recurrent or new primary tumors. A person who has had at least one BCC or SCC is at a higher risk of developing a second tumor; careful vigilance and frequent skin checks are necessary.

Malignant melanoma demands some special consideration regarding treatment, as regional lymph node involvement may be high and subclinical, and the relatively strong metastatic potential of these tumors must be taken into account in treatment planning. A therapeutic node dissection is employed in stage III (large and/or deep primary lesion) patients, whether or not the nodes are clinically involved. Specific guidelines have been established for the accepted surgical margin, depending on thickness and size of the primary lesion. Patients undergoing a prophylactic or definitive groin dissection for a melanoma of the lower extremity are prone to lymphedema, and complex lymphedema evaluation and therapy are indicated. Most patients are fitted with a compression garment. Patients with enlarged regional nodes have a greater than 85% chance of having hematogenous dissemination of their cancer, and the survival rate at 10 years is less than 10%.

The response rates of metastatic melanoma to chemotherapy are encouraging, and many trials are being conducted to determine optimal drugs and dose scheduling. Immunotherapy and gene therapy have been studied in melanoma more than in other tumors, with varying degrees of patient response and success. All of the approaches are really experimental but can provide palliation and relief of distressing symptoms. Unfortunately, cures are few once the disease has metastasized to distant areas. This drives and underscores the importance of the intense research that is carried out into melanoma.

BCC and SCC are treated with chemotherapy and other methods when the disease is extensive or unresectable, or when there are local or distant metastases. Healthcare practitioners can do much to assist the patient in treatment planning and decision-making. It is of note that, because of the common location of tumors on the head and neck and exposed areas, and the sometimes cosmetically disfiguring surgery that is required for their removal, psychosocial intervention is important to total patient care. Noncomplicated surgical removal does not usually require rehabilitation intervention, except where function is compromised or the surgery is extensive. Caution should be utilized when applying manual stretching techniques, massage, heat or electrical stimulation to areas of previous surgery or when using exercise techniques. The surgical site should be examined carefully.

Like lung cancer, skin cancer is largely preventable. Healthcare practitioners should assist in efforts to educate the public in limiting sun exposure and reducing their exposure to chemical carcinogens that can cause skin tumors.

REFERENCES

Buster KS, Tou Z, Fouad M et al 2012 Skin cancer risk perceptions: a comparison across ethnicity, age, education, gender, and income. J Am Acad Dermatol 66(5):771–779

Friedman RJ, Rigel DS, Nossa R et al 1995 Basal cell and squamous cell carcinoma of the skin. In: Murphy GP, Lawrence WL, Lenmhard E (eds) American Cancer Society Textbook on Clinical Oncology, 2nd edn. American Cancer Society, Atlanta, GA, pp. 330–342

Globocan 2008 Melanomas of the skin in males and females. www-dep.iarc.fr/GLOBOCAN_frame.htm

Korner A, Coroiu A, Martins C et al 2013 Predictors of skin self examination before and after a melanoma diagnosis: the role of medical advice and patient's level of education. Int Arch Med 6(1):8

McNaughton SA, Marks GC, Green AC 2005 Role of dietary factors in the development of basal cell carcinoma and squamous cell carcinoma of the skin. Cancer Epidemiol Biomarkers Prev 14(7):1596–1607

Mentzel T 2011 Sarcomas of the skin in the elderly. Clin Dermatol 29(1):80–90

Na CR, Wang S, Kirnser RS 2012 Elderly adults and skin disorders: common problems for non-dermatologists. South Med J 105(11):600–606

Siegel RS, Nashanham M, Amedin J 2013 Cancer statistics 2013. CA Cancer J Clin 63(1):11–30

Stevenson D, Ahmed J 2005 Lentigo melanoma: prognosis and treatment options. Am J Clin Dermatol 6(3):151–164

Swetter SM, Geller AC, Kirkwood JM 2004 Melanoma in the older person. Oncology 18(9):1187–1196

Syrigos KN, Tzannov I, Katirtzoglov N et al 2005 Skin cancer in the elderly. In Vivo 19(3):643–652

Testori A, Stanganelli I, DellaGrazia L et al 2004 Diagnosis of melanoma in the elderly and surgical implications. Surg Oncol 13(40):211–221

Chapter 38
Neoplasms of the prostate

STEPHEN A. GUDAS

INCIDENCE

Prostate cancer is the most common male cancer in the US, accounting for approximately 32% of all newly diagnosed cancers in men (Siegel et al., 2013). It is also the second leading cause of cancer deaths in men in the United States of America, accounting for 13% of all male cancer deaths (Koys & Bubley, 2001; Calabrese, 2004). In 2005, it is estimated that there were 238 590 new cases of prostate cancer diagnosed in the US, with 29 720 deaths (Siegel et al., 2013). The rates of prostate cancer vary between different populations (Table 38.1), and there are factors that may lead to familial clustering of cases (Gronberg, 2003). The median age of onset is 70 years, making it a distinct geriatric problem; the incidence increases for each decade after the age of 50. It is a curious fact that the incidence of prostate cancer peaked in the mid 1990s and has decreased slightly since that time (Brawley, 2012). This is rather constant across cultures and countries, although the incidence of frank prostatic cancer is low in Japan, for example. With the aging of the population, it is expected that the incidence of prostate cancer will rise.

Although the exact etiology of prostate cancer is unknown, there appears to be a hormonal relationship as many tumors respond to orchiectomy, implying that testosterone augments cancer growth in men. Cancer of the prostate has been found to occur at a disproportionately higher rate in certain industrial workers – those who work with cadmium, tire and rubber, and sheet metal (Carter, 1989). Familial factors may play a role but this has not been fully elucidated.

CLINICAL RELEVANCE

Almost 60% of prostate cancer patients will have clinically localized cancer at diagnosis, making cure a real possibility. Frequently, resectable tumors are asymptomatic or patients have a few symptoms of urinary tract obstruction, such as difficulty in initiating and/or stopping micturition. In the absence of infection, marked bladder symptoms should warrant a search for prostate cancer. If the clinical presentation is advanced, there will be symptoms of bladder outlet obstruction and anuria, uremia, anemia and anorexia will ensue. Patients are very ill at this juncture and most will have sought medical attention.

The digital rectal exam still finds most primary prostate cancerous tumors. Approximately 50% of palpable nodules in the prostate are proven to be carcinomas. The prostate-specific antigen (PSA) is a prostate marker that is useful in the early detection of prostate cancer (Catalona et al., 1991; Stenman et al., 2005). PSA levels are determined after a nodule is palpated on digital examination. If the level of PSA is above 10 ng/ml, there is a 66% chance that a subsequent biopsy will be positive. PSA levels are widely used as a screening tool for the general geriatric male population, but the PSA is a prostate specific antigen, not a prostate cancer specific antigen, and thus can be elevated in other conditions (Heinzer & Steuber, 2009). A baseline PSA should be taken in men after the age of 50 and repeated at intervals. Continued investigation will be necessary to determine the true value of both screening and clinical staging procedures (see Fig. 38.1 for a representation of staging for prostate cancer). Prostatic acid phosphatase (PAP) is used to detect metastatic disease, as elevated levels signify spread to at least the lymph nodes (Syrigos et al., 2005).

Prostate carcinoma, like breast and lung cancer, spreads both lymphatically and hematogenously, with

Table 38.1 **Worldwide variation in rates of prostate cancer deaths, 2010**	
Country	Crude Rate Per 100 000 Population
Australia/New Zealand	27.4
Canada	22.5
China	0.9
Ecuador	11.46
Egypt	1.57
Iraq	1.5
Republic of South Africa	9.5
United Kingdom	33.5
United States of America	22.8

Source: Cancer Mondial, 2013.

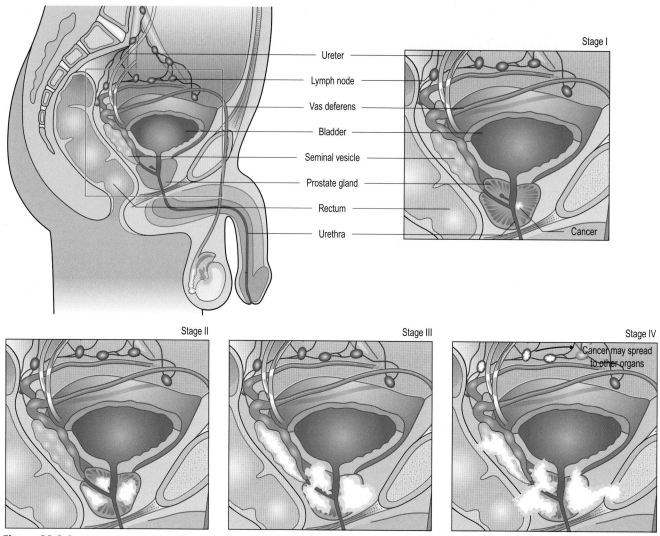

Figure 38.1 Prostate cancer staging. Drawing showing a side view of normal male anatomy and close-up views of stage I, stage II, stage III and stage IV cancer. As prostate cancer progresses from stage I to stage IV, the cancer cells grow within the prostate, through the outer layer of the prostate into nearby tissue and then to lymph nodes or other parts of the body. *(With permission from the National Cancer Institute. Original drawing by Terese Winslow.)*

the regional lymphatics involved in over 60% of cases at diagnosis. Most patients who die of prostate cancer have relatively successful local tumor control. Metastatic disease develops in the vast majority of fatal cases and, as in breast cancer, the favored site is the bone. Similarly to tumors of the chest or chest wall, Batson's vertebral plexus of veins allows easy access to the axial skeleton. In total, 70% of patients develop bony metastases, most commonly in the sacrum, pelvis, lumbar spine and femur (Winell & Roth, 2005). The osseous metastases may cause considerable pain and disability, making management of these patients a challenging clinical problem. For reasons that are not entirely clear, the metastases are usually osteoblastic rather than osteolytic, and occasionally mixed patterns are seen. For this reason, pathological fracture through metastatic lesions is seen much less frequently in prostate carcinoma than in metastatic breast or lung cancer. Bony pain, however, may be severe and out of proportion to the extent of bone involvement or the number of bones involved.

Spinal involvement may lead to epidural spinal cord compression (Benjamin, 2002). As in breast and lung cancer, this complication has increased markedly, partly because of the fact that patients are living longer with spinal disease, long enough to develop the complication. Epidural spinal cord compression is treated in the same way as compression arising from other primary tumors; full spinal cord rehabilitation efforts are employed, as tolerated by the patient. Surgery plus radiation therapy was found to be better than radiation alone in allowing patients to remain ambulatory and continent.

Other distant organs may be involved, usually late in the disease course, with the lungs, liver and pleura the most common sites (Hall et al., 2005). Occasionally, prostate cancer can spread beyond the regional pelvic lymph nodes to other lymphatics, such as lumbar, para-aortic and even mediastinal and chest nodes. Patients with widespread metastatic disease from prostate cancer are quite debilitated and appear older than their stated age.

THERAPEUTIC CONSIDERATIONS

Although, at present, there is no cure for patients with extensive bone or visceral metastases, surgery, radiation therapy, hormonal therapy and chemotherapy have all been used to combat this disease with varying degrees of success. A radical prostatectomy through the retropubic route is the surgical method of choice; this involves resection of the prostate gland, seminal vesicles and a section of the bladder neck. At the time of this procedure, pelvic lymph nodes are removed and sampled for tumor involvement. Although pelvic lymphadenectomy is not therapeutically curative when spread is present, it offers palliation and allows for precise staging, as these nodes are the first sites of metastatic disease in the majority of cases. A laparoscopic approach to the pelvic node dissection can be employed in patients with suspected node involvement but for whom radical prostatectomy is not an option. A nerve-sparing procedure is employed, in which the capsular and periprostatic nerves are spared, and offers a greater chance for preserving potency in many patients. In the past, impotence was an almost certain operative sequel in radical prostatectomy. Even in older individuals preservation of sexual function can be an important issue that needs to be addressed so that appropriate psychosocial intervention can be begun, if desired.

Highly focused modern radiotherapeutic techniques enable a large dose of radiation (60–70 Gy) to be delivered to the patient with relatively little morbidity. Pelvic lymph nodes can also be irradiated. However, the major role of radiation therapy is still to control bone pain from metastases, at which it is extremely effective. Patients can also undergo a surgical or chemical orchiectomy with good local or systemic control of disease for 2–3 years (Pienta & Smith, 2005). The 10-year mortality for high risk prostate cancer treated with radiation therapy alone is 30%; combining radiation with androgen deprivation therapy increases this significantly (Payne & Huges, 2012). A wide variety of chemotherapeutic agents have been employed and it is currently accepted that chemotherapy increases survival in patients with hormone-refractory prostate carcinoma. Current regimens employ docetaxel, mixantrone and zolendromic acid. No schedule of drugs is uniformly efficacious and research in this area continues. Cancer cells exist in complex humeral microenvironments that afford multiple therapeutic targets. Bisphosphonates, which inhibit osteoclast action, have been shown to be effective in hormone-refractory prostate cancer (Pienta & Smith, 2005).

It appears that both radiation therapy and surgery are equally effective, especially in early disease. For large tumors, with expected spread beyond the prostate gland, biological recurrence is seen in 90% of patients at the end of 3 years. On occasion, the clinical course of prostate cancer is indolent and carries a slow decline in function and mobility. There will be comorbidities in the elderly and extensive bony lesions notoriously lead to general debilitation.

In terms of rehabilitation, it is important to remember that patients with prostate cancer, even the elderly, will generally survive for more than 1–2 years and that therapeutic intervention, designed to maximize function and mobility, are standard in patient management. For patients who undergo surgical treatment, it is important to begin gentle exercises and assume the erect bipedal posture as soon as possible because postoperative pain encourages hip/trunk flexion, which may develop into contractures. Severe spinal involvement may lead to restricted motion and a bedfast condition, and even turning and positioning may require assistance. Most patients are elderly and, as mentioned previously, they will have concomitant diseases that themselves influence function. Light range of motion exercises and ambulation with appropriate assistive devices, usually a walker, can both be used and should be encouraged in all patients. Examples of appropriate exercises are active shoulder abduction and flexion, scapular mobilization and active hip flexion and knee flexion from supine. Although bony lesions are usually osteoblastic, lytic lesions may occur and fractures are treated accordingly. Orthotic devices to stabilize the spine in extensive disease tend not to be tolerated well in the elderly and weight and pressure of a brace may actually aggravate symptoms and bone pain in some patients. Degenerative joint disease of the spine may complicate the clinical picture. Transcutaneous electrical nerve stimulation (TENS) can be used on occasion for pain control, lessening the amount of narcotics needed for effective analgesia.

Hospice care in terminal disease is paramount to excellent patient care. Men dying of prostate cancer enrolled in a hospice were less likely to receive high intensity care, i.e. ICU admissions, inpatient stays or emergency department visits (Bergman et al., 2011).

In summary, in the US, prostate carcinoma ranks as number one for incidence and number two for cancer deaths in men. With the possibility of diagnosing the illness in its early stages, when it is confined to the prostate itself and therefore curable by surgery/radiation, many more survivors of prostate cancer will be found among the elderly. New developments need to be specifically applied to elderly patients with advanced prostate cancer (Mukherji et al., 2013). Optimal care of the older patient with recurrent prostate cancer now involves more of a decision process (Kessler & Flaig, 2012). The unique needs of the older population must always be considered in treatment choices. Prostate cancer is an example of a cancer that demonstrates both an increase in survival rates and the length of survival time. Healthcare practitioners will need to respond with appropriate interventions and treatments to assure that this trend continues.

REFERENCES

Benjamin R 2002 Neurologic complications of prostate cancer. Am Fam Physician 65(9):1834–1840

Bergman J, Seigal CS, Lorenz KA et al 2011 Hospice use and high intensity care in men dying of prostate cancer. Arch Intern Med 171(3):204–211

Brawley W 2012 Trends in prostate cancer in the United States. J Natl Cancer Inst Monogr 2012(45):152–156

Calabrese DA 2004 Prostate cancer in older men. Urol Nurs 24(4):258–264

Cancer Mondial 2013 International Agency for Cancer Research. www-dep.iarc.fr/

Carter BS 1989 Epidemiologic evidence regarding predisposing factors to prostate cancer. Prostate 16:187–194

Catalona WJ, Smith DS, Ratliff TL et al 1991 Measurement of prostate-specific antigen in serum as a screening test for prostate cancer. N Engl J Med 324:1156–1160

Gronberg H 2003 Prostate cancer epidemiology. Lancet 361:859–864

Hall WH, Jani AB, Ryu JK et al 2005 The impact of age and comorbidity on surgical outcomes and treatment patterns in prostate cancer. Prostate Cancer Prostatic Dis 8(1):22–30

Heinzer H, Steuber T 2009 Prostate cancer in the elderly. Urol Oncol 27(6):668–672

Kessler ER, Flaig TW 2012 Optimal management of recurrent prostate cancer in older patients. Drugs Aging 29(11):871–873

Koys J, Bubley GJ 2001 Prostate cancer in the older man. Oncology 15:1113–1119

Mukherji D, Pexano CJ, Shamseddine A et al 2013 New treatment developments applied to elderly patients with advanced prostate cancer. Cancer Treat Rev 39(6):578–583

Payne HA, Hughes S 2012 Radical radiotherapy for high risk prostate cancer in older men. Oncologist 17(Suppl 1):9–15

Pienta J, Smith DC 2005 Advances in prostate cancer chemotherapy: a new era begins. Cancer J Clin 55(5):300–318

Siegel RS, Nashanham M, Amedin J 2013 Cancer statistics 2013. CA Cancer J Clin 63(1):11–30

Stenman UH, Abrahamson PA, Ari G 2005 Prognostic value of serum markers for prostate cancer. Scand Urol Nephrol Suppl 216:64–81

Syrigos KN, Karapanagiotov E, Harrington KJ 2005 Prostate cancer in the elderly. Anticancer Res 25(6c):4527–4533

Winell J, Roth AJ 2005 Psychiatric assessment and symptom management in elderly cancer patients. Oncology 19(11):1479–1490

Cardiopulmonary disease

Chapter 39

Exercise considerations for aging adults

PAMELA REYNOLDS

CHAPTER CONTENTS

INTRODUCTION

All exercise requires the coordinated function of both the heart and lungs, as well as the peripheral and pulmonary circulations, to transport nutrients and exchange the oxygen required to support muscular contraction and movement. Age-related cardiovascular and pulmonary changes have been described earlier (see Chapters 6, 7 and 9). This chapter primarily presents an overview of endurance or aerobic exercise considerations for normal age-related changes. Other chapters discuss appropriate exercise interventions for specific cardiovascular and pulmonary pathologies (see Chapters 42–45) as well as additional information related to muscle strengthening (see Chapter 16).

The availability of oxygen and the body's ability to utilize it during physical activity is a key performance factor of therapeutic exercise and related interventions. The Fick equation, $\dot{V}O_2 = CO \times a - vo_2$, concisely represents this concept, where $\dot{V}O_2$ represents the volume of oxygen/min/unit of body weight that is utilized during a specific activity; CO is cardiac output; and a–vo$_2$ is arteriovenous difference. $\dot{V}O_{2(max)}$ is the maximum amount of oxygen that the body can obtain and utilize for any physical activity. This can also be described as a person's physical fitness level or functional capacity. The amount of oxygen that the body can obtain and effectively utilize is dependent on two factors: (i) the delivery of oxygen-rich blood to metabolically active tissues, especially muscles; and (ii) the ability of these tissues to extract and utilize the delivered oxygen. The delivery factor or central component is dependent on CO, which is a product of heart rate (HR) and stroke volume (SV). The peripheral component is represented by the arteriovenous difference (a–vo$_2$), or the difference between the oxygen content of the arterial blood entering the metabolically active tissue and the amount of oxygen left in the venous blood that is returned to the heart. Cardiopulmonary dysfunctions are usually a result of impairments in the delivery system (McArdle et al., 2011).

EXERCISE CONSIDERATIONS

When developing an exercise program or prescription, it is important to consider the following:

- medical screening or clearance
- informed consent
- baseline functional capacity
- consideration of the mode, intensity, frequency and duration
- gradual progression
- safety
- motivation
- regular reevaluation.

SCREENING AND INFORMED CONSENT

Aging has some immutable factors that increase a person's risk for exercise. Many disorders do not demonstrate significant clinical signs during regular daily activities but they may become evident during exercise. The American College of Sports Medicine (ACSM, 2010) identifies men and women as having low cardiovascular disease if they are asymptomatic and have one or less risk factor listed in Table 39.1. Note that age is a positive risk factor for men ≥45 years and women ≥55 years. Men and women who are asymptomatic and have two or more cardiovascular risk factors are categorized as having moderate risk. Any individual who has known or symptomatic cardiovascular, pulmonary, of metabolic disease or has one or more of the symptoms listed in Box 39.1, is considered at high risk for cardiovascular disease.

After establishing risk category, the recommendation for medical examination and need for physician supervision during graded exercise testing can be determined. See Figure 39.1 for this information from the ACSM.

For the elderly in the moderate-risk category only, who plan to engage in moderate exercise training, medical screening is not necessary. Moderate exercise training

Table 39.1 Atherosclerotic cardiovascular disease (CVD) risk factor thresholds for use with ACSM risk stratification

Positive Risk Factors	Defining Criteria
Age	Men ≥45 yr, Women ≥55 yr
Family history	Myocardial infarction, coronary revascularization, or sudden death before 55 yr of age in father or other male first-degree relative, or before 65 yr of age in mother or other female first-degree relative
Cigarette smoking	Current cigarette smoker or those who quit within the previous 6 months or exposure to environmental tobacco smoke
Sedentary lifestyle	Not participating in at least 30 min of moderate intensity (40%–60% $\dot{V}O_2R$) physical activity on at least 3 days of the week for at least 3 months
Obesity[a]	Body mass index ≥30 kg/m² *or* waist girth >102 cm (40 inches) for men and >88 cm (35 inches) for women
Hypertension	Systolic blood pressure ≥140 mmHg and/or diastolic ≥90 mmHg, confirmed by measurements on at least two separate occasions, *or* on antihypertensive medication
Dyslipidemia	Low-density lipoprotein (LDL-C) cholesterol ≥130 mg/dl (3.37 mmol/l) *or* high density lipoprotein (HDL-C) cholesterol <40 mg/dl (1.04 mmol/l) *or* on lipid lowering medication. If total serum cholesterol is all that is available use ≥200 mg/dLl (5.18 mmol/l)
Prediabetes	Impaired fasting glucose (IFG) = fasting plasma glucose ≥100 mg/dl (5.50 mmol/l) but <126 mg/dl (6.93 mmol/l) *or* impaired glucose tolerance (IGT) = 2-hour values in oral glucose tolerance test (OGTT) ≥140 mg/dl (7.70 mmol/l) but <200 mg/dl (11.00 mmol/l) confirmed by measurements on at least two separate occasions

Negative Risk Factor	Defining Criteria
High-serum HDL cholesterol	≥60 mg/dl (1.55 mmol/l)

Note: It is common to sum risk factors in making clinical judgments. If HDL is high, subtract one risk factor from the sum of positive risk factors, because high HDL decreases CVD risk.
[a]Professional opinions vary regarding the most appropriate markers and threshold, for obesity; therefore, allied health professionals should use clinical judgment when evaluating this risk factor.

Box 39.1 *Symptoms or signs suggestive of cardiopulmonary disease*

1. Pain, discomfort (or other angina equivalent) in chest, neck, jaw, arm or other areas that may be ischemic in nature
2. Shortness of breath at rest or with mild exertion
3. Dizziness or syncope
4. Orthopnea or paroxysmal nocturnal dyspnea
5. Ankle edema
6. Palpitations of tachycardia
7. Intermittent claudication
8. Known heart murmur
9. Unusual fatigue or shortness of breath with usual activities

From ACSM, 2010 Guidelines for Exercise Testing and Prescription, 8th edn, with permission from Lippincott, Williams & Wilkins.

entails activities requiring three to six METs (metabolic equivalents). However, although training at this level may be designated as screening 'not necessary', it should not be deemed inappropriate. Examination and evaluation should always guide a clinician's decisions in this area (ACSM, 2010). It is also important to identify the medications that a patient is taking. Regular use of cardiovascular drugs, tranquilizers, diuretics and sedatives can affect the physiological response to exercise.

Patient/clients who are receiving skilled therapeutic rehabilitation services regularly sign informed consent forms before treatment. Informed consent is an important ethical and legal consideration, particularly for health promotion services that may not be covered by insurances. The participant should know the purposes and risks associated with an exercise program and testing.

BASELINE FUNCTIONAL CAPACITY

Establishing a baseline functional capacity is essential for those who intend to participate in an exercise program. As the individual progresses through the exercise program, comparison of the initial exercise test with subsequent tests will provide feedback regarding the individual's success in the program. Such assessments have been shown to play a significant role in decreasing attrition rates in exercise programs.

The selection of a graded exercise test should take into consideration the purpose of the test, desired outcome and the individual being tested. A graded exercise test protocol must effectively challenge the patient/client but not be too aggressive. Tests can be categorized into single-stage and multistage tests. An example of a single-stage exercise test is the 6 minute walk test. It requires a measured course. A seldom used indoor corridor is recommended, with cones indicating turning points. The measure is the distance walked in 6 minutes. The person may use an assistive device and rest as often as necessary during this cycle of time (Roy et al., 2013). Multistage exercise tests include treadmill and cycle ergometer. The Naughton–Balke, modified Balke (Table 39.2) and modified Bruce treadmill protocols (Table 39.3) are recommended for deconditioned

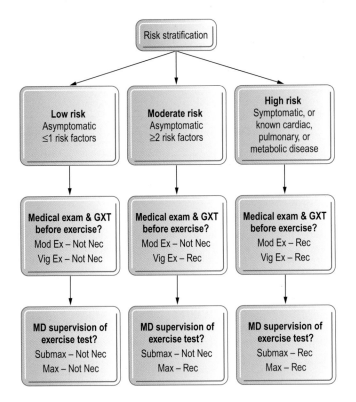

Mod Ex:
Moderate intensity exercise: 40–60% of $\dot{V}o_{2max}$; 3–6 METs; 'an intensity well within the individual's capacity, one which can be comfortably sustained for a prolonged period of time (~45 minutes)'

Vig Ex:
Vigorous intensity exercise: >60% of $\dot{V}o_{2max}$; >6 METs; 'exercise intense enough to represent a substantial cardiorespiratory challenge'

Not Nec:
Not Necessary: reflects the notion that a medical examination, exercise test and physician supervision of exercise testing would not be essential in the preparticipation screening; however, they should not be viewed as inappropriate

Rec:
Recommended: when MD supervision of exercise testing is 'Recommended', the MD should be in close proximity and readily available should there be an emergent need

Figure 39.1 Exercise testing and testing supervision recommendation based on risk stratification. GXT, graded exercise test. *(Reproduced with permission from ACSM's Exercise Guidelines for Exercise Testing and Prescription, 8th edn. Lippincott Williams & Wilkins, Philadelphia, PA; 2010, Figure 2.4, p. 32.)*

individuals with cardiovascular or pulmonary disease (ACSM, 2010; Watchie, 2010).

Heart rate, blood pressure, respiratory rate and possible electrocardiogram (ECG) responses should be recorded minimally at rest, immediately upon completion of testing and until the person regains their pretest or resting measures. It is also highly recommended that vital signs be monitored throughout the stages of the test.

CONSIDERATIONS FOR EXERCISE PRESCRIPTION

In 1995, the Centers for Disease Control (CDC) and the ACSM recommended that 'every US adult should

Table 39.2 Naughton–Balke and modified treadmill protocols

	Speed (mph)	% Grade	Time (min)	METs
Naughton–Balke treadmill protocol	3 (constant)	2.5	2	4.3
		5	2	5.4
		7.5	2	6.4
		10	2	7.4
		12.5	2	8.4
		15	2	9.5
		17.5	2	10.5
		20	2	11.6
		22.5	2	12.6
Modified Balke treadmill protocol	2	0	3	2.5
	2	3.5	3	3.5
	2	7	3	4.5
	2	10.5	3	5.4
	2	14	3	6.4
	2	17.5	3	7.4
	3	12.5	3	8.5
	3	15	3	9.5

From ACSM, 2010, Guidelines for Exercise Testing and Prescription, 8th edn, with permission from Lippincott Williams & Wilkins. METs, metabolic equivalents

Table 39.3 Modified Bruce treadmill protocols

Stage		Speed MPH	Elevation	METs
M	S	Duration = 3 minutes each stage		
1		1.7	0%	2
2		1.7	5%	3
3	1	1.7	10%	5
4	2	2.5	12%	7.
5	3	3.4	14%	10
6	4	4.2	16%	13
7	5	5.0	18%	16
8	6	5.5	20%	19
9	7	6.0	22%	22

M, modified Bruce protocol; S, standard Bruce protocol; METs, metabolic equivalents

accumulate 30 minutes or more of moderate-intensity physical activity on most, preferably all, days of the week' (Pate et al., 1995). In 1996, the Surgeon General's Report, *Physical Activity and Health* (US Department of Health and Human Services, 1996), advised that: 'Significant benefits can be obtained by including a moderate amount of physical activity (e.g. 30 minutes of brisk walking or raking leaves, 15 minutes of running or 45 minutes of playing volleyball) on most, if not all, days of the week. …Additional health benefits can be gained through greater amounts of physical activity.'

Each element of an exercise prescription is designed specifically for the individual related to their goals and unique attributes. The FITT principle of exercise prescription includes *Frequency* (F), *Intensity* (I), *Time* or duration (T), and *Type* (T) or the mode of exercise to be performed. The objective of the exercise training may include cardiovascular (aerobic) fitness, muscular strength and endurance, neuromuscular fitness to improve balance and agility, flexibility and/or improving body composition.

Frequency

Frequency refers to the number of exercise sessions per week that are included in the exercise prescription. It depends on a person's initial functional capacity. The ACSM (2010) recommends an exercise frequency of 3–5 times per week for individuals who have a higher functional capacity and can tolerate a greater exercise intensity. However, the Surgeon General and other US government agencies recommend physical activity on most days of the week. The frequency of exercise for those with a low functional capacity should be more frequent, even daily. Multiple brief daily sessions are advised for patient/clients with an aerobic capacity of less than three METs.

Intensity

Prescribing the appropriate exercise intensity is the most difficult challenge in designing an exercise program. The two most common methods for prescribing and monitoring exercise intensity are HR and rating of perceived exertion (RPE). Because there is a linear relationship between HR and percent functional capacity ($\dot{V}_{O_2}$), HR is used to set an exercise intensity range. Exercise intensities of 60–80% are generally recommended for the younger population. However, in the elderly, an exercise intensity of 40% of the HR reserve has demonstrated aerobic and functional training adaptations (Pate et al., 1995; ACSM, 2010).

One of the oldest and easiest methods of computing intensity is to use the percent of maximum HR (zero to age-predicted maximum). Age-predicted maximum HR is calculated by subtracting the person's age from 220, with a potential adjustment of ± 10–15 beats per minute (bpm). However, this is a very conservative method that is especially inaccurate at lower intensity target ranges. Therefore, the Karvonen method is recommended for setting exercise intensity range; this uses the HR reserve, which is the difference between resting HR and maximum HR. If the results from a graded exercise test are available, then the maximum HR achieved in this test is utilized as the maximum HR. If not, the age-predicted maximum HR formula is used (ACSM, 2010). The calculation of the target HR range for exercise intensity ranging from 40% to 60% in an individual of 70 years with a resting HR of 60 bpm is illustrated in Box 39.2.

Box 39.2 Calculating target heart rate range with the Karvonen method

Maximal heart rate	220	
Subtract age	−70	
Equals	150	
Subtract resting heart rate	−60	
Equals heart rate reserve	90	90
Multiply by % intensity	×40	×60
Equals	36	54
Add back resting heart rate	+60	+60
Target heart rate range for 40–60%	96 bpm to 114 bpm	

Table 39.4 Borg's original and revised rating of perceived exertion (RPE)

Original Category RPE Scale		Revised Category–Ratio Scale	
Value	Description	Value	Description
6		0	Nothing at all
7	Very, very light	0.5	Very, very weak
8		1	Very weak
9	Very light	2	Weak
10		3	Moderate
11	Fairly light	4	Somewhat strong
12		5	Strong
13	Somewhat hard	6	
14		7	Very strong
15	Hard	8	
16		9	
17	Very hard	10	Very, very strong
18		•	Maximal
19	Very, very hard		
20			

From Borg, 1982. Scales © American College of Sports Medicine, with permission from Lippincott Williams & Wilkins.

Individuals with cardiovascular disease are frequently taking medications, such as digoxin or beta blockers, that blunt the HR response to exercise. Measures such as Borg's RPE can also be used to prescribe intensity (see Table 39.4). RPE is a widely used measure, which quantifies the subjective sensation of physical exertion. It correlates closely with several measurable variables such as peak $\dot{V}_{O_2}$ and percentage HR reserve. It can be used to prescribe intensity, especially when a person is taking a medication that alters the cardiopulmonary response to exercise. The original category RPE scale is numbered from 6 to 20. Although the numbering system may appear unusual, it correlates HR with a specific number.

For instance, the number '11', described as 'fairly light' exertion, generally corresponds to a HR of 110. An RPE of 11–16 associates closely with exercise intensities of 50–75%. Numerous studies have demonstrated reproducible results among a wide variety of individuals using this scale. The newer category–ratio scale, numbered 0–10, was designed with the perception that exercise intensity appears to increase as a power function rather than a linear progression. It allows for more fine tuning for subjective responses to small increases in objective exercise intensity. Whichever method is used, it is critical that all individuals are educated in its application to ensure that ratings are reliable and valid.

Duration (Time)

Duration is inversely proportional to intensity. A conditioning response is the result of the interaction of intensity and duration of exercise. The lower the intensity, the longer the duration needs to be. Exercise duration is either measured by total calorie expenditure or by the amount of time the physical activity is performed. The latter mode is obviously the simplest method for individuals to track. The Surgeon General's Report (1996), ACSM and the American Heart Association (ACSM, 2010) recommend a minimum of 150 accumulated minutes of physical activity per week. Duration of one physical activity session must be at least 10 minutes in duration to be included.

Mode of Exercise (Type)

Cardiovascular or aerobic fitness activities are classified into two groups: continuous or sustained activities and discontinuous or intermittent exercise. Any activity that requires work from large muscle masses for a prolonged period of time will elicit an exercise training response from the cardiovascular and pulmonary system. Discontinuous or intermittent exercise activities are often required for those with low functional capacities or any condition that limits performance, such as chronic obstructive lung disease, intermittent claudication, moderate cardiovascular disease and orthopedic limitations. Examples of a continuous and intermittent walking protocol are illustrated by the Senior's Walking Exercise Program in Tables 39.5 and 39.6 (Reynolds, 1991).

PROGRESSION OF PHYSICAL ACTIVITY

The rate of exercise progression depends on several factors including the individual's functional capacity, medical status, age, activity preference and individual goals. Any element of the FITT framework may be increased as a means of progression. ACSM recommends gradually increasing the duration of minutes per session over the first 4–6 weeks. Then intensity can be gradually advanced upward. Older adults and very deconditioned individuals may require slower and longer progression. Table 39.7, from the ACSM Guidelines (2010), offers an example of exercise progression using intermittent exercise for persons with a functional capacity less than and greater 4 METs. All progression of the exercise prescription should be accomplished gradually to avoid musculoskeletal injuries and debilitating fatigue.

Table 39.5 Seniors' walking exercise program protocol: continuous walking protocol[a]

	Time (min)	Frequency (times/week)
Walk	45–50	3
Walk	34–38	4
Walk	27–30	5
Walk	23–25	6
Walk	17–19	8 (or twice a day, 4 times a week)

From Reynolds, 1991, with permission from Wolters Kluwer.
[a]1. At the start of the walking program, do not allow the client to walk for longer than the time indicated on the exercise test.
2. To increase the client's motivation and sense of control, the client should choose how often (frequency) they will exercise per week.
3. The client should determine how long they would like to walk and set that as the time goal.
4. Expect to progress at a rate of 2–5 min/week until the time goal has been achieved.

Table 39.6 Seniors' walking exercise program protocol: intermittent walking protocol[a]

Stage	Exercise (min)	Rest (min)	Total Exercise (min)
1	2	1	6
2	3	1	9
3	4	1	12
4	5	1	15
5	6	1	18
6	7	1	21

From Reynolds, 1991, with permission from Wolters Kluwer.
[a]Repeat each walk/rest cycle three times. Do not progress to the next stage until three cycles can comfortably be completed within set exercise tolerance parameters. Recommended frequency, 5–7 times per week.

Parameters for progression that have guided this author for over 10 years involve monitoring the patient/client's HR, blood pressure and respiratory rate/rhythm/pattern during exercise and through recovery, in conjunction with related signs and symptoms such as pain, sweating and fatigue. Progression in the exercise program is advised when the individual recovers their near-resting HR and blood pressure within 5 minutes, and respiratory rate and effort within 10 minutes. Although the latter measure may seem long, it is especially necessary for patients with respiratory pathologies. Resting or baseline respiratory effort for patient/clients with respiratory pathologies is often 1+ on the dyspnea scale (see Table 39.8). Any exercise program will increase their dyspnea level, which should never be allowed to go above 3+. Because the respiratory system is already compromised, return to baseline will take longer.

Exercise participants should be strongly encouraged and taught to monitor their HR, blood pressure and respiratory effort and share the information with their

Table 39.7 Example of exercise progression using intermittent exercise

Week	% FC	Total Min at % FC	Exercise Bout (min)	Rest Bout (min)	Repetitions
Functional Capacity ≥4 METs					
1–2	50–60	15–20	3–10	2–5	3–4
3–4	60–70	20–40	10–20	Optional	2

Week	% FC	Total min at % FC	Exercise Bout (min)	Rest Bout (min)	Repetitions
Functional Capacity <4 METs					
1–2	40–50	10–20	3–7	3–5	3–4
3–4	50–60	15–30	7–15	2–5	2–3
5	60–70	25–40	12–20	2	2

From ACSM, 2010 Guidelines for Exercise Testing and Prescription, 8th edn, with permission from Lippincott, Williams & Wilkins. Continue with two repetitions of continuous exercise, with one rest period or progress to a single continuous bout. MET, metabolic equivalent; FC, functional capacity

Table 39.8 Assessing dyspnea

Dyspnea Scale[a]	Interpretation[b]
1 Light, barely noticeable	0 Breathing normally 1+ Noticeable only to individual but not observer
2 Moderate, bothersome	2+ Use of accessory muscles noted by observer
3 Moderately severe, very uncomfortable	3+ Only able to speak in two to three words between breaths
4 Most severe or intense dyspnea ever experienced	4+ Unable to speak and must stop activity

[a]From ACSM, 2010 Guidelines for Exercise Testing and Prescription, 8th edn.
[b]From Reynolds, 2000; referred to by colleagues as author's 'Talk Test'.

Box 39.3 *Guidelines for termination of an exercise session*

These signs and symptoms are general indicators of exercise intolerance:

1. Severe breathlessness: only able to speak in two- to three-word sentences
2. Drop in heart rate of ≥10 bpm with an increased or continuous steady workload
3. Drop in systolic blood pressure of ≥20 mmHg while exercising
4. Light-headedness, dizziness, pallor, cyanosis, confusion, ataxia
5. Loss of muscle control or fatigue
6. Onset of angina, tightness or severe pain in chest, arms or legs
7. Nausea or vomiting
8. Excessive rise in blood pressure: systolic blood pressure ≥220 mmHg or diastolic blood pressure ≥110 mmHg
9. Excessively large rise in heart rate of ≥50 bpm with low-level activity
10. Severe leg claudication: 8/10 on a 10/10 pain scale
11. ECG abnormalities: ST-segment changes and multifocal premature ventricular contractions ≥30% of complexes
12. Failure of any monitoring equipment

therapist. Minimally, an individual should know how to monitor their pulse and breathing. They should also be aware of the signs of exercise intolerance. Guidelines to ending an exercise session are listed in Box 39.3. Maintaining an activity log, such as the one in Form 39.1, provides useful feedback to both the participant and health professional.

Progress is recognized as an increase in the individual's $\dot{V}_{O_{2(max)}}$ or an increase in the MET level of activity. Increased distance, speed, repetition and weights all indicate improved exercise or workload tolerance. This improved response can be verified when retesting the patient using the same pretest protocol. An individual having a positive training response will achieve the established workloads at a lower HR and systolic blood pressure. There have been some observations that the older adult with cardiac disease may experience a greater relative improvement in response to an exercise program than their younger counterparts. A possible explanation is that, because exercise has not been part of their regular physical activity for several years, there is a greater percentage of improvement from their baseline (Williams, 1996).

COMPONENTS OF AN EXERCISE SESSION

An exercise training session has four distinct phases: warm-up, stretching; conditioning (aerobic, resistance, neuromuscular); and, cool down. Sometimes recreational activities are added between the stimulus and cool-down phase. The beginning warm-up phase usually lasts for 5–10 minutes. The purpose is to facilitate the transition from rest to exercise. It reduces susceptibility to musculoskeletal problems, which is especially important in the elderly. Activities include low to moderate intensity cardiovascular and muscular endurance exercises. Stretching is a separate distinct phase of the exercise session, which is performed for 10 minutes either after warm-up or cool-down phase.

The activities in the conditioning phase are specific to the FITT principle of *Frequency* (F), *Intensity* (I), *Time or*

Name _____

Date _____

Time of day _____

Heart rate before exercise _____

Heart rate after exercise _____

Heart rate 5 min after exercise _____

Blood pressure before exercise _____

Blood pressure after exercise _____

Blood pressure 5 min after exercise _____

Exercise activity and minutes of activity _____

Pain (Y = yes; N = no). If yes, where? _____

Fatigue, tiredness _____

Weakness _____

Sweating (amount?) _____

Shortness of breath? How long? _____

Rating of perceived exertion after exercise (RPE) _____

Other comments _____

Form 39.1 Prototype activity log to be used by patients with cardiovascular disease in order to record specific exercise considerations before and after exercising

---

Box 39.4 *General recommendations when initiating an exercise training program for elderly patients with cardiac disease*

Warm-up: 5–10 min of stretching and light activity involving the large muscle groups before each session

Intensity: 50–80% of peak oxygen uptake attained at the most recent exercise test, corresponding to 60–85% of the peak heart rate at same test

Frequency: participation 3–5 days/week

Duration: 20–40 min of aerobic exercise broken up into shorter periods, allowing for 1- to 2-min rest intervals when appropriate

Mode: upper and lower extremity exercise using treadmill walking, leg ergometry and arm ergometry

Cool-down: 5–10 min of activity similar to warm-up

Flexibility: 10–15 min of static stretching 'of the muscles of each major body section', including head and neck, shoulders, chest, trunk, hips, legs, knees and ankles

Resistive training: 12–15 repetitions of a modest work load (25% of body weight for larger muscle groups, such as the quadriceps femoris muscle, and 10% of body weight for smaller muscle groups, such as the triceps muscles), 4–8 stations, 2–3 sessions/week; always performed after the regular exercise session to provide for adequate warming of various muscle groups and to reduce likelihood of injury

From Williams, 1996, with permission from the American Physical Therapy Association.

duration (T), and *Type* (T) or the mode of exercise. This phase can last for 20–60 minutes. When both endurance and resistive training are part of an exercise program, they are usually done on alternate days of the week and not on the same day.

Cool-down is an important component of a safe program for both healthy individuals and patient/clients with disease. It decreases exercise-induced circulatory changes, including returning HR and blood pressure to baseline. It also facilitates the dissipation of body heat produced by exercise and attenuates venous return, reducing the potential for post-exercise dizziness and hypotension. This phase lasts for 5–10 minutes and usually includes exercise with diminishing intensity and stretching (ACSM, 2010).

In summary, Williams (1996) offers an example of a well-rounded exercise training program for older adults with cardiac disease (Box 39.4). His recommendations incorporate all of the considerations that have been discussed in this section.

CONCLUSION

Motivating and maintaining exercise participation is difficult to achieve. Research has demonstrated a greater than 50% dropout rate from most supervised exercise programs after 6 months (US Department of Health and

Human Services, 2000). Exercise approaches that highlight organization and safety but focus more on the individual personal goals have better program compliance. This approach also assumes that the participant's commitment to exercise is a personal one and an opportunity for self-expression (Prochaska & DiClemente, 1982). The goal is to encourage safe progression of exercise activity to an unsupervised environment based on education and enjoyment.

REFERENCES

ACSM (American College of Sports Medicine) 2010 ACSM's Exercise Guidelines for Exercise Testing and Prescription, 8th edn. Lipincott Williams and Wilkins, Philadelphia, PA

Borg GA 1982 Psychophysical basis of perceived exertion. Med Sci Sports Exerc 14(5):377–381

McArdle WD, Katch FI, Katch VL 2011 Essentials of Exercise Physiology, 4th edn. Lipincott Williams and Wilkins, Philadelphia, PA

Pate RR, Pratt M, Blair SN et al 1995 Physical activity and public health: a recommendation from the Centers for Disease Control and Prevention and the American College of Sports Medicine. JAMA 273:402–407

Prochaska J, DiClemente C 1982 Transtheoretical therapy, toward a more integrative model for change. Psych Theory Res Pract 19:276–288

Reynolds P 1991 Seniors walking exercise program. Focus Geriatr Care Rehabil 4:8

Reynolds PJ 2000 Cardiopulmonary Considerations for Evaluation and Management of the Older Adult (Monograph for Home Study Course). American Physical Therapy Association: Section on Geriatrics, Alexandria, VA

Roy SH, Wolf SL, Scalzitti DA 2013 The Rehabilitation Specialist's Handbook, 4th edn. FA Davis Co., Philadelphia, PA

US Department of Health and Human Services 1996 Physical activity and health: a report of the Surgeon General. US Department of Health and Human Services, Centers for Disease Control and Prevention, and National Center for Chronic Disease Prevention and Health Promotion, Atlanta, GA

US Department of Health and Human Services 2000 Healthy People 2010: Understanding and Improving Health. USDHHS, Washington, DC

US Department of Health and Human Services 2008 Physical Activity Guidelines for Americans. Available at: www.health.gov/PAGuidelines/pdf/paguide.pdf. Accessed January 2013

Watchie J 2010 Cardiovascular and Pulmonary Physical Therapy: A Clinical Manual, 2nd edn. Saunders Elsevier, St Louis, MO

Williams MA 1996 Cardiovascular risk-factor reduction in the elderly patients with cardiac disease. Phys Ther 76:469–480

Chapter 40

Clinical development and progression of coronary heart disease

PAMELA REYNOLDS

CHAPTER CONTENTS

INTRODUCTION

Globally, cardiovascular diseases (CVDs) were the number one cause of death (30%) in 2008. CVDs include: coronary heart disease, cerebrovascular disease, peripheral artery disease, congenital and rheumatic heart disease, deep vein thromboses and pulmonary embolisms. In low- and middle-income countries, CVDs are disproportionately high, at about 80% of all deaths; and they affect men and women equally. By 2030, it is projected that deaths from CVD will remain high and continue to be the single leading cause of death. About 45% of CVD deaths are due to coronary heart disease (WHO, 2013). The purpose of this chapter is to detail the causes and clinical implication of coronary heart disease (CHD), which are diseases that affect the blood vessels of the heart. The other CVDs are addressed separately in other parts of this text.

CHD can begin early in the young adult and become progressive until it becomes clinically evident in middle to late adulthood (Watchie, 2010). Recognition of early subclinical onset of CHD was discovered by Enos and colleagues in 1953. They autopsied 300 apparently healthy soldiers killed in the Korean War and found 77.3% of them had visible blockages in their coronary arteries. As a result of this work, the medical community now differentiates coronary artery disease (CAD) from coronary heart disease (CHD). In CAD, there are obstructions that limit blood flow in the coronary arteries, however, not enough to significantly impair the function of the cardiac muscle. The term CHD indicates not only that there is obstruction in the coronary arteries, but also permanent damage to the cardiac muscle, limiting its function (Hillegass et al., 2011).

Myocardial ischemia results from a deficient blood supply to the heart muscle because of either obstruction or constriction of the coronary vessels. Underlying this deficiency is an imbalance between the oxygen supply and demand of the myocardial muscle cells. The majority of diseased coronary arteries have fixed obstructions

in the form of atherosclerotic lesions that lead to chronic stable angina symptoms. When blood flow becomes more restricted, angina symptoms increase in frequency and intensity leading to acute coronary syndrome (ACS). Clinical presentations of ACS include sudden death, unstable angina leading to an acute myocardial infarction, which are classified by the presence or absence of specific ECG changes in at least two leads. These changes are classified as either ST elevation myocardial infarction (STEMI) or a non-ST elevation myocardial infarction (non-STEMI or NSTEMI) (Watchie, 2010; Hillegass et al., 2011).

However, ischemia can also be caused by spasms of the coronary artery walls, also known as Prinzmetal's angina. Both atherosclerosis and vasospasms are equally capable of reducing the supply of blood and therefore of oxygen to the myocardial muscle cells. Hypertension can also damage the coronary arteries.

Ischemia produces major changes in two of the important functions of a myocardial cell: electrical activity and contractility. Alteration in electrical activity generates many of the electrocardiogram (ECG) arrhythmias. Impairment of myocardial contractility affects the function of the left ventricle and results in a reduced ejection fraction (the amount of blood pumped out with each heartbeat) and decreased cardiac output, which further compromises the blood supply to the coronary arteries.

CAUSES OF CORONARY ARTERY DISEASE

The Framingham Heart Study has led to the identification of risk factors and acceptance of their role in the development and progression of CVD (Wilson et al., 1987). Risk factors for developing coronary heart disease are discussed in Chapter 39. The most significant and modifiable risk factors in the causation and acceleration of atherosclerotic disease are cigarette/tobacco smoking, hypertension, hypercholesterolemia and physical inactivity. Nicotine increases the sensitivity of low-density lipoprotein (LDL) receptors and increases the levels of fibrinogen circulating in the blood. Persons who quit smoking can reduce their risk of developing CAD by half in 1 year. In 15 years, risk for CAD is equalized with nonsmokers (Goodman, 2009). Hypertension appears to be an independent risk factor in the development of CAD. Efforts to lower blood pressure have been more effective in reducing stroke morbidity and mortality than in decreasing heart attacks (Hillegass et al., 2011). When total blood serum cholesterol level reaches more than 200 mg/dl a person is at greater risk for heart disease. The risk doubles when cholesterol exceeds 240 mg/dl and the ratio of total cholesterol to high-density lipids (HDL) exceeds 4.5 (Goodman, 2009). The Centers for Disease Control and Prevention report that physical inactivity is the most prevalent risk factor for developing CHD (Hillegass et al., 2011).

Heredity, gender and age are non-modifiable risk factors. Some other factors that may influence development of CHD include body habitus (obesity), diet, hyperglycemia, diabetes mellitus, stress and personality type. Also, more recent studies indicate that male gender is no longer considered to be a differentiating risk factor. Male risk is higher until females reach menopause, then the risk is equal (Hillegass et al., 2011). Atherosclerosis and vasospasm causes of CHD are detailed further in this chapter.

ATHEROSCLEROSIS

Coronary arteries have three layers. The outer layer or adventitia provides the support for the artery and is composed primarily of collagen fibers. The middle layer or media has multiple layers of smooth muscle. As demand for blood flow in the coronary arteries changes, this muscular layer is able to make adjustments in the diameter of the vessels. The intima or inner layer is comprised of endothelium and variable amounts of collagen, elastic fibers and some isolated smooth muscle cells (Hillegass et al., 2011).

Development and progression of atherosclerosis is a complex process in which lipid deposits are irregularly distributed in the intima and endothelium layers of the larger and medium coronary arteries. The arterial endothelium is especially permeable to macromolecules the size of low-density lipoprotein (LDL). Fatty streaks in the intima layer of the artery are the first clinical evidence of atherosclerosis. These lesions contain lipid-laden macrophages and smooth muscle cells. Eventually the accumulation of lipid-laden macrophages grows so large that the endothelium stretches and begins to separate, leading to cell injury; and bearing the intima and underlying connective tissue to the circulation. Platelets then accumulate around this injured area and a thrombus is formed, which is the sclerotic element of the atherosclerotic lesion. The arterial walls continue to thicken through the buildup of lipids, macrophages, T lymphocytes, smooth muscle cells, extracellular matrix, calcium and necrotic debris. The growth of the atherosclerotic plaques and thickening of the arterial walls are responsible for the narrowing of the blood vessel, which ultimately leads to end organ ischemia (Goodman, 2009; Cassady & Cahalin, 2011; Hillegass et al., 2011).

The clinical outcomes of atherosclerosis can be improved by removing or reversing a single or group of risk factors. In particular, alteration of diet, reduction of blood cholesterol levels, treatment of hypertension and cessation of smoking are the major targets to prevent the progression of atherosclerotic disease. Physical activity has been shown to reduce the negative effects of some of these factors. Exercise allows an individual to attain or maintain a higher metabolic rate, which allows better caloric intake tolerance – one can enjoy a few more calories without gaining weight. Reduction of blood cholesterol and blood pressure along with successive reductions or elimination of reliance on blood pressure-lowering medications are other benefits of exercise (ACSM, 2010). The general rehabilitation exercise considerations presented in Chapter 39 are all applicable to individuals with atherosclerosis.

VASOSPASM

Prinzmetal's angina is an atypical or variant angina that causes myocardial ischemia and chest pain. It is a variant angina in which there is a transient increase in vasomotor tone or vasospasm. It occurs primarily at rest and often without any precipitants. Unlike the other types of angina, the exercise capacity in those with variant angina is preserved. There is also a tendency for the pain to occur at about the same time each day. Arrhythmia or conduction disturbances may accompany episodes of this variant angina. Considering that up to one-third of variant angina sufferers have no atherosclerotic disease of the coronary vessels, the current theory of pathogenesis is this variant angina is caused by the vasospasm of one or more of the coronary arteries. Vasospasms are not isolated to variant angina; they are also seen in individuals with typical angina and acute myocardial infarction (AMI). Unlike other forms of angina, an episode of variant angina actually causes ST-segment elevation on an ECG. Similar to typical angina, Prinzmetal's again can be quickly relieved by nitroglycerin or other vasodilators (Cassady & Cahalin, 2011; Hillegass et al., 2011).

CLINICAL COURSE OF CORONARY HEART DISEASE

SUDDEN DEATH

Sudden cardiac death is death that occurs within an hour of onset of symptoms of the initial presentation of acute coronary syndrome. Frequently, a patient with CHD is diagnosed during an autopsy for a sudden unexplained death. Sudden cardiac death occurs in about 40% of patients with CHD (Watchie, 2010; Hillegass et al., 2011).

CHRONIC STABLE ANGINA

The term 'angina pectoris' describes paroxysmal or spasmodic chest pain, which is usually caused by myocardial ischemia. It is typically precipitated by exertion or excitement. Stable angina is characterized by episodic chest pain that usually lasts for 5–15 minutes, is provoked by exertion or stress; and is relieved by rest or sublingual nitroglycerin. The pain almost always has a retrosternal component and commonly radiates into the neck, jaw and shoulders and down the left or the left and right arms. Radiation to the back is also possible. Additional symptoms, such as light-headedness, palpitations, diaphoresis, dyspnea, fatigue, nausea or vomiting, may accompany the pain. Females and elderly individuals are more likely to present with atypical symptoms. The specific ECG changes seen with ischemia are usually indicated by ST-segment depression of more than 1 mm, which also occurs in about 50% of cases during an acute attack (Goodman, 2009; Hillegass et al., 2011).

ACUTE CORONARY SYNDROME (ACS)

The term *acute coronary syndrome* is used to describe a patient who presents to the emergency room with symptoms of either unstable angina or an evolving AMI. This diagnostic terminology was adopted to expedite patient management; and decrease myocardial damage and associated morbidity and mortality. Patients with ACS are classified in one of three categories: unstable angina, ST elevation myocardial infarction (STEMI) or a non-ST elevation myocardial infarction (non-STEMI or NSTEMI).

Unstable Angina

Unstable angina represents a clinical state between stable angina and AMI. It is also referred to as crescendo or preinfarction angina. The clinical definition of unstable angina includes any of the following subgroups: (i) exertional angina of recent onset, usually within the past 4–8 weeks (which means that all newly diagnosed angina is essentially unstable); (ii) angina of worsening character, either with increasing severity of pain, increasing duration of pain, increasing frequency of pain or increasing requirement for nitroglycerin; and (iii) angina at rest. Also included within this group of unstable angina is postinfarction angina, which, as its name suggests, occurs after an AMI. It is important to remember that it can occur within days or weeks of an acute infarction or even months to years later (occurring after an angina-free period dating from the AMI). Those who experience angina after successful coronary artery bypass surgery comprise another group of individuals who are considered unstable. Unstable angina is thought to be caused by a progression in the severity and extent of coronary atherosclerosis, coronary artery spasm or bleeding into non-occlusive plaques in the coronary artery. It eventually results in complete occlusion of the artery (Grimes, 2007; Hillegass et al., 2011).

Acute Myocardial Infarction (AMI): STEMI and Non-STEMI

Insufficient blood flow to an area of the myocardium for longer than 20 minutes will evoke symptoms of an acute myocardial ischemia or infarction. The vast majority of people with AMI have CHD, but there is no universal agreement about exactly what precipitates the acute event. Current concepts concerning the immediate cause of AMI include the interaction of multiple trigger factors: progression of the atherosclerotic process to the point of complete occlusion; hemorrhage at the site of an existing, narrowing coronary artery embolism; coronary artery spasm; and thrombosis at the site of an atherosclerotic plaque (American Heart Association, 2005).

The classic symptom of AMI is retrosternal chest pain, which is usually the same as angina pain but lasts for more than 15–30 minutes. Individual variation in the site and radiation of the pain, and also in the nature and severity of the pain, is very common (Fig. 40.1). Associated features such as dyspnea, diaphoresis, palpitations, nausea and vomiting are common accompaniments but not all are present all of the time. The degree of heart muscle damage and extent of infarction is usually independent of the presence of associated features or the severity of the pain. A long duration of pain often indicates more damage. AMIs in elderly patients, as opposed to those in younger individuals, are likely to present with no pain or with a noncardiac type of pain or altered mental status. Longitudinal studies indicate that up to 25% of myocardial infarctions are not recognized clinically but are diagnosed later in routine ECGs performed for unrelated conditions. In addition, individuals with diabetes are more susceptible to silent (painless) myocardial infarction (Goodman, 2009; Watchie, 2010).

An acute myocardial infarction is usually categorized according to the presence or absence of ST segment elevation in the individual's ECG. A STEMI is associated with development of a Q wave on the ECG 24–48 hours after the ACS began. A myocardial infarction that develops Q waves used to be known as transmural MI, because it involved the full thickness of the ventricular wall. A NSTEMI does not develop a Q wave on the ECG. It was formerly known as a non-transmural or subendocardial MI because it did not involve the full wall of the ventricle. However, current evidence using magnetic resonance imaging has demonstrated that the Q waves develop on the ECG as a result of the size of the infarction, not the depth of the mural involvement (Grimes, 2007; Hillegass et al., 2011).

Like ischemia, infarction produces changes in the electrical depolarization and contractility of myocardial cells. These functions are important and derangement in one or both of them can cause the common complications of AMI. During the first few hours after the onset of pain there are areas of infarction interspersed with or surrounded by areas of ischemia; therefore, in the early phases, infarction is not a completed process. These ischemic areas can be saved by the early reperfusion with thrombolytic agents and percutaneous transluminal coronary angioplasty (PTCA). However, the person must receive immediate emergency care either via ambulance or in an emergency room. Localization of the AMI is important for prognosis, as the type and incidence of complications vary with the location and size of infarction (Watchie, 2010; Hillegass et al., 2011)

The physical examination can be quite normal. Mild to moderate increases in pulse rate are common despite the fact that inferior infarcts are usually associated with bradycardia. The pain and the activation of the sympathetic nervous system can cause elevation of blood pressure. However, if left ventricle function is impaired by the pain, hypotension is more likely. Abnormal S3 and S4 heart sounds can usually be auscultated. New systolic murmurs may cause great concern as they can indicate that there is muscle damage affecting the cardiac valves or causing regurgitation or that rupture of the septum has occurred.

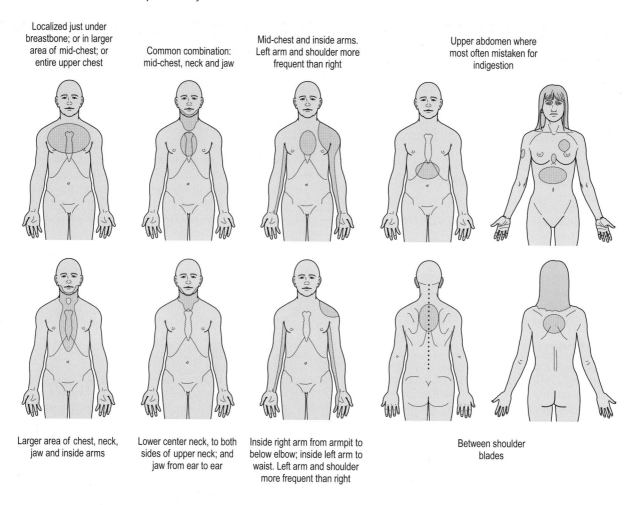

Localized just under breastbone; or in larger area of mid-chest; or entire upper chest

Common combination: mid-chest, neck and jaw

Mid-chest and inside arms. Left arm and shoulder more frequent than right

Upper abdomen where most often mistaken for indigestion

Larger area of chest, neck, jaw and inside arms

Lower center neck, to both sides of upper neck; and jaw from ear to ear

Inside right arm from armpit to below elbow; inside left arm to waist. Left arm and shoulder more frequent than right

Between shoulder blades

Most common warning signs of heart attack

- Uncomfortable pressure, fullness, squeezing or pain in the center of the chest (prolonged)
- Pain that spreads to the throat, neck, back, jaw, shoulders, or arms
- Chest discomfort with light-headedness, dizziness, sweating, pallor, nausea, or shortness of breath
- Prolonged symptoms unrelieved by antacids, nitroglycerin, or rest

Atypical, less common warning signs (especially women)

- Unusual chest pain (quality, location, e.g. burning, heaviness; left chest), stomach or abdominal pain
- Continuous midthoracic or interscapular pain
- Continuous neck or shoulder pain
- Isolated right biceps pain
- Pain relieved by antacids; pain unrelieved by rest or nitroglycerin
- Nausea and vomiting; flu-like manifestation without chest pain/discomfort
- Unexplained intense anxiety, weakness, or fatigue = breathlessness, dizziness

Figure 40.1 Early warning signs of a heart attack. (*Reproduced from Goodman, 2009, in Goodman CC, Fuller KS. Pathology: Implications for the Physical Therapist, 3rd edn. WB Saunders, Philadelphia, PA, with permission from Elsevier.*)

Arrhythmias such as tachycardias, ventricular ectopy, bradycardias and atrioventricular blocks are commonly seen in AMI and are the major manifestations of the disruption of the electrical depolarization of the myocardial cells and the specialized conducting system. The major result of impaired contractility is the failure of the left ventricular pump. Heart failure usually develops if 25% of the left ventricular myocardium is damaged. Cardiogenic shock is also common and involves more than a 40% impairment of left ventricular function. If the papillary muscles of the mitral valve are involved, acute mitral valve regurgitation may develop and cause acute pulmonary edema and hypotension. Rupture of

the myocardial wall or ventricular septum, resulting from autolysis in the infarcted area, can also occur and cause cardiac tamponade or an acutely-acquired ventricular septal defect. Both of these conditions can present as sudden death after AMI (American Heart Association, 2005).

REHABILITATION CONSIDERATIONS FOR THE PERSON WITH ANGINA

Differentiating angina pain from non-angina and musculoskeletal pain is challenging. The person experiencing the angina initially denies it and passes it off as a

Table 40.1	**Differential diagnosis of chest pain**			
Descriptor (Questions to Ask)	Angina	Other Cardiac (e.g. Pericarditis)	Musculoskeletal (e.g. Subacromial Bursitis)	Gastrointestinal
Symptoms	Nonfocal, dull, vague	Sharp, cutting, difficulty swallowing	Intense, constant, dull, sometimes throbbing, vague onset	Vague onset, symptoms ↑ related to food consumption
Location	Anything above the waist (classic: substernal/ LUE/jaw)	Substernal and may radiate to neck, upper back, upper traps, left arm	Anterolateral shoulder region	
CV Exercise	Symptoms ↑	Symptoms ↓ or no effect	Symptoms ↑ with motion of involved UE, especially overhead movements	May exacerbate symptoms (e.g. peptic ulcer), but often no effect
Rest	Symptoms ↓; may awaken from sleep	No effect	Symptoms ↓; sleep delayed	No effect; may awaken from sleep
Body position/ ROM	No effect	Symptoms ↓ in quadruped, leaning forward, sitting upright. Symptoms ↑ by trunk rotation/side bending	Symptoms ↑ with lying on involved side	Symptoms ↑ with head down positioning (e.g. GERD)
Deep breath/ cough	No effect	Symptoms ↑ with any activity that causes chest wall to move	No effect	No effect
Palpation	No effect	Painful over left, anterior/ lower chest wall	Painful over bursa; area may be warm/swollen	No effect
Nitroglycerine	Symptoms ↓	No effect	No effect	No effect
Other		History of fever/chills, recent MI, complains of weakness	Relief with heat, non-steroidal anti-inflammatory agents	Relief with antacids

Excerpted from Malone, 2006: Tables 6–9; pp. 163–164.
UE, upper extremity; ROM, range of motion; MI, myocardial infarction; GERD, Gastroesophageal Reflux Disease

musculoskeletal pain. It is commonly described as pressure, squeezing or tightness in the substernal area. However, there are other individuals whose angina presents in atypical areas such as the jaw, neck, epigastric area or back. Table 40.1 presents some guidelines for differential diagnosis between angina and other chest pain caused by other cardiac issues, musculoskeletal pain or the gastrointestinal system.

Angina can be quantified for evaluation purposes in two ways. First, the rate pressure product (RPP), also called the double product, is closely correlated with the myocardial oxygen requirement. It is calculated by multiplying the heart rate by the systolic blood pressure. When these measures are calculated at the onset of angina symptoms or ECG instability (ST-segment depression 1 mm), it is referred to as the angina threshold. A person with stable angina usually develops symptoms at a consistent level of the RPP. Exercise training programs can therefore be designed to keep the person from reaching the anginal threshold by closely monitoring heart and systolic blood pressure. Second, the subjective experience of the intensity of angina can be graded on an Angina Rating Scale (see Table 40.2) (ACSM, 2010; Hillegass & Temes, 2011).

An individual known to have angina should always carry nitroglycerin medication with him or her. When angina symptoms begin, one tablet of nitroglycerin should

Table 40.2	**Angina rating scale**
0	No angina
1	Light, barely noticeable
2	Moderate, bothersome
3	More severe, very uncomfortable (preinfarction pain)
4	Most severe or intense pain ever experienced (infarction pain)

Source: ACSM, 2010; Hillegass & Temes, 2011.

be taken every 5 minutes. If the angina pain is not relieved after three tablets or 15 minutes, emergency care should be sought immediately.

DIAGNOSTIC TESTS

Electrocardiography is an important diagnostic test for an AMI. However, only 50% of AMIs show diagnostic changes on the initial ECG. The classical AMI produces a progression of ECG changes that include ST-segment elevation, T-wave inversion and development of significant Q waves. Both the pain and ECG changes resolve with relief of the ischemia and infarction.

Damage to cardiac muscle cells results in the release of enzymes into the bloodstream. Both the American College of Cardiology and the American Heart Association state that troponin levels show the best specificity and sensitivity for the diagnosis and prognosis of AMI. Serum levels increase within 3–12 hours of the onset of chest pain, reach peak levels in 24–48 hours and decrease to baseline in 5–14 days. Previously, the diagnostic standard was to monitor increases of creatinine phosphokinase–myocardial band (CK–MB), which occur within 3–12 hours after chest pain starts, peak within 24 hours and decrease to baseline in 2–3 days. However, the sensitivity and specificity are not as high as for troponin levels. Serial blood testing for cardiac enzyme levels in the setting of suspected AMI is now routine and is especially useful when ECG changes are nonspecific or absent. CK–MB may also be elevated after cardiac surgery and cardiopulmonary resuscitation (Grimes, 2007).

AMIs nearly always produce an impairment in left ventricle pumping ability. The greater the area of damage, the more likely it is that symptoms will be clinically apparent. Echocardiography is a form of ultrasound that is used to identify abnormalities in wall motion of regional cardiac muscles and also to observe the function of the cardiac valves. Its primary use is in the detection of complications of AMI that may need surgical intervention, such as rupture of the myocardial wall or valve damage. It is also used after AMIs to determine the extent of impairment to cardiac function (Watchie, 2010).

THE RETURN TO PHYSICAL ACTIVITY

Early mobilization of individuals after an AMI, using a symptom-limited rehabilitation approach, is very important in the postinfarction period. In the acute setting, the physician determines the upper limits of exercise while considering the deconditioning effects of bedrest and lack of exercise. For individuals who are asymptomatic and do not show signs of ischemia, tolerance of exercise is more important than exercising at a specific heart-rate intensity. Box 39.3 in the previous chapter presents guidelines for termination of an exercise session and these should be followed.

The American College of Sports Medicine (ACSM) offers general criteria for exercising, starting initially in the in-patient setting. A frequency of two to four times per day for early mobilization is recommended for the first 3 days. Then two times a day beginning on day 4 concurrent with increased duration. The ACSM guideline for intensity suggest that the rate of perceived exertion on the Borg scale (from 6–20) should be less than 13. The value of 13 is described as 'somewhat hard'. For the post-MI and congestive heart failure, the heart rate should remain less than 120 beats per minute (bpm) or the resting heart rate plus 20 bpm (the arbitrary upper limit). The intensity post surgery should be resting heart rate plus 30 bpm (arbitrary upper limit). The intensity of exercise post myocardial infarction may be to tolerance if asymptomatic. The duration of exercise can be intermittent, with bouts lasting 3–5 minutes. Rest periods or slower walking may be taken at the patient's discretion, lasting 1–2 minutes and should be shorter than the exercise of duration. A ratio of 2:1 is recommended for exercise/rest. When the individual reaches duration of 10–15 minutes of continuous exercise, then exercise intensity can be increased as tolerated (ACSM, 2010).

CONCLUSION

Atherosclerosis leads to the development of CAD and ischemic CHD. Angina is a symptom of myocardial ischemia. Angina pectoris is a retrosternal symptom, and other complaints of pain to the neck, jaw, shoulders and upper extremities result from myocardial anoxia, usually precipitated by exertion or excitement. Angina is commonly denied and dismissed as a musculoskeletal complaint. Appropriate therapeutic exercise training programs must be designed to prevent the patient from reaching the angina threshold. If angina pain is not relieved within 15 minutes, emergency care should be sought because of the likelihood of suffering ACS. Progressively increasing myocardial ischemia will ultimately lead to an ACS. Much like angina, the classic symptom of AMI is retrosternal pain; however, in AMI, the pain lasts for more than 15–30 minutes without relief from rest or sublingual nitroglycerin. It is crucial to seek medical attention early because of the possibility of reversing the ischemia and preventing further infarction. AMI can cause conduction problems that result in arrhythmias and ventricular fibrillation and, possibly, left ventricular failure. It is important to resume physical activity with caution.

REFERENCES

ACSM (American College of Sports Medicine) 2010 ACSM's Exercise Guidelines for Exercise Testing and Prescription, 8th edn. Lippincott Williams & Wilkins, Philadelphia, PA

American Heart Association 2005 Guidelines for Cardiopulmonary Resuscitation and Emergency Cardiovascular Care. Part 8: Stabilization of the patient with acute coronary syndromes. Circulation 112: IV89–IV110

Cassady SL, Cahalin LP 2011 Cardiovascular pathophysiology. In: DeTurk WE, Cahalin LP (eds) Cardiovascular and Pulmonary Physical Therapy: An Evidence-Based Approach, 2nd edn. McGraw-Hill Medical, New York, NY, pp. 135–163

Enos W, Holmes R, Beyer J 1953 Coronary disease among United States soldiers killed in action in Korea. JAMA 256(12):1090–1093

Goodman CC 2009 The cardiovascular system. In: Goodman CC, Fuller KS (eds) Pathology: Implications for the Physical Therapist, 3rd edn. Saunders Elsevier, Philadelphia, PA, pp. 367–471

Grimes K 2007 Heart disease. In: O'Sullivan S, Schmitz T (eds) Physical Rehabilitation: Assessment and Treatment, 5th edn. FA Davis, Philadelphia, PA, pp. 589–641

Hillegass E, Watchie J, McColgon E 2011 Ischemic cardiovascular conditions and other vascular pathologies. In: Hillegass E (ed) Essentials of Cardiopulmonary Physical Therapy, 3rd edn. Saunders Elsevier, St Louis, MO, pp. 47–83

Hillegass E, Temes W 2011 Intervention and prevention measures for individuals with cardiovascular disease, or risk of disease. In: Hillegass E (ed) Essentials of Cardiopulmonary Physical Therapy, 3rd edn. Saunders Elsevier, St Louis, MO, pp. 598–637

Malone DJ 2006 Cardiovascular diseases and disorders. In: Malone DJ, Bishop-Lindsay KB (eds) Physical Therapy in Acute Care: A Clinician's Guide. Slack Inc., Thorofare, NJ, pp. 139–209

Watchie J 2010 Cardiopulmonary pathology. In: Cardiovascular and Pulmonary Physical Therapy, 2nd edn. Saunders Elsevier, St Louis, MO, pp. 72–155

Wilson PWF, Castelli WP, Kannel WB 1987 Coronary risk predictions in adults (The Framingham Heart Study). Am J Cardiol 59(14):G91–G94

World Health Organization (WHO) 2013 Cardiovascular disease. Available at: www.who.int/mediacentre/factsheets/fs317/en/index.html. Accessed February 2013

Chapter 41

Cardiac arrhythmias and conduction disturbances

PAMELA REYNOLDS

CHAPTER CONTENTS

INTRODUCTION

Cardiac rhythm originates from and is controlled by specific areas within the heart itself. These areas are called intrinsic pacemakers and are responsible for the propagation of electrical impulses that generally travel from the right atrium to the apex of the heart, and activate both atria and ventricles in the process. Although these impulses can pass from cardiac muscle cell to adjacent cardiac muscle cell, there is a preferential tract that they follow along specialized conducting tissue situated within the myocardium that minimizes conduction time. This pathway is detailed in Figure 41.1.

The primary intrinsic pacemaker is the sinoatrial (SA) node, situated at the junction of the superior vena cava and the right atrium. Electrical impulses travel from the SA node through the atria to the atrioventricular (AV) node, which sits on the right side of the interatrial septum. The rate of SA node discharge is controlled by the autonomic nervous system. Sympathetic stimulation increases the firing rate whereas parasympathetic activity (vagal stimulation) lowers the rate (Weiderhold, 1988; Mammen et al., 2004; Hillegass, 2011).

The depolarization of the atria corresponds to the P wave on the electrocardiogram (ECG). The impulse conduction is slowed as it traverses the AV node, allowing time for atrial contraction to be completed before ventricular contraction. This slowing or delay corresponds to the P–R interval on the ECG. After passing through the AV node, the impulse passes into the bundle of His, down the interventricular septum and then divides into the right and left bundle branches that supply impulses to the right and left ventricles respectively. The ventricular depolarization corresponds to the QRS complex on the ECG. The ST segment and T wave on the ECG are produced by ventricular

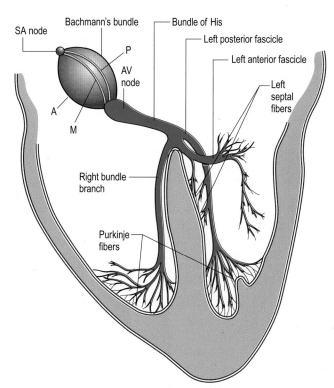

Figure 41.1 The conduction system. A, M and P are the anterior, medial and posterior interatrial tracts. *(From Goldman MJ 1979 Principles of Clinical Electrocardiography, 10th edn. Lange Medical Books, Los Altos, CA, with permission.)*

repolarization. Specifically, the ST segment is the absolute refractory period in which no depolarization of the ventricles can occur. T-wave repolarization is also known as the relative refractory period. During this time, the ventricles can be stimulated to contract but the heart is still electrically unstable, and depolarization in this period can progress to ventricular tachycardia (Weiderhold, 1988).

Each wave, segment and interval has certain normal characteristics, which are identified in Figure 41.2. Variances are usually indicative of different heart impairments. For instance, changes in the ST segment and T wave classically demonstrate some type of myocardial ischemia. Depression of the ST segment by more than 0.1 mm is generally indicative of ischemia and may also produce symptoms of angina. T-wave inversion is usually a sign of ischemia and/or an evolving myocardial infarction. Other abnormalities are discussed in the text that follows.

Many areas of the heart can depolarize spontaneously and rhythmically. The rate of ventricular contraction will be controlled by the area with the highest frequency of discharge. The SA node normally has the highest rate and therefore the ventricles will follow the rate set by the SA node. The normal cardiac cycle is termed normal sinus rhythm because it originates in the SA node and is conducted along the normal electrical pathway of the heart (Malone, 2006; Hillegass, 2011). Disturbances to cardiac rhythm and conduction are classified in several ways, for example: (i) heart rate; (ii) site of origin for the delay or block; (iii) whether rhythm is regular or irregular; (iv) mechanism of the arrhythmia; and (v) the ratio of atrial to ventricular depolarization (P waves–QRS complexes).

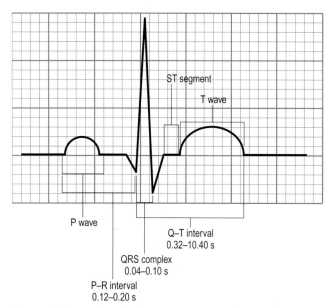

Figure 41.2 Graphic of ECG with all wave segments identified. Normal P–R interval measures between 0.12 seconds and 0.20 seconds. The normal duration for the QRS interval is between 0.04 seconds and 0.10 seconds. Normal R–R intervals are regular and equally distanced; if irregular, the distance between the shortest and longest is <0.12 seconds. Normal values for the Q–T interval depend on the heart rate. A normal ST segment is elevated or depressed by <1 mm. *(From Hillegass E 2011 Electrocardiography. In: Hillegass E (ed) Essentials of Cardiopulmonary Physical Therapy, 3rd edn. Saunders Elsevier, St Louis, MO, figure 9–18, p. 339, with permission.)*

BASIC RHYTHM DISTURBANCES AND IMPLICATIONS

Abnormal cardiac rhythms can arise in the atrial muscle, the junctional region between the atria and ventricles or in the ventricular muscle. These arrhythmias may be slow and sustained (bradycardias), occur as early single beats (extrasystoles or ectopic beats) or be sustained and fast (tachycardias). Rhythm disturbances may decrease cardiac output and potentially lead to orthostatic hypotension and possibly heart failure. If the ventricular rate is too fast, the volume of blood pumped with each contraction decreases. When the heart beats too slowly, the contractions are not adequate to supply the body's demands. In the normal adult, heart rates between 40 and 160 beats per minute (bpm) are usually well tolerated, as physiological adaptations are able to maintain an adequate cardiac output and blood pressure. However, problems can arise in those with significant vascular disease if the heart rate drops below 50 bpm or goes above 120 bpm. These alterations to rate can cause tissue ischemia, with the heart being especially susceptible.

Heart rate can be determined from an ECG through several methods. The gridlines on the ECG paper indicate time on the horizontal axis and electrical voltage on the vertical axis. The paper is set up in millimeters. One millimeter on the horizontal axis equals 0.04 seconds and 0.1 mV on the vertical axis. Heavier dark lines section the ECG paper into 5 mm by 5 mm larger boxes representing 0.2 seconds horizontally and 0.5 mV vertically (Weiderhold, 1988; Hillegass, 2011) (Fig. 41.3). Heart rate can be calculated by counting the number of R waves in a 6-second strip and multiplying by 10. Another way to estimate the heart is to memorize these triplicates: '300, 150, 100' and '75, 60, 50'. Then find an R wave that falls on one of the heavy black lines, count the number of large boxes to the next R wave, counting off heavy black lines with the triplicates between the two R waves (Weiderhold, 1988; Watchie, 2010; Hillegass, 2011) (Fig. 41.4).

Different areas of the heart are able to initiate the depolarization sequence if the SA node fails or, if conduction is blocked, another area will fire a depolarizing impulse and keep the heart beating. These secondary sites have lower depolarization frequencies than the SA node to avoid competition between pacing sites. As the heart is controlled by whichever site is discharging most frequently, the SA node with a rate of about 70 bpm is the primary site of impulse initiation. If the SA node fails, control will be assumed by a focus either in the atrial muscle or around the AV node (junctional region). Both of these have spontaneous depolarization frequencies of 40–60 bpm. If these fail, or conduction through the bundle of His is blocked, a ventricular focus will take over, with a rate of about 30–40 bpm (Weiderhold, 1988; Mammen et al., 2004). Therefore, the major mechanisms that cause bradyarrhythmias are either depression of SA node activity or blocks within the conducting system. In either situation, a supplementary pacemaker takes over to control the heart rate. If these supplementary pacemaker cells are located above the bifurcation of the bundle of His, the rate will be adequate enough to maintain cardiac output. Any bradyarrhythmia that causes hemodynamic compromise of the heart muscle requires urgent medical intervention.

Junctional impulses can arise from the AV node or above the bifurcation of the bundle of His. The impulse then spreads retrogradely or backwards through the atria and antegradely towards the ventricles. Depending on the site of origin and the conduction velocity of the impulse, and the refractory periods of the atria and ventricles, activation of the atria may occur before, during or after depolarization of the ventricle.

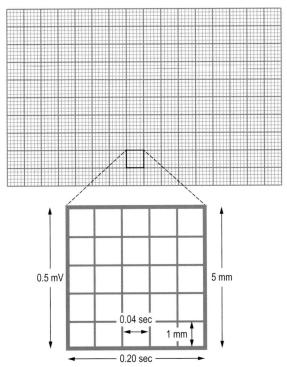

Figure 41.3 Electrocardiogram paper displays time on the horizontal axis. Each small box represents 0.04 seconds, and each large box represents 0.20 seconds. The vertical axis changes are measured in millimeters. Each small box represents 1 mm, each large box represents 5 mm.

Any part of the heart can depolarize earlier than it should and, if it initiates a heartbeat, this is called an extrasystole or ectopic beat. Atrial ectopic beats cause abnormally shaped P waves on the ECG, whereas junctional ectopic beats may have no P wave or a P wave immediately before or after the QRS complex, depending on the site of the ectopic focus within the junctional region. The QRS complexes for atrial and junctional ectopic beats have the same configuration as in normal SA rhythm. Ectopic beats arising in the ventricles do not travel down the normal bundle branches. Therefore, they evoke abnormally shaped QRS complexes, frequently referred to as wide and bizarre, which are easily recognized on an ECG tracing.

Tachycardia refers to a clinical state in which the heart rate is over 100 bpm. Regardless of whether an ectopic focus is within the atria, the junctional (AV nodal) region or the ventricles, it can fire rapidly and repeatedly causing a sustained tachycardia. Bradycardia refers to a heart rate that is less than 60 bpm. Urgent treatment is needed if there is hemodynamic compromise of the cardiac muscle or rhythms develop that have the potential to become life-threatening (Malone, 2006; Collins & Dias, 2009; Watchie, 2010; Hillegass, 2011).

The following discussion of the most common types of rhythm disturbance will be categorized according to the anatomical site of the disturbance: supraventricular (atrial), junctional or ventricular. Each will then be divided into the type of arrhythmia: slow, fast or ectopic. Conduction blocks are discussed separately as a cause of bradycardia.

ATRIAL ARRHYTHMIAS

SINUS ARRHYTHMIA

In sinus arrhythmia, the vagal nerves and changes in respiration can alter the rate of SA node discharge. The ECG is normal except for the variable lengths of the R–R intervals (Fig. 41.5). Variations are common, especially with changes in the rate of respiration. This rhythm is very prevalent in young people and tends to decline

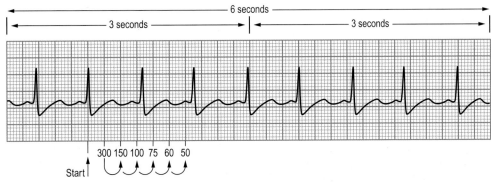

Figure 41.4 Heart rate can be calculated by counting the number of complexes in a 6-second strip and multiplying the result by 10 (particularly useful in very irregular rhythms) or by dividing 300 by the number of large squares between two R waves. To find the specific rate when the second R wave falls between two large squares, determine the difference between the two large squares on either side of the R wave (e.g. in the ECG shown 100 − 75 = 25 and divide this number by 5 (the number of small boxes in a large square); then multiply the result by the number of small boxes between the lesser number and the R wave (e.g. in the ECG shown 5 × 3 = 15) and add this result to the value of the lesser of the two large squares (75) yielding a HR of 90.

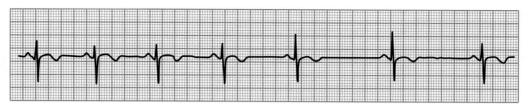

Figure 41.5 Sinus arrhythmia consisting of normal P–QRS–T configuration with increasing and decreasing intervals between the QRS complexes. *(From Thys D, Kaplan J 1987 The ECG in Anesthesia and Critical Care. Churchill Livingstone, New York, with permission.)*

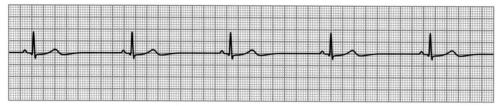

Figure 41.6 Sinus bradycardia with a rate of about 35 bpm.

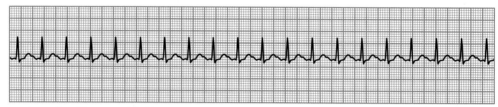

Figure 41.7 Sinus tachycardia with a rate of 150 bpm.

with aging. No treatment is required (Weiderhold, 1988; Mammen et al., 2004; Watchie, 2010; Hillegass, 2011).

SINUS BRADYCARDIA

Sinus bradycardia is a regular sinus rhythm but with a SA node rate below 60 bpm (Fig. 41.6). The ECG has normal P waves and P–R intervals and a 1:1 conduction ratio between the atria and ventricles, but an atrial rate of less than 60 bpm. It represents a suppression of the SA node discharge rate, usually in response to normal physiology in athletes, during sleep and with stimulation of the vagus nerve. It may be drug-related, especially from the use of narcotics, beta blockers and calcium-channel blockers. Pathologies that may produce a bradycardia rhythm include acute myocardial infarction, increased intracranial pressure, hypersensitivity of the carotid sinus and hypothyroidism. If evidence of hemodynamic compromise is present, then treatment is needed. Drug treatment can be useful in the short term; however, in those with symptomatic recurrent or persistent bradycardia, internal cardiac pacing is indicated (Weiderhold, 1988; Mammen et al., 2004; Watchie, 2010; Hillegass, 2011).

SINUS TACHYCARDIA

Sinus tachycardia is an acceleration of the SA node impulse discharge rate (Fig. 41.7). The ECG has normal P waves and P–R intervals and a 1:1 conduction ratio between the atria and ventricles. It only differs from normal sinus rhythm in that the rate is over 100 bpm. SA tachycardia is a normal expected response to increasing exercise intensity. It may also result from a normal

physiological response, as seen in infants, children and adults with emotions, especially anxiety. It may be drug-related, for example from the use of atropine, epinephrine (adrenaline), alcohol, nicotine and caffeine. It may also reflect a pathological process such as fever, hypoxia, anemia, hypovolemia or pulmonary embolism. In many of these conditions the increased rate is the result of the heart increasing cardiac output in an attempt to meet the increased circulatory demands. Treatment of the underlying condition is indicated, especially in those with preexisting cardiac disease, as increased cardiac output may further exacerbate any heart problems (Weiderhold, 1988; Mammen et al., 2004; Larry & Schaal, 2006; Watchie, 2010; Hillegass, 2011).

SUPRAVENTRICULAR TACHYCARDIA

Supraventricular arrhythmias include any rhythm in which the depolarizing impulse occurs above the level of the AV node. These rhythms all have a normal QRS complex following depolarization. Supraventricular tachycardia (SVT, also known as paroxysmal atrial tachycardia) is a regular rapid rhythm that arises from any site above the bifurcation of the bundle of His (Fig. 41.8). Sensations of palpitations and light-headedness are common with SVT. In those with coronary heart disease, angina pain and dyspnea may occur because of the rapid heart rate. SVT also commonly occurs in those with poor left ventricular function, heart failure and pulmonary edema. Treatment includes discontinuation of any causative drugs, use of a variety of antiarrhythmic medications to control rate and the use of vagal maneuvers (such as carotid sinus massage, Valsalva maneuver, holding breath and coughing or

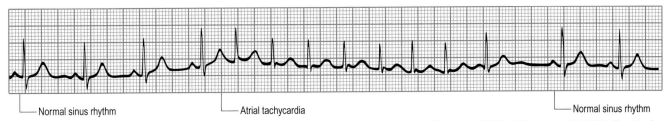

Normal sinus rhythm   Atrial tachycardia   Normal sinus rhythm

Figure 41.8 Paroxysmal atrial tachycardia, also known as supraventricular tachycardia (SVT). *(From Phillips RE, Feeney MK 1990 The Cardiac Rhythms, 3rd edn. WB Saunders, Philadelphia, PA, p. 154, with permission.)*

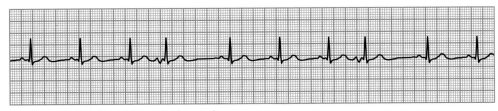

Figure 41.9 Sinus rhythm with PACs in the 4th and 8th complexes.

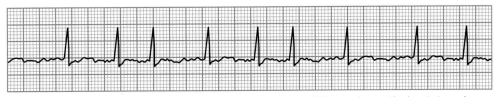

Figure 41.10 Atrial fibrillation – there are no P or T waves present between the QRS complexes. Rhythm is irregular, as noted by unequal distances between QRS complexes.

gagging) to slow the atrial rate. The physician may also perform a synchronized cardiac conversion, especially with an unstable patient with hypotension, pulmonary edema or severe chest pain (Weiderhold, 1988; Mammen et al., 2004; Larry & Schaal, 2006; Hillegass, 2011).

PREMATURE ATRIAL CONTRACTIONS

Premature atrial contractions (PACs) originate from ectopic pacemakers located anywhere in the atrium other than the SA node (Fig. 41.9). The ECG shows ectopic P waves that appear sooner than the next expected sinus beat. The ectopic P wave has a different shape and/or direction to a normal P wave. The ectopic P wave will not be conducted if it reaches the AV node during the absolute refractory period but it will be conducted with delay (longer P–R interval) during the relative refractory period. PACs that are conducted through the AV node, bundle of His and the bundle branches will have typical QRS complexes. PACs may appear at any age and are often seen in the absence of heart disease. It is generally believed that stress, fatigue, alcohol, tobacco and caffeine may precipitate PACs. Frequent PACs are seen in chronic lung disease, ischemic heart disease and digitalis toxicity. Treatment involves cessation of precipitating causes and management of underlying disorders. If the PACs produce symptoms or sustained tachycardias, drug therapy should be implemented, with the aim of suppressing the PACs (Weiderhold, 1988; Mammen et al., 2004; Larry & Schaal, 2006; Malone, 2006; Hillegass, 2011).

ATRIAL FIBRILLATION

Atrial fibrillation is one of the most common arrhythmias. It occurs when there are multiple areas of the atrial myocardium continuously discharging and contracting (Fig. 41.10). The atria literally twitch or quiver erratically. Depolarization and contraction are so disorganized and irregular that the atria quiver rather than contract uniformly. The atrial rate is usually above 400bpm, whereas the ventricular rate is slower because it is limited by the AV node refractory time. The ECG shows fibrillatory atrial activity instead of P waves and an irregular ventricular response (Weiderhold, 1988; Mammen et al., 2004; Larry & Schaal, 2006; Collins & Dias, 2009; Hillegass, 2011).

There are primarily two problems with atrial fibrillation. First, the atria do not depolarize and, consequently, there is no contraction of the atria. Contraction of the atria can add as much as 30% to the ventricular volume, therefore, without it, cardiac output can decrease by up to 30%. Cardiac output is usually not affected in individuals who have a ventricular response of less than 100bpm; however, in an individual with a resting heart rate of more than 100bpm or who exercises, signs of hemodynamic compromise may quickly be demonstrated. Second, there is a danger of blood coagulating in the fibrillating atria; a mural thrombus may form and subsequently lead to an embolus. In total, 30% of all patients with atrial fibrillation develop emboli (Watchie, 2010; Hillegass, 2011).

Atrial fibrillation can occur as either a paroxysmal burst or as a sustained rhythm. Advancing age, rheumatic

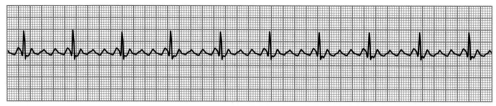

Figure 41.11 Atrial flutter waves are occurring at a rate of 4 per QRS complex.

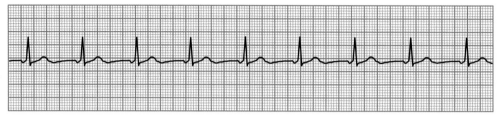

Figure 41.12 Junctional rhythm. Note the absence of P waves.

heart disease, congestive heart failure and hypertension are conditions in which atrial fibrillation commonly occurs. Treatment depends on the overall condition of the patient. Drugs can be used in the more stable patient. Response is best in those in whom the atrial fibrillation is treated shortly after onset. In individuals who become hemodynamically compromised, cardiac conversion or a pacemaker are other treatment choices (Weiderhold, 1988; Mammen et al., 2004; Watchie, 2010; Hillegass, 2011).

ATRIAL FLUTTER

The exact mechanism involved in the development of atrial flutter is unknown but the problem seems to involve a small area of the atrium only (Fig. 41.11). The ECG characteristics include a regular atrial rate of 250–350 bpm and sawtooth-shaped flutter waves in place of P waves. Atrial flutter rarely occurs in the absence of pre-existing heart disease. Incidence is highest in those with coronary artery disease, or acute myocardial infarction, but it can also be a complication of congestive cardiomyopathies, myocarditis, mitral valve disease, pulmonary embolus, blunt chest trauma and dioxin toxicity. Atrial flutter can occur as a transient arrhythmia between SA rhythm and atrial fibrillation. Treatment consists of cardiac conversion or medical therapy depending on the clinical status of the patient (Weiderhold, 1988; Mammen et al., 2004; Larry & Schaal, 2006; Malone, 2006; Collins and Dias, 2009; Hillegass, 2011).

JUNCTIONAL RHYTHM

Under normal circumstances, the SA node discharges at a faster rate than the AV node, so the pacemaker at the AV junction is overridden. If the SA node discharge is slow or fails to reach the AV node, a junctional escape beat (Fig. 41.12) may occur, usually at a rate of 40–60 bpm. Generally, these escape beats do not conduct back into the atria, so a QRS complex without a P wave is seen on the ECG. However, if the impulse generated by the AV node or junctional tissue is reflected back to the atria, it

may be seen as an inverted P wave before, during or after the ventricular contraction. Whenever there is a long enough pause before an impulse reaches the AV node, the junctional pacemaker can elicit a junctional beat. Sustained junctional escape rhythms may be seen with congestive heart failure, dioxin toxicity or myocarditis. (Malone, 2006; Watchie, 2010; Hillegass, 2011).

JUNCTIONAL TACHYCARDIA

An enhanced junctional impulse may override the SA node and produce either an accelerated junctional rhythm (rate 60–100 bpm) or a junctional tachycardia with rates greater than 100 bpm. The P waves are absent. Accelerated junctional rhythm or junctional tachycardia can occur with hyperventilation, coronary artery disease, dioxin toxicity, caffeine or nicotine sensitivity, overexertion and emotional factors. If the enhanced rhythm is sustained and produces symptoms of hemodynamic compromise or ischemia, therapy for the underlying cause is required. Acute therapy to increase the SA rate may also be needed. At higher rates, it is difficult to differentiate SVT from junctional tachycardia because, if the P wave is present, it is lost in the QRS complex and not visualized (Weiderhold, 1988; Mammen et al., 2004; Hillegass, 2011).

VENTRICULAR ARRHYTHMIAS

PREMATURE VENTRICULAR CONTRACTIONS

Premature ventricular contractions (PVCs) are impulses that arise from single or multiple areas within the ventricles. The ECG shows a premature, widened and often bizarre QRS complex with no preceding P wave (Fig. 41.13). The ST segment and T wave of the PVC are opposite in direction to the major QRS deflection. Most PVCs do not affect the SA node discharge and it will therefore trigger the next impulse after the refractory period. If conducted to the atria, a PVC will cause a retrograde (inverted) P wave. PVCs are common, even

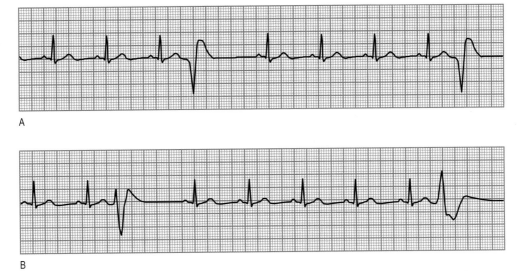

Figure 41.13 Premature ventricular contractions. (A) Sinus rhythm with unifocal PVCs in the 4th and 9th complexes. (B) Sinus rhythm with multifocal PVCs: the 3rd and 9th PVCs look different because they are generated from different ectopic foci.

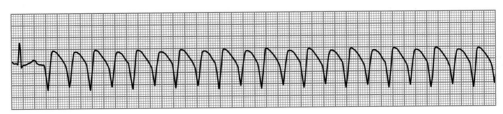

Figure 41.14 Ventricular tachycardia.

in those without heart disease. They occur frequently in individuals with ischemic heart disease and are universally found in those with acute myocardial infarction. This highlights the underlying electrical instability of the heart and the added risk of developing ventricular tachycardia. Other common causes of PVCs include congestive heart failure, hypoxia, dioxin toxicity, caffeine or nicotine sensitivity, and hypokalemia. Treatment of PVCs is important in those with acute myocardial ischemia or infarction where maintenance of cardiac output is critical. The treatment of chronic ectopy depends on balancing the underlying heart disease, the origin of the ectopy and the presence of symptoms against the risks of side-effects from antiarrhythmic drugs (Weiderhold, 1988; Mammen et al., 2004; Larry & Schaal, 2006; Malone, 2006; Collins & Dias, 2009; Hillegass, 2011).

VENTRICULAR TACHYCARDIA

Ventricular tachycardia is the occurrence of three or more beats from a ventricular ectopic pacemaker at a rate of more than 100bpm (Malone, 2006; Watchie, 2010; Hillegass, 2011). The ECG findings are wide QRS complexes because of aberrant conduction, heart rates greater than 100bpm (usually 150–200bpm), a regular rhythm and a constant QRS axis. Ventricular tachycardia can occur in a non-sustained manner, usually as short bursts of a few seconds that then spontaneously terminate, or in a sustained fashion with longer episodes (Fig. 41.14) with symptoms of hemodynamic instability.

The latter requires immediate treatment. A danger with sustained ventricular tachycardia is that it can deteriorate into ventricular fibrillation. Ventricular tachycardia is rare in individuals without underlying heart disease. Ischemic heart disease and acute myocardial infarction are the most common causes of ventricular tachycardia. Unstable patients are treated with cardiac conversion, whereas more stable patients receive intravenous antiarrhythmic drugs (Weiderhold, 1988; Mammen et al., 2004; Malone, 2006; Watchie, 2010; Hillegass, 2011).

VENTRICULAR FIBRILLATION

Ventricular fibrillation is the totally disorganized, erratic depolarization and contraction of the ventricular myocardium so that no effective ventricular or cardiac output occurs. The ECG shows a fine to coarse zigzag pattern with no detectable P waves or QRS complexes (Fig. 41.15). There is no blood pressure or pulse detectable in ventricular fibrillation. In an awake and responsive person, an ECG pattern of ventricular fibrillation is usually a result of loose-lead artifact or electrical interference. Ventricular fibrillation is the most common complication of severe ischemic heart disease, with or without acute myocardial infarction. It can occur suddenly without preceding hemodynamic deterioration or after a period of left ventricular failure and/or circulatory shock. Other etiologic factors include dioxin toxicity, blunt chest injury, hypothermia, severe electrolyte abnormalities and myocardial irritation from

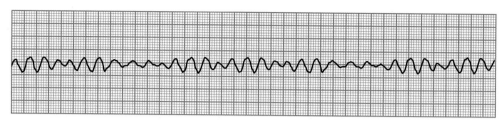

Figure 41.15 Ventricular fibrillation.

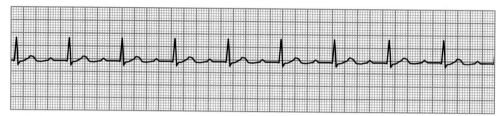

Figure 41.16 Sinus rhythm with first-degree heart block. Note the P wave is greater than 0.20 seconds in length from the beginning of the QRS complex.

intracardiac catheter or pacemaker wires. Treatment is immediate defibrillation; several attempts may be necessary. Antiarrhythmic medications are used as adjuncts to cardiac conversion (Weiderhold, 1988; Mammen et al., 2004; Malone, 2006; Collins & Dias, 2009; Watchie, 2010; Hillegass, 2011).

CONDUCTION DISTURBANCES

SA NODE BLOCK

In normal sinus rhythm, the SA node discharge traverses the atria and paces the heart. SA node block can occur when the impulses are either delayed or have their propagation blocked. The block can be divided into first-, second- and third-degree types. First-degree block results from a delay in impulse conduction out of the SA node to the atria. With second-degree block, some impulses get through whereas others do not. Third-degree block is when the SA node discharge is completely blocked, meaning that no P waves originate from the SA node. SA node block can result from myocardial disease, especially acute inferior myocardial infarction. Drug toxicity and myocarditis can also cause this type of block. Treatment is dependent on the underlying cause, the associated arrhythmias and whether hemodynamic compromise is present. Specific drugs can increase SA node discharge and aid conduction. Recurrent or persistent bradycardia, especially if symptomatic, may require an artificial cardiac pacemaker (Weiderhold, 1988; Mammen et al., 2004).

FIRST-DEGREE AV BLOCK

First-degree heart block is characterized by a delay in AV conduction. In other words, after the SA node discharges, it takes longer for the impulse to reach the AV node. Although each impulse is conducted to the ventricles, the rate is slower than normal, leading to prolongation of the P–R interval by more than 0.20 seconds (or more than five small boxes on the ECG tracing; Fig. 41.16).

It is occasionally found in normal hearts but is more commonly seen with acute myocardial infarction, drug toxicity and myocarditis. Generally, nerve conduction velocity is known to slow with the aging process; first-degree heart block may be a functional result of this decrease. Generally, first-degree heart block is relatively benign. No treatment is required unless more serious conduction disturbances are also present (Weiderhold, 1988; Mammen et al., 2004; Malone, 2006; Collins & Dias, 2009; Watchie, 2010; Hillegass, 2011).

SECOND-DEGREE AV BLOCK

Second-degree AV blocks are subdivided into Mobitz I (or Wenckebach) and Mobitz II blocks. The Wenckebach phenomenon describes the progressive lengthening of the P–R interval, a dropped beat and repetition of the cycle (Fig. 41.17). There is progressive prolongation of AV conduction and the P–R interval until an atrial impulse is completely blocked by a refractory AV node. After the dropped beat, which is seen as a P wave not followed by a QRS complex, the AV conduction returns to normal and the cycle repeats itself with either the same (fixed) or a different (variable) conduction ratio. This block is usually transient and can be associated with an acute myocardial infarction, dioxin toxicity, myocarditis or cardiac surgery. It is usually benign and asymptomatic (Malone, 2006; Collins & Dias, 2009). Specific treatment is not required unless the ventricular rate is slow enough to reduce cardiac output and produce signs of hemodynamic compromise (Weiderhold, 1988; Mammen et al., 2004; Malone, 2006; Hillegass, 2011).

In the Mobitz type II form of second-degree block, one or more beats may not be conducted at a single time and the P–R interval remains constant before and after the nonconducted atrial beats. There are more P waves than QRS complexes (Fig. 41.18). This type of block frequently occurs with bundle-branch (or fascicular) problems and the QRS complexes are consequently widened. Type II block means that there is structural damage to the conducting system, which is usually permanent

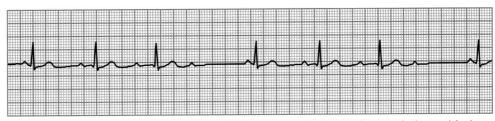

Figure 41.17 Second-degree AV heart block type I (Wenckebach's). Notice how the P waves become farther and farther away from the QRS complex until it fails to elicit a QRS complex. This is occurring after each 4th P wave.

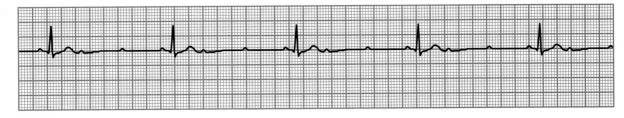

Figure 41.18 Second-degree AV heart block type II (Mobitz II). P waves are occurring at regular intervals, but do not always elicit a QRS wave or ventricular contraction.

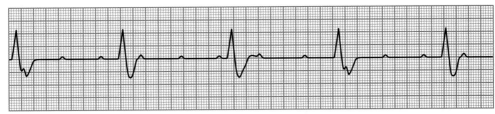

Figure 41.19 Third-degree heart block, also known as complete heart block. The rhythm of the P waves and QRS complexes are independent of each other.

and may proceed suddenly to complete heart block, especially in the setting of acute myocardial infarction. Emergency treatment is required if the ventricular rate is slow enough to produce symptoms of hemodynamic compromise. In most cases, especially those that occur in conjunction with acute myocardial infarction, insertion of permanent cardiac pacemakers is usually indicated (Weiderhold, 1988; Mammen et al., 2004; Malone, 2006; Hillegass, 2011).

THIRD-DEGREE (COMPLETE) AV BLOCK

In third-degree AV block, none of the impulses initiated above the ventricles is through the normal AV conduction system. The ventricles are paced by ectopic impulses generated somewhere in the ventricles and at a slower rate than the atrial rate, which continues to originate from the SA node (Fig. 41.19) (Malone, 2006; Hillegass, 2011). If the block occurs at the level of the AV node, a junctional pacemaker (rate 40–60 bpm) takes over. The resultant QRS complexes are narrow, as the rhythm originates before the bifurcation of the bundle of His. When the block occurs below the AV node, a ventricular rhythm at a rate of less than 40 bpm drives the ventricles. This is usually inadequate to maintain cardiac output. The QRS complexes are wider than normal. Blocks of the SA and AV nodes develop frequently in patients with acute myocardial infarction. Although most are transient, they may persist for several days.

Blocks that originate below the bifurcation of the bundle of His indicate structural damage to the distal conducting system and are seen with extensive acute anterior myocardial infarction. External pacing or drugs may be used in the short term to accelerate the ventricular escape rhythm until insertion of a pacemaker can be completed (Weiderhold, 1988; Mammen et al., 2004; Malone, 2006; Hillegass, 2011).

BUNDLE-BRANCH BLOCKS (FASCICULAR BLOCKS)

Bundle-branch or fascicular blocks can include one, two or all three fascicles. As illustrated in Figure 41.1, the bundle of His bifurcates into the right bundle branch and left bundle branch, which almost immediately divides into the left anterior and posterior branches. The block occurs when one of the three major conduction pathways below the AV node and bundle of His has an obstruction to the passage of the depolarization impulse. It can be recognized by a widening of the QRS complex and an interval length of more than 0.11 seconds (Fig. 41.20). Conduction blocks in the fascicles can be caused by a wide variety of conditions, such as ischemia, cardiomyopathies, valvular heart problems (especially aortic), myocarditis, cardiac surgery and degenerative processes that affect the conduction tissue (Weiderhold, 1988; Mammen et al., 2004; Larry & Schaal, 2006).

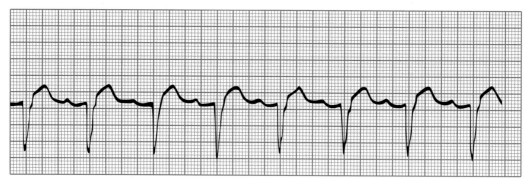

Figure 41.20 Bundle-branch block demonstrating a wide QRS complex with a normal sinus rhythm. *(From Cohen M, Michel TH 1988 Cardiopulmonary Symptoms in Physical Therapy Practice. Churchill Livingstone, New York, p. 157.)*

REHABILITATION CONSIDERATIONS FOR INDIVIDUALS WITH CARDIAC ARRHYTHMIAS AND CONDUCTION DISTURBANCES

The underlying reason for an irregular heart rate cannot be determined by palpation of a pulse. As discussed in the previous sections, some irregularities in rate can be relatively benign, whereas others can lead to potentially lethal arrhythmias. It is imperative that the etiology of the underlying arrhythmia be identified and understood to enable the development of an appropriate treatment plan, either through a prudent chart review or by contacting the physician. It is irresponsible to treat all individuals with cardiovascular disease with the same cardiac precautions. Exercise progression should be response and symptom guided (Weiderhold, 1988; Mammen et al., 2004; Larry & Schaal, 2006; Watchie, 2010; Hillegass, 2011).

Atrial arrhythmias without conduction disturbances are generally less serious than ventricular arrhythmias. Any individual with an arrhythmia that leads to hemodynamic compromise and decreased cardiac output should be monitored closely for signs of exercise intolerance. (See Box 39.3 for guidelines for termination of an exercise session.)

CONCLUSION

The most common cardiac arrhythmias and conduction disturbances have been described. Some of these abnormalities are more serious than others. Differentiating between the less serious and the potentially life-threatening arrhythmias cannot be completely assured by taking a pulse and auscultating heart sounds. A thorough cardiac evaluation is therefore essential. Before beginning an exercise program for a patient with known cardiac pathology, it is important that the therapist understands the implications of the patient/client's cardiac arrhythmias so that they are treated neither too aggressively nor undertreated.

Acknowledgement

The author would like to acknowledge Diann C. Cooper, MSN, RN, BC, for assistance with creation and development of the ECG drawings.

REFERENCES

Collins SM, Dias KJ 2009 Cardiac system. In: Paz JC, West MP (eds) Acute Care Handbook for Physical Therapists, 3rd edn. Saunders Elsevier, St Louis, MO, pp. 1–46

Hillegass E 2011 Electrocardiography. In: Hillegass E (ed) Essentials of Cardiopulmonary Physical Therapy, 3rd edn. Saunders Elsevier, St Louis, MO, pp. 331–364

Larry JA, Schaal SF 2006 Dysrhythmias and selected conduction defects. In: ACSM's Resource Manual for Guidelines for Exercise Testing and Prescription, 5th edn. Lippincott Williams & Wilkins, Philadelphia, PA, pp. 289–302

Malone DJ 2006 Cardiovascular diseases and disorders. In: Malone DJ, Bishop-Lindsay KB (eds) Physical Therapy in Acute Care: A Clinician's Guide. Slack Inc., Thorofare, NJ, pp. 139–209

Mammen BA, Irwin S, Tecklin JS 2004 Common cardiac and pulmonary clinical measures. In: Irwin S, Tecklin JS (eds) Cardiopulmonary Physical Therapy: A Guide to Practice, 4th edn. Mosby–Yearbook, St Louis, MO, pp. 177–244

Watchie J 2010 Cardiopulmonary assessment. In: Cardiovascular and Pulmonary Physical Therapy, 2nd edn. Saunders Elsevier, St Louis, MO, pp. 222–297

Weiderhold R 1988 Electrocardiography: The Monitoring Lead. WB Saunders, Philadelphia, PA

Chapter 42
Heart failure and valvular heart disease

CHRIS L. WELLS

CHAPTER CONTENTS

INTRODUCTION

Despite the increase in diagnostic procedures and medical management, heart disease continues to be one of the most common causes of morbidity and mortality in the United States of America. The rise in life expectancy, increases in hypertension, obesity, diabetes mellitus and sedentary lifestyles are all contributing to the increasing cardiovascular disease. This chapter will briefly discuss heart failure and valvular disease.

HEART FAILURE

Heart failure (HF) is defined as the inability of the heart to pump blood at a sufficient rate to meet the metabolic demands of the body. HF can be the result of many different diseases; therefore, it is important to complete a thorough history taking and evaluation of the patient with HF to identify the underlying pathology and any factors that exacerbate the HF. The heart may compensate for years before the patient reaches a level of dysfunction that leads to the clinical presentation of HF. In many cases, it is an acute event that places additional stress on the heart, beyond its ability to circulate a sufficient blood flow, leading to clinical HF. Exacerbation or progression of other chronic diseases, such as renal insufficiency, infections, cardiac arrhythmias, uncontrolled hypertension or diabetes, and poor dietary consumption, can precipitate the insidious onset of clinical signs and symptoms associated with HF (see Chapters 41 and 46).

HF can be categorized in many ways. The Heart Failure Society of America describes two types of HF. HF with reduced left ventricular function, which is commonly associated with a dilated ventricle, is referred to as systolic HF where the myocardial contraction is ineffective in circulating blood forward into the pulmonary and systemic circulations. In HF with preserved left ventricular function, also known as diastolic dysfunction, the ventricles do not relax to allow for sufficient filling. The patient with HF can be clinically present in an acute or a chronic medical state. Finally, HF can present as predominately left HF or right HF, or as biventricular failure (Lindenfeld et al., 2010).

Heart failure, a clinical syndrome, is associated with symptoms of shortness of breath with exertion and rest, fatigue and tiredness, and signs of abnormal heart rate, elevation in respiratory rate, pulmonary rales, pleural effusions, jugular vein distension, peripheral edema and hepatomegaly. The heart has structural or functional changes that lead to its inability to pump blood at a sufficient rate to meet the metabolic demands of the body (Lindenfeld et al., 2010; Shiba & Shimokawa, 2011). The body attempts to compensate by increasing sympathetic nervous system (SNS) activity which increases heart rate and contractility to improve cardiac output. This increase in the SNS also leads to increased oxygen demand and additional inflammation and stress that eventually will further impair heart function (Barnes et al., 2011).

Congestive heart failure (CHF) is a common clinical term used to describe a cluster of signs and symptoms associated with HF. When cardiac pump function is inadequate to meet the circulatory demands of the body, the body attempts to decrease the volume of blood the heart has to circulate, which leads to fluid retention. Fluid leaves the vascular system and is stored in various parts of the body, hence the term 'congestive heart failure'. When the left ventricular pump function is impaired, excess fluid is stored in the pulmonary interstitium to decrease the workload of the left ventricle. Left ventricular dysfunction is commonly associated with an increase in stress to the right ventricle. Right ventricular myocardial dysfunction leads to an increased blood volume in the venous system and liver which is associated with jugular vein distention, peripheral edema, hepatomegaly and abdominal ascites.

CAUSES OF VENTRICULAR FAILURE

To understand heart failure, it is important to understand the basic cardiac cycle. Blood flows from the venous system and the pulmonary capillary beds into the right and left atria respectively. Once there is a sufficient volume and, therefore, enough pressure in the atria, the atrioventricular, tricuspid and mitral valves will open to allow filling of the ventricles. When the atria contract another 15–20% of the blood volume is delivered into the ventricles and the atrioventricular valves close. The right and left ventricles then begin to contract, generating enough force to open the semilunar, pulmonic and aortic valves and eject blood into the pulmonary circulation for gas exchange and into the systemic circulation to meet the metabolic demands of the body's cells.

Coronary artery disease, which leads to myocardial impairment, is one of the most common causes of HF (McKenna et al., 2012); however, there are many other diseases, such as valvular lesions, viral infections, myocardial dysfunction and pulmonary disease that can also lead to the development of HF. In older adults coronary artery disease and aortic valvular disease are the most common causes of HF (McKenna et al., 2012; Vasques et al., 2012). Along with the diagnosis, it is important to identify factors that exacerbate HF or lead to an uncompensated state, such as excessive fluid consumption, arrhythmias, systematic infection and kidney failure. Understanding the pathology and contributing factors can aid in the delivery of prompt and appropriate medical intervention and patient education.

The most common cause of right ventricular failure (RVF) is left ventricular pump dysfunction. Failure to pump blood forward into the aorta leads to a backflow of blood and an increase in pressure within the left atrium and eventually within the pulmonary system. The right ventricle is not anatomically designed to pump under elevated pressure, which leads to RVF. Right HF may also result from pulmonary hypertension caused by a pulmonary disease such as emphysema and from a pulmonary embolism. Finally, RVF can also be the result of mitral or tricuspid valve disease, restrictive or hypertrophic cardiomyopathies and viral or idiopathic myocarditis.

Left ventricular failure (LVF) leads to lower systemic cardiac output. It can be caused by the long-term adverse effects of hypertension, aortic or mitral valve disease and coronary artery disease. Coronary artery disease can cause pump dysfunction because of the long-term subtle effects of myocardial ischemia or because of an acute ischemic event, such as an abrupt rupture of an atherosclerotic plaque, which leads to a myocardial infarction. Less frequently, LVF may also occur because of a systemic condition such as septic shock. During this critical medical state, the left ventricle attempts to increase cardiac output to meet the high oxygen demand of the body. The stress from this physiological imbalance may lead to the left ventricle being unable to meet the body's needs, resulting in LVF.

CONTRIBUTING FACTORS

There are several factors that can lead to HF. These factors can either increase the body's needs or further decrease cardiac output. Cardiac arrhythmias such as atrial fibrillation can decrease cardiac output in the presence of myocardial pump dysfunction. Atrial fibrillation is a common arrhythmia in older adults and is one of the most common arrhythmias associated with HF. With atrial fibrillation, the atria do not contract as a unit and therefore the ventricles do not receive the last 15–20% of blood volume,

causing the loss of the 'atrial kick'. In the presence of pump dysfunction, atrial fibrillation may lead to a loss of filling which also results in an insufficient stretch of the ventricular myocardium. This consequence is a further decrease in cardiac output. The compensatory mechanism for the loss of the atrial kick is an increase in heart rate, which further impairs filling, increases oxygen demand and decreases output (Trigo & Fischer, 2012). Others types of arrhythmias may exacerbate HF depending on the severity of the pump dysfunction and how the arrhythmia affects myocardial perfusion, ventricular filling time and cardiac output. In general, with tachycardiac rhythms there is an increase in myocardial oxygen demand and a decreased output by shortening the filling time. With bradycardiac rhythms there is sufficient filling time but the rate may not be sufficient to maintain output. Finally, arrhythmias generated from the ventricles can directly lead to insufficient filling and contraction of the ventricles.

Acute myocardial ischemia and infarction are some of the leading causes of HF in the older adult. Coronary artery disease is associated with inflammation and arterial thrombosis and plaque formation, which leads to narrowing of the lumen diameter. This decreases blood flow to the myocardium that eventually impairs the tissue. When oxygen demand exceeds supply, myocardial cells can become injured or die leading to myocardial pump dysfunction and eventually HF.

Improper utilization of medications and poor dietary choices can also precipitate HF. The discontinuation of medications such as diuretics and beta blockers, which are commonly used to manage blood pressure and volume status, can lead to the development of HF. Overuse of beta blockers can lead to an insufficient heart rate to supply sufficient output. Improper prescription/administration and monitoring of the therapeutic levels of medications like antiarrhythmics and calcium-channel blockers can also contribute to HF. In the presence of impaired myocardial function, increased consumption of sodium or large amounts of fluids can lead to fluid overload and HF.

In cases of anemia, the heart tries to compensate by increasing cardiac output to meet oxygen demands. When there is myocardial pump dysfunction, the heart may not be able to sustain this increased stress. Anemia and the increased workload may lead to further ischemia and precipitate HF. Anemia is a common comorbidity in the elderly and is a probable factor to manage during the postoperative period (van Veldhuisen et al., 2011). The therapist must consider the increase in oxygen demand during functional mobility training in an individual with both anemia and heart disease. It is therefore important to monitor laboratory results and vital signs closely.

Individuals with pulmonary disease such as interstitial pulmonary fibrosis, chronic obstructive disease and vascular disease can lead to HF. Often the progression of lung disease leads to vascular changes within the lungs which may lead to pulmonary arterial hypertension (PAH). The increase in pulmonary arterial pressure causes stress on the right ventricle which cannot sustain the increased workload and eventually fails. The failure of the right ventricle will likely lead to left ventricular dysfunction and failure.

CLINICAL MANIFESTATIONS

The most common symptoms associated with HF are dyspnea, fatigue and exercise intolerance. Dyspnea and tachypnea can be related to many factors, including pulmonary vascular congestion and an increased work of breathing. Other factors include a decrease in cardiac output to meet peripheral tissue demand, disuse atrophy, alterations in skeletal muscles and renal dysfunction. The patient will report a progressive shortness of breath with exertion, to dyspnea at rest, as pump dysfunction progresses (Shiba & Shimokawa, 2011; McKenna et al., 2012). Box 42.1 describes the signs and symptoms associated with right and left HF; however, it is important to note that it is uncommon to see isolated unilateral HF. Box 42.2 describes the signs and symptoms associated with systolic and diastolic HF.

Fatigue and exercise intolerance associated with HF are still currently under investigation to better understand this complex clinical disorder. Exercise intolerance is defined as 'the reduced ability to perform activities that involve dynamic movement of large muscles because of symptoms of dyspnea or fatigue' (Downing & Balady, 2011). The failing heart has a limited ability to increase cardiac output on demand. A rise in stroke volume and heart rate is blunted, leading to a depressed cardiac output and a response that is insufficient to meet the rise in metabolic demand. Heart rate response is also reduced with age, which in some individuals can also contribute to the limited cardiac response in the elderly.

In HF there are several factors that limit exercise tolerance which are linked to vascular and peripheral abnormalities. There is a reduction in blood flow to skeletal muscles because of the increase in vasoconstriction, elevation of the renin–angiotensin system and the impaired endothelial mechanism regulating peripheral blood flow (see Chapter 9). There is also a decrease in blood distribution to active muscles when compared with healthy individuals. The skeletal fiber makeup in patients with HF is also altered; there is a reduction in type I fibers and an increase in type II fibers, which reduces the aerobic capacity of the individual. There is also a further reduction to type IIa fibers when compared to type IIB. There is a reduction in mitochondria and oxidative enzymes that leads to lactate production, which leads to reduced work capacity. Finally, in response to the skeletal metabolic acidosis that occurs in the early phase of exercise, there is a further increase in vasoconstriction that amplifies exercise intolerance (Downing & Balady, 2011).

The therapist needs to keep in mind that there is a poor link between the resting ejection fraction, which is the percentage of blood flow ejected upon contraction, and exercise tolerance. Ejection fraction (linked to prognosis and mortality, exercise tolerance and therefore rehabilitation potential) appears to be more related to the heart's ability to respond to the increase in metabolic demand by increasing stroke volume and heart rate than by the resting value for left ventricular ejection fraction (Smart et al., 2012).

THERAPEUTIC INTERVENTION

The number of cases of HF continues to rise as life expectancy increases and there are medical and surgical advances in managing heart disease. The first line of intervention is in the prevention of heart disease by reducing the associated risk factors, such as smoking, hypertension, diabetes and obesity. The American Heart Association recommends that everyone should participate in at least 30 minutes daily of moderately intense activity, eat sensibly and maintain a proper body weight. Medical management includes the proper treatment of hypertension, dyslipidemia, hypercholesterolemia and diabetes. Diuretics can be used to lower blood volume along with beta blockers and angiotensin-converting enzyme (ACE) inhibitors to treat hypertension. When pump dysfunction becomes significant, inotropic medications like dobutamine and milrinone can be used to improve cardiac function; antiarrhythmics are also helpful in the management of HF. The use of pacemakers and implantable cardiac defibrillators are options that have

---

Box 42.1 *Common Signs and Symptoms of Right and Left Heart Failure*

RIGHT HEART FAILURE	LEFT HEART FAILURE
Peripheral edema	Orthopnea
Pitting edema	Paroxysmal nocturnal dyspnea
Ascites	Exercise intolerance with fatigue and weakness
Jugular vein distention	Pulmonary rales
S3 heart sound	Dyspnea of exertion
Hepatojugular reflux	Dry, non-productive cough in supine
Abdominal discomfort/anorexia	Unexplained mental status changes

---

Box 42.2 *Common Signs and Symptoms of Systolic and Diastolic Heart Failure*

DIASTOLIC HEART FAILURE

Right Ventricle	Left Ventricle
Jugular vein distension	Dyspnea
Liver engorgement	Tachycardia
Peripheral edema	Dry cough
Weight gain	Wheezing
Anorexia	Rales
	S3 heart sound
	Systolic murmur
	Hypoxemia
	Orthopnea

SYSTOLIC HEART FAILURE

Dyspnea	Fatigue and exercise intolerance
Desaturation	Angina
Cyanosis	Exertional dyspnea
Tachypnea	Narrow pulse pressure
Hypoxia	Decrease in mental status
	Decrease in urination
	Cool, pale diaphoresis

shown success in the management of serious arrhythmias. Surgical management is appropriate to correct valvular dysfunction, and coronary artery bypass grafting can be carried out to restore myocardial perfusion. More recently the implantation of ventricular assist devices for long-term use, referred to as destination therapy, is becoming more widespread for the management of older adults with HF (Lietz, 2010).

Exercise has become a key component in the medical management of HF. Many studies have documented improvements in aerobic capacity and muscle performance with exercise in subjects with HF. There are improvements in the peripheral abnormalities for patients who participate in a routine exercise program. Improvement in the strength and endurance of respiratory muscles have also been documented and is associated with a decreased level of dyspnea with exertion. Finally, there is an improvement in the quality of life (Downing & Balady, 2011; Smart et al., 2012; Mentz et al., 2013).

VALVULAR DISEASE

The heart has four valves, which function to keep blood flowing in a unidirectional manner with myocardial contraction. The opening and closing of the valves operates on the principles of volume/pressure. As blood returns to the heart via the venous system, the atria fill while all of the valves are closed. Once there is a sufficient volume within the atria, the increased pressure opens the atrioventricular (tricuspid and mitral) valves. The tricuspid valve separates the right atrium and right ventricle, and the mitral valve is located between the left atrium and left ventricle. When the atria contract, the atria finish filling the ventricles, then the valves close. The ventricles contract to generate a pressure that is sufficient enough to overcome the pressure within the pulmonary trunk and aorta. At that time, the semilunar valves (pulmonic and aortic) open to eject blood from the right and left ventricles respectively.

The atrioventricular valves have several components that can be damaged, resulting in various clinical signs and symptoms. The annulus is composed of fibrous rings that provide a secure attachment for the leaflets, or cusps. The space at the edge of the annulus where the leaflets insert is referred to as the commissure. The leaflets are made of a strong fibrous material and function as doors that allow unidirectional blood flow in the presence of a pressure gradient. The margins of the leaflets are thin and are stabilized by the chordae tendineae cordis, strong fibrous cords that originate from the papillary muscle and insert into the leaflet margins. When myocardial contraction occurs, the papillary muscles contract as well, making the chordae tendineae cordis taut. It is this relationship that prevents the leaflets from inverting and causing a backwards flow of blood through the heart (see Fig. 42.1).

The semilunar valves are similar in function but are structurally different from the atrioventricular valves. There are three cusps per valve; they have a concave-convex shape, with the convexity facing the ventricles. After the ventricles begin to relax, there is a tendency for the blood to flow backwards toward the ventricles. The concavities of the cusps fill with blood and the pressure from this blood secures the approximation of the cusps. The pulmonic valve is a more delicate structure than the aortic valve, which must be rugged to function under the high pressure that exists.

Valvular dysfunction is commonly categorized by the alteration in blood flow across the valve, valvular stenosis or regurgitation. A stenotic valve describes the narrowing of the opening of the valve. This condition interferes with the flow of blood through the valve and places an increased oxygen demand on the myocardium. Over time, a stenotic valve will cause hypertrophy and dilatation of the chambers. Regurgitation, which is also referred to as a valvular insufficiency, is defined as backflow of blood across the valve, leading to an enlargement of the cardiac chamber before the dysfunctional valve. In either situation, the end result is an increase in oxygen demand, myocardial ischemia and eventually heart failure. The two dysfunctions are not mutually exclusive of one another; a valve can be categorized as stenotic and insufficient.

CAUSES OF VALVULAR DISEASE

Valvular dysfunction has many causes depending upon the valve in question and the age of the individual. Worldwide, rheumatic heart disease (RHD) is the leading cause of valvular disease, but with the aging population in industrial countries the leading cause of valvular dysfunction is degenerative (Vahanian et al., 2011). The most common valvular dysfunctions are mitral regurgitation (MR) and aortic stenosis (AS). There is an increased incidence of valvular disease with aging, with the incidence at 2% for individuals less than 65 years of age and slightly over 13% for individuals over 75 years of age (Vahanian et al., 2011). Other causes of valvular dysfunction include infectious endocarditis, trauma, dilated cardiomyopathy, myocardial infarction, pulmonary hypertension,

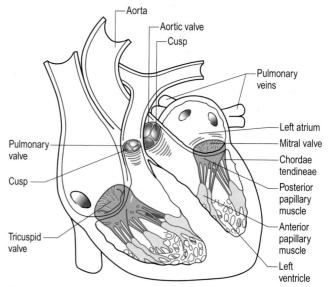

Figure 42.1 Structure of the cardiac valves. (*From Myers R 1995 Saunders Manual of Physical Therapy Practice. WB Saunders, Philadelphia, PA, p 196, with permission from Elsevier.*)

congenital anomaly and HF. The following sections will discuss AS and MR but tricuspid and pulmonic valvular disease can also be present and can lead to right atrial enlargement, right ventricular hypertrophy, pulmonary hypertension and HF.

Many individuals with valvular dysfunction will be asymptomatic until myocardial function is significantly impaired such that cardiac output is no longer maintained at an appropriate level. With a sound understanding of normal cardiopulmonary physiology the therapist can have a better understanding of how a stenotic or insufficient valve will adversely affect cardiac function. Patients with asymptomatic AS commonly develop symptoms within 5 years. With a better understanding of cardiac function (Spaccarotella et al., 2011), the therapist will be more skilled in detecting the signs and symptoms of progressive valvular disease thus becoming a productive member of the healthcare team in the management of patients' health and wellbeing.

Aortic stenosis is a clinically significant valvular dysfunction because of the impact on left ventricular function and associated mortality rates. The prevalence ranges from 2% to 7% for individuals greater than 65 years of age and is associated with a survival rate less than 30% for individuals with severe symptomatic AS. Thirty-three percent of patients over 75 years of age refuse surgery or are not considered surgical candidates. They have up to a 60% 2-year mortality (Spaccarotella et al., 2011). The narrowing of the aortic valve leads to increased pressure across the valve, left ventricular hypertrophy and an increase in myocardial oxygen demand. This leads to increased coronary vascular resistance and, consequently, to a decrease in myocardial perfusion. Hypertrophy is commonly accompanied with subaortic stenosis leading to further narrowing of the left ventricle outflow track. This increases afterload or resistance to eject blood forward and further increases myocardial strain and coronary artery compression. With the oxygen demand and supply mismatch the individual may experience angina, suffer a myocardial infarction or develop ventricular arrhythmias. During exercise, the left ventricle may not be able to increase stroke volume to demand which may result in a drop in systolic pressure, ventricular arrhythmias and syncope. Over time, the heart's attempts to compensate begin to fail with dilatation and myocardial ischemia. The left atria dilates, which leads to the onset of atrial fibrillation and eventually to HF. The individual commonly presents with dyspnea upon exertion (Chrysohoou et al., 2011; Spaccarotella et al., 2011). Aortic stenosis is typically underestimated or managed in the early stages of dysfunction and patients usually present for medical care when the AS is severe and the patient is experiencing HF, angina, a presyncopal or syncopal episode, or progressive shortness of breath (Spaccarotella et al., 2011; Vahanian et al., 2011).

Mitral regurgitation is the most common valvular disease in the US and second reported in Europe (Vahanian et al., 2011). Mitral regurgitation can be classified as an anatomical abnormality or a functional diseased valve. Anatomical MR is also referred to as organic and is most commonly caused by the progression of mitral valve prolapse (MVP), which is defined as a leaflet failing to close

to the other leaflets at the plane of the mitral annulus. Rheumatic heart disease and a congenital valve deformity stenosis are the second and third causes of anatomical MR. Congenital deformity is commonly associated with infectious endocarditis and atrioventricular septal defect. Functional MR is underdiagnosed and most likely associated with left ventricular dysfunction related to ischemia, infarction and cardiomyopathy (Spaccarotella et al., 2011; Vahanain et al., 2011). Mitral regurgitation leads to left atrial enlargement, pulmonary hypertension and right HF, as well as eccentric left ventricle hypertrophy as the heart attempts to maintain cardiac output.

CLINICAL MANIFESTATIONS

The signs and symptoms of valvular dysfunction vary according to which valve is malfunctioning and the severity of the malfunction. The ultimate key is the degree to which the malfunction affects cardiac output. Valvular disease can be clinically detected by the alteration in normal heart sounds and the presence of abnormal heart sounds (Fig. 42.2). Exercise intolerance increases as the heart's compensatory mechanisms fail to maintain an efficient cardiac output to meet the metabolic demand of the body. The increase in volume and pressure within the left atrium, either from stenosis or regurgitation, causes an increase in pulmonary vascular resistance and eventually leads to the signs and symptoms of right HF. Patients may present with progressive dyspnea, orthopnea and paroxysmal nocturnal dyspnea, and rales upon auscultation. In the case of acute valvular dysfunction, the patient may rapidly develop pulmonary edema and respiratory failure, requiring mechanical ventilation of the patient. Aortic stenosis is commonly associated with angina, a presyncopal episode or syncope, arrhythmias and signs of CHF, as described previously.

THERAPEUTIC INTERVENTIONS

Often, medical intervention is initiated when the patient presents with the adverse consequences from valvular dysfunction. Medical treatment will focus on the management of angina, CHF, cause of dyspnea, arrhythmias and syncopal episodes. Patients will commonly be prescribed beta blockers, calcium-channel blockers and/or

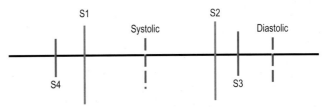

Figure 42.2 This graph represents the normal and common abnormal heart sounds that can be heard across one cardiac cycle. Normal heart sounds: S1 represents the closure of the atrioventricular valves; S2 represents the closure of the semilunar valves. Abnormal heart sounds: S3 is referred to as a ventricular gallop; S4 is referred to as an atrial gallop. Murmurs: systolic can be associated with stenosis of one of the semilunar valves or insufficiency of one of the atrioventricular valves; diastolic can be associated with stenosis of one of the atrioventricular valves or insufficiency of one of the semilunar valves.

diuretics to manage hypertension. Antiarrhythmic medications, such as digoxin or amiodarone, may be used to control atrial and ventricular arrhythmias. An implantable pacemaker and/or automatic implantable cardiac defibrillator may be necessary to control arrhythmias that are life-threatening or impair ventricular function.

There are several invasive procedures that can be considered to correct the valvular dysfunction. Percutaneous balloon valvuloplasty is a nonsurgical approach for stenosis. A catheter is positioned across the lumen of the valve and inflated to decrease the stenosis. For mitral stenosis, another nonsurgical option is a percutaneous mitral commissurotomy, in which the leaflet of the valve is cut via a catheter. In both of these options, there is a risk of restenosis and complications of valvular regurgitation (Figulla et al., 2011).

When medical management has reached its maximal benefit or when ventricular function is impaired or myocardial ischemia needs to be resolved, surgical intervention is the therapy of choice (Figulla et al., 2011; Vahanian et al., 2011; Scandura et al., 2012; Szabo et al., 2012). Depending on the valve involved, the patient's anatomy and the surgeon's training, a mediastinal or anterior thoracotomy may be the surgical approach. Valve replacement is the surgical gold standard for MR and AS, although 33% of individuals with AS and a similar figure for severe MR, particularly functional MR, are not candidates for traditional surgical intervention (Markar et al., 2011; Spaccarotella et al., 2011).

There are many factors that must be considered when the surgeon and patient are determining if the valve should be repaired or replaced and what type of procedure should be done. Some of these factors may include the age of the patient, the risk associated with the use of anticoagulation, the risk of infections and the extent of the anatomical disorder of the valve and the function of left ventricle. If the valve needs to be replaced, it must be decided whether the replacement should be a mechanical or biological valve. Age, past medical history and lifestyle all contribute to the decision regarding the type of valve replacement that is used (Markar et al., 2011; Spaccarotella et al., 2011; Vahanian et al., 2011).

There are increasing surgical options for AS. Surgeons are performing mini invasive procedures, referred to as transapical approach, where the individual does not undergo a complete sternotomy but a 2- to 3-inch (50–80mm) incision of the sternal body is made or a mini anterior thoracotomy with a transection of the sternum is made to repair or replace the aortic valve. This decreases the risk of wound complications and increases the recovery and hospital discharge rates. Individuals with higher surgical risks may undergo a transvascular aortic valve implantation (TAVI). In a TAVI, the approach is commonly through the femoral artery. A bovine pericardial valve is mounted on a balloon expandable stent which is placed with the native valve (Sapien valve) or porcine pericardial valve mounted in a self-expanding stent that extends into the ascending aorta (CoreValve ReValving System) (Webb et al., 2012). The 1-year survival rate for individuals who undergo TAVI is 73–79 % compared to 62% for those who are medically managed (Figulla et al., 2011).

Finally, individuals who are not candidates for a tradi-tional surgical procedure may be offered an aortic valve bypass (AVB) procedure where a left ventricle aortic conduit is surgically implanted from the left ventricle to the descending aorta through a thoracotomy. It is reported that 65–70% of cardiac output goes through the bypass and there can be as much as a 40% increase in stroke volume (Szabo et al., 2012).

The prescription of an exercise program and functional rehabilitation will be dependent upon the type of valvular disease, its severity and the function of the left ventricle. The therapist needs to work closely with the cardiologist to develop hemodynamic parameters as guidelines to monitor the patient during the rehabilitation process. Exercise is contraindicated in a patient with severe aortic or mitral valve disease (particularly aortic stenosis) who is symptomatic at rest. For individuals who undergo invasive or surgical management of their valvular disease the rehabilitation can typically be more progressive. Upper extremity precautions related to a sternotomy and hemodynamic parameters may require the therapist to instruct the individual in modified functional mobility and to monitor vital signs closely.

CONCLUSION

With the increase in the number of older adults there is expected to be a continued rise in the number of individuals with coronary heart disease, HF and valvular disease which will require rehabilitation services across the healthcare spectrum. The therapist needs to have the skill set to accurately complete a comprehensive evaluation and prescribe a safe and effective rehabilitation program with the goal to promote wellness and healthy living, and minimize functional limitation and disability. It is important to identify the precipitating causes of HF; early detection of valvular dysfunction and prompt medical intervention can preserve heart function. It is important that the therapist is an active member of the patient's healthcare team to ensure that screening for hypertension, education to reduce other cardiac risk factors and appropriate medical referrals are sought. The therapist is therefore a vital member of the healthcare team, providing services across the spectrum of preventive and rehabilitative medicine to optimize the patient's quality of life in the community.

REFERENCES

Barnes MM, Dorsch MP, Hummel SL et al 2011 Treatment of heart failure with preserved ejection fraction. Pharmacotherapy 31(3):312–331

Chrysohoou C, Tsiachris D, Stefanadis C 2011 Aortic stenosis in the elderly: challenges in diagnosis and therapy. Maturitas 70:349–353

Downing J, Balady GJ 2011 The role of exercise training in heart failure. J Am Coll Cardiol 58(6):561–569

Figulla L, Neumann A, Figulla HR 2011 Transcatheter aortic valve implantation: evidence on safety and efficacy compared with medical therapy: a systematic review of current literature. Clin Res Cardiol 100:265–274

Lietz K 2010 Destination therapy: patient selection and current outcomes. J Cardiac Surg 25:462–471

Lindenfeld J, Boehmer JP, Collins SP et al 2010 Executive summary: HFSA 2010 comprehensive heart failure practice guideline. J Cardiac Failure 16(6):475–539

McKenna C, Walker S, Lorgelly P et al 2012 Cost-effectiveness of aldosterone antagonists for the treatment of post-myocardial infarction heart failure. Value Health 15:420–428

Markar SR, Sadat U, Edmonds L et al 2011 Mitral valve repair versus replacement in the elderly population. J Heart Valve Dis 20:265–271

Mentz RJ, Schulte PJ, Fleg JL et al 2013 Clinical characteristics, response to exercise training and outcomes in patients with heart failure and chronic obstructive pulmonary disease: findings from Heart Failure – A Controlled Trial Investigating Outcomes of Exercise TraiNing (HF_ACTION). American Heart Journal 65(2):193–199

Scandura S, Ussia GP, Caggegi A et al 2012 Percutaneous mitral valve repair in patients with prior cardiac surgery. J Cardiac Surg 27:295–298

Shiba N, Shimokawa H 2011 Chronic kidney disease and heart failure: bidirectional close link and common therapeutic goal. J Cardiol 57:8–17

Smart NA, Meyer T, Butterfield JA et al 2012 Individual patient meta-analysis of exercise training effects on systemic brain natriuretic peptide expression in heart failure. Eur J Prevent Cardiol 19:428–437

Spaccarotella C, Mongiardo A, Indolfi C 2011 Pathophysiology of aortic stenosis and approach to treatment with percutaneous valve implantation. Circ J 75:11–19

Szabo TA, Toole JM, Payne KJ 2012 Management of aortic valve bypass surgery. Semin Cardiothorac Vasc Anesth 16(1):52–58

Trigo P, Fischer GW 2012 Managing atrial fibrillation in the elderly: critical appraisal of dronedarone. Clin Intervent Aging 7:1–13

Vahanian A, Iung B, Himbert D et al 2011 Changing demographics of valvular heart disease and impact on surgical and transcatheter valve therapies. Int J Cardiovasc Imaging 20:1115–1122

Van Veldhuisen DJ, Anker SD, Ponikowski P et al 2011 Anemia and iron deficiency in heart failure: mechanisms and therapeutic approaches. Nature Rev Cardiol 8:485–493

Vasques F, Lucenteforte E, Paone R et al 2012 Outcome of patient aged ≥ 80 years undergoing combined aortic valve replacement and coronary artery bypass grafting: a systematic review and meta-analysis of 40 studies. Am Heart J 164:410–418

Webb J, Rodes-Cabau J, Fremes S et al 2012 Transcatheter aortic valve implantation: a Canadian Cardiovascular Society Position Statement. Can J Cardiol 28:520–528

Chapter 43

Cardiac pacemakers and defibrillators

CHRIS L. WELLS

CHAPTER CONTENTS

INTRODUCTION

The heart has specialized cells called conduction cells which generate an electrical impulse that alters the resting membrane of the myocardial tissue. This leads to myocardial contraction and the ejection of blood. As well as the conduction system, the myocardium also possesses other electrical properties that facilitate cardiac function. The myocardium has automaticity and excitability; this allows an electrical impulse to be self-generated and able to be depolarized if a stimulus is present. If an impulse reaches a sufficient threshold, the myocardium will depolarize and conduct this electrical impulse throughout the myocardium, which leads to myocardial contraction. Finally, in the all-or-none principle, which is specific to cardiac muscle, if an electrical impulse is sufficient, complete depolarization and full contraction of the myocardium occurs.

In the presence of a cardiac disease or disorder, and through the natural process of aging, there is an increased incidence of dysfunction of the conduction system. This dysfunction may be benign and not disrupt general heart function or it can have life-threatening consequences. The type of conduction dysfunction, its rate and occurrence or frequency determines the clinical significance of the arrhythmia. The bottom line for the clinician is how the arrhythmia affects myocardial perfusion and what happens to cardiac output. For example, in the presence of ischemic heart disease, a fast conducting rhythm, such as supraventricular tachycardia (SVT), rapid ventricular rate or atrial fibrillation, will decrease the diastolic filling time, which leads to a decline in myocardium perfusion and further ischemia, resulting in a vicious cycle. The same tachycardiac arrhythmias can lead to a decrease in cardiac output because of the decrease in filling time. In the presence of myocardial or pump dysfunction, the ventricles rely on volume to improve the contractile force, which is known as the Frank–Starling law. However, with the decrease in the filling time caused by a fast conduction rate, there is a decrease in the volume entering the ventricles leading to a loss of myocardial stretch. The end result is a decrease in contractility. Bradycardiac rhythms allow sufficient time for ventricular filling but the rate may be too slow to maintain the cardiac output needed to meet the metabolic demands of the body. The loss of cardiac output is associated with the following common clinical signs and symptoms: light-headedness, dizziness, visual disturbances, altered mentation, syncope and increased risk of falls. The frequency with which arrhythmia occurs can also disrupt perfusion and cardiac output, particularly in cardiac dysfunction.

Cardiac arrhythmias may be temporary or permanent, depending on the etiology. Transient arrhythmias may be caused by significant alterations in electrolytes. This may result from gastrointestinal distress because of nausea, vomiting and diarrhea, or from the use of medications, such as diuretics and potassium supplements. Transient arrhythmias may also be caused by myocardial hypersensitivity resulting from heart catheterization, open heart procedures, myocardial infarct or trauma. More permanent arrhythmias may be caused by ischemic disease that directly impairs the cells of the conduction system. This may lead to various conduction arrhythmias, such as heart blocks, atrial or ventricular bradycardia or tachycardia. Heart failure (HF) is commonly associated with atrial fibrillation and abnormal ventricular electrical conduction or ectopy. Aging may also lead to a significant loss of conduction cells, which may lead to such conduction dysfunction as sick sinus syndrome. Arrhythmias can be managed via technology, including pacemakers and defibrillators. They are discussed below.

PACEMAKERS

Over 400 000 people in the United States of America and 1 million worldwide undergo pacemaker implantation annually for the management of arrhythmias (Wilkoff et al., 2009). There has been a rise in use of permanent pacemakers because there has been an expansion in the indication for pacemaker placement (Cutro et al., 2012). Permanent pacemakers have been shown to improve the quality of life, oxygen consumption and exercise tolerance, decrease hospital admissions and mortality rates and improve survival of patients with life-threatening arrhythmias and HF (Houthuizen et al., 2011; Crozier & Smith, 2012; Cutro et al., 2012).

Pacemaker devices have become very sophisticated in their programming features, which has expanded their use for various diseases and patient populations (Cutro et al., 2012). Pacemakers basically function by sensing or detecting the intrinsic electrical activity of the heart and deliver an electrical impulse in the absence of intrinsic activity. When the intrinsic conduction system fails the pacemaker delivers an electrical impulse that causes an action potential. This leads to depolarization and contraction of the myocardium and the ejection of blood from the heart into the systemic and pulmonary circulations.

There are specific indications for utilization of a pacemaker, including sinus node dysfunction and atrioventricular heart blocks, which is an ineffective communication between atrial and ventricular conduction pathways. Sinus node dysfunctions are commonly associated with bradycardia, periods of lack of conduction and brady–tachy syndrome in which the heart rate varies from very slow to very fast (Beyerbach & Rottman, 2012). Pacemakers may also be used to control atrial arrhythmias such as atrial fibrillation, other tachyarrhythmias, and the presence of a block of the ventricular bundle branches (Beyerbach & Rottman, 2012). (For a discussion on cardiac arrhythmias and conduction disturbances, readers are referred to Chapter 41.) More recently pacemakers have become accepted as part of optimal medical care for patients with HF (Houthuizen et al., 2011).

TEMPORARY AND PERMANENT PACEMAKERS

Pacemakers can be classified as temporary or permanent. In the case of an acute dysfunction of the conduction system, a temporary pacer may be used to stabilize the patient's rhythm and hemodynamics. It is common practice for the surgeon to place pacer wires on the epicardial surface of the heart (atrial, ventricle or both) during an open-heart procedure because a patient can often have transient arrhythmias after heart surgery; these can result from the myocardium becoming irritable from the trauma of surgery, imbalances of electrolytes, disruption of the acid–base balance and alterations of blood gases. Depending upon the type of open heart surgery, the patient may suffer from sinus node dysfunction leading to atrial fibrillation (which is the most common postoperative arrhythmia), junction arrhythmia and idioventricular arrhythmias (Misiri et al., 2012). The wires are passed transthoracically and secured to the anterior chest wall. In an urgent situation, the heart can be temporarily paced via transcutaneous electrode pads. Finally, a temporary pacemaker can be initiated using a transvenous approach, typically through the jugular or subclavian vein. These electrode wires are then attached to an external pacemaker device which is programmed to stabilize the patient's rhythm with the goal to achieve an adequate cardiac output and blood pressure.

If it is determined that the disturbance of the patient's conduction system is irreversible and interferes with heart function, a permanent pacemaker will be implanted with the patient's consent. The pacemaker will be individually programmed to meet the conduction needs so that efficient cardiac function can be maintained.

DETAILS OF PERMANENT PACEMAKER FUNCTION

The pacemaker comprises two components. The first component is the pulse generator that contains the electronic program and the energy system that generates the electrical stimuli. The device is implanted underneath the skin in the right or left pectodeltoid area or subpectoral in patients who are very thin, to prevent erosion of the skin. The second component of the pacemaker is the lead or wire that senses the activity of the native conduction system and delivers the impulse to the myocardium. The leads for permanent pacemakers are typically attached to the endocardium of the right atrium and right and/or left ventricle via the transvenous approach. Leads can be placed using an epicardial approach at the time of an open-heart procedure.

There are three approaches to lead placement for a permanent pacer. In single chamber pacing there is one pacing lead that is either placed in the wall of the right atrial or right ventricle. Dual chamber pacing has two pacing leads, most commonly in the right atria and right ventricle. Finally there is biventricular pacing; this approach is referred to as cardiac resynchronization therapy (CRT) in which the right ventricle is paced via the endocardial approach and the other pacing wire is advanced through the coronary sinus to pace the left ventricle epicardially (Beyerbach & Rottman, 2012).

The program within the pacemaker generator can sense the intrinsic activity of the conduction system and delay the release of an electrical impulse. In the absence of intrinsic activity, the generator can deliver an electrical impulse that causes the depolarization of the myocardium. There are three general modes for pacing the heart. In a fixed-rate or asynchronous mode, the pacemaker paces the heart at a constant rate, regardless of intrinsic electrical activity or physiological need. This mode does not respond to the metabolic needs of the body and the patient reaches an exercise plateau quickly. Because of this limitation, a fixed mode is not commonly used. The second mode is referred to as the demand or inhibited mode. In this mode, when the pacemaker senses the intrinsic activity it inhibits the generator from releasing its electrical stimuli. In the absence of intrinsic activity, the pacemaker generates a pulse. The third mode is the triggered or synchronous mode that paces when the conduction system fails to pace; this mode also paces in unison with the conduction system when it senses intrinsic activity.

PACEMAKER UNIVERSAL REFERENCE SYSTEM

There is a universal reference system that is used to describe the function of the pacemaker. This is very important and enables any clinician who is working with the patient to have a basic understanding of the pacemaker. The details of the generic pacemaker code are shown in Table 43.1. The first letter of the code represents the chambers in which the pacemaker will pace. The second position of the code tells the clinician where the pacemaker senses conduction system activity. The third letter of the code represents how the pacer will respond to the activity

Table 43.1	**Generic codes for pacemakers**
Position	**Codes**
I (pacing chamber)	O, A, V, D (A + V)
II (sensing chamber)	O, A, V, D (A + V)
III (response to sensing)	O, I, T, D (T + I)
IV (programmability)	O, R, S, M, C, V
V (multisite pacing)	O, A, V, D (A + D)

A, atrium; C, communicating; D, dual; I, inhibited; M, multi; O, none; R, rare; S, simple; T, triggered; V, ventricle

that it senses. The fourth and fifth positions of this coding system are less frequently used. The fourth code refers to the programming. With the rate program (R) feature, the pacer can sense an increase in physiological demand, such as occurs during exercise. This is achieved by either sensing changes in thoracic impedance or movement because of increased respiratory rate or sensing changes in blood gases. When the pacemaker senses the increase in metabolic needs, it paces at a faster rate. The fifth code position refers to the chamber in which the pacemaker can 'tachypace' the heart in an attempt to control atrial and/or ventricular tachycardias.

Two of the more common types of pacemaker are the VVI and the DDDR. A VVI pacer is one that will pace the ventricle (V), sense conduction activity within the ventricle (V) and, if intrinsic activity is detected, inhibit the release of an electrical stimulus (I). A DDDR pacemaker is a device that paces and senses activity within both the atria and ventricles, and that can pace or hold pacing depending on the activity of the conduction system within the atria and ventricles. It can internally increase the pacing rate when the metabolic demand is higher (Zaidan et al., 2005).

Cardiac Resynchronization Therapy (CRT) has become part of optimal medical management for patients with HF. Pacemaker management is indicated for patients with New York Heart Association Functional Classification III or IV with left bundle branch block (Cutro et al., 2012). HF is associated with a decrease in myocardial contractility; disturbance in coordination of atrial to ventricle activation, and many patients suffer from left bundle-branch block (Houthuizen et al., 2012). These impairments lead to delay in electrical conduction and impaired myocardial contraction leading to the heart's inability to eject a sufficient volume of blood to meet the body's needs. The goals of CRT pacing are to optimize the atrioventricular delay to improve ventricular preload and resynchronize the depolarization of the ventricles that should lead to a more effective contraction of the ventricles. Clinically, CRT is also referred to as biventricular pacing or 'Bi-V' pacing. The positive effects of Bi-V pacing include an improvement in interventricular and intraventricular depolarization, contractility and cardiac output, which results from improvements in the wall motion of the ventricles, particularly the intraventricular septum. It also decreases mitral regurgitation by stabilizing the intraventricular septum and the restrictive pattern of the heart (Houthuizen et al., 2011). Several studies have documented improvements in the quality of life, exercise tolerance and

ejection fraction, a 40% reduction in the death rate and decreased hospitalization rates (Beyerbach & Rottman, 2012; Cutro et al., 2012; Houthuizen et al., 2011). There is still a need for large randomized studies to fully understand the role CRT plays in HF management, especially in the older patient, but many smaller studies have reported a decrease in metabolic cost, remodeling of the ventricle improvement in mitral valve function, decrease in ventricle chamber dimensions and a decrease in hospitalization and mortality (Beyerbach & Rottman, 2012; Houthuizen et al., 2011). Cost effectiveness of CRT requires the patient to survive at least 3–4 years post implantation and with the increased complication rate in the older patient it is unknown if CRT is both cost-effective and a clinically effective procedure for patients older than 70 years of age (Cutro et al., 2012).

There are several complications related to the utilization of pacemakers that the clinician should be aware of when caring for a patient. During the implant procedure, the patient may experience a pneumothorax, hemothorax or cardiac tamponade. It is possible for the leads to be displaced, resulting in pacemaker dysfunction; malplacement of the lead may also stimulate the diaphragm or cause other cardiac dysrhythmias. The patient may also develop a hematoma, infection or skin erosion at the site of the pacemaker generator (Woodruff & Prudente, 2005).

Pacemaker dysfunction can be classified according to three categories. 'Inappropriate sensing' means that the pacemaker is either undersensing or oversensing. In undersensing, the pacemaker does not detect the intrinsic activity of the conduction system, which leads to improper pacing. When a pacemaker is oversensing, it does not appropriately detect the lack of conduction activity and inhibits the pacemaker from actually firing an impulse. This is clinically more critical as the patients will be more symptomatic because of the loss of conduction, contraction and cardiac output. 'Loss of capture' means that the pacemaker does not generate a strong enough impulse to cause myocardial depolarization. This may be caused by battery failure, lead dysfunction, an increase in the capture threshold because of fibrosis and necrosis at the lead site, or the use of certain medications. Finally, 'failure to fire' means that the pacemaker fails to release an impulse when it should. This can be caused by a failure of the lead, battery failure or oversensing. The clinician needs to understand the program of the pacemaker and monitor the patient's vital signs and symptoms in order to be able to detect any pacemaker dysfunction and make the appropriate referral.

THERAPEUTIC INTERVENTION

Established data is scarce on rehabilitation in individuals with pacemakers. The following section includes the author's recommendations, which are based upon years of experience and unpublished protocols at the University of Maryland Medical System.

Specific care must be taken when the therapist is treating a patient with a temporary pacemaker. The clinician should understand the reason for the use of the pacemaker and how reliant the patient is on the pacemaker. Before mobilizing the patient, the clinician needs to ensure that the connections of the pacer leads are secure and that the wires and temporary pacemaker are handled with care. It is crucial that the clinician monitors the patient's vital signs and responses to any activity. It is helpful for the therapist to document if there is an increase or decrease in pacing reliance based upon the activity and the intensity of the activity.

When the patient no longer needs temporary pacing, either because there is medical stability of the cardiac rhythm or because there has been a placement of a permanent pacemaker, it is important that the patient is monitored after the removal of the temporary transthoracic epicardial leads. There is a risk of epicardial bleeding when the leads are removed, which is done at the bedside before the patient is discharged from hospital. The clinician should monitor the patient for signs of tamponade or pericardial inflammation. The signs and symptoms of cardiac tamponade include tachycardia, a decrease in systemic arterial blood pressure, diminished heart sounds, dyspnea, orthopnea and jugular venous distension. The adverse effects of inflammation include pain, hypotension, diminished heart sounds and tachycardia.

The protocol for rehabilitation after the placement of a permanent pacemaker varies from facility to facility. Typically, the involved upper extremity is immobilized for the first 24 hours to decrease pain, protect against bleeding or the development of a hematoma at the site of the generator implant, and to decrease the risk of lead displacement. It is safe for the patient to ambulate even if he or she needs to use an assistive device. If a hematoma does not develop, range of motion (ROM), strengthening and functional training can be resumed within the tolerance of the individual. If a hematoma does develop, the patient may experience neurological symptoms because of compression of the brachial plexus. The upper extremity may be immobilized until there are signs that the bleeding has stopped and the hematoma is stable. Some physicians will instruct the patient to avoid resistive overhead activities for 2 weeks after implantation, but active ROM and activities of daily living are safe to resume. It is important that treatment guidelines be established between the rehabilitation service and the electrophysiology department to maximize the patient's recovery.

Before working with a patient who has a permanent pacemaker, the therapist should know which mode of pacing has been programmed into the device because the mode affects a patient's cardiovascular tolerance to exercise. Exercise tolerance is dependent on the underlying disease, the type of pacemaker and the degree to which the patient is dependent on the pacer to maintain cardiac output. Patients with fixed-rate pacemakers are unable to elevate their heart rate to accommodate higher demand, so the therapist must recognize this limitation and adjust the treatment plan accordingly. A pacemaker set on dual mode, for example the DDDR pacemaker, allows the patient's heart rate to vary according to demand. Such a patient would not be expected to have an exercise limitation because of the existing conduction abnormality. Exercise tolerance is also dependent on the patient's level of fitness. It is also important to evaluate the cardiovascular response to exercise to ensure that the patient is tolerating the exercise and that the pacer is working appropriately. Finally, the clinician should talk to the patient to make sure that the pacemaker is appropriately inspected for proper function and to assess battery life.

There are special concerns that the physical therapist must consider when working with a patient who has a pacemaker. Modalities such as transcutaneous electrical nerve stimulation (TENS), shortwave and microwave diathermy, neuromuscular stimulators and ultrasound should not be used in the region of the pacemaker (Woodruff & Prudente, 2005). Superficial heat and cold should be safe to use once the surgical incision has healed, but the tissue directly over the generator should be insulated for protection. If there are any questions regarding the use of a modality or specific rehabilitation technique, the cardiologist should be consulted. The therapist should also be aware that the muscular activity of pectorals, abdominals and the diaphragm can lead to artifacts, which can result in inappropriate sensing (oversensing) and underpacing. Therefore, it is important for the therapist to continue to monitor the patient's vital signs, symptoms and heart rate regularity when new exercises are introduced or the intensity is increased. If the patient complains of light-headedness or presents with syncope, low blood pressure and decreased tolerance to activity, the patient should be referred to the cardiologist to assess the function of the pacemaker.

DEFIBRILLATORS

When a patient has a history of presyncope, syncope, cardiac arrest, HF or heart disease, with documented significant ventricular arrhythmia, an implantable cardiac defibrillator (ICD) may be the intervention of choice. Approximately 300000 ICDs were implanted in 2009 worldwide (Misiri et al., 2012) and since 2008 there has been a 5% increase in utilization of ICDs (Cutro et al., 2012). The purpose of this cardiac device is to recognize the life-threatening arrhythmias of ventricular tachycardiac or fibrillation and deliver a strong enough electrical impulse (shock) to depolarize the entire myocardium, in the hope that the sinus node will resume control as the primary pacemaker.

In general, the use of ICDs decreased the mortality rate by 30–40% over 3 years for patients with HF, but the effectiveness of ICDs in the older adult is more complex. Often older adults with HF have other comorbidities, which increases the risk of death from non-life-threatening arrhythmias. Competing deaths may be related to pneumonia, renal failure and stroke. The older adult with HF is more likely to have a shortened life expectancy than the younger adult with HF. The median life expectancy of a 75-year-old adult with HF is approximately 2 years. This shortened life expectancy decreases the efficiency of ICD utilization for the older adult. For patients over the age of 80 years ICD is considered unwarranted due to increased risks associated with implantation and complications (Cutro et al., 2012).

Most ICDs function in the following manner. The ICD monitors the heart rate and rhythm for abnormalities. It is programmed to detect a preset rate and, if that rate is exceeded, the device is activated. There is a delay in the response of the defibrillator to provide a chance for the abnormal rhythm to convert back to a normal rhythm.

Table 43.2	**Generic codes for ICDS**
Position	**Codes**
I (shock chamber)	O, A, V, D (A + V)
II (antitachycardia pacing chamber)	O, A, V, D (A + V)
III (tachycardia detection)	E, H
IV (antibradycardia pacing chamber)	O, A, V, D (A + V)

A, atrium; D, dual; E, electrogram; H, hemodynamic; O, none; V, ventricle

If the arrhythmia continues beyond the delay, the generator charges, takes a second look at the rhythm and delivers an electrical shock if the abnormality is still present. The goal is to depolarize the myocardium and return the patient's heart to a more stable rhythm.

An implanted cardiac defibrillator may simply be a device that responds to ventricular tachycardia or fibrillation, or it may be combined with pacemaker functions. The generic codes for ICDs are shown in Table 43.2. In patients with brady–tachy arrhythmias, the pacemaker/ICD can be programmed to pace at a minimal rate when the rate becomes too slow. When the rate becomes too fast, the pacemaker will attempt to over-pace the heart to recapture or control the rhythm and then slow the rate down again. This is referred to as 'tachypacing'. If this program does not work, the ICD may deliver a low-level shock (5–10J) in an attempt to convert the rhythm to a more stable rate. If this is unsuccessful or the generator interprets the rhythm as ventricular tachycardia or fibrillation, the ICD will fire a more significant shock (30–50J) to convert this life-threatening rhythm to a more stable rhythm (Cannon & Prystowsky, 2004). The use of a pacemaker/ICD has been shown to improve survival, exercise tolerance and quality of life and decrease hospitalization for patients with HF (Cutro et al., 2012).

The ICD is also comprised of a generator and leads. The generator is commonly inserted in the left or right pectodeltoid area. The endocardial lead is placed in the right ventricular apex via a transvenous approach (Stevenson et al., 2004). When there is also a pacemaking program, leads are placed in the right atria and possibly the left ventricle for pacing function.

A subcutaneous defibrillator has recently been approved for use in Europe and New Zealand. This device is implanted subcutaneously and positioned in the axilla with no intracardiac or epicardial components. Opposed to transvenous leads, a parasternal lead is used to sense arrhythmia and delivers a shock (Crozier & Smith, 2012). The advantage of this device over a traditional ICD is that there is a decrease in implantation complications, which for the older adult may be significant enough to consider use of such a device. More research will need to be conducted to fully understand the clinical effectiveness and efficacy of this new device.

THERAPEUTIC INTERVENTION

It is important that a therapist is aware when working with a patient who has an ICD. In the acute phase, the immobilization of the upper extremity and restoration of arm function follows the same guidelines as described above for pacemakers. If the ICD generator is implanted in the abdominal wall, the patient should be instructed in proper body mechanics to protect the incision. It is also helpful to teach the patient splinting so that pain caused by movement and coughing can be decreased.

The patient and therapist should know the rate at which the generator becomes activated as well as the length of time of the delay. One of the goals of therapy is to determine what are safe activities and proper resistance or workloads for exercise, so that a high enough heart rate is achieved to provide benefit from the exercise but not high enough to activate the ICD. The therapist can provide the electrocardiophysiologist with vital information in setting the heart rate boundaries for the ICD.

The therapist should recognize that there are psychological effects in almost 90% of patients with ICDs. These patients suffer from depression and anxiety, and will self-limit and therefore decrease their quality of life because they are fearful of the firing of the ICD. There is an elevated fear of death and a change in body image, which may interfere with intimate relationships. There is also a loss of control and increase in self-doubt and helplessness (Schermann & Keung, 2005; Crozier & Smith, 2012). Providing education about exercise, self-monitoring and the function of the ICD is important. It is also important that the clinician make sure that the patient is undergoing routine check-ups to ensure that the ICD is working appropriately to prevent false firing and sense appropriately, and that the battery is active.

If the patient's heart rate rises above the preset rate, the patient should sit down and be instructed to cough or perform a Valsalva maneuver. These maneuvers may cause vagal stimulation, which may result in a decrease in heart rate and prevent a shock. The therapist should monitor the patient's vital signs and notify the cardiologist if the defibrillator delivers a shock. The clinician may feel the shock if in contact with the patient at the time of defibrillation but it will not be harmful. Complications involved in the use of an ICD are similar to the complications discussed above for pacemakers.

CONCLUSION

Disturbance or dysfunction of normal heart conduction can result in decreased cardiac output, which leads to symptoms of light-headedness, altered vision or mentation and syncope, and balance/fall dysfunction. Temporary and permanent conduction problems may be treated by inserting a pacemaker or, in cases of life-threatening arrhythmias, an ICD. These devices can improve the patient's safety, tolerance for exercise and participation in work and recreational activities and can therefore improve quality of life. In such circumstances, the therapist must be aware of certain treatment concerns and must know the type and basic programming parameters of pacing or shock delivery before exercising a patient. Vital signs should be monitored during exercise to determine the patient's tolerance. To prevent harm, the clinician should know the relative and absolute contraindications of various modalities in a patient who has a pacemaker and/or ICD implanted.

REFERENCES

Beyerbach DM, Rottman JN 2012 Pacemakers and implantable cardioverter defibrillators. http://emedicine.medscape.com/article/162245

Cannon D, Prystowsky E 2004 Evolution of implantable cardiovertor defibrillators. J Cardiovasc Electrophysiol 15(3):375–385

Crozier I, Smith W 2012 Modern device technologies. Heart Lung Circ 21:320–327

Cutro R, Rich MW, Hauptman PJ 2012 Device therapy in patients with heart failure and advanced age: too much too late? Int J Cardiol 155:52–55

Houthuizen P, Bracke FA, van Geler BM 2011 Atrioventricular and interventricular delay optimization in cardiac resynchronization therapy: physiological principles and overview of available methods. Heart Failure Rev 16:263–276

Misiri J, Kusumoto F, Goldschlager N 2012 Electromagnetic interference and implanted cardiac devices: the nonmedical environment (Part 1). Clin Cardiol 35(5):276–280

Schermann M, Keung E 2005 The year in clinical electrophysiology. J Am Coll Cardiol 4(5):790–795

Stevenson W, Chaitman B, Ellenbegen K et al 2004 Clinical assessment and management of patients with implantable cardioverter devices presenting to a nonelectrophysiologist. Circulation 110:3866–3869

Wilkoff BL, Love CJ, Byrd CL 2009 Transvenous lead extraction: Heart Rhythm Society expert consensus on facilities, training, indications, and patient management. (Document endorsed by the American Heart Association.) Heart Rhythm 6:1085–1104

Woodruff J, Prudente L 2005 Update on implantable pacemakers. J Cardiovasc Nurs 20(4):261–268

Zaidan J, Atlee J, Belott P et al 2005 Practice advisory for perioperative management of patients with cardiac rhythm management devices: pacemakers and implantable cardioverter defibrillators. Anesthesiology 103(1):186–198

Chapter 44

Invasive cardiac procedures

CHRIS L. WELLS

CHAPTER CONTENTS

INTRODUCTION

Invasive procedures for the treatment of cardiac pathologies, such as catheterization, angioplasty and bypass surgery, have become commonplace over the past 40 years. Over 4.5 million invasive cardiac procedures are completed annually in the United States of America (CDC National Center for Health Statistics, 2012) and there have been many advances in the surgical management of cardiac disease, with significant advancements in minimally invasive cardiovascular procedures. The age and number of comorbidities of elderly patients have increased the complexity of the procedures performed; unfortunately, however, these factors affect outcomes such as a return to prior level of function and quality of life. This chapter will briefly discuss the various invasive procedures for the management of heart disease, particularly coronary artery disease.

CATHETERIZATION

Cardiac catheterization remains the gold standard procedure in the diagnosis of cardiac function and cardiac disease (see Fig. 44.1 for a description of the clinical name of the pressures within each of the chambers of the heart and their average values). A right heart catheterization (RHC) can be used to assess the volume and pressures within the cardiopulmonary system and is completed by placing a catheter within the right side of the heart, typically via the internal jugular, femoral or brachial veins. This catheter can measure how much blood is returning to the heart, referred to as preload, by recording the pressure within the right atrium, which is clinically referred to as central venous pressure. The physician can measure the function of the right ventricle and pulmonary vascular system by measuring the volume and pressure through the right ventricle and into the pulmonary trunk (pulmonary arterial pressure). The balloon at the end of the catheter can be inflated and used to indirectly measure the preload of the left side of the heart (pulmonary capillary wedge pressure). This procedure can also be used to estimate blood gases, cardiac output and function of the tricuspid and pulmonic valves and to detect septal defects. Finally, RHC can be used to diagnose pulmonary hypertensive diseases, assess extent and location of embolism, take a tissue biopsy and evaluate the responsiveness to medications used to improve heart function and decrease pulmonary hypertension.

A left heart catheterization (LHC) is commonly used to diagnose coronary atherosclerosis; this helps to determine the state of perfusion of the myocardium. The catheter is passed into the arterial system through the femoral or brachial artery. At the time of the coronary arteriography, a ventriculography can be completed for assessment of left ventricular function, including description of wall motion

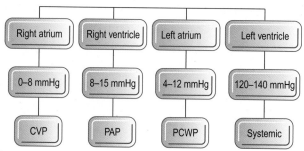

Figure 44.1 This illustration defines the clinical name of the pressures within each of the chambers of the heart and their average values. CVP, central venous pressure; PAP, pulmonary arterial pressure; PCWP, pulmonary capillary wedge pressure.

and function of the mitral and aortic valves and measurement of the ejection fraction, blood gases, the blood volume of the left ventricle, and cardiac output. Heart catheterization can also be used to assess the health of the extracardiac major blood vessels of the body (DiMario & Sirtaria, 2005). More recently transcatheter aortic valve replacements are being performed for individuals who are not candidates for surgical intervention for the traditional median sternotomy approach for aortic valve replacement (Webb et al., 2012). Clinical trials are underway that are investigating mitral valve repairs via percutaneous catheter as well (Rogers & Franzen, 2011).

THERAPEUTIC INTERVENTION

Activity restrictions will vary depending on whether a patient has a RHC or a LHC. If the patient undergoes only a RHC, once the catheter is removed from the vein, pressure is applied to the site for 2–5 minutes to ensure that bleeding has stopped. The patient is then allowed out of bed and can resume activities as tolerated and as medically indicated. After undergoing a LHC, direct pressure is applied for 5–20 minutes or until the bleeding has stopped after which a pressure dressing is applied and the limb immobilized. The physician may insert a vascular plug or a suture to seal the puncture site of the artery but the patient will typically need to be on bedrest. If the femoral artery is the site for catheterization, the patient will be on bedrest for 4–6 hours. If the brachial artery is the site for the LHC, the patient may be allowed out of bed in 2–4 hours but the extremity will need to be elevated and immobilized for 4–6 hours. When the patient and the extremity are permitted to be mobilized, it is important for the clinician to inspect the arterial site for bleeding or the development of a hematoma before and after the therapeutic intervention. If bleeding persists or a hematoma has developed, it is critical to notify the physician in order to control the bleeding and assess the artery for the development of an aneurysm. The therapist should also complete a motor and sensory examination to determine if there are any focal deficits, particularly involving the femoral or median nerve distribution depending the arterial approach. There is also the risk of renal dysfunction because of the dye that is used during the arteriography, which may lead to peripheral edema, muscle weakness, changes in mental status and heart failure, which the therapist will need to assess and adjust the rehabilitation plan.

PERCUTANEOUS CORONARY INTERVENTION (PCI) ANGIOPLASTY

Percutaneous coronary intervention (PCI) – previously referred to as a percutaneous transluminal angioplasty (PTCA) or angioplasty for short – may be performed in the cardiac catheterization laboratory when a diagnosis of coronary atherosclerosis has been confirmed. For a noncalcified discrete lesion involving the proximal artery of one or two vessels, PCI with or without stent placement is a common medical option for management of coronary disease (Wu et al., 2011). Heart function and comorbidities, such as diabetes mellitus and acute myocardial infarction (MI), particularly ST segment elevated MI, should also be

taken into account when the specific invasive procedure is selected (Kalesan et al., 2012).

By performing a PCI, it may be possible for the cardiologist to open the occluded artery and restore blood flow. A guide wire and catheter are inserted using the same procedure as in LHC. The guide wire is advanced through the atherosclerotic lesion and a dilatation catheter balloon is inserted over the guide wire. The balloon is then inflated, with the goal of redistributing the atherosclerotic plaque. The result is an enlargement of both the lumen and the overall diameter of the vessel. The balloon is then deflated and an angiography repeated to assess the effectiveness of the PCI. The patient is typically administered heparin or bivalirudin to decrease the risk of thrombus formation and nitroglycerin may be administered into the coronary artery to prevent vasospasm. The PCI can be repeated if necessary or be performed on other involved arteries. The catheter sheath may not be removed immediately after the procedure in order to have rapid access if the patient experiences angina or signs suggesting ischemia or vasospasm.

Although PCI is a minimally invasive procedure and is associated with an approximate acute success rate of 90% (Tresukosol et al., 2010), the procedure is associated with several complications. Venous thrombosis and embolization may occur, causing a cerebrovascular accident (CVA) or occlusion of another coronary vessel creating further ischemia or infarction. During the procedure, there is a risk of perforating or dissecting the coronary artery, which could lead to tamponade or MI. Tamponade or artery dissection requires emergency surgical intervention to stop bleeding and preserve myocardial function. The catheter can also cause life-threatening arrhythmia, bleeding or infection, and the development of a pseudoaneurysm may occur at the entrance site of the catheter, usually the femoral artery. Percutaneous coronary intervention is associated with a complication rate of 4.1%; in total, 29% of these complications are from arterial dissection. The restenosis rate has been reported to be 4% to 40% and, of patients who suffer from restenosis, the arterial closure leads to MI in up to 50% of cases, with mortality rates reported between 20 and 40%. Approximately 20% of patients will require surgical intervention (Heir et al., 2010).

Despite the advances in medical technology, there is a 30% chance of restenosis within the first year after a PCI. Restenosis within the first 6 months post-PTCA is associated with cell proliferation, macrophage infiltration, platelet agitation and neovascularization that leads to narrowing or occlusion of the coronary artery. After 6 months, it is believed that restenosis is caused by further progression of the coronary artery disease (Heir et al., 2010).

STENTS

The use of an endovascular stent in PCI has been associated with a decreased rate of restenosis and reinfarction compared with the use of a PCI alone. The benefit of stents is that a larger lumen can be achieved and there is a decrease in elastic recoil of the artery (Kalesan et al., 2012). These stents may also be placed after a PCI when there is an acute restenosis. In the US, over a million PCI procedures are completed annually with over half of the individuals also receiving an intra-arterial coronary stent

(Centers for Disease Control and Prevention 2012). The stent is guided into place across the atherosclerotic plaque over the guide wire. Once in position, the stent either self-expands or a balloon is inflated to disrupt the lesion and dilate the coronary artery to restore myocardial perfusion.

There are two basic types of stents used today to manage coronary artery disease: bare metal stents and drug-eluting stents, which are used 75% of the time (CDC, 2012). The implantation of a stent decreases the reocclusion rate, referred to as in-stent stenosis, and reinfarction rate when compared to angioplasty alone (Guagliumi et al., 2011; Kalesan et al., 2012). A stent can be coated with heparin or another drug that actively interrupts the development of restenosis. Thus, drug-coated or drug-eluting stents can be covered with such drugs as sirolimus or rapamycin. Sirolimus actually decreases endothelial function and affects platelet physiology (Lemos et al., 2003) and rapamycin inhibits cell proliferation (Arjomand et al., 2003). Drug-eluting stents are associated with a decrease in early restenosis and reinfarction and improvements in mortality rates compared to bare metal stents. Bare metal stents have a decrease in late restenosis, 1 year after implant, especially if the patient has recently experienced an ST segment elevation myocardial infarction (Douglas et al., 2009; Kalesan et al., 2012). Along with a drug-eluting stent, the patient is typically placed on an anticoagulation medication for 6–12 months to decrease risk of thrombosis formation and aspirin indefinitely to reduce incidence of future MI. If stenosis occurs, angina symptoms will return and further intervention is required to stabilize myocardial function. This may include inserting another stent, PCI, atherectomy, laser or radiation therapy or coronary artery bypass.

ATHERECTOMY

There are four general types of atherectomy procedure that can be used to debulk or remove a thrombosis or atherosclerotic plaque and restore coronary blood flow. Atherectomy can be used independently or in conjunction with PCI or stent deployment. The primary function of the atherectomy is to mechanically remove the plaque. A directional atherectomy (side-cutting) is best used when the lesion is located at a bifurcation or is eccentric and complicated. The rotational atherectomy uses a circular abrasive method and an atherosclerotic extraction device with cutting blades at the end of the endovascular instrument to debulk the artery. Laser has been successfully used to vaporize tissue in the case of 'in-stent' stenosis. Finally, a cutting balloon angioplasty, which is an atherotomy as opposed to an atherectomy, excises the lesion and dilates the artery by using a balloon catheter with a microsurgical blade (Guagliumi et al., 2011). Atherectomy as well as PCI is associated with the possibility of microembolic activity that can result in arterial occlusion of distal smaller arteries leading to other ischemic sites.

LASERS

The atherosclerotic lesion can be managed by an ablative laser atherectomy procedure. Direct ablation by laser is indicated for a lesion in a saphenous vein graft, in aorta–coronary artery ostial stenosis, for a fibrotic or calcified lesion, for a lesion that affects a diffuse area or in-stent

restenosis. Based upon the cellular makeup of the plaque, the correct wavelength can vaporize the lesion. The most common complication of this application of lasers is perforation of the vessel, which may occur at a 5–10% rate (Topaz et al., 2009).

Lasers are also being used to conduct the Maze procedure (see below) for the treatment of atrial fibrillation and transmyocardial revascularization. These procedures will be briefly discussed later in this chapter.

RADIATION

Intracoronary radiation, also known as brachytherapy, is being utilized to manage restenosis of treated coronary artery disease. The use of isotopes inhibits smooth muscle proliferation, delays the healing process and prevents the remodeling of the treated arteries. When brachytherapy is used in stent restenosis, there is a reduction of future restenosis by 50% (Price et al., 2007).

THERAPEUTIC INTERVENTION

The therapeutic intervention during the acute phase after a catheterization procedure is similar to that described above for a LHC. Because the patient has been diagnosed with coronary artery disease and there is the risk of restenosis, it is important that the clinician educates the patient on the importance of compliance with routine medical check-ups and the use of medications, and the patient is able to recognize the signs and symptoms related to myocardial ischemia and MI. In the long term, it is important that the patient begins to minimize his or her cardiac risk factors, such as cessation of smoking, management of hypertension and diabetes, proper diet and weight management, and participate in a regular exercise program. Patients with heart disease benefit from cardiac rehabilitation where they are monitored during exercise, provided with valuable education, and develop a network of social support.

CORONARY ARTERY BYPASS SURGERY

In the presence of multivessel coronary disease, complex diffuse lesions, left main arterial disease, multivessel disease with left ventricular dysfunction and in patients with diabetes, coronary artery bypass graft (CABG) surgery is the invasive procedure of choice and is the most common cardiac surgical procedure performed (Sundt, 2013). The purpose of performing CABG surgery is to restore perfusion to viable myocardium by diverting blood around the atherosclerotic plaque to perfuse the myocardium distal to the occlusion.

Typically, the surgical approach is a median sternotomy, particularly for a multivessel bypass procedure. For isolated left anterior descending artery (LAD) blockages, CABG procedures are being carried out using a small anterior thoracotomy approach, referred to as a minimally invasive direct coronary artery bypass (MIDCAB) or keyhole CABG. See below for more details on MIDCAB procedures.

The vascular tissue that is harvested for the bypass procedure can be either arterial or venous in nature. Traditionally, the saphenous vein has been used to bypass the lesion by making an anastomosis of the vein to the aortic root and to a point distal to the lesion or stenosis.

The vein is sutured in the reverse direction to prevent the valves within the veins from obstructing blood flow. Other sources of grafts or conduits continue to be investigated because the saphenous vein graft (SVG) has a modest rate of stenosis. In total, 15% of SVGs will become occluded within the first year because of hyperplasia and accelerated atherosclerosis and 50% are occluded within 10 years (Holzhey et al., 2012).

The left, right or both internal thoracic (mammary) arteries (IMA) are common grafts for bypassing the left anterior descending artery and right coronary artery, respectively. The left mammary artery, which has a 71% patency rate 15 years after the surgical procedure (Locker et al., 2012), is most commonly used because the use of the right mammary artery or both IMA is associated with sternal wound complications (Cahalin et al., 2011). Other arteries of the torso, such as the right gastroepiploic and inferior epigastric arteries have been employed as conduits but are not commonly used because of the difficulty in harvesting the arteries. In a large meta-analysis, it has been reported that there is an increase in long-term survival when a multiartery bypass procedure is performed when compared to left IMA and SVG, despite being more difficult surgically (Locker et al., 2012). The radial artery is also a common arterial source, but the surgeon must assure sufficient blood flow to the hand and it is a challenge to avoid sensory loss.

Traditionally, when undergoing this procedure, the patient is placed on cardiopulmonary bypass (CPB) to stop the heart and allow the CABG surgery to be completed. The CPB circulates blood to allow for full cardiopulmonary support while the heart is not beating and the grafts are sutured in place. This is a necessary procedure based upon the size and location of the coronary arteries, hemodynamic stability and left ventricular function. Unfortunately, there are adverse effects associated with CPB, particularly in the geriatric population. With the use of CPB there is a diffuse systemic inflammatory response with association of increased activation of platelets, coagulation and fibrinocytes activity. The aorta is manipulated in order to go onto CPB which is associated with increased embolic activity that increases risk for stroke and MI (Cooper et al., 2012). These adverse effects include higher incidence of perioperative or postoperative stroke, postoperative MI and deaths (Afilalo et al., 2012; Cooper et al., 2012). The following risk factors are associated with increased surgical complications and the surgeon should consider completing the CABG off CPB if medically appropriate to improve the individual's outcomes: age, diabetes mellitus, renal insufficiency, decreased left ventricular function, peripheral arterial disease and chronic obstructive pulmonary disease (Cooper et al., 2012).

Certain risks are involved when a patient is undergoing a CABG. The surgery may be complicated by MI, arrhythmia, incisional and sternal infections, and failure to wean from mechanical ventilation, bleeding, stroke or acute renal failure. The procedure also carries a 1–3.6% mortality rate, which can be higher in patients with postoperative complications or in patients with coexisting disease like diabetes, declining left ventricular function and untreated heart failure. New onset of atrial fibrillation after open heart procedure like CABG is associated with increased length of hospital stay, and higher short- and long-term mortality rates. The older adult has an increased risk of developing postoperative atrial fibrillation, along with history of prior stroke, history of hypertension and peripheral arterial disease and longer CPB time (Kaw et al., 2011).

MINIMALLY INVASIVE DIRECT CORONARY ARTERY BYPASS

Depending upon the blood vessels that are occluded, the stability of the patient and the function of the heart, the surgeon may opt to perform the bypass through a small anterior thoracotomy, referred to as minimally invasive direct coronary artery bypass (MIDCAB). The goals of a thoracotomy approach are to decrease the surgical trauma caused by a median sternotomy, improve recovery and reduce the length of the hospital stay and can be completed without CPB support. The MIDCAB is performed through a small anterior thoracotomy incision in the left fourth or fifth intercostal space. Typically, the left IMA is the conduit of choice to bypass the left anterior descending artery.

Commonly the left internal mammillary artery (sometimes called the internal thoracic artery) is used to bypass an occlusion involving the LAD. This approach has more recently been combined with the PCI procedure which has permitted surgeons to address multivessel disease, especially for individuals who were at high complication risks for a standard CABG. This combined approach to surgically managing CAD is referred to as a hybrid procedure. The approach that is used depends on the involved arteries, heart function, stability of the conduction system, the need for cardiopulmonary bypass support and the surgeon's training (Afilalo et al., 2012; Holzhey et al., 2012). The other benefit of a MIDCAB is that the procedure can be performed without cardiopulmonary bypass support and aortic manipulation that results in a decrease in mortality, stroke and postoperative MI (Afilalo et al., 2012; Cooper et al., 2012).

THERAPEUTIC INTERVENTION

Patients who undergo a median sternotomy approach to cardiac surgery are commonly instructed in sternal precautions with the goal to modify the use of the upper extremities to reduce sternal wound complications. The clinician needs to be aware there is insufficient published evidence on what these precautions should be to prevent wound complications while restoring function in the early postoperative period. Sternal precautions vary from facility to facility and can be individualized for each surgeon with a facility. Commonly the precautions include weight lifting limitations, range of motion (ROM) restrictions, particularly elevation above shoulder height, and restriction in basic functional mobility and activities of daily living. There have been no published reports that have linked the performance of range of motion, the use of upper extremities, or performance of functional activities and sternal wound complications. Risk factors associated with surgical complications include obesity, surgical use of bilateral internal mammillary arteries, diabetes mellitus, prolonged mechanical ventilation and prolonged CPB time just to name a few (Cahalin et al., 2011).

With little consensus on sternal precautions, the information provided in this section is the clinical advice from this author. Commonly, the incisions are covered with only a dry dressing in the immediate postoperative phase and in the presence of a draining wound. The sternal wound may remain covered until the patient is weaned from mechanical ventilation support. If the saphenous vein or radial artery are harvested, the involved extremity will typically be ice-wrapped for 24–48 hours to control edema. Female patients with larger breasts have an increased risk of wound complication so it is advised that a bra is worn to decrease tension on the incision.

In terms of shoulder ROM, when a median sternotomy is the surgical approach, ROM is performed within the tolerance of the patient, allowing unilateral and bilateral flexion and abduction above shoulder height to tolerance. Commonly external rotation combined with abduction above 90° degrees is painful and not tolerated. If a patient has various risk factors that are associated with wound complications the surgeon or the therapist may want to consider limiting humeral elevation to shoulder height.

Acute care rehabilitation includes restoring functional mobility, increasing ambulation tolerance and preparing for discharge. Strengthening and functional mobility exercises are also performed within the patient's tolerance, using proper body mechanics to protect the sternum and incision. Using the upper extremities for functional mobility and activities of daily living should be modified to facilitate approximation of the surgically fractured site of the sternum and reduce tissue tension.

Mobility should be initiated as soon as the patient is alert and hemodynamically stable. Out-of-bed activities may begin as early as 3–6 hours in the postoperative period, but commonly begins 12–24 hours postsurgically. Transfers out of bed are typically tolerated with a side-lying to sit transfer and using the nondependent arm to push up while using the dependent arm to splint the sternum

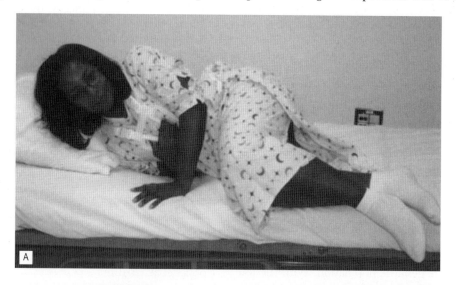

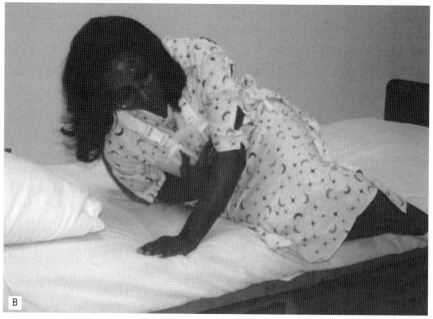

Figure 44.2 (A and **B)** These photographs illustrate how the patient is instructed to progress out of bed using a heart hugger. Please note that the patient is using the right upper extremity to splint the chest wall and that the elbow is held tightly against the rib cage to prevent the patient from abducting the arm.

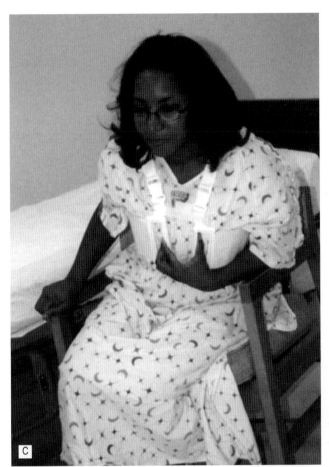 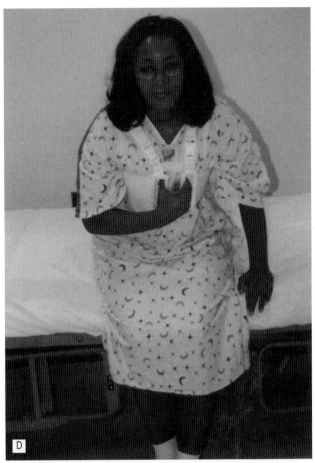

Figure 44.2 (C) During scooting it is important to remind the patient to keep the upper extremities in front of the trunk. **(D)** The upper extremity(-ies) can be used to move from 'sit' to 'stand' but the patient should visually check to make sure that their hand(s) is properly placed in front of the trunk before pushing. This patient is using an external device (heart hugger) to assist in splinting the chest wall.

(see Fig. 44.2). The lower extremities should not be moved off the bed until the patient is fully side-lying to reduce the activation of the abdominal muscles thus reducing tension to the inferior position of the sternal wound.

The role of the rehabilitation therapist is to instruct the patient how to modify activities to protect the sternum and restore basic functional mobility. Typically, to perform basic functional mobility like supine to sit, scooting, and sit to stand transfers, an individual increases their mechanical advantage by extending the humerus behind the trunk to increase the mechanical advance. This position of the upper extremity is painful and not tolerated by most patients after open heart procedures. The author makes the following recommendations when training basic mobility: for scooting in and out of a chair or bed and performing a sit to stand transfer the upper extremities can be used to unilaterally weight-bear or to assist in the standing motion within the patient's tolerance. Patients can be instructed to weight-bear onto the elbow to create a weight shift and can use the contralateral arm to push to help scoot the pelvis. For sit to stand transfers the arms can be placed on their knees, or on the armrest of the chair to push up to standing. It is safe to allow the patient to use an assistive device for gait training if necessary. In the case of manual wheelchair propulsion, the patient is instructed to avoid extreme shoulder extension.

The period of time a patient is advised to comply with sternal precautions is also variable, with ranges averaging 4–8 weeks. More recently, surgeons may stabilize the sternum with a plate opposed to wires, particularly if the patient is at significant risk of sternal wound complications and for patients who perform manual labor (Cahalin et al., 2011). These patients are commonly placed on precautions for 2–4 weeks. Certain activities like heavy overhead lifting, pushups, or bench press exercises may be restricted for 4–6 months after surgery for a patient with sternal wires.

At the University of Maryland Medical Center, patients are classified as moderate risk for sternal complications if they have a significant history of poorly controlled diabetes, a history of type I diabetes of greater than 10 years, history of systemic corticosteroid use, moderate truncal obesity, or if the surgeon used bilateral IMA grafts. Other moderate-risk patients are those with comorbidities such as spinal cord injury or lower extremity amputation that would require partial or full weight-bearing as tolerated for the upper extremities in order to permit mobility. These patients may be placed in a device that approximates the upper rib cage, such as a sheet wrapped around the thorax or a 'heart-hugger' device, to increase the stability of the sternum. Once the sternum is stabilized, functional mobility can be instructed as described above. The clinician should routinely inspect the incision for healing and assess the patient for sternal stability. Figure 44.2 describes mobility training in patients using moderate sternal precautions.

Patients who have undergone a thoracotomy procedure commonly do not have any ROM or mobility restrictions but are allowed to perform activities within their tolerance. Splinting across the surgical site helps to decrease pain and improves the patient's willingness to cough, participate in deep breathing exercises and initiate mobility training.

The goal for discharge is to achieve medical stability, restore functional mobility and complete all the education necessary within 3–5 days of surgery. Rehabilitation during the acute phase of recovery should also address pulmonary care, functional restoration and patient education. Instruction in the use of the incentive spirometer, splinting and coughing techniques, and early ambulation should be emphasized to reduce the risk of atelectasis or pneumonia. It is recommended that patients ambulate at least three times a day with a goal of ambulating for at least 10 minutes in each session. Patient education should include cardiac risk factors (e.g. cessation of smoking, control of blood glucose levels and increased activity level), the proper use of medications and the need for a sensible diet or following a prescribed heart healthy diet. Postoperative education should also include a home exercise program that includes increasing walking tolerance to 30 minutes a day at a light to moderate intensity for 5 days a week over the next 6 weeks of recovery. The patient and family should be instructed as to which signs and symptoms to monitor so that any postoperative complications can be identified and promptly addressed. Finally, it is common that patient education also includes the following instructions: avoid lifting more than 10–20 lb (4.5–9 kg), avoid driving and sit in the back seat of the vehicle to protect against the activation of the front airbags if an accident should occur. Sexual activities can resume when patient has sufficient energy, experiencing no angina or sternal pain. Modification of sexual positions may improve the patient's tolerance until complete bone healing has occurred.

Outpatient cardiac rehabilitation should begin 2–6 weeks postoperatively and typically consists of 24–36 visits with electrocardiogram and vital sign monitoring during exercise. The goal of this phase of rehabilitation is to raise the patient's tolerance to the point where 40–60 minutes of aerobic exercise at moderate intensity can be completed. Once the surgeon has confirmed that the sternum is healed, the patient can begin weightlifting using light to moderate weights. Questions regarding return to work and recreational activities are entertained at this time. If the patient is returning to a job that requires physical labor, the clinician should design a work-hardening program to enable the patient to successfully re-enter the workforce and decrease the risk of work-related injuries.

VALVULAR PROCEDURES

There are many factors that must be considered when the surgeon and patient are determining if a valve should be repaired or replaced and what type of procedure should be done. Some of these factors may include the age of the patient, the risk associated with the use of anticoagulation, the risk of infections and the extent of the anatomical disorder of the valve and the function of the left ventricle. If the valve needs to be replaced, it must be decided whether the replacement should be a mechanical or a biological valve. Age, past medical history and lifestyle all contribute to the decision regarding the type of valve replacement that is used (Markar et al., 2011; Spaccarotella et al., 2011; Vahanian et al., 2011).

There are several invasive procedures that can be considered to correct valvular dysfunction. Percutaneous balloon valvuloplasty is a nonsurgical approach for stenosis. A catheter is positioned across the lumen of the valve and inflated to decrease the stenosis. For mitral stenosis, another nonsurgical option is a percutaneous mitral commissurotomy, in which the leaflet of the valve is cut via a catheter. In both of these options, there is a risk of restenosis and complications of valvular regurgitation (Figulla et al., 2011).

When medical management has reached its maximal benefit or when ventricular function is impaired or myocardial ischemia needs to be resolved, surgical intervention is the therapy of choice (Figulla et al., 2011; Vahanian et al., 2011; Scandura et al., 2012; Szabo et al., 2012). Depending on the valve involved, the patient's anatomy and the surgeon's training, a mediastinal or anterior thoracotomy may be the surgical approach. Valve replacement is the surgical gold standard for MR and AS, although 33% of individuals with AS (and a similar figure for severe MR, particularly functional MR) are not candidates for traditional surgical intervention (Markar et al., 2011; Spaccarotella et al., 2011).

There are increasing surgical options for AS. Surgeons are performing mini invasive procedures, referred to as a transapical approach. The individual does not undergo a complete sternotomy. A 2- to 3-inch incision of the sternal body is made or a mini anterior thoracotomy with a transection of the sternum is made to repair or replace the aortic valve. This decreases the risk of wound complications, increases the recovery rate and hospital discharge rates. Individuals who have higher surgical risks may undergo a transvascular aortic valve implantation (TAVI). In a TAVI the approach is commonly through the femoral artery where either a bovine pericardial valve is mounted on a balloon-expandable stent that is placed with the native valve (Sapien valve) or a porcine pericardial valve is mounted on a self-expanding stent that extends into the ascending aorta (CoreValve ReValving System) (Webb et al., 2012). The 1-year survival for individuals who undergo TAVI is 73–79% compared to 62% for those who are medically managed (Figulla et al., 2011). Finally, individuals who are not candidates for traditional surgical procedures may be offered an aortic valve bypass (AVB) procedure where a left ventricle aortic conduit is surgically implanted from the left ventricle to the descending aorta through a thoracotomy. It is reported that 65–70% of cardiac output goes through the bypass and there can be as much as a 40% increase in stroke volume (Szabo et al., 2012).

THERAPEUTIC INTERVENTION

The rehabilitation of the patient who has undergone valvular repair or replacement is similar to that of patients who have undergone myocardial revascularization (see the discussion above on immediate post-CABG rehabilitation). Patients who are placed on anticoagulation therapy should be educated to be cautious when participating in contact recreational sports and vigorous weight-lifting activities. They should also be educated on the importance of follow-up medical check-ups to monitor anticoagulation levels and the signs and symptoms of bleeding. The clinician and the patient should also monitor for the return of symptoms, especially if the valve was repaired as opposed to replaced, suggesting the repair has failed or additional valve dysfunction has developed.

CRYOMAZE PROCEDURE

Atrial fibrillation is the most common cardiac arrhythmia and the prevalence increases with age, heart failure, mitral and aortic valve disease, and after open heart procedures (Veasey et al., 2011). This is an irregular conduction rhythm that interferes with proper filling of the ventricles and increases the risk of thrombus formation within the atrium, which increases the risk of stroke. Over 2.6 million individuals in US and 4.4 million in Europe were living with atrial fibrillation in 2010 and the arrhythmia is associated with 12% of strokes (Williams et al., 2010; CDC Division of Heart Disease and Stroke Prevention, 2013).

Atrial fibrillation is associated with higher mortality and morbidity rates with open heart procedures, especially mitral valve surgery and CABG (Kaw et al., 2011; Veasey et al., 2011). The pattern of depolarization within the left atria is commonly predictable in atrial fibrillation and abnormal conduction within the left ventricle. With this in mind, it is possible to disrupt the pathway of depolarization within the atria, with emphasis on the left atrium, to ablate the arrhythmia and restore normal sinus rhythm. The Maze procedure involves making surgical incisions or lesions with a cold laser in a precise pattern to create alleys that allow only one-way atrial depolarization to occur (Chen et al., 2012). The Maze procedure can be performed alone through an anterior thoracotomy or, more commonly, performed at the time of the open heart procedure for those individuals with a history of atrial fibrillation. Along with the Maze procedure the surgeon can excise the appendage of the left atrium to reduce the risk of thrombus formation (Williams et al., 2010; Chen et al., 2012).

In the acute phase of recovery, it is not uncommon for the patient's heart to revert back into atrial fibrillation because the myocardial tissue is irritated and inflamed (Veasey et al., 2011; Chen et al., 2012). It is important for the clinician to monitor and be able to recognize the signs and symptoms of atrial fibrillation. Typically, for the first 3 months after the procedure, the patient will be placed on antiarrhythmic medication to decrease the risk of developing atrial fibrillation.

TRANSMYOCARDIAL REVASCULARIZATION

A patient who suffers from disabling angina that is nonresponsive to medical therapy and is not a candidate for a PCI or complete revascularization (CABG), because of diffuse distal coronary disease, may be a candidate for transmyocardial revascularization (TMR). Although TMR continues to be performed as an isolated procedure, more recently surgeons are more likely to perform a TMR in conjunction with a CABG or valvular procedure (Tavris et al., 2012). The TMR procedure involves the use of a laser to create small transmural channels within the myocardium, primarily the left ventricle wall. When the left ventricle is fully distended with blood and depolarization has begun, a laser is fired through the myocardium. The laser makes a 1 mm channel through the wall of the left ventricle and the laser beam is absorbed by the blood in the chamber. Several channels are made through the myocardium. Direct pressure is applied to the epicardial surface to stop bleeding into the pericardial sac. A suture may also have to be placed at the entrance of the laser to control bleeding (Horvath, 2004; Yang et al., 2004).

The exact mechanism that enables TMR to improve myocardial perfusion is still unknown. There are two accepted theories that address the mechanics for relieving angina. One theory involves laser-induced angiogenesis in which more collateral circulation develops, which increases perfusion to the myocardial tissue. The second theory involves the decrease in angina symptoms because the laser causes denervation of the myocardial tissue that is causing the angina state. There is literature to support both theories, but further clinical studies need to be conducted in this area (Bridges et al., 2004; Horvath, 2004).

THERAPEUTIC INTERVENTION

The rehabilitation process regarding mobility will depend upon the approach that was used to perform the TMR. A key clinical factor for the clinician to understand is that patients are not completely revascularized and may continue to experience myocardial ischemia and angina. The rehabilitation progress typically has to be altered for patients undergoing TMR compared to those who undergo a complete revascularization. The exercise prescription typically includes lower intensities, interval exercises and short duration because there still may be a state of impaired overall myocardial perfusion. In this patient population, it is important that the clinician monitor for the signs and symptoms of myocardial ischemia and educate the patient for safe self-monitoring during exertion and exercise. Rehabilitation should focus on functional strengthening and functional activities, for example walking, to promote independence. Patient education should also include work simplification and energy conservation. There have been no reported differences in mortality rates between individuals who undergo CABG versus CABG plus TMR (Tavris et al., 2012). More research is needed to determine if individuals who undergo TMR have an improved functional mobility and quality of life.

VENTRICULAR RECONSTRUCTION

When the ventricle becomes dilated as a consequence of ischemic heart disease or develops an aneurysm as a result of a large transmural myocardial infarction, it is unable to generate sufficient contraction to maintain cardiac output and the patient develops heart failure. Ventricular reconstruction has been used to resect an aneurysm that is the result of a MI or reconstruction can be performed to reduce the size of a globally dilated ventricle. The surgeon may consider a procedure to reconstruct the ventricle to restore its shape, and improve the efficiency of muscle contraction. Ventricular reconstruction has been combined with CABG and mitral valve repair. The results appear mixed in that the combined CAGB and reconstruction has not demonstrated improvement in survival (Zembala et al., 2010). This surgical intervention, along with repair of the mitral valve, has shown improvement in survival for individuals with ischemic cardiomyopathy. It has been reported that there is an improvement in contractility and decrease in oxygen consumption (Shudo et al., 2010; Dor et al., 2011).

This procedure is commonly performed via a median sternotomy, consequently the patient would follow the protocol of sternal precautions for the particular institution or surgeon. The rehabilitation should focus on functional restoration and improved activity tolerance and the clinician should be monitoring for and educating the patient on the signs and symptoms of heart failure. Typically the rehabilitation process will need to be a slow progression with close professional monitoring.

VENTRICULAR ASSIST DEVICES

Recently there has been an incredible increase in the use of ventricular assist devices (VAD), with changes both in engineering design and the clinical use of VAD for the management of heart failure. No longer is the use of VADs only for the younger individual or the individual waiting for transplant. More older adults are undergoing VAD implantation either as a bridge to transplantation or as destination therapy. Destination therapy means that the individual is not a candidate for heart transplantation and the VAD will serve as their final management option for heart failure. In 2010 Thoratec, Inc. received FDA approval for using the HeartMate II VAD for destination therapy, and other devices are in various approval stages with the FDA for destination use. Destination therapy is an area of increasing use according to INTERMAC, which is the national registry for mechanical circulatory support for heart failure. This particularly increases the management options for the older adult with heart failure.

The design and operation of the devices have also significantly changed. Although pulsatile VADs such as Thoratec pVAD have continued to be used, particularly for biventricular failure, the more common type of device provides nonpulsatile circulation. A nonpulsatile VAD such as the HeartMateII (see Fig. 44.3), HeartWare and Jarvik 2000 circulate blood continuously, as opposed to mimicking the filling and ejecting of blood like the native heart. This design has led to smaller devices

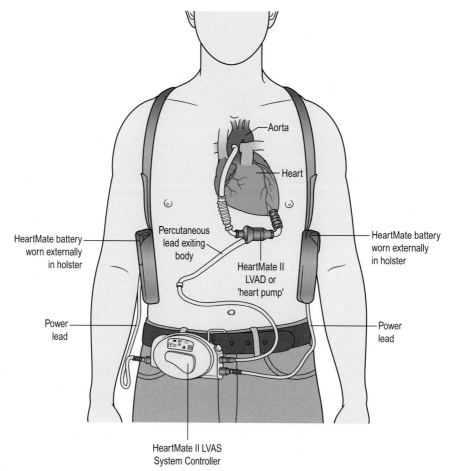

Figure 44.3 The HeartMate II is an example of a nonpulsatile ventricular assist device (VAD) that supports the left ventricle. The position of the VAD within the body and its interface with the cardiovascular system is shown, along with the actual pump, its cannulas that continuously circulate blood from the left ventricle through the pump and back to the ascending aorta. *(From Thoratec Corp., Pleasanton, CA. Available: www. Thoratec.com., with permission.)*

and high durability (Mitter & Sheinberg, 2010). The changes in VAD design have led to smaller-stature individuals being able to be implanted with a VAD for long-term use. The change in how the VAD circulates blood has also resulted in a reduction in strokes (Mitter & Sheinberg, 2010).

THERAPEUTIC INTERVENTION

With the increased utilization of nonpulsatile VADs there are changes in the considerations for vital sign monitoring for these individuals. Depending upon the speed that the VAD is programmed to circulate blood, the patient may no longer have an appreciable pulsatile flow to their blood within the arterial system, meaning the clinician may not be able to find a peripheral pulse to monitor heart rate and blood pressure without more advanced equipment. The clinician and patient need to be comfortable and reliable in using a subjective scale, such as the rate of perceived exertion scale, to assess tolerance. The clinician will also need to track the power utilization and pump outputs to determine clinical stability.

All VADs have a set of alarms that will sound if there is a problem in VAD function. Consequently, as part of the postimplantation recovery phase, the rehabilitation clinician will be working with the VAD team and patient to monitor the patient and function of the VAD and respond appropriately to any alarm that may be activated. Prior to working with patients being supported by a VAD, the clinician needs to complete any training and demonstrate competency, as defined by the facility and the device's manufacturers, to ensure that they understand how the device functions, what the various alarms mean, and what the appropriate sequence of actions should be when an alarm goes off.

The general rehabilitation of patients who have undergone a VAD implantation is very similar to that of patients who have undergone a CABG procedure, although for some VADs the surgical approach will be a thoracotomy. For most, sternal precautions will need to be addressed as well as training the patient to move while managing the VAD. The clinician needs to remember that the VAD is supporting left ventricular function and so cardiac output should be stable; this should allow the patient to participate in an aggressive rehabilitation program to restore function, improve activity tolerance, permit a possible return to work and improve quality of life (Wells, 2013).

CONCLUSION

In the evaluation and treatment of cardiac pathology, various invasive techniques exist. Some are only minimally invasive, whereas others require extensive surgical techniques. Care providers must be aware of the specific invasive techniques used and their associated precautions. Immediate postoperative wound care is a concern for all of these techniques. In most cases, rehabilitation should commence within 24 hours of surgery. The goal of care is to return the patient to as normal a lifestyle as possible within weeks to months and within the limits of individual cardiac and coexisting pathologies.

REFERENCES

Afilalo J, Rasti M, Ohayon SM 2012 Off pump vs. on pump coronary artery bypass surgery: an updated meta-analysis and meta-regression of randomized trials. Eur Heart J 33:1257–1267

Arjomand H, Turi Z, McCormick D et al 2003 Percutaneous coronary intervention: historical perspectives, current status, and future directions. Am Heart J 146:787–796

Bridges CR, Horvath KA, Nugent WC et al 2004 The Society of Thoracic Surgeons practice guidelines series. Transmyocardial laser revascularization. Ann Thorac Surg 77:1494–1502

Cahalin LP, LaPierm TK, Shaw DK 2011 Sternal precautions: is it time for change? Precautions versus restrictions: a review of literature and recommendations for revision. Cardiopulm Phys Ther J 22(1):4–13

CDC National Center for Health Statistics 2012 FastStats: Inpatient surgery. [Online] Available at: www.cdc.gov/nchs/fastats/insurg.htm. Accessed March 2013

CDC Division of Heart Disease and Stroke Prevention 2013 Atrial fibrillation fact sheet. [Online] Available at: www.cdc.gov/dhdsp/data_statistics/fact_sheets/fs_atrial_fibrillation.htm. Accessed March 2013

Chen Y, Maruthappu M, Nagendran M 2012 How effective is unipolar radiofrequency ablation for atrial fibrillation during concomitant cardiac surgery? Interact Cardiovasc Thorac Surg 14:843–847

Cooper EA, Edelman JJB, Wilson MK 2012 Off pump coronary artery bypass grafting in elderly and high risk patients: a review. Heart Lung Circ. 20:694–703

DiMario C, Sirtaria N 2005 Coronary angiography in the angioplasty era: projections with a meaning. Heart 91:968–976

Dor V, Filippo C, Alexandrescu C et al 2011 Favorable effects of left ventricular reconstruction in patients excluded from the surgical treatments for ischemic heart failure (STICH) trial. J Thorac Cardiovasc Surg 141(4):905–906

Douglas PS, Brennan JM, Anstrom KJ et al 2009 Clinical effectiveness of coronary stents in the elderly: results from 262,700 Medicare patients in ACC-NCDR. J Am Coll Cardiol 53(18):1629–1641

Figulla L, Neumann A, Figulla HR 2011 Transcatheter aortic valve implantation: evidence on safety and efficacy compared with medical therapy. A systematic review of current literature. Clin Res Cardiol 100(4):265–276

Guagliumi G, Sirbu V, Musumeci G et al 2011 Strut coverage and vessel wall response to a new-generation Paclitaxel-Eluting stents with an ultrathin biodegradable abluminal polymer. Circ Cardiovasc Intervent 3:367–375

Heir JS, Gottumukkala V, Singh M et al 2010 Coronary stents and noncardiac surgery: current clinical challenges and conundrums. Prevent Cardiol 13:8–13

Holzhey DM, Cornely JP, Rastan AJ 2012 Review of a 13-year single center experience with minimally invasive direct coronary artery bypass as the primary surgical treatment of coronary artery disease. Heart Surg Forum 15(2):E61–E68

Horvath K 2004 Mechanisms and results of transmyocardial laser revascularization. Cardiology 101:37–47

Kalesan B, Pilgrim T, Heinimann K et al 2012 Comparison of drug-eluting stents with bare metal stents in patients with ST-segment elevation myocardial infarction. Eur Heart J 33:977–987

Kaw R, Hernandez AV, Masood I et al 2011 Short- and long-term mortality associated with new onset atrial fibrillation after coronary artery bypass grafting: a systematic review and meta-analysis. J Thorac Cardiovasc Surg 141:1305–1312

Lemos P, Lee C, Degertelem M et al 2003 Early outcome after Sirolimus-eluting stent: implantation of patients with acute cardiac syndrome. J Am Coll Cardiol 41(11):2093–2099

Locker C, Schaff HV, Dearani JA 2012 Multiple arterial grafts improve late survival of patients undergoing coronary artery bypass graft surgery: analysis of 8622 patients with multivessel disease. Circulation 126:1023–1030

Markar SR, Sadat U, Edmonds L et al 2011 Mitral valve repair versus replacement in the elderly population. J Heart Valve Dis 20:265–271

Mitter N, Sheinberg R 2010 Update on ventricular assist devices. Curr Opin Anaesthesiol 23:57–66

Price MJ, Glap H, Teirstein PS 2007 Intracoronary radiation therapy for multi-drug resistant in-stent restenosis: Initial clinical experience. Catheter Cardiovasc Intervent 69(1):132–134

Rogers JH, Franzen O 2011 Percutaneous edge to edge MitraClip therapy in the management of mitral regurgitation. Eur Heart J 32:2350–2357

Scandura S, Ussia GP, Caggegi A 2012 Percutaneous mitral valve repair in patients with prior cardiac surgery. J Cardiac Surg 27:295–298

Shudo Y, Sakaguchi T, Miyagwaw S et al 2010 Impact of surgical ventricular reconstruction for ischemic dilated cardiomyopathy on restrictive filling pattern. Gen Thorac Cardiovasc Surg 58:399–404

Spaccarotella C, Mongiardo A, Indolfi C 2011 Pathophysiology of aortic stenosis and approach to treatment with percutaneous valve implantation. Circ J 75:11–19

Sundt TM 2013 CABG information. The Society of Thoracic Surgeons. [Online] Available at: www.sts.org/patient-information/adult-cardiac-surgery/cabg-information. Accessed December 2013

Szabo TA, Toole A, Payne KJ et al 2012 Management of aortic valve bypass surgery. Semin Cardiothorac Vasc Anesth 16(1):53–58

Tavris DR, Brennan JM, Sedrakyan A et al 2012 Long term outcomes after transmyocardial revascularization. Ann Thorac Surg 94:1500–1508

Topaz O, Polkampally PR, Mohanty PK et al 2009 Excimer laser debulking for percutaneous coronary intervention in left main coronary artery disease. Lasers Med Sci 24(6):955–960

Tresukosol D, Sudjarituk S, Pornratanarangsi S et al 2010 Early and intermediate outcomes of left main coronary intervention. J Med Assoc Thailand 93(1):21–28

Vahanian A, Iung B, Himbert D et al 2011 Changing demographics of valvular heart disease and impact on surgical and transcatheter valve therapies. Int J Cardiovasc Imaging 27:1115–1122

Veasey RA, Segal OR, Large JK 2011 The efficacy of intraoperative atrial radiofrequency ablation for atrial fibrillation during concomitant cardiac surgery: the surgical atrial fibrillation suppression (SAFS) study. J Intervent Cardiac Electrophysiol 32:29–35

Webb J, Rodès-Cabau J, Fremes S et al 2012 Transcatheter aortic valve implantation: a Canadian Cardiovascular Society Position Statement. Can J Cardiol 28:520–528

Wells CL 2013 Physical therapy management of patients with ventricular assist devices: key considerations for the acute care physical therapist. Phys Ther J 93:266–278

Williams ES, Hall B, Traub D et al 2010 Catheter ablation of atrial fibrillation in the elderly. Curr Opin Cardiol 26:25–29

Wu C, Dyer AM, King III SB et al 2011 Impact of incomplete revascularization on long term mortality after coronary stenting. Circ Cardiovasc Intervent 4:413–421

Yang E, Barsness G, Gerth B et al 2004 Current and future treatment strategies for refractory angina. Mayo Clinic Proc 79(10):1284–1292

Zembala M, Michler RE, Rynkiewicz A et al 2010 Clinical characteristics of patients undergoing surgical ventricular reconstruction by choice and by randomization. J Am Coll Cardiol 56(6):499–507

Chapter 45

Pulmonary diseases

CHRIS L. WELLS

CHAPTER CONTENTS

INTRODUCTION

Lung disease can be classified based on its clinical characteristics. It is common to classify pulmonary diseases as obstructive, restrictive (also known as pulmonary fibrosis), vascular, infectious, disease of the pleural lining and cancers. As the population ages, it is anticipated there will be an increased burden to societies in the management of pulmonary diseases (Valente et al., 2010; Akgun et al., 2012). This chapter will briefly discuss obstructive, restrictive and infectious diseases, their clinical presentation and therapeutic interventions.

Chronic obstructive pulmonary disease (COPD) is a generic term to describe many lung pathologies that result in the trapping or retention of air upon exhalation. Emphysema and chronic bronchitis are two common obstructive diseases that affect people in the sixth decade of life. Asthma and cystic fibrosis are also considered to be obstructive lung diseases; they are typically diagnosed early in life, although asthma can develop across the lifespan.

Pulmonary fibrosis refers to diseases that cause a scarring of the lung tissue, for example interstitial pulmonary fibrosis and occupational lung diseases such as silicosis, farmer's or coal worker's pneumoconiosis and sarcoidosis. The result of the scarring causes a restriction or reduction of the lung's compliance, which is the ability of the lung to expand upon inspiration.

When a lung disease results in the destruction of the massive pulmonary vascular bed, pulmonary hypertension develops within the pulmonary system. Pulmonary hypertension in the elderly can be the result of a long-standing progressive obstructive or restrictive lung disease, stenosis of the mitral valve, which causes a chronic rise in pressure in the pulmonary vascular bed, or a pulmonary embolism.

CHRONIC OBSTRUCTIVE PULMONARY DISEASE

EMPHYSEMA AND CHRONIC BRONCHITIS

The two most common diseases classified as a COPD are emphysema and chronic bronchitis. Up to 16% of people worldwide have COPD, which is believed to be significantly underestimated (American Lung Association, 2010; Akgun et al., 2012). It is projected the COPD will become the third leading cause of death by 2020 (Valente et al., 2010).

Emphysema is defined as irreversible anatomical enlargement of the airspaces that are distal to the terminal bronchioles (Fig. 45.1). There is destruction of the acini, which are the functional units of the lung where gas exchange occurs in individuals without fibrosis. Emphysema can be classified based on the location of the anatomical disruption. Centrilobular emphysema is the type of emphysema most commonly associated with smoking and involves the enlargement and destruction of the first- and second-order respiratory bronchioles with the alveoli remaining intact. It most commonly affects the upper lobes and results in a mismatch between ventilation and perfusion. Panacinar emphysema is commonly found in the elderly and in patients who have a genetic form of emphysema called α1-antitrypsin deficiency. This form of emphysema affects all of the respiratory bronchioles in a uniform pattern. Paraseptal emphysema involves the peripheral secondary lobules and is not typically associated with progressive end-stage disease but with an increased risk and incidence of pneumothorax. Finally, paracicatricial emphysema is characterized by irregular enlargements of the acini with fibrosis, usually adjacent to a previous pulmonary lesion (Hogg, 2004).

Emphysema is the second most common of the obstructive diseases. There is a definite increase in the incidence of

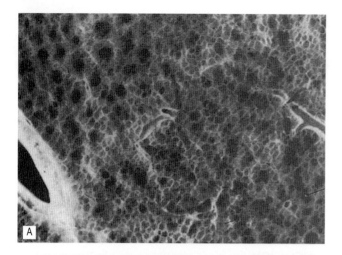

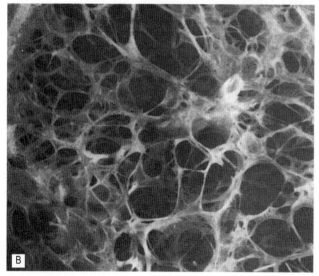

Figure 45.1 Comparison of normal lung tissue **(A)** with the pathological changes observed in lung tissue damaged by emphysema **(B)**. *(From Heard B 1969 Pathology of Chronic Bronchitis and Emphysema. Churchill Livingstone, London, with permission.)*

emphysema in the fifth decade and a continued increase into the seventh decade with the prevalence exceeding 100 cases per thousand (Akgun et al., 2012). Because the lungs have a vast amount of surface area to allow for sufficient gas exchange, many individuals will be asymptomatic in the early stages of the disease unless the activity level is at a high intensity; under such conditions, emphysema may contribute to the fatigue and shortness of breath that individuals relate to deconditioning, the aging process, or other comorbidities (Valente et al., 2010). The level of disability or functional limitation is dependent on the extent of lung destruction, not the type of emphysema, age, number or severity of comorbidities and level of function (Vorrink et al., 2011; Messer et al., 2012).

Chronic bronchitis is a leading COPD disease and is twice as common in women, with a reported prevalence of 57.7 per thousand (Valente et al., 2010). Chronic bronchitis and emphysema are treated as one long continuum, with chronic bronchitis clinically presenting with a persistent productive cough that produces sputum for more than 3 months per year for at least two consecutive years in the absence of another definable medical cause for the sputum production, such as pneumonia. The disease is associated with hyperplastic glands and an increase in goblet cells of the epithelial lining. There is a marked decrease in the ratio of goblet cells to ciliated cells, leading to hypersecretion of mucus, which overwhelms the mucociliary clearance (Fig. 45.2). The end result is overproduction and retention of sputum, which causes airway obstruction, inflammation of the respiratory bronchioles, narrowing or occlusion of the small airways from mucus plugs and hypertrophy of the smooth muscle, resulting in an increased risk of pulmonary infections (American Lung Association, 2010).

Contributing Factors

Several contributing factors have been linked to emphysema and chronic bronchitis, the most common of which is cigarette smoking. Smoking increases the aggregation of neutrophils and alveolar macrophages, which begin

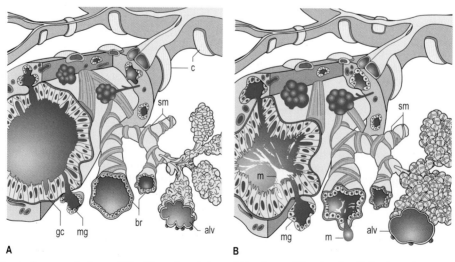

Figure 45.2 Comparison of a normal airway **(A)** with a chronic bronchitic airway **(B)**. alv, alveoli; br, bronchi; c, cartilage; gc, goblet cell; m, mucus; mg, mucus gland; sm, smooth muscle. *(From Des Jardins T 1984 Clinical Manifestations of Respiratory Disease. Year Book Medical Publishers, Chicago, IL, with permission. Redrawn by Kenneth Axen.)*

the immune response to rid the body of foreign materials. One theory suggests that emphysema is the result of an imbalance between the protective antiprotease enzymes that protect the delicate structures of the lungs and the protease enzymes that lyse or break down tissue. This imbalance leads to the loss of the elastic recoil of the lung architecture. The small airways depend upon the adjacent elastic tissue of the parenchyma to recoil and assist with expiration and to provide airway stability to allow for effective inspiration. Another theory currently under examination is the role that smoking plays in the observed elevated rate of apoptosis or cell death of the alveolar cells, followed by the failure to repair the structures to a functional state. There is also an increase in platelet and neutrophil aggregation, which destroys the small capillary beds. This leads to a decrease in the gas exchange function of the lungs and pulmonary hypertension (Higenbottam, 2005; Provinciali et al., 2011).

Exposure to air pollutants and occupational factors is also associated with an increased incidence of emphysema and chronic bronchitis. There is an increased incidence in the development and progression of COPD as the number of respiratory infections increases. The increased frequency and dose exposure to systemic steroids, for example prednisone, has also been linked to the progression of COPD.

Finally, age and genetic factors have also been linked to the development of COPD. With the increase in the age of the population there has been a significant rise in the prevalence of COPD (Akgun et al., 2012; Rycroft et al., 2012). There is a genetic link with a predisposition to emphysema and chronic bronchitis, with a reported association with a decrease in the level of alpha-1-antitrypsin (Akgun et al., 2012). This enzyme is a protease inhibitor which protects tissue from enzymes of inflammatory cells, such as neutrophil elastase. With the reduction in alpha-1-antitrypsin there is an increased rate of cellular breakdown. Within the lungs this leads to emphysema.

Clinical Manifestation

Emphysema and chronic bronchitis can exist without evidence of clinically significant obstruction or functional limitations. However, by the time that the patient presents to the healthcare provider with symptoms, extensive irreversible lung damage is present. COPD results in a limitation of airflow. The lumen size of the bronchioles is decreased because of smooth muscle proliferation and contraction, and because of bronchial edema resulting from inflammation. With the loss of lung parenchyma, there is a reduction in the elastic recoil of the airways, leading to dilatation of the distal airways and early airway closure. The end result of these changes in structure within the lungs is an increase in the ease with which air can enter the lungs during inspiration, which is referred to as an increase in compliance. Unfortunately, the changes also result in the closure or collapse of the fragile airways upon exhalation, leading to air becoming trapped in the distal respiratory bronchioles and acini. This presents clinically as hyperinflation of the lung. The hyperinflation causes shortening of the inspiratory muscles and a flattening of the diaphragm. This leads to compensatory changes in the chest wall called barrel chest deformity, which is

an increase in the anterior–posterior dimension and rib angle. These musculoskeletal changes lead to a decline in the mechanical effectiveness of the diaphragm and other respiratory muscles to support the increased demands of ventilation.

The clinical presentation of patients with COPD has an insidious onset and goes undiagnosed for many individuals. Common symptoms are nonspecific and include chronic cough, dyspnea, possible sputum production and high-pitched wheezing. With the progression of the disease there is an increased work of breathing and a reduction in activity level (Vorrink et al., 2011). Upon auscultation, there are diminished normal breath sounds and high-pitched wheezing, particularly associated with exertion. There is an elongated expiratory phase because the patient tries to slow down the change in airway pressure during expiration to minimize the degree of air trapping or obstruction. Accessory respiratory muscles are commonly hypertrophied and there is a decrease in the excursion of the diaphragm as the lungs hyperinflate. On percussing over the intercostal spaces, there is hyperresonance. With exertion, there is a marked increase in muscle recruitment, both for inspiration and expiration. Shortness of breath is the leading cause of exercise intolerance.

Patients who have a mismatch between ventilation and perfusion have the clinical presentation of desaturation because of the disruption of gas exchange. There may be areas of the lung where there is good blood flow through the pulmonary capillaries but poor ventilation. There may also be areas with an increase in the dead space in patients with COPD, which means that there is sufficient ventilation occurring in areas of the lungs where the capillary bed has been destroyed or pruned. This mismatch between ventilation and perfusion leads to hypoxia and the retention of carbon dioxide.

Examination of pulmonary function tests in patients with COPD reveals a classic pattern. Patients have a marked reduction in the ability to expel air rapidly, measured by the forced expiratory volume in 1 second (FEV_1) and forced vital capacity (FVC). The decline in FEV_1 is associated with the degree of dyspnea or shortness of breath. Exercise limitations because of dyspnea are associated with a FEV_1 of less than 50% of the predicted value for age, height and weight (Barnes & Fromer, 2011). When the patient is dyspneic at rest, the FEV_1 may be as low as 25% of the predicted value. There is also a marked increase in total lung capacity and residual volume, which clearly represents the increased compliance of the lung and the degree of air trapping or obstruction (see Fig. 45.3). It is recommended by the American Association of Respiratory Care and COPD Foundation that questionnaires should be commonly used on all adult patients to identify risk factors for COPD and simple hand-held spirometer or peak flow meters to motor airflow. For those individuals with risk factors and low expiratory flow a high-quality spirometry testing should be completed (Barnes & Fromer, 2011).

Although the majority of patients with COPD have mixed features of both emphysema and chronic bronchitis, there are certain clinical signs and symptoms that are associated more with emphysema than with chronic bronchitis. With emphysema, there is a long history of

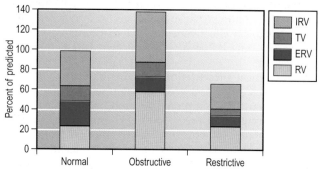

Figure 45.3 The effects of obstructive (COPD, emphysema) and restrictive (pulmonary fibrosis) pulmonary diseases on lung volumes. ERV, expiratory reserve volume; IRV, inspiratory reserve volume; RV, residual volume; TV, tidal volume.

dyspnea on exertion and little sputum production. These patients favor a posture of forward trunk flexion; this is to fixate their upper extremities so that accessory muscle recruitment is increased and the influence of gravity is decreased. The patient with emphysema is more likely to practice pursed lip breathing or grunt during expiration to keep the airways open. The patient will present with an elevated minute ventilation (respiratory rate × tidal volume), which aids in maintaining a sufficient arterial oxygen concentration at least through the early to mid-stages of the disease. In addition, a patient who suffers predominantly from emphysema will have an underweight to cachectic appearance (Hogg, 2004; American Lung Association, 2010).

In contrast, a patient who suffers predominantly from chronic bronchitis usually presents with a long history of a chronic and productive cough. Initially, the productive cough may occur only during the winter months; however, as the disease progresses in duration, frequency and severity, there is excessive sputum production and mucopurulent infections. By the time the patient experiences exertional dyspnea, there is a severe degree of airway obstruction. These patients have a tendency to be overweight and cyanotic, with a lower minute ventilation than patients with emphysema (Hogg, 2004).

As these diseases progress to end-stage, there will be further declines in lung function. The destruction of the respiratory bronchioles and acini lead to additional difficulties with proper ventilation, an increased airway resistance and a significant increase in the work of breathing. The disruption of the capillary bed within the lung causes a rise in pulmonary pressure and places a strain on the right ventricle. Over time, the patient will develop cor pulmonale, or right heart failure, which is associated with peripheral pitting edema, ascites and enlargement of the liver, jugular vein distension and anorexia.

Therapeutic Intervention

Smoking cessation is instrumental in the care of patients with COPD. Cessation leads to a decrease in the rate of loss of FEV_1. Importantly, cessation also means the avoidance of people or places where there is the risk of exposure to second-hand smoke. Behavioral modification training should also focus on weight management and healthy eating, developing coping strategies to minimize

anxiety attacks, controlling responses to stress and learning breathing strategies to control dyspnea.

Beyond behavioral modifications there are many pharmacological options to assist in the management of the disease and the associated symptoms. Short- and long-acting β_2-agonists or bronchodilators such as albuterol can be used to minimize bronchospasm and decrease wheezing and airway resistance. Anticholinergic drugs, such as atrovent, can block bronchoconstriction; xanthine-derived medications, such as theophylline, also produce bronchodilation and accelerate the mucociliary transport system and limit the inflammatory response. Corticosteroids, such as prednisone or flovent, are used for their anti-inflammatory benefits. Considerations need to be made when prescribing these medications to older adults due to pharmacokinetic and pharmacodynamic differences due to effects of aging. It is critical for patients with lung disease to receive a flu shot annually to decrease the risk of infection. When a patient has a history of recurrent infections, antibiotics play a critical role not only in the treatment of a recurrent infection but also as part of prophylactic care (Valente et al., 2010; Abbatecola et al., 2011; Jen et al., 2012).

These patients may also benefit from airway clearance techniques, including postural drainage, percussion and assistive breathing techniques, mobilization, or the use of an oscillating device to mobilize secretions. Finally, supplemental oxygen is used to correct hypoxemia and minimize secondary pulmonary hypertension. Oxygen therapy has been shown to reduce the level of dyspnea, decrease pulmonary hypertension, reduce the incidence of cardiac arrhythmias and improve quality and quantity of life. In the patient who presents with hypercapnia and respiratory insufficiency, bilevel positive airway pressure (BiPAP) ventilation has become recognized as an effective device in the management of patients with progressive disease. The ventilator provides positive airway pressure to decrease the work of inspiration and minimize the air trapping, which can reduce the retention of carbon dioxide.

Pulmonary rehabilitation has become a widely accepted intervention in the care of patients with COPD, with the ultimate goal of improving quality of life. The therapy program should consist of a comprehensive educational program to address such issues as nutrition, weight management, pathology and medical management, including the proper use of medications, work simplification and coping strategies. The program should stress and progress aerobic tolerance and include weight training to improve the muscular strength and endurance of the upper body; this will increase the effectiveness of the accessory respiratory and antigravity muscles in maximizing breathing and promoting functional mobility. The exercises should be functional and weight-bearing in nature to aid in the management of osteopenia and osteoporosis, which are very common in this patient population. Oxygen saturation should be monitored closely and supplemental oxygen adjusted to provide sufficient perfusion to support aerobic training. With training, the majority of patients with COPD will improve their exercise capacity, and note a decrease in the perception of dyspnea, an increase in self-control and a marked improvement in quality of life (Barnes & Fromer, 2011; Burtin et al., 2011; Nagarajan et al., 2011).

There are surgical options for the treatment of emphysema and chronic bronchitis. In the presence of a large bulla, which is a large airspace that is no longer contributing to gas exchange and is compressing adjacent tissue, surgical resection of this tissue (bullectomy) can be performed. Volume reduction surgery is an option for patients with emphysema, in which about 20% of dysfunctional lung tissue is surgically removed to decrease hyperinflation and improve ventilation and perfusion. Finally, lung transplantation has become a viable option for patients with end-stage COPD who have maximized medical therapy (Nathan et al., 2004).

The prognosis for patients with COPD varies depending upon the degree of obstruction, the presence of hypercapnia, the level of hypoxemia, functional mobility, body mass index, the recurrence of infections and country that the individual resides in; the 1-year mortality rate for all disease levels was reported at 27.7% and 5.1% in Canada and Sweden respectively (Rycroft et al., 2012). It is generally accepted that a FEV_1 of less than 25% is associated with a 50% mortality rate within 2 years. In chronic bronchitis, the prognosis is dependent upon age, smoking and the degree of airway obstruction. The 10-year survival rates for individuals with COPD over the age of 50 years is less than 30%, approximately 50% and 63% stratified by severe, moderate and mild disease (Shavelle et al., 2009).

PULMONARY FIBROSIS

Pulmonary fibrosis is the name for the hundreds of pulmonary pathologies that result in a restriction of the lungs. The ability of the patient to increase the volume of air in the lungs, or lung compliance, diminishes as the disease progresses; the compliance of the chest wall also decreases because of the decrease in range of motion of the chest wall, ribs and thoracic spine. Pulmonary fibrosis can be caused by autoimmune diseases, such as rheumatoid arthritis, lupus and scleroderma, or can result from occupational exposure, such as farmer's lung, silicosis and black lung. Pulmonary trauma, fat embolism and infection are associated with the development of acute respiratory distress syndrome, which for a small portion of individuals may result in pulmonary fibrosis. Other diseases, for example interstitial pulmonary fibrosis, are idiopathic in nature and for others the disease has been linked to the adverse effects of medications.

OCCUPATIONAL DISEASE

There is a subset of pulmonary interstitial disorders that result from the inhalation of inorganic dusts (pneumoconioses), organic particles (hypersensitivity pneumoconioses) and industrial gases, fumes and smoke. Fifteen percent of adult onset asthma has been linked to occupational exposure. These occupational lung diseases are associated with a chronic inflammatory process and fibrogenesis that leads to destruction of the alveolar capillary membrane. The end result is arterial hypoxemia (Noble et al., 2010; Schmidt & Flaherty, 2011; Wynn, 2011).

Pneumoconioses involves the permanent deposition of inorganic material (coal, asbestos, silica, beryllium, etc.) within the pulmonary system. The risk of developing pulmonary fibrosis is related to the duration and intensity of exposure and the size and water solubility of the particles. There is a long latency between exposure and disease, sometimes as long as 20–40 years, which may place the onset of disease in the fifth to seventh decades of life.

If the inorganic materials are able to get beyond the ciliary structures of the nasal passage and mucociliary blanket, they may cause an inflammatory process within the air spaces and interstitium, resulting in lung injury. Hyperplasia and proliferation of pulmonary epithelial cells characterize the immune response, which is accompanied by fibroblastic proliferation and collagen and protein deposition.

Hypersensitivity pneumonitis, or external allergic alveolitis, is an immunologically mediated disease that is typically associated with sensitivity from repeated exposure to an antigen. Further exposure results in an inflammatory response that involves the distal airways and alveoli. There are numerous agents that can be the impetus for developing hypersensitivity pneumonitis; these include moldy hay or grains, fungi from water reservoirs, bird serum, feathers and excreta, mining dust and pharmacological products such as gold, amiodarone and minocycline. The inflammatory response persists beyond the exposure time and leads to permanent lung damage. There is infiltration of macrophages and lymphocytes, and epithelioid granuloma formation, which eventually leads to obliteration of the bronchioles because of scarring. If the disease progresses into the chronic phase, the granulomas disappear and are replaced by fibrotic tissue formation and destruction of the architecture of the lung (Harari & Caminati, 2010).

ACUTE RESPIRATORY DISTRESS SYNDROME

Acute respiratory distress syndrome (ARDS) is an acute lung injury that results in bilateral pulmonary infiltrates, severe refractory oxygenation, noncardiac pulmonary edema and an increase in lung stiffness (i.e. a decrease in compliance). It has been suggested that ARDS is the severest form of pulmonary edema, in which diffuse alveolar involvement proceeds to promote further injury. ARDS is associated with high mortality and morbidity rates; 60-day mortality rates have decreased but still remain at 22–35%. Mortality is associated with severity of hypoxia, age over 60 years, liver or renal dysfunction or failure, exposure to tobacco smoke and alcohol use (Mann & Early, 2012; Matthay et al., 2012).

The most common cause of ARDS is a bacterial or viral infection but it can also be the result of sepsis from a nonpulmonary infection, aspiration, major trauma, blood transfusions, or pancreatitis. Diffuse alveolar disease is the hallmark picture of ARDS. Whatever the source, the injury is either to the alveolar membrane or vascular endothelium. This leads to increased permeability and a shift of protein-rich exudate into the alveoli. Subsequently there is pulmonary edema and hypoxemia (Mann & Early, 2012; Matthay et al., 2012).

This heterogeneous disorder changes over time. The initial phase (exudate phase) is characterized by pulmonary edema, hemorrhage and hyaline membrane formation. Clinically, there is a rapid onset of respiratory failure that is refractory to supplemental oxygen. The second phase involves cellular proliferation, with an elevation in the number of neutrophils and other inflammatory cells. This phase is characterized by diffuse alveolar disease (DAD); this is associated with cellular necrosis, epithelial hyperplasia and further inflammation, which leads to destruction of the delicate structures of the lung. The third phase is fibroproliferation, which is the result of chronic inflammation whereby injured lung tissue is replaced with fibrotic tissue. Beyond the destruction of terminal bronchioles and alveoli, there is also obliteration of the pulmonary capillaries, leading to pulmonary hypertension and, eventually, right heart failure (Mann & Early, 2012).

Treatment includes identifying and treating the underlying cause, mechanical ventilation, steroids, sedation and paralytics to reduce oxygen consumption needs, and extracorporeal membrane oxygenation (ECMO). Prescription of mechanical ventilation is still under debate, with most agreeing that the use of positive end-expiratory pressure is critical for gas exchange and to reduce further lung injury from positive mechanical ventilation; there are reports that the use of lower tidal volumes with elevated respiratory rates is also beneficial (Matthay et al., 2012; York & Kane, 2012).

IDIOPATHIC PULMONARY FIBROSIS

The onset of idiopathic pulmonary fibrosis (IPF) occurs in mid to late life with high mortality and morbidity rates. There is variability in the progressive rate of IPF and has a 20–30% 5-year survival rate (Harari & Caminati, 2010; Noble et al., 2010). There is an increased incidence with males and increasing age. Risk factors also include a history of smoking (Noble et al., 2010). Idiopathic pulmonary fibrosis can be associated with usual or desquamative interstitial pneumonia. Usual interstitial pneumonia (UIP) is characterized by patchy, non-uniform and variable destruction of interstitial tissue. There is a minimal inflammatory component to this disease, involving collagen deposition that thickens the alveolar septum. Desquamative interstitial pneumonia (DIP) is another form of IPF that presents with little fibrosis but a significant inflammatory response, with an accumulation of alveolar macrophages within the alveolar spaces and interstitium. The initial injury appears to damage the alveolar and epithelial cells, causing inflammatory cells to release cytokines, tumor necrosis factor and platelet-derived growth factor. These inflammatory chemicals result in smooth muscle proliferation, degradation of the alveoli and the proliferation of fibroblasts and an increase in collagen deposition. With IPF there appears to be abnormal responses during the inflammatory and fibroblastic proliferation phase of healing that leads to advanced scarring and alveolar destruction (Noble et al., 2010; Wynn, 2011).

Clinical Manifestation

Despite the range of etiologies that result in pulmonary fibrosis, patients present with a similar clinical picture of a variable rate of progressive decline, exertional dyspnea, a nonproductive cough that worsens with exertion and severe cyanosis. Along with severe dyspnea, patients generally experience severe desaturation with exertion. There is a decrease in normal breath sounds and the development of rales and clubbing of the nail beds. The breathing pattern is typically shallow with an elevated rate and there is a reduction of rib cage mobility, leading to a marked increase in the work of breathing. Anorexia, malaise and muscle weakness are also common clinical signs. Finally, pulmonary fibrosis is commonly associated with pulmonary hypertension and right heart failure (Markovitz & Cooper, 2010).

Conventional chest radiography reveals diffuse infiltrates, and honeycombing develops in the later stages of pulmonary fibrosis. When pulmonary function tests are examined, there is a decrease in lung volume, especially vital capacity (VC) and total lung capacity (TLC), a decrease in the gas exchange ability of the respiratory system (diffusion capacity; measured using the diffusing capacity of the lung for carbon monoxide [DLCO] test) and a decreased pulmonary compliance with a normal FEV_1–FVC ratio (see Fig. 45.3). A ventilation–perfusion mismatch occurs as ventilation declines and is associated with severe hypoxia. It has also been documented that there is skeletal muscle dysfunction (e.g. a reduction in type 2 muscle fibers) in patients with pulmonary fibrosis which is linked to disuse atrophy, adverse effects of medication therapy and the untoward effects of a prolonged elevated level of inflammatory markers (Markovitz & Cooper, 2010).

Therapeutic Intervention

The best defense against pneumoconiosis is prevention; this is achieved with the use of proper respiratory filter devices and appropriate ventilation in the work area. Management includes the use of corticosteroids to minimize the inflammatory response and monitoring the progression of the disease with radiological studies, pulmonary function tests and exercise testing. Medications that inhibit the immune response are also utilized in the treatment of IPF. Cyclophosphamide impairs the function of neutrophils, eventually decreasing fibroblast and collagen proliferation. Azathioprine and cyclosporin (ciclosporin) suppress the production and maturation of T and B cells involved in the immune response. With the progression of the disease, medical care may include the use of supplemental oxygen and prostacyclin drugs for the treatment of right heart failure resulting from pulmonary hypertension. Non-invasive mechanical ventilatory support may be helpful to decrease the work of breathing, improve oxygen delivery and allow for rest periods. In the presence of isolated pulmonary fibrosis, lung transplantation should be considered on a case-by-case basis (Harari & Caminati, 2010).

Pulmonary rehabilitation can also be beneficial for patients with pulmonary fibrosis with improvement in 6-minute walk distance, decrease in dyspnea levels and improvement in quality of life. Once again, the ultimate goal is to improve the quality of life. An educational and exercise program, similar to that described in the COPD section, should be provided for this patient population but the clinician should expect the rehabilitation progress to be much slower than with COPD patients. It is important that the exercise program be tailored to the individual patient with pulmonary fibrosis (Markovitz & Cooper, 2010). The program should include stretching exercises to maintain chest wall mobility and, in the presence of pulmonary hypertension, interval exercises. Prescribed rest times are essential to decrease the strain on the right ventricle. The rehabilitation prescription should also include aerobic training, functional muscle strength and endurance training. These patients typically require high levels of supplemental oxygen to prevent severe hypoxia so the rehabilitation clinician will need to work closely with the pulmonologist and respiratory therapist to prescribe the proper supplemental oxygen delivery systems and oxygen prescriptions. The disease progression is generally aggressive, so work simplification training is also valuable and the program should be focused on maintaining functional mobility.

The prognosis is generally poor for patients with pulmonary fibrosis because of refractory hypoxemia, right heart failure and the increased risk of bronchogenic carcinoma in patients who smoke and those with occupational exposure pulmonary fibrosis. In ARDS, the mortality rate is as high as 60%, but has been decreasing to 22–35%, with a higher death rate in older patients (Matthay et al., 2012). In general, the mean survival time in cases of pulmonary fibrosis is 2–5 years but this will vary based on the aggressiveness and type of disease, duration of symptoms and response to therapy (Harari & Caminati, 2010; Noble et al., 2010).

PULMONARY HYPERTENSION

Secondary pulmonary hypertension can be the sequela of a congenital heart defect, collagen vascular disease, lung disease, COPD and pulmonary fibrosis, hypoxia, thromboembolic disease and left heart failure resulting from cardiomyopathy and valvular disease. As pulmonary disease progresses to the point where the pulmonary capillary bed becomes affected, pulmonary pressure begins to rise. Pulmonary hypertension can be defined as a mean pulmonary arterial pressure that is greater than 25 mmHg at rest and greater than 30 mmHg during exercise.

A significant amount of the lung parenchyma must be involved to cause pulmonary hypertension because the reserve capacity of the lungs is so vast. As the intrinsic obstructive lung disease progresses, the disruption of capillary beds and destruction of the gas exchange area of the parenchymal tissue leads to hypoxia and vasoconstriction, producing pulmonary hypertension. Precapillary arteries and arterioles also become less distensible and constricted. With pulmonary fibrosis, for example in collagen vascular disease, the scarring of the airways and capillaries causes a decrease in compliance and arterial hypertension. The consequences of abnormal and chronic vasoconstriction include intimal proliferation, smooth muscle hypertrophy and changes in the endothelium that lead to a decrease in the diameter of the arterial lumen and vascular remodeling. With end-stage heart disease there is an increased production of endothelin1 and thromboxane A2 and reduction in nitric oxide leading to smooth muscle cell

hypertrophy and hyperplasia. These changes, along with venous congestion, lead to elevation in pulmonary arterial pressures (Mikus et al., 2011; Akgun et al., 2012).

If the pulmonary pressure is not relieved, the pulmonary vascular system becomes less distensible and blood is shunted to the larger vessels, which causes a ventilation–perfusion mismatch. To compensate for the elevated pulmonary vascular resistance and to maintain cardiac output, the right ventricle hypertrophies. Over time, the myocardium dilates and is unable to maintain efficient blood flow through the lungs for gas exchange, leading to heart failure (Mikus et al., 2011).

Clinical Manifestation

The progression of dyspnea and the early onset of fatigue are typically the first symptoms of pulmonary hypertension, although many patients associate this with aging and deconditioning. Patients may begin to complain of presyncopal symptoms or may experience syncope. Chest pain, muscle fatigue, hypoxemia and hemoptysis are other common symptoms related to pulmonary hypertension. As the patient develops cor pulmonale, the signs and symptoms of right heart failure become present, which include jugular vein distension, peripheral edema and hepatic congestion. (See Chapter 42 for descriptions of the signs and symptoms of heart failure.)

Upon examination, the right ventricle may be palpable in the lower left sternal or subxiphoid area and abnormal heart sounds are present, including S4 gallop and a split S2 sound. As the disease progresses, S3 gallop can be heard, indicating advanced right heart failure. Abnormal valvular heart sounds may also be audible, including a systolic ejection click and tricuspid murmur. The electrocardiogram (ECG) is consistent with right ventricular hypertrophy and changes in the T wave. As the disease progresses, there will be clear signs of right heart failure, in most cases including jugular vein distension, hepatic congestion, peripheral edema, ascites and systemic hypotension (Higenbottam, 2005).

Therapeutic Intervention

The treatment of pulmonary hypertension involves treating the primary cause of it. Drugs to decrease strain on the right side of the heart, such as digitalis and diuretics, and supplemental oxygen therapy to treat the hypoxemia may be effective. Continuous intravenous prostacyclins, for example Flolan and Iloprost, may decrease pulmonary hypertension by vasodilatation when infused into the pulmonary arterial system. The most common positive effects of the intravenous use of prostacyclins are an improvement in exercise tolerance and a decrease in symptoms experienced at rest and with exertion. Endothelin receptor antagonists, such as bosentan, reverse the effects of endothelin, and sildenafil (Viagra) and tadalafil (Cialis) are vasodilators also used in the management of pulmonary hypertension. Anticoagulation medications may be used to decrease the risk of thromboembolic events because of polycythemia, which may develop as a compensatory mechanism to offset hypoxemia. In the case of heart failure, ventricular assist devices may be used to manage, and in some cases reverse, the levels of pulmonary hypertension (Mikus et al., 2011).

Rehabilitation for patients with pulmonary hypertension typically focuses on functional mobility. It is also important to review job simplification and energy conservation in these patients. Patients typically tolerate an interval aerobic program, particularly a walking program. Exercises that isolate muscle groups, such as cycling, are usually less well tolerated because of local muscle fatigue. It is important that the therapist prescribe an exercise intensity that is sufficient for the patient to experience the benefits of exercise without causing abnormal responses to exertion. These patients should be monitored closely for signs of chest discomfort, lightheadedness or excessive fatigue. The therapist should also educate the patient about the adverse signs and symptoms that indicate distress and progression of the disease. It is also vital that the therapist works directly with the physician to establish safe parameters for functional mobility activities (see Box 39.4 and Tables 39.4–39.7 for guidelines).

PULMONARY EMBOLISM

Pulmonary embolism is closely linked to the presence of blood clots or thrombi in the peripheral venous system, known as deep vein thrombosis (DVT). Pulmonary embolism is the third leading cause of cardiovascular deaths and has a 10 per 1000 cases incidence in older adults versus 1 per 1000 cases in young adults (Geersing et al., 2012). Typically, the source of the embolism originates from a DVT in the upper legs or pelvis. Small emboli may present little compromise to a healthy individual but may cause severe respiratory failure in an older individual with a reduced reserve of the cardiopulmonary systems. In the elderly, there are several risk factors that should be part of the clinician's screening process, including previous DVT or pulmonary embolism, surgery, malignancy, hormonal therapy, obesity, venous stasis, immobility, cerebrovascular accident (CVA), recent trauma and heart failure (Geersing et al., 2012; McLenon, 2012). In the older adult PE are underdiagnosed, with up to 40% of PE found at autopsy in older adults (Geersing et al., 2012).

Clinical Manifestation

The most pronounced clinical presentation in cases of pulmonary embolism includes unexplained dyspnea of rapid onset, pleuritic chest pain and hypotension with no obvious cause. The presence of hemoptysis indicates pulmonary hemorrhage or infarction (McLenon, 2012).

During evaluation, it is important to develop a differential diagnostic list and proceed with testing to enable a clinical diagnosis to be formulated. The differential diagnosis may include the following conditions: acute myocardial infarction (MI), asthma, pneumothorax, congestive heart failure (CHF), acute pulmonary edema, pleurisy, pericarditis, musculoskeletal trauma to the chest wall, sepsis, tamponade and aortic dissection. Risk factors associated with PE and prognosis include age > 80, male gender, history of cancer, heart failure, chronic lung disease, previous DVT or PE, renal or liver disease, recent trauma or surgery (Geersing et al., 2012).

Upon physical examination there may be a low-grade fever, cyanosis, tachycardia, jugular vein distension, tachypnea and hypotension. Upon auscultation, there may be a pleural rub and a split of the S2 heart sound may be heard over the pulmonic valve. The degree of respiratory compromise is dependent on the size of the pulmonary embolism and the preexisting cardiopulmonary reserves. An echocardiogram may be suggestive of right heart strain or ischemia and the ECG may demonstrate T-wave inversion.

Clinical Intervention

The key to appropriate medical care is the identification of patients who are at high risk and implementation of effective prophylactic treatment. Treatment includes prevention such as early mobilization and the use of graduated compression devices and TED stockings. The use of intermittent pneumatic compression stockings provides peripheral pumping to encourage venous return and reduce venous stasis. Many patients will be prescribed anticoagulants for the prevention and treatment of DVT formation. In patients who cannot take anticoagulants, an inferior vena cava filter may be placed to decrease the risk of a pulmonary embolism occurring from a lower extremity or pelvic thrombus. Thrombolytic therapy has also been used successfully to break down the DVT or pulmonary embolism, but is associated with a risk of hemorrhage (McLenon, 2012). Finally, pulmonary endarterectomy has become a viable surgical option to remove the emboli from the pulmonary artery or arteries. It is performed through a sternotomy and can be complicated by persistent hypoxia and prolonged mechanical ventilation as well as management of heart failure.

The prognosis for a patient suffering from a pulmonary embolism is dependent upon the size of the pulmonary embolism, the underlying compromise of the cardiopulmonary system and the promptness of medical care. Mortality rate for PE has been reported to be as high as 30% if untreated and 80% of unexplained hospital deaths were related to undiagnosed PE. There is a 10% 1-year mortality for individuals in the first year after diagnosis of PE. Mortality can be as high as 40% within 5 years in individuals who stopped anticoagulation therapy (Geersing et al., 2012; Ouellette & Mosenifar, 2013).

PULMONARY INFECTIONS

PNEUMONIA

The pulmonary system has two primary mechanisms to manage the presence of foreign matter that may precipitate a pulmonary infection. The upper airway warms and humidifies the air and the mucociliary cells aid in the entrapment of particles in this conductive system of the lungs. If particles enter the lung, there is an immune response that attacks the foreign material and removes it. When one or both of these mechanisms is impaired, there is an increased risk of developing a pneumonia, which is defined as an acute inflammation of the lungs, causing the small bronchioles and alveoli to become plugged with fibrous exudate.

Pneumonias can be classified based on several parameters: (i) by the etiology underlying the infection, including bacterial, viral and fungal sources; (ii) as typical or atypical, based on the incidence of the infection in a given population or location; and (iii) by the site in which the infection occurs, with acquired pneumonias referring to infections obtained in the community and nosocomial pneumonias defined as infections that occur during the hospitalization of the patient. With the increase in admissions to such facilities as long-term care or nursing homes, acquired infections may be subdivided into community-acquired and institutionally-acquired pneumonia. However the infection is classified, there are common risk factors that contribute to the susceptibility of developing pulmonary infections (see Box 45.1) Acquired pneumonias account for 650000 annual hospital admissions and has a prevalence of 14 out of 1000 cases. This number is doubled for nursing home residents where aspiration-related pneumonias have a 2–4 times incident rate (Akgun et al., 2012).

When a pathogen enters the respiratory system and is able to multiply and overwhelm the preventive function of the immune system, an infection begins and the inflammatory process is activated along with a further response from the immune system. This vicious cycle continues, leading to the progression of edema and the aggregation of red and white blood cells, which begins to interfere with the ability of the lungs to ventilate and participate in diffusion.

Clinical Manifestation

The typical clinical presentation for pneumonia includes fever and a productive cough with sputum that is usually yellowish-green or a rust color. In most cases there is also an elevation in the white blood cell count and a positive sputum culture identifying the infectious agent. The patient may report an increased level of fatigue and weight loss. If a substantial amount of lung tissue is involved, the patient may also present with dyspnea, tachycardia and tachypnea, and hypoxemia with desaturation upon exertion. The elderly patient may present with atypical signs and symptoms, including delirium, failure to thrive, malaise and increased risk of falls. The clinician also needs to closely monitor vital signs and assess for changes over time, be aware of decreased appetite,

increased incidence of incontinence and decreased functional mobility and activity tolerance (Akgun et al., 2012).

The diagnosis of pneumonia is based on a series of clinical findings, including a positive chest radiograph showing infiltration or consolidation of the infected segment along with clinical symptoms. The clinician should also be aware of the patient's oral motor control. In patients with poor motor control (such as hypotonic state of the musculature of the face and neck, poor phonation and difficulty with motor planning and execution), the clinician should have a heightened concern for aspiration pneumonia.

Clinical Intervention

The primary focus of care should be prevention, which includes proper cleaning of rooms and equipment and compliance with good hand washing. Emphasis should be placed on mobilizing patients to decrease the incidence of atelectasis and muscle atrophy. In patients who cannot participate in some form of exercise or mobilization, methods to increase the minute ventilation, a program of assisted repositioning and assisted breathing and coughing techniques should be employed. Proper seating should be achieved to minimize aspiration. Good dental hygiene is important and all high-risk patients should receive an annual flu vaccine.

Once the diagnosis of pneumonia has been made, treatment should include the administration of the correct medications based on the suspected pathogen. Typically, the patient is placed on a wide-spectrum antibiotic. If the signs and symptoms do not resolve or become recurrent, a sputum culture should be tested. Airway clearance techniques, such as traditional or modified chest physical therapy or other techniques to promote the mobilization of sputum, increase lung volumes and assist in effective cough should be implemented. Mobilizing the patient is also vital to increase ventilation and diffusion of the lungs, and to promote increases in minute ventilation.

Prognosis is dependent upon many factors, including age and the presence of other comorbidities such as smoking, COPD, diabetes mellitus, heart failure and decreased mental status. The need for mechanical ventilation only increases mortality rates. The pathogen's sensitivity to medication will affect the outcome, including the patient's level of function (Akgun et al., 2012).

TUBERCULOSIS

With the increase in the number of patients who are living with an impaired immune system because of human immunodeficiency virus (HIV) infection and acquired immunodeficiency syndrome (AIDS), transplantation, a general increase in life expectancy, substance abuse and homelessness with malnutrition, infection with *Mycobacterium tuberculosis* is on the rise. In 2011 there were a reported 8.7 million cases of tuberculosis worldwide and 1.4 million deaths (Zumla et al., 2013).

As a primary infection, tuberculosis is an airborne-acquired infection of the lungs. It is spread when a person has sufficient exposure to an infected individual and is commonly transmitted through coughing or sneezing. The risk of infection is dependent on exposure, concentration of the mycobacterium and the health of the immune system. The incubation period is 2–12 weeks. The disease can be reactivated or a secondary infection can occur when the patient's immune system is further compromised because of illness or aging. The site of infection can be the lungs or elsewhere in the body (Zevallos & Justman, 2003).

Clinical Manifestation

During the primary infection, most patients are asymptomatic. If there are signs and symptoms, they are similar to the clinical presentation of pneumonia, with a nonproductive cough and fever. Lymph nodes are enlarged and the patient may experience chest wall or pleuritic pain if the pleural lining is involved. Rales may be heard in the area of infection over the infected segments of the lungs, along with bronchial breath sounds if there is consolidation. Radiographs are abnormal, showing atelectasis and usually cavitations in the upper lobes. There is scarring of the lungs, with a loss of tissue function.

Secondary infections are associated with a cough that becomes increasingly productive as the disease progresses, night sweats, weight loss, low-grade fever and sometimes pleuritic pain. There are subtle inspiratory rales, a decrease in tactile fremitus and breath sounds over areas of pleural thickening and cavitation. The signs and symptoms of extrapulmonary disease are dependent upon the particular tissue that is infected (Zumla et al., 2013).

Clinical Intervention

The best intervention is again prevention, including the use of universal precautions, general healthcare for high-risk groups and screening. If a skin test is positive, individuals should undergo a year of treatment to minimize the risk of a secondary infection. During the primary infection, respiratory isolation is important to minimize the spread of the disease and clinicians should comply with the use of personal protective equipment. Patients are usually given rifampin and isoniazid for 1 year to suppress the infection. Further medical or surgical intervention will depend on the site and severity of the extrapulmonary infections. It is important that treatment of tuberculosis be effective since undertreatment leads to drug-resistant disease, reported present in some 300000 individuals, which increases health risk and cost (van der Werf et al., 2012; Zumla et al., 2013).

PULMONARY ONCOLOGY

Lung cancer is a leading cause of cancer-related deaths in the United States of America despite the advances in diagnostic and medical therapies. As part of the medical workup, it is important to obtain an accurate history of tobacco use and occupational exposures that increase the risk of developing lung cancer. The incidence of lung cancer increases with age with mean diagnosis at the age of 70, and over 50% of cases present to the medical system already with metastatic disease (Akgun et al., 2012).

Lung carcinomas are divided into small cell and non-small cell cancers. Small cell carcinomas are linked to smoking and there is a high incidence of metastasis at the time of diagnosis, either to bone or the brain. The non-small cell carcinomas include squamous cell cancer, adenocarcinoma and large cell cancer. Non-small cell cancer

constitutes 85% of lung cancer diagnoses. The lung can be the primary site of the cancer or secondary to metastatic cancer from another site, such as breast or colorectal cancer (Akgun et al., 2012).

Clinical Manifestation

In many instances, the diagnosis of lung cancer is made during routine testing for another elective procedure. In other cases, the patient may seek medical attention because of a persistent cough, hoarseness, hemoptysis, dull ache in the thorax, fatigue and progressive shortness of breath (Akgun et al., 2012). A thorough interview may reveal sleep disturbances, night sweats and unintentional weight loss. Diagnosis is made by abnormal findings on radiographic studies and is confirmed with a biopsy.

Clinical Intervention

As for many of the diseases briefly discussed in this chapter, prevention is the first line of treatment. Smoking cessation and decreasing exposure to chemicals and particles are vital. Routine medical screening, such as mammograms and colonoscopies, has had a huge impact on the early detection and treatment of cancer in general. Medical management may include radiation, chemotherapy or surgical resection. The treatment that is offered to the patient will depend on the type and staging of the tumor. Prognosis is improving but, once again, is dependent on the type of cancer, time of detection and responsiveness to medical therapies. Therapy may involve a spectrum of care, including general strength and conditioning, pain management, functional mobility restoration after surgery and end-of-life issues. Lung cancer deaths account for more cancer-related deaths than breast, prostate and colon cancer combined. Eight percent of all lung cancer deaths are of individuals over 65 years of age (Akgun et al., 2012).

CONCLUSION

This chapter briefly discussed the three major categories of intrinsic lung disease that can impair activity tolerance and diminish quality of life. Clinically, these diseases present with a constellation of signs and symptoms that facilitate diagnosis and management. In the elderly, emphysema is so prevalent after the fifth decade of life that it is important for the therapist to be very familiar with the clinical characteristics of both emphysema and chronic bronchitis, and the management of obstructive lung disease. Rehabilitation involving education, strengthening and aerobic exercise is an effective intervention for patients with obstructive disease. The therapist should also be able to modify the rehabilitation process for patients with pulmonary fibrosis and pulmonary hypertension. The ultimate goal of a comprehensive plan of care is to improve functional mobility and quality of life.

REFERENCES

Abbatecola AM, Fumagalli A, Bonardi D et al 2011 Practical management problems of chronic obstructive pulmonary disease in the elderly: acute exacerbations. Curr Opin Pulmon Med 17(suppl1):S49–S54

Akgun KM, Crothers K, Pisani M 2012 Epidemiology and management of common pulmonary diseases in older persons. J Gerontol A Biol Sci Med Sci 67A(3):276–291

American Lung Association 2010 State of lung disease in diverse communities. [Online] Available at: www.lung.org/assets/documents/publications/solddc-chapters/copd.pdf. Accessed December 2013

Barnes TA, Fromer L 2011 Spirometry use: detection of chronic obstructive pulmonary disease in the primary care setting. Clin Intervent Aging 6:47–52

Burtin C, Decramer M, Gosselink R et al 2011 Rehabilitation and acute exacerbations. Eur Respir J 38:702–712

Geersing GJ, Oudega R, Hoes AW et al 2012 Managing pulmonary embolism using prognostic models: future concepts for primary care. Can Med Assoc J 184(3):305–311

Harari S, Caminati A 2010 Update on diffuse parenchymal lung disease. Eur Respir Rev 116(19):97–108

Higenbottam T 2005 Pulmonary hypertension and chronic obstructive pulmonary disease. Proc Am Thorac Soc 2:12–19

Hogg J 2004 Pathophysiology of airflow limitation in chronic obstructive pulmonary disease. Lancet 364:709–721

Jen R, Rennard SI, Sin DD 2012 Effects of inhaled corticosteroids on airway inflammation in chronic obstructive pulmonary disease: a systematic review and meta-analysis. Int J COPD 7:587–595

McLenon M 2012 Acute pulmonary embolism. Crit Care Nurs Q 35(2):173–182

Mann A, Early GL 2012 Adult respiratory distress syndrome. Missouri Med 109(5):371–375

Markovitz GH, Cooper CB 2010 Review series: rehabilitation in non COPD: mechanisms of exercise limitation and pulmonary rehabilitation for patients with pulmonary fibrosis/restrictive lung disease. Chron Respir Dis 7:47–62

Matthay MA, Ware LB, Zimmerman GA 2012 Acute respiratory distress syndrome. J Clin Invest 122(8):2731–2741

Messer B, Griffiths J, Baudouin SV 2012 The prognostic variables predictive of mortality in patients with an exacerbation of COPD admitted to the ICU: an integrative review. Q J Med 105:115–126

Mikus E, Stepanenko A, Krabatsch T et al 2011 Reversibility of fixed pulmonary hypertension in left ventricular assist device support recipients. Eur J Cardiothorac Surg 40:971–977

Nagarajan K, Bennett A, Agostini P et al 2011 Is preoperative physiotherapy/pulmonary rehabilitation beneficial in lung resection patients? Interact Cardiovasc Thorac Surg 13:300–302

Nathan S, Edwards L, Barnett S et al 2004 Outcomes of COPD lung transplant recipients after lung volume reduction surgery. Chest 126(5):1569–1574

Noble PW, Barkauskas CE, Jiang D 2010 Pulmonary fibrosis: patterns and perpetrators. J Clin Invest 122(8):2756–2763

Ouellette DR, Mosenifar Z 2013 Pulmonary embolism. [Online] Available at: http://emedicine.medscape.com/article/300901-overview. Accessed December 2013

Provinciali M, Cardelli M, Marchegiani F 2011 Inflammation, chronic obstructive pulmonary disease and aging. Curr Opin Pulmon Med 17(suppl):S3–S10

Rycroft CE, Heyes A, Lanza L et al 2012 Epidemiology of chronic obstructive pulmonary disease: a literature review. Int J COPD 7:457–494

Schmidt SL, Flaherty KR 2011 Clinical year in review I: interstitial lung disease, occupational and environmental lung disease, education of residents and fellows and pediatrics. Proc Am Thorac Soc 8:389–397

Shavelle RM, Paculdo DR, Kush SJ et al 2009 Life expectancy and years of life lost in chronic obstructive pulmonary disease: findings from the NHANES III follow-up study. Int J COPD 4:137–148

Valente S, Pascuito G, Bernabei R et al 2010 Do we need different treatments for very elderly COPD patients? Respiration 80:357–368

van der Werf MJ, Langendam MW, Huitric E et al 2012 Multidrug resistance after inappropriate tuberculosis treatment: a meta-analysis. Eur Respir J 39:1511–1519

Vorrink SNW, Kort HSM, Troosters T et al 2011 Level of daily physical activity in individuals with COPD compared with healthy controls. Respir Res 12:33–42

Wynn TA 2011 Integrating mechanisms of pulmonary fibrosis. J Exper Med 208(7):1339–1350

York NL, Kane C 2012 Trends in caring for adult respiratory distress syndrome patients. Dimensions Crit Care Nurs 31(3):153–158

Zevallos M, Justman J 2003 Tuberculosis in the elderly. Clin Geriatr Med 19:121–138

Zumla A, Raviglione M, Hafner R et al 2013 Tuberculosis. N Engl J Med 368:745–755

Blood vessel changes, circulatory and skin disorders

UNIT CONTENTS

Chapter 46

Diabetes

BARBARA J. EHRMANN

CHAPTER CONTENTS

INTRODUCTION

Diabetes mellitus is a prevalent disease, especially among the elderly. In the last 15 years alone, the prevalence of diagnosed diabetes cases has increased by 82%, mostly because of the increase in obesity. Age-related changes involving decreased insulin sensitivity in the peripheral tissues and reduced insulin control of hepatic glucose output, coupled with physical inactivity and increased obesity, contribute to higher incidences of abnormal glucose tolerance in the older population.

It is estimated that the prevalence of diabetes for all age groups worldwide was 8.3% in 2011 and will be 9.9% in 2030. The International Diabetes Federation (2013) reports the total number of people with diabetes in 2013 to be 382 million and has estimated that this number will rise to 582 million in 2035. The increasing proportion of individuals who are older than 65 years of age is an important demographic influence.

Diabetes is more prevalent in certain populations, for example Native American/Native Alaskans, Hispanic/ Latino Americans and African Americans. Approximately 25.8 million people in the United States of America, or 8.3% of the total US population, have diabetes mellitus. Of those aged 65 or above, 10.9 million, or 26.9%, have diabetes. It is estimated that one-third of these individuals are unaware of their disease. Further, it is estimated that 79 million adults have impaired glucose tolerance (IGT), or prediabetes, a condition that often precedes diabetes mellitus. Diabetes mellitus is a serious disease that causes a wide range of complications. In 2007 the total cost of diabetes in the US was $174 billion, $40 billion of which resulted from indirect costs because of disability, work loss or premature mortality (National Diabetes Fact Sheet, 2011).

CLASSIFICATION AND DIAGNOSIS OF DIABETES MELLITUS

Diabetes mellitus is characterized by hyperglycemia. There are four clinical classes of diabetes including type 1, type 2, other specific types of diabetes (genetic defects in ß-cell function or insulin action, disease of exocrine pancreas, drug- or chemically induced diabetes) and gestational diabetes mellitus (GDM). For the purposes of this chapter, discussion will focus on type 1 and type 2 diabetes (see Table 46.1).

In 2009, the American Diabetes Association (ADA) modified the diagnostic criteria for the classification of impaired fasting glucose (IFG) to include both fasting glucose and hemoglobin A_{1c} (A_{1c}) levels. A_{1c} or glycosylated hemoglobin is a measure of blood sugar control which measures a person's average glucose level over the previous 2–3 months. This shows the amount of glucose that is attached to the red blood cells, which is proportional to the amount of glucose in the blood.

There are three ways to diagnose diabetes, each of which must be confirmed on a subsequent day unless there are definitive symptoms of hyperglycemia, such as excess thirst and urination (polydipsia and polyuria), and unexplained weight loss accompanied by increased or normal food intake. The criteria for the diagnosis of diabetes include the following: (i) fasting plasma glucose (FPG) of greater than 126 mg/dl (fasting is defined as no caloric intake for at least 8 hours); (ii) 200 mg/dl or higher on an oral glucose tolerance test (OGTT) with 75 g of glucose; (iii) A_{1c} of 6.5% higher (used for diagnosis of type 2 diabetes only). FPG is the preferred test for diagnosing diabetes in nonpregnant adults. Other common presenting symptoms of diabetes include poor wound healing, fatigue, vaginal yeast infections and blurred vision (American Diabetes Association, 2013a).

Table 46.1 **Comparison of type 1 and type 2 diabetes**		
	Type 1 Diabetes	**Type 2 Diabetes**
No. of diabetics (%)	2–5	90–95
Onset of disease	Abrupt	Insidious
Age of onset	Less than 35 years	Greater than 35 years
Symptoms at onset	Often ketoacidosis	May be asymptomatic
Requiring insulin	Yes	In 25% of cases
Risk for ketoacidosis	Yes	Rare
Body type	Thin or normal	80% are overweight
Suspected cause	Autoimmune reaction with islet cell destruction	Insulin resistance/poor insulin secretion
Genetic predisposition	Yes	Yes

Hyperglycemia that is not sufficient to meet the diagnostic criteria for diabetes is categorized as IFG, IGT or prediabetes. IFG is defined as a FPG between 100 mg/dl and 125 mg/dl. IGT is defined as an OGTT between 140 mg/dl and 199 mg/dl. Prediabetes, type 2, is also diagnosed with an A_{1c} between 5.7 and 6.4% (American Diabetes Association, 2013a).

TYPES OF DIABETES MELLITUS

TYPE 1

Type 1 diabetes is caused by autoimmune destruction of the insulin-producing ß-cells of the pancreatic islets, resulting in insulin deficiency. As a result, these patients have an absolute need for insulin therapy. The age of onset of type 1 diabetes is most commonly during childhood or young adulthood, although it can begin at any age. In the absence of insulin replacement, patients with type 1 diabetes develop severe hyperglycemia and metabolic acidosis, which results from the excess production of ketones, by-products of fat breakdown in the absence of insulin. Diabetic ketoacidosis (DKA) is a medical emergency.

TYPE 2

Of all individuals with diabetes, 90–95% have type 2 diabetes. This has historically been a disease of adults, with its incidence increasing with each decade of aging. However, type 2 diabetes is increasingly being diagnosed in children and adolescents. Type 2 diabetes is associated with obesity, a family history of diabetes, a previous history of gestational diabetes, IGT and physical inactivity. Other factors associated with type 2 diabetes are race/ethnicity, with African Americans, Hispanic/Latino Americans, Native Americans and some Asian Americans and other Pacific Islanders being at particularly high risk. Type 2 diabetes is regarded as being a metabolic disorder that is linked to a modern lifestyle involving stress, excess caloric intake (particularly fat) and inadequate physical activity. From a metabolic perspective, these patients generally have the twin defects of sluggish secretion of insulin following meals (leading to poor overall insulin production with long duration) and peripheral insulin resistance (reduced cellular uptake and utilization of insulin).

METABOLIC SYNDROME

An elevated fasting glucose is one of several risk factors that is known to increase an individual's risk of developing heart disease, stroke and diabetes. These risk factors, grouped together, are called the 'metabolic syndrome'. Other characteristics include obesity, particularly abdominal fat, hyperlipidemia and hypertension. The criteria for metabolic syndrome are met by having any three of the following risk factors, as recently defined by the American Heart Association and International Diabetes Federation: (i) an elevated waist circumference (abdominal obesity); (ii) an elevated triglyceride level of 150 mg/dl or greater; (iii) a reduced high-density lipoprotein (HDL – 'good cholesterol') level of less than 40 mg/dl for men and less than 50 mg/dl for women; (iv) an elevated blood pressure of 130/85 mmHg or higher; and (v) an elevated fasting glucose of 100 mg/dl or higher (Alberti et al., 2009). Fifty-two percent of males and 54% of females in the US over the age of 60 met the criteria for metabolic syndrome for the years 2003–2006 (Ervin, 2009).

THERAPEUTIC INTERVENTION

NEWLY DIAGNOSED DIABETES

Patients newly diagnosed with diabetes mellitus have a special need for comprehensive education. Diabetes self-management education is an integral component of medical care. The onset of diabetes can be precipitated by physical and emotional stress and other illnesses and, usually, the diabetic state persists. In addition, certain medications, most notably oral or parenteral steroid therapy, can trigger the onset of diabetes mellitus or upset metabolic control in a previously diagnosed patient.

MEDICAL TREATMENT

Diet and exercise are the cornerstones of the treatment of type 2 diabetes mellitus and many individuals with diabetes can control their blood glucose by following a careful diet and exercise program, losing excess weight and taking oral hypoglycemic agents (medications that lower plasma glucose levels). A meta-analysis of 27 studies found reductions in A_{1c} with aerobic and/or resistance training (Snowling & Hopkins, 2006). Generally, it is not necessary to increase food intake before exercise of short duration or low intensity. Exercise of moderate intensity may be preceded by consuming 10–15 g of carbohydrate, although this is often unnecessary.

Among adults with diagnosed diabetes, about 14% take both insulin and oral medications, 12% take insulin only, 58% take oral medications only and 16% take neither insulin nor oral medications (American Diabetes Association, 2013b).

Glycemic control in patients with type 1 and 2 diabetes is most often measured using levels of blood glycosylated hemoglobin, or hemoglobin A_{1c} (A_{1c}), in addition to self-monitoring of blood glucose. The A_{1c} level reflects the mean blood glucose concentration over the previous 6–12 weeks. The ADA's current glycemic goal for nonpregnant adults is a value of less than 7.0% (compared with a normal nondiabetic range of 4–6%).

The ADA recommends that blood pressure in patients with diabetes should be less than 140/80 mmHg. Lipid goals for patients with diabetes include a low-density lipoprotein (LDL) level of less than 100 mg/dl, triglyceride level less than 150 mg/dl and HDL level greater than 50 mg/dl (<1.1 mmol/l) (American Diabetes Association, 2013b).

INSULIN THERAPY FOR TYPE 1 DIABETES

Therapy for individuals with type 1 diabetes always includes insulin. Insulin is given by subcutaneous injection or with an insulin pump, which also delivers insulin subcutaneously. Combinations of rapid-, short-, intermediate- or long-acting insulin are used, such as Humalog, Regular, NPH and glargine respectively. In most centers, patients with type 1 diabetes are treated with two or three doses per day of rapid- or short-acting insulin combined with intermediate-acting insulin. Cross-sectional studies have not documented improved control with an increasing number of insulin injections per day, showing that the number of injections alone is not sufficient to achieve optimal glycemic control. The method of using long-acting insulin (glargine) combined with rapid-acting insulin (Humalog), given before meals and snacks, provides greater flexibility but requires a knowledge of carbohydrate counting and the use of an insulin–carbohydrate ratio. Because blood glucose can fluctuate widely in patients with type 1 diabetes, it is recommended that blood glucose be monitored several times a day, before meals and at bedtime, and insulin doses adjusted accordingly.

TREATMENT OF TYPE 2 DIABETES

Oral treatment options for patients with type 2 diabetes are diverse. Control can be achieved with diet and exercise therapy, especially if weight loss is achieved in an overweight patient. However, most type 2 patients also require some pharmacological treatment, either oral hypoglycemic medication or insulin. Oral medications include the sulfonylureas (e.g. glyburide, glipizide, chlorpropamide) and meglitinides, which increase insulin release; thiazolidinediones (rosiglitazone, pioglitazone) and biguanides (metformin), which increase target tissue sensitivity to insulin and reduce glucose production in the liver; acarbose, which slows down the absorption of carbohydrate through the intestine; and prandial glucose regulators (repaglinide), which are taken with meals and help to increase insulin release. These medications can be used alone or in combination.

Another injectable drug can be used to treat type 2 diabetes. Exenatide is a new class of drug known as an incretin memetic. Incretins, such as glucagon-like peptide (GLP-1), are produced in the small intestine and released in response to meals. GLP-1 stimulates insulin secretion and suppresses glucagon release. Exenatide is used in type 2 diabetics to increase insulin secretion when oral medications are not enough.

The United Kingdom Prospective Diabetes Study (UKPDS) showed that good glycemic control in patients with type 2 diabetes results in a reduction in the risk of microvascular disease (UKPDS, 1998). Specifically, a 1% fall in A_{1c} was associated with a 35% reduction in microvascular complications (retinopathy, nephropathy and neuropathy). Based on the results of the UKPDS, normoglycemia is now the goal for most patients with type 2 diabetes. Although insulin may be considered for initial therapy in type 2 diabetes, especially if the patient presents with a very elevated A_{1c} level, it is most often used when hyperglycemia persists despite the use of oral hypoglycemic agents.

HYPOGLYCEMIA

The main adverse effect of insulin or oral therapy is hypoglycemia (low blood glucose). In a patient with diabetes, symptoms of hypoglycemia generally have a rapid onset and occur when blood glucose is less than 70–80 mg/dl (Table 46.2). A severe reaction can occur below 60 mg/dl. A patient may complain of shakiness and sweating or other symptoms caused by increased epinephrine (adrenaline) release, such as tachycardia and anxiety. Deprivation of glucose in the central nervous system causes blurred vision, weakness, confusion, slurred speech and, potentially, seizure and coma, with permanent neurological damage. Symptoms of hypoglycemia may be blunted in a patient with long-standing diabetes, especially the early warning signs of nervousness, tremor and sweating. The initial symptom in patients with long-standing diabetes mellitus may be confusion.

In a diabetic patient, hypoglycemia occurs because of too much insulin (or oral medications), insufficient food intake (relative to insulin or medication dose) or increased physical activity (again, relative to insulin dose). Treatment of hypoglycemia must be prompt. Mild hypoglycemia can usually be quickly reversed by ingesting something containing sugar. Handy sources of

Table 46.2	**Comparison of diabetic complications**		
	Hyperglycemia with Diabetic Ketoacidosis (DKA)	**Hyperglycemia, Hyperosmolarity, Nonketosis, Coma**	**Hypoglycemia**
Precipitating factors	Absence of insulin	Illness, infections, steroid use, burns	Excessive exogenous insulin, decreased oral intake, stress
Onset	Gradual	Gradual	Abrupt
Initial effect	Lethargy	Lethargy	Agitation, shakiness
Skin	Hot, dry	Warm	Clammy, diaphoretic
Serum glucose levels	>300 mg/dl	>300 mg/dl	<70 mg/dl
Hydration	Increased thirst, polyuria, dehydration	Rapid volume depletion with increased thirst; initial polyuria progressing to decreased urine output	Unchanged
Cardiopulmonary symptoms	Rapid deep breathing		Tachycardia
Early CNS symptoms	Headache		Headache, blurred vision, slurred speech
Late CNS symptoms	Confusion, coma, death	Confusion, coma, death	Confusion, coma, (rarely) death
Metabolic acidosis	Elevated serum acetone and ketone bodies in urine, fruity breath	No	No
GI symptoms	Abdominal pain	Abdominal pain	Hunger
Intervention required	Insulin, fluid and sodium bicarbonate replacement	Insulin, fluid and electrolyte replacement	4 oz (120 ml) juice, half a nondiet soda, two glucose tablets or two to four hard candies

CNS, central nervous system; GI, gastrointestinal

sugar include 4 oz (120 ml) of orange juice, half a non-diet soda, a few hard candies, two glucose tablets or two single-spoon-size packets of sugar. Patients with a hypoglycemic episode should monitor their blood sugars carefully in the hours following the episode. Severe hypoglycemic reactions can require intravenous glucose or an intramuscular glucagon injection. These are also necessary if the patient is obtunded and cannot safely be given oral glucose because of the risk of aspiration. A therapist who has treated a patient for a severe hypoglycemic reaction should always notify the physician. Hypoglycemia caused by sulfonylureas can be prolonged and has a higher risk of mortality than that caused by insulin. Patients can require short-term hospitalization.

EXERCISE AND DIABETES

Individuals without diabetes can maintain stable blood glucose levels during exercise. However, physical activity can have a marked effect on blood glucose in a person with diabetes. Exercise increases glucose use by muscles and improves muscle sensitivity to insulin. A regular program of exercise may lower the requirements for insulin or oral medication. These are desirable effects but it should be recognized that exercise can increase the risk of hypoglycemia. About 30 minutes of interval or continuous exercise can decrease blood glucose regardless of fitness level.

Glucose control does not always improve with exercise, so the effect must be evaluated for each patient. Patients should increase their blood glucose self-monitoring during exercise. This is especially important for patients on insulin or oral medications. At the beginning of an exercise program, particularly with type 1 diabetic patients, blood glucose levels should be checked before exercise, every 15–30 minutes during exercise and after stopping exercise. Blood glucose should continue to be checked frequently, as levels can continue to fall for up to 24 hours after exercising. Blood glucose self-monitoring data can be used to assess a patient's response to physical activity and improve performance.

HYPERGLYCEMIA

In type 1 diabetes, exercising during insulin insufficiency can promote a hyperglycemic response and place the individual at risk for metabolic acidosis. Additional insulin may have to be administered and exercise deferred if the glucose level is higher than 250 mg/dl and ketones are present in the urine. Caution should be used if blood glucose is greater than 300 mg/dl and no ketosis is present. Patients with type 1 diabetes should ingest additional carbohydrate if glucose levels are below 100 mg/dl. With type 2 diabetes, the upper value for deferring exercise is higher (300 mg/dl) because ketosis is far less common and is unlikely to be provoked by

Table 46.3   Precautions to take during exercise if diabetic

Physical Feature	Precaution
Hypoglycemia	Exercise 45–60 minutes after eating; may need to increase dietary intake before and during exercise; keep sugar supplements handy; be aware of delayed onset (up to 24 hours)
Insulin levels	Exercise 1 hour after injections; monitor glucose levels carefully; avoid exercise during peak insulin activity; use caution when injecting insulin over an exercising muscle
Cardiovascular functioning	Be aware that vital signs may not be an accurate indicator of exercise tolerance; utilize perceived exertion scale and note dyspnea with exertion; do not exercise with resting claudication
Proliferative retinopathy	Avoid isometrics, Valsalva maneuvers, head-jarring
Autonomic nervous system dysfunction	Be alert to signs of cardiac denervation syndrome (heart rate unresponsive to activity level); orthostatic hypotension; inability to perceive presence of angina or myocardial infarction; poor heat compensation
End-stage renal disease	Stay hydrated
Peripheral neuropathy	Wear proper footwear; avoid repetitive stresses; monitor distal extremities closely

exercise. Occasionally, especially in elderly type 2 individuals, a medical crisis of severe hyperglycemia and cellular dehydration may develop, often in response to the physiological stress of infection, burns or illness. These individuals may progress to a hyperglycemic, hyperosmolar, nonketotic coma. Because of the absence of ketosis, the diagnosis may be overlooked and, in this population, treatment delay can easily result in mortality (see Table 46.2). Proper hydration during exercise is essential.

If exercise substantially lowers blood glucose, particularly if it drops into the range where hypoglycemia is a risk, then some of the following strategies should be considered. The most fundamental options are either to reduce insulin (or the oral medication dose) on exercise days or to take a supplemental snack before exercise (Table 46.3). One approach is to reduce the insulin dose by approximately 20%. The glucose response to exercise will provide additional information when making this decision. If weight loss is a goal, it is desirable to avoid supplemental caloric intake. It is also important to consider the timing of exercise with respect to the timing of insulin or oral medication administration and meals. Exercise should be done at least 1–2 hours after meals and vigorous exercise should be undertaken when insulin levels are near the lower range. This might be in the morning, before injection, or four or more hours after injection of regular insulin. Also, consideration should be given to the site of the insulin injection. Insulin injected over an exercising muscle is absorbed more quickly and this translates into more potent glucose-lowering effects. Because of this, if exercising within 30 minutes of injection, a patient should be advised to use the abdomen, not the arm or thigh, for the subcutaneous injection of insulin (Table 46.3). Exercise should include a standard warm-up and cool-down period, as in nondiabetic individuals.

It is common for a patient initially referred for rehabilitation to have a relatively low fitness level that requires a cautious and gradual introduction to exercise. Before increasing the usual patterns of physical activity or starting an exercise program, patients with diabetes should undergo a detailed medical evaluation and, if indicated, appropriate diagnostic studies such as an electrocardiography, graded exercise test or radionuclide stress testing. The presence of micro- and macrovascular complications should be screened for as some may be worsened by the exercise program. Identification of areas of concern will allow the formulation of an individualized exercise program that can minimize the patient's risk.

DIABETIC COMPLICATIONS

Diabetes is a systemic disorder and the function of every organ system in the body can be affected (Table 46.4). The following discussion emphasizes the diabetic complications that have particular relevance to rehabilitation (see Table 46.3).

Several recent trials, including the Diabetes Control and Complications Trial (DCCT) and the UKPDS, have shown that improved glycemic control in patients with type 1 and type 2 diabetes mellitus significantly reduces the risk of development, or slows the progression, of the microvascular complications of diabetes (retinopathy, nephropathy and neuropathy). The risk of microvascular complications is highest if the A_{1c} is above 12% but is also increased at all values above the non-diabetic range (DCCT, 2010).

The data on the effect of glycemic control on the development of macrovascular disease in patients with type 2 diabetes are less clear. However, a recent meta-analysis of 13 prospective cohort studies showed that, for every one percentage point increase in A_{1c}, the relative risk for any cardiovascular event is 1.18 (Selvin et al., 2004). Clinically, this means that patients with poor glycemic control, as reflected by elevated A_{1c} levels, have a higher risk of having a cardiovascular event than someone with better glycemic control.

CARDIOVASCULAR FUNCTIONING

In total, 60–70% of deaths among individuals with diabetes are due to heart disease or stroke (National

Table 46.4	**Diabetes timeline**		
Complication	**Incidence**	**Prevention**	**Screening**
Progression from IGT (prediabetes) to diabetes	40–50% of those with IGT will develop type 2 diabetes within 10 years	Lifestyle changes (diet, exercise, behavior modification), pharmacological intervention (metformin, acarbose, troglitazone)	Consider FPG or 2-hour OGTT in those <45 years with BMI >25 kg/m² and other risk factors and those ≥45 years. Repeat screen every 3 years
Nephropathy	Occurs in 20–40% of patients with diabetes; develops slowly over 15–25 years	Optimize blood glucose control (goal HbA$_{1c}$ of <7%); lower blood pressure	Annual test for microalbuminuria after ≥5 years' duration of type 1 diabetes and after diagnosis in type 2 diabetes using spot urine microalbumin–creatinine ratio. If found, treat with an ACE inhibitor or an ARB. May require protein restriction
Retinopathy	Occurs in 80% of type 1 diabetics after 15 years' duration; occurs in 10–20% at diagnosis with type 2 diabetes; and 60% develop after 20 years	Optimize blood glucose control (goal HbA$_{1c}$ of <7%); lower blood pressure	An initial dilated and comprehensive eye examination within 5 years of onset of type 1 diabetes and shortly after diagnosis in type 2 diabetes. Repeat examination annually
Neuropathy/delayed wound healing	Occurs in 60–70% of patients with diabetes; symptoms such as numbness and tingling occur 10–20 years after diabetes has been diagnosed; increased risk of foot ulcer or amputation in diabetes of ≥10 years' duration	Optimize blood glucose control (goal HbA$_{1c}$ of <7%)	Annual foot examination to identify high-risk foot conditions. Examination involves a Semmes–Weinstein 5.07 monofilament examination, tuning fork, palpation and visual examination
Cardiovascular disease	60–75% of diabetics die from cardiovascular causes: incidence of CVD is 2–3 times higher in diabetic men and 3–4 times higher in diabetic women, after adjusting for age and other risk factors	Optimize blood glucose control (goal HbA$_{1c}$ of <7%); lower blood pressure; treat dyslipidemia if present; with or without aspirin, and smoking cessation	Frequent blood pressure monitoring. Intervention with lifestyle modifications if BP >120/80 mmHg. If systolic pressure ≥140 mmHg or diastolic pressure ≥ 80 mmHg, should receive pharmacologic therapy along with lifestyle changes. Lipids should be checked at least annually (goal: LDL <100 mg/dl; TG <150 mg/dl; and HDL >50 mg/dl)

ACE, angiotensin-converting enzyme; ARB, angiotensin-receptor blocker; BMI, body mass index; CVD, cardiovascular disease; FPG, fasting plasma glucose; HbA$_{1c}$, hemoglobin A$_{1c}$; HDL, high-density lipoprotein; IGT, impaired glucose tolerance; LDL, low-density lipoprotein; OGTT, oral glucose tolerance test; TG, tryglycerides

Diabetes Fact Sheet, 2011). Diabetic patients who are at high risk for underlying cardiovascular disease include those above 35 years of age, those above 25 years of age with type 2 diabetes of more than 10 years' duration, those above 25 years of age with type 1 diabetes of more than 15 years' duration, those with additional risk factors for coronary disease and those with microvascular disease, peripheral vascular disease or autonomic neuropathy. Diabetic patients who are at high risk for underlying cardiovascular disease may need to undertake a graded exercise test if they are about to begin a moderate to high-intensity physical activity program. Patients who have nonspecific ECG changes in response to exercise, or who have nonspecific ST- and T-wave changes on the resting ECG, may require additional tests. Clinical judgment must be used when assessing the need for exercise stress testing in patients planning to participate in low intensity forms of physical activity such as walking (American Diabetes Association, 2004).

DELAYED WOUND HEALING

Delayed wound healing is a complication of diabetes that is related to poor metabolic control, arterial insufficiency, neuropathy and other factors. In total, 5–10% of diabetic patients have had past or have present foot ulceration. Individuals at greatest risk are men who have had diabetes for more than 10 years, who have poor glucose control or who have cardiovascular, retinal or renal complications. Diabetic foot ulcers are a principal cause of the high rate of lower extremity amputations in diabetics, which is 1–3 times higher than in nondiabetic individuals. Prevention of foot ulcers is the best therapy, and prevention starts with a careful foot and lower extremity examination along with an aggressive program of patient education. Patients must be taught to monitor closely for blisters and other potential damage to their feet, both before and after exercise. Proper footwear is important, especially for patients with peripheral neuropathy.

The use of silica gel or air midsoles, as well as polyester or blend socks to prevent blisters and keep feet dry, may minimize trauma to feet during exercise (Larsen et al., 2003; American Diabetes Association, 2013b).

NEUROPATHY

Neuropathy is found in approximately 60–70% of individuals with diabetes, with sensory loss being more prevalent than motor loss (see Chapters 32 and 33) (National Diabetes Fact Sheet, 2011). Sensory loss typically presents in a stocking/glove pattern. Patients who are unable to perceive the touch of a Semmes–Weinstein 5.07 monofilament on the plantar surface of the foot are at high risk for ulceration. Decreased proprioceptive input may cause balance and motor deficits that typically affect the smaller intrinsic muscles of the feet, thus altering foot structure and pressure dynamics. Patients with insensitive feet (see Chapter 49) are at increased risk for callus or blister formation and this can be the trigger event that leads to serious infection (see Chapter 50), ulcer formation (see Chapter 48) and loss of limb or life (see Chapter 47). The education of patients should include recommendations against walking barefoot and suggestions that water temperatures be tested with the elbow, and daily foot inspections should be made. Although walking is the form of exercise that many older people prefer, a diabetic patient with a marked neuropathy or foot deformity may be exposed to an increased risk of foot ulceration with a walking program. These individuals may benefit more from a non-weight-bearing type of exercise, such as cycling or swimming. Prescription footwear with orthotics may alleviate some of the risk. Medicare has authorized payments for podiatry visits and specialized footwear for diabetic individuals. When a transtibial amputation does occur, 60% of diabetic patients lose the remaining leg within 5 years. Smoking significantly compounds the problem (American Diabetes Association, 2004).

Physical therapists who are treating orthopedic problems should document a concomitant diagnosis of diabetes, as this may help to justify extended interventions. The healing of a foot ulcer can take weeks to months and a multidisciplinary approach is necessary to optimize conditions.

VASCULAR COMPLICATIONS

Vascular complications are the leading cause of death among individuals with diabetes, as they are at an increased risk for coronary artery disease, stroke and peripheral vascular disease (PVD) and often have coexisting hypertension and dyslipidemia. An examination of the feet of a diabetic should assess for the presence of cold feet, a decrease or absence of the dorsalis pedis and posterior tibial pulses, atrophy of subcutaneous tissues and hair loss, all of which are suggestive of PVD. An ankle brachial pressure index (ABPI) can also be obtained. A positive ABPI indicates the need for further vascular assessment.

Symptomatic PVD often presents as intermittent claudication resulting in a burning cramping sensation, usually in the calf, that is caused by activity-induced ischemia. These symptoms can be difficult to distinguish from painful diabetic peripheral neuropathy. Some patients may have significant arterial disease yet remain asymptomatic because of low levels of activity, and the demands of rehabilitation may unmask these problems. Physical rehabilitation should emphasize a graded program of exercise to encourage collateral circulation to the limbs. This entails encouraging patients to exercise the involved muscles to the point of pain but to avoid persisting once ischemia begins. For calf claudication, heel lifts, toe taps, toe raises and ankle circles may be good exercises. It usually takes about 3 months for symptomatic relief through collateral circulation to occur. If the PVD has progressed to the point of constant pain and resting claudication in the foot, all lower extremity exercises are contraindicated. This is because such individuals are at risk for limb loss and require surgical revascularization. Whenever PVD is present, individuals should consult with a physician before using any over-the-counter medications for the foot (American Diabetes Association, 2004).

AUTONOMIC NEUROPATHY

In total, 60–70% of individuals with diabetes have mild to severe nervous system damage (National Diabetes Fact Sheet, 2011). Autonomic neuropathy develops in the sympathetic and parasympathetic nervous systems of 20–40% of those with long-term diabetes. Exercise programs for diabetic patients with autonomic neuropathy should proceed cautiously. Autonomic neuropathy can result in distal anhidrosis, leading to poor heat dissipation as a result of the decreased sweating in the extremities. Patients with this symptom should avoid overheating when exercising. Genitourinary autonomic dysfunction leads to impotence and the risk of urinary infections. Gastrointestinal disturbances include constipation and diarrhea.

Some individuals with autonomic involvement may present with significant cardiac autonomic neuropathy. These individuals do not perceive anginal pain and may be at risk for 'silent' myocardial infarction. Cardiac arrhythmias are not uncommon. Cardiac denervation syndrome (also referred to as cardiac autonomic neuropathy), a result of autonomic dysfunction, produces a heart rate that is typically around 80–90 beats per minute and is unresponsive to activity levels, beta blockers and antiarrhythmics. If a sustained grip, holding one's breath or a Valsalva maneuver produce no changes in vital signs, cardiac denervation syndrome may be present. The inability of the cardiovascular system to augment cardiac output places such individuals at risk for postural hypotension. Whenever cardiac autonomic changes are present, monitoring vital signs to assess exercise tolerance may not always produce accurate information. Individuals in this state should have thorough cardiac workups before their activity levels are increased. If cardiac neuropathy is present, during exercise, emphasis should be placed on perceived exertion rates (RPE), dyspnea and other observed symptoms of distress and not simply on pulse and blood pressure.

A 2003 study concluded that percent heart rate reserve (%HRR) is an excellent indicator of percent Vo_2 reserve (%Vo_2R). There was a similar relationship between RPE and %Vo_2R (Colberg et al., 2003). Exercise warm-ups and cool-downs should be stressed. Patients prone to orthostatic changes may benefit from minimizing changes in position during rehabilitation, wearing compressive stockings and ensuring an adequate fluid intake (American Diabetes Association, 2004).

RETINOPATHY

Retinopathy is a frequent complication of diabetes. About 80% of type 1 diabetics will have some diabetic retinopathy after 15 years of disease, and 60% of patients with type 2 diabetes will develop some degree of retinopathy after 20 years. Further, 20% of type 2 diabetics have some degree of retinopathy at diagnosis (Larsen et al., 2003). Although most cases of retinopathy are of the nonproliferative variety (with only mild background changes in vision), some patients progress to proliferative retinopathy, which is the leading cause of blindness in adults aged from 20 to 74.

In patients with active proliferative diabetic retinopathy (PDR), strenuous activity may lead to vitreous hemorrhage or tractional retinal detachment. Patients with active PDR should avoid physical activity that involves straining, jarring, jogging, high-impact aerobics or Valsalva-like maneuvers. Patients with moderate to severe nonproliferative diabetic retinopathy (NPDR) should also limit activities such as heavy lifting, Valsalva maneuvers, boxing and highly competitive sports (American Diabetes Association, 2004).

NEPHROPATHY

Diabetic nephropathy occurs in 20–40% of patients with diabetes and is the leading cause of end-stage renal disease, accounting for 44% of new cases (National Diabetes Fact Sheet, 2011). The earliest sign of diabetic nephropathy in type 1 diabetes is persistent albuminuria in the range of 30–299 mg over 24 hours (microalbuminuria). Microalbuminuria is also a marker for the development of nephropathy in type 2 diabetes, as well as a marker for increased cardiovascular disease risk. Controlling blood pressure has been shown to reduce the development of nephropathy. Blood pressure should be carefully monitored during exercise. The ADA has not developed specific physical activity recommendations for patients with microalbuminuria or overt nephropathy. Patients with nephropathy may have a reduced capacity for physical activity leading to self-limitation of activity level. However, there is no need for specific exercise restrictions for those with diabetic kidney disease (Larsen et al., 2003; American Diabetes Association, 2013b).

In 2008, a total of 202 290 people with diabetes underwent dialysis or kidney transplantation (National Diabetes Fact Sheet, 2011). For patients on dialysis therapy, fluid replacement is a crucial issue that must influence the scheduling of exercise and rehabilitation. In addition, patients are given heparin during infusions and any wound care that is performed within 24 hours of dialysis should minimize aggressive debridement. Exercise programs should incorporate anticoagulant precautions, such as guarding against skin trauma caused by weights, hand placement or jarring, especially at intravenous sites, and there should be renewed vigilance against falling.

CONCLUSION

Diabetes is a common and chronic disease that includes multisystem involvement. Many patients with diabetes mellitus need medical and rehabilitative care because of complications resulting from the diabetes or from other illness. It is important that the healthcare provider be aware of the significant influence that diabetes has on rehabilitation.

REFERENCES

Alberti KGMM Eckel RH, Grundy SM et al 2009 Harmonizing the metabolic syndrome. Circulation 120:1640–1645
American Diabetes Association 2004 Physical activity/exercise and diabetes. Diabetes Care 27(Suppl 1):S58–62
American Diabetes Association 2013a Diagnosing diabetes and pre-diabetes. (Accessed at www.diabetes.org/diabetes-basics/prevention/pre-diabetes/December 2013)
American Diabetes Association 2013b Standards of medical care in diabetes. Diabetes Care 36(Suppl 1):S11–66
Colberg SR, Swain DP, Vinik AI 2003 Use of heart rate reserve and rating of perceived exertion to prescribe exercise intensity in diabetic autonomic neuropathy. Diabetes Care 26(4):986–990
DCCT (Diabetes Control and Complications Trial) 2010. http://clinicaltrials.gov/ct2/show/NCT00360815
Ervin RB 2009 Prevalence of metabolic syndrome among adults 20 years of age and over, by sex, age, race and ethnicity, and body mass index: United States, 2003–2006. National Health Statistics Report, no. 13
International Diabetes Federation 2013 IDF Diabetes Atlas, 6th edn. Key Messages. [Online] (Accessed at www.idf.org/diabetesatlas December 2013)
Larsen PR, Kronenberg H, Melmed S et al (eds) 2003 Williams Textbook of Endocrinology, 10th edn. WB Saunders Elsevier, Philadelphia, PA
National Diabetes Fact Sheet 2011. [Online] (Accessed at www.cdc.gov/diabetes/pubs/pdf/ndfs_2011.pdf December 2013)
Selvin E, Marinopoulos S, Berkenblit G et al 2004 Meta-analysis: glycosylated hemoglobin and cardiovascular disease in diabetes mellitus. Ann Intern Med 141(6):421–431
Snowling NJ, Hopkins WG 2006 Effects of different modes of exercise training on glucose control and risk factors for complications in type 2 diabetic patients. Diabetes Care 29(11):2518–2527
UKPDS (United Kingdom Prospective Diabetes Study) 1998. (Accessed at www.dtu.ox.ac.uk/ukpds_trial/index.php December 2013)

Chapter 47

Amputations

JOAN E. EDELSTEIN

CHAPTER CONTENTS

INTRODUCTION

Amputation is the removal of a bodily segment. Geriatric patients are much more likely to have lower, than upper, limb amputations. Peripheral vascular disease, with or without diabetes, is the leading cause of amputation in the United States of America; dysvascular amputations are likely to increase (Fletcher et al., 2002). Trauma, congenital anomaly and cancer are other etiologies. Older people with amputations due to these causes usually have years of experience accommodating their lifestyles to cope with the interference with walking and other daily activities imposed by amputation. Nevertheless, insidious musculoskeletal, neuromuscular, integumentary and cardiopulmonary changes associated with aging are troublesome to older adults with amputations, regardless of cause, because of the added stress on remaining tissues that limb anomaly and a prosthesis impose.

CLASSIFICATION OF AMPUTATIONS

Anatomic location is one way of classifying amputations. Partial foot amputations are very common among those with peripheral vascular disease. The levels include phalangeal, ray and transmetatarsal amputations. Removal of one or more phalanges compromises late stance. If an entire toe, including the proximal phalanx, is absent, then the longitudinal arch of the foot will flatten because the insertion of the plantar aponeurosis has been disrupted. A ray pertains to a metatarsal and its phalanges. Ray amputation interferes with late stance and the longitudinal arch; in addition, the foot will be narrowed. Transmetatarsal amputation has major negative effects on late stance, foot support and balance; the patient tends to lean backwards on the heel. In all instances of partial foot amputation, the patient should be fitted with a shoe that has a rocker sole to aid late stance and an arch support. The shoe insert for the individual with ray amputation must have a longitudinal segment to prevent the narrowed foot from sliding in the shoe.

Syme's amputation involves surgical removal of the entire foot, except for the calcaneal fat pad. The fat pad is sutured to the distal tibia and fibula. The patient should have a Syme's prosthesis, which replaces the shape and basic function of the foot. Syme's and partial foot amputations provide good support and sensory feedback because the patient can stand on the distal end of the amputation limb (end-bearing).

Transtibial (below-knee) amputation is the most common site for major (that is, proximal to the ankle) lower-limb amputation (Fletcher et al., 2002). Retaining the anatomic knee enables the individual to sit and walk reasonably well. Geriatric patients with transfemoral (above-knee) amputation have poorer functional capacity, and generally rely on a wheelchair for community travel. Ankle, knee and hip disarticulations are uncommon, particularly among older adults.

The older person with bilateral amputations due to vascular disease generally sustained one amputation prior to the second one. The presence of diabetes accelerates loss of the contralateral limb, so anyone with an amputation due to diabetes must be taught proper care of the residual and contralateral limbs. (See the discussion of education and prevention in Chapter 46, Diabetes).

RELATED CONDITIONS

Those who sustain dysvascular amputation often have other vascular disease, including cardiovascular disease that compromises their ability to tolerate vigorous exercise. Severe cardiovascular disease, in which the patient has dyspnea at rest, contraindicates prosthetic fitting. Cerebrovascular disease is a frequent concomitant. Hemiparesis, usually ipsilateral, is not uncommon. Paresis does not preclude prosthetic use, particularly if the amputation antedated the stroke. When peripheral vascular disease in one limb is severe enough to lead to amputation, circulation in the opposite limb is also compromised. Individuals may complain of intermittent claudication after a short walk. Prosthetic fitting reduces stress on the remaining limb. The remaining foot is vulnerable to pressure sores, which can lead to amputation. Vigilant foot inspection and hygiene, as well as suitable footwear, are essential.

Peripheral vascular disease associated with diabetes is often accompanied by obesity, visual impairment, proprioceptive and tactile loss, and renal dysfunction, all of which complicate prosthesis use. Severe arthritis in the lower limbs or the hands hampers prosthetic donning and use.

TESTS AND RELATED DIAGNOSES

In addition to tests of the peripheral vascular system, including angiography and Doppler ultrasound, the patient with an amputation should be investigated for sensory diminution. Tactile sensation may be graded with a 10g filament, while proprioception can be judged with balance testing. Heart rate and blood pressure should be monitored to keep the rehabilitation program at a challenging level without overstressing the patient.

The amputation limb requires daily inspection to identify any incipient ulceration. A patient who has had recent amputation should have the surgical scar examined to ascertain whether healing is proceeding satisfactorily. Amputation limbs at or above the transtibial level are measured longitudinally and circumferentially. The longer the amputation limb the more efficient the gait. The proximal circumferential measurement of the transtibial limb is taken at the fibular head. For the transfemoral limb it is taken at a fixed distance below the greater trochanter. Additional distal measurements are taken at 4-cm intervals. Consistent circumferential measurements indicate that edema has subsided and the patient is ready for a prosthesis.

Motor power and joint excursion in all limbs and the trunk should be assessed periodically. Weakness interferes with the ability to maintain sitting balance, transfer from bed to wheelchair, stand and manage a prosthesis. Hip and knee flexion contractures compromise prosthetic alignment and the patient's ability to stand and walk with a prosthesis. The clinician should ask the patient about the presence and intensity of phantom (awareness of the missing body part) sensation and pain, which is highly prevalent (Ephraim et al., 2005). Many modalities reduce pain intensity.

The history should also include inquiry regarding the individual's functional level prior to surgery. The person with bilateral amputation who could not use a unilateral prosthesis is unsuited for bilateral prostheses. Cognitive assessment is essential because dementia contraindicates prosthetic fitting. Other factors that influence rehabilitation include environmental features, such as the number of steps at the entrance and within the home, and the patient's vocational and avocational interests. For example, someone who enjoyed golfing prior to surgery may benefit from a prosthetic foot that accommodates to the sloping terrain of a golf course.

CLINICAL RELEVANCE: MOBILITY AND REHABILITATION

Preprosthetic rehabilitation involves measures designed to improve the health of the amputation limb and interventions that increase the individual's independence. The goals of treating the amputation limb are to reduce postoperative pain, foster healing, stabilize limb volume, and prevent complications, particularly contractures and skin disorders. The patient should be guided toward increasing self-care, including dressing, grooming, personal hygiene, maneuvering in bed and various transfers, such as from bed to wheelchair, from wheelchair to toilet and standing. Some older individuals with unilateral amputation can negotiate short distances with a walker or a pair of crutches and the remaining leg. These activities should not be performed unless the patient is wearing a clean sock and a well-fitting shoe on the intact foot.

Most people with unilateral amputation or bilateral transtibial amputation receive prostheses (see Chapter 70, Prosthetics). Rehabilitation aims to enable the individual to don and use the prosthesis safely, either as the sole mode of locomotion or as an alternative to wheelchair mobility, particularly indoors. A preparatory prosthesis for balance during transfers or for cosmetic value may be considered. The clinic team, consisting of physician, physical therapist and prosthetist, should select the prosthetic components that will provide the patient with the best opportunity to accomplish meaningful activities and that are within the individual's functional capacity. Medicare guidelines to prosthetic prescription (HCFA, 2001) are based on prediction of the function of individuals with unilateral amputation:

Level 0: Patient does not have the ability or potential to ambulate or transfer safely with or without assistance and a prosthesis does not enhance their quality of life or mobility.
Level 1: Patient has the ability or potential to use a prosthesis for transfer or ambulation on level surfaces at fixed cadence; a typical limited or unlimited household ambulator.
Level 2: Patient has the ability or potential for ambulation with the ability to traverse low-level environmental barriers such as curbs, stairs, or uneven surfaces; a typical community ambulator.
Level 3: Patient has the ability or potential for ambulation with variable cadence; a typical community ambulator with the ability to traverse most environmental barriers and may have vocational, therapeutic, or exercise activity that demands prosthetic use beyond simple locomotion.
Level 4: Patient has the ability or potential for prosthetic ambulation that exceeds basic ambulation skills, exhibiting high impact, stress, or energy levels, typical of the prosthetic demands of the child, active adult, or athlete.

THERAPEUTIC INTERVENTIONS

EARLY CARE

Reducing postoperative edema has the triple benefit of diminishing pain, fostering healing, and stabilizing limb volume by promoting resorption of interstitial fluid. Elastic bandage or other modality is used until limb girth stabilizes. Most patients can learn to apply elastic bandage to a partial foot, Syme's or transtibial amputation limb, but it is exceedingly difficult for a person of any age to wrap a transfemoral amputation limb. Regardless of amputation level, the elastic bandage loosens as the patient moves in bed or transfers into and out of the wheelchair. Consequently, the bandage must be reapplied several times a day. Elastic shrinker socks are easier to apply and can be used at the transtibial and transfemoral levels, although suspension on the thigh is difficult to maintain. As limb volume reduces, successively smaller socks are needed.

Elastic bandages and shrinker socks are the least effective ways of controlling edema. A rigid plaster dressing applied at the time of surgery is a much more effective way to control edema, particularly for transtibial amputation (Van Velzen et al., 2005). Unless signs of infection are evident, the dressing is left in place until the time of suture removal. An aluminum or plastic pylon and a prosthetic foot can be attached to the rigid dressing to create an immediate postoperative prosthesis, although this modification is rarely used with older patients. Plaster dressings are more difficult to apply, require suspension from a waist belt, and usually prevent inspection of the operative wound. Sometimes the distal portion of the dressing over the scar is cut so that the plaster can be removed for wound inspection, then replaced easily. Alternatively, a removable rigid dressing can be used, and it, too, allows viewing the wound. Removal of the plaster requires a cast cutter.

The Unna semirigid dressing is zinc oxide, calamine, gelatin and glycerin in a gauze bandage. It is easy to apply and remove, adheres to the skin and thus requires no waist belt, and promotes healing; it is well suited to amputations at every level, including transfemoral (Wong & Edelstein, 2000). The dressing remains on the limb until the sutures are removed. The semirigid dressing by itself cannot support a pylon and foot. After removal of the rigid or semirigid dressing, most patients wear a shrinker sock to resolve residual edema.

ADDITIONAL CARE

In addition to stabilizing amputation limb volume, other interventions that focus on the amputation limb are those that reduce phantom pain, including ultrasound, transcutaneous electrical nerve stimulation (TENS), bilateral resistive exercise, and percussive massage. An educational program and peer support may help the patient accept the phenomenon of phantom sensation. Contractures can be prevented by encouraging the patient to adopt alternate positions rather than remain seated. A bivalved plaster or a canvas knee splint and a wheelchair knee support retard development of a knee flexion contracture. Resistive exercises should emphasize hip and knee extension. After it has healed, the scar can be massaged to prevent adherence.

Interventions that enable the patient to resume self-care and mobility foster independence. Most patients receive a wheelchair. It should promote good sitting posture. The seat should have a firm foundation and a proper cushion to distribute pressure. A lumbar support to overcome the sling-back effect of a flexible backrest is helpful. The brakes must be operative. Leg amputation shifts one's center of gravity posteriorly. Consequently, either a special model of wheelchair having posteriorly offset wheels should be obtained or a pair of adapters should be bolted to the rear wheels of a standard wheelchair. The wheelchair will then have an increased base of support, preventing upset of the wheelchair and its occupant when ascending steep ramps. The person with unilateral amputation should have a wheelchair with swing-out footrests so that the remaining foot and the prosthesis can be supported. The individual with bilateral amputations who is not a candidate for prostheses will have a less difficult time transferring if the wheelchair does not have footrests. Removable armrests facilitate transfers.

The physical therapist should demonstrate the safest way of transferring into and out of the wheelchair and the most efficient ways of maneuvering it. The home may require modification to accommodate the wheelchair, such as rearranging furniture to create a pathway and removing throw rugs and saddle boards at doorways to ease rolling the wheelchair. If the wheelchair cannot fit through the bathroom door, then a commode and alternative bathing facilities will be needed.

Exercises that improve the flexibility, coordination and strength of the hands, shoulders and trunk are important. All patients with unilateral amputation should be taught how to inspect and clean the foot and need a suitable sock and shoe. Peer support helps many patients and their families cope with the emotional and practical problems associated with amputation.

REHABILITATION

Prosthetic rehabilitation begins with assessment to ascertain whether the prosthesis fits well and that all components function properly. The basic program emphasizes donning the prosthesis, transfer into and out of chairs, standing balance and walking, as well as instruction in care of the amputation limb and the prosthesis. Some older adults can climb stairs and ramps, drive a car and engage in a wide range of recreational activities once they become used to the prosthesis.

Applying a partial foot prosthesis generally involves slipping the prosthesis into the shoe, donning the appropriate sock, making sure that it is not wrinkled, and finally inserting the foot into the shoe. The sequence for dressing when one has the usual transtibial prosthesis is to put the sock and shoe on the prosthetic foot, drape the trouser around the prosthesis, don the amputation limb sock, insert the amputation limb into the socket, and secure any straps or other fastenings. Some people prefer to don the amputation limb sock and the socket liner and then enter the socket. The entire sequence can be performed while sitting. If the prosthesis has distal pin suspension, the patient applies a silicon sheath to the amputation limb, one or more socks, then inserts the covered amputation limb into the socket, matching the pin to its hole at the base of the socket.

Donning the transfemoral prosthesis can begin while the patient sits. The person applies the amputation limb sock, bringing its proximal margin to the groin, removes the suction valve from the prosthetic socket, then places the thigh in the socket. At that point the patient stands and pulls the distal end of the sock through the valve hole in order to smooth superficial tissues into the socket. The patient tucks the sock end into the socket, installs the valve and fastens the belt around the torso. If the prosthesis has total suction suspension, the easiest method is to lubricate the thigh, insert it into the socket while sitting or standing, and install the valve.

Teaching the patient to move safely from various chairs to the standing position and back again is the most critical aspect of prosthetic rehabilitation for the older adult. Regardless of amputation level, a patient has the easiest time moving from an armchair with a firm seat, such as the wheelchair. Both feet should be on the floor, with the sound foot placed slightly posterior. Initially, the patient may use the armrests to assist in rising.

Balancing with a prosthesis may begin at the parallel bars or at the side of a sturdy table. The latter approach prevents the individual from forming the habit of pulling, rather than pushing, on the supporting structure. The therapist should guide the patient in shifting from side to side, forwards and backwards, and diagonally while maintaining upright posture. Eventually the patient should be able to shift weight without holding onto a support. Advanced balancing exercises include stepping on a low stool with the sound foot, thus prolonging weight-bearing on the prosthesis.

Gait training may involve the use of a cane, forearm crutch, or a walker, depending on the patient's ability to master balance exercises. Proper adjustment of the assistive device and instruction in its use are essential to promote safe walking. The two-wheeled walker enables faster gait than a four-wheeled aid (Tsai et al., 2003). The goals of gait training are safety, symmetrical step length, and equal time spent on each leg. Older adults who wore transfemoral prostheses walked faster when the knee unit was locked, even though the appearance of the gait was abnormal (Devlin et al., 2002). Patients should practice walking on various surfaces, such as smooth flooring, carpets and grass.

People who can walk safely on level surfaces should have an opportunity to climb stairs and ramps. The easiest task is ascending stairs that have a handrail on the contralateral side. Most individuals with transtibial or more distal amputations ascend and descend in a foot-over-foot manner, alternating feet on each step. In contrast, people with transfemoral prostheses ascend leading with the sound foot and descend leading with the prosthesis. A few exceptionally agile individuals learn to descend in a foot-over-foot pattern. Stair climbing by those who wear bilateral transfemoral prostheses is exceedingly rare. They may choose to ascend and to descend seated on the buttocks. Maximal assistance is often necessary. Two handrails may be facilitative, or an electric stair seat may be appropriate. Ramps pose a problem for those who wear prostheses, because most prosthetic feet have limited ranges of dorsiflexion and plantarflexion. Diagonal (sideways) climbing may be more practical for older adults.

Driving a car involves two concerns, namely transferring into and out of the car and operating the vehicle. The individual with a right amputation naturally has an easier time entering the passenger side, at least in the US. (The opposite obviously applies to motor vehicles with left-hand steering wheels.) With a left prosthesis, the patient should first sit sideways on the passenger's seat and then lift the prosthesis to the forward-facing position while pivoting on the buttocks. Operating an automobile that has automatic transmission is easier for the individual with left amputation. The adult with a right prosthesis may choose to cross the left leg so that the sensate left foot moves the accelerator and brake pedals. Others install an extension to the accelerator so that the left foot can reach it comfortably. Individuals with transtibial amputation often require no special adaptation or equipment for driving.

CONCLUSION

Amputation in an aging adult usually results from peripheral vascular disease. Key assessment factors include sensory evaluation and measurement of joint excursion and motor power. Preprosthetic care should focus on controlling edema of the amputation limb and fostering resumption of self-care. Prosthetic training begins with assessment of the fit and function of the prosthesis. Basic care includes teaching the patient to transfer from one seat to another and to standing, as well as walking with or without assistive devices. Environmental modifications facilitate household ambulation. Some older patients with amputations resume full independence, including driving a car and participating in recreational activities.

REFERENCES AND FURTHER READING

Devlin M, Sinclair LB, Colman D et al 2002 Patient preference and gait efficiency in a geriatric population with transfemoral amputation using a free-swinging versus a locked prosthetic knee joint. Arch Phys Med Rehabil 83:246–249

Ephraim PL, Wegener ST, MacKenzie EJ et al 2005 Phantom pain, residual limb pain, and back pain in amputees: results of a national survey. Arch Phys Med Rehabil 86:1910–1919

Fletcher DD, Andrews KL, Hallett JW et al 2002 Trends in rehabilitation after amputation for geriatric patients with vascular disease: implications for future health resource allocation. Arch Phys Med Rehabil 83:1389–1393

HCFA Common Procedure Coding System 2001. US Government Printing Office, Washington, DC, ch 5.3

Tsai HA, Kirby RL, MacLeod DA et al 2003 Aided gait of people with lower-limb amputations: comparison of 4-footed and 2-wheeled walkers. Arch Phys Med Rehabil 84:584–591

Van Velzen AD, Nederhand MJ, Emmelot CH et al 2005 Early treatment of trans-tibial amputees: retrospective analysis of early fitting and elastic bandaging. Prosthet Orthot Int 29:3–12

Wong CK, Edelstein JE 2000 Unna and elastic postoperative dressings: comparison of their effects on function of adults with amputation and vascular disease. Arch Phys Med Rehabil 81:1191–1198

Chapter 48

Wound management

RICHARD MOWRER

CHAPTER CONTENTS

INTRODUCTION

The integument (the skin) is a vital organ. When a person sustains an injury to the integument, a break has occurred in the protective barrier between the organs/underlying tissues and the outside environment. This principle is crucial to the survival of the older adults especially, because chronic dermal wounds occur frequently in the elderly (Zhao et al., 2010). The body's ability to heal is altered by various health problems – diabetes mellitus, circulatory problems, hypertension and chronic obstructive pulmonary disease (COPD). Normal age-related changes in skin also affect the rate and quality of healing (see Chapter 50), and there may be additional risk factors including inadequate nutrition, limited mobility and muscle atrophy.

WOUNDS AND THE HEALING PROCESS

The normal healing process has three phases (Stillman, 2005). In phase one the inflammatory response is activated, which is the body's natural response to injury. This inflammatory response extends from injury to 4–6 days after injury. The process follows a normal sequence of events, including vasoconstriction, fibrin clots, vasodilatation and the presence of neutrophils and macrophages that remove bacteria and debris. Initially after injury, transudate leaks out of the blood vessels to fill the interstitial space, leading to localized edema and, thus, slowing the bleeding. Next, blood vessels reflexively constrict to assist with reducing blood loss. Platelets aggregate and become 'sticky'; this plugs up the lymphatic tissue, causing greater edema. The platelets release growth factors that control cell growth, differentiation and metabolism. Finally, chemotactic agents are released to attract cells that are necessary to fight infection and repair the wound. As the chemotactic agents attract new healing cells, the vasoconstriction changes to vasodilatation, allowing these cells to reach the site of the injury. Vasodilatation results in localized redness, swelling and warmth, which are characteristics of inflammation. Fluid seeping from the wound, containing macrophages, white blood cells (WBC) and neutrophils, is called exudate; it is yellow/cream colored and more viscous than transudate. Pain is also usually present (Mowrer, 2004).

Phase two, the proliferative phase, occurs approximately 7 days after injury. This phase includes the utilization of growth factors, endothelial cells, fibroblasts, new blood vessels and collagen. The growth factors also generate keratinocytes, which are involved in re-epithelialization. The inflammatory and proliferation phases usually overlap, with no definitive marker for when one ends and the other begins. There are four crucial events of the proliferative stage:

1. Angiogenesis is the formation of new capillaries; these capillaries tie into loops that bring nutrition and blood to the injured site (this does not happen in areas of ischemia).
2. Granulation tissue is formed as dead tissue is removed and the capillary network 'fills in' the space. This tissue serves as a latticework for new epithelium to grow on.
3. Fibroblasts lay down a fibrous network in which myofibroblasts (complete with actin) begin to pull the edges of the wound together.
4. The wound contracts: keratinocytes begin to migrate across the wound bed and growth factors act to produce proliferation of new epithelial growth, also known as re-epithelialization.

In phase three, the remodeling phase, there is no longer an open wound. During this phase, connective tissue becomes better aligned and tensile strength increases. After the re-epithelialization process has completely covered the wound surface, the maturation phase begins; this means the 'new skin' begins to thicken and mature. The new skin is primarily scar tissue that is formed by randomly laid down collagen. This collagen will eventually need to be 'remodeled' so that it can work in conjunction with the surrounding tissue, i.e. move or become

341

Table 48.1	**Wound classification systems**	
Wound Type	**Classification**	**Characteristics**
Pressure ulcers	Stage I	Nonblanchable erythema of intact skin, the heralding lesion of skin ulceration
	Stage II	Partial-thickness skin loss involving epidermis and/or dermis; ulcer is superficial and presents clinically as an abrasion, blister or hollow crater
	Stage III	Full-thickness skin loss involving damage or necrosis of subcutaneous tissue that may extend down to, but not through, underlying fascia; ulcer presents clinically as a deep crater, with or without undermining of the adjacent tissue
	Stage IV	Full-thickness skin loss with extensive destruction, tissue necrosis or damage to muscle, bone or supporting structures (e.g. tendon or joint capsule)
	Unstageable	Full-thickness loss in which actual depth is completely obscured by slough and/or eschar
	Suspected deep tissue injury – depth unknown	Purple or maroon localized area of discolored intact skin or blood-filled blister due to damage of underlying soft tissue from pressure and/or shear
Burns	First-degree	Involves the superficial epidermal layer; skin is pink or red, dry and painful, and sheds within a week without residual scar
	Second-degree	Involves the epidermis and the dermis; wound is immediately blistered and wet, local edema is present; if superficial, will heal within 2–3 weeks and will not scar if not infected or unduly traumatized; if deep, may require skin grafting to achieve optimal healing
	Third-degree	Involves the entire thickness of the skin; wound varies in color from white to black and may present with dark networks of thrombosed capillaries that do not blanch with pressure; surface is usually dry, but may be wet; these wounds require skin grafting for closure if more than 1 in (2.54 cm) in diameter
	Burns are also designated, at times, by partial- and full-thickness; first- and second-degree burns are synonymous with partial-thickness. Full-thickness burns are those in which the entire epidermis has been destroyed. Parts of the dermis may also be destroyed, along with injury into the subcutaneous structures	
Venous, arterial, and traumatic wounds	Partial-thickness	Penetration into the epidermis or into the beginning of the dermis
	Full-thickness	Penetration into the subcutaneous tissue, muscle or bone

mobile. This process can take up to 2 years to complete (Stadelmann et al., 1998).

WOUND CLASSIFICATION

Wounds are generally classified according to the predominant underlying cause. Common categories include arterial insufficiency, venous insufficiency, pressure ulcers, neurotrophic ulcers, traumatic wounds and burns. There are several wound classification systems. Table 48.1 presents the classification systems for pressure ulcers (NPUAP, 2007) burns, and venous, arterial and traumatic wounds that are not included in the other classifications. The Wagner (1981) system is another important assessment tool for the classification of ulcer stages (Table 48.2).

Table 48.2	**Wagner classification system of ulcer stages**
Stage	**Description**
0	Intact skin
1	Superficial ulcer involving skin only
2	Deep ulcer involving muscle and, perhaps, bone and joint structures
3	Localized infection; may be abscess or osteomyelitis
4	Gangrene, limited to forefoot area
5	Gangrene of the majority of the foot

Physical History

Name: _____ Date: _____

Brief history: _____

_____

_____

_____

Past Medical History:

Major illness:

Cardiovascular:	Coronary disease _____	Angina _____	Malignancies: _____
	Congestive heart failure _____	Arrhythmia _____	_____
	Myocardial infarct _____	Hypertension _____	_____
	Hypercholesterol _____	_____	_____
	Other _____	_____	Operations: _____
Pulmonary:	COPD _____	Pneumonia _____	_____
	TB _____	Asthma _____	_____
	Other _____	_____	Injuries: _____
Diabetes mellitus:	Insulin-dependent _____	_____	_____
	Noninsulin-dependent _____	_____	Hospitalizations: _____
Vascular:	Claudication _____	Rest pain _____	_____
	Varicose veins _____	DVT _____	_____
	Other _____	_____	_____
Musculoskeletal:	Arthritis _____	Muscle weakness _____	Medications: _____
	Fractures _____		_____
Gastrointestinal:	Peptic ulcer disease _____	Cirrhosis _____	Allergies: _____
	Bleeding _____	Hepatitis _____	_____
	Pancreatitis _____	Other _____	_____
Genitourinary:	Kidneys _____	_____	Social history:
	Bladder _____	_____	Occupation _____
	Other _____	_____	Smoking _____
Hematology:	Anemia _____	Bruisability _____	Alcohol _____
	Sickle cell anemia _____	_____	Drugs _____
	Bleeding tendency _____	_____	Family history: _____
Neurological:	TIA _____ Stroke _____	RIND _____	_____
	Other _____	_____	_____

Family physician: _____

Other physicians _____

_____

COPD, chronic obstructive pulmonary disease; DVT, deep vein thrombosis; RIND, reversible ischemic neurological deficit; TB, tuberculosis; TIA, transient ischemic attack

Form 48.1 Sample form for taking a patient history.

EVALUATING THE PATIENT

Evaluation of a patient with a wound should be completed by a multidisciplinary team (physician, nurse, physical therapist and social worker, and nutritionist). The physical therapist plays an important role and must have expertise in dealing with the integumentary system and the classification of wounds to establish a plan of care that optimizes wound homeostasis and healing. It is important to remember to treat the patient, not the wound.

When initiating the evaluation, the following elements should be included (see Forms 48.1, 48.2 and 48.3):

- Obtain a thorough medical history; a patient's past medical history may predispose them to a non-healing wound (e.g. diabetes mellitus or peripheral vascular disease).

Physical Assessment

General: Alert_____   Oriented_____   Height_____   Weight_____

Vital signs: Temperature_____   Pulse_____   Respiration_____   BP _____
                  RN_____

HEENT: Normal_____   Abnormal_____   _____

Neck: JVD_____   Node_____   Bruits_____   Thyroid_____

Heart: Regular_____   Irregular_____

Lungs: Clear_____   Rhonchi_____   Rales_____   Wheezes _____

Abdomen: Tenderness_____   Masses_____   Hernias_____   Organs_____

Extremities: Edema _____   Cyanosis_____   Clubbing _____
                  Other_____

Pulses (0–4+):   (R)   Radial _____ Femoral _____ Popliteal _____ Dorsalis pedis _____ Post-tibial _____
                  (L)   Radial _____ Femoral _____ Popliteal _____ Dorsalis pedis _____ Post-tibial _____

Description of wound: _____
_____
_____
_____

Impression: _____
_____
_____
_____

Plan: _____
_____
_____
_____MD

BP, blood pressure; HEENT, head, ears, eyes, nose, throat; JVD, jugular vein distension; L, left; R, right

Form 48.2 Sample physical assessment form.

- Encourage the patient's primary care physician to evaluate the patient's medical status extensively (e.g. assess blood sugars, albumin, hemoglobin, wound cultures, if necessary, and medications).
- Assess the patient's physical mobility; contractures may predispose a patient to pressure ulcers and immobility limits a patient's ability to change positions in bed or a chair.
- Assess the integument. Is it well hydrated? Is there good turgor?
- Assess nutrition. What and how much is the patient eating?
- Assess the patients support surface. What type of bed, chair and shoes does the patient use regularly?
- Review the patient's personal care (hygiene).
- Assess peripheral pulses, i.e. ankle brachial pressure index (ABPI) (see Table 48.3).
- Assess the wound:
  - specific location of the wound;
  - size of the wound (length, width, depth);

Name: _____

Date: _____

Pulses: (R) Post-tibial _____ Dorsalis pedis _____ Popliteal _____

 (L) Post-tibial _____ Dorsalis pedis _____ Popliteal _____

Location: _____

_____

Type of wound: _____

_____

_____

Stage: _____

Partial/full thickness: _____

_____

Size/depth: _____

_____

Exposed tendon: _____

Exposed bone: _____

Color: _____

_____

Percent of necrosis: _____

_____

_____

Drainage: _____

_____

_____

Odor: _____

_____

Undermining: _____

_____

_____

Periwound condition: _____

_____

_____

_____

Assessment: _____

_____

_____

_____

Plan: _____

_____

_____

_____

_____

_____

Form 48.3 Sample wound evaluation form.

- wound classification
- wound odor;
- percentage of necrotic tissue, slough and granulation tissue;
- drainage (amount, odor, color, consistency);
- presence of undermining or tunneling;
- wound color;
- periwound condition;
- girth measurements (when applicable).

ABPI PROCEDURE

ABPI is measured using Doppler ultrasound, a hand-held device that utilizes sound waves to determine blood flow, and a blood pressure cuff. This is a quantitative way to measure blood flow without invasive testing. With the Doppler ultrasound, a whooshing sound is heard, either biphasic (two sounds) or monophasic (one sound). The ultrasound device should be held at a 45° angle to the artery, against the direction of flow (gel will need to be utilized). The blood pressure of the brachial artery is taken as 'normal' and the maximum cuff pressure at which the pulse can just be heard with the Doppler ultrasound is recorded. This is repeated on the lower extremity (usually

Table 48.3	**Interpretation of ABPI values**	
ABPI	**Interpretation**	**Possible Vascular Interventions**
1.1–1.3	Vessel calcification	ABPI not valid measure of tissue perfusion
0.9–1.1	Normal	None needed
0.7–0.9	Mild to moderate insufficiency	Conservative interventions normally provide satisfactory wound healing
0.5–0.7	Moderate arterial insufficiency with intermittent claudication	May perform trial of with conservative care, physician may consider revascularization
<0.5	Severe arterial insufficiency, rest pain	Wound is unlikely to heal without revascularization, limb-threatening arterial insufficiency
≤0.3	Rest pain and gangrene	Revascularization or amputation

From Myers B 2004 Wound Management: Principles and Practice. Prentice Hall, Pearson Education, Upper Saddle River, NJ, p 211, with permission.

the dorsalis pedis). The blood pressure of the lower extremity is divided by that of the upper extremity to give the ABPI. In the presence of diabetes mellitus, the arteries may be calcified, therefore the measurements will be altered and unreliable. If this is the case, an arteriogram is indicated. If Doppler ultrasound is not available, pulses will need to be assessed using palpatory skills or vascular studies.

TYPES OF ULCERS

In order to intervene appropriately in the treatment of ulcers, it is crucial to be able to distinguish between the various different types (Table 48.4). (See Chapter 9, Effects of aging on vascular function.)

Venous

Venous insufficiency, defined as a disturbance in the forward flow of blood in the lower extremities, may progress to increased hydrostatic pressure, venous hypertension and, ultimately, dermal ulceration (Fig. 48.1). Signs and symptoms of venous disease are hemosiderin staining, a purple hue that covers the skin (Fig. 48.2), coupled with a 'heavy feeling' in the legs and edema. Venous wounds are usually found in the lower leg in the proximity of the medial malleoli. These wounds present with large surface areas and have shallow edges. Many patients will complain of increased pain with prolonged lower extremity dependence, such as standing or sitting, with relief upon elevation of the involved limb.

The wound bed will be wet with a mixture of viable and nonviable tissues. An ABPI of >0.8 will present in the venous wound, as will palpable pulses. Palpating pulses in the edematous lower extremity can be difficult. In this

Table 48.4	**Clinical typing of ulcers**			
	Pressure	**Venous**	**Arterial**	**Neuropathic**
Location	Bony prominences	Medial aspect lower leg/ ankle; superior to medial malleolus	Between toes, tips of toes; around lateral malleolus; over phalangeal heads	Plantar aspect of foot; metatarsal; heads; heels; altered pressure points; site of repetitive trauma
Wound appearance	Presence of redness, tunneling/undermining, maceration, induration, pain and odor; necrotic tissue may be present	Irregular wound margins; ruddy base (color); shallow depth; moderate to heavy exudate; granulation present	Pale or necrotic base; granulation absent or minimal; minimal exudate; gangrene/ necrosis; infection	Even, well-defined wound margins; variable depth; variable exudate; variable extent of necrotic tissue; granulation present
Surrounding skin	Erythema; possible induration; cellulitis	Erythema; possible induration; cellulitis; hemosiderin stains	Erythema; possible induration; cellulitis	Erythema; possible induration; cellulitis; callus frequently present
Pain	Frequent pain	Minimal unless infected or desiccated	Frequently painful	Usually painless
Prevention	Education; identify at-risk patients; improve tissue tolerance; protect against pressure	Patient education; no smoking; adequate nutrition; skin care; optimize venous return; take medications; constant compression	Patient education; no smoking; take medications; diabetes control; avoid leg crossing, cold, moisture; professional foot care; well-fitting footwear; pressure reduction	Patient education; no smoking; take medications; control diabetes; avoid cold, moisture, extreme temperatures, external heat; daily foot care; appropriate footwear

instance, it may be beneficial to seek a noninvasive vascular study through the patient's referring physician or the medical director.

Patients with venous insufficiency are frequently significantly overweight. Therefore, it is important to include a weight loss program or consult a dietician for the comprehensive management of venous disease.

The etiology includes valvular incompetence of lower extremity veins, obstruction of the deep venous system, congenital absence or malformation of valves in the venous system and regurgitation from the deep to the superficial venous system via the venous perforators that connect the deep and superficial venous systems. Inadequate pulmonary function will augment the problem because of a weak 'pulmonary pump'. The pulmonary pump functions via deep breathing, forcing the diaphragm against the abdominal cavity and increasing the pressure on the venous system, which increases the flow of blood. Additionally, the deep veins are surrounded by calf muscles that act as pumps by squeezing the veins and forcing the blood proximally. Paralysis or atrophy (possibly caused by a sedentary lifestyle) will impair this pump. This demonstrates the importance of exercise, specifically aerobic exercise, for patients with open wounds. Failure of the muscle pump is usually coupled with venous dysfunction, i.e. the veins fail to function and/or the one-way valves stop working. The veins become distended, with the increased internal pressure from the backflow of blood and subsequent increase in pressure in the capillaries leading to a 'cuff-like' pressure around the wound that limits oxygen and nutrients reaching the tissues. Proteins and fluids migrate out of the vein walls and flood the interstitial tissues, leading to edema and hemosiderin staining.

The treatment of venous insufficiency involves four major areas: (i) control of underlying medical and nutritional disorders; (ii) education of the patient; (iii) control of edema; and (iv) topical therapy to reduce bacterial load, control drainage and promote granulation tissue formation.

Arterial

Arterial insufficiency is defined as insufficient arterial perfusion of an extremity or particular location (Fig. 48.3). It may be caused by arteriosclerosis, trauma, rheumatoid arthritis, diabetes mellitus, Buerger's disease or atherosclerosis. The ABPI will be >0.8, signifying arterial involvement. Any edema is localized or can be associated with an infection.

Pain is a significant symptom associated with arterial insufficiency. The pain may be described as intermittent claudication, which is pain during fast/prolonged ambulation or cramping of the muscles of the lower extremity on climbing many steps. This results from inadequate blood flow to the musculature of the lower extremity; the muscles begin to cramp, secondary to loss of oxygen perfusion and subsequent fuel usage. Ischemic rest pain is another type of problem that is positional in nature, i.e. during sleeping, when the legs are flat on the bed, blood flow is decreased, leading to pain. Often patients will

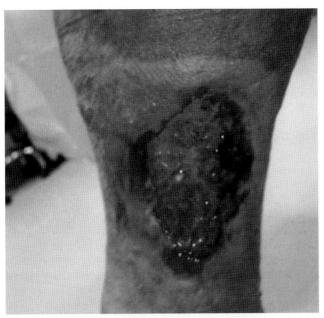

Figure 48.1 Venous wound: medial calf, large wet granular wound.

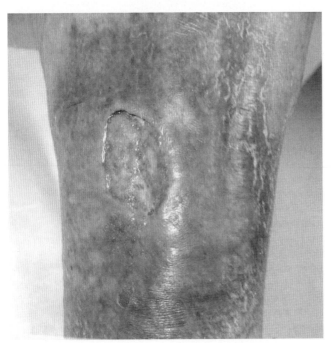

Figure 48.2 Venous wound: significant hemosiderin staining and edema.

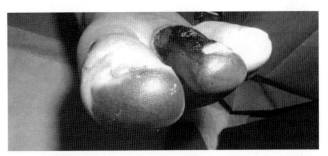

Figure 48.3 Arterial wound: note capillary occlusion in great toe and line of demarcation at the base of the second toe.

describe a 'pain in my feet (or legs) that wakes me up, I need to walk around for a little while before it goes away'. Often these patients will sleep with their legs dangling over the side of the bed or even in a recliner to allow gravity to assist with circulation. A final type of pain that is reported by patients is an intractable pain that is not managed or decreased in response to analgesia.

There are a few simple tests that can be used to assess perfusion: (i) check to see whether peripheral pulses are absent or diminished (the ABPI is a useful measure); (ii) check for a decrease in skin temperature; (iii) check for a delayed capillary refill time (more than 3 seconds); and (iv) check color – is there pallor on elevation or rubor?

Treatment of arterial insufficiency involves seven major focuses: (i) control any underlying medical and nutritional disorders; (ii) educate the patient on controlling risk factors, such as smoking, high blood pressure and cholesterol management, as well as utilization of proper footwear; (iii) manage the pain; (iv) control edema; (v) encourage ambulation and/or exercise to tolerance; (vi) use topical therapy; and (vii) carry out daily skin checks of sensitive areas, especially toes and feet.

Ulceration and gangrene (Fig. 48.4) are physical representations of significant peripheral vascular disease (PVD). These types of wounds require vascular surgery to bypass the blockages in the lower extremity arterial system and increase blood flow. A physician may prescribe anticoagulants and other medications to increase blood flow to the lower extremities; however, this may only be a temporary solution to the underlying problem.

Neuropathic

Neuropathic ulcers (also referred to as neurotrophic or diabetic ulcers) have a direct correlation with peripheral neuropathy. Peripheral neuropathy is defined as an altered function in the extremities that may involve a diminished or absent sensation in response to touch, pain or temperature, an absence of sweating, foot deformities and altered gait and weight-bearing.

Causes of peripheral neuropathy include damage to sensory, motor and autonomic nerves of the lower extremities (see Chapter 32). Gradual paralysis of the intrinsic muscles of the foot leads to muscle imbalances, atrophy and instability of the foot during stance. This, in turn, leads to increased pressure and shearing forces on the metatarsal heads of the feet. The foot itself can also change in shape, leading to hammer toes, hallux valgus or hyperextension of the great toe, all of which change the

weight-bearing forces on the plantar aspect of the foot. Patients begin walking on bones and skin that do not have sufficient padding to withstand the shearing/pressure forces.

Additionally, autonomic neuropathy increases the risk of ulceration secondary to impaired sweating mechanisms, increased callus formation and impaired blood flow. Impaired sweating mechanisms decrease the elasticity of skin, leading to greater 'overgrowth' of skin or callous formation and increased pressure at the point of 'overgrowth'. In turn, the callous formation develops a reduced or altered blood flow, decreasing the body's ability to heal itself. This affects the bones, resulting in a loss of calcium from the bone and fractures because of bone softening. The foot changes shape, often resulting in the appearance of a 'rocker bottom foot' or Charcot's foot (Figs 48.5 and 48.6).

Physical examination of the patient should include: (i) palpation of peripheral pulses; (ii) notation of skin temperature; (iii) notation of skin color; (iv) assessment of capillary refill (less than 3 seconds); and (v) assessment of motor, sensory and autonomic neuropathy. Clinicians must also determine if the neuropathic ulceration has exposed (or tunnels down to) bone. In these instances, radiographic studies will be needed to rule out osteomyelitis. As already noted, ABPI assessment of the diabetic patient may be unreliable because of calcification of the arteries.

Treatment of neuropathic ulcers involves six major areas: (i) control of underlying medical and nutritional

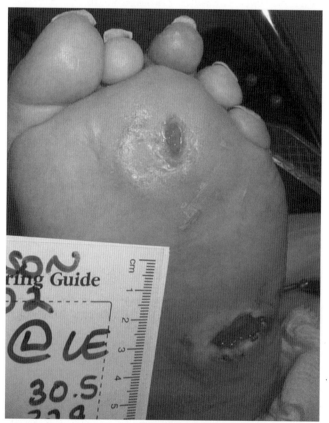

Figure 48.5 Neuropathic ulcer and Charcot's foot with hammer toes and pes planus deformity or 'rocker bottom'.

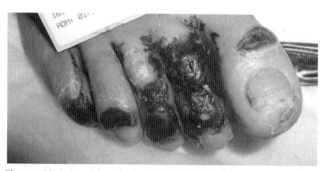

Figure 48.4 Arterial wound: significant necrotic tissue involved in all toes. This resulted in a transmetatarsal amputation.

disorders; (ii) patient education; (iii) cessation of smoking; (iv) good control of diabetes; (v) off-weighting of the affected area coupled with good wound care to assist in wound healing; and (vi) use of innovative ointments and procedures to assist wound healing, including growth factors, synthetic skin grafting and hyperbaric oxygen. At this stage a referral may be needed to a prosthetist/orthotist for custom-molded shoes or inserts. Keeping the callus thin

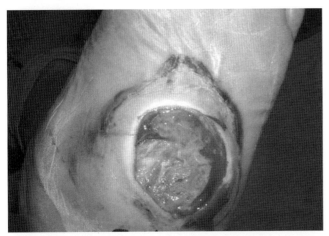

Figure 48.6 Neuropathic ulcer with 'rocker bottom foot'.

by filing or sharp debridement will maintain good skin integrity in the periwound skin and promote contraction of wound edges. Keeping the wound moist, free from bacterial colonization and devoid of nonviable tissue are fundamental for the care of diabetic/neuropathic wounds.

Pressure

Pressure ulcers are a serious problem that can affect patients regardless of their living environments. Pressure ulcers lead to pain, longer hospital stays and slower recovery. They are lesions that usually develop over bony prominences and are caused by unrelieved pressure, resulting in damage to underlying tissue. The four main risk factors for developing pressure ulcers are shear, moisture, impaired mobility and malnutrition. In 2007 the National Pressure Ulcer Advisory Panel (NPUAP) redefined pressure ulcers, including the original four stages and adding two stages on deep tissue injury and unstageable pressure ulcers (see Box 48.1).

The staging system for pressure ulcers classifies the degree of tissue damage. It is important to note that pressure ulcers do not necessarily progress from stage I to stage IV, and they do not heal from stage IV to stage I, i.e. documenting reverse staging is a misnomer. Reverse staging implies that the tissue reforms with all of its original components. New tissue formation is scar tissue and not the normal epidermis/dermis organization. The treatment

---

Box 48.1 *National pressure ulcer advisory panel: stages defined*

A pressure ulcer is localized injury to the skin and/or underlying tissue, usually over a bony prominence, as a result of pressure, or pressure in combination with shear. A number of contributing or confounding factors are also associated with pressure ulcers; the significance of these factors is yet to be elucidated.

PRESSURE ULCER STAGES/CATEGORIES

Category/stage I: non-blanchable erythema

Intact skin with non-blanchable redness of a localized area usually over a bony prominence. Darkly pigmented skin may not have visible blanching; intact skin with non-blanchable redness of a localized area usually over a bony prominence. Darkly pigmented skin may not have visible blanching; its color may differ from surrounding area. The area may be painful, firm, soft, warmer or cooler as compared to adjacent tissue. Category I may be difficult to detect in individuals with dark skin tones. May indicate 'at risk' persons.

Category/stage II: partial-thickness loss

Partial-thickness loss of dermis presenting as a shallow open ulcer with a red–pink wound bed, without slough. May also present as an intact or open/ruptured serum-filled or serosanguineous-filled blister. Presents as a shiny or dry shallow ulcer without slough or bruising*. This category should not be used to describe skin tears, tape burns, incontinence associated dermatitis, maceration or excoriation.

Category/stage III: full-thickness tissue loss

Full-thickness tissue loss. Subcutaneous fat may be visible but bone, tendon or muscle are *not* exposed. Slough may be present but does not obscure the depth of tissue loss. *May* include undermining and tunneling. The depth of a Stage III pressure ulcer varies by anatomical location. The bridge of the nose, ear, occiput and malleolus do not have (adipose) subcutaneous tissue and Stage III ulcers can be shallow. In contrast, areas of significant

*Bruising indicates deep tissue injury.

adiposity can develop extremely deep Stage III pressure ulcers. Bone/tendon is not visible or directly palpable.

Category/stage IV: full-thickness tissue loss

Full-thickness tissue loss with exposed bone, tendon or muscle. Slough or eschar may be present. Often includes undermining and tunneling. The depth of a Stage IV pressure ulcer varies by anatomical location. The bridge of the nose, ear, occiput and malleolus do not have (adipose) subcutaneous tissue and these ulcers can be shallow. Stage IV ulcers can extend into muscle and/or supporting structures (e.g. fascia, tendon or joint capsule) making osteomyelitis or osteitis likely to occur. Exposed bone/muscle is visible or directly palpable.

ADDITIONAL CATEGORIES/STAGES FOR THE UNITED STATES OF AMERICA

Unstageable/unclassified: full-thickness skin or tissue loss – depth unknown

Full-thickness tissue loss in which actual depth of the ulcer is completely obscured by slough (yellow, tan, gray, green or brown) and/or eschar (tan, brown or black) in the wound bed. Until enough slough and/or eschar are removed to expose the base of the wound, the true depth cannot be determined; but it will be either a Stage III or IV. Stable (dry, adherent, intact without erythema or fluctuance) eschar on the heels serves as 'the body's natural (biological) cover' and should not be removed.

Suspected deep tissue injury – depth unknown

Purple or maroon localized area of discolored intact skin or blood-filled blister due to damage of underlying soft tissue from pressure and/or *shear*. The area may be preceded by tissue that is painful, firm, mushy, boggy, warmer or cooler as compared to adjacent tissue. Deep tissue injury may be difficult to detect in individuals with dark skin tones. Evolution may include a thin blister over a dark wound bed. The wound may further evolve and become covered by thin eschar. Evolution may be rapid, exposing additional layers of tissue even with optimal treatment.

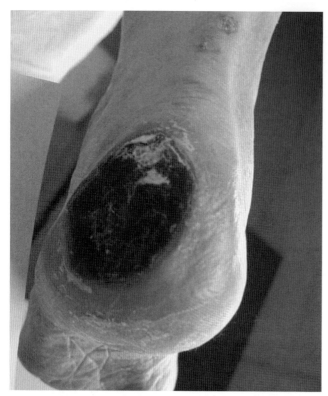

Figure 48.7 Left posterior/lateral heel ulcer. Note the 100% non-viable tissue (necrotic) covering.

of pressure ulcers involves six major areas: (i) control of underlying medical and nutritional disorders; (ii) management of tissue loads; (iii) ulcer care; (iv) topical therapy, i.e. enzymatic/autolytic debridement; (v) management of bacterial colonization and infection; and (vi) education. In terms of the management of tissue loads, it is paramount in the treatment of pressure ulcers to keep pressure off the wound bed. Patients with heel ulcerations (Fig. 48.7) will benefit from pressure relief provided by many different types of off-weighting boots, such as the multipodus splint and/or the RIK boot™ (KCI Products, Boulder, CO). Paralyzed patients will need consistent weight-shifting when sitting and lying, as well as proper cushioning in wheelchairs and mattresses (Fig. 48.8).

Individuals with limited mobility should always be assessed for additional factors that increase the risk of developing pressure ulcers. These factors include immobility, incontinence, nutritional factors and altered levels of consciousness. The multidisciplinary team should adopt a validated risk assessment tool such as the Braden Scale or the Norton Scale (Forms 48.4 and 48.5). The results recorded on these scales should be documented and used periodically to reassess the patient's risk.

THERAPEUTIC INTERVENTION

A wide variety of interventions are used by physical therapists to treat patients with chronic dermal wounds (Tables 48.5 and 48.6). When physical therapy intervention is utilized, the two primary goals are: (i) to directly amplify the body's natural healing processes, and (ii) to eliminate factors that block the activity of the body's natural healing processes.

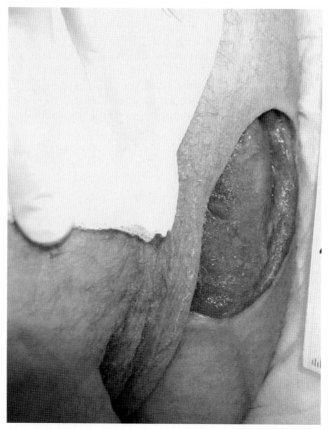

Figure 48.8 Right ischial tuberosity pressure ulcer, full thickness.

Hydrotherapy, the oldest known modality of physical therapy, is crucial for the cleansing of wounds. Over the years, hydrotherapy has taken various forms, such as whirlpools, water piks and pulsatile lavage. The combination of water, heat and agitation is successful in cleansing, softening necrotic tissue, assisting with the debridement process and removing residues left after the application of topical agents (see Table 48.6).

Compression therapy is the primary modality used to control edema (Stillman, 2005). Edema is a major factor in the lack of healing of lower extremity ulcers complicated by venous insufficiency. Compression devices assist in decreasing interstitial fluid. The pressure shift encourages the movement of fluid and proteins from the interstitial spaces into the veins and lymphatics. Compression therapy also increases the efficiency of the muscle pump, as well as physically approximating the valves of the veins. Compression therapy can be provided by a variety of devices including intermittent/sequential compression pumps, custom-made elastic stockings, Unna boots, elastic bandages and ready-made elastic stockings. The goal is to provide sufficient compression to stimulate fluid resorption. The compression found in elastic garments ranges from 8 mmHg to 60 mmHg. Numerous multilayer and multiday (usually 5–7 days) compression bandages, with a compression approaching 40 mmHg, are on the market today. The challenge for the patient with these dressings is not to get them wet, i.e. the patient must cover the leg for showering. Pressures greater than 40 mmHg may occlude blood flow, so caution is necessary if arterial insufficiency

Patient's name:				Evaluator's name:		Date of assessment:	

	1	2	3	4
Sensory perception: ability to respond meaningfully to pressure-related discomfort	**1. Completely limited:** unresponsive (does not moan, flinch or grasp) to painful stimuli because of diminished level of consciousness or sedation OR a limited ability to feel pain over most of body surface	**2. Very limited:** responds only to painful stimuli; cannot communicate discomfort except by moaning or restlessness OR has a sensory impairment that limits the ability to feel pain or discomfort over half of the body	**3. Slightly limited:** responds to verbal commands but cannot always communicate discomfort or need to be turned OR has some sensory impairment that limits ability to feel pain or discomfort in one or two extremities	**4. No impairment:** responds to verbal commands; has no sensory deficit that would limit ability to feel or avoid pain or discomfort
Moisture: degree to which skin is exposed to moisture	**1. Constantly moist:** skin is kept moist almost constantly by perspiration, urine etc.; dampness is detected every time patient is moved or turned	**2. Moist:** skin is often, but not always, moist; linen must be changed at least once a shift	**3. Occasionally moist:** skin is occasionally moist, requiring an extra linen change approximately once a day	**4. Rarely moist:** skin is usually dry; linen changed only at routine intervals
Activity: degree of physical activity	**1. Bedfast:** confined to bed	**2. Chairfast:** ability to walk severely limited or nonexistent; cannot bear own weight and/or must be assisted into chair or wheelchair	**3. Walks occasionally:** walks occasionally during day but for very short distances, with or without assistance; spends majority of each shift in bed or chair	**4. Walks frequently:** walks outside the room at least twice a day and inside room at least once every 2 hours during waking hours
Mobility: ability to change and control body position	**1. Completely immobile:** does not make even slight changes in body or extremity position without assistance	**2. Very limited:** makes occasional slight changes in body or extremity position but unable to make frequent or significant changes independently	**3. Slightly limited:** makes frequent, though slight, changes in body or extremity position independently	**4. No limitations:** makes major and frequent changes in position without assistance
Nutrition: usual food intake pattern	**1. Very poor:** never eats a complete meal; rarely eats more than one-third of any food	**2. Probably inadequate:** rarely eats a complete meal and generally eats only about one-half of any food offered;	**3. Adequate:** eats over one-half of most meals; eats a total of four servings of protein (meat, dairy products) each day;	**4. Excellent:** eats most of every meal; never refuses a meal; usually eats a total of four or more servings of meat and dairy

(Continued)

Form 48.4 Braden Scale for predicting pressure-sore risk.

				products; occasionally eats between meals; does not require supplementation
	offered; eats two servings or less of protein (meat or dairy products) per day; takes fluids poorly; does not take a liquid dietary supplement OR is NPO and/or maintained on clear liquids or IV for more than 5 days	protein intake includes only three servings of meat or dairy products per day; occasionally takes a dietary supplement OR receives less than optimum amount of liquid diet or fed by tube	occasionally refuses a meal but will usually take a supplement if offered OR is on a tube feeding or TPN regimen, which probably meets most of nutritional needs	
Friction and shear	1. **Problem:** requires moderate to maximum assistance in moving; complete lifting without sliding against sheets is impossible; frequently slides down in bed or chair, requiring frequent repositioning with maximum assistance; spasticity, contractures or agitation leads to almost constant friction	2. **Potential problem:** moves feebly or requires minimum assistance; during a move, skin probably slides to some extent against sheets, chair, restraints or other devices; maintains relatively good position in chair or bed most of the time but occasionally slides down	3. **No apparent problem:** moves in bed and chair independently and has sufficient muscle strength to lift up completely during move; maintains good position in bed or chair at all times	
				Total score

From Braden BJ, Bergstrom N 1987 A conceptual schema for the study of the etiology of pressure sores. Rehabil Nurs 12:8–12, with permission.
IV, intravenously; NPO, nothing by mouth; TPN, total parenteral nutrition

Form 48.4 (Continued)

	Physical condition		Mental condition		Activity		Mobility		Incontinent		Total score
	Good	4	Alert	4	Ambulant	4	Full	4	No	4	4
	Fair	3	Apathetic	3	Walks with help	3	Slightly limited	3	Occasionally	3	3
	Poor	2	Confused	2	Chairbound	2	Very limited	2	Usually (urine)	2	2
	Very bad	1	Stupor	1	Bed	1	Immobile	1	Doubly	1	1

Name: Date:

From Norton D, McLaren R, Exton-Smith AN 1962 An investigation of geriatric nursing problems in the hospital. National Corporation for the Care of Old People (now the Centre for Policy on Ageing), London, with permission.

Form 48.5 Norton scale.

Table 48.5 Therapeutic interventions

Treatment	Used For	Clinical Applications	Physiological Response
Hydrotherapy/ pulsatile lavage	Neurotrophic, venous, arterial, pressure and diabetic ulcers; burns; acute trauma	Cleanse; debride; soak off dressings	Superficial heat/cold; micromassage; increased moisture
Ultrasound	Neurotrophic, venous, arterial and diabetic ulcers	Debride; promote clean wound bed	Increase microcirculation; edema absorption; superficial/deep heat
Compression	Venous, arterial and diabetic ulcers; burns	Reduce edema	Decrease venous hypertension; increase venous return
Electrical stimulation	Neurotrophic, venous, arterial, pressure and diabetic ulcers; burns; acute trauma	Debride; decrease infection and pain; increase circulation; promote closure	Increase circulation; bactericidal effects; increase fibroblast activity; decrease edema
Pulsed electromagnetic fields	Venous, arterial, pressure and diabetic ulcers; acute trauma	Reduce pain and edema	Edema reduction; increase transport of cutaneous oxygen

is suspected and the use of compression on arterial wounds is dependent upon the ABPI and the amount of edema. An ABPI should also be performed to rule out concomitant arterial issues. In general practice, the compression stocking is donned before getting out of bed and removed before bedtime. One common problem in the geriatric population is the inability to pull on the compression stocking. In these cases, compression pumps are a great help in fluid resorption. Compression stockings should be replaced every 9–12 months, depending upon wash/wear times, because they tend to lose their compressive qualities over time. Patients tend to neglect replacing them (usually because of cost) and this can lead to reoccurrence.

Ultrasound (non-thermal) has been found to be effective in enhancing wound healing, particularly when venous insufficiency is a major factor. The 3-MHz unit has been proposed to be the most effective frequency because most energy is absorbed by the superficial tissues. Ultrasound has been found to enhance the body's ability to move from the inflammatory to the proliferative phase of wound healing. It has also been associated with less dense and more resilient scar tissue. Ultrasound must be administered through a medium such as hydrogel or a hydrogel sheet. The treatment can be administered either

along the periphery or directly over the wound bed (see Table 48.6 for parameters).

Electrical stimulation has been advocated over the years for the enhancement of wound healing, regardless of the underlying cause. Some studies have shown the effectiveness of electrical stimulation in enhancing wound healing (Zhao et al., 2010; Recio et al., 2012). High voltage electrical stimulation has been shown to alter the pH of wound chemistry and facilitate a decrease in inflammation. Current protocols result in removal of nonviable tissue from the wound bed.

Sussman (1998) advocates the following parameters:

- Settings for the inflammatory phase of healing:
  - negative polarity;
  - 100–128 pulses per second (pps);
  - 100–150 V;
  - 60 minutes for 5–7 days/week.
- Settings for the epithelialization phase of healing:
  - alternating current: 3 days positive, 3 days negative etc.
  - 64 pps;
  - 100–150 V;
  - 60 minutes for 5–7 days/week.

Table 48.6 **Treatment suggestions**	
Hydrotherapy	
Whirlpool	10–20 minutes per treatment session (daily); temperature 92–99°F (33–37°C)
Pulsatile lavage	10–30 minutes in entirety, periodic placement of tube throughout the wound; room temperature saline solution
Ultrasound	
3 MHz pulsed (partial-thickness wounds) and 1 MHz (full-thickness wounds)	0.5–1.5 W/cm² for 1 min/cm² of wound; pulsed, 20–40% duty cycle; use hydrogel medium or conductive gel; use over the wound or around the wound periphery
Compression	
Sequential/intermittent	Ideally, patient is supine with lower extremity elevated; use a pressure at least 20 mmHg below the diastolic reading of the blood pressure taken in the treatment position; treat for a minimum of 1 hour; treat in morning if possible; follow with static compression wrap
Static	Wrap bandage from metatarsophalangeal joints to two fingers below the fibula head; be certain to apply equal pressure; overlap bandage by at least two-thirds with each wrap; cover with protective stocking or additional elastic wrap
Electrical stimulation (high-voltage pulse current)	Initially (−) polarity, 50–80 pps, 100–150 V; after five visits (or when wound is clean), (+) polarity, 80–100 pps, 100 V; electrode placement: dispersive pad proximal, foil electrode with saline-soaked or conductive hydrogel pad placed directly into the wound
Pulsed electromagnetic fields	
Thermal	5 minute warm-up (5/10 cycles); 20 minute treatment (10/12 cycles); 5 minute cool down (5/10 cycles); treat once per day
Nonthermal	
Acute wound	30 minute cycle, cycle 6
Chronic wound	45 minute cycle, cycle 4; treat once per day

Utilization of a hydrogel-impregnated or saline-soaked gauze as a wound contact conductor is optimal. Petrolatum-based products will impede the efficacy of electrical stimulation. The dispersive pad (which should be larger than the wound-contact pad) should be placed proximal to the wound surface. The pads should be placed close together for shallow wounds and further apart for deeper or undermining/tunneling wounds.

Pulsed electromagnetic fields are a relatively new entity in wound care. Solid-state equipment generates radio waves into the tissues, creating an electrical charge. The specifications include using radio waves with a frequency of 27.12 MHz. To date, conclusive scientific evidence for the efficacy of pulsed electromagnetic fields in wound care has not been established, although several clinical trials have been completed in the US (see Table 48.6 for parameters).

Total contact casting is used primarily in the treatment of patients with neuropathic plantar ulcers that are classified as grades I and II. The goal of this treatment is to remove weight-bearing forces from inflamed tissues and immobilize them so that healing can occur. Following the application of a total contact cast, a patient must be instructed in partial weight-bearing with an appropriate assistive device. Generally, these patients have altered sensation, which makes an exact fit of the cast crucial. The cast is generally reapplied every 1–2 weeks; however, loosening of the cast, large amounts of drainage or damage to the cast requires premature removal. In some cases, a bivalve cast is appropriate. The patient must understand that the bivalve cast is not to be removed until bedtime.

Currently, there are many skin substitutes available on the market for increasing the wound healing rate. These skin substitutes have all of the components of normal skin, including all 21 growth factors, except for hair follicles and sweat glands. They are applied by a physician and are accompanied with strict protocols for dressing changes.

Additional products for treatment of neuropathic ulcers are specific mediums containing the dominant skin growth factor (Stillman, 2005). These prostaglandin growth factors play a large role in wound healing. Currently, a few products on the market use topical applications of growth factors. There are currently a few products available, such as Regranex™ (Ortho-McNeil, Somerville, NJ), that use topical application of growth factors. This gel-type medium is an expensive product but has been successful in speeding up the closure of different types of wounds. A clean granulating wound bed is necessary to increase the effectiveness of the gel. They have biological activity similar to that of endogenous platelet-derived growth factor, which includes promoting the chemotactic recruitment and proliferation of cells involved in wound repair and enhancing the formation of granulation tissue. A clean granulating wound bed is necessary to increase the effectiveness of the gel. Regranex™ has biological activity similar to that of endogenous platelet-derived growth factor, which includes promoting the chemotactic recruitment and proliferation of cells involved in wound repair and enhancing the formation of granulation tissue.

The wound VAC® (vacuum-assisted closure) device has significantly decreased the healing time for pressure ulcerations. In this technique, a special sterile sponge-type dressing is cut slightly smaller than the diameter of the wound. This is covered with an occlusive dressing and hooked to a suction unit with a canister/reservoir to collect wound fluid. The wound VAC is then used to wick all of the air and fluid away from the wound bed. Blood flow at the wound surface is increased and the wound edges are pulled together. This author has found it a very effective adjunct to traditional wound-healing methods (see www.kci1.com for further information).

All members of the wound care team should be aware of the importance of nutrition and recognize that adequate calories and protein, vitamins A, C and E, zinc, glucosamine (Stillman, 2005) and the amino acids arginine and glutamine (MacKay & Miller, 2003) are important for proper wound healing.

HYPERBARIC OXYGEN (HBO)

The definition of hyperbaric oxygen is a treatment in which 100% oxygen (O_2) is delivered to a patient at greater than two times the normal atmospheric pressure at sea level. The goal is to increase the partial pressure of oxygen in plasma. HBO is applied in a chamber with the patient in it and the increased pressure and O_2 improves oxygenation of the blood which enhances wound healing. Chambers can also be multi-place walk-in, where multiple patients can be treated simultaneously.

Oxygen (O_2) is often utilized during the inflammatory and repair phases of wound healing. Its presence is essential to O_2-dependent neutrophils, macrophages and fibroblasts. The presence of O_2 assists not only with control of infection via release of endotoxins to kill bacteria, but also increases the effectiveness of antibiotics. HBO enhances angiogenesis via stimulation of growth factors and collagen matrices.

Indications are numerous and include but are not limited to:

- Infected wounds
- Traumatic wounds: crush injuries, compartment syndrome
- Compromised skin grafts
- Radiation and thermal burns
- Non-healing wounds: diabetic, vascular insufficiency ulcers and chronic non-healing ulcers of any etiology.

HBO is often utilized when traditional management of wounds is ineffective. The introduction of increased oxygenation not only kills off bacteria but lowers the overload on the immune system and healing can begin. Consequently the increase in angiogenesis and decreased bacterial load lead to greater percentages of skin graft adherence and increased healing rates of damaged tissue due to irradiation and burns.

Patients with diabetes can also benefit from HBO, as greater O_2 delivery to starving tissues results in an improved opportunity for angiogenesis. However, the diabetic patient should have a Doppler (ABPI) score of at least 0.5 in order to consider a trial. Additionally, transcutaneous oxygen pressure (TcPO$_2$) measures the amount of O_2 in the skin. It is a noninvasive method to quantify skin oxygenation and is particularly useful for evaluation of cutaneous ischemia in advanced stages of arteriopathy of the lower limbs.

Diabetic Foot Ulcer

The ulcer must be categorized as Wagner 3 or 4 (see Table 48.2) and TcPO$_2$ should also be assessed.

Hyperbaric therapy is an expensive procedure but has had excellent results in treatment of chronic wounds (Kaur et al., 2012). In addition to the cost of the therapy, there are side-effects to HBO, including but not limited to:

- Ear and sinus barotrauma
- Myopia
- Aggravation of congestive heart failure
- Oxygen seizures
- Pulmonary barotrauma
- Chronic obstructive pulmonary disease (COPD).

Contraindications include pneumothorax, as well as medications that may combine adversely with HBO to cause additional medical issues. These medications must be evaluated by the patient's physician. Additional requirements before HBO can be considered and include:

1. Arterial insufficiency: vascular surgery, if appropriate, must be done before HBO can be considered. If the patient is not a surgical candidate, than HBO may be considered. Vascular testing must be done to ascertain blood flow status. TcPO$_2$ should also be assessed.
2. Soft radionecrosis: any body part that has received radiation, regardless of how long it has been, and has a non-healing ulcer, may be considered for HBO.

Chronic Osteomyelitis

A wound must have a minimum of 6 weeks of conservative antibiotic care (PO or IV) to the wound, as well as a positive bone scan or X-ray, before consideration of HBO therapy.

Preservation of Failing or Failed Flap or Graft

Wounds that have led to amputations or partial-thickness or full-thickness skin grafts that are now either dehiscing, or showing tissue death, also qualify for HBO. The sooner HBO is started after failure has been noted, the better the expected response.

THE ROLE OF EXERCISE IN WOUND CARE

Aerobic exercise, has a positive effect on wound healing. Emery et al. (2005) found that 1 hour of aerobic exercise at 70% of the maximum heart rate, three times a week, increased wound healing in healthy individuals. The mean healing time was 29.2 days in the exercise group compared with 38.9 days in the nonexercise group. The authors theorized that exercise may increase blood flow to the skin and skin oxygen tension. The subjects in this report were healthy older men and women; the authors suggest further research including patients with comorbidities.

Finally, it is important for all medical providers to treat the patient as a whole. It is likely that the patient's wound has had other physiological, musculoskeletal or biomechanical effects that require expertise. It is important to treat the entire patient, not just the open wound area. This is ethically correct as well as financially sound.

CONCLUSION

Effective intervention for wound care requires thorough examination and evaluation and an individualized treatment plan established by a multidisciplinary team. The team must coordinate a plan that focuses on removing factors that contribute to nonhealing status and choosing an intervention that will foster healing. This plan may require multiple revisions before healing is achieved. When healing has been attained, the patient, family and caregivers must be educated in continued care and prevention. Clinicians who frequently treat open wounds must continually keep up to date on new products, dressings and techniques for the effective healing of wounds.

Acknowledgements

Special thanks to Drs Michael Flood and Mark Evans for their continued hard work and dedication to their patients. They were invaluable in this chapter's development.

Pam Unger wrote this chapter in the first edition of this text.

REFERENCES

Emery CF, Kiecolt-Glaser JK, Glaser R et al 2005 Exercise accelerates wound healing among healthy older adults: a preliminary investigation. J Gerontol A Biol Sci Med Sci 60:1432–1436

Kaur S, Pawar M, Banerjee N et al 2012 Evaluation of the efficacy of hyperbaric oxygen therapy in the management of chronic nonhealing ulcer and role of periwound transcutaneous oximetry as a predictor of wound healing response: a randomized prospective controlled trial. J Anaesthesiol Clin Pharmacol 28:70–75

MacKay D, Miller A 2003 Nutritional support for wound care. Altern Med Rev 8:359–377

Mowrer R 2004 Wound Care for Older Adults: Implications for the Physical Therapist Assistant. American Physical Therapy Association, La Crosse, WI, pp. 14–15

NPUAP (National Pressure Ulcers Advisory Panel) 2007 NPUAP Pressure Ulcer Stages/Categories. www.npuap.org/resources/educational

Recio A, Fetter C, Schneider A et al 2012 High-voltage electrical stimulation for the management of stage III and IV pressure ulcers among adults with spinal cord injury: demonstration of its utility for recalcitrant wounds below the level injury. J Spinal Cord Med 35:58–63

Stadelmann W, Digenis A, Tobin G 1998 Physiology and healing dynamics of chronic cutaneous wounds. Am J Surg 176(Suppl 2A):26–38

Stillman RM 2005 Wound Care. www.emedicine.com/med/topic2754.htm

Sussman C 1998 Electrical stimulation. www.medicaledu.com/estim.htm

Wagner F 1981 The dysvascular foot: a system for diagnosis and treatment. Foot Ankle 2:64–122

Zhao M, Penninger J, Isseroff R 2010 Electrical activation of wound-healing pathways. Adv Skin Wound Care 23:567–573

Chapter 49

The insensitive foot

JENNIFER M. BOTTOMLEY

CHAPTER CONTENTS

INTRODUCTION

Insensitivity of the foot is the usual end result of numerous pathological conditions that affect the elderly. Chronic diseases such as diabetes mellitus, Hansen's disease, peripheral vascular disease, Raynaud's disease, deep vein thrombosis, spinal cord injury (e.g. spinal stenosis, tumors), peripheral nerve injuries, hormonal imbalances and vitamin B-complex deficiencies produce breakdown of the microvascular structures with diminution of sympathetic nerve endings and somatic sensory receptors leading to neuropathic conditions of the foot. These pathologies lead to a decrease in circulatory and peripheral nerve integrity, which results in edema, discoloration, diminished skin status, increased pain, absence of sensation and, ultimately, a decrease in functional mobility (Birke, 2002; Jeffcoate & Harding, 2003; Driver et al., 2010).

Typical warning signs such as changes in gait patterns and pain associated with foot pathologies are absent in the insensitive foot. Repetitive stress, coupled with the loss of protective sensation, is the primary cause of foot ulcerations. The lack of a warning system for pain and abnormal stress on the plantar surface of the foot predispose the neuropathic foot to injury and ulceration (Boulton, 2012). However, if the mechanism of injury and the risk factors are recognized (Table 49.1), foot ulcerations are preventable and treatable (Bottomley, 2012).

Neuropathic changes in the insensitive foot include progressive distal polyneuropathy, ischemic mononeuropathy, amyotrophy and neuroarthropathy (Boulton, 2012). A combination of sensory, autonomic, and motor neuropathies of the foot results in symmetrical or asymmetrical loss of perception of pain and temperature. Sympathetic denervation can lead to a progressive mixed-fiber neuropathy with a loss in light touch and vibratory sensation and motor loss in the intrinsic muscles of the foot (Birke, 2002; Jeffcoate & Harding, 2003). Characteristic foot deformities such as hyperextension of the metatarsophalangeal joints, clawing of the toes and distal migration of the adipose cushions (fat pads) under the heel and metatarsal heads result in abnormal weight-bearing patterns and increased plantar pressures (Lemaster et al., 2003). Tissue damage to the insensitive foot may result from continuous pressure that causes ischemia or from concentrated high pressure, heat or cold, repetitive mechanical stress, or infection of the tissues (Driver et al., 2010).

Amyotrophic changes result from a lack of nourishment to the musculature. There is progressive weakening and wasting of muscles accompanied initially by an aching or stabbing pain and resulting in the total loss of muscle function due to atrophy, paresthesia, paralysis, and loss of sensory input (Jeffcoate & Harding, 2003).

Table 49.1 Risk factors in the neuropathic foot

Risk Factor	Possible Injury
Loss of protective sensation	Absence of pain-warning input
High plantar pressures	Ulcers occurring at peak pressure sites
Autonomic neuropathy	Dehydrated inelastic skin
Previous ulceration or amputation	Concentration of stress over scar or lesion
Foot deformities	Increased local pressures
Neuropathic fractures	Increased plantar pressures and foot instability
Abnormal foot function	Abnormal load application
High activity level	Increased cumulative stress
Vascular disease	Devitalized tissue susceptible to injury, poor healing
Inadequate footwear or foot care	Decreased protection, instability, poor hygiene
Visual loss	Inappropriate assessment of environment, inability to inspect feet
Poor insulin regulation	Complications of diabetes

Neuropathic arthropathy results from joint erosions, unrecognized fractures, demineralization and devitalization of the bones and articulations of the foot. Typically, these changes result from routine weight-bearing activities in the absence of normal protective proprioceptive and nociceptive functions of the peripheral sensory system. In the limb with intact sensation, pain inhibits functional activities and further trauma to the joints so that the hypertrophic or reparative phases of callus formation can commence. In the insensate limb; however, the injured part is repeatedly traumatized, leading to increased hyperemia and resorption of damaged bone (Pai & Ledoux, 2011; Resnik & Borgia, 2011).

Loss of sensation in the joints and bones of the foot predisposes the neuropathic foot to bony destruction. Midtarsal fractures or dislocations and hypertrophic bone formation may lead to a Charcot's deformity, which is the collapse of the foot into severe rocker-bottom foot deformity. Charcot's fracture is evidenced by swelling and increased temperature in the area of bone involvement (Frykberg & Belczyk, 2008). Clinically, neuropathic fractures should be suspected in all patients with signs of inflammation in the absence of an open wound. Differential diagnosis includes: cellulitis, osteomyelitis, pyarthrosis and reflex sympathetic dystrophy.

EVALUATION OF THE NEUROPATHIC FOOT

Regular and comprehensive screening of the neuropathic foot is essential for early identification of risk factors that may predispose an elderly individual to injury (Form 49.1). The foot screening is a brief examination to identify the history of any previous ulceration, motor weakness, sensory dysfunction, or deformities that would predispose the foot to local areas of high stress. Circulatory status, color, temperature, general condition and the presence of edema or skin lesions should be assessed. Based on the foot screening, the relative risk of foot complications can be determined for each individual (Bottomley, 2012).

The level of sensory loss that places an individual at risk for foot injury is referred to as loss of protective sensation. The use of nylon monofilaments calibrated to bend at 10g of force (Semmes–Weinstein monofilaments) is a precise method of determining loss of sensation. The inability to feel a monofilament of 5.07g has been determined to be the level at which loss of protective sensation occurs (Birke, 2002). A risk classification scheme identifies the individuals most likely to benefit from protective footwear and education (Box 49.1).

EVALUATING SENSATION AND NEUROLOGICAL INVOLVEMENT

Protective sensation, as defined by Nawcozenski and Birke, is 5.07g of pressure using the Semmes–Weinstein monofilaments. Specific evaluation of the entire plantar surface of the foot determines areas of sensory loss that are vulnerable to breakdown (Birke, 2002; Van Schie, 2005).

Vibratory and temperature sense are diminished very early in the process of peripheral vascular disease, and that loss compromises proprioception, kinesthesia and awareness of temperature gradients.

The neurological examination requires a reflex hammer, a tuning fork (128cps) and Semmes–Weinstein filaments. Testing for vibratory, proprioceptive, temperature and protective sensation should be done with the patient's eyes closed. Distinguish the boundaries of any hyper- or hypoesthesia and determine whether these patterns are symmetrical or asymmetrical. The absence or presence of sweating should be noted. Reflexes to be tested include the patellar reflex and the ankle jerk. As the ankle jerk is increasingly difficult to elicit with increasing age; it may appear to be absent. To aid eliciting this reflex, gently pronate and dorsiflex the foot putting tension on the Achilles tendon and gently tap the tendon. Test for the Babinski reflex to determine whether there is a superficial plantar response. To determine if there is clonus, forcibly dorsiflex the foot at the ankle and clonus will be initiated at end range. To test for loss of balance, have the individual stand with eyes closed and feet close together and compare this to the same stance with the eyes open (Romberg's sign) (Chantelau et al., 2007; Kruse et al., 2010; Ites et al., 2011).

Muscle strength should be tested in all lower extremity muscles using a graded manual muscle test. Again, symmetry should be noted. Gait evaluation is a helpful adjunct to muscular evaluation to determine unsteady gain patterns, foot-drop or the presence of a 'steppage' gait. Range of motion and joint mobility should be evaluated and any deformities (e.g. Charcot joints, hammer, claw, or mallet toes, hallux abductus valgus) should be noted, as these abnormalities are usually indicative of intrinsic foot muscle weakness. Trophic nail changes should also be evaluated (Driver et al., 2010).

The Semmes-Weinstein monofilament instrument is a reproducible and accurate way to test sensation, and is reliable in predicting which individuals are at risk for ulceration due to loss of protective sensation. The Carville group from the G.W. Long Hansen's Disease Center in Carville, LA, measured protective sensation using the Semmes–Weinstein monofilaments and found that individuals who could not feel the 5.07 monofilament were at greater risk for skin breakdown than those who could feel this level of stimulation. They demonstrated that 5.07 was the threshold of protective sensation. Standardization of sensory testing is crucial in evaluation, so that adequate protective measures can be taken to prevent feet at risk from developing ulcers (Birke, 2002; Boulton, 2012).

EVALUATION OF CIRCULATORY STATUS

Vascular evaluation should include the palpation and grading of the femoral, popliteal, dorsalis pedis and posterior tibial pulses, and the observation of other clinical signs and symptoms indicating vascular compromise in the lower extremities. These include intermittent claudication, foot temperature (i.e. cold feet), nocturnal and rest pain (including pain relieved by dependency), blanching on elevation, delayed venous filling time after elevation, dependent rubor, atrophic skin, absence of hair growth and presence of gangrene. Any lesions

_____

Date: _____

Name: _____

Address: _____

Phone: ( ) _____

Sex: ____ Date of birth: _____

Language or communication problems: No   Yes   (describe) _____

Primary doctor/podiatrist: _____

Address: _____

Phone: ( ) _____

Subjective Data

Medical history: _____

1. Do you have:
   - Arthritis _____
   - Circulatory problems _____
   - Heart disease _____
   - Diabetes mellitus _____
   - Kidney problems _____
   - High blood pressure _____
   - Foot problems _____
   - Eye problems _____
   - Thyroid problems _____
   - Hearing problems _____
   - Vertigo _____
   - Dizziness _____
   - Fractured (Fx) hip _____

2. Did you have an injury in the:

		Left leg		Right leg	
		Sprain	Fx	Sprain	Fx
No					
Yes	Hip				
	Knee				
	Ankle				
	Foot				
	Back				

3. Are you experiencing any leg pain?

		Left leg	Right leg
No			
Yes	Hip		
	Knee		

4. Are you experiencing any foot pain?

		Left leg	Right leg
No			
Yes	Aching		
	Burning		
	Stabbing		
	Nail pain		
	Shoe pain		
	Metatarsal heads		
	Toes		

(Continued)

Form 49.1 Foot-screening evaluation guide

Pain increased:

	Left leg	Right leg
When standing		
When walking		
When wearing shoes		
In the morning		
In the afternoon		
At other times (describe)		

Objective Data

1. Ambulates without assistance?   No   Yes
2. Ambulates with assistive devices?   No   Yes

Cane	
Walker	
Crutches	
Other	

3. Falls?   No   Yes   (describe) _____

4. Distance ambulated?   Home   One block   Two blocks   Five blocks   1 mile   Unlimited

5. Regular exercise?   No   Yes

6. Examination of feet (remove shoes and stockings)

	Left foot		Right foot	
	Unacceptable	Acceptable	Unacceptable	Acceptable
Cleanliness of foot?				
Socks/stockings a good fit?				
Proper fitting shoes? ___	Short		Short	
___	Long		Long	
___	Narrow		Narrow	
___	Worn down		Worn down	
Shoe wear: Heel ___				
Sole ___				
Lateral counter ___				

7. Problems

• Bunions

	Left foot	Right foot
HAV		
Taylor		

		Left foot					Right foot				
		I	II	III	IV	V	I	II	III	IV	V
• Calluses	Spin										
	Pinch										
	IPK										
	Sub										
	Shear										
• Corns	Metatarsal heads										
	Heloma molle										
	Heloma duram										
• Involuted nails											
• Ingrown toenails											
• Nail trophic changes											

(Continued)

Form 49.1 (Continued)

• Circulatory problems

	DPP: 0		PTP: 0			DPP: 0		PTP: 0	
	1+ 2+ 3+		1+ 2+ 3+			1+ 2+ 3+		1+ 2+ 3+		
• Toe clubbing										
• Toe deformities: Hammer										
Claw										
Mallet										
Overlap										
Hallux										
	I	II	III	IV	V	I	II	III	IV	V

	Left leg	Right leg
• Foot/ankle deformities		
• Dermatitis (PI) fungus infection		
• Dry scaly skin		
• Edema — Foot		
Ankle		
Extremity		

• Infection (describe): _____

• Other: _____

Foot Screening Evaluation

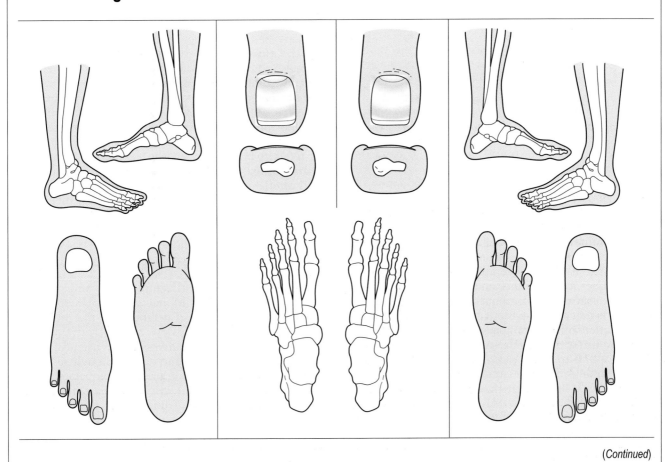

(Continued)

Form 49.1 (Continued)

Comments: _____

_____

_____

_____

Assessment: _____

_____

_____

_____

Recommend:
- None
- Refer to orthotics clinic   Date: _____   Time: _____
- Refer for shoes
- Refer to pediatrist
- Refer to podiatrist
- Educated in: _____
- Orthotics fabricated: Date: _____   Time: _____

- 2-month follow-up: Date: _____   Time: _____
- 6-month follow-up: Date: _____   Time: _____

DPP, distal pedal pulse; HAV, hallux abductus valgus; IPK, interphalangeal keratosis; IP, interphalangeal; PTP, posterior tibial pulse

Form 49.1 (Continued)

Box 49.1 *Risk classification*

0 No loss of protective sensation
1 Loss of protective sensation with no deformity or history of ulcer
2 Loss of protective sensation with deformity but no history of ulcer
3 Loss of protective sensation with history of ulceration

---

or areas of hyperkeratosis or discoloration should be observed and documented (Young et al., 2011).

To differentiate an organic disorder such as blockage of the lumen of the vessel from a vasospastic condition, temporary dilation of the vessel in question is a useful vascular test. This is accomplished by using an arterial tourniquet for 3 minutes and then releasing it. The perfusion distal to the tourniquet should increase if the condition is due to vasospasm (Chantelau et al., 2007).

Observation of blanching and filling times is accomplished by using the Buerger–Allen vascular assessment (see Forms 49.2 to 49.4). A stopwatch is used to determine the time it takes the veins in the distal part of the foot to fill with blood after they have been drained by elevating the leg. Basically, this is a means of appraising the general circulation in the foot. The arterial blood being pumped into the dependent leg diffuses into the arterioles, the capillaries and the venules, and then into the veins of the foot. The time of venous filling is subject to several variables: arterial blood pressure, the caliber of the arteries, the volume of blood reaching the capillary bed of the foot with each thrust of the heart and the rate of venous return. A filling time of up to 20 seconds indicates reasonably good collateral circulation. A venous filling time longer than 20 seconds is indicative of a compromised peripheral vascular system and of venous insufficiency (Young et al., 2011).

Rubor of the skin should be noted. Dependent rubor is a reddish-blue color of the toes and forefoot caused by reduced blood flow in the capillaries. When there is diminished arterial flow, peripheral resistance drops with arterial capillary dilatation and maximum oxygen extraction by the tissues. With dependency, this is exaggerated. The actual degree of rubor can be noted when measuring venous filling time. Maximum rubor is usually evident in 2–3 minutes; it manifests as a dusky red color when severe ischemia is present (Peters et al., 2001).

The evaluation of skin temperatures and circumferential measures are additional means of assessing circulatory insufficiency and determining the presence of infection.

Skin temperature measurements are useful if the circulatory problem is asymmetrical, although test results may be variable because of ambient temperature. In an individual with peripheral vascular disease, the extremities are often cool to the touch, and in the presence of infection, there may be hot spots. The use of a skin temperature monitoring device to obtain precise temperature measures is helpful, but the therapist can also evaluate skin temperature by touch, rating it cold, cool, warm or hot (Young et al., 2011).

PATIENT:_____ AGE:_____ SEX:_____ RM no.: _____

DIAGNOSIS: _____ Physician: _____

DATE INITIAL EVALUATION:_____ Therapist: _____

	RIGHT LEG	LEFT LEG
APPEARANCE:	_____	_____
SKIN INTEGRITY:	_____	_____
SKIN TEMPERATURE:	_____	_____
EDEMA PRESENT:	0 □ +1 □ +2 □ +3 □	0 □ +1 □ +2 □ +3 □

CIRCUMFERENTIAL:

	Right	Left
□ Metatarsal heads	_____	_____
□ Arch	_____	_____
□ Ankle	_____	_____
□ Supramalleolar	_____	_____
□ Mid-calf	_____	_____
□ Subpatellar	_____	_____

PULSES:

Dorsal pedalis	0 □ +1 □ +2 □ +3 □	0 □ +1 □ +2 □ +3 □
Post-tibialis	0 □ +1 □ +2 □ +3 □	0 □ +1 □ +2 □ +3 □
Popliteal	0 □ +1 □ +2 □ +3 □	0 □ +1 □ +2 □ +3 □
Femoral	0 □ +1 □ +2 □ +3 □	0 □ +1 □ +2 □ +3 □

SENSORY TESTING:

Vibratory sense:	□ PRESENT □ DIMINISHED □ ABSENT	□ PRESENT □ DIMINISHED □ ABSENT

Protective sensation:

1 = 0.1 g (4.17 for normal)
2 = 10 g (5.07 protective sense)
3 = 75 g (6.10 loss protective sense)
4 = No protective sensation

	Right	Left
Dorsum:	1 □ 2 □ 3 □ 4 □	1 □ 2 □ 3 □ 4 □
Plantar digit 1:	1 □ 2 □ 3 □ 4 □	1 □ 2 □ 3 □ 4 □
Plantar digit 3:	1 □ 2 □ 3 □ 4 □	1 □ 2 □ 3 □ 4 □
Plantar digit 5:	1 □ 2 □ 3 □ 4 □	1 □ 2 □ 3 □ 4 □
Metatarsal head 1:	1 □ 2 □ 3 □ 4 □	1 □ 2 □ 3 □ 4 □
Metatarsal head 3:	1 □ 2 □ 3 □ 4 □	1 □ 2 □ 3 □ 4 □
Metatarsal head 5:	1 □ 2 □ 3 □ 4 □	1 □ 2 □ 3 □ 4 □
Proximal head 3:	1 □ 2 □ 3 □ 4 □	1 □ 2 □ 3 □ 4 □
Arch:	1 □ 2 □ 3 □ 4 □	1 □ 2 □ 3 □ 4 □
Heel:	1 □ 2 □ 3 □ 4 □	1 □ 2 □ 3 □ 4 □

STRENGTH:

	Right		Left
		Anterior tibialis:	
		Extensor hallucis longus:	
		Flexor hallucis longus:	
		Posterior tibialis:	
		Peroneus longus:	
		Gastrocnemius/soleus:	
		Intrinsics (strong/weak/ atrophied)	

DEFORMITIES:

	Right	Left
Hammer/claw:		
Bony prominence:		
Drop-foot:		
Charcot's foot:		
Hallux limitus:		
Rear/forefoot varus:		
Plantar flexed first:		
Equinus:		
Amputation:		

FOOTWEAR: □ Standard □ Special Describe _____

□ Adequate □ Inadequate Describe _____

Blanching/filling times: _____ Elevated _____ Horizontal _____ Dependent _____

TREATMENT RECOMMENDATIONS:[b]

□ Buerger–Allen exercises Cycles _____ Times/day _____ Modified Yes/no

□ Patient education □ Skin care □ Footwear □ Orthotics

[a]Buerger–Allen evaluation form created by: Jennifer M. Bottomley, PT, MS, PhD © 1996.
[b]Refer to Buerger–Allen treatment flow sheet for initial blanching/filling times etc.

Form 49.2 Buerger—Allen Initial Evaluation form[a]

PATIENT: _____ AGE: _____ SEX: _____ RM no.: _____ MD: _____
DIAGNOSIS: _____ Initial evaluation: _____ F/U evaluation: _____
TOTAL NO. TREATMENTS: _____ Therapist: _____

	RIGHT LEG	LEFT LEG
APPEARANCE:		
SKIN INTEGRITY:		
SKIN TEMPERATURE:		
EDEMA PRESENT:	0☐ +1☐ +2☐ +3☐	0☐ +1☐ +2☐ +3☐

CIRCUMFERENTIAL:

	Right	Left
☐ Metatarsal heads		
☐ Arch		
☐ Ankle		
☐ Supramalleolar		
☐ Mid-calf		
☐ Subpatellar		

PULSES:

	Right	Left
Dorsal pedalis	0☐ +1☐ +2☐ +3☐	0☐ +1☐ +2☐ +3☐
Post-tibialis	0☐ +1☐ +2☐ +3☐	0☐ +1☐ +2☐ +3☐
Popliteal	0☐ +1☐ +2☐ +3☐	0☐ +1☐ +2☐ +3☐
Femoral	0☐ +1☐ +2☐ +3☐	0☐ +1☐ +2☐ +3☐

SENSORY TESTING:

Vibratory sense:
- ☐ PRESENT / ☐ DIMINISHED / ☐ ABSENT (Right)
- ☐ PRESENT / ☐ DIMINISHED / ☐ ABSENT (Left)

Protective sensation:

1 = 0.1 g (4.17 for normal)
2 = 10 g (5.07 protective sense)
3 = 75 g (6.10 loss protective sense)
4 = No protective sensation

	Right	Left
Dorsum:	1☐ 2☐ 3☐ 4☐	1☐ 2☐ 3☐ 4☐
Plantar digit 1:	1☐ 2☐ 3☐ 4☐	1☐ 2☐ 3☐ 4☐
Plantar digit 3:	1☐ 2☐ 3☐ 4☐	1☐ 2☐ 3☐ 4☐
Plantar digit 5:	1☐ 2☐ 3☐ 4☐	1☐ 2☐ 3☐ 4☐
Metatarsal head 1:	1☐ 2☐ 3☐ 4☐	1☐ 2☐ 3☐ 4☐
Metatarsal head 3:	1☐ 2☐ 3☐ 4☐	1☐ 2☐ 3☐ 4☐
Metatarsal head 5:	1☐ 2☐ 3☐ 4☐	1☐ 2☐ 3☐ 4☐
Proximal head 5:	1☐ 2☐ 3☐ 4☐	1☐ 2☐ 3☐ 4☐
Arch:	1☐ 2☐ 3☐ 4☐	1☐ 2☐ 3☐ 4☐
Heel:	1☐ 2☐ 3☐ 4☐	1☐ 2☐ 3☐ 4☐

STRENGTH:

	Right	Left
Anterior tibialis:		
Extensor hallucis longus:		
Flexor hallucis longus:		
Posterior tibialis:		
Peroneus longus:		
Gastrocnemius/soleus:		
Intrinsics (strong/weak/atrophied)		

DEFORMITIES:

	Right	Left
Hammer/claw:		
Bony prominence:		
Drop-foot:		
Charcot's foot:		
Hallux limitus:		
Rear/forefoot varus:		
Plantar flexed first:		
Equinus:		
Amputation:		

FOOTWEAR: ☐ Standard   ☐ Special   Describe _____
☐ Adequate   ☐ Inadequate   Describe _____

TREATMENT RECOMMENDATIONS:[b]
☐ Buerger–Allen exercises   Cycles _____   Times/day _____   Modified   Yes/no
☐ Patient education   ☐ Skin care   ☐ Footwear   ☐ Orthotics

[a] Buerger–Allen evaluation form created by: Jennifer M. Bottomley, PT, MS, PhD © 1996.
[b] Refer to Buerger–Allen treatment flow sheet for initial blanching/filling times etc.

Form 49.3 Buerger—Allen Follow-up Evaluation form[a]

Patient: _____ Age: _____ Sex: _____ Rm no.: _____ Therapist initials: _____

Diagnosis: _____ Diabetes: _____

Wound: ☐ Present ☐ Not present ☐ Describe _____ ☐ Pvd ☐ Amputee ☐ Cardiac ☐ Htn

Buerger–Allen protocol: _____ Cycles _____ Times/day _____ Modified _____

Parameter	Initial evaluation	Follow-up	Follow-up	Follow-up	Notes
Date/therapist initials					
Resting heart rate (supine)					
Blood pressure (supine)					
Respiratory rate (supine)					
Plantar skin temperature	L: ___ R: ___	L: ___ R: ___	L: ___ R: ___	L: ___ R: ___	
Dorsal pedalis pulse left	0☐ +1☐ +2☐ +3☐	0☐ +1☐ +2☐ +3☐	0☐ +1☐ +2☐ +3☐	0☐ +1☐ +2☐ +3☐	
Dorsal pedalis pulse right	0☐ +1☐ +2☐ +3☐	0☐ +1☐ +2☐ +3☐	0☐ +1☐ +2☐ +3☐	0☐ +1☐ +2☐ +3☐	
Post-tibialis pulse left	0☐ +1☐ +2☐ +3☐	0☐ +1☐ +2☐ +3☐	0☐ +1☐ +2☐ +3☐	0☐ +1☐ +2☐ +3☐	
Post-tibialis pulse right	0☐ +1☐ +2☐ +3☐	0☐ +1☐ +2☐ +3☐	0☐ +1☐ +2☐ +3☐	0☐ +1☐ +2☐ +3☐	
Edema (supine)	0☐ +1☐ +2☐ +3☐	0☐ +1☐ +2☐ +3☐	0☐ +1☐ +2☐ +3☐	0☐ +1☐ +2☐ +3☐	
Circumferential measures					
Metatarsal heads	L: ___ R: ___	L: ___ R: ___	L: ___ R: ___	L: ___ R: ___	
Arch	L: ___ R: ___	L: ___ R: ___	L: ___ R: ___	L: ___ R: ___	
Ankle (figure of eight)	L: ___ R: ___	L: ___ R: ___	L: ___ R: ___	L: ___ R: ___	
Supramalleolar	L: ___ R: ___	L: ___ R: ___	L: ___ R: ___	L: ___ R: ___	
Mid-calf	L: ___ R: ___	L: ___ R: ___	L: ___ R: ___	L: ___ R: ___	
Subpatellar	L: ___ R: ___	L: ___ R: ___	L: ___ R: ___	L: ___ R: ___	
Blanching time elevated					
Filling time horizontal					
Filling time dependent					

[a] Jennifer M. Bottomley, PT, MS, PhD © 1996.
Pvd, peripheral vascular disease; Htn, hypertension

Form 49.4 Burger–Allen Treatment Flow sheet[a]

Circumferential measurements of the lower leg and foot also aid in the assessment of an individual with peripheral vascular involvement. Edema is often present when the peripheral vascular system is involved because of the inability of the involved vessels to efficiently remove waste materials from the interstitial tissues. This edema will increase in the dependent position, owing to gravity. Measurement of circumference can be accomplished by using a measuring tape around the metatarsal heads, the midfoot, in a figure of eight around the ankle and incrementally every 3 inches up the lower leg from the malleolar level to the subpatellar level.

Another means of determining the degree of edema is volume displacement. Using a bucket of water with a ruler taped to the inside, measure the amount of water that is displaced when the lower extremity is submerged. This method provides an objective and reproducible means of assessing edema in the lower extremity (Chantelau et al., 2007).

EVALUATION OF WOUND STATUS

In the presence of foot lesions it is helpful to grade the lesion for objective monitoring. Wagner's classification grades vascular dysfunction from 0 to 5, as follows (also see Box 49.1):

Grade 0 Foot: The skin is without ulceration. No open lesions are present, but potentially ulcerating deformities, such as bunions, hammer toes and Charcot's deformity, may be present. Healed partial-foot amputations may also be included in this group.
Grade 1 Foot: A full-thickness superficial skin loss is present. The lesion does not extend to bone. No abscess is present.
Grade 2 Foot: An open ulceration is noted; it is deeper than that of grade 1. It may penetrate to tendon or joint capsule.
Grade 3 Foot: The lesion penetrates to bone, and osteomyelitis is present. Joint infection or plantar fascial plane abscess may also be noted.
Grade 4 Foot: Gangrene is noted in the forefoot.
Grade 5 Foot: Gangrene involving the entire foot is noted. This condition is not salvageable by local procedures.

In the presence of ulceration, objective documentation of wound size is best accomplished by tracing the wound on sterilized X-ray film or by photographing it on line-graphed film. This is helpful in monitoring improvement or decline in wound status (Resnik & Borgia, 2011).

THERAPEUTIC INTERVENTIONS

PREVENTIVE MANAGEMENT

A management plan for the patient presenting with a neuropathic foot is based on the risk classification scheme. Patients in risk categories 1 through 3 are given education in foot inspection, skin care and selection of footwear. Footwear recommendations are dependent on level of risk and on the specific needs of each individual. For example, patients in category 1 benefit from a shoe with a leather (or other compliant material) upper and a toe-box

that accommodates the shape of the foot. A cushioned insole may be added. Category 2 and 3 patients may need customized insoles and shoe modifications appropriate for their deformities (Driver et al., 2010). Once a patient is assigned a level of risk through the screening process, a program of routine follow-up is recommended: once a year for risk 0, twice yearly for risk 1, every 3 months for risk 2, and monthly for those in the risk 3 category.

TREATMENT OF PLANTAR ULCERS

The treatment of choice for plantar ulcers is a total contact cast. In total-contact casting, foam padding encloses the toes; felt pads provide protection over the malleoli, tibial crest, posterior heel and navicular tuberosity; and local padding provides relief at the ulcer site. The initial cast should be changed within the first week to prevent injury due to an improper fit, as edema resolves.

The effectiveness of walking casts in healing diabetic and non-diabetic foot ulcers has been demonstrated in numerous studies. Walking casts promote plantar wound healing by (1) reducing plantar pressures, (2) reducing leg edema and (3) protecting the affected area from traumatic re-injury (Lemaster et al., 2003; Driver et al., 2010; Bottomley, 2012; Boulton, 2012).

Not every patient will accept, or is a candidate for, a walking cast. Infection and fragile skin are contraindications for casting. For these cases, alternatives to casting should be employed. A walking splint is a posterior cast secured to the leg by an elastic wrap. The shell is made of plaster reinforced by fiberglass taping, and relief for the posterior heel and plantar lesion is provided by adhesive-backed padding (Boulton, 2012).

The ulcer relief (cut-out) sandal is another device that can be used as an alternative to casting for patients with plantar lesions. The foot bed of molded plastazote is cut out, or cut in relief, to reduce pressure beneath the plantar lesion (Boulton, 2012).

PREVENTION AND TREATMENT

The challenge is to prevent re-ulceration. The patient must be provided with temporary protective footwear during healing and protective footgear following the healing of the ulceration and then gradually allowed to resume activities, avoiding those that may have contributed to the ulcer formation. A sandal molded from thermoplastic materials is an acceptable device during this critical period. Individuals who resume activity too quickly after a period of casting or other immobilization by protective footwear are at risk of developing a neuropathic fracture.

The best way to monitor progress is by comparing temperature differences between the involved and uninvolved foot. Temperatures increase by as much as one degree due to stress-induced inflammation. A skin-surface temperature monitor can by employed to evaluate differences in temperature between the inflamed and the non-inflamed areas of the foot. The patient must be aware that the first sign of injury to the bones of the foot may be swelling and warmth (Birke, 2002; Young et al., 2011).

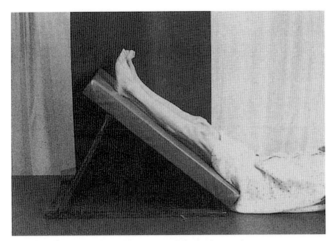

Figure 49.1 Buerger–Allen protocol: legs elevated.

When the ulcer site is fully healed, footwear is progressed to modified shoes fitted with accommodative orthotics. With mild deformities, molded insoles are added to extra-depth shoes or sneakers. For healed forefoot ulcers, a rocker sole is applied to the sole of the shoe to assist with push-off. If the foot is significantly shortened or deformed, custom shoes may be required. Custom shoes are made by pedorthists or orthotists over plaster models of the patient's feet and extra depth is incorporated in the shoe to accommodate a soft, molded interface beneath the foot (Pai & Ledoux, 2011).

Charcot fractures often result in serious foot deformities. Acute Charcot fractures may require surgery or long periods of immobilization in a cast. Additional immobilization and temperature monitoring are required. The length of time of casting and immobilization varies based on the individual rate of healing. Custom shoes are prescribed for the individual when there is no longer a difference in skin temperature between the fractured and the uninvolved foot (Boulton, 2012).

Buerger–Allen Exercise Protocol

Buerger–Allen exercises are performed according to the protocol displayed in Figures 49.1–49.3 (Young et al., 2011). The individual lies supine with the legs elevated at an angle of 45° until blanching occurs or for a maximum time of 3 minutes (Fig. 49.3). Active pumping and circling of the feet and isometric quadriceps and gluteal contractions are performed for the first minute or more in the elevated position. Once the blanching has occurred, the subject sits up and hangs the lower leg over the edge of the bed (Fig. 49.2). (Note: If the individual is subject to orthostatic hypotension, the legs should be held horizontally between elevated and dependent positions.) While the legs are in the dependent position, the individual is encouraged to actively plantarflex, dorsiflex and circle the foot. This position is maintained for a minimum of 3 minutes, or until rubor has occurred. Finally, the individual lies supine with the lower extremities flat for 3 minutes (Fig. 49.3). Again, active contraction of the leg muscles is performed for at least 1 minute in this position. One note of caution: in the presence of severe physiological compromise of the cardiovascular system, I

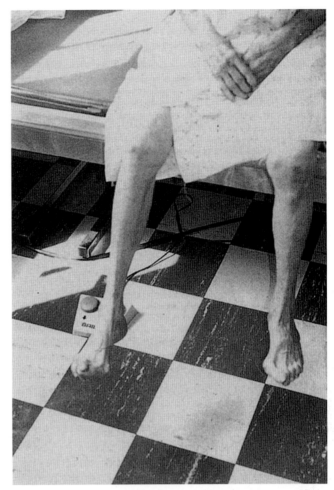

Figure 49.2 Buerger–Allen protocol: legs dependent.

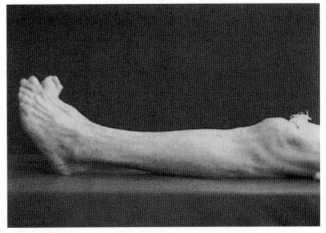

Figure 49.3 Buerger–Allen protocol: legs horizontal.

recommend assuming the supine position between phases to prevent the consequences of orthostatic hypotension. The entire sequence is repeated three times in each session. If peripheral neuropathy is present and active muscle contraction is not possible, the clinician can passively plantarflex and dorsiflex the foot in each of the respective positions to increase blood flow, which is facilitated by the pumping action of the surrounding musculature.

CONCLUSION

The insensitive foot, which results from various pathological conditions, is far too common and problematic for aging persons. The key to good care is proper evaluation, which leads to appropriate therapeutic intervention. Several evaluation tools are presented and total-contact casting, protective footgear, and the Buerger–Allen exercise routine are described. In conjunction with patient education, which is crucial for prevention, effective care can mitigate the deleterious effects of the insensitive foot.

REFERENCES AND FURTHER READING

Birke JA, Pavich MA, Patout Jr CA et al 2002 Comparison of forefoot ulcer healing using alternative off-loading methods in patients with diabetes mellitus. Adv Skin Wound Care 15(5):210–215

Bottomley JM 2012 Footwear: the foundation for lower extremity orthotics. In: Lusardi MM, Nielsen CC (eds) Orthotics and Prosthetics in Rehabilitation, 3rd edn. Butterworth/Heinemann Publishers, Boston, MA

Boulton AJ 2012 Diabetic foot – what can we learn from leprosy? Legacy of Dr Paul W. Brand. Diabetes Metab Res Rev 28(suppl1):3–7

Chantelau E, Richter A, Ghassem-Zadeh N et al 2007 'Silent' bone stress injuries in the feet of diabetic patients with polyneuropathy: a report on 12 cases. Arch Orthop Trauma Surg 127(3):171–177

Driver VR, Fabbi M, Lavery LA et al 2010 The costs of diabetic foot: the economic case for the limb salvage team. J Vasc Surg 52(Suppl 3):17S–22S

Frykberg RG, Belczyk R 2008 Epidemiology of the Charcot foot. Clin Podiatr Med Surg 25(1):17–28

Ites KI, Anderson EJ, Cahill ML et al 2011 Balance interventions for diabetic peripheral neuropathy: a systematic review. J Geriatr Phys Ther 34(3):109–116

Jeffcoate WJ, Harding KG 2003 Diabetic foot ulcers. Lancet 361(9368):1545–1551

Kruse RL, LeMaster JW, Medsen RW 2010 Fall and balance outcomes after an intervention to promote leg strength, balance, and walking in people with diabetic peripheral neuropathy: "Feet First" randomized controlled trial. Phys Ther 90(11):1568–1579

Lemaster JW, Reiber GE, Smith DB et al 2003 Daily weight-bearing activity does not increase the risk of diabetic foot ulcers. Med Sci Sports Exerc 35(7):1093–1099

Pai S, Ledoux WR 2011 Visoelastic properties of diabetic and non-diabetic plantar soft tissue. Ann Biomed Eng 39(5):1517–1527

Peters EJ, Lavery LA, Armstrong DG et al 2001 Electric stimulation as an adjunct to heal diabetic foot ulcers: a randomized clinical trial. Arch Phys Med Rehabil 86(6):721–725

Resnik L, Borgia M 2011 Reliability of outcome measures for people with lower-limb amputations: distinguishing true change from statistical error. Phys Ther 91(4):555–565

Van Schie CH 2005 A review of the biomechanics of the diabetic foot. Int J Low Extrem Wounds 4(3):160–170

Webber SC, Porter MM 2010 Reliability of ankle isometric, isotonic, and isokinetic strength and power testing in older women. Phys Ther 90(8):1165–1175

Young D, Schuerman S, Flynn K et al 2011 Reliability and responsiveness of an 18 site, 10-g monofilament examination for assessment of protective foot sensation. J Geriatr Phys Ther 34(2):95–98

Chapter 50
Skin disorders

RANDY GORDON

CHAPTER CONTENTS

INTRODUCTION

As the skin ages many structural and functional changes naturally occur, including flattening of the dermal–epidermal junction. In the epidermis, the following occur: the number of Langerhans cells, responsible for immune recognition, decreases by 20–50%; the number of melanocytes, responsible for protective pigmentation, also declines; and the size and shape of keratinocytes begins to vary (Yaar & Gilcrest, 2001). The dermis is characterized by a decrease in thickness cellularity, a decrease in vascularity and a degeneration of elastic fibers.

Photoaging, skin changes that result from chronic exposure to ultraviolet radiation, potentiates an average 20% age-related loss of dermal thickness. The number of mast cells, fibroblasts and specialized nerve endings is diminished with age. Between ages 10 and 90 years, about one-third of the cutaneous sensory nerve-end organs are lost, which may contribute to a 20% increase in cutaneous pain threshold.

In general, hair follicles and sebaceous and eccrine glands decrease in number. During adulthood, there is a 15% loss of eccrine glands and a diminished output by the remaining glands, which, compounded by the reduced cutaneous vascularity, increases the risk of heatstroke, especially in dry heat. The loss of hair bulb melanocytes accounts for the graying of hair, which is substantial in 50% of individuals by the age of 50. Subcutaneous fat, an insulator that helps with thermoregulation, provides shock absorption and protects the body from trauma, decreases with age. The body's overall proportion of fat, however, usually increases and is redistributed to the thighs and abdomen (Habif, 2004; *Merck Manual*, 2011).

Many of the protective functions of the skin are decreased with age. Functional changes in aging skin include: (a) altered permeability, (b) diminished sebum production, (c) decreased inflammatory and immunological responsiveness and (d) attenuated thermoregulation with decreased sweating. Wound healing and sensory perception are impaired, elasticity is reduced and vitamin D production is decreased.

In addition to these normal changes, known as intrinsic aging, other changes take place in response to cumulative ultraviolet irradiation. These changes include: (a) atrophy of the epidermis, (b) epidermal dysplasia and atypia, (c) a further decrease in the number of Langerhans cells, (d) increased and irregular distribution and activity of melanocytes, (e) dermal elastosis (deposits of abnormal elastic fibers) and (f) further decreases in inflammatory and immunological responsiveness (Habif, 2004; *Merck Manual*, 2011).

GENERAL PRINCIPLES

When evaluating a patient with a skin disorder, it is important to ascertain which topical home remedies and other products, such as alcohol or detergents, are being applied, as these products often exacerbate the primary skin condition. It is essential to take a full medical history, with particular emphasis on medications. The chronicity of the condition and whether others in the patient's environment have a similar condition may also provide clues to the diagnosis (Wolff et al., 2005).

Management of skin conditions must be tailored to the patient's physical capabilities and circumstances. Limitations in movement of the geriatric rehabilitation patient can make application of topical treatments difficult. Remedies commonly used in younger patients, such as oil in bath water, may be quite dangerous for the elderly. To avoid errors, treatment regimens should be as simple as possible. Moreover, the elderly are two to three times more likely to experience adverse reactions to antihistamines and corticosteroids, drugs frequently used to treat skin disorders. These drugs should be prescribed reluctantly and always with clear written instructions. See Table 50.1 for examples of topical corticosteroid preparations.

Most dermatological agents are applied topically, and the choice of a base for the active ingredient is important. Ointments – greasy preparations containing little water – are most useful for treating conditions in which the skin is dry, scaly or thickened. In general, a medication in an ointment base is better absorbed, and therefore more potent, than the same medication in a cream or lotion vehicle. Creams – semisolid emulsions of water in oil – are more cosmetically appealing, but can be drying, and are thus useful for treating exudative conditions. However, most creams contain stabilizers or preservatives that can induce allergic sensitization. Lotions and sprays, usually suspensions of fine powder in an aqueous base, are useful for the evaporative cooling and drying of the skin and are preferred on hair-bearing areas because of their ease of application. Powders are useful for absorbing moisture from weepy or intertriginous skin. Soaks and compresses, which are very drying as they evaporate, are soothing and thus appropriate for highly exudative and vesicular lesions.

Topical steroid medications are commonly used in the treatment of dermatological conditions. Numerous preparations are available, which are classified by their potency. Certain basic principles should be emphasized. Overuse of topical steroids can result in local side-effects, including: (a) skin atrophy, (b) telangiectasia, (c) hypopigmentation and (d) tachyphylaxis, or reduced efficacy over time. Side-effects increase with higher potency drugs and longer duration of use. Only mild-potency topical steroids

should be used on delicate skin, such as the face, genitalia and intertriginous areas. Finally, application of topical steroids over a large area of the body may results in systemic absorption, which can lead to possible adrenal suppression and other adverse sequelae.

TREATMENT OF INFECTIONS

VIRAL INFECTIONS

Herpes Simplex

Herpetic infection appears clinically as grouped vesicles on an erythematous base (Elgart, 2002). Vesicles can become pustules and eventually crusts and erosions, with a characteristic punched-out appearance. Herpes simplex virus (HSV) infection can be accompanied by pruritus, burning, or pain. The diagnosis is often made by the clinical presentation of the vesicular rash, and can be confirmed either by the presence of multinucleated giant cells on a Tzank smear or by viral culture.

Herpes simplex eruptions can be either primary or secondary. Secondary eruptions can be provoked by stress, infection, trauma, or ultraviolet radiation. They are most commonly seen in the perioral and anogenital regions; although they can appear in any location.

Herpetic whitlow is a herpes simplex infection of the finger, classically seen in healthcare workers as a result of inoculation by a patient's lesions. In the immunocompetent host, HSV is a self-limited infection that does not necessarily require treatment; this is often the case with perioral herpes. If treatment is desired, as in genital herpes, 400 mg three times a day, or 200 mg of oral acyclovir five times a day is effective (treat for 10 days for primary infection, 5 days for recurrent infection). When indicated, acyclovir can be used for the chronic suppression of HSV (400 mg twice daily). Neither the need for nor the proper increased dosage of acyclovir has been established conclusively in immunocompromised individuals. Patients who do not respond to the recommended dose of acyclovir may require a higher oral dose, intravenous acyclovir, or may be infected with an acyclovir-resistant HSV strain, requiring IV Foscarnet (Wolff et al., 2005). Patients may be treated with 5 mg/kg of intravenous acyclovir every 8 hours for 14 days, or 400 mg five times a day for 14 days.

Herpes Zoster

Varicella-zoster virus (VZV) infection, more commonly known as shingles, is a human herpes virus that infects 98% of the adult population, and is caused by the reactivation of the dormant varicella virus in the dorsal root ganglia (Wolff et al., 2005). Although it may occur at any age, elderly patients are at greater risk (Elgart, 2002). Individuals who have never been exposed to varicella may contract it from someone with active herpes zoster. Other factors that predispose patients to a zoster eruption include: (a) immunosuppressive drugs, (b) corticosteroids, (c) malignancies, (d) local irradiation and (e) surgical trauma.

One possible consequence of herpes zoster infection is postherpetic neuralgia (PHN), for which the incidence, duration and severity increase with age. Uncommon complications include: (a) encephalitis, (b) ophthalmic disease

Potency	Compound	Formulation
Very high	Clobetasol proprionate	Cream or ointment 0.05%
	Halobetasol proprionate	Cream or ointment 0.05%
High	Betamethasone diproprionate	Cream or ointment 0.05%
	Betamethasone valerate	Ointment 0.1%
	Fluocinonide	Cream or ointment 0.05%
	Halcinonide	Cream or ointment 0.1%
Medium	Betamethasone valerate	Cream 0.1%
	Fluocinolone acetonide	Cream or ointment 0.025%
	Hydrocortisone valerate	Cream or ointment 0.2%
	Triamcinolone acetonide	Cream, ointment, or lotion 0.1% or 0.025%
Low	Hydrocortisone	Cream, ointment, or lotion 2.5% or 1.0%

Table 50.1 **Examples of topical corticosteroid preparations**

Adapted from Habif TP, 2004 Clinical Dermatology: A Color Guide to Diagnosis and Therapy, 4th edn. Mosby, Philadelphia, PA, pp. 958–959.

when the first branch of the trigeminal nerve is involved, (c) facial paralysis and taste loss when the second branch of the trigeminal nerve is involved (Ramsay–Hunt syndrome), (d) motor neuropathies, (e) Guillain–Barré syndrome and (f) urinary or fecal retention when sacral nerves are involved. Transmission may occur by direct contact with lesions, and occasionally by airborne droplets. Patients may be contagious several days before the exanthum appears.

The clinical presentation of herpes zoster infection is sometimes preceded by prodromal symptoms of pain, pruritus or paresthesia along the affected dermatome. Fever, chills, malaise and gastrointestinal symptoms can also occur. Usually, red papules appear along a dermatome within 3 days. These rapidly progress to grouped vesicles on an erythematous base that may become hemorrhagic or pustules. After about 5 days, the vesicle formation ceases and crusts form. Gradual healing occurs over the next 2–4 weeks, sometimes resolving with pigmentary disturbances or scarring. Disseminated herpes zoster infection can occur in patients with underlying malignancy or immunodeficiency and is a potentially life-threatening infection that requires hospitalization and intravenous acyclovir (10 mg/kg every 8 hours).

Not all cases of herpes zoster require treatment. Ideally, treatment should be started within 24–72 hours of the onset of symptoms. Two antiviral drugs are currently available: 800 mg of acyclovir four times a day for 7–10 days (note that a much higher dose is needed than for herpes simplex) or 500 mg of famcyclovir three times a day for 7 days. Other antivirals are currently undergoing testing. Antiviral therapy has been shown to hasten the resolution of the acute disease. However, its role in decreasing the incidence of postherpetic neuralgia is controversial.

In addition, the use of systemic steroids has been in and out of favor in recent years. Certainly antiviral therapy has a more favorable side-effect profile and, if systemic steroids are prescribed, they must be used with care in the elderly. Topical soaks for 20 minutes four times daily with an astringent solution such as Burow's solution (aluminum acetate) can help to dry vesicles and soothe affected areas. Crusted lesions are no longer infectious. Analgesics are commonly required to treat them.

It should be kept in mind that vesicle fluid is contagious to those who have never had varicella and to immunocompromised individuals. Thus, caregivers should wear gloves to avoid direct contact with the lesions, and pregnant women should strictly avoid contact. Immunization with VZV vaccine may boost humoral and cell-mediated immunity, and decrease the incidence of zoster in populations with declining VZV-specific immunity (Wolff et al., 2005).

FUNGAL INFECTIONS

Superficial fungal infections may be caused by yeast or dermatophytes. Deep fungal infections of the skin are rare, and occur mainly in severely immunocompromised patients. Dermatophytes are molds that require keratin for nutrition and must live on stratum corneum, hair, or nails to survive. Human infections are caused by *Epidermophyton*, *Microsporum* and *Trichophyton* spp. These infections differ from candidiasis in that they are rarely, if ever, invasive. Transmission is person-to-person, animal-to-person and (rarely) soil-to-person. The organism may persist indefinitely. Most people do not develop clinical fungal infections; those who do may have impaired T-cell responses from an alteration in local defenses (e.g. due to trauma, with vascular compromise) or from primary (hereditary) or secondary (e.g. diabetes, HIV) immunosuppression.

Tinea

Tinea is a superficial dermatophyte infection of the skin and is classified by anatomical location: tinea pedis (foot), tinea cruris (groin), tinea manuum (hand), tinea corporis (body) and tinea unguium or onychomycosis (nails). Tinea cruris characteristically spares the genitalia, as opposed to candidiasis, which involves the scrotum and penis in men and the vulva in women. Tinea capitis, or fungal infection of the scalp, is rare in older adults. Heat and moisture may predispose the skin to fungal infection. Tinea manifests clinically as scaly patches or plaques with annular or serpiginous, often slightly raised, borders. Varying degrees of erythema and pruritus may be present. Tinea pedis and tinea manuum may present as diffuse scaling of the plantar or palmar surfaces. Often one hand and two feet are affected. Tinea pedis may also present with toe-web maceration. Nails are also commonly involved, showing thickening and yellow discoloration of the nail plate, onycholysis (separation of the nail plate from the nail bed) and hyperkeratotic debris under the nail plate. Greenish discoloration indicates pseudomonal superinfection of the nail. When fungal infections are mistakenly treated with topical steroids, initial improvement may be noted in scaling and inflammation. However, fungal organisms flourish and infected areas may enlarge (tinea incognito). The infection can invade the hair follicle, resulting in a deeper infection known as Majocchi's granuloma.

Diagnosis of a fungal infection is confirmed by culture or by direct visualization under a microscope of fungal hyphae collected from scales and bathed with potassium hydroxide. Most cutaneous dermatophyte infections can be treated with a 4-week course of topical antifungal medication. Patients should be instructed to continue topical treatment for at least 1 week longer than symptoms persist to avoid discontinuing treatment prematurely. Affected areas should be kept as dry as possible, particularly the groin and toe-web spaces.

The exceptions to topical treatment are tinea unguium and tinea capitis, which may require oral antifungal agents. The drug of choice approved for the treatment of cutaneous dermatophyte infection of the scalp is griseofulvin. A dose of 10 mg/kg per day of ultramicrosized griseofulvin for 6 weeks to several months is common. Short-term terbinafine, itraconazole and fluconazole have been shown to be comparable in efficacy and safety.

Drug interactions may occur. Carefully monitoring the complete blood count and liver function is recommended, particularly if risk for hepatitis exists or treatment lasts longer than 3 months. In patients with both tinea pedis and onychomycosis, recurrence of tinea pedis is common if the nails are not treated concurrently, often necessitating indefinite topical treatment (*Merck Manual*, 2011).

Candidiasis

Candida albicans, the most frequent cause of candidiasis, thrives in warm moist areas such as the groin, the axilla and the inframammary regions. Diabetic and immunosuppressed patients, as well as those receiving systemic antibiotic therapy that reduces competing surface bacteria, are at increased risk for infection. The organism may be carried asymptomatically in the bowel, mouth and vagina.

Cutaneous candidal infection is characterized by beefy red, often moist, plaques with satellite pustules and papules. Unlike tinea cruris, candidiasis involves the skin of the genitalia. Oral candidiasis, or thrush, presents as creamy white plaques on the tongue, palate or buccal mucosa that cannot be easily scraped off.

Perleche, or angular cheilitis, is a candidal infection of the corners of the mouth, characterized by erythema, fissures and white exudate. Predisposing factors are dental malocclusion, poorly fitting dentures and deep folds at the corners of the mouth, with consequent retention of saliva and food particles in the affected area.

Candida paronychia is an infection of the skin proximal and lateral to the nails, characterized by erythema, tenderness and swelling, with separation of the nail plate from the adjacent nail folds. This condition is chronic and should be distinguished from acute paronychia, which is usually bacterial in origin. Frequent immersion of the hands in water is a predisposing factor. Confirmation of cutaneous candidiasis infection is by culture or potassium hydroxide preparation. Topical antifungal medication is usually effective, and attempts should be made to keep affected areas clean and dry.

BACTERIAL INFECTIONS

Impetigo

Impetigo is a superficial bacterial infection of the skin that is most commonly caused by either *Staphylococcus aureus* or Group A β-hemolytic streptococcus (*Streptococcus pyogenes*, or GAS) (Elgart, 2002). In the early stages of infection, vesicles or pustules break down to form golden-colored crusts that often adhere to the underlying skin. The infection can occur on previously normal intact skin or it may present as a superinfection of a primary skin disorder (e.g. eczema, neurodermatitis, herpes zoster), in which breaks in the cutaneous barrier allow bacteria to penetrate.

In managing impetigo, a skin swab should be collected for culture and to determine sensitivity. Focal or localized lesions can be treated topically with mupirocin (Bactroban) ointment applied three times a day. More extensive impetigo requires systemic antibiotics, such as antistaphylococcal penicillin, amoxicillin/clavulanate (Augmentin), cephalosporins or macrolides. Wet lesions can be soaked in an astringent (such as Burow's solution) that also has antimicrobial properties.

Folliculitis

Infection of the hair follicle is manifested by follicular-based erythematous papules and pustules. Lesions can be either superficial or deep (Elgart, 2002). Areas of predilection are the scalp and extremities, although the eruption can occur anywhere. Sweating and occlusion, such as under a splint, predispose to folliculitis; however, as long as therapy has been initiated, exercise and splints are not contraindicated in patients with folliculitis.

The most common causative organism is *S. aureus*. However, Gram negative organisms (such as *Pseudomonas aeruginosa*, which causes hot-tub folliculitis), *C. albicans* and *Pityrosporum ovale* can also be pathogenic.

Because of the variety of potentially causative organisms, it is advisable to send pustule contents for culture and determination of sensitivity. However, given that most cases are caused by *S. aureus*, it is reasonable to empirically begin antistaphylococcal medications, and adjust treatment pending culture results. Mild cases can be treated with topical anti-staphylococcal antibiotics, such as erythromycin, clindamycin or mupirocin. Clindamycin 1% gel or lotion applied to the affected area for 7–10 days is generally effective (*Merck Manual*, 2011). Antibacterial soaps, such as Hibiclens, pHisoHex and Dial, help to maintain a lower bacterial count in predisposed patients.

Pityrosporum folliculitis occurs mainly on the trunk and is often associated with diabetes mellitus, antibiotic therapy or immunosuppression. Treatment is with a 2-week course of selenium sulfide 2.5% lotion applied daily for 10 minutes and then washed off. Topical antifungal creams may also be required.

Erysipelas

Erysipelas is a superficial infection of the skin caused by Group A or Group C hemolytic streptococci. The organism may enter the skin through minor cuts, wounds, or insect bites. Lesions of erysipelas are characterized by hot, edematous, erythematous plaques with well-defined, often rapidly advancing, margins. Vesicles and bullae may be present and can even be hemorrhagic. Fever, malaise and lymphadenopathy accompany cutaneous infection. The face is the most common location for erysipelas, but infection can occur anywhere. Treatment is with oral or intravenous anti-streptococcal antibiotics such as penicillin or erythromycin (in penicillin-allergic patients). A typical outpatient regimen is 250–500 mg four times a day for 2 weeks. Clinical judgment and continuous evaluation of the clinical course determine the treatment setting and route of administration of antibiotics. Because infection continues to spread during the first 12–24 hours of oral therapy, patients with facial lesions often require hospitalization and intravenous antibiotics to prevent the complication of cavernous sinus thrombosis. The treatment of choice for lower-extremity erysipelas is penicillin V 500 mg orally four times a day for not less than 2 weeks. In severe cases, penicillin G 1.2 million units IV every 6 hours is indicated, which can be replaced by oral therapy after 36–48 hours (*Merck Manual*, 2011).

Cellulitis

Cellulitis is a deeper bacterial infection of the skin, most commonly caused by group GAS and occasionally by *S. aureus* or Gram negative organisms (*Merck Manual*, 2011). It may occur as a complication of an open wound, a venous ulcer, tinea pedis, or it can develop on intact skin, particularly on the legs. Clinically, it presents as rapid-onset erythema, tenderness, swelling and warmth. Fever and lymphadenopathy may also occur. Treatment is with oral or intravenous antibiotics, depending upon the severity of infection and the concurrent health of the patient. Streptococcal cellulitis is best treated with penicillin. However, if *S. aureus* is suspected or the causative agent is unclear, broader coverage antibiotics, such as dicloxacillin or cephalexin, should be instituted and adjusted according to the clinical response. Methicillin-resistant *S. aureus* (MRSA) has emerged as a nosocomial as well as a community-acquired pathogen and has a higher associated morbidity and mortality. Oral therapy is usually adequate with dicloxacillin 250 mg or cephalexin 500 mg four times a day for mild infections. Levofloxacin 500 mg once a day or moxifloxacin 400 mg once a day works well for patients who are unlikely to adhere to multiple daily dosing schedules. For more serious infections, oxacillin 1 g IV every 6 hours is given (*Merck Manual*, 2011). Patients with diabetes mellitus or peripheral vascular disease need close monitoring and perhaps intravenous therapy. Diabetic patients are more likely to have Gram negative, anaerobic and mixed microbial infections. The treatment of any underlying predisposing condition should also be undertaken. If the cellulitis does not respond to antimicrobial therapy, drug resistant organisms or an alternative diagnosis should be considered. Recurrent leg cellulitis is prevented by treating concomitant tinea infections.

Swelling, pain and open lesions may necessitate modification or temporary suspension of physical rehabilitation. Cellulitis is not a frank contraindication to physical exercise. Clinical judgment must be used and the effects of disuse weighed against the need for rest. It is important to avoid aggravating the condition.

TREATMENT OF INFESTATIONS

Scabies

Scabies is an intensely pruritic eruption caused by the *Sarcoptes scabiei* mite. The female mite burrows into the skin and deposits eggs, which hatch into larvae in a few days. Scabies is easily transmitted by skin-to-skin contact and can be readily spread between residents of the same household, nursing home, or institution. Pruritus is caused by a hypersensitivity reaction, so infestation has usually been present for weeks before it manifests clinically. Pruritus is severe and often worse at night. The clinical hallmark of a scabies infection is the burrow, which is a linear ridge, often with a tiny vesicle at one end; however, these lesions may be obscured by scratching.

Other cutaneous signs of scabies are papules, nodules and vesicles. Lesions are characteristically found in the interdigital web spaces, the flexor aspects of the wrists, the axilla, the umbilicus, around the nipples and on the genitalia. The skin is almost always excoriated and lesions are susceptible to secondary impetiginization. In elderly and physically or mentally disabled patients scabies may present less typically because of the inability to scratch and is often a long-standing infestation. The condition may mimic eczema or exfoliative dermatitis. Widespread hyperkeratotic and crusted lesions may be present.

The diagnosis is confirmed by observation of the scabies mite, eggs, or excretions in a skin scraping placed in mineral oil and examined under a microscope. A typical patient has only 10–12 adult female mites at one time, so confirmation of scabies is not always possible and diagnosis is often presumptive.

Several antiscabitic creams and lotions are effective in treating scabies. The two most commonly used are 5% permethrin cream and 1% lindane lotion or cream. Lindane, particularly if overused, can have neurotoxic side-effects. Mite resistance to lindane has developed in North America, Latin America, South America and Asia. Permethrin is the drug of choice and is thought to be a safer treatment for infants and pregnant women.

Successful treatment requires the treatment of all close personal contacts. In an inpatient or residential facility, all clinical staff, patients, selected visitors and their household contacts should be treated. The infestation can be subclinical for weeks, so infested contacts may be asymptomatic. Medication should be applied to the entire body, from the neck down (the head is also treated in infants). Particular attention should be paid to applying the cream or lotion under the fingernails and to the external genitalia. The medication should be washed off 8 hours later and, at that time, all clothing and linens should be washed in hot water, dry-cleaned or placed in a hot dryer. This process should be repeated 1 week later to kill any newly hatched larvae.

Unlike lindane, permethrin has the advantage of killing scabies eggs as well as the mites and larvae, therefore requiring only one application. However, two applications are usually performed to ensure comprehensive treatment. It should be understood that pruritus is caused by allergic sensitization and not viable organisms. Pruritus may continue for 1–2 weeks after successful treatment. This can usually be controlled with mild- to mid-potency topical steroids and oral antihistamines. Itching that continues beyond a few weeks may indicate treatment failure, reinfestation or an incorrect diagnosis (Wolff et al., 2005).

Pediculosis

Three species of Pediculosis (lice) infest humans: *Pediculus humanus capitis* (head lice), *Pediculus humanus corporis* (body lice) and *Phthirus pubis* (pubic lice, also known as crab lice). Transmission is by close person-to-person contact or by sharing clothing, hats or combs. Elderly individuals who have poor personal hygiene or who live in an overcrowded environment are at risk for head and body lice. *Pediculosis capitis* presents with scalp pruritus, which can progress to eczematous changes with impetiginization. Localized lymphadenopathy may occur. Examination reveals small, gray-white nits (ova) adherent to hair shafts. Adult lice can occasionally be found. *Pediculosis corporis* should be considered in a patient who presents with generalized pruritus. Secondary eczematous changes, excoriation and impetiginization can occur. Lice and nits are usually not found on the body but rather in the seams of clothing. *Phthirus pubis* is usually spread by sexual contact, but may also be transmitted via clothing or towels. The bases of pubic hairs should be examined for lice and nits in a patient complaining of pubic pruritus.

Head lice are treated with 1% lindane shampoo, which is applied for 4 minutes and then washed off. Treatment should be repeated once in 7–10 days. Close contacts should also be examined and treated. Combs and brushes should be soaked in lindane shampoo for 1 hour. The presence of nits after appropriate treatment does not signify treatment failure. They can be removed from the hair with a fine-tooth comb dipped in vinegar.

Body lice are treated by washing the affected clothing in hot water, dry-cleaning them or placing them in a hot dryer and then ironing the seams. Alternatively, the clothing can be disinfected with an insecticidal powder such as DDT 10% or malathion 1%. If lice or nits are found on the skin, the patient can wash with lindane shampoo as above. Pubic lice are treated identically to head lice, with local application of lindane shampoo. In all forms of infestation, pruritus and dermatitis can be treated with emollients and topical steroids, and impetiginization may require antibiotics.

TREATMENT OF INFLAMMATORY SKIN CONDITIONS

Pruritus

Pruritus, or itching, is a common complaint that can cause significant discomfort, and is one of the most common reasons for consultation with a dermatologist. It can occur in the presence or absence of objective cutaneous findings; associated skin eruptions may be causative (primary) or secondary. Patients who complain of pruritus should be examined for inconspicuous primary skin lesions because some pruritic skin diseases, such as bullous pemphigoid and scabies, may show little, if any, cutaneous signs initially.

Systemic disorders associated with generalized pruritus without primary skin lesions include liver and renal disease, Hodgkin lymphoma, polycythemia vera, mycosis fungoides, iron deficiency anemia, leukemias, parasitosis (usually of the gastrointestinal tract) and psychiatric disease. Some drugs (e.g. barbiturates or narcotics) can also cause itching without a skin eruption.

Disorders rarely associated with itching include diabetes mellitus, hyperthyroidism, hypothyroidism (where pruritus is usually secondary to xerosis) and solid malignancies. The most common cause of pruritus is xerosis (dry skin) and, regardless of cause, most patients complaining of pruritus benefit from treatment for xerosis (see the following section). Oral antihistamines can be helpful in some cases but should be used cautiously in the elderly.

If no skin disease is evident, patients should be examined for evidence of systemic disorders such as lymphadenopathy, hepatosplenomegaly, jaundice and anemia. Appropriate laboratory tests for screening include a complete blood count, erythrocyte sedimentation rate, electrolytes (including urea nitrogen and creatinine), urine glucose, thyroid function tests and liver function tests. If indicated by history or physical examination, a chest radiograph may be obtained or stools tested for occult blood, ova and parasites. When itching begins suddenly and is severe and unrelenting, an underlying disease should be strongly suspected and laboratory evaluation should be thorough (*Merck Manual*, 2011).

Xerosis

Xerosis (dry skin) is quite common in the elderly and it is the most common cause of pruritus. Symptoms are often worse in the winter when central heating decreases the humidity indoors and the skin is exposed to cold and wind outdoors. Patients should be advised to avoid very hot baths or showers, as well as irritants such as harsh detergents and topically applied alcohol. Emollients should be applied liberally and frequently, especially immediately after bathing when the skin is still moist. Severely dry skin may become inflamed (see Asteatotic dermatitis).

TREATMENT OF DERMATITIS

Often used interchangeably with the term eczema, dermatitis indicates a superficial inflammation of the skin caused by exposure to an irritant, allergic sensitization, genetically determined factors or a combination of these factors. Pruritus, erythema and edema progress to vesiculation, oozing, crusting and scaling. Eventually, the skin may become lichenified (thickened and with prominent skin markings) from repeated rubbing or scratching (*Merck Manual*, 2011).

Allergic Contact Dermatitis

Allergic contact dermatitis (ACD) is a type IV cell-mediated hypersensitivity reaction. The consequence is dermatitis. The primary symptom is intense pruritus; pain is usually the result of excoriation or infection. Acute lesions tend to be vesicular, whereas chronic contact dermatitis appears scaly and lichenified. Clues to an allergic contact dermatitis are a bizarre shape or location or linear arrangement of lesions. Common contact allergens include nickel, fragrance additives, preservatives in cosmetics or medications, rubber, lanolin, chromates (used in tanning leather), topical antibiotics (especially neomycin, which is used, for example, on chronic ulcers) and topical anesthetics (e.g. benzocaine).

Treatment consists of identifying and removing the causative agent and applying mid- to high-potency topical steroids. Wet-to-dry dressings and soaks, such as Burow's solution, soothe and dry acute vesicular lesions and promote healing. Pure petrolatum has no fragrances or preservatives and is advised when a fragrance or preservative allergy is suspected or when the allergen is unknown. If contact dermatitis is suspected and a causative agent is not apparent by history and physical examination, patch-testing, usually performed by a dermatologist, can aid in making a diagnosis. All cutaneous allergies should be documented on the patient's chart because systemic exposure (e.g. via oral medication) to chemically related compounds may result in severe systemic allergic reactions.

Irritant Contact Dermatitis

Unlike allergic contact dermatitis, irritant contact dermatitis (ICD) is not immune-mediated. Given enough contact with an irritant, any patient may develop dermatitis. Common irritants are soaps and detergents. Although the elderly have a less pronounced inflammatory response to most irritants than younger patients, chronic irritant dermatitis is a common occurrence in the elderly. Clinical manifestations are identical to those of allergic contact dermatitis, and treatment is similar.

Atopic Dermatitis

Atopic dermatitis, commonly referred to as eczema, is a chronic pruritic condition that is commonly associated with other concurrent conditions, such as asthma, allergic rhinitis and xerosis. Atopic dermatitis is often referred to as 'the itch that rashes', underscoring pruritus as the hallmark of this condition. Atopic dermatitis rarely begins in adulthood and usually improves with age. However, it can be exacerbated by environmental factors, for example the dry environment that occurs in winter as a result of central heating, woolen clothing, harsh detergents and prolonged bathing. Treatment centers on altering habits to avoid these factors and aggressively using emollients and mid-potency topical steroids.

Lichen Simplex Chronicus

Also known as neurodermatitis, lichen simplex chronicus is a localized pruritic eruption that results from chronic scratching and rubbing, eventuating in a scratch–itch–scratch cycle. Clinically, lesions appear erythematous or hyperpigmented, lichenified and scaly. High-potency topical steroids are often required to break the cycle. Steroid-impregnated tape, such as flurandrenolide (Cordran), applied at bedtime or after bathing and left in place for up to12 hours, also protects the lesions from being scratched. When symptoms improve, the potency of the steroid and the frequency of use can be reduced. Topical doxepin relieves pruritus and also helps break the cycle, but systemic absorption and drowsiness sometimes limit its use. If applicable, lesions can be covered with dressings, such as an Unna boot, to prevent the patient from scratching. More nodular lesions are termed prurigo nodularis, or picker's nodules.

Asteatotic Dermatitis

When skin becomes excessively dry and scaly, fissures and excoriation allow environmental irritants to penetrate and further worsen the condition, adding inflammation to dryness. This commonly occurs on the lower legs and is characterized by scaly erythematous plaques with a cracked porcelain appearance, which are caused by superficial fissures and crust. Treatment consists of the aggressive use of emollients and, initially, the additional use of a low- to mid-potency topical steroid ointment.

Stasis Dermatitis

Stasis dermatitis, commonly seen in the aging population, occurs in the context of chronic venous hypertension. Scaling and erythema are seen on a background of edema, varicosities and hemosiderin hyperpigmentation. At times, stasis dermatitis may be confused with cellulitis, but it is usually chronic and bilateral. When severe and chronic, the condition may induce sclerosis, beginning around the ankles and progressing proximally (termed lipodermatosclerosis). Another complication of severe venous stasis is ulceration. Successful treatment of stasis dermatitis is contingent upon treating the underlying venous hypertension with leg elevation and compression therapy, if not contraindicated by concomitant arterial disease. Low-potency topical steroids and emollients relieve the dermatitis component and the frequently associated pruritus. Potential contact allergens, such as neomycin, should be avoided (*Merck Manual*, 2011).

Seborrheic Dermatitis

Seborrheic dermatitis is a common scaly erythematous eruption of the central part of the face (particularly eyebrows, glabella, eyelids and nasolabial folds), postauricular and beard areas, body flexures and scalp, where it is known in lay terms as dandruff. The central chest and interscapular areas can also be affected. Seborrheic dermatitis affecting the eyelids causes blepharitis and, sometimes, associated conjunctivitis.

Seborrheic dermatitis is especially prevalent among patients with neurological conditions, particularly Parkinson's disease, facial nerve injury, poliomyelitis, syringomyelia and spinal cord injury. Neuroleptic drugs with parkinsonian side-effects can also bring about seborrheic dermatitis. Severe seborrheic dermatitis has been found with increased frequency in individuals infected with human immunodeficiency virus (HIV).

Although still a controversial theory, an inflammatory response to an overgrowth of the normally resident lipophilic yeast *Pityrosporum ovale* is thought to be the cause. Treatment focuses on suppressing inflammation by means of a mild-potency topical steroid such as hydrocortisone or on killing the yeast with a topical antifungal such as ketoconazole. Topical ketoconazole also exerts some anti-inflammatory effects. Seborrheic dermatitis of the scalp responds to shampoos containing selenium sulfide, zinc pyrithione, salicylic acid and tar. Ketoconazole 2% shampoo and mild topical steroid solutions can also be helpful. In some patients, ketoconazole cream or other topical imidazoles applied twice daily for 1–2 weeks induce a remission that lasts for months. For eyelid margin seborrhea, a dilution of 1-part baby shampoo to 9-parts water is applied with a cotton swab.

Intertrigo

Intertrigo is an inflammation of intertriginous skin, resulting from irritation, friction and maceration. It appears as moist, erythematous and scaly areas in the flexures. Patients may complain of pruritus or soreness. Contributing factors include obesity, poor hygiene, hot weather, irritating or occlusive products applied locally and clothing made of synthetic fabrics that do not breathe. Secondary yeast or dermatophyte infection is common and should be treated with an antifungal cream. Treatment should focus primarily on eliminating the contributing factors mentioned above. The affected areas should be kept as dry as possible. A low-potency topical steroid such as hydrocortisone is used initially to decrease inflammation and allow restoration of an intact skin barrier. Lotrisone, a commonly prescribed combination antifungal and topical steroid cream, should not be used for this condition because the steroid that it contains (betamethasone diproprionate) is too strong for use on intertriginous skin.

TREATMENT OF PSORIASIS

Psoriasis is a common chronic papulosquamous condition that follows an unpredictable waxing and waning course. It usually commences in individuals from 16 to 22 years of age, but can also initially occur later in life. The cause of psoriasis is not known, although a genetic predisposition has been noted. Clinically, psoriasis is characterized by well-demarcated pink plaques with adherent thick silvery or micaceous scales. Areas of predilection are the extensor surfaces of both upper and lower extremities, the scalp, the gluteal cleft and the penis.

Psoriatic plaques commonly occur in areas of trauma, such as scars or burns. This is referred to as the isomorphic response or Koebner phenomenon. Nails are often involved, often as pitting of the nail plate, areas of yellowish discoloration known as oil spots, onycholysis (separation of the nail plate from the nail bed) and subungual debris. Psoriatic arthritis accompanies skin lesions in 5–8% of patients. Factors that exacerbate psoriasis include: (a) stress, (b) streptococcal infection, (c) a cold climate and (d) certain medications, for example, beta blockers, antimalarials, nonsteroidal anti-inflammatory drugs, lithium and alcohol. Systemic steroids should be used with care and tapered slowly in a psoriatic patient, as a severe flare can occur with abrupt discontinuation. Psoriatic variants include: (a) inverse psoriasis of intertriginous areas, (b) guttate psoriasis, (c) pustular psoriasis and (d) erythrodermic psoriasis.

Treatment is focused on control of the condition, rather than a cure. In the elderly, keeping the patient comfortable and functional is optimal. The most commonly prescribed medications are the topical steroids. In general, mid- to high-potency steroids are a mainstay of treatment. The vitamin D-derived calcipotriene (Dovonex) ointment is often effective and lacks the side-effects of atrophy, tachyphylaxis and (rarely) adrenal suppression resulting from systemic absorption associated with long-term topical steroid use. A maximum of 100g can be used per week and it is contraindicated in patients with hypercalcemia, vitamin D toxicity, or renal stones. Tar-containing bath additives, shampoos and ointments are good adjunctive therapy, although they can be messy and baths are often not feasible for patients who are elderly or disabled. Treatment of a coexisting streptococcal infection often results in improvement of the psoriasis. Emollients should also be used liberally.

Other treatment modalities used by dermatologists include anthralin, phototherapy, oral retinoids or methotrexate. An important advance has been the development of a group of drugs called biologic response modifiers or biologics, such as etanercept (Enbrel) or adalimumab (Humira). They differ significantly from traditional drugs used to treat psoriatic arthritis in that they target specific components of the immune system instead of broadly affecting many areas of the immune system. Biologics may be used alone but are commonly given along with topical medications (*Merck Manual*, 2011).

TREATMENT OF DRUG ERUPTIONS

Drug eruptions can present in a wide variety of clinical manifestations. Adverse drug reactions are found in 10–20% of all hospitalized patients and are the cause of hospitalization in 3–6% of admissions (*Merck Manual*, 2011). Eruptions typically appear 1–10 days after starting a drug and last for up to14 days after discontinuation of the drug. Rarely, drug eruptions can occur after weeks, months, or even years of using a medication. The drugs most commonly implicated are: (a) penicillins, (b) sulfonamides, (c) cephalosporins (10% cross-reactivity with penicillins), (d) anticonvulsants, (e) blood products, (f) quinidine, (g) barbiturates, (h) isoniazid and (i) furosemide (Lasix). However, any medication, including over-the-counter preparations and sporadically used drugs, can cause eruptions.

The most common morphology is the morbilliform, or maculopapular, eruption, which is a symmetrical pruritic eruption of coalescing erythematous macules and papules distributed on the trunk and extending peripherally onto the extremities. Other forms of drug eruptions are urticaria, photosensitivity, lichenoid drug eruption, vasculitis and fixed-drug eruption. A fixed-drug eruption is characterized by a single or a few localized red-to-violaceous round plaques that resolve with hyperpigmentation and recur in the same location when medications are withdrawn and reintroduced. Treatment of a drug eruption requires discontinuation of the culprit drug. Medium-potency topical steroids, antihistamines and antipruritic lotions, such as calamine and Sarna lotion, give symptomatic relief.

Potentially life-threatening drug eruptions requiring hospitalization, especially in the elderly, are: (a) exfoliative erythroderma, (b) anticonvulsant hypersensitivity syndrome, (c) erythema multiforme major (Stevens–Johnson syndrome) and (d) toxic epidermal necrolysis. These are real dermatological emergencies, requiring hospitalization and supportive care.

Exfoliative erythroderma is characterized by generalized erythema and scaling. The inability to maintain fluid balance, regulate electrolytes and body temperature, and high-output cardiac failure are potential complications. Anticonvulsant hypersensitivity syndrome is a multi-organ reaction that occurs with phenobarbital, carbamazepine and phenytoin, all of which cross-react with each other. In addition to cutaneous findings, which can be of any type, fever, lymphadenopathy, hematological abnormalities and hepatitis are seen. Other organs can also be affected.

In erythema multiforme major, the pathognomonic target lesions, which have red peripheries and cyanotic or bullous centers, are accompanied by erosion of the mucous membranes. This can sometimes be seen on a continuum with toxic epidermal necrolysis, which is characterized by a tender skin eruption that rapidly progresses to blistering and sloughing of skin. Applying lateral force to the skin causes the overlying epidermis to shear off (Nikolsky's sign). This condition carries a 50% mortality rate and requires patients to be treated in a hospital burn unit.

TREATMENT OF URTICARIA

Urticaria, or hives, is characterized by pruritic, edematous and, usually, erythematous papules and plaques, often surrounded by a red halo (flare). Urticaria results from the release of histamine, bradykinin, kallikrein and other vasoactive substances from mast cells and basophils in the superficial dermis, resulting in intradermal edema caused by capillary and venous vasodilatation and occasionally caused by leukocyte infiltration (*Merck Manual*, 2011). Angioedema or deeper subcutaneous swellings may accompany urticaria. Typically, individual lesions last no longer than 24 hours. If lesions are longer-lasting, urticarial vasculitis or other diagnoses should be considered.

Urticaria has a variety of causes, the most common of which is an allergic reaction to foods (e.g. strawberries, nuts, shellfish) or drugs (e.g. penicillin, contrast dye). Physical factors, such as cold, pressure or sunlight, emotional stress or infections (e.g. dental abscess, streptococcal upper respiratory infection, parasitic infection), can also induce urticaria. Certain medications, such as aspirin and narcotics, can cause direct nonimmunological degranulation of mast cells, which results in urticaria. Bullous pemphigoid (see below) can initially mimic urticaria. Urticaria usually resolves spontaneously within days to a few weeks. If lesions continue to appear for more than 6 weeks and if no allergen can be identified, a workup for systemic disease is warranted. Whenever possible, the causative agent should be identified and eliminated. Oral antihistamines are the mainstay of treatment. Topical steroids and antihistamines are ineffective. In the case of anaphylaxis or laryngeal edema, emergency resuscitation measures should be undertaken, including the administration of epinephrine (adrenaline), support of blood pressure and maintenance of a patent airway (*Merck Manual*, 2011).

DIFFERENTIAL DIAGNOSIS AND TREATMENT OF BULLOUS DISORDERS

Bullous eruptions in an elderly patient can range from those caused by benign physical factors to life-threatening immune-mediated bullous disorders. A flattening of the dermal–epidermal junction with aging results in increased skin fragility and susceptibility to blistering. Edematous skin is even more likely to develop blisters. The following is a partial list of diagnoses to consider.

Burns

Chemical, thermal and ultraviolet-light injury can result in blisters in affected areas. A diagnosis can usually be made after taking a patient history. Treatment is supportive, employing cool soaks for thermal and ultraviolet burns, as well as antibiotic ointments, such as silver sulfadiazine and protective dressings. Nonsteroidal anti-inflammatory drugs, such as aspirin or indomethacin, can also be beneficial in the early treatment of sunburns.

Contact Dermatitis

As discussed above, an acute contact dermatitis can result in such serious inflammation and edema that it leads to frank vesiculation. Clues to contact dermatitis are a linear arrangement of vesicles, odd-shaped lesions and sharply demarcated lesions. Treatment is outlined above (see under Dermatitis).

Bullous Impetigo

This superficial staphylococcal infection presents as flaccid bullae that easily rupture, leaving yellowish crusts.

Treatment is with anti-staphylococcal antibiotics, such as 250–500 mg of dicloxacillin four times a day.

Bullous Pemphigoid

This is a chronic, immunologically mediated, bullous disorder characterized by tense bullae on normal or erythematous skin. Pruritus is common and mucous membrane involvement occurs in approximately 20–50% of cases. Bullous pemphigoid can have a pre-bullous phase that presents as urticaria or pruritus without distinct skin lesions. Men and women are equally affected and most patients are over 60 years of age at the onset of disease. Diagnosis is made by skin biopsy followed by routine pathology and immunofluorescence. Immunofluorescence reveals immunoglobulin G (IgG) and complement (C3) deposits at the dermal–epidermal junction of perilesional skin. Traditionally, bullous pemphigoid has been treated with systemic corticosteroids and immunosuppressive therapy. The combination of minocycline and nicotinamide has been shown to be effective in some patients. Consultation with a dermatologist is strongly advised.

Pemphigus Vulgaris

Much less common than bullous pemphigoid, pemphigus vulgaris is another chronic immunologically mediated bullous disease that presents with flaccid rather than tense bullae. Often, only ruptured bullae (erosions and crusts) are present. Mucous membranes are almost always affected and may sometimes be the only manifestation of the disease. Again, the diagnosis is made by skin biopsy and immunofluorescence, which shows IgG and C3 deposited on the surface of keratinocytes. Before the advent of corticosteroids, pemphigus vulgaris was universally fatal. Today, it is treated aggressively with corticosteroids and other immunosuppressive agents, leading to long-lasting remissions.

TREATMENT OF PURPURA

Purpura result when blood extravasates into cutaneous tissue. Purpura can be classified as a disorder of hemostasis, increased fragility of blood vessels and their supporting connective tissue, vasculitis (inflammation of blood vessels) or pigmented purpura.

Purpura can be a manifestation of bleeding disorders, such as idiopathic thrombocytopenic purpura (ITP), thrombotic thrombocytopenic purpura (TTP), disseminated intravascular coagulation (DIC), liver disease, thrombocythemia or bone marrow dysfunction secondary to leukemia or drugs. Anticoagulants, such as heparin and coumadin, aspirin or nonsteroidal anti-inflammatory drugs, can also be associated with purpura, usually in response to an injury to the skin. Often in patients with other dermatitides, such as drug eruptions, skin may become purpuric. Treatment is directed at correcting the underlying cause.

Fragility of Blood Vessels

The most common cause of this purpura is actinic (Bateman's) purpura (*Merck Manual*, 2011). The combination of aging and chronic sun damage leads to degeneration of the collagen that surrounds and supports small vessels. Incidental trauma often results in slowly resolving purpuric macules. Chronic corticosteroid administration can produce similar changes.

Vasculitis

Palpable purpuric papules should point to the possibility of vasculitis, although lesions of vasculitis need not always be palpable. Causes of vasculitis include: (a) drug allergy, (b) bloodborne infection (e.g. streptococcus, meningococcemia, viral hepatitis and endocarditis), (c) serum sickness, (d) collagen vascular diseases and (e) cryoglobulinemia. Wegener's granulomatosis and polyarteritis nodosa are examples of vasculitis involving larger medium-sized vessels. When vasculitis is present in the skin, it is important to rule out systemic involvement with a urinalysis, renal and liver function tests, and a stool guaiac test. Whenever possible, treatment is directed at the underlying condition. Treatment is generally supportive, although some forms of vasculitis, particularly those with systemic involvement, may require treatment with corticosteroids, other anti-inflammatory or immunosuppressive drugs.

Pigmented Purpura

In this disorder, there are several idiopathic purpuric eruptions, unrelated to any the systemic disease, that primarily affect the lower legs. Lesions may be predominantly red to purple (of recent onset) or brown to golden-brown (chronic hemosiderin deposits). No treatment is necessary or very effective.

CONCLUSION

Age-related changes occur in the structure and function of the skin. Viral, fungal and bacterial infections of the skin, as well as infestations and inflammatory conditions, may occur. The use of some common treatment interventions can be affected by the advanced age of the patient and so precautions must be taken. The proper care of the skin of an aging individual is confounded by coexisting pathologies; thus, effective patient education and monitoring of this patient population by primary and rehabilitation health professionals is critically important.

REFERENCES

Elgart ML 2002 Skin infections and infestations in geriatric patients. Clin Geriatr Med 18(1):89–101
Habif TP 2004 Clinical Dermatology: A Color Guide to Diagnosis and Therapy, 4th edn. Mosby, Philadelphia, PA
Merck Manual 2011. In: Porter RS, Kaplan JLet al (eds) The Merck Manual, 19th edn. Merck Laboratories, Inc., Whitehouse Station, NJ
Wolff K, Johnson RA, Suurmond D 2005 Fitzpatrick's Color Atlas and Synopsis of Clinical Dermatology, 5th edn. McGraw-Hill, New York
Yaar M, Gilchrest BA 2001 Skin aging: postulated mechanisms and consequent changes in structure and function. Clin Geriatr Med 17(4):617–630

UNIT SEVEN

Aging and the pathological sensorium

UNIT CONTENTS

Chapter 51

Functional vision changes in the normal and aging eye

BRUCE P. ROSENTHAL • MICHAEL FISCHER

CHAPTER CONTENTS

DEMOGRAPHICS

The World Population Clock showed 7 069 054 252 in one instant on 28 February 2013. The world population total is expected to rise to over 11 billion by 2050 (US Census Bureau, 2013) (see Table 51.1).

The 21st century has continued to experience a dramatic increase in the aging population throughout the United States of America as well as the world. The number of individuals aged 85 and older, as well as centenarians, will grow significantly for the first time in history. The upswing in aging in developed as well as developing nations reflects a similar increase in aging. Many of these factors include healthcare management, decrease in fertility rates, increase in chronic diseases, health and diet awareness campaigns, training of medical and ancillary personnel, early diagnosis and early treatments. These dynamics in turn have translated into an increase in the 'old old' worldwide, especially where half of the world's oldest of the old reside: China, the US, India, Japan, Germany and Russia. (The National Eye Institute distinguishes between the old and the oldest old, for research and policy purposes, as people age 85 and over.)

One of the more remarkable worldwide statistics is that by 2030, nearly 24% of all older Japanese are expected to be at least 85 years old (National Institute on Aging, 2011).

The increased aging population, throughout the world, will translate into greater numbers of persons developing age-related eye diseases. There is a 1.8% (3 377 037) rate of vision disability in the age group of 18–64 years (192 699 903). This increases to 36.6% (14 658 874) in the 65 years and over population of 40 086 253 (United States Census Bureau, 2012) (see Table 51.2 and Fig. 51.1).

The dramatically aging demographic shift converts into greater numbers of individuals who will experience changes in vision as a result of the normal aging process. These changes range from a decrease in the ability to focus on the printed page (presbyopia), to the reduction in the production of tear fluid, to a need for greater illumination when reading. By 2020, there will also be an increased cohort who will experience a significant loss of vision from pathological eye conditions such as macular

Table 51.1 **Projected increase in global population between 2005 and 2030, by age**	
Age	Increase
0–64	21%
65+	104%
85+	151%
100+	400+%

Table 51.2 **Prevalence of adult vision impairment and age-related eye disease in the United States of America[a]**	
Total population ≥40	142 648 393
All vision impairment	4 195 966
Blindness	1 288 275
Myopia ≥1.0 diopters	34 119 279

Based on 2010 US Census populations.
[a]Estimated number of cases by vision problem : age ≥40 years.

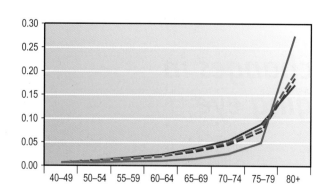

Figure. **51.1** US prevalence rates for all vision impairment, 2010. *(Data from Prevent Blindness America: Vision Problems in the US. Available at: www .visionproblemsus.org/index.html. Accessed December 2013.)*

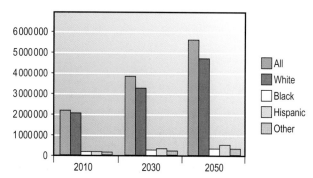

Figure. 51.2 Projected change in US incidence of AMD, 2010–2050. *(Source: National Eye Institute.)*

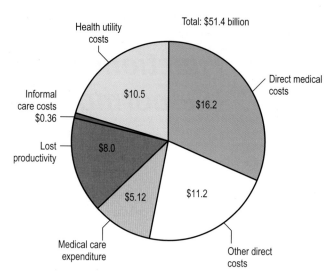

Figure. 51.3 The annual economic impact ($bn) of adult vision problems in the United States of America. *(Based on The Silverbook: Vision loss. [Online] http://www.silverbook.org/category/80; and Prevent Blindness America 2007 The Economic Impact of Vision Problems. Prevent Blindness America, Chicago, IL.)*

Table 51.3 **Characteristics of falls and injuries sustained among older adults with AMD over a 12-month period**

	No. falls	Percent
All falls	102	100
Injurious falls	64	63
Injury sustained		
Soft-tissue injury	55	86
Fracture	4	6
Head trauma	5	8

Excerpted from Wood et al., 2011, Table 2.

degeneration (Fig. 51.2), diabetic retinopathy, glaucoma, stroke and cataract. This will translate into an increase in persons with visual impairment, blindness and low vision.

VISION-RELATED HEALTHCARE COSTS

The annual burden to the US economy of age-related macular degeneration (AMD), cataract, diabetic retinopathy, glaucoma, refractive errors, visual impairment and blindness in adults age 40 and older was estimated in 2007 at $35.4 billion – $16.2 billion in direct medical costs, $11.1 billion in other direct costs and $8 billion in lost productivity (see Fig. 51.3).

VISION IMPAIRMENT AND FALLS

Vision impairment has been found to be one of the leading causes of falls in the elderly, along with functional decline and depression. One study found that visual field loss was associated with a 6-fold risk of frequent falls (Wood et al., 2011).

Ramrattan et al. (2001) found that visual field loss, most commonly associated with glaucoma and stroke, was associated with a six-times risk of falling. Macular degeneration has been one of the eye diseases closely studied with regards to falls. Wood et al. (2011) found that persons with AMD reported a fall in 54% and more

than two falls in 30% of the cohort studied. Of those falling, 63% of the falls reported resulted in injury. In another study on AMD, Soubrane et al. (2007) found that there was double the rate of falls in a population of persons as well as a quadrupled need for help with activities of daily living (ADLs).

The LALES study (Los Angeles Latino Eye) study followed 3202 Latino adults between 2004 and 2008. Decreased central vision from conditions such as macular degeneration and diabetic retinopathy and peripheral vision loss from conditions such as glaucoma and stroke resulted in more frequent and more serious falls. Macular degeneration is the major condition resulting in vision loss in Caucasians in the US. Central vision loss increased risk of fall or injury by 2.8 times, while peripheral vision loss increased this risk by 1.4 times. Over a 1-year period, 54% of individuals with AMD reported a fall and 30% reported more than one. Of all reported falls, 63% resulted in an injury (Wood et al., 2011) (see Table 51.3). Researchers concluded that elderly patients' peripheral vision is a large factor in their chances of falling (Patino et al., 2010).

Mogk and Watson (2008) have pointed out that seniors often rely on their vision to compensate for other age-related losses, so that when vision is lost too, they are particularly vulnerable to age-specific functional declines and dangerous falls.

Dual sensory loss, including hearing loss with vision loss, as well as other impairments, further contributes to falls. In the geriatric population, on average, sensory impairment doubles the number of falls, as noted by Harwood (2001; Harwood et al., 2005, 2009). Harwood's suggestions for decreasing the number of falls include 'simple interventions' such as correcting refractive error as well as operating on cataracts.

OTHER CONCERNS ABOUT VISION CHANGES

As noted, there is a sharp increase in the incidence of ocular disease in the seventh, eighth and ninth decade of life. It is, however, important to look at the changes in the visual system of the normal aging eye in order to understand, as well as differentiate these deviations from more serious changes in vision. These changes may be the result of comorbidities such as stroke, ocular pathology such as the complications from diabetes, hypertension, high cholesterol, auto-immune disease, tumors, kidney and heart disease.

Polypharmacy, common in the age group cited, may have serious implications in persons with low vision and may have a profound affect in adversely affecting the visual system. Zagar and Baggarly (2010) in fact point out that individuals with visual impairment have difficulty reading prescription and nonprescription medication information. They may even take the wrong medication or incorrect doses of medication which may result in serious negative consequences, including overdoses or inadequate treatment of health problems. This in turn may lead to emergency room visits or hospitalization.

The majority of individuals with vision loss also report increased anxiety related to medication management and having to rely on companions, or in some cases complete strangers, to obtain necessary drug information. Furthermore, 65% of Americans indicate that if they were to have severe vision loss, they would be most concerned about not being able to properly identify their medications (American Foundation for the Blind, 2004, 2008).

Presbyopia is an eye condition which makes its appearance as one of the earliest signs of aging of the visual system as well as the body. The word presbyopia comes from the Greek word *presbys* (πρέσβυς), meaning 'old', 'elderly', and the Neo-Latin suffix *-opia*, meaning 'sightedness' (Merriam-Webster Online Dictionary, 2013). Presbyopia generally begins in the early 40s and may be evident when the print is blurry, your arms are too short to hold text far enough away and fatigue sets in with prolonged close work as well as with using a computer or electronic device. The ability to accommodate or focus for close work such as reading or intermediate tasks such as the computer is known as accommodation. The near point of vision is the closest that one can accommodate (focus the eye) close

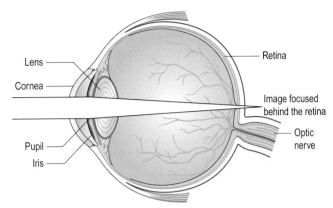

Figure. 51.4 A cross-section of eye showing that the image (of an object, e.g. newsprint) is focused behind the retina when the accommodation begins to decrease. The condition, known as presbyopia, requires corrective lenses to clear up the picture seen. *(Source: National Eye Institute.)*

up. The near point of the eye is generally considered to be about 3 in (7 cm) at age 10 moving out to about 6 in (16 cm) at age 40 and 39 in (1 meter) at age 60. As a result, a person from age 40 to 45 may require corrective lenses to read at a 'normal' reading distance, of 14–18 in (35–45 cm) (Fig. 51.4). The distance will depend on the length of one's arms as well, since the further from the eye the print is held, the less the accommodative demand required for reading. The accommodative demand is also dependent upon the near visual task. It is normally accompanied by a convergence of the eyes to keep them directed at the same point, sometimes termed the accommodation convergence reflex (Bhola, 2006).

Distance, font size and contrast may also affect the accommodative demand. A computer, for example, is generally placed at 24 in (60 cm) or greater from the eye, while an electronic or digital device may be held at a closer distance. The font and the contrast will also allow an increase in the working demand with a decrease in the accommodative demand.

The mechanical system that regulates the flexibility of the human lens to become more convex (accommodate) for close work requires not only the lens but the ciliary body and the zonules (tiny guy wires in the insert connecting the lens to the ciliary body which help to make the lens more convex to see close up) (see Figs 51.5 and 51.6).

AGE-RELATED EYE DISEASES

The most prevalent age-related eye diseases include:

- AMD and other conditions of the retina
- Cataracts
- Glaucoma
- Diabetic retinopathy
- Optic atrophy
- Visual field loss resulting from stroke, ischemia and tumors.

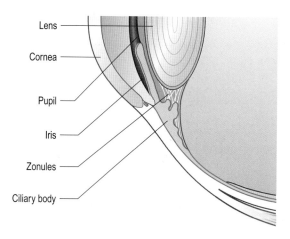

Figure. 51.5 Cross-section showing the lens and the zonules (at the bottom of the lens), which appear as tiny wires that connect to a structure known as the ciliary body. (*Source: National Eye Institute.*)

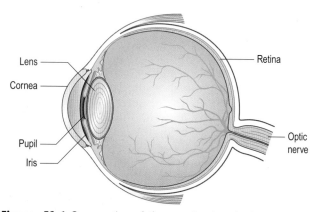

Figure. 51.6 Cross-section of the eye showing the lens. The lens has the ability to accommodate (become more convex) for seeing clearly at near (e.g. reading as well as seeing the computer). The decreasing flexibility, known as presbyopia, is on one the first indicators of the aging process in the body. (*Source: National Eye Institute.*)

AGE-RELATED MACULAR DEGENERATION (AMD)

AMD is a leading cause of vision loss in the US (Fig. 51.7). AMD may result in a destruction of the macula, the critical zone of the retina that provides the highest resolution for sharp, central vision needed to see objects clearly.

The macula is the small central portion of the retina that subtends an area of 20° of the visual field at 13 in (33 cm) from the eye. This 20° area is used to evaluate the integrity of the visual function with the use of a grid (the Amsler grid) that is 20 × 20 squares with each subtending an angle of 1° at that distance. Figure 51.8 illustrates a normal-appearing Amsler compared to an Amsler grid that has been impacted by a significant loss from AMD.

But the macula is integral for the quality of the central vision and color vision, as well as fine detail. The center of the macular, the fovea, has the highest density of receptors and is responsible for being able to

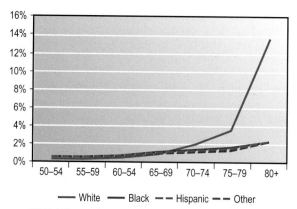

Figure. 51.7 US prevalence rates for age-related macular degeneration, 2010. (*Source: National Eye Institute.*)

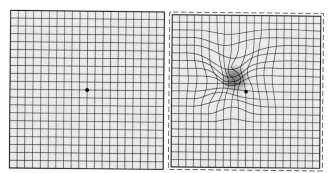

Figure. 51.8 Normal and abnormal Amsler grid. (*Source: National Eye Institute.*)

read newsprint or the print on a prescription bottle. The macula has the highest density of the color receptors in the eye. The macula also plays an important role in regulating the ability to adapt to changes in conditions of illumination.

The retina is a complex structure that includes the photoreceptors (rods and cones) as well as the RPE (retinal pigment epithelial layer). The RPE, which cannot regenerate, plays a role in removing debris from the eye. Damage to the macula from the debris (also known as drusen) affects central vision and may result in blurring, distortion and loss of areas of vision (scotomas).

AMD is an umbrella term that includes dry and wet AMD. As noted in the statistics, it is a major cause of visual impairment in Caucasians throughout the world. The wet type of AMD is considered to be more destructive to visual function. But new treatments have been developed that preserve the vision. The treatment for wet AMD may involve anti-VEGF (vascular endothelial growth factor) injections.

Low vision remediation includes the prescription of low vision devices (see section on LV devices). It is also important to include a discussion on the use of anti-oxidants, including vitamin C, zinc and copper, as well as lutein and omega-3 in the treatment of AMD.

CATARACTS

Cataracts are the most common age-related eye condition. They are best described as a clouding of the

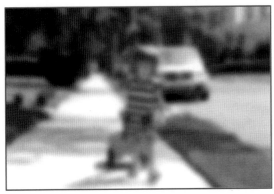

Figure. 51.9 Simulation of cataract. *(Courtesy of Bruce Rosenthal.)*

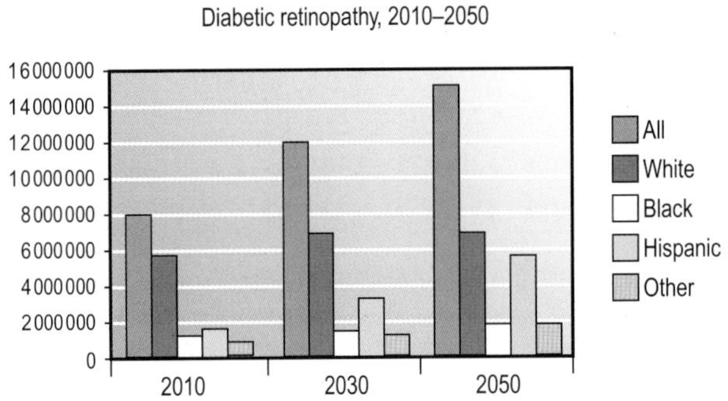

Diabetic retinopathy, 2010–2050

Figure. 51.10 Projected change in US incidence of diabetic retinopathy, 2010–2050. *(Source: National Eye Institute.)*

normally clear lens of the eye. The changes may range from an early opacification that causes little or no interference to vision to dense cloudiness, which results in marked visual impairment. The rate of progression of cataracts varies from person to person as well as between the right and left eye of the same individual.

A cataract is most common in age-related changes in the structure of the lens of the eye which manifests itself with symptoms that include: blurry vision, disability glare and difficulty when trying to read, for example, the highway signs when driving (see Fig. 51.9). The prevalence of cataracts increases with age, but may also be related to systemic pharmacological treatment of systemic conditions, such as the use of corticosteroids, as well as trauma.

Cataract surgery in the absence of other ocular pathologies, such as AMD, will result in a return to normal visual functioning. Treatment involves replacement of the normal lens with intraocular lenses by means of non-invasive stitchless surgery. New implant lens replacements have been complemented with multifocal implants. Patients will, however, have decreased vision following surgery when another pathological condition exists, such as AMD. Cataract surgery is generally performed when visual function, as well as visual efficiency, is reduced. Pre-existing conditions, particularly wet AMD, complicate the situation and necessitate a discussion with the ophthalmologist on the risks and benefits.

Symptoms of cataracts may include glare sensation to oncoming headlights of automobiles, a reduction of vision when wearing sunglasses, the need to shade the eyes when going outdoors in the sun, glare from fluorescent ceiling lights or bright reading lamps, or difficulty seeing street or highway signs.

GLAUCOMA

Glaucoma is a major health concern since vision loss may be progressive without evidence of pain. It is one of the most common age-related conditions that may result in serious vision loss when undiagnosed or not treated. The eye pressure generally ranges from 10 to 20 mmHg. The loss of the visual field from glaucoma can be profound and affect mobility, peripheral and night vision

when the pressure is elevated or compromised, with other compounding factors including the thickness of the cornea.

The analogy of a drain outflow being affected can illustrate why vision can be lost from a 'clogged' drainage system in the eye. Aqueous fluid is continuously produced and drained by the trabecular meshwork which in turn drains the aqueous into the venous drainage in the eye. Obstruction of the aqueous fluid through the drainage trabecular meshwork may result in fluid build-up. The increase in the intraocular pressure without adequate drainage through the canal of Schlemn may damage the optic nerve. Damage to the optic nerve may affect quality of life, ADLs and, especially, mobility under conditions of poor illumination. Glaucoma is a very complex eye disease that was formerly thought to be the result of elevated eye pressure only. But new models have shown that the corneal thickness plays a role in destroying cells in the optic nerve with pressure heretofore thought to be normal. Progressive optic nerve loss from glaucoma may impair night vision, mobility and functioning in poorly lit or even crowded environments.

Treatment includes eye drops as well as surgical intervention. Despite the best efforts, longevity may result in a severe decrease in contrast and the usable visual field. Low vision coping interventions may include new glasses, improved lighting, or even prisms for mobility.

DIABETIC RETINOPATHY

Diabetic retinopathy is the leading cause of blindness in American adults. The increase of diabetic retinopathy in the Caucasian, black, and especially Hispanic populations will be dramatic over the next 35 years. Diabetic retinopathy is the result of changes in the blood vessels of the retina. Individuals with diabetic retinopathy develop porous and leaky blood vessels that affect the photoreceptor layer (light-sensitive) tissue at the back of the eye. Diabetic retinopathy is treated with laser photocoagulation (PR) or steroids. The laser therapy preserves vision on one hand and destroys the peripheral or night vision on the other. Diabetes and diabetic retinopathy is predicted to be a major health crisis over the next 50 years (see Fig. 51.10 and Table 51.4).

Table 51.4	**Increase in diabetic retinopathy**				
Year	All	White	Black	Hispanic	Other
2010	7 685 237	5 251 907	826 102	1 194 231	412 997
2030	11 350 006	6 384 275	1 191 481	2 939 136	835 113
2050	14 559 464	6 374 626	1 547 724	5 254 328	1 382 786

Source: www.nei.nih.gov/eyedata/diabetic.asp#4.

REFRACTIVE ERROR

There are many 'normal' changes in the refraction of the eye that require correction across the lifespan, including myopia, hyperopia and astigmatism. Eyeglass corrections may correct for myopia and hyperopia, as well as incorporating the astigmatic correction as well.

Correction may include distance, intermediate, or reading lenses, bifocals and progressive lenses, contact lenses and laser correction.

Myopia, also known as nearsightedness, is a common type of refractive error where close objects appear clear, but distant objects appear blurry. Concave or minus lenses are used in the correction of myopia. Hyperopia, also known as farsightedness, is a common type of refractive error where distant objects may be seen more clearly than objects that are near. Convex or plus lenses correct for hyperopia. Astigmatism is unequal curvature of the cornea or induced by changes in the lenses of the eye (the eye is similar to the shape of a football or spoon).

The correction of refractive error, in the absence of ocular pathology, will generally restore distance, intermediate (e.g. seeing the computer) or near vision.

VISUAL FUNCTION IN THE AGING PROCESS

The eye is a unique structure that has many components, which comprise the multiple visual functions. Changes in each of these individualistic functions may affect normal aging, as well as the aging eye. The most important constituents of visual function include visual acuity, visual field, contrast sensitivity, color vision, binocularity, depth perception, sensitivity to light, stereo acuity, glare and fixation. Any of these functions, affected by disease or the aging process, may significantly impact the ability to manage ADLs, including the ability to travel independently or maintain one's own affairs.

VISUAL ACUITY

Visual acuity is a single aspect of vision but perhaps the most synonymous with visual health, since it is the standard measurement for vision testing in the US. Dr Herman Snellen is credited with introducing the modern 'eye testing' system in 1862. It has survived and remains in place to this day. The Snellen fractions, 20/20, 20/30, 20/200, relate to the ability to identify a letter (optotype) of a certain size at a specific distance.

It is based on the ability of an individual to resolve the detail of a target: 20/20 vision indicates that one has the ability to resolve or distinguish a target that is 5 minutes of arc at a distance of 20 feet (6 m) with detail of 1 minute of arc. The 20 foot test distance was selected because it is considered optical infinity. Theoretically, an object placed at this distance from the eye requires no accommodation.

Visual acuity may be measured at closer distances (10 feet [3 m] or less) when the vision, as noted, is decreased from ocular pathology. Accurate functional acuity measurement may demand the use of specialized vision charts that record visual acuity to 20/800 or less. Vision below that may be designated as CF ('counts fingers') or HM ('hand motion'). 'Light perception' indicates the ability to see a light source, while 'light projection' indicates the position of the projected light. This information may be very beneficial in orienting one's self in space.

Visual Fields and Assessment

Visual fields are another very important measure of visual function. The visual fields provide significant functioning of the peripheral vision and central vision. Visual fields are important in monitoring the progression of visual field loss in conditions such as glaucoma, ischemic optic nerve diseases and retinitis pigmentosa. The extent of the visual field is important in helping to understand issues of mobility in progressive eye diseases as well as those from stroke, brain tumors and head trauma.

Visual fields may be an important indicator in predicting injuries from falls. Methods used to determine the extent of the visual field involvement include: observational assessment; the confrontation test (a cursory test of being aware of the examiner's hands while fixating in the straight ahead position); utilization of a computer, which requires the ability to detect a moving object in the field while fixating straight ahead; and an automated perimeter.

Visual field measurement involves assessing the extent of the visual field in all directions while the patient monocularly fixates in the straight-ahead position. The normal visual field, for each eye, when looking in the straight-ahead position, is approximately 60° degrees to the nasal side, 90° to the temporal side, 50° superior, and 70° inferior.

Visual fields will help to reveal any depression in sensitivity, constriction, or scotomas (areas of no vision). The scotoma may be relative (sensitive to certain stimuli but not others), or absolute (corroborate no sensitivity to a stimulus – black holes). The visual field will also locate and define the shape of the scotoma, as well as any sector or field cut.

Measurement of the visual field following a stroke may require modification or simplification of the testing procedure to obtain the extent of the visual field involvement due to cognitive deficits. The National Institutes of Health Stroke Scale or NIH Stroke Scale (NIHSS) (Table 51.5) is a tool used by healthcare providers to objectively quantify the impairment caused by a stroke. The NIHSS is composed of 11 items, each of which scores a specific ability between a 0 and 4.

Table 51.5 National Institutes of Health Stroke Scale

Score	Test Results
0	No vision loss
1	Partial hemianopia or complete quadrantanopia; patient recognizes no visual stimulus in one specific quadrant
2	Complete hemianopia; patient recognizes no visual stimulus in one half of the visual field
3	Bilateral blindness, including blindness from any cause

Source: www.ninds.nih.gov/doctors/NIH_Stroke_Scale.pdf.

Legal Blindness

Visual acuity and visual field are two extremely important benchmarks in disability determination in the US and elsewhere in the world. The designation of 'legally blind' may provide eligibility for disability benefits, an extra income tax deduction, as well as training and reimbursement to maintain one's position at work. An individual who satisfies the definition of legal blindness is also entitled to services from a state 'commission for the blind and visual handicapped', free talking books from the Library of Congress, operator-assisted telephone service, handicapped parking privileges and increased access to public transportation, including door-to-door services provided by some states.

The definition for the determination of legal blindness in the US is:

Legally blind: A best-corrected visual acuity of 20/200 (6/60) or less in the better eye with best optical or contact lens correction or a visual field of 20 degrees or less in the widest meridian of the better eye with best correction.

The World Health Organization (10th Revision) International Statistical Classification of Diseases, Injuries and Causes of Death defines *low vision* as visual acuity of less than 20/60 (6/18), but equal to or better than 20/200 (6/60), or corresponding visual field loss of less than 20° in the better eye with best possible correction. The WHO also defines *blindness*, which is a visual acuity of less than 20/400 (6/120), or corresponding visual field loss to less than 10° in the better eye with best possible correction (WHO, 2010, 2013).

There are other very important definitions that are used in the US when discussing vision loss:

Vision impairment refers to conditions encompassing the continuum from blindness to partial sight and is defined as having 20/40 or worse vision in the better eye even with eyeglasses. Those with the least degree of vision impairment may still face challenges in everyday life. People with vision worse than 20/40 cannot obtain an unrestricted driver's license in most US states.

Low vision or *partial vision sight* (Silverstone et al., 1999) refers to a significant reduction of visual function that cannot be corrected to the normal range by ordinary glasses, contact lenses, medical treatment and/or surgery. (New treatments are helping to change some of this definition, e.g. anti-VEGF).

Blindness (Silverstone et al., 1999) is defined as no usable vision with the exception of light perception.

CONTRAST SENSITIVITY FUNCTION (CSF)

Contrast sensitivity is a measure of how much a pattern must vary in contrast to be seen while visual acuity measures how big an object must be to be seen. Contrast sensitivity is increasingly recognized as an important factor influencing the quality of vision. In fact it is considered in certain circumstances to be more important than visual acuity or the visual field (e.g. dim restaurants).

A decrease in the contrast sensitivity function can lead to a loss of spatial awareness and mobility as well as an increase in the risk of accidents. Contrast sensitivity may also affect the ability to: walk down steps, recognize faces, drive at night or in the rain, find a telephone number in a directory, read instructions.

Various charts have been designed for the measurement of the contrast sensitivity function (Arditi, 2005; Haymes et al., 2006; Sayan et al., 2008) in response to another method of monitoring visual function, especially in progressive eye disease. CSF is associated with ocular pathological conditions such as a cataract, AMD, diabetic retinopathy, glaucoma and optic nerve degenerations. Improvement in contrast is essential for safe mobility as well as managing ADLs at home or in the office. There are many strategies that may enhance or increase the CSF. The use of absorptive lenses and filters that are in the orange (527 nm) or yellow–orange range (527 nm), for example, may be beneficial for persons with AMD.

Contrast along with shape, color and texture are keys to identifying items. High contrasting color for the edges of steps, as well as train or subway platforms, are good safety measures. Safety measures in the home may also include outlining the bathtub with contrasting colors. Textures may include the use of 'hi mark' (marking liquid), black felt tip pens may be used to mark medicine bottles or appliance settings. Lighting sources throughout the home, including night lights, will also serve to reduce injuries when the CSF is decreased.

Access to increasing contrast when reading has taken a quantum leap with the advent of the electronic book, smart phone and improvements in computer monitor and television screen resolution. But it is the ability to change print to a white on black ground that can significantly improve reading efficiency.

Automotive engineering has significantly improved lighting systems that now enhance the ability to see under conditions of poor illumination. Simple tasks such as reading menus under conditions of poor illumination can be enhanced with portable xenon pen lights.

Binocularity is a common component of aging for many persons affected with the significant loss of vision in one or both eyes. The loss may be due to ocular disease such as macular degeneration, glaucoma, or field loss following a stroke or tumor. Outside as well as indoors, mobility training may be recommended when balance is affected.

GLARE SENSITIVITY

Glare sensitivity is generally classified as either discomfort glare or disability glare. Disability glare is the common type of glare encountered by an oncoming headlight at night and may be the result of a media opacity in the cornea or as a result of a developing cataract. But uncorrected refracted error such as myopia, hyperopia, or astigmatism may be the source of glare as well.

Discomfort glare may be experienced, for instance, when skiing or on the beach. Older individuals are generally more sensitive to glare as well as the ability to recover or adapt quickly when exposed to a glare source (Rea, 2000).

COLOR VISION

Macular degeneration and other retinal diseases may have an effect on color vision. The color receptors (the cones) are densely packed in the macula when compared to the peripheral area of the retina. Color perception will therefore be seriously affected when there is damage, such as a macular scar, or edema (e.g. diabetic macular edema) to the central retinal receptors.

Changes in color perception may result in injury when it affects the ability, for example, to see the color of traffic lights. Being able to discriminate and match colors when getting dressed, as well as distinguishing whether fruit is ripe or food is cooked, is affected as well by central visual field loss.

It has been established that the ability to see color declines with 'normal' aging as a result of changes in absorption of light by the ocular media including the lens as well as the reduction in the pupillary aperture of the eye. Acquired color vision loss in older persons differs from congenital (present at birth) defects in which altered characteristics of cone photopigments lead to color confusion. One way of classifying acquired color defects is Kollner's rule (Schwartz, 2011) that pertains to the progressive nature of color vision loss that is secondary to eye disease. This rule states that lesions in retinal diseases and media changes give rise to blue–yellow defects, whereas lesions in the inner retina including the optic nerve, visual pathways and visual cortex give rise to red–green defects.

Individuals with cataracts, that have only a nuclear yellowing, commonly have a blue–yellow confusion, as do individuals with AMD. Other individuals with optic neuritis (inflammation of the optic nerve) may report a red–green defect. Medications or combinations of drugs affect the perception of color. Drugs that alter perception of colors includes sedatives, antibiotics and antipsychotics.

DARK ADAPTATION

Dark adaptation, or the ability, to adjust to new levels of illumination, such as going from the outdoors to the indoors, may be very apparent and debilitating from retinal diseases (e.g. macular degeneration, macular edema, diabetic and hypertensive retinopathy). Adapting to changes in lighting levels is exemplified by the effect of a camera flash into the eye or entering a dark movie theatre. The response time in adapting, especially for elderly, may result in a fall from an object not obvious in the environment. Absorptive lenses and filters may be beneficial in minimizing the adaptation time as well as enhancing the contrast. Stereoacuity vision loss may often result in the vision being much poorer in one eye. This disparity between the two eyes may manifest itself in such tasks as threading a needle or tying shoelaces.

CHANGES IN THE AGING EYE

Aging may affect the muscle innervation to the eyelids, which in turn may have serious consequences as well as permanent and possibly blinding damage to the eye. A common eyelid alteration in the elderly is *entropion*. Entropion is a condition in which the eyelid turns inward (generally the lower lid) and may result in the eyelashes rubbing against the cornea. An abrasion to the epithelium and deeper layers of the cornea can result in serious damage, including scarring of the cornea. There is a sensation of discomfort as a result of the eyelashes rubbing against the front surface (epithelial layer) of the cornea. *Ectropion* is a turning out of the eyelid (generally lower) and can be manifested by drying out of the cornea, excessive tearing and keratitis, also resulting in inflammation of the cornea.

Blepharoptosis (also known as ptosis) is a drooping of the upper eyelid when there is a dysfunction of one or both upper eyelid elevator muscles. The result is a narrowing of the palpebral fissure (space between the eyelids) when the eyelid is open. The clinical significance is the obstruction in being able to see. Ptosis surgical intervention is often recommended as well as nonsurgical intervention which involves holding up the lid with a 'ptosis' crutch or tape. Precautions, however, must be taken when there is extensive exposure of the corneal surface, by supplementation of artificial tears.

Other age-related physiological changes include the thinning and yellowing of the conjunctiva. The corneal surface tends to dry out as tear production decreases and the tear film loses stability during the aging process. In addition, dry environments, especially in the winter or on airplanes, will often exacerbate the condition.

The tear film is actually three layers with an outer lipid layer, aqueous layer and mucin layer. The tear film protects and lubricates the cornea and conjunctiva. However, tear production (lacrimation) will often decrease with advancing age as a result of a decrease in production of the watery fluid from the lacrimal gland.

Artificial tears, as well as plugging up the drainage canal (puncta), will often result in greater comfort and less irritation to the eye.

Starting at about the age of 20, the pupillary aperture may decrease about 2.5 mm across the lifespan. The reduction in size can be clinically significant under lowered levels of illumination. In addition, mobility at night as well as reading (e.g. the menu in the restaurant) may be impacted by the resulting loss of light through the decreased pupil.

The density and weight of the lens of the eye (also known as the crystalline lens) increases with age. The lens become yellower (brunescent) in color and demonstrates fluorescence. Other physiological changes include a decrease in the number of RPE (retinal pigment epithelial) cells in the posterior pole of the eye.

IMPACT OF VISUAL LOSS ON ADLS AND EMOTIONAL STATUS

Depression may also be a symptom of age-related vision loss that severely impacts ADLs. In a study by Horowitz et al. (2005) of new applicants for recent vision loss rehabilitative services, 7% had current major depression and 26.9% met the criteria for subthreshold depression. Patients with wet AMD reported 45% worse vision-related functioning, 13% worse overall wellbeing, 30% more anxiety and 42% more depression than those without the disease. They also reported a doubled fall rate and a quadrupled need for assistance with ADLs.

Campbell et al. (1999) and Carabalese et al. (1993) reported that vision impairment is associated with higher than normal risk of depression. Depression may affect the ability to drive, read, cross a street; see the traffic signs and lights, read the temperature on the oven, as well being able to distinguish steps. Reinhardt et al. (2005) found, however, that depression is not an inevitable consequence of vision impairment. Whether a person with vision loss becomes depressed seems more related to the impact the vision loss has on a person's functioning rather than to the actual severity of vision loss.

The clinical literature on the issue of depression and visual impairment indicates that depression is a common emotional reaction to vision loss. Horowitz and Reinhardt (2000) assert that it is wrong to see depression as an essential part of the grieving process before adjustments could be made to cope with vision loss. The majority of adults with vision loss and adults who experience other chronic illnesses do not suffer from depression and it is important to recognize that depression is a serious disease that can be treated. However, a significant subgroup of older adults who are visually impaired are affected by depression which can have significant impact on functional ability, rehabilitation experiences and general quality of life.

DRIVING AND VISION LOSS

Telling a patient that 'you are no longer able to legally drive is often, as Horowitz describes, 'a challenging turning-point for older disabled adults' (Horowitz et al., 2002). Changing status to former driver can influence not only mobility, but also social ties, the ability to work, and one's sense of independence and public safety. This will be a major challenge and a trying transition for the aging population.

Horowitz et al. (2002) found that older drivers faced with vision problems are generally reluctant to discuss driving-related issues with others – only half talk about it with a family member, and only a quarter talk with a physician. However, the majority said that their doctors, spouses, or children would be most likely to influence their driving decisions.

THE LOW VISION EVALUATION

The low vision examination enables the low vision clinician to assess the magnitude of the effect of the eye disease on the amount of the vision loss. The examination also helps to develop a treatment plan in order to prescribe the appropriate optical, non-optical, electronic and digital strategies as well as triage to other members of the vision rehabilitation team. The members of the vision rehabilitation team may require the expertise of the vision rehabilitation therapist, orientation and mobility instructor, social worker, as well as the occupational or physical therapist. The orientation and mobility instructor may be assigned to facilitate the ability to navigate independently in one's environment. The social worker, psychologist, or psychiatrist may be required to address many of the issues noted, including depression, anger, isolation, family dynamics and independence. The ultimate objective is to maximize visual potential and quality of life.

The evaluation is the most important step in assessing the need for corrective lenses and adaptive low vision devices. They can be not only beneficial in restoring the ability to resume many of the activities that have been difficult if not impossible but to begin the rehabilitation process to facilitate independence.

The low vision examination integrates modern technology into the evaluation, as well as the treatment plan. Diagnostic equipment, including new fundus photography of the posterior portion of the eye, is valuable in helping patients, family and caregivers understand the underlying frustrating causes that impact on the vision loss. The new technological innovations have also helped to maximize vision with the ability to enlarge as well as make objects bolder.

A low visual examination, by an optometrist or ophthalmologist, with expertise in the care of the partially sighted, is therefore an essential step in the early adjustment to vision loss. It is especially important for persons who are under some of the recent treatments for conditions such as AMD or diabetic retinopathy, where the vision may actually improve over time.

The low vision evaluation is an eye examination that has been modified to investigate visual function in persons with pathological vision loss. The evaluation includes a very detailed functional history, including the activities of daily living, measurement of distance and near visual acuity, external evaluation (e.g. lids, pupillary reflexes), subjective and objective evaluation, tests of visual function, as well as the prescription of distance, intermediate and near prescriptive lenses or low vision optical and non-optical devices.

The case history provides information on patient objectives as well as the need for medical and psychosocial counseling, mobility, rehabilitation and training, or surgical intervention. The areas that are investigated include: medical history, ocular history including past diagnosis and treatment including surgery, laser, eye medications, or other treatments, psycho-social history, as well as a task analysis. The task analysis will explore and detail activities of daily living, such as seeing the microwave dials, the food on the plate, reading a label on a prescription bottle, the ability to see the numbers on the telephone, ability to travel independently, as well as other distance and near tasks, lighting considerations, as well as job activities. Near tasks are especially important and may include a discussion of the ability to read the newspaper, seeing prices and labels, to being able to fill a syringe or write a check. But the use of electronic devices has become an integral part of day-to-day living. The new digital world has provided a fresh approach to coping with activities such as managing a check book, calling on the telephone, or reading digitally, whether it is an enlarged bold font or voice output.

The clinician should have an impression of the patient's objectives and goals, whether or not they are realistic, and the patient's reaction to the vision loss and a sense of what can be done on the first visit. That is, the examiner should sense what can and cannot be covered during the initial evaluation without fatiguing the patient.

Distance and near visual acuity is evaluated using specialized eye charts at a distance and near. The idea is to establish useable vision in both eyes. Traditional eye charts are not sensitive enough to evaluate the vision. External evaluation, which follows visual acuity measurement, includes pupillary position, size and responses, and position of the lids, eyes and orbits. Refraction is essential in determining the best correction for the patient at distance and near. It is also important to determine an intermediate correction, whether it is looking at the computer screen, digital pad, or portable telephone.

A visual field analysis is one of the most important tests of visual function. The use of static and automated perimetry, as well as integrating new technology such as microperimetry with the optical coherence tomographer, helps establish the extent of the visual field loss and the ability to travel independently. But visual field analysis will also help to determine whether persons affected from conditions such as stroke or a tumor may benefit from the application of optical solutions, including the use of prisms for mobility.

The low vision evaluation also determines the appropriate low vision devices (for examples see Bakker, 2005) to help achieve the patient objectives. These include the prescription of a very strong reading lens (also known as high plus or microscopic reading lenses) and hand and stand magnifiers. The recommendation for hand and stand magnifiers (magnifiers that sit on the page) has changed with an understanding that enhancement of contrast conditions requires the use of good task lighting. One of the best new light sources includes the use of xenon. Halogen is too bright and hot, and constitutes a burn and fire hazard (Government of Western Australia Fire and Rescue Service, 2012).

The patient with a distance objective such as independent travel may benefit from a hand-held or spectacle-mounted telescopic. But newer and future technologies, such as a head-borne computer with GPS, may help to facilitate independent travel.

Filters and absorptive lenses, as previously noted, play an important role when there are complaints of glare,

light sensitivity, or poor contrast. The patient's own prescription that is incorporated in the absorptive lenses will further enable the clarity as well as absorb harmful UVB, blue light and IR.

Very high magnification as well as enhanced contrast is especially essential in profound loss of vision as well as a profound loss in the CSF. The prescription of table-mounted (in-line) and portable electronic magnification has provided the ability not only to increase magnification to 35–40× but the ability to reverse polarity, that is to be able to put white letters on a black background or black letters on a white background. The new smart cell phones and digital reading devices also improve quality of life for patients with low vision.

CONCLUSION

The increased incidence of visual impairment in older persons engenders the need for additional services and trained professionals. Major impediments to managing visual impairment in patients include the escalating cost of healthcare service delivery, and limited coverage for services. Low vision rehabilitation helps to optimize patients' visual potential, as well as assist them in coping with depression, and ultimately to improve their quality of life.

REFERENCES

American Foundation for the Blind 2004 Comments on prescription drug information accessibility. Available at: www.afb.org/Section.asp?SectionID=3&TopicID=329&DocumentID=2454. Accessed July 2010

American Foundation for the Blind 2008 Access to drug labels survey report. Available at: www.afb.org/Section.asp?SectionID=3&TopicID=135&DocumentID=4520. Accessed February 2013

Arditi A 2005 Improving the design of the Letter Contrast Sensitivity Test. Invest Ophthalmol Vis Sci 46(6):2225–2229

Bakker R 2005 Household tips for people with low vision. Available at: www.environmentalgeriatrics.com/pdf/handouts/household_tips_low_vision.pdf. Accessed December 2013

Bhola R 2006 Binocular vision. The University of Iowa Department of Ophthalmology & Visual Sciences. Available at: http://webeye.ophth.uiowa.edu/eyeforum/tutorials/BINOCULAR-VISION.pdf. Accessed February 2013

Campbell V, Crews E, Moriarty D et al 1999 Surveillance for sensory impairment, activity limitation, and health-related quality of life among older adults – United States, 1993–1997. MMWR CDC Surveill Summ 48(8):131–156

Caraballese C, Appollonio I, Rozzini R et al 1993 Sensory impairment and quality of life in a community elderly population. J Am Geriatr Soc 41(4):401–407

Government of Western Australia Fire and Rescue Services 2012 Halogen downlights and fire safety. Available at: http://en.wikipedia.org/wiki/Halogen_lamp. Accessed December 2012

Harwood G, Else V, Ranhoff A et al 2009 Prevalence of vision, hearing, and combined vision and hearing impairments in patients with hip fractures. Scand J Caring Sci 23(4):635–643

Harwood R 2001 Visual problems and falls. Age Ageing 30(Suppl 4): 13–18

Harwood R, Foos A, Osborn F et al 2005 Falls and health status in elderly women following eye cataract surgery: a randomized controlled trial. Br J Ophthalmol 89:53–59

Haymes SA, Roberts KF, Cruess AF 2006 The Letter Contrast Sensitivity Test: clinical evaluation of a new design. Invest Opthalmol Vis Sci 47(6):2739–2745

Horowitz A, Boerner K, Reinhardt JP 2002 Psychosocial aspects of driving transitions in elders with low vision. Gerontechnology 1:262–273

Horowitz A, Reinhardt J 2000 Mental health issues in visual impairment: research in depression, disability, and rehabilitation. In: Silverstone B, Lang M, Rosenthal B (eds) The Lighthouse Handbook on Vision Impairment and Vision Rehabilitation, Vol. II. Vision Rehabilitation. Oxford University Press, New York, pp. 1089–1109

Horowitz A, Reinhardt JP, Kennedy GJ 2005 Major and subthreshold depression among older adults seeking vision rehabilitation services. Am J Geriatr Psychiatry 13(3):180–187

Merriam-Webster Online Dictionary 2013. [Online] Available at: www.merriam-webster.com/dictionary/presbyopia. Accessed 28 February 2013

Mogk LG, Watson G (eds) 2008 Special issue on age-related macular degeneration. J Vis Impairment Blindness 102(10):581–659

National Institute on Aging 2011 Why population aging matters: a global perspective. Trend 3: Rising numbers of the oldest old. Available at: www.nia.nih.gov/health/publication/why-population-aging-matters-global-perspective/trend-3-rising-numbers-oldest-old. Accessed December 2013

Patino C, McKean-Cowdin R, Azen S, Los Angeles Latino Eye Study Group 2010 Central and peripheral visual impairment and the risk of falls and falls with injury. Ophthalmology 117(2):199–206

Ramrattan RS, Wolfs RC, Panda-Jonas S et al 2001 Prevalence and causes of visual field loss in the elderly. Age Ageing 30(Suppl 4):13–18

Rea MS 2000 IESNA Lighting Handbook, 9th edn. Illuminating Engineering Society of North America, New York

Reinhardt J, Horowitz A, Sussman-Skalka C 2005 Depression, vision loss and vision rehabilitation. [Online] Available at: www.lighthouse.org/services-and-assistance/social-services/depression-vision-loss-and-vision-rehabilitation. Accessed December 2013

Sayan D, Foss A, Grainge M et al 2008 The importance of acuity, stereopsis, and contrast sensitivity for health-related quality of life in elderly women with cataracts. Invest Ophthalmol Vis Sci 49(1):1–6

Schwartz S 2011 Visual Perception: A Clinical Orientation, 4th edn. McGraw-Hill, New York

Silverstone B, Lang M, Rosenthal B et al 1999 The Lighthouse Handbook on Vision Impairment and Vision Rehabilitation. Oxford University Press, New York

Soubrane G, Cruess A, Lotery A et al 2007 Burden and health care resource utilization in neovascular age-related macular degeneration: findings of a multicountry study. Arch Ophthalmol 125(9):1249–1254

United States Census Bureau 2012 Population estimates. [Online] Available at: www.census.gov/popest/data/national/totals/2012/. Accessed February 2013

United States Census Bureau 2013 US and World Population Clock. [Online] Available at: www.census.gov/main/www/popclock.html. Accessed February 2013

WHO 2010 International Statistical Classification of Diseases and Related Health Problems 10th Revision (ICD-10). Visual disturbances and blindness (H53-H54). Available at: http://apps.who.int/classifications/icd10/browse/2010/en#/H53-H54. Accessed February 2013

WHO 2013 Visual impairment and blindness. [Online] Available at: www.who.int/mediacentre/factsheets/fs282/en/. Accessed February 2013

Wood JM, Lacherez P, Black AA et al 2011 Risk of falls, injurious falls, and other injuries resulting from visual impairment among older adults with age-related macular degeneration. Invest Ophthalmol Vis Sci 52(8):5088–5092

Zagar M, Baggarly S 2010 Simulation-based learning about medication management difficulties of low-vision patients. Am J Pharm Educ 74(8):146

Chapter 52
Functional changes in the aging ear

KATIE L. MCARTHUR • STEPHEN E. MOCK

CHAPTER CONTENTS

INTRODUCTION

Aging is a gradual process. It does not happen suddenly but rather in such a way that most people sense a slow deterioration of sensory and motor skills over time. The aging process causes both structural and functional changes to occur in the body. Twentieth- and twenty-first century science and technology have led to many advances that have improved both quality of life and life expectancy, thus enabling the average human to live longer and better. If a person lives into or beyond the sixth or seventh decades of life, one must anticipate that modifications of mind and body will occur. Areas such as cognition, circulation, coordination and vision can be affected. Another area that is frequently affected by aging is the inner ear.

AGING WITHIN THE INNER EAR STRUCTURES

Hearing loss associated with the aging process is commonly termed 'presbycusis', which comes from the Greek *presbys* (πρέσβυς) 'elder' and *akusis* or 'hearing'. Thus, presbycusis can be directly translated as 'hearing in the elderly'. Both auditory and vestibular structures within the inner ear can be adversely affected by presbycusis. In fact, according to several past studies, hearing deficits associated with the aging process may begin in some individuals as early as 30 years of age and can be progressive, such that by the age of 65, approximately one-third of persons, both male and female, will suffer from significant hearing loss. These figures can rise to almost two-thirds for those people over the age of 80 (Christensen et al., 2001; NIDCD, 2002).

Within the aging process in humans, hearing loss can occur secondary to changes within the outer, middle or inner ear structures, within the brain itself, or sometimes because of changes in multiple areas of the auditory system (Martin & Jerger, 2005). When a hearing loss occurs within the outer or middle ear system, it is termed a conductive hearing loss because the conduction of the sound waves to the inner ear structures is disrupted. Conductive hearing loss is often medically or audiologically treatable and may be secondary to such problems as excessive buildup of cerumen or ear wax within the ear canal, fluid build-up within the middle ear cavity, perforations of the tympanic membrane, ossicular chain dysfunction or the effects of Paget's disease on bone tissue. These conductive problems can usually be diagnosed within a comprehensive audiological evaluation and appropriate treatment measures can be initiated.

Hearing deficits within the inner ear system are termed sensorineural in nature. This type of hearing impairment is traced to deficiencies within the inner ear or eighth cranial nerve structures. Unlike conductive hearing loss, sensorineural hearing loss is rarely treatable by medical or surgical intervention and is therefore considered to be a permanent condition. Degenerative changes within the auditory structure of hair cells and nerve fibers within the inner ear are the primary culprit. Although genetic changes secondary to the aging process can be a potential cause of presbycusis, the most common reason for age-related changes in hearing sensitivity is associated with exposure to the intense noise levels of day-to-day living. These exposures may be industrial or recreational in nature with the interrelationship between intense noise and hearing loss well documented over the years (NIDCD, 2008). Since the 1970s, the Occupational Safety and Health Administration (OSHA, 2002) has published and enforced guidelines on hearing conservation and protection in industrial settings (Center for Disease Control and Prevention, 2013). However, industrial noise is not the only potential cause of a noise-induced hearing loss, as many noise sources within the home environment can also be loud enough to potentially affect hearing. Individual susceptibility is also a factor in determining the effects of noise on an individual. Other possible causes of sensorineural hearing loss include: vascular changes within the inner ear, including diabetic-type changes; ototoxicity; viruses that may affect the cochlea and eighth nerve tumors or lesions.

Hearing loss related to changes within the cerebral cortex of the brain is termed central hearing loss. Understanding and interpreting speech is a complex task. Unfortunately for some individuals, their outer, middle and inner ears as well as the eighth nerve may be functional, but the brain itself may fail in interpreting the signals sent by the auditory system. It is the auditory system that allows us to 'hear' sounds, but it is the brain that allows for the 'interpretation' of speech. Some people may exhibit central problems secondary to traumatic head injury, tumor or stroke and thus present difficulty in interpreting or understanding speech. The degree of injury and the area of the brain affected usually dictate the prognosis for improvement or recovery in these instances. However, a category termed 'central auditory processing disorders' also falls into the realm of central hearing loss. These problems are quite common across the ages but are most commonly present in older individuals. With a central auditory processing problem, the person may exhibit difficulty understanding

or interpreting speech sounds when extraneous stimuli, such as background noises, are present. As one ages, structural and cortical chemical changes in the brain can occur. These changes can be exacerbated by factors such as overall health, genetics and environment. As the age-related decline of the brain occurs, auditory processing problems may become more evident. However, in some instances, therapeutic or rehabilitative measures may be available to inhibit or counteract these processing difficulties (Murphy et al., 2006).

Lastly, the condition of auditory neuropathy warrants mention. Within the evaluation of hearing loss, it can sometimes be found that, despite the presence of minimal measured hearing loss, the patient experiences very poor speech understanding in background noise situations. This condition is now able to be identified by enhanced auditory test measures, but auditory neuropathy presents significant challenges for successful rehabilitation of this auditory deficit (Hain & Micco, 2003; Roush, 2008).

SIGNS AND SYMPTOMS OF HEARING LOSS

Hearing loss is a common anomaly, especially among older individuals. However, hearing loss is also insidious and not always apparent to the individual, the family or primary care physician, who may be asked for an opinion. In general, people over the age of 50 should undergo a comprehensive auditory evaluation in order to determine a hearing baseline for future comparisons. However, numerous research studies generated by hearing professionals (Kochkin, 2009) continue to define the hearing-impaired as an underserved population for treatment. One of the primary reasons for this finding is a

lack of desire or understanding of the symptoms of hearing impairment. In fact, it is commonly felt that hearing loss, especially in its early stages, will more commonly be noted by family or friends, rather than by individuals themselves. For example, a family member may notice the television volume is increased or the individual must frequently ask others to repeat themselves.

Although hearing-impaired individuals may experience symptoms differently, some of the more common subjective signs of hearing impairment include: (1) inability to clearly understand all or parts of conversations; this problem may be exacerbated when background noise is present; (2) frequent requests for repetitions or clarifications; (3) individual withdrawal from conversations or social situations; (4) a need to request others to raise their voices; (5) a perception that people 'mumble', rather than speak distinctly; (6) a perception of the voice of the hearing-impaired speaker as being too loud or too soft; (7) end-of-the-day fatigue secondary to a necessity of straining to hear (UCSF, 2013).

PRESBYCUSIS

As previously noted, hearing loss associated with aging is termed presbycusis. Although some may continue to think of presbycusis as a factor of aging alone, it is actually the outcome of several variables that can occur within an individual's lifespan (Rosenhall, 2001). These variables may include, but are not limited to, metabolic, vascular or renal diseases, inflammations, infections, medications, head trauma, nutritional deficits and hereditary factors. However, exposure to intense noise levels over time continues to be the most common factor in precipitating the hearing decline related to aging. In a classic study published in 1962 by Rosen et al., individuals living in a relatively noise-free environment in the Sudan showed significantly less hearing loss when compared across the ages to people living in industrialized societies. As a result of this and other studies, attempts continue to educate people about the effects of loud noise on their hearing and the importance of using hearing protective devices when exposed to such noise.

The hearing loss associated with presbycusis is usually insidious and is initially noted not as a significant and sudden decrease in hearing, but rather as a problem in understanding speech. Sound will become distorted secondary to outer and inner hair-cell damage. Many patients with presbycusis will present with the complaint of 'I hear but cannot understand'. This initial complaint is usually a result of a decrease in hearing within the high frequency range of the inner ear cochlea. At birth the normal human ear is thought to be functional within a frequency range of 20 to 20 000 Hz. However, as the individual ages, the cochlear hair-cell function begins to diminish, especially in the higher frequencies. The cochlear change deprives the inner ear of a critical connection to the cerebral cortex. If the auditory signal is unable to reach the brain, interpretation will be lacking, resulting in a deficit or loss of auditory function. The greater the amount of hair-cell damage, the greater the amount of hearing loss and the greater the handicap imposed on the individual. Unfortunately, no medical or surgical treatments are presently available to remediate the vast majority of inner ear hearing loss. Although ongoing laboratory studies present hope in such areas as hair-cell regeneration and temporal bone transplant, it will probably be many years before such dramatic innovations are readily available. At present, the best hope for alleviation of inner ear hearing loss lies with electroacoustic devices that can assist the hearing-impaired. The most common of these is the hearing aid.

TINNITUS

The expression of someone's 'ears ringing' is not only a common phrase, but a true inner ear condition. The condition is referred to as tinnitus, and it affects as many as 50 million Americans (Kochkin et al., 2011). Tinnitus is most often described by patients as a ringing sound, but others classify it as 'crickets', roaring, hissing, whooshing, whistling, or even a chirping sound. The description also varies among patients in relation to the sound quality, duration and intensity of the perception. In most instances, tinnitus is a subjective sensation and, therefore, audible only to the individual suffering from the condition. However, there are rarer instances in which tinnitus is audible to others. This condition is termed 'objective tinnitus' and is generally related to spasms within the middle ear musculature or changes in blood flow or increased blood turbulence in the area of the ear. It should be noted that tinnitus is not a disease itself, but rather a symptom of another condition. The American Speech–Language–Hearing Association (1997–2013) has classified some of these triggering mechanisms to include hearing loss, noise trauma, head and neck injury/trauma, disease such as Menière's disease, ototoxic medication and other health-related problems to include otosclerosis, impacted cerumen, ear infections, middle ear tumors and temporomandibular joint dysfunction.

The impact of tinnitus will vary among patients, and so the management of the condition will vary from patient to patient as well. Most tinnitus sufferers are undisturbed by the condition, but some can suffer psychologically (American Tinnitus Association, 2013). It is not uncommon for patients suffering from an intractable tinnitus to develop feelings of anxiety, lack of energy and concentration, general fatigue or even clinical depression. These problems usually develop when patients ascertain that the tinnitus condition is beyond their control and hence becomes a negative fixture within their everyday lives. Some patients will develop such fearful reactions that they may withdraw from what had previously been their everyday lifestyle.

Despite extensive research, there is not presently a cure that will silence tinnitus. Various forms of medical treatment have been attempted without significant success to this time. However, despite the lack of cure, tinnitus can be managed in many situations by treating the underlying causes or by attempting to alter the patient's perception of the condition. Some treatment management methods include: medical treatment of the underlying issues, alternative or non-medical methods

of remediation, sound therapy, hearing aids, education and counseling, or combinations of these options.

Alternative methods for treating tinnitus have included such disciplines as acupuncture, hypnosis, homeopathy, magnets, and vitamins and herb supplementation. A study conducted by Meehan, Eisenhut and Stephens in 2004 showed that of all the varied alternative methods for managing tinnitus, only hypnosis significantly improved patient relaxation and wellbeing. Also, there are no FDA-approved medications for treating tinnitus. Some tinnitus suffers may be prescribed medications to treat accompanying depression, sleeping disorders, or anxiety. It should also be mentioned that several prescription drugs label tinnitus as a potential adverse effect of the medication (Fausti, 2004; Mayo Clinic, 1998–2013).

By presenting external noise to the tinnitus patient's ears, sound therapy is used to help decrease the perceived intensity of the tinnitus (Jastreboff & Jastreboff, 2004). White noise, music and soothing sounds like rolling waves or mountain winds are most commonly used for this type of therapy. A patient can listen to these external sounds by either wearing a device, such as a hearing aid with tinnitus treatment, or just listening to these sounds through an external speaker. Amplification from hearing aids has proven to help alleviate patients' stress towards their tinnitus by simply adding additional sound to their environment, secondary to their hearing deficit (Kochkin et al., 2011; Newman et al., 2011). The use of hearing aids combined with the addition of external sounds has proven so effective that some hearing aid manufacturers are presently including sound therapy options in their hearing aids. Folmer and Carroll (2006) reported that ear-level-worn hearing instruments can help patients with chronic tinnitus by reducing their perception to the tinnitus and/or facilitating the habituation process.

Finally, education and counseling also need to be key components for the management of tinnitus. It is important for patients to know what mechanisms may trigger their tinnitus. Once individuals become more knowledgeable about the tinnitus condition, they may become less fearful towards the condition itself. This in turn may prepare them to move forward into an appropriate treatment paradigm (Tyler, 2006). Other counseling tools such as cognitive behavioral therapy and tinnitus retraining therapy may also attempt to guide the patient to accept, rather than react negatively towards, their tinnitus condition (Jastreboff, 2007).

EVALUATION OF THE HEARING-IMPAIRED ADULT

No rehabilitative process can be effective without a comprehensive identification program. The current protocol for initial auditory evaluation is based upon both traditional and modern procedures. The purposes of a hearing evaluation include diagnosing conductive versus inner ear lesions, determining the need for medical or surgical referral, creating a course of rehabilitation, determining the need for site-of-lesion evaluation and determining the extent of disability. The two professions primarily involved in inner ear evaluation and treatment are otolaryngology and audiology. The otolaryngologist or ear, nose and throat specialist is a physician who is skilled in the medical treatment of auditory disease or dysfunction. Over the years, many auditory conditions that were once thought to be permanent have been found to be treatable through medical or surgical techniques. Although reversal of inner ear aging patterns has not yet been accomplished, ongoing research, including genetic modification practices, continue to show promise for the regeneration of hair-cell tissue or recovery of hair-cell damage (Ryals & Rubel, 1988; Mizutarik et al., 2013).

Audiology is the other profession involved with inner ear impairment. An audiologist is a nonphysician specialist involved with the evaluation, diagnosis and treatment of hearing and balance problems that cannot be managed medically. It is usually the realm of the audiologist to initiate and complete the comprehensive testing process necessary to identify any problem and develop a course of realistic treatment of inner ear dysfunction. The initial aspect of the auditory evaluation includes such time-tested measures as otoscopic examination and tuning-fork testing. These procedures can act as a screening mechanism to allow the professional audiologist to determine, within a reasonable degree of certainty, whether a hearing loss is present and whether it can be localized within the conductive or inner ear mechanism.

Following these initial screening procedures, the audiologist may use two other traditional hearing measures: pure-tone audiometry and speech audiometry. In pure-tone audiometry hearing thresholds are obtained at several frequencies. In pure-tone air-conduction testing, the entire auditory system is evaluated, whereas in pure-tone bone-conduction testing, only the inner ear reserve is evaluated. By comparing air conduction thresholds with bone conduction thresholds, the clinician can determine, among other things, if medical referral is indicated.

The pure-tone test results are supplemented by speech audiometry. Using speech signals to evaluate the auditory system is a tradition that has been ongoing since the earliest days of auditory testing. Speech testing cannot only be used to validate and confirm the reliability of pure tones, but also to estimate the presence or absence of any distortion that may be present within the auditory system, secondary to hair-cell damage.

Other diagnostic measures that are routinely applied include acoustic immittance testing, which is an objective measure of the peripheral auditory system and which can provide efficient information regarding that system. Pure tone, speech and acoustic immittance evaluations coupled with otoscopy and tuning-fork testing are considered the bedrock of the auditory evaluation. However, these tests can be supplemented with other measures to provide additional diagnostic and site-of-lesion information. Additional evaluations may include:

1. Auditory brainstem response (ABR) evaluation, in which an auditory evoked potential is generated and extracted from ongoing electrical activity in the cochlear and higher auditory pathways. The ABR information can be used in several different ways to include auditory threshold determination, site of lesion detection and evaluation of functional hearing loss. The ABR can also be valuable in such areas as newborn hearing screening and intraoperative monitoring of surgical patients.
2. Electrocochleography (ECOG), which allows for the recording of electrical potentials within the inner ear. The presence or absence of potentials has become extremely useful in the identification and diagnosis of Menière's disease and acoustic neuropathy.
3. Otoacoustic emissions (OAEs), which are thought to reflect sound potentials that are generated within the inner ear. These sounds are either not present or disappear with inner ear damage. Although not used extensively with the adult population, OAEs have proven to be invaluable in the early detection of hearing loss in infants. When performed by a licensed physician or audiologist, these diagnostic services are recognized and covered for reimbursement by Medicare and most third-party insurances.

REMEDIATION OF HEARING LOSS

At this time there is no cure for hearing loss, although extensive research is currently underway to attempt to regrow damaged hair cells in the inner ear (Mizutarik et al., 2013). Until such time that this research can be integrated into the treatment repertoire, people with hearing loss will continue to seek management of their hearing deficits through amplification and/or aural rehabilitation. As most individuals are aware, hearing loss can leave people feeling very isolated within social gatherings. For the elderly individual, hearing loss may also come to symbolize the physical and emotional changes that occur with age. In a classic study conducted by Bess et al., in 1989, it was dramatically demonstrated that hearing loss in the elderly can have significant ramifications in both physical and psychosocial functions.

Amplification, whether it is a conventional or digital hearing aid, cochlear implant, or a surgically implanted, bone-anchored device, has drastically improved over the years. The past century has seen significant improvement in the treatment of the hearing impairment. It was not too many years ago that the 'ear trumpet' offered what was thought to be the biggest hearing improvement since a hand cupped behind the ear. Technology quickly advanced to electronic hearing aids that started off as big, bulky, body devices that served only to amplify sound, to the hearing instruments of today, which are small, digital and fully computer-programmable. However, it is important to note that, despite the tremendous technological advances that have been made, the instrumentation continues to be termed 'hearing aids' and not 'hearing cures'. Current hearing aids are not a panacea, although research continues in the hope that hearing impairment may someday be eradicated.

At present, personal hearing instruments continue to be the treatment of choice for sensorineural hearing loss.

When a patient sees an audiologist for hearing aid evaluation, he or she is first evaluated to determine the presence and degree of the hearing deficit. If a hearing loss is present, the provider must determine if the patient is a hearing aid candidate. The patient can then decide on style, color, technology level and accessory options. Today's hearing aids are so sophisticated that they can communicate wirelessly with one another to provide speech discrimination benefits, especially in the presence of background noise. Present hearing aid technology also allows for interaction with Bluetooth cellular phones, as well as for streaming signals from radio, television and various other music-playing devices. Hearing aids are able to be computer-programmed specifically to each hearing loss by adding gain or volume to the specific frequencies that are impaired within the patient's inner ears. The amount of gain added to each frequency is dependent upon the severity of the hearing loss at that specific frequency. The higher the technology level of the hearing aid, the greater the amount of fine tuning that can be programmed into the instrument for ultimate results.

Some people perceive hearing aids to be costly, so not all patients with hearing loss will opt to spend money on this form of hearing loss management. A less-expensive option is for the patient to purchase a personal amplifier device. The major difference between these devices and hearing aids is that personal amplifiers cannot be specifically programmed to a patient's hearing deficit. Personal amplifiers, like early generation hearing aids, cannot be programmed to the patient's specific loss, but rather they amplify all sounds within the speech spectrum to an equal degree. A volume control is the only means for increasing or decreasing the sound level of the stimulus. Also, there is an acoustic limit as to how much amplification these devices can provide, so a person with a severe to profound hearing loss may receive little to no benefit from this form of amplification.

Cochlear implants and bone-anchored hearing aids have become increasingly utilized for many individuals with hearing impairment. However, these devices are generally utilized for specific populations. Cochlear implants are primarily used for those individuals who suffer from profound hearing loss and who are not able to significantly benefit from traditional or digital-processing hearing aids. A cochlear implant is a surgically implanted electronic device that is inserted into the cochlea and utilizes electrodes to stimulate various portions of the inner ear to transmit the proper coding signals to the auditory nerve and into the higher auditory pathways of the brain. Bone-anchored hearing aids amplify sounds via bone vibration and send auditory signals directly to the inner ear, bypassing the outer and middle ear. A surgically implanted abutment is used for this type of sound transmission. Bone-anchored hearing aids are suited for those patients who have developed middle ear disorders with chronic aural drainage and who are unable to successfully wear ear-level hearing instruments due to the potential of occlusion of the instrument by the aural discharge. The bone-anchored instrument can also be used successfully with patients suffering from ear canal malformations or atresia.

Aural rehabilitation is another individual treatment option that patients can utilize, but it is most successful when used in conjunction with personal hearing aids. Patients can participate in either group or individual aural rehabilitation classes, or they can choose to complete such classes at home. Some programs are now computer-based, and patients can investigate strategies within such areas as lip- or speechreading, auditory training and the development of communication strategies. Aural rehabilitation has become so technologically advanced that it is now offered as a smart phone application. However, no matter which form of aural rehabilitation is utilized, it is important that patients and their families learn from these training sessions to enhance their overall communication skill level to more effectively deal with their communication handicap.

DIZZINESS AND AGING

According to Desmond and Touchette (1998), dizziness is the most common reason for primary care physician visits for patients over the age of 75, and almost 80% of these visits were found to be directly related to inner ear dysfunction. Dizziness, or the loss of orientation of the body in space, can be an extremely frightening experience to the older adult. Individuals are used to being in control of their bodies and doing what they want, when they want; however, the dizzy patient may no longer be able to control spatial orientation. In addition, the person's fright may be complicated by concern that the dizziness is a symptom of a serious problem, such as a heart attack or stroke. The potential causes of dizziness may be many and varied, and it is, therefore, imperative that a comprehensive examination be completed to determine the correct paths for evaluation and treatment of any condition.

As the aging process continues, older adults may expect their balance to become less secure. Like audition, the number of sensory nerve fibers serving the vestibular and balance systems diminish with age. In addition, circulatory changes within the inner ear and within the lower extremities of the body can also contribute to balance dysfunction. These problems can be further exacerbated when deficiencies within the visual system, arthritis, circulation or the central nervous system are present.

EVALUATION OF THE DIZZY PATIENT

There are several evaluative methods that may be utilized to aid in the diagnosis of the vestibular patient. Although no tests can be considered foolproof, the following tools in the hands of a competent practitioner can go a long way towards obtaining a correct diagnosis and pointing the patient toward relief or recovery. The diagnostic procedures are as follows:

1. Historical intake – The case history provided by the patient may be the most valuable tool available to

the diagnostician. Important considerations within the historical information include the onset and description of the condition, the patient's belief as to causation and other associated symptoms.

2. Electronystagmography (ENG) – The ENG is a battery of eye movement tests, the results of which are recorded through the use of electrodes placed close to the orbits of both eyes. Videonystagmography (VNG) is a similar procedure in which the patient's eye movements are recorded by the use of an infra-red video camera mounted within goggles that the patient wears. One particular portion of the ENG examination, termed caloric testing, can help determine if one inner ear is working more effectively than the other, thus causing a vertiginous condition.

3. Rotation testing – The use of auto-rotation or the rotary chair is another means of determining if the inner ears and the visual system are working together. Some instances of dizziness or imbalance can be motion-provoked such that the eyes and the ears cannot easily integrate the information that is sent to them. The result may be feelings of dizziness or imbalance. Some associated nausea or even vomiting may be present. Auto-rotational testing can be either computerized or non-computerized. However, in both instances, the patient is asked to focus on a fixed object as the head is moved either horizontally or vertically for a short period of time. In the rotary chair examination, the patient is secured and seated in a chair that is programmed to change direction in order to precipitate eye movements.

4. Dynamic posturography – Dynamic posturography is an evaluation of postural stability. In the computerized version, the patient stands on a platform and is secured by a safety harness. The patient is usually advised to visually focus on a target. The platform is then programmed to move in various directions while pressure gauges within the platform measure the body's sway via weight shift information. Dynamic posturography attempts to assess not only the visual–vestibular interactions of the patient but also the somatosensory signals that are received by the brain from the muscles and joints of the lower extremities. Computerized dynamic posturography is an expensive tool that may not be readily available in all areas. However, a sensory organization of the balance procedure that utilizes components of the traditional 'Foam and Dome' techniques that have been in place within balance laboratories for many years can be a surprisingly comparative and cost-effective means of substituting for the computerized procedures.

5. Vestibular evoked myogenic potential (VEMP) – The VEMP is a procedure that utilizes an evoked response computer, a sound generator and surface electrodes that are placed on the neck of the patient to measure whether structures within the inner ears are in working order. The saccule, one of the inner ear otolith organs that help to provide spatial orientation information to the body, is particularly targeted by the VEMP evaluation, although the vestibular nerve and central connections are also evaluated. VEMP is becoming more popular over time and, as research efforts into VEMP expand, it is thought that the procedure will become more utilized and useful. At present VEMP can be used to obtain diagnostic information about Menière's disease, BPPV, vestibular neuritis and central vestibular disorders, as well as more obscure conditions of the vestibular system. For additional information on balance and balance testing, the reader is referred to Chapter 59.

CONCLUSION

The aging process frequently results in changes to the inner ear structures of hearing and balance. These changes may present significant quality of life issues, not only to the affected individuals but to their families as well. Although evaluation of these patients may be challenging, both traditional and advanced technology methods are now available to aid in differential diagnosis. Remedial procedures are progressing; however, few 'cures' for inner ear damage are available at this time. Ongoing research efforts continue to provide hope for a future in which hearing and balance disorders can be eradicated.

REFERENCES

American Speech–Language–Hearing Association 1997–2013 Tinnitus triage guidelines. [Online] Available at: www.asha.org/aud/Articles/Tinnitus-Triage-Guidelines. Accessed December 2013

American Tinnitus Association 2013. http://ata.org

Bess FH, Lichtenstein ML, Logan SA et al 1989 Hearing impairment as a determinant of function in the elderly. J Am Geriatr Soc 37:123–128

Center for Disease Control and Prevention 2013 Noise and hearing loss prevention. [Online] Available at: www.cdc.gov/niosh/topics/noise. Accessed December 2013

Christensen K, Frederiksen H, Hoffman HJ 2001 Genetic and environmental influences on self-reported reduced hearing in the old and oldest old. J Am Geriatr Soc 49(11):1512–1517

Desmond AL, Touchette DT 1998 Balance disorders. Micromedical Technologies, Chatham, IL

Fausti SA 2004 Audiologic assessment. In: Snow JB (ed) Tinnitus: Theory and Management. BC Decker, Lewiston, NY, pp. 310–313

Folmer RL, Carroll JR 2006 Long-term effectiveness of ear-level devices for tinnitus. Otolaryngol Head Neck Surg 134:132–137

Hain TC, Micco A 2003 Cranial nerve 8: vestibulocochlear nerve. In: Goetz CG, Pappert EJ (eds) Textbook of Neurology, 2nd edn. WB Saunders, Philadelphia, PA

Jastreboff PJ 2007 Tinnitus retraining therapy. In: Langguth B, Hajak G, Kleinjung A (eds) Progress in Brain Research, vol. 166. Tinnitus: Pathophysiology and Treatment. Elsevier, Amsterdam, pp. 415–423

Jastreboff P, Jastreboff M 2004 Tinnitus retraining therapy. In: Snow JB (ed) Tinnitus Treatment and Management. BC Decker, Hamilton, Ontario

Kochkin S 2009 Marke trak VIII: 25 year trends in the hearing health market. Hearing Rev 16(11):12–31

Kochkin S, Tyler R, Born J 2011 Marke trak VIII: the prevalence of tinnitus in the United States and the self-reported efficacy of various treatments. Hearing Rev 18(12):10–26

Martin JS, Jerger JS 2005 Some effects of aging on central auditory processing. J Rehabil Res Dev 42:25–44

Mayo Clinic 1998–2013 Drugs and supplements. [Online] Available at: www.mayoclinic.com/health/druginformation/DrugHerbIndex. Accessed December 2013

Meehan T, Eisenhut M, Stephens D 2004 A review of alternative treatments for tinnitus. Audiol Med 2(1):74–82

Mizutarik K, Fujioka M, Hosoya M et al 2013 Notch inhibition induces cochlear hair cell regeneration and recovery of hearing after acoustic trauma. Neuron 77(1):58–69

Murphy DR, Daneman M, Schneider BA 2006 Why do older adults have difficulty following conversations. Psychol Aging 21:49–61

Newman CW, Sandridge SA, Bea SM et al 2011 Tinnitus patients do not have to 'just live with it'. Cleve Clin J Med 78:312–319

NIDCD (National Institute on Deafness and Other Communicative Disorders) 2002 United States Department of Health and Human Services, Publication NO-97-4235

NIDCD (National Institute on Deafness and Other Communicative Disorders) 2008 United States Department of Health and Human Services, Publication NO-97-4233

Occupation Safety and Health Administration (OSHA) 2002 Hearing Conservation Publication 3074

Rosen S, Bergman M, Plester D 1962 Presbycusis study of a relatively noise-free population in the Sudan. Transcripts Otologic Soc 50:135–152

Rosenhall U 2001 Presbycusis-hearing loss in old age. Lakartidningen 98(23):2802–2806

Roush P 2008 Auditory neuropathy spectrum disorder: evaluation and management. Hearing J 61(11):36–41

Ryals BM, Rubel EW 1988 Hair cell regeneration after acoustic trauma in adult Coturnix quail. Science 240(4860):1774–1776

Tyler RS 2006 Neurophysiological models, psychological models and treatments for tinnitus. In: Tyler RS (ed) Tinnitus treatment. Thième, New York, pp. 1–22

UCSF Medical Center 2002–2013 Hearing loss signs and symptoms. [Online] Available at: www.ucsfhealth.org/conditions/hearing_loss/signs_and_symptoms.html. Accessed December 2013

Chapter 53

Considerations in elder patient communication

SARA HAYES • NIALL MCGRANE

CHAPTER CONTENTS

INTRODUCTION

In order for healthcare professionals to deliver optimal treatment to older adults, the barriers to communication that often present in this population must be considered and overcome through mutually understandable, accurate and satisfying communication between the healthcare professional and older adult. The healthcare professional should identify what communication skills are necessary to reach each older adult. They must be familiar with the person's sensory assessment so that they can be aware of any hearing or visual deficits.

Knowledge of a person's educational level and reading ability is also necessary to determine how to most effectively present information concerning treatment and self-care. Inadequate health literacy is common among elderly patients. Such people often have an array of communication problems that may affect treatment outcome. Cognitive dysfunction may present as a short-term or long-term barrier to optimal communication between the healthcare professional and older person. Bell-McGinty et al. (2002) recommend that relatives should be encouraged to participate in patient interviews or education sessions, with patients' consent, to ensure that patients have understood essential information. Creative written patient education materials should be used. Cultural differences should also be considered and an effort to understand and adapt to them should be made.

CULTURAL CONSIDERATIONS

To ensure that the older person is fully informed, healthcare professionals must provide accurate information to each of their patients regarding their treatment. Healthcare professionals must communicate in a manner in which the patient can understand. Language is the most obvious barrier to communication but healthcare professionals must consider more than just language as a barrier to informing their patients. Each individual's personal history, cultural and religious beliefs, myths and customs regarding health, diet and exercise can affect how healthcare is received and provided. There are three cultures interacting with each encounter: the culture of the older person, the culture of the healthcare professional and the culture of medicine.

The trends in migration in today's world make it necessary for healthcare professionals to be aware of each older person's cultural, ethical and religious backgrounds. In 2010 the estimated number of international migrants was 214 million – 3.1% of the total world population. Approximately 8% of this total is made up of refugees. Former countries of emigration, such as Spain, Italy and Ireland, have become preferred destinations. By 2050 it is projected that 2.4 million individuals will migrate to developed regions annually (United Nations Department of Economic and Social Affairs, 2011). The ramifications of these UN findings are that healthcare professionals will almost certainly treat people from a different cultural background from their own.

A lack of understanding can frustrate both the older adult and the healthcare professional. Both verbal and nonverbal communication can be used to increase understanding. There are differences in both with diverse cultures and an understanding of these can greatly aid communication. Language and respect are closely linked. Several languages include honorifics, and an older person could be insulted quite easily if the wrong word is used. Many cultures have a great respect for older people and the appropriate term should be used.

Often older adults will not ask for explanations or question healthcare professionals when they do not fully comprehend what they have been told. This can be due to many reasons, including different cultural ones. Older people may not want to admit that they do not understand. They do not want to be perceived as ignorant or perhaps they do not want to insult the healthcare professional by implying that their explanation was poor. In this author's experience the most common reason is that they believe the healthcare professional is too busy and that they do not want to waste their valuable time by asking silly questions. They believe that there are more important things for the healthcare professional to be doing.

Attitudes towards health, diet and exercise are influenced by culture and religion. These attitudes and beliefs can have positive and/or negative impacts on patients' wellbeing (Koenig et al., 2012). Diet plays a major role in culture. No custom is more universally shared than the ritual of eating a meal together. This ritual symbolizes family traditions, close friendships and sentiments, and results in definitive dietary and cultural practices and habits, which are often passed from generation to generation. A clinician may not be aware of all the cultural intricacies of their patient's diet but some knowledge and awareness must be sought when managing a patient whose culture is different from their own.

Religious beliefs also impact health and healthcare. There have been well-documented cases of parents relying on prayer or faith healing instead of seeking healthcare for their children, leading to their death. Nearly seventy thousand sick or disabled people travel to Lourdes in France each year with the hope of being healed despite the Catholic Church recognizing only 66 miracles since 1858 (Plunkett, 2002).

A lack of understanding can lead to the confusion of one or both parties. Confusion on the part of the patient can lead to misunderstanding of the presenting condition or non-adherence with treatment. Patients are more likely to be adherent to treatment if their provider communicates well (Zolnierek & Dimatteo, 2009). When patients do not follow a prescribed treatment regimen, they are sometimes described as being 'not compliant'. Compliance is understood to mean the act of conforming or yielding, and a tendency to yield readily to others, especially in a weak or subservient way. Adherence is a preferred term which is used within healthcare and effective adult patient education, and is defined as 'a mutually agreed-upon course of action'.

LITERACY

Collins Dictionary defines literacy as: (i) the ability to read and write and (ii) the ability to use language proficiently. They define illiteracy as (i) unable to read and write; (ii) violating accepted standards in reading and writing; and (iii) uneducated, ignorant, or uncultured. It is necessary to define culture and Collins's definition is: (i) the total of the inherited ideas, beliefs, values, and knowledge, which constitute the shared bases of social action; (ii) the total range of activities and ideas of a group of people with shared traditions, which are transmitted and reinforced by members of the group; (iii) a particular civilization at a particular

period; (iv) the artistic and social pursuits, expression and tastes valued by a society or class, as in the arts, manners, dress, etc.; (v) the enlightenment or refinement resulting from these pursuits; and (vi) the attitudes, feelings, values and behavior that characterize and inform society as a whole or any social group within it. Knowledge is defined as: (i) the facts, feelings or experiences known by a person or group of people; (ii) the state of knowing; (iii) awareness, consciousness, or familiarity gained by experience or learning; (iv) erudition or informed learning; and (v) specific information about a subject.

The definitions of both culture and knowledge do not mention the ability to read or write. One can be rich in both culture and knowledge without the ability to read or write. It has been reported that there are approximately 6909 languages in the world today and very few of these have even been written down (Lewis, 2009). Eleven languages each have over 100 million mother-tongue speakers and these account for approximately 51% percent of the world's population (Lewis, 2009). The inability to read or write is often based on individual circumstances and has nothing to do with intelligence. Today's standard of education may not have been available years ago and an older person may not have had the same educational opportunities that are available to today's youth. Healthcare providers will encounter people who cannot read or write and although this medium of communication is closed this does not mean that the person lacks intelligence. Providers must be aware that low literacy is associated with several adverse health outcomes (Dewalt et al., 2004).

Alternative forms of communication must be explored if a person is illiterate. Take-home instructions, a major part of treatment for medications, exercises or diet, must be provided in an understandable form. If not, adherence will be affected. Logs and diaries of health behavior, if prescribed, must be issued in a format that an illiterate person can complete. The involvement of family members and carers is of vital importance in these situations.

ECOLOGICAL FRAMEWORK

Hamadeh (1987) describes an excellent example of a practitioner of Western medicine who recommended going beyond what some consider to be customary practice in order to understand his patient and the patient's situation. He used what he described as the Ecological Framework approach to generate hypotheses about the patient's responses. Hamadeh described several levels of analysis: (i) the individual level, in which psychological problems, stress and depression may all be factors that contribute to a poor response; (ii) the family level, in which the factors affecting the patient's illness include family myths and beliefs about disease and the family's experience with the medical profession; and (iii) the cultural level, in which factors affecting illness behavior may be misunderstood by healthcare providers unless they are aware of the larger context of the patient's background, which includes knowledge of the economic, social and religious factors affecting the patient's life.

Hamadeh offers a list of pertinent questions to be asked when a healthcare provider is new to a community and wishes to better understand the community and its patients (Hamadeh, 1987):

1. What is the community's understanding of good health?
2. When is a member considered to be ill?
3. What are common explanations for causes of illness in the community?
4. What usual modes of treatment and alternative healthcare systems are available?
5. How much is the patient considered responsible for illness, cure or prevention?
6. Who is the medical decision-maker in the family?
7. What are the attitudes towards death and dying?

Analyzing a patient with a background different to one's own with this framework and asking these seven questions will go a long way to improving understanding, enhancing communication and increasing adherence to treatment. This in turn will lead to improved outcomes.

SUPPORTING AUTONOMY

To understand and treat elderly people who have lived a traditional life within their particular culture, healthcare professionals should learn about their traditions and relate to them with understanding and acceptance. The way in which educators and healthcare professionals approach individuals must be respectful and honour their culture.

Is it ethical to keep on insisting on behavioral change when individuals demonstrate that they understand the intentions of the caregiver but they do not wish to change? A patient's autonomy must be respected and encouraged. Autonomy in relation to healthcare means encouraging individuals to make choices about how to behave, providing them with the information they need to make choices, and respecting the choices they make (Deci & Ryan, 2012). Informed decisions regarding their treatment and their behavior can only be made by the patients. The attitude of the professional can have a great impact on the acceptance of a course of action, depending on whether rigid adherence is required and expected, or whether a course of action toward change is recommended and mutually agreed upon. The attitude of the provider can greatly affect the likelihood that a change in behavior or lifestyle will occur, therefore an autonomy-supportive stance should be taken.

SELF-EFFICACY

Perceived self-efficacy is defined as people's beliefs about their capabilities to produce designated levels of performance that exercise influence over events that affect their lives (Bandura, 1994). The belief that one can master change in behavior and the belief that one can master an individual task, be it an exercise program or an individual exercise, are equally important examples of self-efficacy. Self-efficacy is modifiable and can influence health status, motivation and adherence across many aspects of health.

To achieve optimal disease management goals, the healthcare professional should facilitate older people enhancing their self-efficacy (Marks et al., 2005). Each individual who presents for treatment brings with them a unique and complex background and it is important to consider that each person also has a unique personality and may respond to treatment situations in a different manner. According to Bandura (1994), there are four main sources of influencing self-efficacy. The first, mastery experience, influences self-efficacy by building on previous success. Health professionals should remind older people of previous success they have had with healthcare behavior. The second, vicarious experience or modeling, influences self-efficacy by seeing people similar to oneself succeed. An example of this is the results from a study published in 2001, a peer-led fall prevention program proved to be more successful than a professionally-led one (Waters et al., 2011). Older people should be used as role-models for older patients. Any handouts or visuals should include pictures of older people completing target behaviors, for example, prescribed exercises. The third, social persuasion, is the easiest and most readily available source of influence for healthcare professionals. Verbally persuading older people that they possess the capabilities to master tasks is likely to mobilize greater effort and increase self-efficacy. The role that physiological factors play is the fourth and final source of influence. Reducing stress reactions and altering negative emotional proclivities and misinterpretations of physical states will influence self-efficacy. How normal emotional and physical responses to stress are interpreted and perceived is an important aspect of increasing self-efficacy. Informing patients about realistic perceptions of normal physiological responses and educating them on their condition and prognosis will also increase their self efficacy.

There are published tools to measure self-efficacy for numerous different conditions; however, health professionals must be aware of methodological limitations of many of these tools (Frei et al., 2009). Bandura believes that general self-efficacy scales are limited, and provides guidance on how best to construct them (Bandura, 1997, 2006).

IMPAIRMENT OF SENSORY FUNCTION

HEARING IMPAIRMENT

It is important to consider the negative effects of sensory impairment on communication between healthcare professionals and older adults. Loss of hearing may have a significant impact on rehabilitation (this is described in detail in Chapter 52). In older adults, the presence of hearing loss may lead to disengagement and paranoia if impairments are severe and continue for any length of time. Additionally, loss of hearing may create a sense of loneliness and isolation, and result in emotional distress because of anxiety or depression. Certain behavioral compensations by an older person may lead a healthcare professional to suspect a hearing loss. These compensations are listed in Box 53.1.

VISUAL IMPAIRMENT

An additional sensory impairment that leads to communication difficulties is the loss of vision (presbyopia and various visual pathologies are described in Chapter 51). Loss of vision is often a main inhibitory factor to safe physical mobility and independent self-care among older adults. Simple compensations can be used to assist individuals with visual loss, for example increasing print size and using bold print in all printed materials, including medical and personal history forms and prescribed self-care programs. Glare should be minimized and sans serif font and bold primary colors should be used for all written materials.

It is not uncommon for older adults to have both hearing and visual loss, which leads to typical behaviors such as squinting, frowning or grimacing during conversation. Often individuals with this type of impairment rely more on touch for reassurance. Many older adults with visual and hearing impairments tend to mobilize by 'furniture crawling' using the tactile feedback from surrounding surfaces to compensate for their other sensory losses. At times, they appear to be distrusting or withdrawn. Additionally, they may worry about being awkward and may exhibit a reluctance to communicate. This may lead to fearful behavior, even during normal activities, placing them at an increased risk of social isolation. Methods that help in communication with older adults who have visual or hearing impairments or both are shown in Box 53.2.

IMPAIRMENT OF LANGUAGE

Aphasia is defined as partial or complete loss of language function (Berthier et al., 2011). It is a common consequence of stroke or brain injury among older adults and it may affect one or more areas of communication, including speaking, understanding spoken words, reading and writing (Brady et al., 2012). Aphasia may be described as expressive aphasia (difficulty producing spoken or written language) or receptive aphasia (difficulty understanding the spoken or written word). Variation in the severity of expressive impairments may range from the individual experiencing occasional word-finding difficulties to having no effective means of communication (Brady et al., 2012).

When working with people with aphasia it is important for healthcare professionals to liaise with the speech and language therapist (SALT) within the service. Based on a thorough assessment of the person's language function the SALT will advise the members of the multidisciplinary team on the most appropriate methods of communication to be used with the person. Firstly, it is imperative to establish if the person has a consistent 'yes/no' response. Following this, the healthcare professional should establish the person's strongest modality of communication, i.e. speaking, writing, picture pointing, drawing, or the use of sign language. When this has been ascertained, it should be incorporated into every interaction with the person with aphasia. Additionally, healthcare professionals should ensure that the person with aphasia is able to understand the instructions being given to him/her, e.g. if the person's strongest modality of communication is writing, it may be useful to ask the person some questions and instruct them to write down the answers.

It is crucial to point out progress so that the patient grasps the idea that gains are being made. The healthcare professional should ask questions using verbal and nonverbal communication and encourage patients to answer them to the best of their ability. If an individual cannot find the proper words and becomes frustrated, it is important to express empathy and understanding; however, it is unwise for the healthcare professional to pretend to understand something that has not been comprehended. The healthcare professional should get the person's attention before speaking and should speak according to their ability, avoiding long sentences, rapid speech or difficult and uncommon words. It is helpful to communicate one idea at a time, using clear short sentences and everyday words, and to avoid speaking in a loud voice unless the individual has suffered a hearing loss. Facing the aphasic individual when speaking and using gestures are also useful practices. Family and friends should be educated about the nature of the aphasic person's problems. Family members may find it helpful to attend some therapy sessions in order to learn the most appropriate ways of communicating with the older person and incorporate this into everyday life. It is crucial that healthcare professionals do not discuss the older adult's condition in their presence, as if they were not there. Older adults with aphasia should have every opportunity to hear speech and should be encouraged to participate in social activities in the home and community at whatever level they are able.

IMPAIRMENT OF COGNITION

Cognitive impairment can act as a barrier to effective communication between healthcare professionals and older adults. Participation in a rehabilitation program requires both physical and cognitive resources and healthcare professionals are becoming more aware of the importance of cognition for the success of rehabilitation (Studer, 2007). Cognitive impairment may cause difficulties in orientation, memory, concentration, attention and executive function. It is now widely accepted that the presence of cognitive impairment in older adults has negative implications for functional performance (Grigsby et al., 1998; Bell-McGinty et al., 2002; Cahn-Weiner et al., 2002; Ble et al., 2005; Coppin et al., 2006; Johnson et al., 2007; Nieto et al., 2008; de Bruin and Schmidt, 2010; Voelcker-Rehage et al., 2010; McAuley et al., 2011; Lowry et al., 2012).

Cognitive impairment may present in the clinical setting as a short- or long-term condition among older adults. Many variables may explain short-term cognitive dysfunction, e.g. medication toxicity, depression, nutritional deficiency, anesthesia, allergic reaction, infection or elevated inflammatory markers. Furthermore, hyperthermia and hypothermia, electrolyte imbalance and certain medications may lead to acute short-term states of confusion. Also, an individual may be living alone and the loss of human companionship can result in withdrawal and disengagement from social activities. An older adult may also suffer from short-term confusion, including the distortion of time and space cues, as a result of being in an unfamiliar room and having no familiar objects in view. The hospital schedule is often totally asynchronous with the individual's normal schedule. Long-term cognitive impairment is a common clinical presentation in geriatric inpatient or outpatient healthcare facilities and unfortunately is a significant determinant of the inability to live independently among older adults. There are various common reasons for long-term cognitive dysfunction in older people, including stroke, dementia, white matter abnormalities, traumatic brain injury, developmental disability and degenerative neurological conditions, e.g. Alzheimer's disease, multiple sclerosis and Parkinson's disease.

EXECUTIVE FUNCTION

Executive function (EF) is one aspect of cognition and the deterioration of EF with age is widely accepted (Grigsby et al., 1998; Carlson et al., 1999; Ble et al., 2005; Coppin et al., 2006; Atkinson et al., 2007; Johnson et al., 2007; Liu-Ambrose et al., 2009; Liu-Ambrose et al., 2010; Schneider-Garces et al., 2010; Kraybill & Suchy, 2011; Mirelman et al., 2012). The rationale for this inverse relationship between EF and age relates to the fact that the prefrontal regions of the brain, which mediate EF, undergo the most significant age-related degeneration (Zimmerman et al., 2006; Hillman et al., 2008; Eggermont et al., 2009; Turner & Spreng, 2012). Age-related functional and structural changes in the brain, such as cortical thinning, white matter changes and reduction in hippocampal activation, lead to inefficient processing and, therefore, executive dysfunction (ED) (Park & Reuter-Lorenz, 2009).

Donovan et al. (2008) characterized EF as the group of cognitive processes responsible for guiding, directing and managing cognitive, emotional and behavioral functions, during novel tasks such as organizing thoughts and activities, prioritizing tasks, managing time efficiently and decision-making. This definition is meaningful for clinical interpretation by healthcare professionals working with older people. For example, an older adult who demonstrates deficits in organizing his or her activities may experience difficulty in correctly self-administering a prescribed insulin program. The participation in goal-oriented behavior is a crucial element to successful rehabilitation (Wade, 1999; Levack et al., 2006). Difficulty in the prioritization of tasks may compromise the success of rehabilitation, e.g. choosing to engage in sedentary behavior as opposed to engaging in additional self-directed exercise outside dedicated therapy treatment time. Furthermore, people who demonstrate time management deficits may miss arranged appointments with their healthcare professional. Older adults who lack the ability to self-monitor their performance and make appropriate decisions, e.g. recognize that they have parked the wheelchair too far from the bed to conduct a safe transfer (Studer, 2007), may engage in unsafe physical maneuvers in the clinical setting (Hayes et al., 2011). The onus is on healthcare professionals to be aware of the negative effect that ED may have on successful communication with older people.

There is no single comprehensive test for EF. The complex nature of EF and the lack of consensus on a standardized definition of EF make its measurement difficult and possibly contribute to its underevaluation in the clinical setting (Godefroy, 2003). The discrepancies across various theoretical frameworks have resulted in the development of numerous measures of EF, many of which aim to capture its different aspects. The Behavioral Assessment of Dysexecutive Syndrome (BADS) (Wilson et al., 1996) was designed to predict everyday problems arising from ED (Norris & Tate, 2000). The BADS consists of six tests, which are designed to encompass the skills most pertinent to EF, including: set shifting, novel problem-solving, planning and behavioral regulation and judgment and estimation. The Frontal Assessment Battery (FAB) (Dubois et al., 2000) is a popular bedside screening test of EF which takes 5–10 minutes to administer. The BADS and FAB have demonstrated adequate reliability and validity in neurological and older adult populations (Dubois et al., 2000; Norris & Tate, 2000).

There is growing evidence to support the positive effects of aerobic exercise on EF in healthy older adults (Colcombe & Kramer, 2003; Angevaren et al., 2008; Weinstein et al., 2012). Physiologically, aerobic exercise has been shown to have beneficial effects on cognition by promoting increased cerebral blood flow, oxygen extraction and glucose utilization as well as an activation of growth factors that mediate structural changes such as capillary density (Angevaren et al., 2008). A meta-analytic study that examined the impact of aerobic fitness training on cognitive function in healthy but sedentary older adults demonstrated that aerobic training had robust but selective benefits for cognition, the largest of which were benefits for EF, with an effect size of 0.48 (Colcombe & Kramer, 2003).

Various authors have suggested the introduction of alternative treatment strategies as necessary precursors for the effective rehabilitation of physical function in the presence of ED (Zinn et al., 2007; Pahlman et al., 2011, 2012; Wolf et al., 2011). Systematic reviews of acquired brain injury literature have demonstrated compensatory interventions that healthcare professionals may find useful in ameliorating ED (Cicerone et al., 2011; Whyte et al., 2011; Poulin et al., 2012). Compensatory interventions involve the promotion of a person's adaptation to his/her environment and response (Whyte et al., 2011). Cicerone et al. (2011) recommended the use of metacognitive compensatory training for the management of ED post-traumatic brain injury and stroke. Metacognitive training interventions are aimed at improving self-awareness and self-regulation during the execution of everyday tasks. This involves asking older adults with ED to define their performance goals, predict task performance, anticipate difficulties, select a strategy to circumvent difficulties, assess the amount of assistance required to successfully perform the task and self-evaluate performance during rehabilitation. Another compensatory intervention recommended by Cicerone et al. (2011) for the management of ED relates to the application of formal problem-solving strategies to everyday situations, e.g. successful performance of a safe transfer from bed to chair.

Rehabilitation is based to a considerable degree on the attempt to facilitate learning (Pahlman et al., 2011). Shumway-Cook and Woolacott (2007) categorized two types of learning which are required during participation in rehabilitation: procedural and declarative. Procedural learning refers to the acquisition of new skills that can be performed automatically, without attention or EF; declarative learning involves the recall of knowledge that can be consciously recalled and requires awareness, attention and EF (Pahlman et al., 2011). It may be more difficult for people with ED to engage in declarative learning in comparison with procedural learning during rehabilitation (Pahlman et al., 2011; Whyte et al., 2011). Therefore, healthcare professionals should be mindful to implement strategies that facilitate the procedural learning of skills during rehabilitation among older adults with ED.

People with executive dysfunction often lack autonomy. When there is a diagnosis of ED, or if an older adult is unable to go from step one to step two in a procedure in which proper instruction has been given, the family, significant other or caregiver must be taught the procedure.

In the home or in any healthcare setting, the following suggestions can help those who care for people with ED:

- Establish a daily routine, e.g. if the older adult with ED is an inpatient attending a therapy gym, it may be helpful to organize therapy sessions for the same time daily, in the same part of the gym, with the same therapist.
- Use constant verbal cues and positive feedback to guide the older adult during treatment.
- Remove or alter environmental stimuli that seem to trigger problem behaviors, e.g. eliminate background noise by turning off the radio or treating the person on a one-to-one basis as opposed to in a group session.
- If the older adult demonstrates difficulty following instructions, incorporate functional tasks into the treatment session as opposed to isolated exercises, e.g. encourage the person to practice transferring from bed to chair as opposed to providing the person with upper limb and lower limb strengthening exercises in isolation.
- Provide the older adult with clear written instructions in order to enable correct independent practice.
- Encourage the older adult to monitor their own performance during treatment and suggest ways of improving their performance.
- Use checklists to encourage goal-directed behavior, e.g. each step that is required in order to successfully make breakfast.

CONCLUSION

When communicating with older people, many facets of their life must be taken into account. Not only is there an onus on healthcare professionals to identify deficits in communication among older adults under their care, but also to implement appropriate alternative treatment strategies in order to facilitate the optimal success of rehabilitation. Communication deficits result from a variety of sources: cultural differences, language barriers, sensory loss, aphasia, short-term or long term global cognitive impairment, or specific cognitive impairments, including executive dysfunction. An effort must be made by healthcare professionals to understand cultural differences, accommodate for lack of educational opportunities and to overcome physical and cognitive deficits.

REFERENCES

Angevaren M, Aufdemkampe G, Verhaar HJ et al 2008 Physical activity and enhanced fitness to improve cognitive function in older adults without known cognitive impairment. Cochrane Database Syst Rev 16:CD005381

Atkinson HH, Rosano C, Simonsick EM et al 2007 Cognitive function, gait speed decline, and comorbidities: the health, aging and body composition study. J Gerontol Series B: Psychol Sci Social Sci 62A:844–850

Bandura A 1994 Self-efficacy. In: Ramachaudran VS (ed) Encyclopedia of Human Behavior. Academic Press, New York

Bandura A 1997 The Nature and Structure of Self-efficacy. In: Bandura A (ed) Self-Efficacy: The Exercise of Control. Worth Publishers, New York

Bandura A 2006 Guide for Constructing Self-efficacy Scales. In: Pajares F, Urdan TC (eds) Self-Efficacy Beliefs Of Adolescence. Information Age Publishers, Charlotte, NC

Bell-McGinty S, Podell K, Franzen M et al 2002 Standard measures of executive function in predicting instrumental activities of daily living in older adults. Int J Geriatr Psychiatry 17:828–834

Berthier ML, Garcia-Casares N, Walsh SF et al 2011 Recovery from post-stroke aphasia: lessons from brain imaging and implications for rehabilitation and biological treatments. Discov Med 12:275–289

Ble A, Volpato S, Zuliani G et al 2005 Executive function correlates with walking speed in older persons: the InCHIANTI study. J Am Geriatr Soc 53:410–415

Brady M, Kelly H, Godwin J et al 2012 Speech and language therapy for aphasia following stroke. Cochrane Database Syst Rev 16:CD000425

Cahn-Weiner DA, Boyle PA, Malloy PF 2002 Tests of executive function predict instrumental activities of daily living in community-dwelling older individuals. Appl Neuropsychol 9:187–191

Carlson MC, Fried LP, Xue Q et al 1999 Association between executive attention and physical functional performance in community-dwelling older women. J Gerontol 54B:S262–S270

Cicerone KD, Langenbahn DM, Braden C et al 2011 Evidence-based cognitive rehabilitation: updated review of the literature from 2003 through 2008. Arch Phys Med Rehabil 92:519–530

Colcombe S, Kramer AF 2003 Fitness effects on the cognitive function of older adults: a meta-analytic study. Psychol Sci 14:125–130

Coppin AK, Shumway-Cook A, Saczynski JS et al 2006 Association of executive function and performance of dual-task physical tests among older adults: analyses from the InChianti study. Age Ageing 35:619–624

De Bruin ED, Schmidt A 2010 Walking behaviour of healthy elderly: attention should be paid. Behav Brain Funct 6:59–66

Deci EL, Ryan RM 2012 Self-determination theory in health care and its relations to motivational interviewing: a few comments. Int J Behav Nutr Phys Act 9:24

Dewalt DA, Berkman ND, Sheridan S et al 2004 Literacy and health outcomes: a systematic review of the literature. J Gen Intern Med 19:1228–1239

Donovan NJ, Kendall DL, Heaton SC et al 2008 Conceptualizing functional cognition in stroke. Neurorehabil Neural Repair 22:122–135

Dubois B, Slachevsky A, Litvan I et al 2000 The FAB: a Frontal Assessment Battery at bedside. Neurology 55:1621–1626

Eggermont LH, Milberg WP, Lipsitz LA et al 2009 Physical activity and executive function in aging: the MOBILIZE Boston Study. J Am Geriatr Soc 57:1750–1756

Frei A, Svarin A, Steurer-Stey C et al 2009 Self-efficacy instruments for patients with chronic diseases suffer from methodological limitations – a systematic review. Health Qual Life Outcomes 7:86

Godefroy O 2003 Frontal syndrome and disorders of executive functions. J Neurol 250:1–6

Grigsby J, Kaye K, Baxter J et al 1998 Executive cognitive abilities and functional status among community-dwelling older persons in the San Luis Valley Health and Aging Study. J Am Geriatr Soc 46:590–596

Hamadeh G 1987 Religion, magic, and medicine. J Fam Pract 25:561–568

Hayes S, Donnellan C, Stokes E 2011 The measurement and impairment of executive function after stroke and concepts for physiotherapy. Phys Ther Rev 16:178–190

Hillman CH, Erickson KI, Kramer AF 2008 Be smart, exercise your heart: exercise effects on brain and cognition. Nature Rev Neurosci 9:58–65

Johnson JK, Lui L, Yaffe K 2007 Executive function, more than global cognition, predicts functional decline and mortality in elderly women. J Gerontol A Biol Sci Med Sci 62:1134–1141

Koenig H, King D, Carson VB 2012 Handbook of Religion and Health. Oxford University Press, New York

Kraybill ML, Suchy Y 2011 Executive functioning, motor programming, and functional independence: accounting for variance, people, and time. Clin Neuropsychol 25:210–223

Levack WM, Taylor K, Siegert RJ et al 2006 Is goal planning in rehabilitation effective? A systematic review. Clin Rehabil 20:739–755

Lewis MP 2009 Ethnologue: Languages of the World. SIL International, Dallas, TX

Liu-Ambrose T, Katarynch LA, Ashe MC et al 2009 Dualtask gait performance among community-dwelling senior women: the role of balance confidence and executive functions. J Gerontol Series A: Biol Sci Med Sci 64A:975–982

Liu-Ambrose T, Davis JC, Nagamatsu LS et al 2010 Changes in executive functions and self-efficacy are independently associated with improved usual gait speed in older women. BMC Geriatrics 10:1–8

Lowry KA, Brach JS, Nebes RD et al 2012 Contributions of cognitive function to straight- and curved-path walking in older adults. Arch Phys Med Rehabil 93:802–807

McAuley E, Mullen SP, Szabo AN et al 2011 Self-regulatory processes and exercise adherence in older adults: executive function and self-efficacy effects. Am J Prevent Med 41:284–290

Marks R, Allegrante JP, Lorig K 2005 A review and synthesis of research evidence for self-efficacy-enhancing interventions for reducing chronic disability: implications for health education practice (part I). Health Promot Pract 6:37–43

Mirelman A, Herman T, Brozgol M et al 2012 Executive function and falls in older adults: new findings from a five-year prospective study link fall risk to cognition. PLOS ONE 7:1–8

Nieto ML, Albert SM, Morrow LA et al 2008 Cognitive status and physical function in older African Americans. J Am Geriatr Soc 56:2014–2019

Norris G, Tate RL 2000 The Behavioural Assessment of the Dysexecutive Syndrome (BADS): ecological, concurrent and construct validity. Neuropsychol Rehabil 10:33–45

Pahlman U, Gutierrez-Perez C, Savborg M et al 2011 Cognitive function and improvement of balance after stroke in elderly people: the Gothenburg Cognitive Stroke Study in the Elderly. Disabil Rehabil 33:1952–1962

Pahlman U, Savborg M, Tarkowski E 2012 Cognitive dysfunction and physical activity after stroke: the Gothenburg Cognitive Stroke Study in the Elderly. J Stroke Cerebrovasc Dis 21(8):652–658

Park DC, Reuter-Lorenz P 2009 The adaptive brain: aging and neurocognitive scaffolding. Ann Rev Psychol 60:173–196

Plunkett O 2002 The miracles of Lourdes. Student Br Med J 10:1–44

Poulin V, Korner-Bitensky N, Dawson DR et al 2012 Efficacy of executive function interventions after stroke: a systematic review. Top Stroke Rehabil 19:158–171

Schneider-Garces NJ, Gordon BA, Brumback-Peltz CR et al 2010 Span, CRUNCH, and beyond: working memory capacity and the aging brain. J Cogn Neurosci 22:655–669

Shumway-Cook A, Woolocott MH 2007 Motor Control: Translating Research into Clinical Practice, 3rd edn. Lippincott Williams & Wilkins, Philadelphia, PA

Studer M 2007 Rehabilitation of executive function: to err is human, to be aware – divine. J Neurol Phys Ther 31:128–134

Turner GR, Spreng RN 2012 Executive functions and neurocognitive aging: dissociable patterns of brain activity. Neurobiol Aging 33:1–13

United Nations Department of Economic and Social Affairs 2011 International Migration Report 201): A Global Assessment. United Nations, New York

Voelcker-Rehage C, Godde B, Staudinger UM 2010 Physical and motor fitness are both related to cognition in old age. Eur J Neurosci 31:167–176

Wade DT 1999 Goal planning in stroke rehabilitation: why? Top Stroke Rehabil 6:1–7

Waters DL, Hale LA, Robertson L et al 2011 Evaluation of a peer-led falls prevention program for older adults. Arch Phys Rehabil 92:1581–1586

Weinstein AM, Voss MW, Prakash RS et al 2012 The association between aerobic fitness and executive function is mediated by prefrontal cortex volume. Brain Behav Immun 26:811–819

Whyte E, Skidmore E, Aizenstein H et al 2011 Cognitive impairment in acquired brain injury: a predictor of rehabilitation outcomes and an opportunity for novel interventions. Phys Med Rehabil 3:S45–S51

Wilson BA, Alderman N, Burgess P et al 1996 Behavioural assessment of the dysexecutive syndrome. Thames Valley Test Company, Bury St Edmunds, Suffolk

Wolf TJ, Barbee AR, White D 2011 Executive dysfunction immediately after mild stroke. OTJR 31:S23–S29

Zimmerman ME, Brickman AM, Paul RH et al 2006 The relationship between frontal gray matter volume and cognition varies across the healthy adult lifespan. Am J Geriatr Psychiatry 14:823–833

Zinn S, Bosworth HB, Hoenig HM et al 2007 Executive function deficits in acute stroke. Arch Phys Med Rehabil 88:173–180

Zolnierek KB, Dimatteo MR 2009 Physician communication and patient adherence to treatment: a meta-analysis. Med Care 47:826–834

Specific problems

UNIT CONTENTS

Chapter 54

Dysphagia

DARCI BECKER • LISA TEWS

CHAPTER CONTENTS

DEFINITION AND PREVALENCE

For most individuals, eating is a pleasurable and social event that is an important aspect of quality of life. However, for those with dysphagia, the task of eating may be difficult and even lead to serious medical consequences, such as airway obstruction, dehydration, malnutrition, aspiration pneumonia or death.

Dysphagia (pronounced 'dis-fay-ja' or 'dis-fah-zha') is the medical term used when an individual experiences difficulty with or disordered swallowing. Dysphagia is a symptom of underlying pathology, not a primary medical diagnosis.

Dysphagia occurs across the age spectrum, from premature babies to elderly adults. Estimates of prevalence vary, depending on the patient population, setting and criteria used. Rates cited in the literature include:

- 10–25% of all children, 40–70% of premature infants and 70–90% of children with medical/developmental delays (Roche et al., 2011).
- 25–30% of patients admitted to hospitals.
- 61% of adults admitted to acute trauma centers.
- 41% of individuals admitted to rehabilitation settings.
- 30–75% of nursing home residents.

Conditions associated with a high prevalence of dysphagia include stroke, multiple sclerosis, Parkinson's disease, amyotrophic lateral sclerosis, cerebral palsy and tumors of the head and neck or esophagus (American Speech–Language–Hearing Association, 2008).

ETIOLOGY

Dysphagia can be caused by a multitude of conditions (Box 54.1). Medications that reduce saliva production, muscle strength, coordination or alertness level may also affect swallowing function. These may include antipsychotics, anticonvulsants, antihistamines and barbiturates. The risk for dysphagia increases with age. One reason is that natural, healthy aging results in alterations in the swallowing mechanism, known as presbyphagia.

This contributes to a general decline in functional reserve, which increases susceptibility of dysphagia in older individuals when additional stressors, such as acute illness, occur (Ney et al., 2009).

NORMAL SWALLOWING PHYSIOLOGY

The process of deglutition, or swallowing, is typically divided into four stages that overlap and are interdependent.

1. *Oral preparatory stage:* food or liquid is received into the mouth, manipulated and masticated if necessary, and reduced to a consistency ready for swallowing.
2. *Oral phase:* the tongue propels the food or liquid posteriorly toward the pharynx until the pharyngeal swallow is triggered; this typically takes less than 1 second.
3. *Pharyngeal stage:* the pharyngeal swallow is triggered and the bolus is carried through the pharynx; laryngeal closure occurs to protect the airway from aspiration; this stage normally takes 1 second.
4. *Esophageal stage:* esophageal peristalsis carries the bolus through the cervical and thoracic esophagus and into the stomach; food normally reaches the stomach in 5–15 seconds.

For a normal swallow to occur, there must be oral propulsion of the bolus into the pharynx, tongue base to pharyngeal wall propulsion to transport the bolus through the pharynx to the esophagus, airway closure and upper esophageal sphincter opening (Fig. 54.1). Airway closure is achieved when the epiglottis inverts over the entrance to the larynx, directing the bolus toward the esophagus and away from the airway, and when the false and true vocal folds approximate. During the swallow when airway closure is achieved, respiration halts until the swallow is completed.

When one or more of the stages of swallowing is atypical, there is an increased potential for aspiration to occur. Aspiration is defined as the entry of material into the airway *below* the level of the true vocal folds. If no

Box 54.1 *Conditions that may affect the swallowing process*

NEUROLOGICAL/NEUROGENIC

- Pseudobulbar palsy
- Bulbar palsy
- Cerebrovascular accident
- Traumatic brain injury
- Neurovascular disease
- Acute encephalitis
- Acute meningitis
- Seizure disorder
- Peripheral neuropathy
- Transient ischemic attack
- Metastatic cancer

CONGENITAL/PROGRESSIVE NEUROLOGICAL

- Polio
- Postpolio syndrome
- Multiple sclerosis
- Parkinson's disease
- Amyotrophic lateral sclerosis
- Huntington's chorea
- Myasthenia gravis
- Myotonic dystrophy
- Guillain–Barré
- Cerebral palsy
- Tardive dyskinesia

COGNITIVE/PSYCHOLOGICAL

- Globus hystericus
- Right hemisphere dysfunction
- Dementia

MEDICAL/OTHER

- Esophageal reflux
- Decline in functional status/deconditioning
- Radiation therapy (head and neck)

STRUCTURAL

- Head and neck cancer
- Laryngectomy
- Glossectomy
- Esophagectomy
- Hiatal hernia
- Zenker's diverticulum
- Congenital or acquired anomalies
- Burns
- Tracheostomy
- Focal tumors
- Laryngeal trauma/vocal fold injury

SKELETAL AND CONNECTIVE TISSUE

- Lupus
- Scleroderma
- Inflammatory myopathy
- Cervical rheumatoid arthritis
- Cervical osteophyte
- Osteoarthritis
- Cervical spinal cord injury
- Fractures (facial, spinal)
- Contractures

RESPIRATORY

- Chronic obstructive pulmonary disease
- Asthma
- Emphysema

SURGICAL PROCEDURES

- Laryngectomy
- Anterior cervical spine surgery
- Carotid endarterectomy

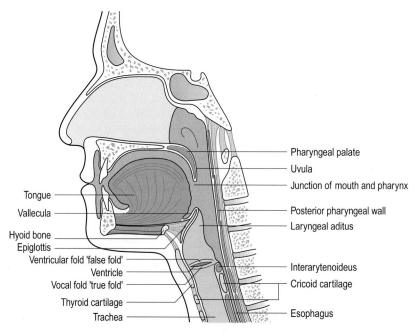

Figure 54.1 Lateral view of the anatomy of the head and neck pertinent to swallowing. *(From Bosma JF, Donner MW, Tanaka E et al. 1986 Anatomy of the pharynx, pertinent to swallowing. Dysphagia 1:24.)*

cough response occurs with aspiration, it is referred to as 'silent aspiration'. Penetration is defined as the entry of material into the laryngeal vestibule which, unlike aspiration, remains *above* the level of the true vocal folds. In the past, both penetration and aspiration have been considered to be pathologic occurrences, not present in those with normal swallowing. Studies continue to affirm that aspiration is not a normal finding in awake individuals, however recent evidence indicates that occasional, high penetration is present in *normal* individuals, particularly with increasing age (Daggett et al., 2006; Allen et al., 2010).

There are many signs and symptoms of dysphagia (Box 54.2). It should be noted that the symptom of gagging is listed in Box 54.2. In some instances, physicians order a swallowing evaluation when an oral motor examination indicates that an individual lacks a gag reflex. Data, however, do not support a relationship between the gag reflex and ability to swallow. Studies have confirmed that individuals with a *normal* gag reflex may exhibit aspiration and, conversely, individuals who *lack* a gag reflex may swallow normally (Leder, 1996, 1997).

In addition to observing patients for signs and symptoms of dysphagia, patients should be monitored for signs of aspiration pneumonia. These include fever, shortness of breath, elevated white blood cell count, hypoxemia and radiographic evidence of an infiltrate in a dependent bronchopulmonary segment. Individuals who aspirate while in a reclined position will tend to have infiltrates located in the posterior segments of the upper lobes. Those who aspirate while in an upright or semi-reclined position, will tend to have infiltrates in the basal segments of the lower lobes (Cavallazzi et al., 2009).

Signs of dysphagia or aspiration may be discovered by any member of the interdisciplinary team. For example, the occupational therapist may observe problems while addressing feeding skills, the dietitian might learn that the patient prefers ground meats, or the nurse might observe that the patient is having difficulty managing secretions or swallowing pills. If dysphagia is suspected, this information should be communicated to the medical team. It is also appropriate for a referral to be made to the speech-language pathologist, as it is their role to evaluate, diagnose and treat oropharyngeal dysphagia.

DYSPHAGIA ASSESSMENT

Swallowing is most commonly evaluated in one of two ways: a clinical (or 'bedside') swallow examination or an instrumental examination.

CLINICAL EXAMINATION

After obtaining a thorough case history, the clinical examination typically includes a physical examination of the swallowing musculature and observations of swallowing ability with test swallows. Recommendations are then made regarding the patient's candidacy for safe oral feeding and, if so, what the safest diet may be. If there is evidence of dysphagia, an instrumental exam is often recommended, as it allows for the assessment of oral, pharyngeal and esophageal structures and functions. It is important to note that 50–60% of individuals who aspirate exhibit silent aspiration. Evidence suggests, therefore, that 40% of patients who aspirate will be undetected if evaluated by a bedside examination alone, even when performed by the most experienced clinicians (Logemann, 1998).

INSTRUMENTAL EXAMINATION

The most common types of instrumental exams performed in the United States of America are the radiographic evaluation (also known as the modified barium swallow evaluation, videofluoroscopic swallow study, or cookie swallow test) and the fiberoptic endoscopic evaluation of swallowing. The purposes of the instrumental exam are to identify the presence and cause of dysphagia, identify any strategies or maneuvers that might eliminate or reduce dysphagia and to determine what therapeutic techniques might be appropriate.

In cases of severe dysphagia, nothing by mouth (NPO) and alternative means of nutrition and hydration may be recommended. Alternative means of nutrition and hydration may also be recommended if dysphagia precludes the ability to maintain adequate nutrition and hydration orally. Alternative sources of nutrition and hydration may be a temporary means, such as intravenous feedings or a nasogastric tube (NG tube). If recovery is anticipated to be more long-term, a gastrostomy tube (G-tube) or jejunostomy tube (J-tube) may be placed. Use of alternative or supplemental means of nutrition and hydration do not always prevent oral intake. In many cases, a hybrid approach in which the patient receives pleasure or therapeutic oral feedings with the speech-language pathologist, in addition to alternative feedings via non-oral routes, is utilized. The use of tube feedings is not without risk. In addition to risks associated with surgical placement of tubes, infection and reflux of feedings are of concern. Studies exploring the use of feeding tubes in specific populations, such as those with advanced dementia, have found that they do not reduce the incidence of aspiration pneumonia or prolong life beyond expected limits (Groher & Crary, 2010).

Whenever possible, the risks and benefits of alternative nutrition sources should be discussed among the patient, family and healthcare team. Individuals have the right to autonomy in making their healthcare decisions and they may not agree to recommendations of NPO status or alternative means of nutrition. If a patient disagrees with recommendations, the healthcare team should ensure the patient has been fully educated on the risks and benefits of all options and, if possible, offer suggestions to minimize risks of dysphagia or aspiration.

DYSPHAGIA TREATMENT

Dysphagia treatment must be individualized. Based on the findings of a swallowing assessment, thickened liquids or diet modifications may be recommended (Table 54.1). Thickened liquids are often prescribed for patients with dysphagia, as they may reduce the incidence of aspiration (Kuhlemeier et al., 2001). Patients, however, often voice dislike of thickeners and may demonstrate reduced or inadequate intake of thickened fluids (Finestone et al., 2001). Use of thickeners may also result in clumps or yield products that lack stability of consistency over time (Dewar & Joyce, 2006).

Modified diet textures, such as pureed or mechanically altered diets, are also commonly prescribed for those with chewing or swallowing difficulties. While institutions may utilize their own diet hierarchies, many have adopted the levels of the National Dysphagia Diet (Table 54.1).

In addition to liquid and diet modifications, postural changes while eating and drinking may be recommended, if they reduce dysphagia and/or aspiration (Table 54.2). It is important that only postural strategies found to be beneficial during an individual's swallowing evaluation be utilized, as all strategies will not benefit all patients with dysphagia.

Dysphagia rehabilitation typically includes a regimen of strengthening exercises, range of motion exercises (ROM) and/or specific swallowing maneuvers (Table 54.3). It is generally developed by the speech-language pathologist and tailored specifically to the deficits of the individual. In some cases, surgical intervention may also be required. There are several additional treatments for dysphagia that are gaining favor and have varying levels of evidence to support their use. These include surface electromyography, a noninvasive method of providing feedback about muscle activity during the swallow (Stepp, 2012); neuromuscular electrical stimulation, electrical stimulation applied via surface electrodes to the neck resulting in muscle contractions (Clark et al., 2009); and respiratory muscle strength training, typically achieved with handheld devices that offer varying amounts of resistance to inspiratory or expiratory airflow (Sapienza & Troche, 2012). The use of free water protocols in those with dysphagia has also become popular; however, evidence on the risks and benefits of such protocols is presently mixed (Coyle, 2011; Langmore, 2011). Free water protocols permit oral water in those with known dysphagia, by following guidelines about when and how water is permitted. To minimize the risk of aspiration pneumonia, such protocols are often employed with strict oral care regimens.

While new fads and dysphagia treatments continually emerge, speech-language pathologists are urged to utilize evidence-based practice (EBP) when treating individuals with dysphagia. EBP requires clinicians to develop treatment plans based on the best available evidence from published literature, as well as considering the patient's wishes and the experiences of the clinician.

Table 54.1 Examples of liquid modifications and dysphagia diets

Liquids:	Thin liquid
	Nectar consistency liquid
	Honey consistency liquid
	Pudding consistency liquid

National Dysphagia Diet Levels

Level I	Dysphagia Pureed (homogeneous, very cohesive, pudding-like; requires very little chewing ability)
Level II	Dysphagia Mechanically Altered (cohesive, moist, semi-solid foods; requires some chewing ability; meats are ground or finely chopped)
Level III	Dysphagia Advanced (foods that are naturally soft and near regular texture; hard, dry, sticky or crunchy foods are excluded)
Level IV	Regular (all foods allowed)

Adapted from the National Dysphagia Diet Task Force 2002.

Table 54.2 Effects of applied posture changes during the swallow

Posture	Effect
Head back	Uses gravity to clear the oral cavity
Chin down	1. Widens valleculae, narrows entrance to larynx 2. Pushes tongue base backward toward pharyngeal wall 3. Puts epiglottis in more protective position
Head rotated to damaged side	1. Increases vocal fold adduction by applying extrinsic pressure 2. Eliminates damaged side from bolus path
Head tilt to stronger side	Directs bolus down stronger side
Lying down on one side	Eliminates gravitational effect on pharyngeal residue
Head rotated	Pulls cricoid cartilage away from posterior pharyngeal wall, reducing resting pressure in cricopharyngeal sphincter

Adapted from Logemann J (1998) Evaluation and Treatment of Swallowing Disorders. Pro-Ed, Austin, TX.

Table 54.3 Exercises, swallowing maneuvers and surgical procedures

Oral Stage of the Swallow

Reduced lip closure	Lip exercises (resistance, ROM)
Reduced cheek tension	Manual pressure
Reduced tongue elevation	Tongue exercises (resistance, ROM)
Reduced tongue lateralization, anterior to posterior movement	Tongue exercises (chewing with gauze, manipulation)
Reduced range of jaw movement	Jaw ROM exercises
Oral awareness	Oral stimulation (taste, temperature, pressure, texture)
Apraxia	Increase oral sensation (pressure/cold/sour)

Pharyngeal Stage of the Swallow

Delayed or absent triggering of the pharyngeal swallow	Thermal/tactile stimulation; suck/swallow; quick downward pressure on tongue; sour bolus
Slow pharyngeal transit	Lee Silverman Voice Treatment
Reduced base of tongue movement	Effortful swallow; super-supraglottic swallow; tongue holding (Masako maneuver); tongue base retraction exercises (yawn, tongue hold, gargle)
Reduced pharyngeal contraction	Falsetto; effortful swallow; effortful phonation of 'eee'
Reduced laryngeal excursion	Super-supraglottic swallow; falsetto; pitch exercises; Mendelsohn maneuver; Shaker exercises
Reduced closure at laryngeal entrance	Super-supraglottic swallow; Mendelsohn maneuver
Reduced laryngeal closure at vocal folds	Supraglottic swallow; adduction exercises; Teflon or gelfoam injection
Cricopharyngeal dysfunction	Mendelsohn maneuver; Shaker exercises; dilatation; myotomy
Aspiration	Shaker exercises

Adapted from Logemann JA 1983 Evaluation and Treatment of Swallowing Disorders. Pro-Ed, Austin, TX.

REFERENCES

Allen JE, White CJ, Leonard RJ et al 2010 Prevalence of penetration and aspiration on videofluoroscopy in normal individuals without dysphagia. Otolaryngol Head Neck Surg 142:208–213

American Speech–Language–Hearing Association (ASHA) 2008 Communication facts: special populations: dysphagia. Available at: www.asha.org/Research/reports/dysphagia/. Accessed December 2013

Cavallazzi R, Vasu TS, Marik PE 2009 Aspiration pneumonitis and aspiration pneumonia. Perspect Swallow Swallow Disord (Dysphagia) 18:25–33

Clark H, Lazarus C, Arvedson J et al 2009 Evidence-based systematic review: effects of neuromuscular electrical stimulation on swallowing and neural activation. Am J Speech Lang Pathol 18:361–375

Coyle J 2011 Water, water everywhere, but why? Argument against free water protocols. Perspect Swallow Swallow Disord (Dysphagia) 20:109–115

Daggett A, Logemann J, Rademaker A et al 2006 Laryngeal penetration during deglutition in normal subjects of various ages. Dysphagia 21:270–274

Dewar RJ, Joyce MJ 2006 Time-dependent rheology of starch thickeners and the clinical implications for dysphagia therapy. Dysphagia 21:264–269

Finestone H, Foley N, Woodbury G et al 2001 Quantifying fluid intake in dysphagic stroke patients: a preliminary comparison of oral and nonoral strategies. Arch Phys Med Rehabil 82:1744–1746

Groher ME, Crary MA 2010 Dysphagia, Clinical Management in Adults and Children. Mosby Elsevier, St Louis, MO

Kuhlemeier K, Palmer J, Rosenberg D 2001 Effect of liquid bolus consistency and delivery method on aspiration and pharyngeal retention in dysphagia patients. Dysphagia 16:119–122

Langmore S 2011 Why I like the free water protocol. Perspect Swallow Swallow Disord (Dysphagia) 20:116–120

Leder SB 1996 Gag reflex and dysphagia. Head Neck 18:138–141

Leder SB 1997 Videofluoroscopic evaluation of aspiration with visual examination of the gag reflex and velar movement. Dysphagia 12:21–23

Logemann J 1998 Evaluation and Treatment of Swallowing Disorders. Pro-Ed, Austin, TX

Ney DM, Weiss JM, Kind AJ et al 2009 Senescent swallowing: impact, strategies, and interventions. Nutr Clin Pract 24:395–413

Roche E, Martorana P, Berkowitz M et al 2011 An oral, motor, medical, and behavioral approach to pediatric feeding and swallowing disorders: an interdisciplinary model. Perspect Swallow Swallow Disord (Dysphagia) 20:65–74

Sapienza C, Troche M 2012 Respiratory Muscle Strength Training: Theory and Practice. Plural Publishing, San Diego, CA

Stepp C 2012 Surface electromyography for speech and swallowing systems: measurement, analysis and interpretation. J Speech Lang Hear Res 55:1232–1246

Chapter 55

Incontinence of the bowel and bladder

SANDRA J. LEVI • TERI ELLIOTT-BURKE

CHAPTER CONTENTS

INTRODUCTION

Bladder and bowel incontinence among older adults is common and often treatable. Unfortunately, embarrassment and inadequate knowledge of treatment options prevent many older adults from reporting incontinence to healthcare professionals. The social consequences of incontinence are profound. Older adults who live at home may reduce or eliminate trips outside the home due to care needs and embarrassment. Moreover, incontinence often precipitates institutional placement. About 13–34% of community-dwelling older adults report urinary incontinence (Komesu et al., 2009) and up to 15% report fecal incontinence (Whitehead et al., 2009). Among residents of nursing homes, over 50% have urinary incontinence (Offermans et al., 2009) and 33–65% (Shah et al., 2012) have some problem with fecal incontinence. Both types of incontinence are much more common in women than men but, in the case of fecal incontinence, the gender ratio decreases with increasing age.

Pelvic floor muscle dysfunction contributes to urinary and fecal incontinence. The pelvic floor contains three layers of muscles that have sphincter, support and sexual functions. Pelvic floor muscle function includes closing the urinary and anal sphincters as well as closing the vaginal opening. Pelvic floor muscles also support the abdominal viscera and aid in sexual function and appreciation in men and women.

INCONTINENCE OF THE BOWEL

NORMAL CONTROL

Incontinence of the bowel is defined as an involuntary loss of stool through the anus that is severe enough to cause hygienic or social problems. In older adults, it may occur as an isolated incident in response to an acute event. Chronic fecal incontinence increases with increasing age.

Sensory and motor mechanisms contribute to the control of defecation. Typically, contractions in the proximal colon move feces into the rectum. The rectum stretches to hold the feces. The internal and external anal sphincters, as well as the puborectalis muscle, play especially important roles in preventing leakage. The internal anal sphincter is a 2–3 mm band of smooth muscle surrounding the anus. It is tonically contracted to keep the anal canal closed, except when it relaxes to allow emptying of the rectum. The external anal sphincter primarily consists of striated muscle; it voluntarily contracts, when needed, to prevent leakage. The puborectalis muscle forms a loop around the posterior aspect of the external sphincter. Contraction of the puborectalis muscle creates an anorectal angle. This angle and the puborectalis muscle assist in preventing defecation.

Defecation is initiated in response to rectal filling. Parasympathetic nerve impulses initiate strong peristaltic waves that move the fecal content along. At the same time, other body actions such as bearing down (i.e. the Valsalva maneuver) and upward and outward contraction of the pelvic floor musculature help to move the feces downward and outward. The final response is voluntary relaxation of the puborectalis muscle and the external anal sphincter.

With increasing age, pelvic floor musculature may weaken. Age-related loss of strength, as well as possible changes in tissue elasticity, may contribute to a decreased resting tone of the anus, particularly in women (Tariq, 2004).

CAUSES OF INCONTINENCE

The causes of fecal incontinence in the elderly are shown in Box 55.1. Fecal impaction, often associated with constipation (Leung & Rao, 2009; Shah et al., 2012), and diarrhea are the most common causes of fecal incontinence and are often treatable. Leakage of stool may also result from loss of sensation or loss of muscle

Box 55.1 *Etiology of fecal incontinence*

- Fecal impaction
- Loss of normal continence mechanism
  - Local neuronal damage (e.g. pudendal nerve)
  - Impaired neurological control
  - Anorectal trauma/sphincter disruption
- Problems that overwhelm normal continence mechanism
- Psychological and behavioral problems
  - Severe depression
  - Dementia
  - Cerebrovascular disease
- Neoplasm (rare)

Adapted from Tariq, 2004, with permission.

tone. Finally, stool loss may occur as a result of changes in the cognitive capacity to interpret sensory signals.

Stool leakage around an obstruction is often found in older adults. Most of these individuals have chronic fecal impaction, often as a result of inadequate fluid intake, chronic laxative abuse and poor bowel habits. Cancer or a benign polyp will sometimes be the cause. Whatever the cause, liquid stool from higher in the colon will leak past the hard immovable obstruction and drain from the anus, despite the best efforts of the patient.

A patient who has a condition that causes loose stool (drugs, inappropriate diet or infection) may suffer involuntary loss of this watery fecal material. For example, antacids containing magnesium, the consumption of dairy products by a person who is lactose intolerant and *Salmonella* infection can cause diarrhea. Loose stool may also be seen in bedridden patients who have poor muscle tone. A change of gravitational force may cause additional physiological and social demands on bedridden patients who are starting transfer and gait activities.

Loss of sensation of the perineum results in the patient not sensing the need for rectal emptying until natural forces have done so, leading to involuntary loss. Such perineal anesthesia may result from spinal cord injury, tumor or stroke, or previous injury including damage occurring during childbirth.

Loss of muscle tone by the muscles of continence may change the balance of forces such that the expulsive force of the colon exceeds any voluntary attempt by the patient to impede such force. Tumor, stroke, spinal cord injury, pudendal neuropathy and surgery frequently precipitate loss of muscle tone.

Patients may lose stool because they lack the cognitive capacity to realize what is happening. Such patients may have forgotten how to properly manage stool (as in dementia) or may not be sufficiently oriented to manage it (as in delirium).

Patients who have a moderate impairment – anatomical, physiological, mental or a combination of these – and who are impeded in some way from establishing a usable stooling position may appear to be incontinent. In addition, individuals with mobility limitations may be prevented from getting to a commode in a timely fashion. Rearranging their environment may make it easier for these patients to manage.

DIAGNOSIS AND THERAPEUTIC INTERVENTION

Multidisciplinary teams, including physicians, physical and occupational therapists, nursing staff and others provide optimal management of bowel and bladder incontinence.

Diagnosis of fecal incontinence begins by obtaining a careful history from the patient and the medical record. The history includes a description of:

- bowel habits, change in habits and fecal consistency (The Bristol Stool Chart provides a classification system for fecal consistency [Lewis & Heato, 1997]);
- bowel frequency, urgency, ability to delay, soiling and ability to distinguish gas from feces;
- emptying difficulties, including straining, incomplete emptying and pain;
- the capacity to access or get on and off the toilet (communication, cognitive and mobility);
- diet, especially fatty foods, caffeine and alcohol intake, and sugary foods;
- medication, chronic medical conditions, obstetrical injury, radiation to prostate or cervix and surgeries in the anorectal area;
- any previous treatment.

The physical examination includes palpation of the abdomen to look for colon distention, a rectal examination, a neurological examination and assessment of mobility, hygiene and mental functioning. Diagnostic tests may include stool cultures, blood tests, a barium enema, radiographic procedures, anal manometry, ultrasonography, electromyography and defecography.

Treatment is guided by the underlying cause and severity of incontinence. Medical management may include dietary management, e.g. increasing fluid and fiber intake (Bliss et al., 2001; Norton et al., 2010). Bowel management and training may involve medication (e.g. loperamide can be used to prevent diarrhea) (Norton et al., 2010) and a toileting schedule (Ouslander et al., 1996). Neuromuscular re-education, including biofeedback, has also shown promising results in some patients (Heymen et al., 2009). Neuromuscular re-education emphasizes strengthening the pelvic floor musculature and training the pelvic floor to properly descend (Hay-Smith et al., 2008). Diarrhea, one of the reversible conditions, should be controlled no matter what its cause. Treatment of fecal incontinence typically requires multiple approaches (Abrams et al., 2010; Norton et al., 2010; Shah et al., 2012).

INCONTINENCE OF THE BLADDER

Many of the points already discussed are important when considering urinary incontinence, which is a much more common occurrence. Urinary incontinence is defined as an involuntary loss of urine that is severe enough to cause social or hygienic problems. The consequences of urinary incontinence are listed in Box 55.2. The enormity of the problem can be seen by examining the direct and indirect costs, as shown in Box 55.3.

NORMAL CONTROL

Urine is stored in the bladder, which stretches during filling. Urine is held in the bladder as long as the pressure in the bladder remains lower than the urethral resistance. Urination occurs when the bladder muscle (detrusor muscle) contracts, forcing urine into the urethra. The pelvic floor muscles surrounding the urethra relax, allowing urine to pass out of the body.

TYPES OF INCONTINENCE

Four distinct types of urinary incontinence can be identified, although, in many cases, these presentations are mixed: urge incontinence, stress incontinence, overflow incontinence and functional incontinence.

Urge incontinence occurs when a patient feels the need to empty the bladder but is unable to get to a toilet before urination occurs. The urge to urinate is often triggered by an external stimulus such as running water or placing a key in the door. In urge incontinence, involuntary loss of urine may be large and post-void residual volume small. Post-void residual volume is measured by having the patient void as completely as possible and then immediately placing a straight catheter into the bladder and measuring the remaining urinary volume. The most common cause of this type of incontinence is an overactive bladder muscle (detrusor instability). It is most prevalent among individuals with diabetes, stroke, Alzheimer's disease, Parkinson's disease and multiple sclerosis.

Stress incontinence occurs when a cough, strain, laugh, sneeze, physical activity or otherwise-initiated Valsalva maneuver causes involuntary loss of urine. In men, the most common cause of stress incontinence is prostatectomy. Trunk flexion exercises and, possibly, the sit-to-stand movement may provoke stress incontinence. At such times, a few drops to a few ounces of urine escape from the bladder. Post-void residual volume is small. This is the most common type of incontinence seen among middle-aged women (Hannestad et al., 2000).

Overflow incontinence occurs when the bladder is overly distended (either because of an outlet obstruction or a bladder anomaly), causing bladder pressure to exceed urethral pressure, no matter what the patient may attempt. Another cause of overflow incontinence is the loss of the bladder sphincter secondary to surgery or injury. Loss of urine occurs in small amounts, but may occur nearly continuously. The post-void residual volume is high (potentially liters). Diabetes, spinal cord injury and an enlarged prostate can all precipitate overflow incontinence.

Functional incontinence occurs when an individual with normal bladder and urethral function has difficulty getting to the toilet before urination occurs. Those with impaired mobility or mental confusion may have this type of incontinence.

DIAGNOSIS AND THERAPEUTIC INTERVENTION

Diagnosis of urinary incontinence begins with a carefully conducted history that includes a description of:

- voiding history;
- urinating difficulties, including straining, decreased flow of stream, intermittent flow, hesitancy;
- irritation symptoms, such as urgency, frequency, urge incontinence;
- communication and cognitive capacity to access a toilet;

Box 55.4 *Reversible causes of urinary incontinence*

DIAPPERS

- **D**elirium or other confusional state
- **I**nfection, urinary tract, symptomatic
- **A**trophic urethritis or vaginitis
- **P**harmaceuticals:
  - Sedative/hypnotics, especially long-acting
  - Alcohol abuse
  - Loop diuretics (e.g. Bumex, Lasix, Edecrin)
  - Anticholinergic agents (e.g. antipsychotics, antidepressants, antihistamines, antiparkinsonian agents, antiarrhythmics, antispasmodics, opiates, antidiarrheal agents)
- **P**sychological disorders (especially depression)
- **E**ndocrine disorders (hyperglycemia or hypercalcemia)
- **R**estriction mobility
- **S**tool impaction

From Frantl JA, Newman DK, Colling J et al., 1996 Agency for Health Care Policy and Research: Managing acute and chronic urinary incontinence. Publication no. 96–0686, with permission.

Box 55.5 *Selected treatment options available to therapists*

- Bladder training, including:
  - Patient education
  - Diet counseling
  - Scheduled voiding
  - Positive reinforcement
  - Urge-suppression techniques
- Pelvic floor muscle retraining, including:
  - Biofeedback
  - Strengthening exercises
  - Endurance exercises
- Transvaginal electrical stimulation

- medications, chronic medical conditions, pelvic or spinal surgery, trauma;
- diet, especially major bladder irritants such as caffeine, alcohol, artificial sweeteners and citric acid;
- any previous treatment.

The patient should be examined to identify any reversible causes of incontinence, as well as any neurological disease, abdominal mass or pelvic organ prolapse. The DIAPPERS mnemonic shown in Box 55.4 is useful for identifying reversible causes of urinary incontinence. Men should also receive a prostate examination. Diagnostic tests may include post-void residual volume and urodynamic tests, urinalysis and culture, cystoscopy, bladder diary and blood tests.

Treatment is guided by the underlying cause and the severity of incontinence. Some causes of urinary incontinence are reversible and easily treated. Medications may be used to prevent unwanted detrusor muscle contractions or to increase muscle tone (DuBeau et al., 2010). Implants can be used to help close the urethra and reduce stress incontinence. Several systematic reviews have demonstrated that pelvic floor muscle training, with or without biofeedback, helps women with stress and urge incontinence (Neumann et al., 2006; Dumoulin & Hay-Smith, 2010). In a systematic review, Choi et al. (2007) concluded that performance of at least 24 daily contractions for at least 6 weeks decreases urinary leakage. Treatment typically requires multiple approaches. Some of the treatment options that are available to physical therapists are listed in Box 55.5.

CONCLUSION

Constant efforts must be made to find and treat reversible causes of incontinence. It must never be assumed that incontinence is a result of aging. Although many people with bowel and bladder incontinence cannot be completely cured, most can be helped significantly if the healthcare team takes the time to think about possible causes and to institute treatment plans based on

careful diagnoses. Often, conservative treatments such as strengthening pelvic floor musculature successfully alleviate incontinence.

REFERENCES

Abrams P, Andersson K, Birder L et al 2010 Fourth International Consultation on Incontinence Recommendations of the International Scientific Committee: evaluation and treatment of urinary incontinence, pelvic organ prolapse, and fecal incontinence. Neurourol Urodynam 29:213–240

Bliss DZ, Jung HJ, Savik K et al 2001 Supplementation with dietary fiber improves fecal incontinence. Nurs Res 50:203–213

Choi H, Palmer MH, Park J 2007 Meta-analysis of pelvic floor muscle training: randomized controlled trials in incontinent women. Nurs Res 56:226–234

DuBeau CE, Kuchel GA, Johnson T et al 2010 Incontinence in the frail elderly: report from the 4th International Consultation on Incontinence. Neurourol Urodynam 29:165–178

Dumoulin C, Hay-Smith J 2010 Pelvic floor muscle training versus no treatment, or inactive control treatments, for urinary incontinence in women. Cochrane Database Syst Rev 1:CD005654

Hannestad YS, Rortveit G, Sandvik H et al 2000 A community-based epidemiological survey of female urinary incontinence: the Norwegian EPINCONT study. J Clin Epidemiol 53:1150–1157

Hay-Smith J, Mørkved S, Fairbrother KA et al 2008 Pelvic floor muscle training for prevention and treatment of urinary and faecal incontinence in antenatal and postnatal women. Cochrane Database Syst Rev 4:CD007471

Heymen S, Scarlett Y, Jones K et al 2009 Randomized controlled trial shows biofeedback to be superior to pelvic floor exercises for fecal incontinence. Dis Colon Rectum 52:1730–1737

Komesu Y, Rogers R, Schrader R et al 2009 Incidence and remission of urinary incontinence in a community-based population of women ≥50 years. Int Urogynecol J 20:581–589

Leung FW, Rao SS 2009 Fecal incontinence in the elderly. Gastroenterol Clin North Am 38:503–511

Lewis SJ, Heato KW 1997 Stool form scale as a useful guide to intestinal transit time. Scand J Gastroenterol 32:920–924

Neumann PB, Grimmer KA, Deenadayalan Y 2006 Pelvic floor muscle training and adjunctive therapies for the treatment of stress urinary incontinence in women: a systematic review. BMC Women's Health 6:1–28

Norton C, Wee Whitehead, Gliss DZ et al 2010 Management of fecal incontinence in adults. Neurol Urodynam 29:199–206

Offermans M, Du Moulin M, Hamers J et al 2009 Prevalence of urinary incontinence and associated risk factors in nursing home residents: a systematic review. Neurourol Urodynam 28:288–294

Ouslander JG, Simmons S, Schnelle J et al 1996 Effects of prompted voiding on fecal continence among nursing home residents. J Am Geriatr Soc 44:424–428

Shah BJ, Chokhavatia S, Rose S 2012 Fecal incontinence in the elderly: FAQ. Am J Gastroenterol 107:1635–1646

Tariq SH 2004 Geriatric fecal incontinence. Clin Geriatr Med 20:571–587

Whitehead WE, Borrud L, Goode PS et al 2009 Fecal incontinence in US adults: epidemiology and risk factors. Gastroenterol 137:512–517

Chapter 56

Iatrogenesis in older adults

JOHN O. BARR • TIMOTHY L. KAUFFMAN

CHAPTER CONTENTS

OVERVIEW

Iatrogenesis is defined as any injury or illness that occurs as a result of medical care (Taber's Cyclopedic Medical Dictionary, 2013). An iatrogenic condition is a state of ill health or adverse effect caused by medical treatment; it usually results from a mistake made in diagnosis or treatment, and can also be the fault of any member of the healthcare team. The risk of iatrogenesis in individuals over the age of 65 is twice as high as that of a younger person (Gurwitz et al., 1994) and iatrogenic complications may be more severe in the elderly (Merck Manual, 2013). A sentinel report from the Institute of Medicine attributed most errors not to negligence or misconduct, but to system-related problems (Institute of Medicine, 1999).

From 2007 to 2009, 708 642 patient safety events were reported to have contributed to the deaths of 79 670 hospitalized Medicare beneficiaries in the United States of America (Healthgrades, 2011). Iatrogenic events have been estimated to affect 65% of nursing home residents annually and are likely to have negative impacts on older individuals residing in assisted living facilities as well (Mitty, 2010). Adverse drug reactions from prescription medications result from incorrect ordering and administration of dosages, and from polypharmacy in the elderly. Other problematic errors may be based on misreading test results, or on the ambiguous presentations of symptoms, a hallmark of aging (Lantz, 2002; Agency for Healthcare Research and Quality, 2004; Mitty, 2010). For 2011, 874 116 adverse event reports for drugs and therapeutic biologic products were received by the Food and Drug Administration, up from 370 240 reports in 2003 (FDA, 2012). It is estimated that 27% of adverse drug events in primary care and 42% in long-term care are preventable (American Geriatrics Society, 2012).

Hospitalization increases the risk for nosocomial infections, transfusion reactions, polypharmacy and immobility. Mobility is critical for well-being and quality of life in the elderly individual. Surgical and medical interventions may lead to complications because of anesthesia or fluid overload (Merck Manual, 2013). Older patients often arrive at hospital without medications or an appropriate list of prescribed drugs, meaning that scheduled doses may be missed for hours or days. Hospitalized older adults are especially at risk for 'cascade iatrogenesis', the development of multiple complications initiated by a seemingly innocuous initial event (Thomlow et al., 2009).

A host of factors augment the risk of the elderly suffering an iatrogenic condition. The presence of multiple chronic diseases increases the possibility that the treatment of one problem may have a negative impact on another. For example, the use of a nonsteroidal anti-inflammatory (NSAID) medication in the treatment of arthritis may exacerbate heart failure or chronic gastritis. Fragmentation of health delivery into many specialties may lead to changes being made in therapeutic interventions without adequate communication among caregivers.

A number of initiatives have been suggested to prevent iatrogenesis, especially in the frail elderly, including: use of case managers to coordinate services; judicious involvement of a geriatric interdisciplinary team for complex cases; consultation with a pharmacist; establishment of specific acute care units for the elderly; and preparation of advance directives, including designation of a proxy for medical decisions (Merck Manual, 2013). In an effort to promote safer healthcare, the Agency for Healthcare Research and Quality has published '20 Tips to Help Prevent Medical Errors', presented in Box 56.1. This fact sheet informs patients and their family members about practical steps that they can take to prevent medical errors, thus ensuring safer healthcare.

An array of both voluntary and mandatory adverse event reporting systems in countries around the world has been summarized, and guidelines for reporting and learning systems have been drafted by the World Alliance for Patient Safety (2005). Not meant to be punitive (which likely would inhibit reporting), these systems are intended to enhance patient safety by facilitating learning from healthcare system failures and by taking action to make corrective changes.

This chapter focuses on iatrogenesis related to adverse drug reactions and immobility, and offers suggestions for proactively preventing these conditions.

Box 56.1   *20 Tips to help prevent medical errors*

WHAT YOU CAN DO TO STAY SAFE

The best way you can help to prevent errors is to be an active member of your healthcare team. That means taking part in every decision about your healthcare. Research shows that patients who are more involved with their care tend to get better results.

Medicines

1. Make sure that all of your doctors* know about every medicine you are taking. This includes prescription and over-the-counter medicines and dietary supplements, such as vitamins and herbs.
2. Bring all of your medicines and supplements to your doctor visits. 'Brown bagging' your medicines can help you and your doctor talk about them and find out if there are any problems. It can also help your doctor keep your records up to date and help you get better quality care.
3. Make sure your doctor knows about any allergies and adverse reactions you have had to medicines. This can help you to avoid getting a medicine that could harm you.
4. When your doctor writes a prescription for you, make sure you can read it. If you cannot read your doctor's handwriting, your pharmacist might not be able to either.
5. Ask for information about your medicines in terms you can understand – both when your medicines are prescribed and when you get them:
   - What is the medicine for?
   - How am I supposed to take it and for how long?
   - What side-effects are likely? What do I do if they occur?
   - Is this medicine safe to take with other medicines or dietary supplements I am taking?
   - What food, drink, or activities should I avoid while taking this medicine?
6. When you pick up your medicine from the pharmacy, ask: Is this the medicine that my doctor prescribed?
7. If you have any questions about the directions on your medicine labels, ask. Medicine labels can be hard to understand. For example, ask if 'four times daily' means taking a dose every 6 hours around the clock or just during regular waking hours.
8. Ask your pharmacist for the best device to measure your liquid medicine. For example, many people use household teaspoons, which often do not hold a true teaspoon of liquid. Special devices, like marked syringes, help people measure the right dose.
9. Ask for written information about the side-effects your medicine could cause. If you know what might happen, you will be better prepared if it does or if something unexpected happens.

Hospital stays

10. If you are in a hospital, consider asking all healthcare workers who will touch you whether they have washed their hands. Hand washing can prevent the spread of infections in hospitals.
11. When you are being discharged from the hospital, ask your doctor to explain the treatment plan you will follow at home. This includes learning about your new medicines, making sure you know when to schedule follow-up appointments, and finding out when you can get back to your regular activities.
    It is important to know whether or not you should keep taking the medicines you were taking before your hospital stay. Getting clear instructions may help prevent an unexpected return trip to the hospital.

Surgery

12. If you are having surgery, make sure that you, your doctor and your surgeon all agree on exactly what will be done.
    Having surgery at the wrong site (for example, operating on the left knee instead of the right) is rare. But even once is too often. The good news is that wrong-site surgery is 100% percent preventable. Surgeons are expected to sign their initials directly on the site to be operated on before the surgery.
13. If you have a choice, choose a hospital where many patients have had the procedure or surgery you need. Research shows that patients tend to have better results when they are treated in hospitals that have a great deal of experience with their condition.

Other steps

14. Speak up if you have questions or concerns. You have a right to question anyone who is involved with your care.
15. Make sure that someone, such as your primary care doctor, coordinates your care. This is especially important if you have many health problems or are in the hospital.
16. Make sure that all your doctors have your important health information. Do not assume that everyone has all the information they need.
17. Ask a family member or friend to go to appointments with you. Even if you do not need help now, you might need it later.
18. Know that 'more' is not always better. It is a good idea to find out why a test or treatment is needed and how it can help you. You could be better off without it.
19. If you have a test, do not assume that no news is good news. Ask how and when you will get the results.
20. Learn about your condition and treatments by asking your doctor and nurse and by using other reliable sources. For example, treatment options based on the latest scientific evidence are available from the Effective Health Care website (www.effectivehealthcare.ahrq.gov/options). Ask your doctor if your treatment is based on the latest evidence.

*Note: the term 'doctor' refers to the person who helps you manage your healthcare.
Adapted with permission from 20 Tips to Help Prevent Medical Errors. Patient Fact Sheet. AHRQ Publication No. 11-0089, September 2011. Agency for Healthcare Research and Quality, Rockville, MD. http://www.ahrq.gov/consumer/20tips.htm.

ADVERSE DRUG REACTIONS

Polypharmacy is a complex multifactorial issue. Individuals aged 65 and over take 33–40% of all prescription medications in the US (Lantz, 2002) and more than 50% of the over-the-counter medicines. Approximately four out of five people in this age group take at least one drug daily (Beyth & Shorr, 2002). Zhan and associates (2001) reported that one out of five people aged 65 or older who lived in the community was taking at least one prescription drug that was inappropriate as determined by an expert panel. These researchers recommend that the following medications be avoided in the elderly: barbiturates, flurazepam, meprobamate, chlorpropamide, meperidine (pethidine), pentazocine, trimethobenzamide, belladonna alkaloids, dicyclomine, hyoscyamine and propantheline.

Age-related physiological changes affect the absorption, distribution, metabolism and elimination of drugs. Stomach changes, such as increased pH or altered motility, may reduce drug absorption. Decreases in total body water and lean body mass, as well as increases in total body fat, can alter drug distribution. Diminution of liver mass and blood flow may alter drug metabolism, and reductions in renal plasma flow and glomerular filtration rate (GFR) decrease drug elimination via the kidney (Beyth & Shorr, 2002).

A complication of type 2 diabetes mellitus is chronic renal failure. Corsonello et al. (2005) reported that chronic renal failure may be unrecognized or 'concealed' and may contribute to an adverse drug reaction (ADR). A standard method for determining renal failure is detection of elevated serum creatinine; however, in the elderly, it may be within the normal range because of the decreased GFR. Thus, renal failure may be 'concealed' and subsequently lead to an ADR, especially in patients using hydrosoluble drugs (sulfonylureas, metformin, digitalis, angiotensin-converting enzyme [ACE] inhibitors, insulin, diuretics, antibiotics such as penicillins and cephalosporins, and NSAIDs). In their study of 2257 hospitalized patients with type 2 diabetes mellitus, more than 16% had concealed renal failure and more than 10% of all patients had ADRs.

Individuals with dementia are especially vulnerable to ADRs because of an increased availability of protein-bound agents (because of loss of lean body mass, and reduced albumin) such as antidepressants and antipsychotics (American Geriatrics Society, 2012). Secondary parkinsonism is often caused by medications, including antipsychotics (Merck Manual, 2013). Tardive dyskinesia is a drug-induced movement disorder that is usually caused by antipsychotics such as haloperidol. It is characterized by abnormal involuntary movements involving the tongue and lips, e.g. chewing motions, and produces a feeling of motor restlessness and not wanting to stay still. As with all ADRs, a change of prescription drugs is helpful, if at all possible. Additionally, antipsychotics, as well as beta blockers, carbidopa–levodopa, diuretics and sedative–hypnotics (benzodiazepines), may cause sleep disturbances in elderly individuals.

In recent years, testosterone replacement has been used to treat secondary hypogonadism and the related male problems of sarcopenia and changes in libido, bone mass and visuospatial cognition. Calof et al. (2005) performed a meta-analysis of clinical trials to evaluate the risks of ADRs in men over the age of 45 who undergo testosterone replacement. They reported that this medical intervention was significantly associated with higher rates of prostate cancer, elevated prostate-specific antigen and prostate biopsies. Hematocrit was also elevated and warrants monitoring in men taking testosterone. There were no significant differences between the testosterone group and placebo group in the frequency of sleep apnea or cardiovascular events.

Quiceno and Cush (2005) have noted that medication-related iatrogenic events may masquerade as rheumatic disorders. Although rare, myopathic syndromes associated with the use of statins include myopathy, myalgia, myositis and rhabdomyolysis. Drugs that induce lupus include procainamide, hydralazine,

methyldopa, quinidine and chlorpromazine. Gout, most commonly produced by underexcretion of uric acid, is associated with ethanol use, diuretics, low-dose salicylate, cyclosporin (ciclosporin), ethambutol, pyrazinamide, levodopa and nicotinic acid. Arthralgias can be the result of anti-infectives (e.g. quinolones and vaccines), biological agents (e.g. interferons and growth factors), supplements (e.g. fluoride and vitamin A), lipid-lowering statins and fibrates, cardiac drugs (e.g. quinidine, propranolol, acetabulol, nicardipine) and hormonal agents (e.g. raloxifene, tamoxifen, letrozole).

The use of medications in the elderly is complex and is associated with iatrogenesis, as noted above. Antidepressant or analgesic medications have also been associated with falls in ambulatory frail elderly individuals (American Geriatrics Society, 2012). However, medications that carry risks of ADRs may also provide benefits. Won et al. (2006) reported that the use of short- or long-acting opioids in nursing home residents was not associated with an increased risk of falls, depression, constipation, delirium, dehydration or pneumonia. They found that the use of pain medications improved functional status and social engagement.

Actions that can be taken to limit drug-related iatrogenesis have been long known, as outlined by Stolley et al. (1991). These include educating patients and staff about drug effects and potential problems; carrying out a formal drug review by a gerontological nurse and pharmacist; and taking an accurate drug history, which includes a thorough assessment of drug allergies, possible drug borrowing and proper drug use by patients.

DECREASED MOBILITY AND DISUSE

Many physical, psychological, pathological and environmental factors can decrease mobility and encourage disuse in older individuals thus promoting further diminutions in cells, tissues and function. Box 56.2 summarizes common causes of decreased mobility in the elderly, some of which are iatrogenic and some are self-selected.

Bedrest may be necessary and beneficial during an illness, but it can also have negative consequences that complicate the return to independence. It may contribute to iatrogenic complications if activity is not resumed as soon as possible after a limiting event. During a prolonged period of decreased mobility, pathophysiological alterations may occur. In review articles involving young and aged adults Nigam et al. (2009) and Knight et al. (2009) reported that deleterious effects of bedrest were found in the musculoskeletal, cardiovascular, respiratory, hematological and integumentary systems. These alterations occur to varying degrees depending on the organ system, the previous level of fitness of the individual and the extent of remaining or permitted mobility. Bedrest-induced alterations can begin within the first 24 hours. A summary of the effects of prolonged bedrest is shown in Box 56.3.

There are challenges in understanding the consequences of bedrest in older individuals because they have diminished physiological reserves secondary to age-related changes and disease processes It is critical that healthcare professionals recognize the negative

Box 56.2 *Causes of decreased mobility in the elderly*

MUSCULOSKELETAL DISORDERS
- Arthritis
- Osteoporosis
- Fractures (especially femur)
- Podiatric problems (bunions, calluses)
- Pain

NEUROLOGICAL DISORDERS
- Stroke
- Parkinson's disease
- Alzheimer's disease

CARDIOVASCULAR DISEASE
- Congestive heart failure
- Coronary artery disease (frequent angina)
- Peripheral vascular disease (with frequent claudication)
- Pulmonary disease
- Chronic obstructive pulmonary disease

ENVIRONMENTAL CAUSES
- Forced immobility
- Inadequate aids for mobility (canes, walkers, appropriately placed railings)
- Being wheelchair-bound
- Stairs and other architectural barriers

OTHER
- Fear of falling
- Malnutrition
- Deconditioning
- Drug side-effects

Box 56.3 *Deleterious effects of prolonged bed rest or disuse*

MUSCULOSKELETAL
- Decreased range of motion
- Decreased joint flexibility
- Development of contractures
- Loss of muscular strength and endurance
- Decreased muscle protein synthesis
- Decreased exercise capacity
- Loss of bone density and strength

CARDIOVASCULAR AND RESPIRATORY
- Decreased ventilation
- Atelectasis
- Pneumonia
- Decreased inspiratory pressure and forced vital capacity
- Decreased cardiac output, stroke volume and peripheral vascular resistance
- Increased resting heart rate
- Increase of orthostatic hypotension

INTEGUMENTARY
- Development of pressure sores
- Skin atrophy
- Skin tears

URINARY AND GASTROINTESTINAL
- Urinary infection
- Urinary retention
- Bladder calculi
- Constipation
- Fecal impaction

NEUROLOGICAL
- Compression neuropathies
- Depression
- Perceptual ability
- Social isolation
- Learned helplessness
- Altered sleep patterns, anxiety, irritability, hostility

METABOLIC
- Negative nitrogen balance
- Loss of calcium
- Decreased insulin sensitivity
- Decreased aldosterone and plasma renin activity

Based on Knight et al., 2009; Nigam et al., 2009; Truong et al., 2009.

consequences of bedrest for the older individual. The return to independence of elderly individuals can be facilitated if all healthcare professionals understand the deleterious consequences of immobility, the relative time frame in which these consequences can develop and the potential value of therapeutic interventions.

The effects of 10 days of bedrest on functional abilities of healthy adults, mean age 67 years, were reported by Kortebein and associates (2008). Knee extensor isotonic strength, stair-climbing power and Vo_2 max were all significantly decreased. The Short Performance Physical Battery and a performance test (5 minute walk, 50-foot walk, 5-step test, functional reach and floor transfer) did not significantly decline. But after the cessation of bedrest, the percentage of inactive time significantly increased. The authors suggested this inactivity may have been due to fatigue, resulting from decreases in aerobic capacity, muscle strength and power. This is an important consideration when rehabilitating older patients after hospitalization especially because these subjects in this study were young–old, healthy community dwellers.

Gill et al. (2004) examined bedrest in community-dwelling individuals over an 18-month period who were at least 70 years old. Each month, the participants were asked if they had stayed in bed for at least half a day because of illness, injury or other problems. Nearly 60% of the nondisabled volunteers had at least one episode of bedrest, lasting an average of 2.8 months. Bedrest was significantly associated with declines in instrumental activities of daily living and social activity, with trends toward diminished physical activity and mobility also noted.

It is important to ascertain the basis for instituting bedrest. Rest is indeed important for individuals who complain of fatigue and tiredness. However, Avlund et al. (2003) determined that community-living individuals who were 'tired' during daily activities at an initial evaluation had greater mobility disability and participated less in strenuous activities at follow-up 18 months later. Gill et al. (2013) studied 284 community dwellers between the ages of 18 and 89 years and found agreement that physical activity was beneficial for physical health and emotional wellbeing. See Box 56.3 for the deleterious effects of bedrest and disuse.

CONCLUSION

Older individuals, especially the frail, are susceptible to the iatrogenic effects of ADRs and the degrading effects of bedrest and immobility. The onset of negative consequences from bedrest can occur within the first 24 hours and may affect the major organ systems and normal physiological functions. Additionally, decreased mobility or disuse caused by an ADR or hospitalization accentuates age-related changes that impair physiological reserve. Management depends on the healthcare provider's awareness of the effects of bedrest and the importance of rehabilitation. Mobility is a critical issue that pertains to all functions and the very quality of life. All members of the rehabilitation team need to be proactive in taking steps to prevent iatrogenesis in older adults and encourage physical activity in order to offset immobility/disuse associated declines.

REFERENCES

Agency for Healthcare Research and Quality 2004 Reducing Errors in Healthcare. Publication No. 00-PO58. Agency for Healthcare Research and Quality, Rockville, MD

Agency for Healthcare Research and Quality 2011 20 Tips to Help Prevent Medical Errors: Patient Fact Sheet. [Online] Available at: www.ahrq.gov/consumer/20tips.htm. Accessed December 2013

American Geriatrics Society 2012 Updated Beers criteria for potentially inappropriate medication use in older adults. J Am Geriatr Soc 60:616–631

Avlund K, Vass M, Hendriksen C 2003 Onset of mobility disability among community-dwelling old men and women: the role of tiredness in daily activities. Age Ageing 32:579–584

Beyth R, Shorr R 2002 Principles of drug therapy in older patients: rational drug prescribing. Clin Geriatr Med 18:577–592

Calof O, Singh A, Lee M et al 2005 Adverse events associated with testosterone replacement in middle-aged and older men: a meta-analysis of randomized, placebo-controlled trials. J Gerontol A Biol Sci Med Sci 60:1451–1457

Corsonello A, Pedone C, Corica F et al 2005 Concealed renal failure and adverse drug reactions in older patients with type 2 diabetes mellitus. J Gerontol A Biol Sci Med Sci 60:1147–1151

Food and Drug Administration 2012 reports received and reports entered into FAERS by year. [Online] Available at: fda.gov/Drugs/GuidanceComplianceRegulatoryInformation/Surveillance/AdverseDrugEffects/ucm070434.htm. Accessed December 2013

Gill DL, Hammond CC, Reifsteck E et al 2013 Physical activity and quality of life. J Prev Med Public Health 46(Suppl 1):S28–S34

Gill TM, Allore H, Guo Z 2004 The deleterious effects of bed rest among community-living older persons. J Gerontol A Biol Sci Med Sci 59:755–761

Gurwitz JH, Sanchez-Cross MT, Eckler MA et al 1994 The epidemiology of adverse and unexpected events in the long-term care setting. J Am Geriatr Soc 42:33–38

Healthgrades 2011 Patient Safety in American Hospitals Study. Healthgrades, Chicago, IL. Available at: www.cpmhealthgrades.com/CPM/assets/File/HealthGradesPatientSafetyInAmericanHospitalsStudy2011.pdf. Accessed December 2013

Institute of Medicine 1999 To Err is Human: Building a Safer Health System. National Academy Press, Washington, DC

Knight J, Nigam Y, Jones A 2009 Effects of bedrest 1: cardiovascular, respiratory and haematological systems. Nurs Times 105(2):16–20

Kortebein P, Symons T, Ferrando A et al 2008 Functional impact of 10 days of bed rest in health older adults. J Gerontol A Biol Sci Med Sci 63:1076–1081

Lantz M 2002 Problems with polypharmacy. Clin Geriatr 10:18–20

Merck Manual 2013 The Merck Manual for Health Care Professionals: Geriatrics: Prevention of iatrogenic complications in the elderly. [Online] Available at: www.merckmanuals.com/professional/geriatrics.html. Accessed December 2013

Mitty E 2010 Iatrogenesis, frailty, and geriatric syndromes. Geriatr Nurs 31(5):368–374

Nigam Y, Knight J, Jones A 2009 Effects of bedrest 3: musculoskeletal and immune systems, skin and self-perception. Nurs Times.net 105:23

Quiceno GA, Cush JJ 2005 Iatrogenic rheumatic syndromes in the elderly. Clin Geriatr Med 21:577–588

Stolley JM, Buckwalter KC, Fjordbak B et al 1991 Iatrogenesis in the elderly: drug-related problems. J Gerontol Nurs 17(9):12–17

Taber's Cyclopedic Medical Dictionary 2013 Twenty-second edition. FA Davis, Philadelphia, PA

Thomlow DK, Anderson R, Oddone E 2009 Cascade iatrogenesis: factors leading to the development of adverse events in hospitalized older adults. Int J Nurs Stud 46(11):1528–1535

Truong A, Fan E, Brower R et al 2009 Bench-to-bedside review: mobilizing patients in the intensive care unit: from pathophysiology to clinical trials. Crit Care 13:216

Won A, Lapane K, Vallow S et al 2006 Long-term effects of analgesics in a population of elderly nursing home residents with persistent nonmalignant pain. J Gerontol A Biol Sci Med Sci 61:165–169

World Alliance for Patient Safety 2005 WHO draft guidelines for adverse event reporting and learning systems: from information to action. Available at: www.who.int/patientsafety/events/05/Reporting_Guidelines.pdf. Accessed December 2013

Zhan C, Sangl J, Bierman AS et al 2001 Potentially inappropriate medication use in the community-dwelling elderly. Findings from the 1996 Medical Expenditure Panel Survey. JAMA 286(22):2823–2829

Chapter 57

Hormone replacement therapy

CHRISTINE STABLER

Chapter Contents

INTRODUCTION

Hormone therapy has been riding the roller coaster of public opinion since 1966 when Robert Wilson published *Feminine Forever* (Wilson, 1966). Touted as the fountain of youth, estrogen used in uncontrolled amounts was thought to revitalize and rejuvenate menopausal women. The tidal wave of interest in estrogen replacement therapy came to an abrupt halt 12–15 years later after the publication of an article that provided the first clinical evidence that estrogen therapy may increase a woman's risk of endometrial cancer (Mack et al., 1976).

Estrogen regained some of its luster 10 years later, with the support of clinical data that demonstrated its efficacy and safety when used in a combined regimen with progesterone. Retrospective analyses demonstrated the protective effects of hormone therapy on the development of osteoporosis, heart disease, Alzheimer's disease and, potentially, colon cancer. These results strengthened support for hormone therapy among clinicians and patients alike (McMichael & Potter, 1980; Colditz et al., 1987). However, this short-lived respite once again came to a grinding halt in July 2002 when the National Heart, Lung and Blood Institute of the National Institutes of Health (NIH) released the unblinded first arm of the first prospective study into the effects of hormone replacement therapy on post-menopausal women (Petitti, 2002).

RESULTS OF THE WOMEN'S HEALTH INITIATIVE

The Women's Health Initiative (WHI) studied almost 50 000 women receiving hormone replacement therapy after menopause. The women were divided into two groups: those with an intact uterus receiving a combination of estrogen and progesterone and those, post hysterectomy, receiving estrogen alone. The estrogen and progesterone arm was stopped in July 2002 because the apparent risks of hormone replacement therapy outweighed any evident benefits. The estrogen-only arm of the study continued for another 2 years before it, too, was prematurely discontinued: it failed to show the protective cardiovascular benefit that the study was designed to demonstrate. In total, 7 of the 8 projected years of the study had elapsed and, although with estrogen alone there was no increase in the risk of breast cancer, a significant increase in the risk of heart disease, blood clots and stroke became evident for women receiving hormone replacement therapy (Anderson & Limacher, 2004). This information was a wake-up call to physicians to carefully analyze what women need in the menopausal years to maintain health and reduce risk.

The WHI was designed to look at the effects of hormone replacement therapy on the risks of breast cancer, heart disease, stroke, blood clotting, osteoporosis and fractures, and colorectal cancers. It did not initially assess the symptoms of menopause, including hot flashes, insomnia, mood changes and genital dryness and atrophy. However, further analysis looked at menopausal quality of life and found that, although women receiving hormone replacement therapy had significant improvements in sleep, physical functioning, body pain, hot flashes and mood swings, overall, there was no significant difference in sexual wellbeing, mental health or vitality. What the study did show was an increased risk of breast cancer that began after 4 years of clinical use and that raised the relative risk by almost 25% in women receiving estrogen plus progesterone. This extrapolated to eight additional breast cancers per year per 10 000 women receiving hormone replacement therapy. In the women receiving estrogen alone, no such increased risk was evident. Concurrent studies published in the *Journal of the American Medical Association* reported that breast cancers that developed after hormone replacement therapy were more aggressive and larger than other breast cancers, and that women with a previous history of breast cancer had a higher rate of recurrence when receiving hormone therapy (Anderson & Limacher, 2004).

Heart disease was also a major factor in the discontinuation of the WHI (Anderson & Limacher, 2004). An increased risk of heart disease was noted in the first year of the study and the relative risk for the development of heart disease rose by 29%, extrapolating to seven more heart attacks per 10000 women using hormone replacement therapy each year. This seemed to hold true for both women receiving estrogen alone and women receiving estrogen and progesterone in combination. Multiple etiologies for these phenomena have been postulated, including an increase in the levels of C-reactive protein and insulin-like growth factor in women receiving oral estrogen. However, this has yet to be proven definitively (Ridker et al., 2003).

The study also found an increased risk of stroke, with an increased relative risk of 41%, which extrapolated to eight more cerebrovascular accidents per 10000 women taking hormone replacement therapy per year. This risk seemed to hold true for all age groups, regardless of any baseline stroke risk such as hypertension, diabetes, previous coronary disease or use of aspirin or lipid-lowering drugs. For women less than 60 years of age, the absolute risk of stroke from standard-dose hormone therapy is rare, about two additional strokes per 10000 person-years of use; the absolute risk is considerably greater for older women (Henderson & Lobo, 2012). A similar and parallel risk was demonstrated for the development of other blood clots: there were approximately 18 more clots per 10000 women per year. The risk for the development of blood clots was greatest in the first 2 years of therapy and decreased, but was still elevated even after 4 years of use.

The Women's Health Initiative Memory Study (WHIMS) was published in May 2003 (Hays et al., 2003) and, contrary to previous beliefs supported by the Nurses Health Study, which identified hormone replacement therapy as a major prevention strategy for dementia, demonstrated an increase in dementia among women using hormone replacement therapy over the age of 65. There were an additional 23 cases of dementia per 10000 women, with no statistical difference in risk regardless of socioeconomic status, educational attainment or use of aspirin. In addition, no protection was afforded for mild cognitive impairment, a less severe form of dementia (Shumaker et al., 1998). Subsequent analyses seem to infer a protective effect for younger women initiating therapy at the onset of menopause (Ryan et al., 2008).

There was some good news in the WHI: osteoporotic fracture risk was reduced by 34%, resulting in five fewer fractures per 10000 women per year. This was the first trial to document a decreased risk of fractures with hormone replacement therapy and not just an improvement in bone density (WHI, 2006). A similar reduction in the risk of colon cancer was demonstrated; after 3 years of hormone replacement therapy, the relative risk of the development of colon cancer was reduced by 37%, resulting in six fewer cancers per 10000 women per year.

LIMITATIONS OF THE WOMEN'S HEALTH INITIATIVE

There were some significant limitations to the WHI that may make interpretation of the data difficult. This was a short study; however, breast cancer, colon cancer, osteoporosis and heart disease may take many years to develop. The average age of new participants in the study was 63 years, and many of these women had spent more than 10 years in menopause before beginning hormone replacement therapy.

Subclinical coronary disease, as well as subclinical breast cancer, may have been present before the initiation of therapy, meaning that some so-called healthy participants were, in fact, more ill than the general population. In addition, women with a high risk of developing the symptoms of menopause, such as hot flashes or osteoporosis, were excluded from the study, resulting in an eligibility bias against benefit. Finally, only one in four of the experimental group was actually taking their hormone replacement therapy at the end of the fifth year of study. These limitations make data interpretation a challenge. Newer subgroup analyses indicate that the use of HRT in healthy women at the onset of menopause may confer even more benefit, with significantly less risk than identified in the WHI (Marjoribanks et al., 2012).

ALTERNATIVE MANAGEMENT OF MENOPAUSE

No other menopausal treatment or regimen has undergone this degree of scrutiny. The assumption that alternative treatments for menopause and their effects are safe is unwise (North American Menopause Society, 2004). We are therefore faced with an aging population of women who are living more of their life in menopause, and a population of patients who are more educated and more consumer-savvy about healthcare. It is up to clinicians to educate themselves about the management of menopause, to talk to patients and allow them to contribute to decision-making with regard to menopausal therapies and to continually reassess the risk of adverse outcomes for patients over their lifetime (Moyer, 2012).

The WHI has provided physicians with a unique opportunity to join with patients to create a designer approach to their menopause management. No two women have the same experiences, risks and needs. The goal of this partnership is to create a fluid approach that continually evaluates risks, symptoms and comorbidities and addresses the specific needs of women as they enter menopause. Special attention must be given to the prevention of heart disease, osteoporosis, memory loss and sexual dysfunction and the development of menopausal symptoms (Moyer, 2012).

The modification of heart disease risk requires lifestyle changes. Risk can be reduced by dietary reduction of saturated fats, exercise, smoking cessation, assumption of ideal body weight and reduction of alcohol consumption. Preexisting conditions such as hypertension, diabetes and hyperlipidemia should be optimally controlled to prevent the development of heart disease. The recognition of the gender differences between men and women in the presentation of heart disease is essential for optimal risk reduction (Mosca et al., 2011).

The prevention of osteoporosis goes beyond hormone replacement therapy. Lifestyle changes such as increasing exercise, smoking cessation, maintenance of an ideal body weight and adequate calcium and vitamin D intake will help to prevent osteoporosis. Other therapeutic devices, such as selective estrogen receptor modulators (SERMs) that mimic the effects of estrogen in bone without affecting the cardiovascular system or breasts, have been proven to prevent osteoporosis. Bisphosphonates have been shown to build damaged bone. Calcitonin, approved since the 1980s in the United States of America, has recently had reports of increased risks of cancer and the efficacy for fracture reduction has not been clearly established. Thus, the European Medicines Agency and others recommend that calcitonin not be used for osteoporosis and fracture prevention (Overman et al., 2013). Unfortunately, natural estrogen analogs have not been found to be as helpful in osteoporosis prevention.

The reduction of menopausal symptoms relies on lifestyle changes such as limiting alcohol and caffeine intake and stress reduction; the wearing of light clothing may also be helpful. Soy supplementation has been shown to reduce mild hot flashes when six to eight servings are taken per day. Selective serotonin reuptake inhibitors (SSRIs), a type of antidepressant, offer moderate relief for women with menopausal symptoms. Estrogen remains the only proven treatment for severe hot flashes and the NIH now recommend short-term use at the lowest effective dose as the ideal treatment for the vasomotor symptoms of menopause (Marjoribanks et al., 2012).

Urogenital atrophy (vaginal dryness) can be treated with lubricants and feminine moisture replacements. The topical use of estrogen in small doses at infrequent intervals is helpful and may limit systemic exposure and therefore risk. Newer delivery systems, such as the vaginal ring with estrogen, have also proven to be quite successful in the reduction of symptomatology.

The WHIMS demonstrated no benefit of hormone replacement therapy in the prevention of Alzheimer's disease in older women. The improvement of memory as women enter menopause relies upon an active lifestyle and the early recognition and treatment of depression and other forms of pseudodementia that may mimic Alzheimer's dementia (Shumaker et al., 1998).

CONCLUSION

Life after the WHI is more complex for physicians and healthcare providers who care for women as they enter menopause. The designer approach to the management of menopause will require education of the clinician, the continued and ongoing risk assessment of the patient, patient participation and the judicious use of lifestyle changes, nonpharmacological interventions, pharmacological treatments and hormone replacement therapy.

REFERENCES

Anderson G, Limacher M 2004 The Women's Health Initiative Randomized Control Trial. JAMA 291(14):1701–1712

Colditz GA, Willett WC, Stampfer MJ 1987 Menopause and the risk of coronary heart disease in women. N Engl J Med 316:1105–1110

Hays J, Ockene J, Brunner R et al 2003 Effects of estrogen plus progestin on health related quality of life. N Engl J Med 348(19):1839–1854

Henderson VW, Lobo RA 2012 Hormone therapy and the risk of stroke: perspectives 10 years after the Women's Health Initiative trials. Climacteric 15(3):229–234

Mack TM, Pike MC, Henderson BE et al 1976 Estrogens and endometrial cancer in a retirement community. N Engl J Med 296:1262–1267

McMichael AJ, Potter JD 1980 Reproduction, endogenous and exogenous sex hormones, and colon cancer: a review and hypothesis. J Natl Cancer Inst 65:1201–1207

Marjoribanks J, Farquhar C, Roberts H et al 2012 Long term hormone therapy for perimenopausal and postmenopausal women. Cochrane Database Syst Rev 7:CD004143

Mosca L, Benjamin EJ, Berra K et al 2011 Effectiveness-based guidelines for the prevention of cardiovascular disease in women – 2011 update: a guideline from the American Heart Association. Circulation 2011 123(11):1243

Moyer VA, on behalf of the US Preventive Services Task Force 2012 Menopausal hormone therapy for the primary prevention of chronic conditions: US Preventive Services Task Force Recommendation Statement. Ann Intern Med 158(1):1–34

North American Menopause Society 2004 Treatment of menopause-associated vasomotor symptoms. Position statement of the North American Menopause Society. Menopause 11:11–33

Overman R, Borse M, Gourlay M 2013 Salmon calcitonin use and associated cancer risk. Ann Pharmacother 47:1675–1684

Petitti DB 2002 Hormone replacement therapy for prevention; more evidence, more pessimism. JAMA 288:99–101

Ridker P, Buring J, Cook N et al 2003 C-reactive protein, the metabolic syndrome, and risk of incident cardiovascular events. Circulation 107:391–397

Ryan J, Scali J, Carriere I et al 2008 Hormonal treatment, mild cognitive impairment and Alzheimer's disease. Int Psychogeriatr 20:47–56

Shumaker SA, Reboussin BA, Espeland MA et al 1998 The Women's Health Initiative Memory Study (WHIMS): a trial of the effect of estrogen therapy in preventing and slowing the progression of dementia. Control Clin Trial 19:604–621

WHI (Women's Health Initiative) 2006 Findings from the WHI Postmenopausal Hormone Therapy Trials. Available at: www.nhlbi.nih.gov/whi/. Accessed March 2006

Wilson RA 1966 Feminine Forever. M. Evans, New York

Chapter 58

Dizziness

SUSAN L. WHITNEY

CHAPTER CONTENTS

INTRODUCTION

Dizziness is a frequently occurring disorder of older individuals that can result in serious functional deficits. Dizziness negatively affects quality of life (White et al., 2005). Older adults often visit their physicians with nonspecific complaints of dizziness; it is the most common complaint of adults over the age of 75 and the third most common complaint in outpatient settings, regardless of age (Kroenke et al., 1992). In a recent national health survey, 35% of persons over the age of 40 reported vestibular dysfunction (Agrawal et al., 2009). People who reported dizziness were 12 times more likely to have reported a fall (Agrawal et al., 2009). As dizziness is a subjective experience, it is difficult to determine whether the patient and the examiner agree on what the symptoms are. The most common new onset cause of dizziness is a change in medication in older persons.

PRESENTATION AND DIAGNOSIS

Dizziness is interpreted differently by various people and is often difficult to describe. Commonly, people complain of a sense of giddiness, floating, lightheadedness or a sensation of being drunk. Table 58.1 includes other common descriptors used by patients to explain their complaints to their practitioners.

Some patients who experience dizziness have nystagmus, which is involuntary rhythmic oscillation of the eyes in either the lateral, superior/inferior direction, often accompanied by a torsional component. The nystagmus usually manifests with a fast and a slow component to the eye movements in opposite directions.

Patients also describe symptoms of vertigo, which is classically defined as an illusion of movement that usually has a rotatory component (Furman et al., 2010). People who experience vertigo often have a sensation of turning. Vertigo has been described as rotational, as translational and as a sense of being tilted. It does not matter whether the patient or their world is spinning, as both are considered to be vertigo. The sensation of vertigo usually indicates an inner ear problem, although occasionally it can be related to an anterior inferior or posterior inferior cerebellar stroke.

Most patients who experience dizziness or vertigo modify their activity levels even when they are not having symptoms. Fear of falling is often associated with the symptoms of dizziness or imbalance in elderly people (Bronstein & Lempert, 2010). They become noticeably less active over time because of the fear of experiencing dizziness or imbalance, especially in unfamiliar environments. This fear leads to inactivity, which can start a downward decline in function. Falls have been related to the most common cause of dizziness, which is benign paroxysmal positional vertigo (BPPV) (Katsarkas, 1999). BPPV can cause people to fall and BPPV may also be caused by a fall (Katsarkas, 1999). The otoconia within the otolith organs can become dislodged with head trauma (Katsarkas, 1999).

Several other disease processes or conditions have been associated with BPPV, including diabetes, migraine, Menière's disease and post viral infection. It is also suspected that BPPV may be caused by damage over time to the otolith production area. Benign paroxysmal positional vertigo runs in families (Gizzi et al., 1998) and has a recurrence rate of approximately 15% per year, increasing to a 40–50% chance of recurrence 3–4 years after the initial episode (Nunez et al., 2000). The spinning is often brought on by a change of head position, most commonly in moving from supine to sitting first thing in the morning or rolling over in bed at night (Whitney et al., 2005). Epley or Semont maneuvers are commonly used to move the otoconia out of the semicircular canal and back into the otolith organ (Epley, 1980, 1992; Semont et al., 1988; Hillier & McDonnell, 2011a; Chen et al., 2012;) There is recent evidence that by moving the otoconia out of the semicircular canal one can decrease the risk of falling (Gananca et al., 2010). Treatment of BPPV has been shown to be highly effective in older persons. Both the Epley and the Semont maneuvers are equally effective at causing the vertigo associated with a change of head position to stop. Two recent practice guidelines

Table 58.1 Common complaints of persons experiencing dizziness

Chief Complaint	Assessed During the History	Assessed During the Physical Exam
Head alignment abnormalities		x
Difficulty controlling their center of mass within their base of support	x	x
Difficulty orienting their bodies to vertical	x	x
Problems with selecting the most appropriate sensory strategies information to make decisions		x
Eye movement abnormalities	x	x
Abnormal motion perception	x	x
Physical deconditioning	x	x
Gait abnormalities	x	x
Swimming sensation in the head	x	x
Imbalance	x	x
Blurred vision	x	x
Tinnitus	x	Sometimes
Aural fullness	x	Sometimes
Hearing loss	x	x
Oscillopsia (an illusory movement of the visual world that occurs with high-frequency head movement)	x	x
Confusion, especially in rich sensory environments	x	
Lightheadedness	x	x
Anxiety	x	Sometimes
Headache	x	
Fatigue	x	x
Falling	x	Sometimes
Clumsiness	x	Sometimes
Fear of falling	x	
Neck pain	x	x

Table 58.2 Common causes of dizziness

Peripheral vestibular disorders	Benign paroxysmal positional vertigo (BPPV)[a]
	Menière's disease
	Endolymphatic hydrops
	Perilymph fistula
	Vestibular neuritis
	Labyrinthitis
	Bilateral vestibulopathy
Central disorders	Cervical vertigo
	Vestibular ocular dysfunction
	Traumatic head injury
	Anterior or posterior inferior cerebellar stroke
	Posttraumatic anxiety symptoms
	Transient ischemic attacks
	Migraines
	Multiple sclerosis
Psychiatric disorders	Panic disorders
	Agoraphobia
	Hyperventilation syndrome
Others	Low blood pressure
	Medication
	Presyncope
	Arrhythmias
	Vertebral artery trauma
	Alternobaric vertigo
	Diabetes mellitus
	Thyroid dysfunction
	Renal disease
	Human immunodeficiency virus
	Syphilitic labyrinthitis
	Epstein–Barr virus
	Brain stem hemorrhage
	Friedreich's ataxia
	Recent diplopia

[a]BPPV is the most common vestibular diagnosis in older persons.

suggest that BPPV is very common in older people but can be 'fixed' with the repositioning maneuvers (Bhattacharyya et al., 2008; Fife et al., 2008). BPPV has been associated with being older, with diabetes and with falling (Bhattacharyya et al., 2008).

There are numerous possible causes of dizziness, as noted in Table 58.2, rendering it impossible to determine the cause without testing. Laboratory and clinical tests that are performed in the attempt to diagnose the cause of the dizziness are included in Table 58.3. Although thorough testing is crucial to obtain an accurate diagnosis, most physical therapists will not have the benefit of such an extensive workup before seeing

a patient. By being aware of the various causes of and tests for dizziness, the physical therapist is more likely to make appropriate clinical decisions about referrals and care. The head thrust or head impulse test is a particularly useful tool for us in the clinical diagnosis of peripheral vestibular disorders (Halmagyi & Curthoys, 1988). One moves the head quickly to both the right or the left, and if the eyes cannot stay focused on a distant

Table 58.3 **Common testing provided to older persons who experience chronic dizziness**

	Tests Commonly Performed by	
	Physician	Physical Therapist
Caloric testing	x	
Rotational testing: assesses the vestibulo-ocular reflex independent of vision and can assess the visual/vestibular interaction	x	
Oculomotor testing: smooth pursuit movements, saccades	x	x
Dynamic visual acuity	x	x
Subjective visual vertical	x	x
Head thrust (impulse) test	x	x
Vestibular evoked myogenic potentials (VEMPs)	x	
Neurological examination	x	x
Optokinetic screening	x	x
Electronystagmography: a test for vestibulo-ocular asymmetry and includes caloric testing, positional testing, and ocular motor function	x	
Audiogram	x	
Electrocochleography	x	
MRI or CT scan	x	
Brain stem auditory evoked potential	x	
Visual evoked potential	x	
Posturography	x	x
Standing and lying blood pressure measures	x	x
Hallpike maneuver	x	x
Fistula test	x	
Romberg/tandem Romberg test	x	x
Electrocardiogram	x	
Holter monitoring	x	
Cervical spine X-rays	x	
Testing for positional nystagmus with Frenzel glasses	x	x
Biochemical metabolic evaluation	x	
Glucose tolerance test	x	
Electroencephalogram	x	

target throughout the rapid head movement, it suggests that the person has a peripheral vestibular disorder (Halmagyi & Curthoys, 1988). If the person exhibits a skew deviation, direction-changing nystagmus in eccentric gaze and a normal head thrust test, there is a 100% sensitivity and 96% specificity for the identification of stroke (Kattah et al., 2009).

DIZZINESS HISTORY

A complete history of a patient's dizziness is essential so that the physical therapist can develop the best individualized exercise program. Some of the common questions that should be asked concern the characteristics of the dizziness, how long the patient has had the symptoms, how the first incident would be described, what makes the symptoms worse or better, any associated otological or neurological symptoms, and the frequency of the incidents or attacks (Whitney & Sparto, 2011). A thorough history of past and present functional activities is also important. Specific activities of daily living (ADLs) may exacerbate the symptoms. This functional history is helpful in designing a treatment program based on symptoms. The Dizziness Handicap Inventory (DHI) (Jacobson & Newman, 1990) provides a numerical score that ranges from 0 to 100 to specify how handicapped the patient perceives himself or herself to be because of the dizziness (see Form 58.1). A 'yes' answer scores 4; 'sometimes' scores 2; and 'no' is 0. The higher the total score, the greater the dizziness handicap. The DHI has also been used to document a patient's self-rating of improvement or lack of progress. High DHI scores (>60) have been related to reported falls in persons with vestibular disorders (Whitney et al., 2004).

The patient with a chief complaint of dizziness will often receive an antidizziness medication, which can decrease the ability of the central nervous system (CNS) to compensate (Peppard, 1986). Most antidizziness medications are depressants of the CNS and may limit the ability of the CNS to adapt to change caused by an insult to or dysfunction in the balance mechanism, or to respond to physical therapy intervention. It is best to provide physical therapy when the patient is on a low dose of vestibular suppressants or none at all. Medication use to suppress dizziness may even slow the process of rehabilitation (Bamiou et al., 2000). Some patients are unable to function without a vestibular suppressant, so removal of vestibular suppressant medication may not be possible.

FUNCTIONAL DEFICITS

Dizziness can severely limit a patient's ability to perform ADLs (Cohen et al., 1995a, 1995b). Each person's dizziness is unique, but common complaints include having difficulty with transitional movements (e.g. rolling, moving from a supine position to sitting, bending over, moving from sitting to standing, and walking while making certain head movements) and with moving quickly. Even standing while moving the head can increase symptoms in some patients. Walking while making head movements is often the most difficult

Name: _____   Date: _____

Instructions: The purpose of this scale is to identify difficulties that you may be experiencing because of your dizziness. Please answer 'yes', 'no' or 'sometimes' to each question. Answer each question as it pertains to your dizziness problem only (Scoring: yes = 4; sometimes = 2; no = 0).

1. Does looking up increase your problem?   _____

2. Do you feel frustrated because of your problem?   _____

3. Do you restrict your travel for business or recreation because of your problem?   _____

4. Does walking down the aisle of a supermarket increase your problem?   _____

5. Do you have difficulty getting into or out of bed because of your problem?   _____

6. Does your problem significantly restrict your participation in social activities such as going out to dinner, going to the movies, dancing or going to parties?   _____

7. Do you have difficulty reading because of your problem?   _____

8. Does performing more ambitious activities like sports, dancing or household chores, such as sweeping or putting dishes away, increase your problem?   _____

9. Because of your problem are you afraid to leave your home without having someone to accompany you?   _____

10. Have you been embarrassed in front of others because of your problem?   _____

11. Do quick movements of your head increase your problem?   _____

12. Do you avoid heights because of your problem?   _____

13. Does turning over in bed increase your problem?   _____

14. Is it difficult for you to do strenuous housework or yard work because of your problem?   _____

15. Are you afraid people may think that you are intoxicated because of your problem?   _____

16. Is it difficult for you to go for a walk by yourself because of your problem?   _____

17. Does walking down a sidewalk increase your problem?   _____

18. Is it difficult for you to concentrate because of your problem?   _____

19. Is it difficult for you to walk around your house in the dark because of your problem?   _____

20. Are you afraid to stay home alone because of your problem?   _____

21. Do you feel handicapped because of your problem?   _____

22. Has your problem placed stress on your relationship with friends or members of your family?   _____

23. Are you depressed because of your problem?   _____

24. Does your problem interfere with your job or household responsibilities?   _____

25. Does bending over increase your problem?   _____

[a]From Jacobson and Newman, 1990, with permission from American Medical Association.

Form 58.1 Dizziness Handicap Inventory (DHI)[a]

activity because the patient is unstable and may feel unsafe.

Often patients complain of having difficulty when movement is perceived within their peripheral vision, or when watching television or reading. A patient may have dizziness when driving or when a passenger in a car. Clinically, it is noted that patients report less dizziness when they themselves are driving. For some older adults, losing the ability to drive can cause significant psychosocial dilemmas.

One characteristic symptom of patients with dizziness is having difficulty walking down the aisle of a grocery or department store because of the input from the person's peripheral vision (Sparto et al., 2004). High contrast colors and shapes in the older person's peripheral vision can cause them to become dizzy. The optic flow as one ambulates can be disorienting and can contribute to increased dizziness, nausea and headaches; thus, people with severe dizziness often limit the amount of time they spend out of the home. Indeed, dizziness has been associated with agoraphobia (fear of leaving one's home) and depression (Jacob et al., 1996). Dizziness is a problem that can limit function even when the dizziness is not present, for the fear of becoming dizzy in a stressful situation is often enough for some people to limit their activities.

Not all patients with dizziness are easily treated. Patients with unilateral vestibular dysfunction often do the best with exercise programs. Hillier and McDonnell suggest that there is moderate to strong evidence that vestibular exercises are 'safe and effective when used with patients with vestibular hypofunction' (Hillier & McDonnell, 2011a). Patients with central vestibular dysfunction have more difficulty with exercise because of CNS involvement, and those with fluctuating symptoms are difficult to treat since they do not have consistent symptoms. Some of the fluctuating disorders, such as Menière's disease and perilymphatic fistulas, may have to be surgically repaired. Dizziness may be decreased or eliminated through surgery, yet some patients continue to experience tinnitus. Tinnitus may be a disabling symptom and has been described as a dull roar or loud noise in the ear. Dizziness can be associated with multiple sclerosis and stroke. In these patients, dizziness can lessen but may not completely resolve as a result of rehabilitation.

People with dizziness often have difficulty explaining their symptoms to family members because there are no externally obvious signs of the disorder. Family members can find it hard to comprehend the physical and psychological effects of dizziness and sometimes cannot understand that the patient may be severely disabled by the condition.

THERAPEUTIC INTERVENTION

Not all older patients with dizziness have balance disorders. There appear to be three categories: those with dizziness, those with balance disorders and those with balance disorders and dizziness. Each of these symptom categories should be treated differently. The treatment program should be based on the functional deficits of the patient.

During the assessment of dizziness, it is important to determine if patients have fallen, and if so, how often, and whether they have had to seek medical intervention for the fall. Finding oneself suddenly and unexpectedly on a lower surface, usually the floor, is often defined as a 'fall'. Frequent falls (more than two within the past 6 months when no environmental hazards were present) are reason for significant concern. These individuals should be treated more frequently in the clinic and should be monitored closely at home by a family member. The patients who fall frequently might benefit from some type of alarm device to notify emergency personnel when a fall occurs.

EXERCISE

In an exercise program for vestibular dysfunction, the patient is asked to perform movements that increase symptoms of dizziness or of being off-balance. The objective is to either challenge their balance or let the patient feel dizzy in a safe environment. How quickly to advance a program is difficult to determine because if the exercises designed to stimulate their dizziness are progressed too rapidly, the patient might get worse, discontinue the exercises and not return for future therapy. A combination of easier and more difficult exercises is often best so that the patient will be successful with at least a few of the exercises. Keeping the number of exercises under five at each visit also helps with compliance.

When designing an exercise program, it is usually important to warn the patient that they will initially and temporarily feel worse because of the exercises. If the patient remains severely dizzy for longer than 20 minutes after the exercises have been completed, the exercises were too difficult and must be modified in terms of intensity or number (Whitney & Sparto, 2011).

It is extremely important to get the patient to progress as quickly as possible while in a safe place so that confidence can be restored. Functional retraining, muscle strengthening, eye and head exercises, and having the patient attempt to perform difficult tasks are components of an individualized exercise program for a patient with vestibular dysfunction (Box 58.1). Dual tasking (walking and thinking) should also be implemented as the patient improves (Redfern et al., 2004; Roberts et al., 2011; Bessot et al., 2012). Often a combination of balance and eye exercises are provided simultaneously with the exercises started in 'safe' positions for the older adult, progressing to situations where their balance is challenged while standing, walking, or even reaching while standing.

Older adults most likely to benefit from a vestibular rehabilitation program include those with unilateral vestibular hypofunction (peripheral vestibular disorders) and those with bilateral peripheral vestibular disorders (Hillier & McDonnell, 2011b). Other patients helped by physical therapy include those with head trauma, cerebellar atrophy or dysfunction, cerebellar stroke and multiple sclerosis. Patients who have been diagnosed with bilateral disorders may continue to improve with physical therapy up to a year after the insult, although the functional result is not as successful as it is in patients with unilateral peripheral disorders. Patients with bilateral disorders often walk with a wide-based gait and may continue to require assistive devices even after intervention (Telian et al., 1991; Minor, 1998; Herdman et al., 2000; Brown et al., 2001; Hillier & McDonnell, 2011b).

It is much more difficult to treat persons with central disorders, anxiety disorders and combined central/peripheral vestibular disorders than those who present with peripheral vestibular dysfunction (Whitney & Rossi, 2000; Whitney & Sparto, 2011). Older patients with dizziness can be helped by rehabilitation (Whitney et al., 2002; Herdman et al., 2003; Cohen & Kimball, 2005).

One of the most important components of the exercise program is getting patients to comply with the prescribed exercise routine on a regular basis. When compliance is an issue, it may be necessary to treat those patients more frequently. Older adults may be fearful of performing exercises alone at home, even though a

Box 58.1 *Exercises for the patient with dizziness*

EXERCISES FOR THE PATIENT WHO EXPERIENCES DIZZINESS WITH TRANSITIONAL MOVEMENTS

- Head movements
- Supine
- Sitting
- Standing
- Walking
- Walking and performing a functional activity
- Functional activities
- Pivots
- Circle and figure-of-eight walking
- Ball toss
- Obstacle course

BALANCE EXERCISES

- Consider the head, foot and arm position plus whether the eyes are open or closed
- Use the Clinical Test of Sensory Organization to help you plan your treatment
- Hip and ankle strategies
- Weight shifts
- Single-leg stance
- Stepping forward and back
- Side stepping
- Standing on foam
- Kicking a ball
- Walking backwards
- Crossovers
- Tandem walking
- Romberg
- Step-ups
- Move objects to different surfaces
- Trace the alphabet
- Heel raises
- Racquetball against the wall
- Walk and carry an object
- Walk in a dark room
- Catch a ball while sitting on a gym ball
- Stepping on a compliant surface
- Ankle 'proprioceptive' boards
- Weight shift with a weight around the waist

- Elastic band exercises while standing on one leg
- Heel walking
- Single-leg stance with kicking a ball on a string
- Bus step-ups
- Stand on one leg and rotate the head
- Functional movements for weight shift like golfing
- Tilt boards
- Toe walking
- Walking and talking
- Walking and counting

EYE MOVEMENTS (CAN BE ASSESSED WITH FRENZEL GLASSES)

- Examples of eye exercises
  - Head stable, eye tracking an object
  - Object stable with the head moving
  - Object and head both moving to track an object
- Eye–head exercises
  - Focus on a card and move head to left and right
  - Track a moving object up and down
  - Focus on a card and move the head up and down
  - Move head and card in the same direction at arm's length
  - Look left and right quickly and focus on an object
  - Look up and at eye level at two cards, head still moving
  - Move head and card up and down
  - Look right and left at the card while it is held in front of you
  - 'Simon Says'
  - Mall walking
  - Play ping-pong
  - Spin in a chair that rotates
  - Laser tag
  - Imaginary target exercise
  - X2 viewing
  - Look up and at eye level at two cards, head still
- Otolith stimulation
  - Bounce on a ball
  - Jump rope
- Benign paroxysmal positional vertigo (BPPV) maneuvers
  - Epley maneuver
  - Semont maneuver
  - Brandt–Daroff exercises
  - Horizontal CRM (canalith repositioning maneuver)

home exercise program always includes very specific instructions for performing the exercises safely.

The exercise most commonly recommended for older adults with dizziness is a walking program. Walking challenges the patients, especially outside the home, and exposes them to a wide variety of visual stimuli. In some older individuals, initiating a walking program may not be possible because they live alone and may be afraid of falling.

Recently the Wii™ virtual reality system has been used for persons with vestibular disorders with some success. It is not yet clear how effective the Wii is, but it is an emerging technology that is being used in clinics to improve balance in persons with dizziness (Meldrum et al., 2012). In addition, the use of a vibrotactile vest has been shown to improve gait in persons with balance and vestibular disorders (Wall et al., 2009). Dynamic gait index scores improved during the time period when persons wore the vest while walking compared to a control condition (Wall et al., 2009).

CONCLUSION

Dizziness is an elusive disorder that can be difficult to diagnose. Older adults present with many different causes of dizziness. These can be central, peripheral, psychiatric, or be based on various systemic diseases. Treatment is best initiated after a thorough medical workup to determine a medical diagnosis. If the cause of the dizziness is vestibular, individually tailored exercise is of great benefit in the recovery of functional skills.

REFERENCES

Agrawal Y, Carey JP, Della Santina CC et al 2009 Disorders of balance and vestibular function in US adults: data from the National Health and Nutrition Examination Survey, 2001–2004. Arch Intern Med 169:938–944

Bamiou DE, Davies RA, Mckee M et al 2000 Symptoms, disability and handicap in unilateral peripheral vestibular disorders. Effects of early presentation and initiation of balance exercises. Scand Audiol 29:238–244

Bessot N, Denise P, Toupet M et al 2012 Interference between walking and a cognitive task is increased in patients with bilateral vestibular loss. Gait Posture 36:319–321

Bhattacharyya N, Baugh RF, Orvidas L et al 2008 Clinical practice guideline: benign paroxysmal positional vertigo. Otolaryngol Head Neck Surg 139:S47–S81

Bronstein AM, Lempert T 2010 Management of the patient with chronic dizziness. Restor Neurol Neurosci 28:83–90

Brown KE, Whitney SL, Wrisley DM et al 2001 Physical therapy outcomes for persons with bilateral vestibular loss. Laryngoscope 111:1812–1817

Chen Y, Zhuang J, Zhang L et al 2012 Short-term efficacy of Semont maneuver for benign paroxysmal positional vertigo: a double-blind randomized trial. Otol Neurotol 33:1127–1130

Cohen H, Ewell LR, Jenkins HA 1995a Disability in Menières disease. Arch Otolaryngol-Head Neck Surg 121:29–33

Cohen H, Kanewineland M, Miller LV et al 1995b Occupation and visual–vestibular interaction in vestibular rehabilitation. Otolaryngol-Head Neck Surg 112:526–532

Cohen HS, Kimball KT 2005 Effectiveness of treatments for benign paroxysmal positional vertigo of the posterior canal. Otol Neurotol 26:1034–1040

Epley JM 1980 New dimensions of benign paroxysmal positional vertigo. Otolaryngol Head Neck Surg 88:599–605

Epley JM 1992 The canalith repositioning procedure: for treatment of benign paroxysmal positional vertigo. Otolaryngol Head Neck Surg 107:399–404

Fife TD, Iverson DJ, Lempert T et al 2008 Practice parameter: therapies for benign paroxysmal positional vertigo (an evidence-based review): report of the Quality Standards Subcommittee of the American Academy of Neurology. Neurology 70:2067–2074

Furman JM, Cass SP, Whitney SL 2010 Vestibular Disorders A Case Study Approach. Oxford University Press, New York

Gananca FF, Gazzola JM, Gananca CF et al 2010 Elderly falls associated with benign paroxysmal positional vertigo. Braz J Otorhinolaryngol 76:113–120

Gizzi M, Ayyagari S, Khattar V 1998 The familial incidence of benign paroxysmal positional vertigo. Acta Otolaryngol 118:774–777

Halmagyi GM, Curthoys IS 1988 A clinical sign of canal paresis. Arch Neurol 45:737–739

Herdman SJ, Blatt P, Schubert MC et al 2000 Falls in patients with vestibular deficits. Am J Otol 21:847–851

Herdman SJ, Schubert MC, Das VE et al 2003 Recovery of dynamic visual acuity in unilateral vestibular hypofunction. Arch Otolaryngol Head Neck Surg 129:819–824

Hillier SL, Mcdonnell M 2011a Vestibular rehabilitation for unilateral peripheral vestibular dysfunction. Cochrane Database Syst Rev 2:CD005397

Hillier SL, Mcdonnell M 2011b Vestibular rehabilitation for unilateral peripheral vestibular dysfunction. Clin Otolaryngol 36:248–249

Jacob RG, Furman JM, Durrant JD et al 1996 Panic, agoraphobia, and vestibular dysfunction. Am J Psychiatry 153:503–512

Jacobson GP, Newman CW 1990 The development of the Dizziness Handicap Inventory. Arch Otolaryngol Head Neck Surg 116:424–427

Katsarkas A 1999 Benign paroxysmal positional vertigo (BPPV): idiopathic versus post- traumatic. Acta Otolaryngol 119:745–749

Kattah JC, Talkad AV, Wang DZ et al 2009 HINTS to diagnose stroke in the acute vestibular syndrome: three-step bedside oculomotor examination more sensitive than early MRI diffusion-weighted imaging. Stroke 40:3504–3510

Kroenke K, Lucas CA, Rosenberg ML et al 1992 Causes of persistent dizziness – a prospective study of 100 patients in ambulatory care. Ann Intern Med 117:898–904

Meldrum D, Glennon A, Herdman S et al 2012 Virtual reality rehabilitation of balance: assessment of the usability of the Nintendo Wii(R) Fit Plus. Disabil Rehabil Assist Technol 7:205–210

Minor L 1998 Gentamicin-induced bilateral vestibular hypofunction. JAMA 279:541–544

Nunez RA, Cass SP, Furman JM 2000 Short- and long-term outcomes of canalith repositioning for benign paroxysmal positional vertigo. Otolaryngol Head Neck Surg 122:647–652

Peppard SB 1986 Effect of drug therapy on compensation from vestibular injury. Laryngoscope 96:878–898

Redfern MS, Talkowski ME, Jennings JR et al 2004 Cognitive influences in postural control of patients with unilateral vestibular loss. Gait Posture 19:105–114

Roberts JC, Cohen HS, Sangi-Haghpeykar H 2011 Vestibular disorders and dual task performance: impairment when walking a straight path. J Vestib Res 21:167–174

Semont A, Freyss G, Vitte E 1988 Curing the BPPV with a liberatory maneuver. Adv Otorhinolaryngol 42:290–293

Sparto PJ, Furman JM, Whitney SL et al 2004 Vestibular rehabilitation using a wide field of view virtual environment. Conf Proc IEEE Eng Med Biol Soc 7:4836–4839

Telian SA, Shepard NT, Smith-Wheelock M et al 1991 Bilateral vestibular paresis: diagnosis and treatment. Otolaryngol Head Neck Surg 104:67–71

Wall 3rd C, Wrisley DM, Statler KD 2009 Vibrotactile tilt feedback improves dynamic gait index: a fall risk indicator in older adults. Gait Posture 30:16–21

White J, Savvides P, Cherian N et al 2005 Canalith repositioning for benign paroxysmal positional vertigo. Otol Neurotol 26:704–710

Whitney SL, Rossi MM 2000 Efficacy of vestibular rehabilitation. Otolaryngol Clin North Am 33:659–661

Whitney SL, Sparto PJ 2011 Principles of vestibular physical therapy rehabilitation. Neuro Rehabil 29:157–166

Whitney SL, Wrisley DM, Marchetti GF et al 2002 The effect of age on vestibular rehabilitation outcomes. Laryngoscope 112:1785–1790

Whitney SL, Wrisley DM, Brown KE et al 2004 Is perception of handicap related to functional performance in persons with vestibular dysfunction? Otol Neurotol 25:139–143

Whitney SL, Marchetti GF, Morris LO 2005 Usefulness of the dizziness handicap inventory in the screening for benign paroxysmal positional vertigo. Otol Neurotol 26:1027–1033

Chapter 59
Balance testing and training

DIANE M. WRISLEY • TIMOTHY L. KAUFFMAN

INTRODUCTION

The medical and sociologic consequences of falls in the older adult are one of the largest worldwide public health issues. It is estimated that 28–35% of persons over 65 years of age fall each year and this increases to 32–42% for persons over 70 years and fatalities are greatest in the over 85 age group (WHO, 2007). Falls in the elderly are multifactorial and have been attributed to medication use, environmental challenges, cardiopulmonary compromise, cognitive changes, frailty and sensory and motor deficits (WHO, 2007; Tom et al., 2013).

Once an older adult falls, changes occur (e.g. fear of falling, decreased mobility, speed, and fluency of movement) that increase their risk of falling. Therefore, it is essential that the geriatric specialist performs a thorough multifactorial balance evaluation and initiates treatment as early as possible. Definitions of key terms concerned with balance are included in Box 59.1.

PHYSIOLOGY OF BALANCE

Balance, the ability to maintain the center of gravity over the base of support within a given sensory environment, is composed of several subcomponents and influenced by several systems. Human balance is a complex neuromusculoskeletal process involving the sensory detection of body motions, integration of sensorimotor information within the central nervous system (CNS), and programming and execution of the appropriate neuromuscular responses. Figure 59.1 summarizes the organization of the human balance system. The brain uses visual, vestibular, and somatosensory systems to determine the body position and movement in space. Although there are age-related changes in these systems, older adults do not display increased postural sway compared with younger adults when standing or walking when they have all three senses available (Woollacott et al., 1986). When older adults are first asked to balance on a posture platform under conditions of minimized somatosensory and visual input, half lose their balance (Woollacott et al., 1986).

Box 59.1 *Definitions of key terms concerning balance*

Balance: the ability to maintain the center of gravity over the base of support within a given sensory environment.

Static balance: the ability to hold a position.

Dynamic balance: the ability to transition or move between positions.

Automatic postural responses: operate to keep the center of gravity over the base of support in response to a stimulus or unexpected perturbation such as a slip or a jostle in a crowd.

Anticipatory postural control: similar to automatic postural control but occurs prior to and in preparation for the perturbation.

Volitional postural control: postural control under conscious control; self-initiated perturbations that are strongly influenced by prior experience and instruction.

Center of gravity: an imaginary point in space, calculated biomechanically from measured forces and moments, where the sum of all the forces equals zero. In a normal person standing quietly, it is located just forward of the spine at about the S2 level.

Base of support: the body surfaces that experience pressure as the result of body weight and gravity. In standing, the base of support is the soles of the feet; in sitting, it is the thighs and buttocks. The narrower the base of support, the more difficult the balance task.

Limits of stability: the limits to which a body can move in any direction without either falling (as the center of gravity exceeds the base of support) or establishing a new base of support by stepping or reaching (to relocate the base of support under the center of gravity).

Balance strategies: stereotypic sequences of muscle activity used to maintain upright posture. The most commonly suggested include the ankle, hip and stepping strategies.

Source: Nashner, 1990; Allison, 1995.

With repeated exposure, however, they are able to learn to maintain their balance on the platform (Woollacott et al., 1986). Interestingly, on further investigation, it was found that the falls correlated positively with subclinical pathologies in either the sensory or the motor systems (Woollacott et al., 1986).

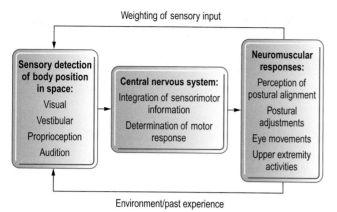

Weighting of sensory input

Sensory detection of body position in space:
Visual
Vestibular
Proprioception
Audition

Central nervous system:
Integration of sensorimotor information
Determination of motor response

Neuromuscular responses:
Perception of postural alignment
Postural adjustments
Eye movements
Upper extremity activities

Environment/past experience

Figure 59.1 The organization of the human balance system.

As sensory changes are common in older adults, the reader is referred to additional chapters in this text on peripheral neuropathies (Chapters 32 and 33) and sensory changes in visual (see Chapter 51), somatosensory (see Chapter 49) and vestibular (see Chapters 52 and 58) systems for further evaluation and treatment techniques for these systems that will affect balance.

The information from the various sensory systems is relayed to the CNS and is integrated in several areas including the vestibular nuclei and the cerebellum prior to the generation of appropriate motor responses. Prioritization of use of sensory information for use by the CNS is most likely based on the availability of a particular sensory modality, the task at hand and past experiences (Peterka, 2002). The CNS then generates the appropriate motor responses to maintain upright body posture. Various balance strategies are thought to maintain balance depending on the speed of perturbation and the support surface. Slow, small perturbations on level surfaces result in muscle activity that is sequenced from distal to proximal (ankle strategy), while perturbations that are larger, faster, or on smaller surfaces result in muscle sequences from proximal to distal (hip strategy) (Nashner, 1994). A stepping strategy is used when the perturbations take the center of gravity outside the base of support or limits of stability and is used to recover balance (Nashner, 1994). Older adults frequently switch from an ankle strategy to a hip strategy during different conditions such as walking on slippery surfaces or with smaller, slower perturbations (Horak, 2006). Use of inappropriate balance strategies may contribute to falls in older adults.

There are many other factors that contribute to the ability to maintain an upright posture. First, musculoskeletal constraints must be met. Adequate range of motion (ROM) must be available, especially in crucial joints such as the ankle and hip. Impaired ROM of the neck or painful syndromes in the cervical muscles may lead to an altered representation of trunk and head movement and therefore cause imbalance. The proper generation of neuromuscular force is also essential to developing the appropriate balance strategies. The ability to sequence the muscles appropriately and the timing of the muscle activity are crucial and are sometimes the most difficult to retrain following injury

(Horak & Shumway-Cook, 1990). When automatic postural responses are examined, older adults demonstrate slowed onset and reversal in normal distal to proximal sequencing of muscle activation compared with younger adults (Woollacott, 1990). Posture or alignment of bony segments can either assist with the production of the balance responses or make it more difficult to generate balance reactions. Maximizing a patient's postural alignment can assist in regaining their ability to generate balance responses (Horak & Shumway-Cook, 1990). Although most of our balance reactions occur at a subconscious level, a patient's cognitive status can influence their ability to generate the balance reactions necessary to maintain an upright posture. If a subject is easily distracted or has slow processing, he or she may not be able to react quickly enough to environmental changes to allow them to stay upright. This may be especially true if there is increased activity in the environment, if the patient is distracted by conversation, or if they are preoccupied (Horak, 2006). Many environmental factors can affect a patient's ability to maintain balance. Decreased or absent lighting, and soft, pliable surfaces decrease the sensory input available to the patient for spatial orientation. Small children or pets underfoot can cause sudden perturbations and make it difficult for a patient to maintain balance, especially if they already have an increased reaction time. Many classifications of medications, ranging from diuretics to CNS suppressants, can also impair a patient's ability to balance (WHO, 2007; Kenny et al., 2011) (see Chapter 12).

BALANCE ASSESSMENT

The last two decades have seen a proliferation of tools for assessing balance. Some of these tools evaluate only one underlying impairment, and some are multidimensional. The tools range from highly technical and expensive to simple and portable. Table 59.1 provides an overview of various tools and the components of balance that they assess. Box 59.2 illustrates 'red flags' or signs and symptoms that indicate that the patient would benefit from further medical workup.

One of the most important areas that requires assessment when working with older adults is their risk of falling. Box 59.3 summarizes the risk factors that have been identified for falling in older adults. The reader is referred to the Guideline for the Prevention of Falls in Older Persons (Kenny et al., 2011) that summarizes the literature on the evaluation and treatment of fall risk in the older adult and provides recommendations.

Although self-report measures do not directly measure impairments, several self-report measures are available to allow the clinician to determine how stable the patient perceives that he or she is, and this will facilitate the clinician's ability to treat and assess for fall risk. Sometimes, patients will perceive that they are more stable than testing reveals. This indicates that they are either performing differently in the clinic or may be taking unnecessary risks at home and need some counseling regarding ways to decrease their fall risk. At other times, patients will perceive that they are less stable than tests reveal. These subjects may have a history of

Table 59.1	**Evaluation tools for assessing balance**
Self-perception scales	Falls Efficacy Scale (Tinetti et al., 1990, 1994b)
	Modified Falls Efficacy Scale (Hill et al., 1996)
	Activities-specific Balance Confidence Scale (Powell & Myers, 1995)
Assessment of sensory components	Sensory Organization Test of Computerized Dynamic Posturography (Monsell et al., 1997)
	Clinical Test of Sensory Interaction and Balance (Shumway-Cook & Horak, 1986)
Assessment of motor components	Functional Reach Test (Duncan et al., 1990)
	Multidirectional Reach Test (Newton, 2001)
	Four Square Step Test (Dite & Temple, 2002)
	Limits of Stability (El-Kashlan et al., 1998)
	Motor Control Test (El-Kashlan et al., 1998)
	Five Times Sit to Stand (Csuka & McCarty, 1985)
Multidimensional assessment	Performance Oriented Mobility Assessment (Tinetti, 1986)
	Physical Performance Scale
	Berg Balance Scale (Berg et al., 1992)
	Balance Evaluation Systems Test (BESTest) (Horak et al., 2009)
Gait assessment	Timed 'Up & Go' (Podsiadlo & Richardson, 1991)
	Dynamic Gait Index (Shumway-Cook & Woollacott, 1995)
	Functional Gait Assessment (Wrisley et al., 2004)
	Gait speed

Box 59.2 _Red flags – urgent referrals to physician for workup_

- Unexplained central nervous system signs – motor, sensory, or cognitive changes
- Unexplained cranial nerve dysfunction
- Unexplained sudden or unilateral hearing loss, especially if accompanied by vertigo
- Two or more falls in the previous 4 weeks
- Inconsistencies in clinical examination

Box 59.3 _Risk factors for falls_

INTRINSIC

- Lower extremity weakness
- Poor grip strength
- Balance disorders
- Functional and cognitive impairments
- Visual deficits
- History of falls
- Gait deficit
- Visual deficit
- Urinary incontinence
- Chronic disease

EXTRINSIC

- Polypharmacy (four or more prescription medications)
- Environmental
- Poor lighting
- Loose carpets
- Limited access to healthcare
- Low income and education levels

Source: WHO, 2007; Kenny et al., 2011.

---

falling and have lost confidence in their balance abilities, causing them to decrease their activity (Kenny et al., 2011). Without intervention, this decrease in activity may lead to greater impairment and more balance problems. Two of the most common self-report measures for balance function are the Falls Efficacy Scale (Tinetti et al., 1990) and the Activities-specific Balance Confidence Scale (Powell & Myers, 1995). Both the Falls Efficacy Scale (test–retest reliability Intraclass Correlation Coefficient [ICC] (2,1) = 0.91) (Tinetti et al., 1990) and the Activities-specific Balance Confidence Scale have been shown to be reliable (test–retest reliability ICC (2,1) = 0.91) and valid. The Falls Efficacy Scale correlates with getting up from a fall and level of anxiety (Tinetti et al., 1990). The modified Falls Efficacy Scale was developed to incorporate higher functional activities. It has high test–retest reliability (ICC = 0.93) and discriminates between older adults with and without a history of falling. Myers et al. (1998) reported that scores on the Activities-specific Balance Confidence scale correlate with physical functioning and falls in community-living older adults. Scores above 80% were strongly correlated with highly functioning community-dwelling older adults; scores between 50% and 80% were correlated with moderate physical functioning seen in older adults in retirement homes or with chronic disease; and scores below 50%

were correlated with low physical functioning of older adults receiving home-care.

Balance impairments can be assessed using single-item balance tools such as the Romberg test, Functional Reach test (Duncan et al., 1990), single limb stance (Bohannon et al., 1984), or tandem stance (Fregly & Graybiel, 1968). They are easy to administer and generally provide a method for quick screening of balance function. The disadvantage is that these tools test only one aspect of balance. Without correlating findings with other tests, this may limit their usefulness in developing a treatment plan. These single-item tests have good reliability. The inability to maintain single limb stance for more than 5 seconds is correlated with increased risk of falls in older adults.

The ability to use sensory information for balance can be assessed using either high or low technology such as the Sensory Organization Testing (SOT) via the Equitest® or the Clinical Test of Sensory Interaction and Balance (CTSIB) or 'Foam and Dome' respectively (Shumway-Cook & Horak, 1986). Each consists of six conditions designed to test whether the patient can utilize visual, vestibular, or somatosensory information for balance. Both the SOT and the CTSIB are reliable and valid (El-Kashlan et al., 1998; Wrisley et al., 2007). The SOT provides an equilibrium score and additional information on motor strategies and the relative reliance on sensory information for balance. The CTSIB is a portable alternative that will provide similar information. Scores achieved on the CTSIB correlate moderately with scores achieved on SOT (Wrisley & Whitney, 2004).

Several multidimensional balance assessments have been developed in order to take into account the many facets of balance in order to predict an individual's risk of falling. One of the primary benefits of multidimensional balance tests is that they assess several aspects of balance that are integrated into a single overall score. This makes them very useful for predicting one's risk of falling, but may make it more difficult to sort out which balance impairments should be addressed in treatment. Overall scores are used to determine fall risk (Tinetti et al., 1986; Duncan et al., 1990; Berg et al., 1995; Shumway-Cook et al., 1997) a functional baseline before intervention, and to quantify the effectiveness of intervention (Rubenstein et al., 2000). The therapist may need to look at the performance of individual test items or perform single-item assessments in order to identify the impairments that need to be treated. The inter- and intrarater reliability of multidimensional tests is good to excellent (Tinetti et al., 1986; Berg et al., 1995).

Walking, a complex balance task, is a very functional means of both assessing and treating balance disorders. During ambulation, the center of gravity is moved outside the base of support, as in a fall. Then there is recovery from the loss of balance by the base of support being reoriented with a step. Gait assessments allow us to measure a patient's ability to integrate balance and to measure balance during mobility. Assessments that appear to be particularly useful for gait are the Dynamic Gait Index (Shumway-Cook & Woollacott, 1995), the Functional Gait Assessment (Wrisley et al., 2004, Wrisley & Kumar, 2010) and the Timed Up and Go Test (Podsiadlo & Richardson, 1991). Functionally, in some settings patients need to be able to walk 1.22 m/s to cross a street safely.

The assessment of an older adult's balance function may include self-perception measures, impairment-based or multidimensional tools, and will be directed by the purpose of the evaluation (e.g. fall risk assessment, diagnosis, or directing intervention). The assessment should include motor, sensory, musculoskeletal and extrinsic factors underlying the balance dysfunction. A thorough balance assessment will guide treatment.

TREATMENT

Treatment of balance disorders is based on the specific impairments (e.g. ROM, strength, decreased sensation, pain, use of sensory inputs, use of motor strategies, etc.)

and functional limitations identified in the evaluation. Balance strategies and the ability to use sensory information for balance can be learned with the appropriate exercise and practice. For balance training, it is important to provide opportunities for patients to practice tasks that allow them to use the necessary balance strategies and, when at all possible, to incorporate the tasks into functional activities, as patients will be more likely to follow through with the exercise and to generalize the tasks they are learning (see Table 59.2A). Safety is important for patients when working on balance. The exercises prescribed need to challenge the patient's balance and therefore are ones that may make them stumble or fall. Upper extremity support changes the sequence of muscle activation so that it originates in the upper extremities. This alteration in the sequence of muscle activity is not usually desirable if the goal of treatment is independent ambulation without an assistive device. For standing exercises, having the patient stand in a corner of the room with a chair in front of them provides a surface on all sides that can catch the patient, minimizing the chance of injury. The American Geriatrics Society/British Geriatrics Society Panel for Prevention of Falls recommends multicomponent exercises including strength, balance coordination and gait training. Their research review indicated benefits were obtained in programs lasting longer than 12 weeks at 1–3 times weekly (Kenny et al., 2011).

Age-related changes in sensory function and pathology of the different sensory systems may lead to patients having difficulty using sensory information for balance. Exercise can assist in training a patient to use a sense they are not using well or train them to compensate with an alternate sense. The general principle used when trying to maximize an individual's ability to use sensory inputs for balance is first to practice activities with all the sensory information available and then gradually to remove sensory information. Table 59.2B illustrates exercises that will stimulate the use of different sensory inputs.

Gait is the act of losing one's balance and then regaining it by taking a compensatory step. This makes it an excellent treatment tool for balance dysfunction because the majority of our patients have a primary goal of ambulation. There are many activities that can be introduced into gait to improve balance. Ambulation with head turns in the yaw and pitch planes, at varying speeds, while negotiating objects, and on compliant surfaces or in varied lighting can all improve balance.

Robinovitch et al. (2013) used video cameras to study falls in long-term care facilities (2013). Falls were attributed to incorrect weight shifting (41%), trip or stumble (21%), loss of support (11%), collapse (11%) and slip (3%). Activities with the greater percentages of falls were forward walking (24%), standing quietly (13%) and sitting down (12%). These results should be considered when evaluating and developing a treatment plan for persons with a history of falls.

EVIDENCE FOR THE USE OF EXERCISE TO TREAT BALANCE

The majority of research on the effectiveness of exercise for balance has focused on older adults at risk of falling. Randomized clinical trials have demonstrated

Table 59.2	**Treatment strategies**	

A	Exercises to improve center of gravity control	Begin with slow weight shifts on a stable surface
		Add upper extremity activities, functional activities
		Progress the activity by:
		    Increasing the distance moved away from the midline
		    Alter the speed of movement
		    Add manual resistance
		    Narrow the base of support
		    Use an unstable surface, i.e. foam, rocker board, 2 × 4, half-roll
		    Add combined head and eye movement
		    Alter vision: dim lighting, close eyes, use opaque glasses

	Exercises that promote use of the ankle strategy	Small, slow perturbations on firm surface, either self- or externally generated Closed chain exercises such as stepping over a 2 × 4, walking Functional activities such as reaching to take objects off shelves, performing upper extremity activities in standing
	Exercises that promote use of the hip strategy	Moderate, rapid perturbations on narrow surfaces either self- or externally generated Tandem standing or walking Single limb support Functional activities such as reaching into the trunk of a car or laundry dryer, ascending and descending stairs
	Exercises that promote the use of the stepping strategy	Large, rapid perturbations either self- or externally generated that require the use of a step; progress from predictable to unpredictable Walking on uneven surfaces Stepping over obstacles

B	Exercises to stimulate the use of somato sensory inputs	Disadvantage vision while providing reliable somatosensory inputs on a stable surface:
		    Sit to and from stand with eyes closed
		    Ambulation with eye and head movements
		    Conflicting visual environments: crowds, striped curtains, moving visual surrounds, virtual reality

	Exercises to stimulate the use of visual inputs	Disadvantage somatosensory input while providing reliable visual cues (stable visual cues with landmarks):
		    Standing or sitting on a compliant surface or rocker board
		    Ambulate with foam boots
		    Instruct in visual fixation

	Exercises to stimulate the use of vestibular inputs	Disadvantage vision and somatosensation while providing reliable vestibular cues (detectable head position): Standing or ambulating on unstable or compliant surface with absent vision, destabilized vision, and inaccurate vision

that exercise improves balance in community-dwelling older adults (Tinetti et al., 1994a; Wolf et al., 1996; Rubenstein et al., 2000). Sherrington et al. (2008) conducted a systematic review with meta-analysis to assess the effectiveness of exercise for preventions of falls in older community and residential care adults. The pooled effect of the 44 trials including 9603 participants showed a 17% reduction in falls and importantly the benefits were greater in persons who exercised over 50 hours in the intervention program. This threshold of 50 hours is more effective in falls reduction if it is achieved within 6 months as opposed to 12 months; thus representing greater intensity over time (Shubert, 2011).

Clemson et al. (2012) reported a significant reduction in falls over 1 year among community dwellers over 70 years of age with two or more falls within the previous 12 months. Their Lifestyle intervention Functional Exercise (LiFE) program consisted of specific balance and strengthening activities that are incorporated into daily living and thus repeated throughout the day, including: 'step over objects'; 'turning and changing direction'; 'shift weight from foot to foot'; 'sit to stand'; 'walk sideways'; 'bend your knees' and other strategies.

In conclusion, several relevant points concerning exercise intervention can be deduced: (i) the optimal type, duration and intensity of exercise for fall prevention remain unclear; (ii) exercise intervention needs to be custom designed; (iii) exercise needs to be sustained – the successful programs lasted for more than 12 weeks; (iv) exercise may be more effective for fall prevention when combined with other forms of intervention such as home modification and education (Kenny et al., 2011).

CONCLUSION

Balance is a complex neuromusculoskeletal process involving sensory, skeletal and motor components. Current research has shown that balance dysfunction is not a normal part of aging, but is often associated with a decline in the neuromusculoskeletal and sensory systems and should be taken seriously by healthcare practitioners working with this population. Functional balance presumes competence in a variety of areas. Healthcare practitioners need to address the sensory, motor and integrative components of balance from both evaluative and training standpoints for the older adult.

Balance in the older adult is not greatly different from balance in the younger adult but the consequences of balance dysfunction may be greater, and the ability of older persons to adapt motor and sensory strategies may be slower. Therefore, one must recognize balance deficits early and implement successful intervention strategies proactively while not restricting the activity of older people. Exercise is effective for improving balance and reducing falls for older persons.

REFERENCES

Allison L 1995 Balance Disorders, 3rd edn. Mosby Year Book, St Louis, MO, pp. 802–837

Berg KO, Wood-Dauphinee SL, Williams JI et al 1992 Measuring balance in the elderly: validation of an instrument. Can J Public Health 83(suppl 2):7–11

Berg KO, Wood-Dauphinee S, Williams JI 1995 The Balance Scale: reliability assessment with elderly residents and patients with an acute stroke. Scand J Rehabil Med 27(1):27–36

Bohannon RW, Larkin PA, Cook AC et al 1984 Decrease in timed balance test scores with aging. Phys Ther 64(7):1067–1070

Clemson L, Fiatarone Singh M, Cumming R et al 2012 Integration of balance and strength training into daily life activity to reduce rate of falls in older people (the LiFE) study: randomised parallel trial. BMJ 345:e552 [Epub 15 August 2012]

Csuka M, McCarty DJ 1985 Simple method for measurement of lower extremity muscle strength. Am J Med 78(1):77–81

Dite W, Temple VA 2002 A clinical test of stepping and change of direction to identify multiple falling older adults. Arch Phys Med Rehabil 83(11):1566–1571

Duncan PW, Weiner DK, Chandler J et al 1990 Functional reach: a new clinical measure of balance. J Gerontol 45(6):192–197

El-Kashlan HK, Shepard NT, Asher AM et al 1998 Evaluation of clinical measures of equilibrium. Laryngoscope 108(3):311–319

Fregly AR, Graybiel A 1968 An ataxia test not requiring rails. Aerospace Med 39:277–282

Hill KD, Schwarz JA, Kalogeropoulos AJ et al 1996 The modified falls efficacy scale. Arch Phys Med Rehabil 77:1025–1029

Horak F 2006 Postural orientation and equilibrium: what do we need to know about neural control of balance to prevent falls. Age Ageing 35(Suppl ii7–ii11)

Horak FB, Shumway-Cook A 1990 Clinical Implications of Posture Control Research. APTA, Alexandria, VA, pp. 105–111

Horak F, Wrisley D, Frank J 2009 The Balance Evaluations Systems Test (BESTest) to differentiate balance deficits. Phys Ther 89:484–498

Kenny R, Rubenstein L, Tinetti M et al 2011 Summary of the updated American Geriatrics Society/British Geriatrics Society clinical practice guideline for prevention of falls in older persons. J Am Geriatr Soc 59:148–157

Monsell EM, Furman JM, Herdman SJ et al 1997 Computerized dynamic platform posturography. Otolaryngol Head Neck Surg 117:394–398

Myers AM, Fletcher PC, Myers AH et al 1998 Discriminative and evaluative properties of the activities-specific balance confidence (ABC) scale. J Gerontol A Biol Sci Med Sci 53(4):M287–M294

Nashner LM, Peters JF 1990 Dynamic posturography in the diagnosis and management of dizziness and balance disorder. Neurol Clin 8(2):331–349

Newton RA 2001 Validity of the multi-directional reach test: a practical measure for limits of stability in older adults. J Gerontol A Biol Sci Med Sci 56(4):248–252

Peterka RJ 2002 Sensorimotor integration in human postural control. J Neurophysiol 88(3):1097–1118

Podsiadlo D, Richardson S 1991 The Timed 'Up & Go': a test of basic functional mobility for frail elderly persons. J Am Geriatr Soc 39(2):142–148

Powell LE, Myers AM 1995 The Activities-specific Balance Confidence (ABC) Scale. J Gerontol A Biol Sci Med Sci 50(1):28–34

Robinovitch S, Feldman F, Yang Y et al 2013 Video capture of the circumstances of falls in elderly people residing in long term care: an observational study. Lancet 381:47–54

Rubenstein LZ, Josephson KR, Trueblood PR et al 2000 Effects of a group exercise program on strength, mobility, and falls among fall-prone elderly men. J Gerontol A Biol Sci Med Sci 55(6):317–321

Sherrington C, Whitney J, Lord S et al 2008 Effective exercise for the prevention of falls: a systematic review and meta-analysis. J Am Geriatr Soc 56:2234–2243

Shubert T 2011 Evidence-based exercise prescription for balance and falls prevention: a current review of the literature. J Geriatr Phys Ther 34:100–108

Shumway-Cook A, Horak FB 1986 Assessing the influence of sensory integration on balance: suggestions from the field. Phys Ther 66(10):1548–1549

Shumway-Cook A, Woollacott M 1995 Motor control: Theory and Practical Applications. Williams & Wilkins, Baltimore, MD

Shumway-Cook A, Baldwin M, Polissar NL et al 1997 Predicting the probability for falls in community-dwelling older adults. Phys Ther 77(8):812–819

Tinetti ME 1986 Performance-oriented assessment of mobility problems in elderly patients. J Am Geriatr Soc 34(2):119–126

Tinetti ME, Williams TF, Mayewski R 1986 Fall risk index for elderly patients based on number of chronic disabilities. Am J Med 80(3):429–434

Tinetti ME, Richman D, Powell L 1990 Falls efficacy as a measure of fear of falling. J Gerontol 45(6):239–243

Tinetti ME, Baker DI, McAvay G et al 1994a A multifactorial intervention to reduce the risk of falling among elderly people living in the community. N Engl J Med 331(13):821–827

Tinetti ME, Mendes de Leon CF, Doucette JT et al 1994b Fear of falling and fall-related efficacy in relationship to functioning among community-living elders. J Gerontol 49(3):140–147

Tom S, Adachi J, Anderson F et al 2013 Frailty and fracture, disability and falls; a multiple country study from the global longitudinal study of osteoporosis in women. J Am Geriatr Soc 61:327–334

WHO 2007 Global Health Report on Falls Prevention. World Health Organization, Geneva Switzerland, pp. 1–47

Wolf SL, Barnhart HX, Kutner NG et al 1996 Reducing frailty and falls in older persons: an investigation of Tai Chi and computerized balance training. Atlanta FICSIT Group. Frailty and Injuries: Cooperative Studies of Intervention Techniques. J Am Geriatr Soc 44(5):489–497

Woollacott M 1990 Postural Control Mechanisms in the Young and Old. APTA, Alexandria, VA, pp. 23–28

Woollacott MH, Shumway-Cook A, Nashner LM 1986 Aging and posture control: changes in sensory organization and muscular coordination. Int J Aging Hum Dev 23(2):97–114

Wrisley DM, Kumar NA 2010 Functional gait assessment: concurrent, discriminative, and predictive validity in community-dwelling older adults. Phys Ther 90(5):761–773

Wrisley DM, Whitney SL 2004 The effect of foot position on the modified clinical test of sensory interaction and balance. Arch Phys Med Rehabil 85(2):335–338

Wrisley DM, Marchetti GF, Kuharsky DK et al 2004 Reliability, internal consistency, and validity of data obtained with the functional gait assessment. Phys Ther 84(10):906–918

Wrisley DM, Stephens MJ, Mosley S et al 2007 Learning effects of repetitive administrations of the sensory organization test in healthy young adults. Arch Phys Med Rehabil 88:1049–1054

Chapter 60

Fracture considerations

TIMOTHY L. KAUFFMAN • CARLEEN LINDSEY

CHAPTER CONTENTS

INTRODUCTION

The fracture of a bone has a profound impact on any member of the aging population, as the consequences may negatively impact independence and can even lead to death (Leslie et al., 2013). Fractures in aging individuals are usually associated with low bone mineral density (BMD) and osteoporosis (see Chapter 18), as defined by the World Health Organization in Box 60.1. It is estimated that there are nearly 9 million osteoporotic-related fractures a year worldwide. One in five females over the age of 50 in developed countries is likely to sustain a hip fracture with associated high morbidity and mortality (WHO, 2007). The proportion of all fractures from osteoporotic bone reported from international community-based populations is 0.716–0.924. These data include males and females aged 50 years and older (Morrison et al., 2013).

In a population study of all persons over age 49 from Manitoba, 5-year survival after hip fracture was 51% females and 36% males. The average first year costs were 23 361 Canadian dollars for hip fractures and total healthcare costs for all incident fractures were $194 million (Leslie et al., 2013). In the US there were about 2 million osteoporotic fractures in 2010 with costs projected to exceed $18 billion (Levis & Theodore, 2012).

A bone fractures when a force or stress is placed upon it that is greater than the bone can withstand. Bone has a tensile strength of approximately 140 MPa (megapascals; one MPa equals 145 pounds per square inch) in the second decade of life, and it decreases to approximately 120 MPa by the eighth decade of life. The fracture threshold for the vertebrae and the epiphyseal areas of the femur is a bone density of less than $1\,g/cm^3$ (Gerhart, 1995). Even though the stiffness and strength of trabecular bone depends on bone density and the direction of loading, trabecular bone appears to be more susceptible to failure from shear rather than compressive loads (Sanyal et al., 2012). The major physical difference between trabecular bone and cortical bone is the increased porosity exhibited by trabecular bone. This porosity is reflected by measurements of the apparent density (i.e. the mass of bone tissue divided by the bulk volume of the test specimen, including mineralized bone and marrow spaces). In the human skeleton, the apparent density of cortical bone is about $1.8\,g/cm^3$, whereas the apparent density of trabecular bone ranges from approximately 0.1 to $1.0\,g/cm^3$

Fragility fractures are usually related to lower BMD; however, urinary markers of bone resorption including collagen cross-linked N, C-telopeptide and free deoxypyridinoline may be predictive of hip fracture independent of bone mass (Garnero et al., 2009). Additionally, the large majority of fractures result from falls and physical interventions are successful but probably not utilized as widely as they should be (see Chapters 15, 16, 58, 59).

NORMAL FRACTURE HEALING

Normal fracture healing can be divided into three overlapping phases. First, there is an immediate inflammatory phase in which there is bleeding resulting from the injury to the bone and surrounding soft tissue, and a hematoma forms (Fig. 60.1A). The bone cells at the fracture line die. The reparative, or proliferative, phase starts shortly after the injury, usually 24–48 hours if a good

---

Box 60.1 *World Health Organization classification of skeletal status*

- *Normal:* Bone mineral density that is not more than one standard deviation below the young adult mean value.
- *Low bone mass or osteopenia:* Bone mineral density that lies between 1 and 2.5 standard deviations below the young adult mean value.
- *Osteoporosis:* A value of bone mineral density that is more than 2.5 standard deviations below the young adult mean value.
- *Severe osteoporosis:* A value of bone mineral density more than 2.5 standard deviations below the young adult mean value and the presence of one or more fragility fractures.

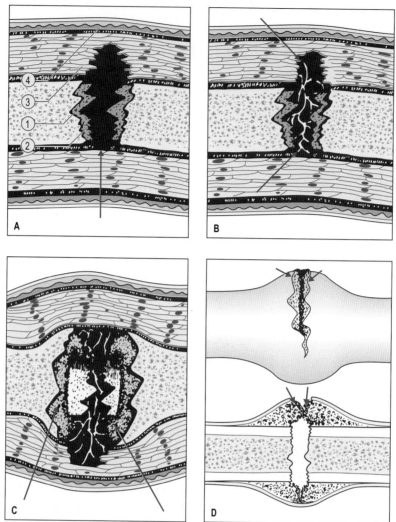

Figure 60.1 Fracture healing. (A) Bleeding occurs from the bone ends, marrow vessels, and damaged soft tissues, with the formation of a fracture hematoma that clots (closed fracture is illustrated). (1, periosteum; 2, haversian systems; 3, muscle; 4, skin.) **(B)** The fracture hematoma is rapidly vascularized by the ingrowth of blood vessels from the surrounding tissues and, for some weeks, there is rapid cellular activity. Fibrovascular tissue replaces the clot, collagen fibers are laid down and mineral salts are deposited. **(C)** New woven bone is formed beneath the periosteum at the ends of the bone. The cells responsible are derived from the periosteum, which becomes stretched over these collars of new bone. If the blood supply is poor, or if it is disturbed by excessive mobility at the fracture site, cartilage may be formed instead and remain until a better blood supply is established. **(D)** If the periosteum is incompletely torn, and there is no significant loss of bony apposition, the primary callus response may result in establishing external continuity of the fracture ('bridging external callus'). Cells lying in the outer layer of the periosteum itself proliferate to reconstitute the periosteum. *(Reproduced from McRae R 2008 Practical Fracture Treatment, 5th edn, by permission of Churchill Livingstone.)*

local blood supply to the fracture exists (Fig. 60.1B). Good reduction and immobilization of the fracture also help the bone during the reparative phase. Osteogenic cell proliferation lifts the fibrous layer of the periosteum from the bone and, somewhat more slowly, the osteogenic cells of the bone marrow cavity also proliferate (Fig. 60.1C). This proliferation gradually forms a collar, or callus, around the fracture line, which usually takes place in 2–4 weeks, but radiographic evidence of external callus formation may not appear until 3–6 weeks. A bone scan usually reveals increased metabolic activity shortly after the fracture and before the callus can be seen on a radiograph (McRae, 2008).

The remodeling phase starts during proliferation as the osteogenic cells begin to differentiate into osteoblasts, which start to form bony trabeculae that bridge the living and dead bone across the fracture line (Fig. 60.1D). Some of the osteogenic cells differentiate into chrondrocytes and form cartilage in the fracture callus, which eventually calcifies, becoming bone. Osteoclasts gradually remove the necrotic bone at the fracture site. The callus, consisting mostly of cancellous bone that has now formed across the fracture site, is fusiform. The cancellous bone is slowly remodeled into compact bone and, finally, the original fracture line is no longer discernible.

FRACTURE REPAIR IN THE AGING INDIVIDUAL

The rate of fracture repair in the aging patient should always be considered to be similar to that of a younger person with early callus formation in 2–4 weeks and bony bridging over the fracture in 6 weeks, as shown on radiographs. However, a host of factors such as degranulating platelets, cytokines, transforming factor-beta, interleukins 1 and 6, prostaglandin E_2 and tumor necrosis factor alpha (Borelli et al., 2012), are crucial to this normal progression. Osteoporotic bone may not heal as well as bone with normal tissue density. The inflammatory response to the injury and the blood supply may be inadequate, and failure to immobilize the fracture site also delays the healing process. Morphogenetic proteins and growth factors in fracture healing and adequate nutrition are crucial. Diabetes and hypovitaminosis, especially vitamins D and C, have deleterious effects on bone repair. Polytrauma, chronic inflammation (Borelli et al., 2012), overall health or frailty as well as impaired cognition can also delay the healing process (see Chapter 18).

In the case of open reduction and internal fixation of a fracture, there is greater risk of further bone injury, called a stress riser, due to the orthopedic hardware. The use of screws and plates may weaken or pull out from bone that is already osteopenic.

SPECIAL FRACTURES IN THE ELDERLY

Not all fractures in the elderly are considered to be complete fractures. Stress fractures, also referred to as insufficiency fractures, occur in areas of repeated trauma when bone remodeling is insufficient to repair the stresses of repetitive loading. Clinically, this is a particular concern when treating a patient who is at risk for increased bone fragility. Orthopedic internal fixation devices can become stress risers and cause increased loosening at the bone–appliance interface (Kim et al., 2011). People with spinal cord injury who have been fitted with a new orthotic device may develop stress fractures due to new movement abilities. The sedentary and overweight elderly, especially with low vitamin D (Breer et al., 2012), are at risk when they start new, strenuous physical activities. Physically, these patients will present with pain, swelling and warmth. Stress fractures or pseudofractures may arise in bone that has faulty mineralization, which is associated with inadequate repair of microtraumas.

Microfractures of the bony trabeculae have been demonstrated. The proclivity of these microfractures to cause pain is unclear. However, they may progress and lead to the silent fractures that are recognized on radiograph but may be old fractures. Despite the radiograph evidence of fracture, a patient can be unaware of having experienced any frank trauma – hence the term 'silent fracture'. This may be one of the causes of the lumbar kyphosis that is seen in some individuals who spend excessive amounts of time sitting.

Occult fractures, also referred to as insufficiency fractures, are best diagnosed with bone scan or magnetic resonance imaging (MRI). This type of fracture is usually intramedullary and undisplaced, and frequently occurs as a result of some minor or major trauma, but radiograph examination is negative. Typically, occult fractures occur in the proximal femur or humerus after a fall, but they have also been reported in the sacrum, acetabulum, calcaneus, tibia and spine. Quickly these patients present with moderate to severe pain and tenderness. There is a concomitant reduction in range of motion and strength and, if in the femur, there is a marked antalgic gait. In nursing and rehabilitation this type of fracture should be treated seriously even if it has not been confirmed on initial radiograph. If pushed too aggressively, complete disruption of bone may occur. Protected ambulation with a walker is requisite while the femoral or pelvic occult fracture heals.

A pathological fracture results from primary or metastatic malignant tumors in bone. These types of fractures usually present as pain without any reported history of trauma; however, at times, metastatic bone disease is found in a patient who is being radiographed because of trauma. Significantly, these patients complain of increased pain at night and of being awakened by the pain. The pain frequently increases with bedrest and the severity increases with time. Those presenting with primary tumors of the breast, prostate, thyroid, kidney, or other organs should be suspected of having metastatic disease if pain complaints fit these descriptions. Standard radiographs are helpful for specific bony sites; however, for diffuse bone metastasis, a nuclear medicine bone scan may be important for a total skeletal evaluation (see Chapter 14).

FUTURE METHODS OF PROMOTING FRACTURE HEALING

As stated above, natural fracture repair in the elderly may not proceed in precisely the same pattern as repair proceeds in younger individuals. However, several medical and physical methods for enhancing bone repair are being investigated. A number of factors have been found that influence fracture repair, including fibroblast growth factor, platelet-derived growth factor, transforming growth factor 13 and bone morphogenic protein. Insulin-like growth factor may stimulate fibroblast proliferation (Glass et al., 2011; Borelli et al., 2012).

Ceramic composites of calcium phosphate have been used for bone grafts. Electrical stimulation and ultrasound at specific parameters are two physical modalities that are currently being used to promote fracture healing. Fracture treatment in the future is likely to involve active intervention to promote healing and thereby reduce morbidity.

THERAPEUTIC INTERVENTIONS

OSTEOPOROSIS-RELATED FRACTURES

Osteoporosis is caused by increased action of osteoclasts (cells that absorb bone) or decreased action of osteoblasts (cells that lay down bone). It affects cancellous (trabecular) bone more than cortical bone. The areas of the human skeleton that are most likely to fracture as a result of osteo-porosis are neck of the femur, vertebral bodies, humerus and wrist (WHO, 2007). A vertebral compression fracture (VCF) is common in an individual with osteoporosis, and it is often the first indication that a person has osteopo-rosis. Estrogen is protective of bone and prevents osteo-porosis, whereas long-term steroid use has the effect of weakening the bone and increasing osteoporosis. Weight-bearing exercise has been shown to be protective of bone strength, and is associated with decreased bone resorp-tion and increased osteogenesis (Kemmler et al., 2013). Postmenopausal women in Western culture are at the highest risk (see Chapters 18 and 57 for further discussion of this subject).

Treatment of someone with an osteoporosis-related fracture consists of promoting healing, preventing defor-mity and facilitating the individual's return to full func-tioning. This type of fracture should not be viewed as an isolated event. It is usually the harbinger of future frac-tures. Thus, prevention of future fractures should be part of the treatment plan (Eisman et al., 2012). In working with a patient who has had a compression fracture, the nurse or therapist should screen carefully for any signs of neurological compromise. By definition, compression fractures do not involve the posterior portion of the ver-tebral body and so do not involve a risk of protrusion of fractured bone into the spinal canal. If neurological signs are present, the client should be referred for stud-ies to determine the presence of burst fracture or fracture dislocation.

PHARMACOLOGICAL INTERVENTIONS TO PROMOTE HEALING

Persons with osteoporotic fractures are likely to be given medications to reduce risk of future fractures. These include bisphosphonates, estrogen, estrogen agonist/antagonist (formerly SERMs), parathyroid hormone, cal-citonin and denosaumab. Strontium renelate is available in Europe but not in the United States of America. These medications may exhibit some potential negative effects and there are reports of jaw osteonecrosis and atypical femoral shaft fractures associated with bisphosphonate use. Bisphosphonates inhibit bone resorption and may cause impaired bone formation which is then responsi-ble for these unusual fractures (Rizzoli et al., 2011).

The nurse or therapist treating someone who is taking bisphosphonates may assist by ensuring that these medi-cations are being taken correctly. They must be taken on an empty stomach with 8 fluid ounces (236.6ml) of water. The individual should be upright after ingestion and should wait 30 minutes before eating. The side-effects of gastrointestinal upset may be worsened if these guidelines are not followed. Another medication that inhibits bone resorption is salmon calcitonin, which is either injected or used as a nasal spray. It may be given to those who cannot take any of the above medications.

PAIN MANAGEMENT

An individual with a vertebral compression fracture (VCF) is likely to have pain with movement and might need instruction in log-rolling (moving with no trunk rotation while rolling). The use of a neoprene lumbosa-cral corset with gel-foam lumbar support, clavicle strap, Spinomed (Pfeifer et al., 2004) or Jewett brace may pre-vent extraneous motion and facilitate mechanically sound trunk muscle use to minimize pain. In our experi-ence, modalities such as gentle manual therapy, postural taping (Bennell et al., 2010), cold, heat and pulsed ultra-sound with high-voltage galvanic electric stimulation are effective in reducing pain during the 6-week acute heal-ing phase (see Chapters 67 and 68). Caregivers also need to be instructed in safe transfers using the pelvis for contact guarding rather than putting any compression through the trunk. They also need to be made aware of bed and chair positioning with spinal alignment such that lumbar lordosis is supported and forward head with kyphotic posture minimized.

Water exercises can be done, as the buoyancy of water provides a comfortable, gravity-free environment, but the client must eventually transition to a land-based program in order to develop strength and polish the skills necessary to live in a gravitational environment (see Chapter 73).

PREVENTION OF FURTHER INJURY

Although the effects of a diet change on bone strength will take longer to be seen, the individual who has suf-fered a fracture may be amenable to changes in diet that will help to prevent future fractures. Referral to a reg-istered dietician is indicated (see Table 60.1 for recom-mended intake for calcium and Table 60.2 for vitamin D) and further information about diet, calcium and patient education can be found in Chapter 18).

All possible measures should be taken to prevent additional fractures and, above all, to avoid falling. A full balance evaluation and then interventions (see Chapters 15, 58 and 59) based upon identified impair-ments need to be implemented as soon as the person is ambulatory. The environment should be inspected for and cleared of fall hazards. A gradual resumption of mobility is necessary to prevent other medical complica-tions such as pneumonia. Indeed, the person should be encouraged to slowly increase his or her participation in the activities of daily living.

At that point, useful instruction must include a dem-onstration of how to perform activities without flex-ing the trunk. Sitting and forward flexion have been shown to increase intervertebral disc pressure and risk of fracture (Sinaki et al., 2002), so these postures are to be avoided. As the individual begins to tolerate sitting, the use of a lumbar support will help to achieve some measure of lordosis in the lumbar spine. A person with a VCF may be given a walker to assist in ambulation, but a four-legged, or pick-up, walker can place strain on the back because the individual must lean forward slightly to reach it, and then must lift it, which puts a great deal of pressure on the intervertebral discs and vertebral bodies. A four-wheeled walker with hand-brakes and a folding seat provides the biomechanical protection nec-essary for the patient with a healing vertebral compres-sion fracture (Shipp, 2009). A walker with front wheels

Table 60.1   Recommended dietary allowance (RDA) for calcium

Age	Male	Female	Pregnant	Lactating
0–6 months[a]	200 mg	200 mg		
7–12 months[a]	260 mg	260 mg		
1–3 years	700 mg	700 mg		
4–8 years	1000 mg	1000 mg		
9–13 years	1300 mg	1300 mg		
14–18 years	1300 mg	1300 mg	1300 mg	1300 mg
19–50 years	1000 mg	1000 mg	1000 mg	1000 mg
51–70 years	1000 mg	1200 mg		
71+ years	1200 mg	1200 mg		

Source: http://ods.od.nih.gov/factsheets/Calcium-HealthProfessional/.
Recommended dietary allowances (RDAs) for calcium
[a]Adequate intake (AI)

Table 60.2   Recommended dietary allowance (RDA) for Vitamin D

Age	Male	Female	Pregnancy	Lactation
0–12 months[a]	400 IU (10 µg)	400 IU (10 µg)		
1–13 years	600 IU (15 µg)	600 IU (15 µg)		
14–18 years	600 IU (15 µg)	600 IU (15 µg)	600 IU (15 µg)	600 IU (15 µg)
19–50 years	600 IU (15 µg)	600 IU (15 µg)	600 IU (15 µg)	600 IU (15 µg)
51–70 years	600 IU (15 µg)	600 IU (15 µg)		
>70 years	800 IU (20 µg)	800 IU (20 µg)		

Source: http://ods.od.nih.gov/factsheets/VitaminD-HealthProfessional/.
[a]Adequate intake (AI)

does not completely solve this problem, as the individual still has to lift the walker for turns and for backing up.

Clinical experience shows that an individual with a history of VCFs remains in a forward-flexed posture as a consequence of using a standard walker. The neurological system, particularly the vestibular system, learns that the 'normal' walking posture involves a forward-flexed trunk. Skeletal muscle lengths may change too, and contribute further to this new 'normal' posture. The person never experiences a truly upright posture and loses control of posterior sway, becoming fearful of standing up straight.

One means of preventing this problem is to have the individual work on exploring his or her limits of posterior stability (see Chapter 59) while standing in a place perceived as providing protection from a backwards fall. The most useful exercises include wide-based squats at a sink counter, or wall slides, in which the person stands with his or her back to a wall, hands lightly on the walker, and moves up and down or side-to-side. Progress can be made toward requiring less and less support from the wall and from the walker. Another helpful exercise is 'wall arches', in which the person faces the wall and reaches upward, by sliding their hands up in front of themselves (see Fig. 60.3 below). Wall slides, in which the person stands with his or her back to a wall, hands

lightly on the walker, and moves up and down and side-to-side, are also very useful. Progress can be made toward requiring less and less support from the wall and from the walker. When the person is ready to progress to trunk-strengthening activities, it is of paramount importance that the clinician understands the importance of maintaining spine neutral position for any abdominal exercises. A striking example of this was demonstrated in a retrospective study in which VCF subjects were divided according to the exercise regimen prescribed by their physician. Those who were prescribed extension exercises had a 16% incidence of new fractures, whereas those who were prescribed spinal flexion exercises (i.e. crunches) had an 89% incidence of new fractures. Fifty-three percent of those who were prescribed combined flexion and extension exercises had new fractures, and 67% of those who were prescribed no exercise at all had new VCFs (Sinaki & Mikkelsen, 1984).

PREVENTION OF FURTHER DEFORMITY

It is important for clinicians to carefully track the degree of spinal deformity when assessing progress and designing an effective exercise program both for individuals recovering from vertebral compression fractures and also for those with risk factors for further vertebral fractures.

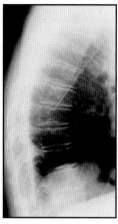
T7 vertebral height loss
with initial fracture

A

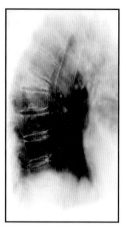
T7 vertebral compression
refracture

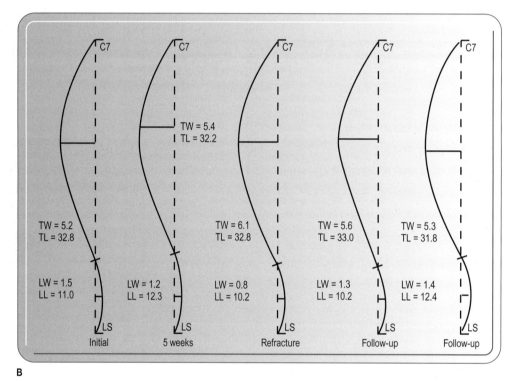

B

Figure 60.2 A 62-year-old woman with osteoporotic vertebral compression fracture, reinjury and recovery. **(A)** Lateral spinal radiographs for a 62-year-old woman with osteoporosis before and after her T7 vertebral refracture (right). **(B)** Flexicurve kypholordosis tracings during her rehabilitation at initiation, 5-week re-examination, immediately post refracture (coinciding with second radiograph), and at two more examinations throughout her rehabilitation. TW = thoracic width (cm); TL = thoracic length; LW = lumbar width; LL = lumbar length. Notice that her kyphosis increased noticeably after the second fracture, and diminished by the time of discharge. *(Reproduced with permission. Carleen Lindsey, PT, MS, GCS 2006.)*

Flexicurve ruler tracings, kyphometer measurement and lateral radiographs have all been shown to be reliable methods for tracking kypholordosis alignment (Greendale et al., 2011). Radiographs of a T7 vertebral compression fracture and subsequent refracture are shown in Figure 60.2A. Flexicurve tracings taken during rehabilitation of the same patient are shown in Figure 60.2B. This visual representation of spinal alignment can also serve as motivational feedback for patients during treatment.

During rehabilitation after a VCF, it is vital to strengthen muscles that have become weak from disuse.

Particular attention should be paid to exercises that encourage extension and upright posture. Of course, consideration must be given, during exercise programs, to restoring the length of tightened muscles and concurrently developing strength in them to provide the necessary stability. It is well documented that contracted muscles require strengthening exercises after they have been stretched, or weakness and instability will prevail in that area.

Various studies that have investigated methods of improving BMD have shown that weight-bearing

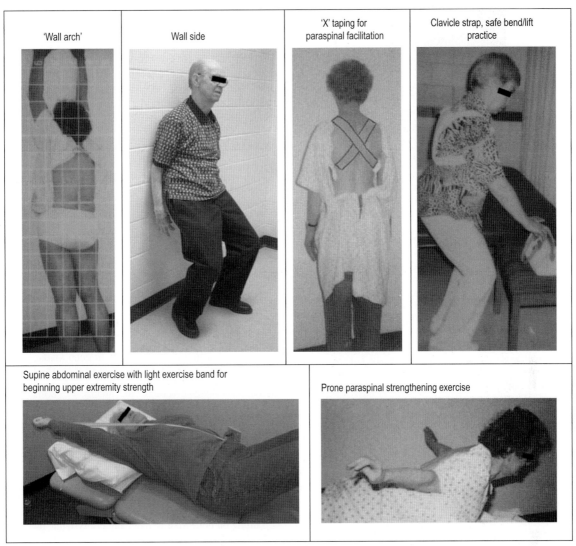

Figure 60.3 Exercises and postural protection for postvertebral compression fracture patients. *(Reproduced with permission. Carleen Lindsey, PT, MS, GCS 2006.)*

exercises improve BMD in the lower extremities and the spine, and weight-training exercises, which include upper and lower extremity resisted exercises, improve BMD in the upper extremities as well as in the spine and lower extremities (Gomez-Cabello et al., 2012; Kemmler et al., 2013). Many studies have also demonstrated that trunk extension exercise is a valuable tool not only for kyphotic deformity prevention but also for limiting spinal bone loss over time (Sinaki et al., 2002). Some abdominal and paraspinal strengthening exercises are included in Figure 60.3. Certain yoga postures may be too extreme and potentially harmful for osteoporotic spines (Sinaki, 2012).

Exercises should be instituted even with people who are not ambulatory because of the positive effects that exercise has on bones. For individuals who are attempting to regain mobility after an episode of bedrest necessitated by an osteoporotic fracture, balance exercises that address the individual's specific impairments and unique needs are necessary. Some generic exercises are included in Box 60.2. They are helpful as general exercises for middle-aged and older people, but it is important to

remember the necessity of tailoring an exercise routine to the idiosyncrasies of the individual.

VERTEBROPLASTY AND KYPHOPLASTY

Kyphoplasty and vertebroplasty (PVP) provide pain relief and functional recovery as measured by the Oswestry Disability Index but there is risk for cement leakage and subsequent fractures, with occurrence nearly the same for both procedures (Han et al., 2011). Klazen et al. (2010) reported no statistical significance for new vertebral fractures at 11.4 months follow-up comparing vertebroplasty with conservative care. The median time before refracture for patients treated with physical therapy including back-strengthening exercises (ROPE) was 60.4 months; for patients treated with PVP, only 4.5 months; and for patients treated with PVP-ROPE, 20.4 months (Huntoon et al., 2008). The results of this study support use of spinal extension exercise and body mechanics training with VCF patients, whether or not they have surgical intervention. A back exercise program after PVP demonstrated significantly better results

Box 60.2 *Exercises for people 55 years old and older*

These exercises are to be gradually increased. Work at your own pace and level of ability. Start with 5 or 10 repetitions and do fewer if you must or more if you can. Slowly increase, by adding two to four or more repetitions every 5–10 days. Progress until you can do approximately 15–25 repetitions of each exercise. Do these exercises at least 3 times a week.

1. *High step:* Hold on to a chair for balance; stand up straight. Raise one foot off the floor so that your knee is as high as your hip. Reverse legs. Try not to lean on the chair too much. As you get stronger, you may be able to raise your leg higher, hold for a count of 5 (less if necessary), and decrease the amount of leaning on the chair. *Purpose*: to increase hip and leg strength and balance.
2. *Side step:* Hold on to a chair for balance; stand up straight. Move one leg out to your side and hold it in the air. Don't bend at the waist. Hold leg up for 5 seconds, or less if necessary. Reverse legs. At first, you may be unable to hold your leg in the air. If so, simply move your foot out to the side. *Purpose*: to increase hip and leg strength and balance.
3. *Stand up–sit down:* This is the key to being independent. Simply stand up, then sit down. To do this, you must get your feet under the front of the chair. Move your center of gravity forward and then up. If necessary, use the chair's arm rest. As you get stronger, decrease the amount of push that you need from your arms. *Purpose*: to improve strength, balance, coordination, and joint motion.
4. *Shoulder shrug:* Sit up or stand up straight. Shrug your shoulders up high and release. Pull your shoulders back. You should feel your shoulder blades pull together. *Purpose*: to strengthen back, stretch chest muscles, and improve posture.
5. *Cervical range of motion:* Sit up or stand up, head erect but not forward. Turn your chin to your left shoulder, then reverse to the right. Lean your ear to your left shoulder, then reverse to the right. Lightly place your finger on your chin and push your chin back. Do not roll your head back as if looking up at the ceiling. *Purpose*: to improve posture, balance, and range of motion.
6. *Walk, walk, walk:* Walk at whatever level of ability you have. If you can walk only 50 feet, start at that level and try to increase the distance and improve your gait speed. Avoid stops and starts. If you are walking longer distances, such as half a mile or longer in 5–10 minutes, do a little stretching before starting. When finishing your walk, cool down by simply walking slowly, stretching and doing a few of these exercises or your favorite ones. *Purpose*: to enhance overall health of muscles, bones, joints, circulation, heart, lungs, digestion, bowels and mind

If you need help getting started or if you have any concerns about your health, show these exercises to your physician.

Reprinted with permission from Kauffman T 1987 Posture and age. Top Geriatr Rehabil 2:13–28. © Aspen Publishers Inc., New York.

at 1 and 2 years on the visual analog pain scale and on the Oswestry Disability Index (Chen et al., 2011). See Chapter 18 for further discussion.

CONCLUSION

Fractures are major problems for aging people and, in the great majority of cases, rehabilitation is a necessary follow-up. Understanding normal fracture healing and the possible factors that alter it will assist in the provision of optimal care. Special fractures such as the occult and insufficiency fractures and also metastatic lesions are requisite considerations in geriatric rehabilitation. Proper therapeutic exercise, balance and gait training, pain control and prevention of further injury facilitate rehabilitation and enable the patient to attain as high a quality of life as is possible.

REFERENCES

Bennell KL, Matthews B, Greig A et al 2010 Effects of an exercise and manual therapy program on physical impairments, function and quality-of-life in people with osteoporotic vertebral fracture: a randomised, single-blind controlled pilot trial. BMC Musculoskelet Disord 11:36

Borelli J, Pape C, Hak D et al 2012 Physiological challenges of bone repair. J Orthop Trauma 26:708–711

Breer S, Krause M, Marshall R et al 2012 Stress fractures in elderly patients. Int Orthop 36:2581–2587

Chen B, Zhong Y, Huang Y et al 2011 Systematic back muscle exercise after percutaneous vertebroplasty for spinal osteoporotic compression fracture patients: a randomized controlled trial. Clin Rehabil 26:483–492

Eisman J, Bogoch E, Dell R et al 2012 Making the first fracture the last fracture: ASBMR task force on secondary fracture prevention. J Bone Min Res 27:2039–2046

Garnero P, Hausherr E, Chapuy M et al 2009 Markers of bone resorprtion predict hip fracture in elderly women: the EPIDOS prospective study. J Bone Min Res 11:1351–1358

Gerhart TN 1995 Fractures. In: Adams W, Beers M, Berkow R (eds) Merck Manual of Geriatrics, 2nd edn. Merck & Co. Inc., Whitehouse Station, NJ, pp. 69–84

Glass G, Chan J, Freiden A et al 2011 TNF-alpha promotes fracture by augmenting the recruitment and differentiation of muscle-derived stromal cells. Proc Nat Acad Sci USA 25:1585–1590

Greendale GA, Nili NS, Huang MH 2011 The reliability and validity of three non-radiological measures of thoracic kyphosis and their relations to the standing radiological Cobb angle. Osteoporos Int 22(6):1897–1905

Gomez-Cabello A, Gonzalez-Aguero A, Casajus JA et al 2012 Effects of training on bone mass in older adults a systemic review. Sports Med 42:301–325

Han S, Wan S, Ning L et al 2011 Percutaneous vertebroplasty versus balloon kyphoplasty for treatment of osteoporotic vertebral compression fracture: a meta-analysis of randomised and non-randomised controlled trials. Int Orthop 35:1349–1358

Huntoon EA, Schmidt CK, Sinaki M 2008 Significantly fewer refractures after vertebroplasty in patients who engage in back-extensor-strengthening exercises. Mayo Clin Proc 83(1):54–57

Kemmler W, Häberle L, von Stengel S 2013 Effects of exercise on fracture reduction in older adults a systematic review and meta-analysis. Osteoporos Int 24(7):1937–1950

Kim D, Tantorski M, Shaw J et al 2011 Occult spinous process fractures associated with interspinous process spacers. Spine 36:1080–1085

Klazen C, Venman A, de Vries J et al 2010 Percutaneous vertebroplasty is not a risk factor for new osteoporotic compression fractures: results from VERTOS II. AJNR Am J Neuroradiol 31:1447–1450

Leslie W, Lix L, Finlayson G et al 2013 Direct costs for 5 years post-fracture in Canada. Osteoporos Int 24(5):1697–1705

Levis S, Theodore G 2012 Summary of AHRQ's comparative effectiveness review of treatment to prevent fractures in men and women with low bone density of osteoporosis: update of the 2007 report. J Manag Care Pharm 18(4b):S3–S15

McRae R 2008 Practical Fracture Treatment, 5th edn. Churchill Livingstone, New York, p 19

Morrison A, Fan T, Sen S et al 2013 Epidemiology of falls and osteoporotic fractures: a systematic review. Clinicoecon Outcomes Res 5:9–18

Pfeifer M, Begerow B, Minne HW 2004 Effects of a new spinal orthosis on posture, trunk strength, and quality of life in women with postmenopausal osteoporosis: a randomized trial. Am J Phys Med Rehabil 83(3):177–186

Rizzoli R, Akesson K, Bouxsein M et al 2011 Subtrocanteric fractures after long-term treatment with bisphosphonates: a European Society on Economic Aspects of Osteoporosis and Osteoarthritis, and International Osteoporosis Foundation Working Group Report. Osteoporos Int 22:373–390

Sanyal A, Gupta A, Bayraktar H et al 2012 Shear strength behavior of human trabecular bone. J Biomech 11:2513–2519

Shipp KM 2009 Physical therapy management of acute vertebral fracture. American Physical Therapy Association Combined Sections Meeting. Las Vegas, NV: APTA

Sinaki M 2012 Exercise for patients with osteoporosis: management of vertebral compression fractures and trunk strengthening for fall prevention. PM R 4:882–888

Sinaki M, Mikkelsen BA 1984 Postmenopausal spinal osteoporosis: flexion versus extension exercises. Arch Phys Med Rehabil 65:593–596

Sinaki M, Itoi E, Wahner HW et al 2002 Stronger back muscles reduce the incidence of vertebral fractures: a prospective 10 year follow-up of postmenopausal women. Bone 30:836–841

WHO 2007 Scientific Group on the Assessment of Osteoporosis at Primary Health Care Level. WHO, Geneva

Chapter 61

Contractures and stiffness

MARK LOMBARDI

CHAPTER CONTENTS

How can we explain the aging of a system built of non-aging elements?

LEONID AND NATALIA GAVRILOVA,
HANDBOOK OF THE BIOLOGY OF AGING (2006, P 9)

INTRODUCTION

Stiffness, or the loss of joint mobility, is a common complaint of sedentary and elderly patients. Stiffness limits numerous functional activities in the daily life of an elderly individual by interfering with the initiation and completion of movement patterns. Decreased activity increases the incidence of frailty (Wilson, 2004). Frail individuals are at a significantly greater risk for poor outcomes in rehabilitation, and have also been reported to have higher levels of markers related to inflammation and clotting than do non-frail individuals. Frail individuals are clinically identified from those individuals having three of the five attributes of frailty: unintentional weight loss, muscle weakness, slow walking speed, exhaustion and low physical activity (Wilson, 2004).

In the elderly, exudation of fibrinogen into extracellular tissue spaces increases with decreased levels of activity, so more fibrin, an elastic filamentous protein, tends to be deposited in the tissue spaces of older persons. Protein aggregation, while widely reported to be a common physiological feature of aging, is not clearly understood. If physical activity is not maintained a complete breakdown of fibrin may not occur, and increased amounts of sticky fibrin may accumulate in the tissue spaces, producing the lesions that restrict movement between adjacent structures. Fibrinous adhesions also form in a localized area following damage to tissues. These fibrinous adhesions, commonly referred to as 'cross-links', occur naturally during periods of immobilization or inactivity (Pickles, 1983).

In many cases, restoration of normal physical activity is sufficient to cause the breakdown of fibrous adhesions. In some cases, when the mass has become consolidated, it may be necessary to intervene with massage, PNF, stretching (using low-load sustained, passive over-pressure), graded mobilization or manipulation techniques under anesthesia.

COMMON CAUSES OF STIFFNESS

Traditionally, the clinician has accepted stiffness to be a natural part of the aging process, perhaps without identifying the actual causes, some of which may be prevented and/or treated. Four common causes of stiffness are:

- biomechanical changes in connective tissue and related structures
- hypokinesis (diminished or abnormally slow movement)
- arthritis (seen in both rheumatoid and osteoarthritis)
- trauma.

BIOMECHANICAL CHANGES IN CONNECTIVE TISSUE AND RELATED STRUCTURES

Changes in the numerous properties of connective tissue and related structures contribute to the onset of stiffness in the elderly; a select few are highlighted here.

Myofibroblasts

Connective tissue cells that produce unusually large amounts of contractile proteins are termed myofibroblasts. When damage occurs in connective tissue, there are two stages of response: cell multiplication and increased cellular secretion. If hyperplasia creates excessive production of actomyosin, the resulting contractile force may be significant enough to prevent normal range of motion in the affected area.

In addition, numerous studies describe the natural loss of muscle mass in the aged. Mayer et al. note that muscle strength decreases gradually between the third and fifth decade of life (Mayer et al., 2011: 359). They describe an 'accelerated, non-linear decrease of muscle mass up to 15% that has been shown to increase to as much as 30% by the 8th decade in sedentary geriatric patients'. Other studies (Watson, 2000; Brennan, 2002) report the rate of muscle mass loss to be more gradual, stating that losses of 3–5% are seen following the sixth decade of life. In their studies, Watson (2000) and Brennan (2002) also reported strength loss as high as 30% per decade after age 60.

Strength loss studies suggest that traditional aerobic and endurance training activities employed in rehabilitation, while effective in the reduction of coronary heart disease, may also contribute to positive changes in both muscle strength and bone density (Wallace & Cumming, 2000; Kean et al., 2004).

Mayer et al. (2011) cite several studies supporting these findings, suggesting that muscle mass may be increased with training intensities ranging from 60% to 85% of a patient's maximum voluntary strength (Mayer et al., 2011). In their research, Mayer et al. cite training effects having a positive effect on the maintenance of muscle strength through gains in muscle mass. Unfortunately, they also report compliance as clinicians' greatest obstacle, noting that current studies show that only 10–15% of the elderly participate in regular training sessions.

Collagen

Collagen is the main supportive protein in skin, tendon, bone, cartilage and connective tissue. A decrease in the elasticity of collagen and volume of ground substance is associated with the aging process. In addition, cross-linking between collagen fibers increases with age, inactivity and trauma, thereby restricting mobility of the connective tissue.

The decrease in ground substance creates a loss of critical interfiber distance which restricts the ability of the fibers to move smoothly over each other. With intervertebral disc disease of the spine, decreased collagen mobility may compromise not only spinal mobility, but also spine length. Changes in the length of the spine may also impair breathing patterns in the geriatric patient (Wilson, 2004).

Contractures, frequently the result of tight joint capsules, fibrotic or short muscles, or other scar tissues, are part fibrous adhesions and part collagenous shortening. Newly developed contractures have a greater portion of fibrinous adhesions, whereas chronic contractures are more collagenous. Normal activity may break down fibrinous adhesions, but collagenous shortening often requires heat, prolonged low-load progressive stretching and possible surgical manipulation.

Hyaluronic Acid

Hyaluronic acid is secreted from the hyaline (articular) cartilage that covers the surface of synovial joints. Compression of the joint enhances this secretion which entraps the synovial fluid among the hyaluronic acid molecules and lubricates the joint during movement. Secretion of hylauronic acid decreases with age, thus causing a diminution in the effectiveness of joint lubrication (Pickles, 1983). Another source of joint stiffness is said to occur as a result of 'articular gelling'. In healthy joints surface-active phospholipids (SAPL) inhibit the 'gelling' process (Hills & Thomas, 1998). What triggers the 'deactivation' of SAPL in the joint is not known.

Cartilage

Cartilage, having no direct blood supply of its own, receives its nutrients from the blood flow in adjacent bones and the synovial fluid in the joint cavity. Chondroblasts secrete a glycoprotein (chondroitin sulfate) into the surrounding matrix and, through osmosis, attract water containing dissolved gases, inorganic salts and other organic materials necessary for normal cartilage cell metabolism. Dehydration of the cartilage occurs with increasing age due to decreased secretion of chondroitin sulfate (Pickles, 1983). Normal loading and unloading of cartilage is necessary for the movement of nutrients in and out of the chondrocytes. Without joint compression, metabolites remain in the matrix and oxygen content is lowered, causing a reduction in glycoprotein secretion and an increase in the collagen precursor, procollagen. This process may convert hyaline cartilage to fibrocartilage. Degeneration of the cartilage is not reversible. However, further deleterious changes in the cartilage can be avoided through initiation of regular activities that promote alternating compression and expansion (relaxation) of the joint resulting in increased nutrition to the cartilaginous tissue.

HYPOKINESIS

Too little, or less than normal movement is termed hypokinesis. Joints or muscles left in a lengthened (extension) or shortened (flexion) state for prolonged periods may develop collagenous adhesions. To reduce the incidence of adhesions, physical activity several times during the day should be encouraged. Patient compliance is one major problem confronting clinicians' successful treatment of their patients (Watson, 2000; Brennan, 2002). Clinicians are encouraged to individualize patient programs, seeking movement patterns that the patient is comfortable with, and interested in, in an effort to increase patient compliance. Recommendations include identifying specific activities (sports, hobbies, life skills) that interest the patient when developing intervention strategies.

ARTHRITIS

Arthritis is reported to be the most common cause of disability in adults aged 18 and over (Kelley et al., 2011). The American Rheumatological Association (Wheeless, 2011) states that for a patient to be diagnosed with rheumatoid arthritis they must report at least 5 of the following 7 conditions or symptoms over a period greater than 6 weeks:

- morning stiffness
- pain on motion, or tenderness in at least one joint
- swelling (soft tissue thickening or fluid, not bony overgrowth alone) in at least one joint

- swelling of at least one other joint (any interval free of joint symptoms between the two joints)
- poor mucin precipitate from synovial fluid
- characteristic histologic changes in synovium
- characteristic histologic changes in nodules.

A recent finding by Kelley et al. states that there are over 46 million adults aged 18 and older reporting that they have a doctor-diagnosed form of arthritis (Kelley et al., 2011). Kelley cites a study by Hootman et al. predicting that this number will increase to more than 67 million by 2030 (Kelley et al., 2011). Arthritis is reported to be comprised of over 100 rheumatic diseases and conditions (Kelley et al., 2011). Currently, osteoarthritis (the most common form of arthritis) as well as systemic and rheumatic arthralgias are the most common causes of decreased flexibility or stiffness in the elderly (Burbank et al., 2002). Commonly identified arthritic areas involve the spine, knees, hips and distal interphalangeal joints of the hand. Complaints of stiffness may be attributed to acute synovitis, minute fragments of articular cartilage in the synovial fluid, inability of the joints to glide smoothly, muscle spasms, osteophytes at the joint margins, stretching of the periosteum, or muscle weakness secondary to disuse.

Polymyalgia rheumatica (PMR) (Dasgupta et al., 2012) is a common systemic arthritis seen in older adults. PMR is characterized by pain, weakness and stiffness in proximal muscle groups, along with swelling, fever, malaise, weight loss and a very rapid increase in the erythrocyte sedimentation rate. Polymyalgia rheumatica is often hard to diagnose given the absence of any specific laboratory test or inflammatory markers. Most primary and secondary providers rely on a corticosteroid response as a 'test of treatment' to establish their diagnosis (Dasgupta et al., 2012). The origin of a patient's complaint of pain is thought to be the result of stimulation of A delta mechanoreceptors and C polymodal nerve endings in the synovium and surrounding tissues (Kean et al., 2004). The most commonly affected areas of the body are the shoulders and hips. The neck, back and pelvis are other commonly cited areas of pain and stiffness. Corticosteroid therapy is effective in the acute phase (Wheeless, 2011). However, following this phase, graded soft tissue mobilization along with graded strengthening exercises may be helpful to the patient in restoring functional range of motion and improved joint nutrition.

TRAUMA

Trauma caused by a significant external force, repetitive internal or external microtrauma, or surgery can produce longstanding soft-tissue changes and scarring.

It is important to focus on how a particular trauma has affected the functional abilities of an elderly person. For example, have the biomechanics of an individual gait pattern been altered by trauma to the pelvic girdle? Decreased mobility of the pelvic girdle may limit the ability of the individual to propel the lower extremity during gait, to shift weight equally, to perform effective arm swing, and to maintain head, neck and trunk in alignment.

CONNECTIVE TISSUE AND STRETCHING TECHNIQUES

The unique qualities of deformation of connective tissues are referred to as viscoelastic properties ('viscous' refers to a permanent deformation characteristic and 'elastic' to a temporary deformation characteristic). The explanation of Cantu and Grodin (1992) is as follows:

- The elastic component of connective issue represents the temporary change when subjected to stretch (spring portion of model). The elastic component has a post-stretch recoil in which all the length or extensibility gained during stretch or mobilization is lost over a short period of time. The elastic component is not well understood but it is believed to be the 'slack' taken out of connective tissue fibers.
- The viscous (or plastic) component represents the permanent deformation characteristic of connective tissue. After a stretch or mobilization, part of the length or extensibility gained remains even after a period of time (hyaluronic cylinder portion of the model). There is no post-mobilization recoil or hysteresis in this component.
- If force is applied intermittently, as in progressive stretching, a progressive elongation may be achieved. If the stress is reapplied to the tissue, the curve looks identical, but starts from a new length. With each progressive stretch, the tissue has some gain in total length that is considered permanent.

In the clinical setting, the above description of the elastic versus viscous deformation is evidenced by range of motion that is measured before intervention, immediately after intervention and 1–2 days later when the patient returns for subsequent treatment. Although the patient may demonstrate an increase in the range of motion (the viscous portion) after intervention, part of that increased range may be lost from the elastic portion of the connective tissue by the time the patient returns for subsequent treatment. Repeated sessions along with an effective home exercise program should result in a overall increase in range of motion and improved function.

Connective tissue, like bone, responds to Wolff's law and adapts in the direction in which the stress is applied. Newly synthesized collagen will be laid down in the direction of the stress applied (Cantu & Grodin, 1992). Therefore, it is critical to focus on effective home exercise programs that enhance optimal postural and movement retraining. An important factor to consider when stretching the connective tissue of the elderly is that the tissue responds optimally to slow and prolonged stretching. The elderly individual requires a longer time to loosen the connective tissue because of changes in biomechanical properties such as decreased ground substance and collagen flexibility. Heating modalities that produce tissue temperatures in the 42.5–45.0°C range in conjunction with prolonged stretching have been shown to produce a residual lengthening of tendons. Collagen fibers have to be heated to 42.5°C or above and have continuous force applied to them for at least 30 minutes. Ultrasound (at 1 MHz with an intensity of 1.0 Watts/cm^2 for 10 minutes) may be used to raise tissue temperature (Johnson, 2010).

POSTURE, STIFFNESS AND MOBILITY

A common and often preventable postural change in the elderly is the forward-flexed posture. This posture exhibits varying degrees of forward-thrust head and shoulders, decreased chest and rib cage mobility, increased kyphosis, elevation of the first rib, decreased flexibility of hips and knees, and a shift in the center of gravity. Functionally, the individual has greater difficulty in performing sit-to-stand motions, walking on uneven services, turning, walking backwards and performing abrupt starts and stops. As posture changes over time, collagenous adhesions increase, with resultant joint structural deformities. Table 61.1 highlights areas where the elderly commonly report stiffness and discomfort that limit functional activities and movements.

PELVIC MOBILITY

Pelvic anterior/posterior tilts and diagonal motions should be assessed with the patient in side-lying, sitting and standing positions. If restrictions exist, identify the tissues involved and perform soft tissue mobilization and stretching techniques. Muscles commonly involved are the psoas major, the quadratus lumborum and the paraspinals. At the same time the therapist is releasing the restriction, the patient can be performing an active movement such as the pelvic tilt, which may assist the release. As in all the following examples, it is important to educate the patient in positions to improve functional movement patterns, as well as to formulate an individualized home exercise program with the patient's input.

TRUNK MOBILITY

Assess the patient's trunk mobility in supine, side-lying, sitting and standing positions. Identify any restrictions in the abdominal muscles, such as the rectus abdominus, internal or external oblique, the transverse abdominus, as well as the lumbar extensors, and combine various trunk motions performed actively by the patient with soft-tissue release techniques to the affected areas.

HIP MOBILITY

Assess the patient in all of the above positions with the patient performing hip motions actively as much as possible. Pay particular attention to restrictions in the gluteal muscles, the rectus portion of the quadriceps, the hip adductors, the tensor fascia latae and the iliotibial band.

KNEE MOBILITY

Assess the knee in the positions described above, focusing on the quadriceps, sartorius, hamstring, gastrocnemius and soleus muscles, as well as the mobility and tracking of the patellae. The hip, knee and ankle should be assessed in isolation as well as in combination, including the trunk and pelvis, because areas of stiffness may involve limitations in muscles and connective tissues that cross over two joints. A thorough examination requires that the patient be assessed in both non-weighted and weighted positions to assess the effects of gravity and balance on strength and muscle endurance.

ANKLE MOBILITY

In addition to assessing motions of the ankle, observe the position of the foot (pronation/supination) and restrictions in the talus/calcaneus and other bones of the foot, particularly in the standing position. Bressel reported preliminary data, from a study looking at ankle stiffness in a small population of stroke patients, and showed ankle stiffness decreases after both prolonged static and cyclic stretching (Bressel & McNair, 2002).

SHOULDER MOBILITY

Assess the shoulder in all the described positions, noting restrictions in the pectoralis major (noted cause of shoulder protraction) and minor (cause of scapula malposition), the rotator cuff muscles (looking for atrophy indicative of injury to the muscle or nerve), the long head of the triceps, the biceps (known source of pain in the shoulder) and the latissimus dorsi. Scapulohumeral and scapulothoracic motions should be evaluated for synchronicity of movement along with motions in the rib cage, sternum, acromioclavicular joint and clavicle.

HEAD AND NECK MOBILITY

Assess all motions and identify restrictions in the scaleni, upper trapezii, levator scapulae, sternocleidomastoids and paraspinals of the cervical area. It is highly recommended that the clinician exercise caution when hyperextending the cervical spine to avoid potential compromise of the vertebral artery in those patients with cervical spondylosis.

Table 61.1 **Areas of stiffness and discomfort and the muscles involved**	
Area of Stiffness and Discomfort	**Key Muscles Involved**
Pelvic girdle and trunk	Psoas, iliacus, quadratus lumborum
Hips	Rectus/hamstrings, internal/external rotators
Knees	Quadriceps, hamstrings
Ankles	Dorsi and plantar flexors, gastrocnemius, soleus, tibialis anterior, plantar fascia
Shoulders	Pectoralis major, pectoralis minor
Rib cage	Intercostals
Neck	Suboccipitals, scalene

RIB CAGE

Identify restrictions in the intercostal muscles, diaphragm and overall mobility of the rib cage. Stiffness or loss of flexibility of the thorax in the aging person can be partially reversed through soft-tissue mobilization and stretching techniques, movement re-education and specifically designed home programs that focus on posture, further resolving connective tissue restrictions. Great caution and individualized attention must be given to each patient because of a high risk for injury due to osteoarthritis, osteoporosis and soft-tissue changes. Improved posture facilitates movement patterns used in the completion of activities of daily living, such as transfers, bed mobility, balance, ambulation and other functional activities.

CONCLUSION

Stiffness, a frequent symptom in geriatric patients is caused by a variety of factors leading to functional declines in posture, mobility, balance, muscle strength and endurance resulting in frailty. Factors identified as contributing to stiffness may be mitigated by proper assessment, application of appropriate heating modalities, progressive therapeutic exercises and manual techniques. Regular slow, prolonged stretching is optimal to increase the length of connective tissues in the geriatric patient.

REFERENCES

Brennan FH 2002 Exercise prescription for active seniors. Phys Sportsmed 30(2):19–26

Bressel E, McNair PJ 2002 The effect of prolonged static and cyclic stretching on ankle joint stiffness, torque relaxation, and gait in people with stroke. Phys Ther 82(9):880–887

Burbank P, Reibe D, Padula CA 2002 Exercise and older adults: changing behavior with the transtheoretical model. Orth Nurs 21(4):51–63

Cantu RI, Grodin AJ 1992 Histology and biomechanics of myofascia. In: Cantu RI, Grodin AJ (eds) Myofascial Manipulation: Theory and Clinical Application. Aspen Publishers, Gaithersburg, MD

Dasgupta B, Cimmino M, Maradit-Kremers H 2012 Provisional classification criteria for polymyalgia rheumatica: a European League Against Rheumatism/American College of Rheumatology collaborative initiative. Ann Rheum Dis 71:484–492

Gavrilova L, Gavrilova N 2006 Reliability theory of aging and longevity. In: Masoro E, Austad S (eds) Handbook of the Biology of Aging, 6th edn. Elsevier, San Diego, CA, pp. 3–42

Hills BA, Thomas K 1998 Joint stiffness and 'articular gelling': inhibition of the fusion of articular surfaces by surfactant. Br J Rheumatol 37(5):532–538

Johnson GS 2010 Soft-tissue mobilization. In: Donatelli RA, Wooden MJ (eds) Orthopedic Physical Therapy, 4th edn. Churchill Livingstone, New York

Kean WF, Kean R, Buchanan WW 2004 Osteoarthritis: symptoms, signs and source of pain. Inflammopharmacology 12(1):3–31

Kelley G, Kelley K, Hootman J et al 2011 Effects of community-deliverable exercise on pain and physical function in adults with arthritis and other rheumatic diseases: a meta-analysis. Arthritis Care Res 63(1):79–93

Mayer F, Scharhag-Rosenberger F, Carlsohn A 2011 The intensity and effects of strength training in the elderly. Deutsch Arztebl Int 21:359–364

Pickles B 1983 Biological aspects of aging. In: Jackson O (ed) Physical Therapy of the Geriatric Patient. Churchill Livingstone, New York

Wallace BA, Cumming RG 2000 Systematic review of randomized trials of the effect of exercise on bone mass in pre- and postmenopausal women. Calcif Tissue Int 67(1):10–18

Watson C 2000 Aging and exercise: are they compatible in women? Clin Orthop Rel Res 372:151–158

Wheeless CR 2011 Wheeless' Textbook of Orthopaedics. [Online] www.wheelessonline.com

Wilson JF 2004 Frailty – and its dangerous effects – might be preventable. Ann Intern Med 6:489–492

Chapter 62

Fatigue

CAROLINE O'CONNELL • EMMA K. STOKES

CHAPTER CONTENTS

INTRODUCTION

Fatigue is hard to define. In the nineteenth century, Beard (1880) referred to fatigue as 'the Central Africa of medicine, an unexplored territory which few men enter'. Unfortunately, fatigue still remains a vague and difficult concept to define. Nevertheless, it is likely that most people will experience fatigue at one or more times in their lives. It can present in a multitude of ways, with a myriad of personal experiences and descriptions, such as mental exhaustion, lack of motivation, physical tiredness and weariness. Increasingly in the older population, fatigue is identified as having consequences both for quality of life and mortality.

FATIGUE: DEFINITIONS AND CONCEPTS

Fatigue is rarely a binary state, i.e. one has fatigue or one does not. At different times, everyone may experience levels of fatigue varying from mild to overwhelming. Within the concepts of fatigue, it is also important to consider a number of other descriptors of fatigue, namely normal, abnormal, peripheral, or central, in addition to the differing dimensions of fatigue. There is a clear distinction between *peripheral* and *central* fatigue. Peripheral fatigue is defined as a reduction in the maximal muscle force or motor output and is commonly due to overexertion, prolonged or strenuous physical activity. Central fatigue conversely refers to the general feeling often described as 'tiredness', 'weakness', 'languor', or 'sleepiness'. This may exist independently or may be due to some underlying psychological or pathological condition, as outlined in Table 62.1. It is accepted that 'normal' fatigue is a state of general tiredness that is the result of overexertion and can be ameliorated by rest. In contrast, 'abnormal' or 'pathologic' fatigue is a state characterized by weariness unrelated to previous exertion levels and is usually not ameliorated by rest. Both peripheral and central fatigue may exist in normal and abnormal states. This discussion focuses on this general tiredness and lack of motivation associated with central fatigue.

Ream and Richardson (1996), in a large-scale concept analysis review of fatigue literature, assimilated the pertinent information on fatigue in its various forms and proposed a clarified definition for the otherwise amorphous concept. The authors suggest 'fatigue is a subjective, unpleasant symptom which incorporates total body feelings ranging from tiredness to exhaustion creating an unrelenting overall condition which interferes with an individual's ability to function to their normal capacity'. Further searches for an adequate definition have added to this explanation and a review of these definitions by Yu et al. (2010) concluded simply that the overall fatigue experienced among older adults is a 'debilitating compromise of quality of life'. Following

Table 62.1	**Common conditions associated with fatigue**
Infections	Rheumatoid arthritis
Sequelae from neurological disorders	Depression
Autoimmune disorders	Lyme Disease, HIV/AIDS, Postpolio Syndrome
Malignancy	Head trauma, Parkinson's disease, stroke
Endocrine disorders	Multiple sclerosis, systemic lupus erythematosus
Hormonal imbalance	Cancer-related anemia, chemotherapy
Cardiac and pulmonary disorders	Thyroid disorders
Postoperative states	Pregnancy
Fibromyalgia	Obstructive sleep apnea, COPD, deconditioning

HIV, human immunodeficiency virus; AIDS, acquired immunodeficiency syndrome; COPD, chronic obstructive pulmonary disease

Box 62.1   *Concepts associated with fatigue*

Decreased mental and physical endurance
Decreased motivation
Depletion of reserves
Fatigability
Inability to rise to the occasion
When healthy, performance that is less that one's expectations
Lassitude

From Krupp, 2003.

a systematic search of the literature relating to fatigue among older people, they identified 15 relevant studies and 3 main aspects of reported fatigue: the lived experience of fatigue, relating factors of fatigue and impact of fatigue on overall health. They cautioned that the complexity of this phenomenon, in terms of its 'ubiquitous nature, heterogeneous etiologies, and multidimensional manifestation imposes real challenges to health professionals in managing this distressing symptom'.

Krupp (2003) suggests that the experience of fatigue reported by a patient may also be interpreted in different ways by different healthcare professionals – physiotherapists, oncologists, nurses, occupational therapists and neurologists. Nevertheless, she goes on to suggest that fatigue can be conceptualized in a number of different ways, included in Box 62.1. Fatigue is not one-dimensional; many authors report the importance of the various dimensions of fatigue. In designing an instrument to measure fatigue, Smets et al. (1995) identified five discernible dimensions of fatigue, which are general fatigue, physical fatigue, reduction in activity, reduction in motivation and mental fatigue.

FATIGUE IN LATER LIFE

Are we more likely to be fatigued when we are older? Does the type of fatigue experienced throughout the course of life change? Does fatigue matter in old age, are we 'supposed' to slow down?

The findings are contradictory: Beutel et al. (2004) observed, in a large sample of women, that all five dimensions of fatigue described above increased gradually over time. However, Watt et al. (2000), investigating the levels of fatigue in people aged 20–79 years in a population-based study, found that most dimensions of fatigue decreased with age among healthy people, compared with an increase with age in the group with disease. Older people living in long-term care facilities may experience more fatigue symptoms (Liao & Ferrell, 2000). In 2007, Wijeratne et al. reported that 27% of people over 60 attending a primary care setting reported fatigue, which they subsequently determined was largely independent of physical or psychological illness. Hence, all people, both ill and healthy alike, old and young, may experience fatigue. The likelihood of experiencing fatigue is increased in people suffering from a range of different medical conditions. These conditions are listed in Box 62.1, many of which can be more common in people over 65 years of age. It is probably more helpful

to focus on what self-reported fatigue or tiredness is associated with, or a predictor of, in later life.

What of the effect of this fatigue? Avlund et al. (1998) note that self-reported tiredness in functional mobility in people aged 70 years is strongly predictive of mortality during the following 10 years, even when disability at baseline is considered. This was echoed 10 years later in a study by Hardy and Studenski (2008) in which self-reported tiredness, as a measure of fatigue, was related to increased mortality over 10 years. The influence of fatigue was shown to be almost as great as that of diabetes or heart disease. The study assessed fatigue with the question 'during the past month, have you felt tired most of the time?' The authors acknowledge that this measure of fatigue may not encompass all aspects of the condition; however, it is a clinically useful and easy-to-administer method to gain an insight into fatigue. Avlund et al. (2002) also noted a predictive association between people aged 75 years who report tiredness in 4 lower limb activities and onset of disability in the following 5 years. This association exists even when other variables associated with onset of disability are considered in the analysis. In this sample, Avlund et al. (2001) also noted that men and women who self-reported tiredness in functional mobility at 75 years of age were twice as likely to be hospitalized in the year prior to follow-up, i.e. at 80 years, and were also more likely to use home help services. Fatigue was determined to be an early indicator of functional decline, as measured by a loss in walking speed, in a 5-year follow-up study of 292 adults aged 75 (Manty et al., 2012).

It is important to take seriously reports of tiredness or fatigue by older people. Hence, measuring fatigue or tiredness in older people and exploring the reasons for its presence are significant because its report may be an early marker of coexisting disease or a decrease in functional reserve. If present, early intervention may prevent functional decline and/or highlight the need for more substantive evaluation.

MEASURING FATIGUE

Owing to the elusiveness of a precise definition of fatigue in the literature, an individual's reported perception of his or her fatigue has become the focus of fatigue measurement. These self-report scales have therefore become widely used. They also have the advantage of being easily understandable by the patient and requiring little prior training by the assessor. They are usually short and readily available. Self-report measures have different structures, from simple unidimensional measures such as the Visual Analog Fatigue Scale (Glaus, 1993) to more complex measures encompassing the multidimensional nature of fatigue, such as the Multidimensional Fatigue Inventory (Smets et al., 1995). Debate continues as to the most useful tool to assess fatigue. The multidimensional measures capture the subtleties of the symptom, perhaps affording more sensitivity to change; however, they often benefit from the addition of a simple linear scale to quickly assess the patient's own evaluation of the impact of the symptom. Among the studies mentioned here, a range of

Table 62.2 **Instruments to measure fatigue**		
Name	Developed By	Populations Validated
Avlund Fatigue Scales	Avlund & Schultz-Larsen (1991)	Older population
Brief Fatigue Inventory	Mendoza et al. (1999)	Cancer patients, general population
Fatigue Assessment Instrument	Schwartz et al. (1993)	General population, various medical conditions
Fatigue Descriptive Scale	Iriarte et al. (1999)	Multiple sclerosis (MS)
Fatigue Impact Scale	Fisk et al. (1994)	General population, MS, hypertension patients
Fatigue Scale	Chalder et al. (1993)	General population
Fatigue Severity Scale	Krupp et al. (1989)	General population, MS, systemic lupus erythematosus, chronic fatigue syndrome, depression
Fatigue Symptom Inventory	Hann et al. (1998)	Cancer patients and general population
Iowa Fatigue Scale	Hartz et al. (2003)	General population, range of different coexisting medical conditions
Multidimensional Fatigue Inventory	Smets et al. (1995)	Radiotherapy patients, chronic fatigue syndrome, psychology and medical students, army recruits
Piper Fatigue Scale	Piper et al. (1989)	Cancer, general population, postpolio syndrome
Visual Analog Fatigue Scale	Glaus (1993)	Cancer and gastrointestinal disease patients, general population

self-report measurement tools have been utilized, from a simple polar question, as used by Hardy and Studenski (2008), to the six-point Avlund Mobility-Tiredness scale (Manty et al., 2012) and the popular Multidimensional Fatigue Inventory (Watt et al., 2000; Beutel et al., 2004), which is further explained below.

Table 62.2 contains some of the commonly used self-report scales, along with the populations in which they have been validated. One particular measure of value for use with older people is the Multidimensional Fatigue Inventory (MFI-20) (Smets et al., 1995). The Multidimensional Fatigue Inventory is a 20-item self-report instrument that acknowledges the comprehensive nature of fatigue. It divides fatigue into the following dimensions: general fatigue, physical fatigue, mental fatigue, reduced motivation and reduced activity. It has been validated in both healthy older people and those with a range of common conditions. The creators found the instrument to have good internal consistency and construct validity (Smets et al., 1995). The MFI-20 is copyrighted on the names of the authors and is reproduced here with permission (Form 62.1). The scoring system and conditions of use are available from Dr E.M.A. Smets, Medical Psychology Academic Medical Center, University of Amsterdam, PO Box 22660, 1100 DD, Amsterdam, The Netherlands, e-mail: e.m.smets@amc.uva.nl.

INTERVENTIONS FOR FATIGUE

To date, there exists no standardized intervention for fatigue. The treatment approaches taken depend largely on the suspected underlying pathology resulting in the fatigue. For example, people with anemia may notice an improvement in fatigue levels following iron supplementation, while it may be appropriate to prescribe medications and support for sleep apnea in other cases. Other pharmacologic interventions suggested for fatigue are insulin to control blood sugar and thyroxine to regulate thyroid function. The link between fatigue and depression may indicate that antidepressive treatment will ameliorate the effects of fatigue. Advice on nutritional support and correct dietary supplements has been demonstrated to reduce self-reported fatigue levels. Increasingly, exercise has been recommended for its role in increasing general fitness levels and thus reducing fatigue. This is supported by findings such as those of Manty et al. (2012) suggesting that fatigue may be an indicator of functional decline. It seems logical then that limiting functional decline may have a positive impact on fatigue. Liu and Latham (2009) note the benefits of physical exercise and resistance training for older people in terms of muscle strength and physical functioning, but the true effectiveness with fatigue is still uncertain. Avlund (2010) suggests that as fatigue is a result of multiple potentially modifiable factors, some of which may be treated or alleviated, a reduction in fatigue may have a resultant reduction in the speed of the aging process. Given the multifaceted nature of self-reported fatigue, clinicians face a challenge to manage the biomedical, physical and psychological perspectives of the condition, while remaining mindful of its close relationship with depression and chronic disease. The role of fatigue in predicting mortality suggests that effective management of fatigue, regardless of its bedfellows or causes, may have a very positive impact on increasing wellbeing into older age.

Instructions

By means of the following statements we would like to get an idea of how you have been feeling lately. There is, for example, the statement:

'I FEEL RELAXED'

If you think that this is entirely true, that indeed you have been feeling relaxed lately, please place an X in the extreme left box; like this:

yes, that is true [X| | |] no, that is not true

The more you disagree with the statement, the more you can place an X in the direction of 'no, that is not true'. Please do not miss out a statement and place one X next to each statement.

1.	I feel fit	yes, that is true	[| | |]	no, that is not true
2.	Physically I feel only able to do a little	yes, that is true	[| | |]	no, that is not true
3.	I feel very active	yes, that is true	[| | |]	no, that is not true
4.	I feel like doing all sorts of nice things	yes, that is true	[| | |]	no, that is not true
5.	I feel tired	yes, that is true	[| | |]	no, that is not true
6.	I think I do a lot in a day	yes, that is true	[| | |]	no, that is not true
7.	When I am doing something, I can keep my thoughts on it	yes, that is true	[| | |]	no, that is not true
8.	Physically I can take on a lot	yes, that is true	[| | |]	no, that is not true
9.	I dread having to do things	yes, that is true	[| | |]	no, that is not true
10.	I think I do very little in a day	yes, that is true	[| | |]	no, that is not true
11.	I can concentrate well	yes, that is true	[| | |]	no, that is not true
12.	I am rested	yes, that is true	[| | |]	no, that is not true
13.	It takes a lot of effort to concentrate on things	yes, that is true	[| | |]	no, that is not true
14.	Physically I feel I am in a bad condition	yes, that is true	[| | |]	no, that is not true
15.	I have a lot of plans	yes, that is true	[| | |]	no, that is not true
16.	I tire easily	yes, that is true	[| | |]	no, that is not true
17.	I get little done	yes, that is true	[| | |]	no, that is not true
18.	I don't feel like doing anything	yes, that is true	[| | |]	no, that is not true
19.	My thoughts easily wander	yes, that is true	[| | |]	no, that is not true
20.	Physically I feel I am in an excellent condition	yes, that is true	[| | |]	no, that is not true

Thank you very much for your cooperation.

© E. Smets, B. Garssen, B. Bonke. Reprinted with permission.

Form 62.1 The multidimensional fatigue inventory (MFI-20)

REFERENCES

Avlund K 2010 Fatigue in older adults: an early indicator of the aging process? Aging Clin Exp Res 22:100–115

Avlund K, Schultz-Larsen K 1991 What do 70 year old men and women actually do? And what are they able to do? From the Glostrup survey in 1984. Aging Clin Exp Res 3:39–49

Avlund K, Schultz-Larsen K, Davidsen M 1998 Tiredness in daily activities at age 70 as a predictor of mortality during the next 10 years. J Clin Epidemiol 51(4):323–333

Avlund K, Damsgaard MT, Schroll M 2001 Tiredness as a determinant of subsequent use of health and social services among nondisabled elderly people. J Aging Health 13(2):276–286

Avlund K, Damsgaard MT, Sakari-Rantala RI 2002 Tiredness in daily activities among nondisabled old people as a determinant of onset of disability. As a predictor of mortality during the next 10 years. J Clin Epidemiol 55:965–973

Beard G 1880 A Practical Treatise on Nervous Exhaustion (Neurasthenia): Its Symptoms, Nature, Sequences, Treatments. William Wood, New York

Beutel ME, Weidner K, Schwarz E et al 2004 Age-related complaints in women and their determinants based on a representative community study. Eur J Obstet Gynecol Reprod Biol 117:204–212

Chalder T, Berelowitz G, Pawlikowska J et al 1993 Development of a fatigue scale. J Psychosom Res 37:147–153

Fisk JD, Pontefract A, Ritvo PG et al 1994 The impact of fatigue on patients with multiple sclerosis. Can J Neurol Sci 21(1):9–14

Glaus A 1993 Assessment of fatigue in cancer and non-cancer patients and in healthy individuals. Support Care Cancer 1(6):305–315

Hann DM, Jacobsen PB, Axxarello LM et al 1998 Measurement of fatigue in cancer patients: development and validation of the fatigue symptom inventory. Qual Life Res 7:301–310

Hardy S, Studenski S 2008 Fatigue predicts mortality among older adults. J Am Geriatr Soc 56(10):1910–1914

Hartz A, Bentler S, Watson D 2003 Measuring fatigue severity in primary care patients. J Psychosom Res 54:515–521

Iriarte J, Katsamakis G, De Castro P 1999 The fatigue descriptive scale (FDS): a useful tool to evaluate fatigue in multiple sclerosis. Mult Scler 5(1):10–16

Krupp LB 2003 Fatigue. Elsevier Science, Philadelphia, PA

Krupp LB, LaRocca NG, Muir-Nash J et al 1989 The fatigue severity scale: application to patients with multiple sclerosis and systemic lupus erythematosus. Arch Neurol 46:1121–1123

Liao S, Ferrell BA 2000 Fatigue in an older population. J Am Geriatr Soc 48(4):426–430

Liu CJ, Latham NK 2009 Progressive resistance strength training for improving physical function in older adults. Cochrane Database Syst Rev 3:CD002759

Manty M, Mendes de Leon C, Rantanen T et al 2012 Mobility-related fatigue, walking speed and muscle strength in older people. J Gerontol A Biol Soc Med Sci 67A(5):523–529

Mendoza TR, Wang XS, Cleeland CS et al 1999 The rapid assessment of fatigue severity in cancer patients: use of the Brief Fatigue Inventory. Cancer 85(5):1186–1196

Piper BF, Lindsey AM, Dodd MJ et al 1989 The development of an instrument to measure the subjective dimension of fatigue. In: Funk SG, Tornquist EM, Champagne MT (eds) Key aspects of comfort: management of pain, fatigue, and nausea. Springer, New York, pp. 199–208

Ream E, Richardson A 1996 Fatigue: a concept analysis. Int J Nurs Stud 33(5):519–529

Schwartz JE, Jandorf L, Krupp LB 1993 The measurement of fatigue: a new instrument. J Psychosom Res 37:753–762

Smets EM, Garssen B, Bonke B et al 1995 The multi-dimensional fatigue inventory (MFI): psychometric qualities of an instrument to assess fatigue. J Psychos Res 39:315–325

Watt T, Groenvold M, Bjorner JB et al 2000 Fatigue in the Danish general population. Influence of sociodemographic factors and disease. J Epidemiol Commun Health 54:827–833

Wijeratne C, Hickie I, Brodaty H 2007 The characteristics of fatigue in an older primary care sample. J Psychosom Res 62:153–158

Yu D, Lee D, Wai Man N 2010 Fatigue among older people: a review of the research literature. Int J Nurs Stud 47:216–228

Chapter 63

The aging wrist and hand

KEVIN J. LAWRENCE

CHAPTER CONTENTS

INTRODUCTION

The wrist and hand are the most important components of the upper extremity. The shoulder, elbow and forearm are utilized to position the wrist and hand for function. Without the wrist and hand the upper extremity would be little more than a club. Hand function is dependent on the coordinated performance of the different tissues of the hand including skin, fingernails, bone, articular cartilage, muscle, tendon, ligament, nerve and vascular tissues. The aging process can have a degenerative effect on all of these tissues and therefore affect function of the wrist and hand. Additionally, certain disease processes and pathologies that affect the hand become much more common with aging.

The aging process can affect all of the tissues that make up the wrist and hand simultaneously. When combined with common pathologies associated with aging the overall effect on hand function can result in a major effect on an individual's ability to carry out normal functional activities of daily life (ADLs). This chapter aims to discuss the aging process as it affects the tissues that make up the wrist and hand and how the changes in these tissues effect function of the hand.

SKIN

There are a number of changes that occur in the skin of the hands of older adults. The layers of the skin, both dermis and epidermis, become thinner and less elastic. This effect is often most obvious on the dorsum of the hand (Watkins, 2011). The skin becomes more vulnerable to injury, especially with shear forces. When the skin of the hand of an older adult is injured it will tend to heal more slowly (Nazarko, 2005). Other conditions that can result in prolonged healing time of skin lesions include diabetes, hypertension, cardiac disease, a history of smoking and those who have had excessive exposure to the sun (Helfrich et al., 2008).

The effects of aging skin have been linked to changes that occur with collagen synthesis. The collagen in skin breaks down more readily and synthesizes less readily, resulting in thinner, more fragile skin. Long-term use of corticosteroids, especially topical corticosteroid use, can also lead to further collagen breakdown and thinning of the skin. These patients bruise very easily and their skin can become more prone to damage. This effect is often most evident on the skin of the dorsum of the hand and forearms.

FINGERNAILS

Fingernail growth diminishes with aging. Often fingernails will become thicker and rougher with a yellow discoloration. Fingernails will become more brittle and more prone to fungal infections (Carmeli et al., 2003). Certain changes in fingernails may be warning signs of underlying disease. Clubbing of the nails may be a sign of longstanding cardiopulmonary disease. Spoon shaped nails may be a sign of longstanding anemia. Beau's lines, deep grooved lines running across the nails may be a sign of past trauma, exposure to severe cold or malnutrition. Muehrcke's lines, white lines under the nail beds, may be a sign of renal disease. Pitting of the nails may be a sign of a connective tissue disorder (Fawcett et al., 2004).

BONE

The aging process of bone involves demineralization of the bone (see Chapters 3 and 18). Demineralization occurs in both males and females; however, this is especially true of elderly females. Demineralization in females has been linked to estrogen deficiency associated with menopause. Bone becomes less ductile and more brittle resulting in a higher incidence of fracture. Postmenopausal females, especially those over 65 years of age and those who have experienced previous fractures related to osteoporosis, are at a higher risk for experiencing future fractures (Tremollieres, 2012).

Any of the bones in the wrist and hand complex are at a greater risk to fracture due to trauma. The distal radius has been reported to be one of the most common fractures experienced by older adults (Obert, 2012). One of the most common ways to fall is forward, landing on an outstretched hand with the forearm in pronation and the wrist extended. Initial contact with the ground forces the scaphoid and lunate into the concave distal radius. This can result in the distal radius fracturing and the distal fragment displacing dorsally. This dorsal displacement is known as a Colles' fracture.

When the individual falls backwards they may impact the ground with the forearm in supination and the wrist in flexion. If the distal radius fractures the distal fragment will displace palmarly. This is known as a Smith's fracture. Both the Smith's and Colles' fractures may result in significant deformity depending on the amount of bone compression and displacement. Either may require surgical intervention and a prolonged period of immobilization. One of the most common complications of the injury is the involvement of the median nerve at or proximal to the carpal tunnel. This can affect median nerve sensation to the lateral four digits and weakness of thumb flexion, opposition and abduction. Diminished or lost sensation to these fingers makes it much more difficult for individuals to perform fine motor control activates and gives them a tendency to drop small objects.

Falling on an outstretched hand can also result in a fracture of the scaphoid, lunate, pisiform or hook of the hamate (Skirven et al., 2011). When the scaphoid fractures, it is often missed on initial radiographs. This can be especially true if the fracture is at the waist of the scaphoid. If this fracture is missed, it can lead to necrosis of the proximal portion resulting in severe wrist pain during upper extremity weight bearing activities, and diminished strength and range of motion. Fractures to the pisiform or hook of the hamate can result in ulnar nerve involvement resulting in diminished strength of pinch and grip.

ARTICULAR CARTILAGE

Articular cartilage is primarily made up of type 2 collagen. This type of collagen is rich in glycosaminoglycans (GAGS). GAGS are hydrophilic and give articular cartilage viscoelastic properties that aid in the ability of articular cartilage to tolerate compressive forces. As articular cartilage ages it tends to lose GAGS and therefore articular cartilage is less resistant to compressive forces (see Chapter 4). The loss of viscoelastic properties leads to articular cartilage breakdown resulting in osteoarthritis.

Osteoarthritis of the wrist and hand is a very common occurrence of the older adult. Stukstette et al. (2011) reported that elderly women (>70 years of age) are twice as likely to have symptomatic arthritic changes effecting the hand than elderly men. The most common joints of the wrist and hand to experience osteoarthritis are the radiocarpal joints, MCP joints, IP joints and the trapezium with the base of the first metacarpal. The DIP joints were the joints most frequently reported to cause pain and reported to be tender with palpation. Osteoarthritis of the DIP joints is often accompanied by the formation of Bouchard's nodes. Bouchard's nodes are calcific spurs that form around the periphery of the joints. Heberden's nodes are the name given to the same nodes that form around the periphery of the PIP joints (Slatkowsky-Christensen, 2010). Osteoarthritis can lead to a significant loss of hand function due to joint stiffness, pain and limited range of motion. Many will also experience diminished strength in the wrist and hand due to disuse atrophy.

Rheumatoid arthritis (RA) in the wrist and hand often affects the older adult. RA is a systemic autoimmune disease that can occur at any age and comes in multiple forms. The effects of RA in the elderly may be long standing or may be a form known as elderly onset rheumatoid arthritis. This form of RA occurs in individuals over the age of 60 and is estimated to comprise between 10% and 30% of all cases of RA (Olivieri et al., 2005). The effects of RA on the hand can range from mild to severe and include pain, swelling, limited range of motion, joint instability and deformity.

Ligaments, tendons and joint capsules are all made up of connective tissue that experiences changes with aging. As connective tissue ages there is an increase in cross links between collagen fibers and degeneration of elastin fibers (Avery & Bailey, 2005). The changes, known as the Maillard reaction, occur with articular cartilage, tendons, ligaments and joint capsules. The result is loss of flexibility, joint stiffness and diminished range of motion and significant loss of wrist and hand function. This process is accelerated in individuals with diabetes mellitus.

MUSCLE

A decrease in muscle strength has been well documented in the literature to occur with aging. The decrease in muscle strength has been attributed to a loss of muscle mass that occurs with aging (Newman et al., 2003; Goodpaster et al., 2006). Jansen et al. (2008) report that both grip and pinch strength decreased for both men and women after the age of 65. In the younger age groups men were found to have greater pinch and grip strength than women. But as age increases, men were found to have a greater decrease in strength. By the time both genders were in the oldest age group, above 85 years of age, the strength of grip and pinch of both genders was about equal (Jansen et al., 2008).

NERVE

Peripheral nerves that innervate the hand undergo significant changes with aging (see Chapter 32). Thakur et al. (2010) reported that both sensory and motor peripheral nerve function diminishes with aging. Sensory receptors are also affected with aging. Shaffer and Harrison (2007) report changes in the function of muscle spindles, Golgi tendon organs, cutaneous receptors and joint proprioceptors. Diminished function of all of these structures can have a significant effect on overall hand function.

Peripheral nerves are also much more likely to become entrapped with aging. The median nerve can become entrapped between the two heads of the pronator teres or at the carpal tunnel. The radial nerve can become entrapped between the two heads of the supinator and the ulna nerve at the elbow or at the tunnel of Guyon (Skirven et al., 2011). These entrapments become more common with aging due to the thickening that commonly occurs in the surrounding connective tissues.

Peripheral neuropathy is a problem of the older adult. Peripheral neuropathy is linked to diminished blood supply of the small blood vessels to myelin sheaths and axons of the most distal nerves of the upper and lower extremities. Peripheral nerve function to the hand can be especially affected for those older adults with diabetes mellitus or alcoholics (Gries et al., 2003). Peripheral neuropathy will affect all the nerves innervating the hand from distal to proximal. The first signs of peripheral neuropathy will be paresthesiae in the fingertips. The paresthesiae will spread proximally over time and can progress to anesthesia, resulting in complete loss of sensation in the area affected. Pain may also be a symptom of peripheral neuropathy to the hand. Often this pain is described as burning in nature. Motor changes with peripheral neuropathy will generally occur from distal to proximal regardless of the nerves involved. The initial result will be weakness of the intrinsic muscles of the hand. In severe cases there could be paralysis of the muscles of the hand resulting in a claw-hand deformity. These individuals will lack the ability to abduct their thumbs adequately to grab cylinder-shaped objects or to extend the IP joints on any of the four medial digits. They will experience weakness in all pinches and grips.

Peripheral neuropathy that affects the autonomic nervous system can affect peripheral blood flow to the hand. This can result in an individual's inability to adjust to changes in temperature and make it more likely to experience a burn at a lower than normal temperature or frostbite at a higher than normal temperature. Effects on the autonomic nervous system can result in anhydrosis leading to dry, cracked skin, which may result in infection.

CONCLUSION

When performing an examination of the hand of an older adult, no matter the primary pathology, the examiner must keep in mind all of these issues of aging. These effects can lead to greater loss of function of the hand than would be experienced with a specific injury or disease for a younger adult. It is essential to consider all aspects of the aging process in order to adequately assess the overall effect of any given pathology and to choose the best intervention for rehabilitation of the aging individual.

REFERENCES

Avery NC, Bailey AJ 2005 Enzymic and non-enzymic cross-linking mechanisms in relation to turnover of collagen: relevance to aging and exercise. Scand J Med Sci Sports 15:231–240

Carmeli E, Patish H, Coleman R 2003 The aging hand. J Gerontology 58A:146–152

Fawcett RS, Linford S, Stulberg DL 2004 Nail abnormalities: clues to systemic disease. Am Fam Phys 69:1417–1424

Goodpaster BH, Park SW, Harris TB et al 2006 The loss of skeletal muscle strength, mass and quality in older adult: the health, aging and body composition study. J Gerontol A Biol Sci Med Sci 10:1059–1064

Gries FA, Cameron NE, Low PA et al 2003 Textbook of Diabetic Neuropathy. Thieme, New York

Helfrich YR, Sachs DL, Voorhees JJ 2008 Overview of skin aging and photoaging. Dermatol Nurs 20:177–183

Jansen CWS, Niebuhr BR, Coussirat DJ et al 2008 Hand force of men and women over 65 years of age as measured by maximum pinch and grip force. J Aging Phys Act 16:24–41

Nazarko L 2005 Consequences of ageing and illness on skin. Nurs Resident Care 7:255–257

Newman AB, Haggerty CL, Goodpaster B et al 2003 Strength and muscle quality in a well-functioning cohort of older adults: the health aging and body composition study. J Am Geriatr Soc 51:323–330

Obert L, Uhring J, Rey PB et al 2012 Anatomy and biomechanics of the distal radius fracture. Chir Main 31:287–297

Olivieri I, Palazzi C, Peruz G et al 2005 Management issues with elderly-onset rheumatoid arthritis. Drugs Aging 22:809–822

Shaffer SW, Harrison AL 2007 Aging of the somatosensory system: a translational perspective. Phys Ther 87:193–207

Skirven TM, Osterman AL, Fedorczyk JM 2011 Rehabilitation of the hand and upper extremity. Elsevier, Mosby

Slatkowsky-Christensen B, Haugen I, Kvien TK 2010 Distribution of joint involvement in women with hand osteoarthritis and associations between joint counts and patient-reported outcome measures. Ann Rheum Dis 69:198–201

Stukstette MJPM, Hoogeboom TJ, de Ruiter R et al 2011 A multidisciplinary intervention for patients with hand osteoarthritis. Clin Rehabil 26:99–110

Thakur D, Paudel BH, Jha CB 2010 Nerve conduction study in healthy individuals: a preliminary age based study. Kathmandu Univ Med J. 31:311–316

Tremollieres F 2012 What patients need to know about bone fracture and its prevention. J Gynecol Obstet Biol Reprod (Paris) 41:F20–F27

Watkins J 2011 Ageing skin, part 1: normal ageing. Pract Nurs 22:250–257

Chapter 64

Overweight and obesity

RICHARD W. BOHANNON

INTRODUCTION

Body composition (adiposity) is generally understood to be the amount of lean body mass relative to fat mass. The National Institutes of Health (NIH) advocates use of body mass index (BMI = [weight (kg)/height(m^2)] to characterize body composition) (NIH, 1998). Although underweight (BMI <18.5 kg/m^2) is a problem for some older adults, overweight and obesity, which the NIH defines as a BMI of 25.0–29.9 kg/m^2 and $\geq$30.0 kg/m^2 respectively (see Table 64.1), are far more prevalent. In the United States of America, between 1999 and 2002, the prevalence of overweight and obesity combined was 39.4% for 60- to 69-year-olds and 25.3% for individuals at least 70 years. Both mean BMI and the prevalence of overweight and obesity are increasing in all Western European countries, Australia, the US and China (Silventoinen et al., 2004).

Numerous untoward consequences are associated with increased body weight. Although overweight may have some survival benefit for adults 70 years or older (Flicker et al., 2010), obesity is associated with an estimated 111 909 excess deaths among older adults in the US (Flegal et al., 2005). Overweight and obesity are also accompanied by numerous comorbidities. The relationship between weight and type 2 diabetes is particularly strong, with Colditz et al. (1995) showing that women experience a 25% increase in the relative risk of diabetes for each added unit of BMI over 22.0 kg/m^2. Other comorbidities accompanying increased body weight in older adults are hypertension, coronary artery disease, stroke, respiratory problems (including sleep apnea), osteoarthritis and some forms of cancer (NIH, 1998).

Although mortality and comorbidities warrant attention, functional limitations accompanying increased body weight are particularly relevant to geriatric rehabilitation. The combination of decreased strength and increased body fat (which typically occur with aging) can render demanding activities, such as standing from a chair or climbing stairs, painful, difficult or impossible (Sarkisian et al., 2000; Larrieu et al., 2004; Bohannon

et al., 2005; Bohannon, 2007). Consequently, it is essential that rehabilitation professionals address the body composition of their patients. Hereafter, some fundamentals of the examination of and interventions for overweight and obesity are covered.

EXAMINATION

Based on its practicality, BMI is recommended by the US Preventative Services Task Force for screening adults for obesity (McTigue et al., 2003). Indeed, the measurement of weight and height, on which BMI is based, is possible for most adults. When height and weight cannot be measured, they can be obtained by self-report. However, the accuracy of BMI may be compromised by the tendency of individuals to underreport weight and overstate height (Niederhammer et al., 2000). Regardless of the source of height and weight information, BMI has limitations. These include the propensity of older adults (particularly women with osteoporosis) to lose stature with age (Sorkin et al., 1999) and the failure of BMI to differentiate between lean body mass and fat mass.

Alternatives to BMI are available. Air displacement plethysmography (Fields & Hunter, 2004) and dual

Table 64.1 **Classification of body weight recommended by the National Institutes of Health**

Classification	BMI (kg/m^2)
Underweight	<18.5
Normal weight	18.5–24.9
Overweight	25.0–29.9
Obese (class I)	30.0–34.9
Obese (class II)	35.0–39.9
Obese (class III)	$\geq$40

Source: NIH, 1998.
BMI, body mass index

energy X-ray absorptiometry provide more specific information about body composition than BMI, but neither is widely available nor portable. Bioelectrical impedance is also more informative regarding body composition (Vilaca et al., 2011), and it is portable. However, it is influenced by hydration and other variables used in its predictive algorithms. Skinfold measurements are relatively easy to obtain, and measurements from a single site (e.g. subscapular) may be sufficient (Garn et al., 1971). The relationship between central adiposity and cardiovascular disease makes waist circumference a useful supplement to BMI (NIH, 1998). Waist circumference should be measured just above the pelvic crest, parallel to the floor, while the tested individual stands. A man is considered to be at high risk of weight-related comorbidities if his waist circumference exceeds 102 cm (40 in); for women the criterion is 88 cm (35 in).

INTERVENTIONS

For older adults who are overweight or obese, even small losses of weight have been shown to be highly advantageous. Larsson and Mattsson (2003), for example, found that obese women who achieved a 10% weight loss realized significant improvements in walking speed, oxygen consumption, pain and perceived exertion. Felson et al. (1992) reported that individuals who achieved a weight loss of 2 or more BMI units (about 5.1 kg) over a 10-year period reduced their likelihood of developing knee osteoarthritis by more than 50%. Given such findings, health professionals should not be shy about engaging older adults about their weight. Patients are generally desirous of advice about diet, assistance with setting weight goals, and recommendations regarding exercise (Potter et al., 2001). Adults with arthritis who receive advice from a health professional to lose weight are more likely than those not receiving such advice to make an effort to lose weight (Mehrotra et al., 2004).

There are five basic strategies that can be used alone or in combination to lose weight. They include: diet, physical activity, behavior therapy, pharmacotherapy and bariatric surgery.

Dietary therapy focuses on reduced daily caloric intake. Low calorie diets (800–1500 kcal/day) can reduce total weight by a mean 8% over a period of 6 months. Unfortunately weight loss thus achieved is usually not sustained (NIH, 1998).

Physical activity is often reduced in overweight and obese older adults. Those who walk less (Tryon et al., 1992) and sit more (Brown et al., 2003) are more likely to be overweight or obese. Aerobic exercise regimens, which serve to increase activity over baseline, are able to produce modest weight losses (3.0 kg for men and 1.4 kg for women) (Garrow & Summerbell, 1995). Such exercise can take many forms, but research indicates that older adults prefer walking as a mode of exercise (McPhillips et al., 1989). Employing a pedometer and having an exercise 'buddy' can be motivational for increasing walking activity (Thomas et al., 2012). For individuals unable to tolerate sufficient walking to achieve a therapeutic beneficial effect, alternatives not entailing full weight-bearing may be indicated. These include recumbent

cycling or aquatic activities. Resistance exercise should also be considered as it can enable older adults to better handle their body weight and to increase their muscle mass and energy expenditure. In lieu of, or in addition to, formal exercise interventions, older adults can expend additional energy by walking rather than driving short distances, taking the stairs instead of the elevator or escalator, and forgoing use of 'labor-saving devices' (Lanningham-Foster et al., 2003).

Behavior therapy is multifaceted, but much of it is directed at altering dietary and exercise habits. Key components include, but are not limited to: training in self-monitoring, self-control, exercise and diet information, stimulus control strategies, reinforcement, problem-solving and goal-setting, behavior modification, family support, stages of change, cognitive restructuring, peer relations and maintenance strategies. Behavior therapy has been described as offering benefits that are supplemental to those provided by other approaches (NIH, 1998).

When more conservative approaches prove insufficient, drugs or surgery may be appropriate. Several drugs, including orlistat and sibutramine, can be prescribed. As part of a comprehensive program they can contribute to weight loss when used for 6 months to a year (NIH, 1998). For patients with severe obesity, bariatric surgery (either open or laparoscopic) is immensely successful in causing weight loss. Weight loss is greatest in the first year or two after surgery and ranges from 20% to 40%. In the Swedish Obese Subjects Study, patients' weight losses were 16.3% after 8 years and 16.1% after 10 years (Sjöström et al., 2004). Bariatric surgery has a powerful effect on some of the comorbidities that tend to accompany obesity. Specifically, diabetes, hypertension and sleep apnea are resolved or improved in the vast majority of cases.

CONCLUSION

Rehabilitation professionals are well positioned to serve older adults who are overweight or obese. Such service first requires the objective documentation of weight status. Thereafter, interventions can be initiated. Although some interventions (e.g. drugs and surgery) are beyond the scope of rehabilitation practice, aspects of diet, exercise and behavior therapy can be incorporated with modest effect. As patients are typically open to such interventions, they should not be overlooked by rehabilitation professionals caring for them.

REFERENCES

Bohannon RW 2007 Knee extension strength and body weight determine sit-to-stand independence after stroke. Physiother Theory Pract 23:291–297

Bohannon RW, Brennan P, Pescatello L et al 2005 Relationship among perceived limitations in stair climbing and lower limb strength, body mass index, and self-reported stair climbing activity. Top Geriatr Rehab 21:350–355

Brown WJ, Miller YD, Miller R 2003 Sitting time and work patterns as indicators of overweight and obesity in Australian adults. Int J Obes 27:1340–1346

Colditz GA, Willett WC, Rotnitzky A et al 1995 Weight gain as a risk factor for clinical diabetes mellitus in women. Ann Intern Med 122:481–486

Felson DT, Zhang Y, Anthony JM et al 1992 Weight loss reduces the risk for symptomatic knee osteoarthritis in women. The Framingham Study. Ann Intern Med 116:535–539

Fields DA, Hunter GR 2004 Monitoring body fat in the elderly: application of air-displacement plethysmography. Curr Opin Clin Nutr Metab Care 7:11–14

Flegal KM, Graubard BI, Williamson DF et al 2005 Excess deaths associated with underweight, overweight, and obesity. JAMA 293:1861–1867

Flicker L, McCaul KA, Hankey GJ et al 2010 Body mass index and survival in men and women aged 70 to 75. J Am Geriatr Soc 58:234–241

Garn SM, Rosen NN, McCann MB 1971 Relative values of different fat folds in a nutritional survey. Am J Clin Nutr 24:1380–1381

Garrow JS, Summerbell CD 1995 Meta-analysis: effect of exercise, with or without dieting, on body composition of overweight subjects. Eur J Clin Nutr 49:1–10

Lanningham-Foster L, Nysse LJ, Levine JA 2003 Labor saved, calories lost: the energetic impact of labor-saving devices. Obes Res 11:1178–1181

Larrieu S, Pérès K, Letenneur L et al 2004 Relationship between body mass index and different domains in older persons: the 3C study. Int J Obes 28:1555–1560

Larsson UE, Mattsson E 2003 Influence of weight loss programmes on walking speed and relative oxygen cost (%VO$_2$ Max) in obese women during walking. J Rehabil Med 35:91–97

McPhillips JB, Pelletera KM, Barreto-Conner E et al 1989 Exercise patterns in a population of older adults. Am J Prev Med 2:65–72

McTigue K, Harris R, Hemphil B et al 2003 Screening and interventions for obesity in adults: summary of evidence for the US Preventive Services Task Force. Ann Intern Med 139:933–949

Mehrotra C, Naimi TS, Serdula M et al 2004 Arthritis, body mass index, and professional advice to lose weight: implications for clinical medicine and public health. Am J Prev Med 27:16–21

Niederhammer I, Bugel I, Bonenfant S et al 2000 Validity of self-reported weight and height in French GAZEL cohort. Int J Obes 24:1111–1118

NIH (National Institutes of Health) 1998 Clinical Guidelines on the Identification, Evaluation, and Treatment of Overweight and Obesity in Adults. NIH, Bethesda, MD, The Evidence Report. NIH Publication No. 98-4083

Potter MB, Vu JD, Croughan-Minihane M 2001 Weight management: what patients want from their primary care physicians. J Fam Pract 50:513–518

Sarkisian CA, Liu H, Gutierrez PR et al 2000 Modifiable risk factors predict functional decline among older women: a prospectively validated clinical prediction tool. J Am Geriatr Soc 48:170–178

Silventoinen K, Sans S, Tolonen H, for the WHO MONICA Project 2004 Trends in obesity and energy supply in the WHO MONICA Project. Int J Obes 28:710–718

Sjöström L, Lindroos A-K, Peltonen M et al 2004 Lifestyle, diabetes, and cardiovascular risk factors 10 years after bariatric surgery. N Engl J Med 251:2683–2693

Sorkin JD, Muller DC, Andres R 1999 Longitudinal change in height of men and women: implications for interpretation of body mass index. Am J Epidemiol 150:969–977

Thomas GN, Macfarlane DJ, Guo B et al 2012 Health promotion in older Chinese: a 12-month cluster randomized controlled trial of pedometry and 'peer support'. Med Sci Sports Exerc 44:1157–1166

Tryon WW, Goldberg JL, Morrison DF 1992 Activity decreases as percentage overweight increases. Int J Obes 16:591–595

Vilaca KH, Paula FJ, Ferriolli E et al 2011 Body composition assessment of undernourished older subjects by dual-energy X-ray absorptiometry and bioelectric impedance analysis. J Nutr Health Aging 15:439–443

ADDITIONAL READING

Sluka K, Turk D 2009. Cognitive-behavioral therapy for older adults with chronic pain. Phys Ther 89(5):470–472

Chapter 65

Frailty in older persons

MARTHA ACOSTA

INTRODUCTION

The concept of frailty usually evokes an image of an older person barely able to stand and/or laboriously walking with an assistive device across the room of an extended care facility. Although the end stages of frailty may have some semblance to this picture, the frailty phenotype is now known to be more variable and modifiable with evidence-based therapeutic interventions. Perhaps most importantly it is possible to identify and reduce the risk for frailty, even amongst the oldest-old population.

Frailty is a distinct and multidimensional clinical syndrome (Fried et al., 2001), and is commonly associated with declining status in physical and functional states that are associated with physiological, social and emotional changes. From this perspective, deteriorating health can result in a loss of reserves in energy, physical ability, cognition and health. When combined, these factors give rise to vulnerability (Rockwood, 2005). However, studies of frail older adults have identified positive benefits from training to functional capacity in areas, including increased gait speed (Chandler et al., 1998: 91), decreased risk of falls (Liu-Ambrose et al., 2004) and improved physical endurance (Ehsani et al., 2003). Even older adults in the ninth decade of life can show increases in muscle strength from resistance exercise training, despite the age-related changes in muscle strength (Fiatarone et al., 1990).

To fully appreciate frailty from a comprehensive framework, it is useful to consider the domains of health that make up the International Classification of Functioning, Disability and Health (ICF) model (Fig. 65.1). In this model, the domains impacting the frail (health) condition can be external and/or internal to the individual. In addition, the model itself can provide an integrated framework with terms that are compatible to those used in frailty language. An analysis of

that compatibility determined that the functional status indicators defined in the classification scheme of the ICF model provided a profile of frailty that reflects the multifactorial aspect of the frail condition (Nash, 2008). Thus, a thorough assessment of all the potential domains that may be involved with a frail older adult is critical. But, preceding a discussion of its multidimensional nature, frailty must first be defined. There is no complete agreement on a standardized definition of frailty, which may explain in part how the image of a person barely able to move through the environment and/or in a certain age category are often the only criteria used to define frailty. An examination of how definitions of frailty have evolved is a starting point in the following discussion. Noting the research studies that have specified frailty criteria will help the clinician determine the most

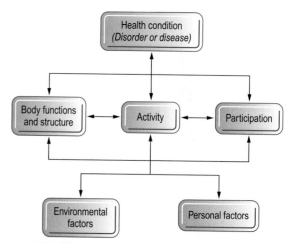

Figure 65.1 The International Classification of Functioning, Disability and Health (ICF) model. *(From World Health Organization (2001) International Classification of Functioning, Disability and Health. Geneva, WHO.)*

appropriate tool to use for screening and/or for patient treatment outcomes.

HISTORICAL PERSPECTIVE

Frailty is typically associated with declining health, functional status and the loss of abilities. A commonly held belief is that frailty is an inevitable part of the aging process. However, some older persons never become frail and some younger persons can be characterized as frail. Reviewing the progression of ideas over time that have lead up to proposed models of frailty will help clarify the definitions-in-progress of frailty used in clinical care and research.

In the early 1970s the term frailty was used synonymously with institutionalization (Abellan van Kan et al., 2008). Then, the concept of failure to thrive, which referred to weight loss with cognitive and functional decline at the end of life, was introduced in the late 1980s (Braun et al., 1988). A practical definition of frailty was reported in 1994 as persons needing help with activities of daily living (ADLs) or at a high risk of becoming dependent (Rockwood et al., 1994). A more multidimensional definition was reported in 1998 that includes 16 variables across four functional domains (physical, cognitive, nutritive and sensory domains) (Box 65.1). If impairments existed in two or more domains, the individual was considered frail (Strawbridge et al., 1998).

Other authors defined frailty as it relates to disability (Campbell & Buchner, 1997). A few years later, the definition included the concept of risk due to instability of health, where frailty leads to an increased risk of disability and death (Rockwood et al., 1999). As the conceptualization of frailty expanded, so did its definitions, which reflected the increased understanding of its multidimensionality.

DEFINING FRAILTY

Frailty research has grown exponentially over the past 20 years. In the majority of studies, multisystem involvement and decreased reserve capacity across all systems are characteristic of the syndrome of frailty. In 2002, Bortz defined frailty as the result of early disease in multiple systems, resulting in impaired muscle strength, mobility, balance and endurance (Bortz, 2002). Similar references to frailty as a biologic syndrome in which reserves and resistance to stressors are diminished, further suggest that the decline in a multiplicity of systems leads to vulnerability for adverse outcomes (Buchner & Wagner, 1992; Lipsitz & Goldberger, 1992). Based on the markers of frailty accepted by several researchers, Fried et al. (2001) formulated a set of frailty criteria (frailty phenotype) including age-related losses in strength, lean muscle mass, balance, endurance, walking performance and low physical activity (Fried et al., 2001). Presence of three or more of these criteria identify a person as being frail (Fig. 65.2).

Fried utilized data from the Cardiovascular Health Study, a prospective, observational study of 5317 men and women 65 years and older recruited from four US communities. This frailty phenotype has demonstrated

Box 65.1 Variables used to assess frailty across four domains

PHYSICAL DOMAIN
- Sudden loss of balance
- Weakness in arms
- Weakness in legs
- Get dizzy or faint when stand up quickly

COGNITIVE DOMAIN
- Difficulty paying attention
- Trouble finding the right word
- Difficulty remembering things
- Forgetting where something was put

NUTRITIVE DOMAIN
- Loss of appetite
- Unexplained weight loss

SENSORY
- Difficulty reading a newspaper
- Recognizing a friend across the street
- Reading signs at night
- Hearing over the phone
- Hearing a normal conversation
- Hearing a conversation in a noisy room

Source: Strawbridge et al., 1998.

predictive validity for adverse outcomes that geriatricians associate with frailty: increased risk for falls, disability, hospitalization and death. Frailty remained an independent predictor of risk for these adverse outcomes even after adjusting for socioeconomic status, health status, clinical and subclinical disease, depressive symptoms and disability status at baseline.

The current literature suggests that frailty is best described as an aggregation of relevant domains into phenotypes. The discussion centers mostly on deciding whether physical, cognitive, social and functional domains should be components of the model for frailty outcomes. An example of this controversy regarding measurement is the concept of disability and whether it is considered a component of the syndrome or an outcome (Abellan van Kan et al., 2010). However, it is widely accepted that frailty is a clinical syndrome resulting from multisystem impairments that are separate from the normal aging process. Grouping these impairments into a phenotype provides a basis for various assessment measures used in research.

The two main phenotypes used in assessments are the phenotype of physical frailty and the multidomain phenotype that includes cognitive, functional and social aspects (Morley et al., 2006: 41). The physical phenotype includes five measurable items (weight loss, exhaustion, weak grip strength, slow walking speed and low energy expenditure) that identify frailty and has consistently predicted poor clinical outcomes. An overall grouping of functional impairments formed the basis for this phenotype (Fried et al., 2001). The multidimensional phenotype includes components such as cognitive impairment, chronic diseases, sensory impairment,

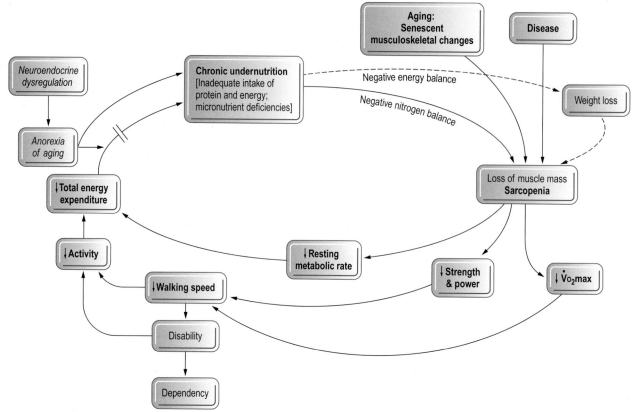

Figure 65.2 Fried's model of frailty.

mood disorders, poor social conditions and support, and disability (Morley et al., 2006).

The physical phenotype based on an operational definition of frailty has been conceptualized as a syndrome with diminished physiologic reserves and resiliency, where a cycle of declining systems results in decreased endurance for exertion, decreased strength, sarcopenia and a negative balance of energy. Within this phenotype, the five measurable characteristics identifying frailty include weight loss, exhaustion, weak grip strength, slow walking speed and low energy expenditure. A person is classified as frail if three or more of the criteria are met. If only one or two criteria are met, the category is labeled intermediate. If no criteria are met, an individual is considered robust. With the data from the Cardiovascular Health Study (4317 community-dwelling adults aged 65 and over) and using these criteria, a 7% prevalence of frailty was found, increasing to 30% in the subgroup 80 years and older (Fried et al., 2001). In the Women's Health and Aging Studies (moderately to severe disabled population of 1002 community-dwelling women aged 65 and over), a 28% prevalence of frailty was identified (Bandeen-Roche et al., 2006). Additionally, in these cohorts the phenotype classification predicted poor clinical outcomes, including falls, hospitalization, development of disability and mortality (Fried et al., 2001).

In addition to the five criteria of the physical phenotype, the multidomain phenotype includes cognitive, functional and social circumstance domains. Addition

of these factors has added value to the predictive capacity of the physical phenotype for projecting poor outcomes. This aggregation of the domains is referred to as expanded model of physical frailty (Abellan van Kan et al., 2010).

In one multidomain model, researchers from the Canadian Study of Health and Aging (CSHA) examined function with regard to comorbidity and disability (Theou et al., 2012). Although considered distinct entities, comorbidity and disability are related conceptually according to the physical phenotype. As reported by Theou et al, results from Fried's study in 2004 indicated the proportion of older women were more frail compared to older men, and had more ADL impairments; men had a higher death rate and reported more chronic conditions. Fewer than 10% of persons who were frail did not experience any comorbidity or disability. Also, ADL limitations and chronic diseases occurred more frequently in the group with the highest levels of frailty (Theou et al., 2012). The presence of chronic diseases will impact clinical management of the older patient and may help explain the higher mortality among men compared to women. The impact of multiple chronic diseases is well known to physical therapists working with the older patient. In the area of cognition, dementia can be considered an outcome or a component of frailty depending on which definition is used. The addition of lower cognitive function to the physical phenotype does slightly increase the prediction of developing disability although there was no effect on mortality as identified in the MacArthur Study of Successful Aging, a longitudinal cohort study (Sarkisian et al., 2008; Avila-Funes et al., 2009). When considering socioeconomics and frailty, a statistically significant association was found between lower health-related quality of life scores and frailty in the Hispanic Established Populations for the Epidemiological Studies of the Elderly (EPESE) (Masel et al., 2009). Similarly, a statistically significant association was found between lower socioeconomic status (SES) and frailty in the Women's Health and Aging Studies. In this cross-sectional analysis of 727 older women, the odds of frailty among women of low SES increased independent of age, race, insurance, smoking status and comorbidities (Szanton et al., 2010). Overall, the multidomain phenotypes have added clinical significance to the assessment process with frail older adults.

In addition to the phenotypes, another approach to operationalizing frailty uses the concept of deficit accumulation whereby a Frailty Index (FI) is constructed. The index is calculated as the proportion of the number of deficits present to the number of deficits counted (Mitnitski et al., 2001; Jones et al., 2004). The index was determined from 92 variables representing a range of disabilities and health conditions. Variables for the frailty index included symptoms, signs, comorbidities, functional impairments, abnormal lab values and disabilities. The summed scores are then stratified to define three levels of frailty: mild, moderate and severe. Clinically the FI gives an overview of health status and permits the risk stratification of potential adverse outcomes. Clinical applications of the FI have been used to describe functional and clinical characteristics of frailty as well as examine differences in health status comparing rural and urban older adults. Hence, the tool assessed the risk of death better than measures of comorbidity, function or cognition.

BIOLOGICAL FOUNDATIONS OF FRAILTY

Factors that underlie the cause of frailty continue to be the subject of geriatric research. Although all the mechanisms involved remain unclear, an essential cause of frailty that has been proposed is a multisystem dysregulation of the neuromuscular, endocrine and immune systems (Ko, 2011). Collectively, these system changes may have synergistic adverse effects greater than the age-related or disease-related individual factors; therefore, it is important to examine this concept in more detail.

Age-related sarcopenia (loss of muscle mass) accelerates after age 50 (Rice et al., 1989; Metter et al., 1997). Loss of muscle mass and strength is reflected in most definitions of frailty. Sarcopenia can be defined in a formal assessment of body composition using dual-energy X-ray absorptiometry that can produce estimates of lean body mass. Absolute values or scores are reported relative to normal gender-specific values and skeletal size, the 'relative skeletal muscle index' (RSMI). Sarcopenia defined by the RSMI is <2 standard deviations below normal in approximately 15% of persons aged 60–69 years and approximately 40% of those over 80 years (Fried et al., 2009). The biological basis for muscle decline includes age-related changes in type I muscle fibers, alpha-motor neurons, growth hormone (GH) production, sex steroid levels, inflammatory markers and physical activity (Fried et al., 2009). However, the age-related loss of muscle mass is modifiable with resistance training in the older adult. This topic will be discussed in more detail later in the chapter.

Although sarcopenia is a central manifestation of frailty, the age-related decline in muscle mass is modulated by several physiologic factors, including hormones, neurologic integrity, nutritional status, physical activity and inflammation (Fried et al., 2009). With regards to the endocrine system, hormones that are crucial to skeletal muscle metabolism include sex steroids and insulin growth factor (IGF-1). Lower levels of these hormones contribute to age-related loss of muscle mass and strength, particularly decreased estrogen in postmenopausal women and testosterone in older men (Poehlman et al., 1995; Morley et al., 1997). In addition, serum levels of the sex hormone dehydroepiandrosterone sulfate (DHEA-S) and IGF-1 are significantly lower in frail versus non-frail older women (Leng et al., 2004). In relation to outcomes, lower levels of IFG-1 are also associated with poor muscle strength, slow walking speed, progressive disability and increased mortality as evidenced in the Women's Health and Aging Study (Cappola et al., 2001, 2003). Future investigations in these modulatory functions will broaden our understanding of frailty.

In common with many other conditions, the immune system has been linked to frailty. Chronic elevation of serum levels of proinflammatory cytokine interleukin 6 (IL-6) which is characteristic of chronic inflammation, is strongly associated with frailty (Leng et al., 2002). Also, IL-6 has been strongly associated with weight loss, increased susceptibility to infections and adverse physiologic effects of sarcopenia. It may also contribute to anemia by interfering with iron metabolism or by directly inhibiting erythropoietin production (Ershler, 2003). Finally, elevated white blood cell (WBC) counts and IL-6 levels were independently associated with prevalent frailty in community-dwelling older women in the Women's Health and Aging Studies (Leng et al., 2007).

The biological and physiological features of frailty indicate multisystem involvement with interactions among systems, rather than a single system. Thus a global approach to the assessment and management of problems affecting frail older adults is warranted.

CONSIDERATIONS FOR ASSESSMENT

As healthcare clinicians, the assessment measures used should be standardized, evidence-based and psychometrically sound. Researchers and therapists strive to develop and test such clinical tools. Although geriatric assessments used by physical therapists are numerous, there are currently no instruments that are specific for measuring and evaluating frailty, either as screening or outcome tools. Considering the challenges with singularly defining the frailty construct, this is understandable. Nevertheless, the issue is being addressed, as noted below.

To understand the scope and scale of the issue, a systematic review (SR) investigated the clinical operational

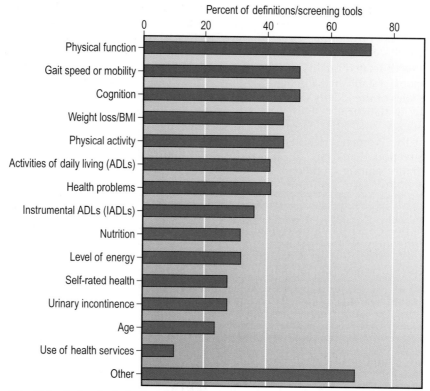

Figure 65.3 Prevalence of identifying factors for frailty in definitions and screening tools.

definitions of frailty, frailty screening instruments and tools to measure the severity of frailty (Sternberg et al., 2011: 1). Inclusion criteria were studies examining community-dwelling adults aged 65 and older who had clinically relevant outcomes (change in functional status, hospitalization or death), articles describing original tools (not subsequent validation studies) and articles that mentioned frailty rather than simply disability. Results of the SR pertaining to definitions and screening criteria are shown in Figure 65.3. Findings indicate the most commonly identified factors for frailty in definitions and screening tools were physical functioning (73%), gait speed (50%) and cognition (50%). Gait speed and cognition are found more often in recent literature compared to factors of ADLs (41%) and IADLs (instrumental activities of daily living) (36%) in earlier studies. These findings can direct the clinician in the absence of a specific frailty instrument by using the identifying factors as a guide to select which standardized assessment tools address the problem areas.

Subsequent to determining the best assessment instrument, establishing the extent of the frail condition will be a key component of the patient's profile at baseline. One way to accomplish this is by stratification using levels of frailty. An FI was operationalized by Jones et al. (2004) with three levels of frailty including mild, moderate or severe. To determine the FI, a standard Comprehensive Geriatric Assessment (CGA) representing impairment, disability and comorbidity burden was scored and summed, thus becoming the FI-CGA levels. The three levels of frailty are: mild (FI-CGA 0–7),

moderate (FI-CGA 7–13) and severe (FI-CGA >13) (Jones et al., 2004). Information on the extent of the frail condition will benefit the clinician in establishing targeted outcomes besides gaining a more robust composite of the impact on future health.

Beyond the patient's status at baseline, monitoring changes in the frail condition will provide necessary information for planning interventions and realistic outcomes. The Clinical Global Impression of Change in Physical Frailty (CGIC-PF) tool is used to evaluate changes in physical frailty (Studenski et al., 2004). The CGIC-PF measures six domains (mobility, healthcare utilization, appearance, self-perceived health, ADL, emotional status and social status). This tool also captures the multidimensional nature of frailty.

A final assessment consideration is the potential predictive capacity of some assessment tools. In one study, three criteria (gait speed, grip strength and repeated chair stands) were added to the original five criteria used by Fried and Rockwood. All three criteria were predictive for identifying frailty, with gait speed being the best indicator of multidimensionality frailty. Adults who walked slower than 0.65 m/s were >20 times as likely to be frail compared to those who walked faster. Individuals with grip strength <25 kg were six times more likely to be frail. When rising from seated position <7 times per 30 seconds people were 14 times more likely to be frail. These three single-item criteria predicted mortality at 6 months, with walking speed as the best predictor for adverse outcomes like mortality, hospitalization or disability (Abellan van Kan et al., 2008).

THERAPEUTIC INTERVENTIONS WITH FRAIL ELDERS

In 2006, an international consensus report described frail older persons as having impairments in balance, mobility, strength, cognition, motor processing, nutrition, endurance (fatigue) and physical activity (Ferrucci et al., 2004). Most of these areas are routinely addressed in physical therapy interventions. Physical activity or regular exercise training can favorably impact several of the frailty criteria, such as muscular weakness, low physical activity, exercise intolerance and slowed motor performance. Confirmation of the benefits of low levels of physical activity, defined as walking at least a mile a week, decreased the risk of developing ADL/IADL impairments as evidenced in the Longitudinal Study of Aging after adjusting for age, gender, comorbidities and baseline disability. These findings provided evidence that engagement in at least low levels of physical activity can slow the progression of ADL and IADL disability (Miller et al., 2000). Additional studies addressing the effects of exercise on non-disease-specific characteristics of frailty suggest the potential for reversal of these traits (Fiatarone et al., 1994; Faber et al., 2006).

Physical activity pertaining to age-related declines in physical function is associated with decrease in measures of exercise tolerance including muscle strength, maximal aerobic capacity and fatigue levels (Walston et al., 2006). However, the idea of endurance/aerobic training for the frail older adult can be unnerving to many clinicians who are not familiar with exercise tolerance capacity in the frail older adult. A more thorough understanding of the impact of aerobic exercise on frailty may alleviate this concern.

Aerobic exercise can alter the frailty phenotype via two mechanisms: increase muscle mass and improvement in maximal oxygen uptake (Vo_2 peak). The maximum rate of oxygen consumption during vigorous exercise (Vo_2 peak) is related to exercise tolerance and submaximal exercise capacity (Liu & Fielding, 2011). In one intervention study, a 9-month program of walking and strength training in frail men and women increased endurance by improving Vo_2 by 14% during peak effort of cardiac output measurements in response to training; the goal was 78% of peak heart rate (Ehsani et al., 2003). Another study demonstrated improved maximal aerobic capacity by 30% among seven healthy elderly (71 ± 2 year) sedentary women after a 12 week regimen of cycle ergometer training (Harber et al., 2009). This study also found an increase in quadriceps muscle mass by 12% with endurance training. In previous studies it had been shown that aerobic exercise did not change muscle size in older adults; however, the percentage of muscle mass in the extremities did increase with aerobic training compared to sedentary older persons (Sugawara et al., 2002).

The effectiveness of progressive resistance strength training in older adults is well documented (Latham et al., 2004: 199). Even into the ninth decade, the reversibility of muscle weakness through strength training has been documented. In an 8-week program of high intensity resistance training, 10 frail, institutionalized adults aged 90 ± 1 year participated in a training program that was adapted from standard rehabilitation principles of progressive resistance training including concentric (lifting) and eccentric (lowering) muscle contractions. At 8 weeks the average strength gain was 174% ± 31% ($P < 0.0001$) from baseline. Improvements in functional mobility accompanied strength gains (Fiatarone et al., 1990). Considering the major level of frailty often seen among nursing home residents, the efficacy of resistance training in this population is especially encouraging, and is a viable option in treatment planning. Beneficial effects of exercise for frail, institutionalized older adults were also confirmed in a systematic review of institutionalized older adults aged 70 years and older (Weening-Dijksterhuis et al., 2011). In this review, authors took a comprehensive approach to address several outcome measures simultaneously, thus although the benefits in muscle strength from progressive resistance training were identified, the training effects based on exercise specificity was less evident. In contrast, a single-blinded randomized controlled trial (RCT) of 22 institutionalized older adults (mean age, 81.5 years) studied the dose–response effect of a free-weight resistance program comparing two intensity training levels on knee extensor muscles (Seynnes et al., 2004: 202). The high-intensity group ($n = 8$) trained at 80% of their 1-repetition maximum (RM) and the low intensity group trained at 40%. Results demonstrated significant improvements in the high-intensity strength training group (80% of 1 RM) for knee extensor strengthening, endurance and the 6-minute walking test with a similar trend for chair-rising and stair-climbing, compared to a low-intensity (40% of 1 RM) group. Findings further identified a strong dose–response relationship between strength gains and resistance training intensity as well as between improved strength and functional outcomes. Thus, to optimize functional performance, a high-intensity resistance training (80% of 1 RM) is preferable. With a free weight-based program that is supervised, this form of higher-intensity resistance training appears to be as safe as lower-intensity training, although it is more effective functionally and physiologically than lower intensity for frail older adults.

Added benefits in areas of motor performance, secondary to resistance training, have been identified. Walking speed improved among healthy and frail elders after resistance training as reported in 14 studies. Also, an increase in distances in the 6-minute walk test were found in six trials in this same systematic review (Latham et al., 2004). Improvements in gait speed specifically among frail older persons living in nursing homes and the community were also seen after 10 weeks of resistance training (Fiatarone et al., 1994; Chandler et al., 1998). Benefits of resistance training for frail older persons are well founded and can contribute to favorable treatment expectations.

Exercise interventions for frail older persons have shown similar benefits with reduction of fall risk. A single fall is known to increase three-fold the chance of nursing home placement, after adjusting for social, cognitive, psychological, functional and medical factors (Tinetti & Williams, 1997). However, the risk of falls was decreased by 57% from baseline after resistance training for 25 weeks in a study of older women aged 75–85 years with low bone mass (Liu-Ambrose et al., 2004).

In addition to the motoric effects of exercise interventions, underlying mechanisms at the cellular level can potentially be affected by exercises. One such mechanism is the immunologic response, which declines with age-related changes in the thymus gland and T cells (Gruver et al., 2007). This was examined in a RCT of frail older nursing home residents where an intervention of functionally oriented endurance and resistance exercise training was provided every 2 hours from 8 am to 4 pm for 5 days a week for 8 months. Results of the study showed no beneficial or detrimental effects on the immune system as measured by changes in lymphocyte subpopulations, activation markers, *in vitro* proliferation and cytokine activity (Kapasi et al., 2003). In a related study among frail older women, researchers investigated the effects of dehydroepiandrosterone (DHEA) combined with exercise on strength, bone mass and physical function. Participants received 50 mg/d DHEA or a placebo for 6 months; they all received calcium and cholecalciferol. The exercise regimen included was a 90-minute program of gentle exercises with chair aerobics or yoga twice weekly. Results indicated improved lower extremity strength and function in those taking DHEA, although no changes were seen in bone mineral density. Also among those taking DHEA supplement, significant increases were found in all levels of hormones, including estradiol, DHEAS, estrone and testosterone (Kenny et al., 2010).

Another area of major concern with frailty is disability in performing ADLs. In Latham's systematic review (41 studies), the risk of ADL disability did not decrease with resistance exercise training (Latham et al., 2004). In contrast, the Cochrane Review of 121 trials found an association between resistance training and reduced ADL disability (Liu & Latham, 2009: 254). It is noted that neither of these two reviews were stratified by severity of frailty. In a RCT of a 6-month home program of combined resistance exercises with balance training and home safety and assistive device evaluations, the intervention group classified as moderately frail had a decrease in functional decline over time as per their disability scores. Disability scores in the intervention and control groups were 2.3 and 2.8, respectively, at baseline; 2.0 and 3.6 at 7 months for the comparison between the groups in change from baseline); and 2.7 and 4.2 at 12 months. This change was not observed in the severely frail adults. Moderate frailty was defined as the inability to rise from a chair with arms folded, or the inability to perform a rapid gait test which requires more than 10 seconds to walk a 3 meter course. Severe frailty was defined as lacking both characteristics or abilities (Gill et al., 2002: 80). In a different study, there was no improvement in the Older American Resources and Services (OARS) ADL score in a group of mild to moderately frail persons secondary to a regimen of balance, resistance and flexibility training (Binder et al., 2002). More recently, the FRASI (Frailty Screening and Intervention) RCT addressed the question of preventing ADL disability in non-disabled, frail, older persons

screened in primary care (Bandinelli et al., 2006). The study built on previous research showed that supervised exercises improved physical performance in older persons and prevented functional decline in persons who already have mild disability. Whether such a program can prevent new disability in frail older persons is yet to be determined.

Designing exercise programs for frail older persons must be relevant to functional activities, particularly in the presence of limited reserve capacity and increased fatigue. As a result of compromised levels in both areas, task specificity may become paramount in improving function, compared to intensity level of exercises (de Vreede et al., 2007). In frail older persons, increases in strength from participating in task-specific exercises have produced results similar to those of resistance exercises (Bean et al., 2003; de Vreede et al., 2004; Manini et al., 2007). Performance of daily tasks in a safe and energy-efficient manner are at the core of achieving independence in self-directed activities. Decreases in muscle strength impact specific functional tasks in areas of mobility over even and uneven surfaces, transfer skills and upright activities requiring good balance skills. Task-specific interventions to address these areas can include weight-shifting exercises, stepping up and over, reaching, stooping and other multidirectional movement exercises. These can be progressed with increasing loads and/or speed of movement (Avers & Brown, 2009). In the frail older person, task-specific training may supersede resistance training alone for improved functional gains (de Vreede et al., 2004).

SPECIAL CONSIDERATIONS

COMMUNITY-DWELLING OLDER PERSONS

Characteristics related to community-dwelling status may potentially impact the risk of developing frailty. In a longitudinal study of 2069 Mexican American adults, factors including access to healthcare, cognitive functioning and neighborhood characteristics had a protective effect with regards to rates of frailty for adults 75+ years of age (Aranda et al., 2011). In contrast, findings of a systematic review have confirmed the positive impact of resistance strengthening exercise programs, revealing gains in muscle strength and walking speed (Latham et al., 2004), improved balance and reduction in falls (Bulat et al., 2007), and increased bone mineral density (Layne & Nelson, 1999). In one longitudinal study, physical activity modified the effect of disability on depression in older adults (Lee & Park, 2008).

Results of studies focusing exercise programs among community-dwelling frail older persons have varied findings, possibly secondary to different levels of frailty. In one RCT, participants with moderate frailty benefited from a 6-month intervention of home-based physical therapy with less functional decline at 12 months. Focus of the intervention was on underlying impairments including balance, muscle strength, transfers and mobility. Similar results were not seen in those with severe frailty (Gill et al., 2002). In another RCT of elderly persons after hospital discharge, there was no effect on rehabilitation outcomes of physical performance after receiving a vitamin D supplementation and a home-based high-intensity quadriceps resistance exercise program (Latham et al., 2003). In regards to this study, it is noted that participants were recently ill, and the authors did generalize findings to the wider population of frail persons based on the study design and the broad characteristics of patients who were recruited for the study. Further research is needed on the impact of levels of frailty on efficacy of interventions.

A cohort study of community-dwelling older adults in the Canadian Study of Health and Aging involved 36 centers (Hubbard et al., 2009) and used a Frailty Index based on 40 variables representing a range of health conditions and disabilities to capture the gradations in health status. Results indicated that persons who participated in high levels of physical activity had a lower risk of death compared to non-exercisers or those who did minimal exercise. Also, the death rates for men and women over 75 years who did exercise were comparable to their peers aged 65–75 who did not exercise. After adjusting for age and sex, there was a greater chance for improving health status in the exercisers compared to non-exercisers. And interestingly, the greatest impact on health status was among those who were the most frail at baseline. The authors noted that they used the definition of frailty based on the Frailty Index (deficit count) rather than the phenotypic definition. They further noted that these results are not applicable to nursing home or residential clients, or those with significant cognitive impairments. Benefits derived were extended to those with a higher number of health deficits at baseline, which offers evidence to support the idea that health prevention in older adults extends longevity in a healthy state.

FRAIL OLDER PERSON WITH BALANCE DEFICITS

A large-scale study of the efficacy of targeted and non-targeted exercises on fall risk and fall-related injuries involved RCTs in the multicenter Frailty and Injuries: Cooperative Studies on Intervention Techniques (FICSIT). With consideration of the variations among interventions with respect to type of exercise, intensity, frequency and duration, the combined multisite outcomes showed a significant decrease (13%) in fall risk for those individuals who engaged in interventions that had exercise as a core component. The risk was further reduced (by 24%) if the exercise intervention included specific balance and walking activities (Province et al., 1995). In another RCT, a group of frail homebound women (≥80 years) who were identified as high risk for falls, received an individualized exercise program (Otago home exercise program) 3 times per week for 12 months and included walking 3 times per week. Results included a significant reduction in fall rates (about one-third) and injurious falls, and significant improvement in balance at 6 months (Campbell & Buchner, 1997).

Tai chi has been shown to lower the risk of multiple falls by 47.5% among certain groups of older adults (Wolf et al., 1996; Li et al., 2005; Voukelatos et al., 2007). An Eastern form of exercise, tai chi also provides numerous health benefits in functional balance, physical performance and reduced fear of falling. In contrast, a 48-week intervention program of intense tai chi did not significantly reduce the risk of falls in a group of older adults (70–97 years) who were classified as frail or becoming frail (Wolf et al., 2003). However, as the researchers have noted, the imprecise definition of transitional frailty used in the study may have contributed to lack of significance. Therefore, the therapist's clinical judgment will still be driven by the patient s' presenting problems, which can range from minimal debility to complex polypharmacy considerations. Tai chi as a stand-alone strategy may be less effective than a multifactorial intervention that combines other traditional clinical approaches in the reduction of fall risk. Given the multifactorial nature of frailty, besides the number of contributing factors to a heightened fall risk, a thorough analysis of all factors involved will be critical to the development of a well-rounded treatment program.

FRAILTY AND INCONTINENCE

The older adult population has the highest prevalence of urinary incontinence and is a reflection of the exponential growth of the aging population worldwide. In a report from the 4th International Consultation on Incontinence, the clinical phenotype used to address frailty included impairments in physical activity, mobility, balance, muscle strength, motor processing, cognition, nutrition and endurance (DuBeau et al., 2010). This report further identified associations that contribute to urinary incontinence with other factors besides age-related changes in muscular, hormonal and structural features. They included comorbidities and impairments (dementia, falls, decreased vision and hearing, dizziness), neurological and psychiatric disorders, and/or medications as important factors associated with urinary incontinence. The overall impact of incontinence frequently involves functional decline secondary to decreased mobility and becoming socially isolated from a fear of urinary accidents in public. Identification of this issue early in the assessment process is critical to planning interventions and outcomes.

Studies have also shown an association between an increased risk of urinary incontinence with ADL and physical performance functional limitations (Cigolle et al., 2007; Huang et al., 2007). For an extensive summary of evidence regarding treatment and management of urinary incontinence, the reader is referred to the 4th International Consultation Report (DuBeau et al., 2010).

FRAILTY AND PARKINSON'S DISEASE

Few research studies are available on frailty and Parkinson's disease (PD). One study does shed light on the prevalence of PD and its relationship to individual frailty criteria and the level of severity of PD (Ahmed et al., 2008). In an observational, cross-sectional analysis of adults with PD, disease severity was measured using the unified Parkinson's disease rating scale (UPDRS). This assessment tool is divided into three sections: the first section addresses mood and intellectual functioning;

the second section evaluates a person's daily functioning (rolling in bed, showering and writing); the third looks at motor ability. Higher scores indicate more severe disease, with results reported on a 0–199 scale. To diagnose frailty, the five components of Fried were used (walking speed, exhaustion, grip strength, weekly caloric expenditure and weight loss). Three or more of the five criteria confirmed frailty. Average age of the population was 70.8 ± 9.2 years. Results of the study indicated that the prevalence of frailty in adults with optimally treated PD was higher than expected (32.6%). The best discriminator between those who met the frailty criteria and those who did not was weekly caloric expenditure. The number of criteria that were positive for frailty increased with the severity of the disease. Also, there was a direct relationship between walk time and the severity of the disease. UPDRS scores ranged from 11 to 75 with the mean score of 35.8 ± 15.0. These scores in combination with the high prevalence (nearly five times higher than the general population) emphasize the importance of proper diagnosis and treatment of frailty in people with PD.

FRAILTY AND CHRONIC DISEASES

Chronic diseases in the older adult play a major role in their health trajectory in later life. There is less time spent in the frail state compared to being disabled because of the higher risk of mortality (Thorpe et al., 2009). In the Cardiovascular Health Study (CHS), among those with comorbidities (comorbidity defined as having two or more of the following nine diseases: myocardial infarction, angina, congestive heart failure, claudication, arthritis, cancer, diabetes, hypertension, chronic obstructive pulmonary disease), 46% were also frail (Fried et al., 2001). The diagnosis of Parkinson's disease was excluded from this study as a condition that could present with frailty characteristics consequential to a single disease. Also in this study, the mean number of comorbid diseases in the frail older adults was approximately 2.1 compared to 1.4 in the non-frail group.

With aging we observed an increased susceptibility to multiple chronic diseases that had no evident 'usual' risk factors. The regulatory network of biological signaling that maintains homeostatic equilibrium is involved as it progressively becomes less efficient. Physiologic dysregulation in multiple systems may contribute to the loss of reserves and vulnerability as well as disease manifestations seen in frail older adults (Fried et al., 2009).

In cohort studies of older adults, chronic diseases that have been associated with frailty include (in descending order of prevalence): hypertension, chronic kidney disease, osteoarthritis, depressive symptoms, coronary heart disease, diabetes mellitus, chronic lower respiratory tract disease, myocardial infarction, rheumatoid arthritis, stroke, peripheral arterial disease and congestive heart failure. From among these diseases there was no association identified between a single disease and frailty (Weiss, 2011).

Related to chronic diseases, other common conditions associated with frailty have been identified. A poor nutritional state in the frail older adult (Semba et al., 2006) together with low activity levels suggested an

energy dysregulation that is also involved in congestive heart failure, diabetes, stroke and chronic lung disease. Anemia and its potential association with frailty is being studied to understand the synergistic interactions with cardiovascular disease as a risk factor for frailty (Weiss, 2011). Heightened inflammation and changes in the immune system likely are responsible for the overall decline in immunologic function in the frail, older adult (Yao et al., 2011). Lastly, an association has been found between frailty and the risk for venous thromboembolism in community-dwelling older adults with intermediate to definite frailty (Folsom et al., 2007).

The multidimensional nature of frailty provides the basis for impaired function in more than one system (Bandeen-Roche et al., 2006; Inouye et al., 2007). The numerous physiologic subsystems suggest there may be several subtypes of frailty (Fried et al., 2005) with several points of entry into the frailty process, such as advanced chronic disease complicated by malnutrition. Analyses of interactions and relationships among these subsystems may require more complex, non-linear models in research (Weiss, 2011). Also, this multifactorial approach to frailty is reflective of impaired homeostasis in several systems.

CONCLUSION

As definitions of frailty have evolved, so have the multiple factors for consideration when assessing and treating the frail older adult. The variability of the multidimensional nature of frailty is well documented. Along that line, knowledge of the cluster of signs and symptoms for early identification of frail or pre-frail status will be paramount in developing appropriate therapeutic interventions. With evidence from the research identifying the benefits of strengthening programs even for the oldest-old, therapists can confidently intervene and expect positive outcomes. The key will be to capture all aspects of frailty at baseline, then apply evidence-based principles of practice. Future studies will direct the way for more specific tools as the older population continues to grow worldwide.

REFERENCES

Abellan van Kan G, Rolland Y, Bergman H et al 2008 The IANA Task Force on frailty assessment of older people in clinical practice. J Nutr Health Aging 12(1):29–37

Abellan van Kan G, Rolland Y, Houles M et al 2010 The assessment of frailty in older adults. Clin Geriatr Med 26(2):275–286

Ahmed NN, Sherman SJ, Vanwyck D et al 2008 Frailty in Parkinson's disease and its clinical implications. Parkinsonism Relat Disord 14(4):334–337

Aranda MP, Ray LA, Soham AS et al 2011 The protective effect of neighborhood composition on increasing frailty among older Mexican Americans: a barrio advantage? J Aging Health 23(7):1189–1217

Avers D, Brown M 2009 White paper: strength training for the older adult. J Geriatr Phys Ther 32(4):148–152 158.

Avila-Funes JA, Amieva H, Barberger-Gateau P et al 2009 Cognitive impairment improves the predictive validity of the phenotype of frailty for adverse health outcomes: the three-city study. J Am Geriatr Soc 57(3):453–461

Bandeen-Roche K, Xue Q-L, Ferrucci L et al 2006 Phenotype of frailty: characterization in the women's health and aging studies. J Gerontol A Biol Sci Med Sci 61(3):262–266

Bandinelli S, Lauretani F, Boscherini V et al 2006 A randomized, controlled trial of disability prevention in frail older patients screened in primary care: the FRASI study. Design and baseline evaluation. Aging-Clin Exp Res 18(5):359–366

Bean JF, Leveille SG, Kiely K et al 2003 A comparison of leg power and leg strength within the InCHIANTI Study: which influences mobility more? J Gerontol A Biol Sci Med Sci 58(8):M728–M733

Binder EF, Schechtman KB et al 2002 Effects of exercise training on frailty in community-dwelling older adults: results of a randomized, controlled trial. J Am Geriatr Soc 50(12):1921–1928

Bortz II WM 2002 A conceptual framework of frailty. J Gerontol A Biol Sci Med Sci 57(5):M283–M288

Braun JV, Wykle MH et al 1988 Failure to thrive in older persons: a concept derived. Gerontologist 28(6):809–812

Buchner DM, Wagner EH 1992 Preventing frail health. Clin Geriatr Med 8(1):1–17

Bulat T, Hart-Hughes S et al 2007 Effect of a group-based exercise program on balance in elderly. Clin Intervent Aging 2(4):655–660

Campbell AJ, Buchner DM 1997 Unstable disability and the fluctuations of frailty. Age Ageing 26(4):315–318

Cappola AR, Bandeen-Roche K et al 2001 Association of IGF-I levels with muscle strength and mobility in older women. J Clin Endocrinol Metabol 86(9):4139–4146

Cappola AR, Xue Q-L et al 2003 Insulin-like growth factor 1 and interleukin-6 contribute synergistically to disability and mortality in older women. J Clin Endocrinol Metabol 88(5):2019–2025

Chandler JM, Duncan PW et al 1998 Is lower extremity strength gain associated with improvement in physical performance and disability in frail, community-dwelling elders? Arch Phys Med Rehabil 79(1):24–30

Cigolle CT, Langa KM et al 2007 Geriatric conditions and disability: the Health and Retirement Study. Ann Intern Med 147(3):156–164

de Vreede PL, Samson MM et al 2004 Functional tasks exercise versus resistance exercise to improve daily function in older women: a feasibility study. Arch Phys Med Rehabil 85(12):1952–1961

de Vreede PL, van Meeteren NL et al 2007 The effect of functional tasks exercise and resistance exercise on health-related quality of life and physical activity. Gerontology 53(1):12–20

DuBeau CE, Kuchel GA et al 2010 Incontinence in the frail elderly: report from the 4th International Consultation on Incontinence. Neurourol Urodyn 29(1):165–178

Ehsani AA, Spina RJ et al 2003 Attenuation of cardiovascular adaptations to exercise in frail octogenarians. J Appl Physiol 95(5):1781–1788

Ershler WB 2003 Biological interactions of aging and anemia: a focus on cytokines. J Am Geriatr Soc 51(3):S18–21

Faber MJ, Bosscher RJ et al 2006 Effects of exercise programs on falls and mobility in frail and pre-frail older adults: a multicenter randomized controlled trial. Arch Phys Med Rehabil 87(7):885–896

Ferrucci L, Guralnik JM et al 2004 Designing randomized, controlled trials aimed at preventing or delaying functional decline and disability in frail, older persons: a consensus report. J Am Geriatr Soc 52(4):625–634

Fiatarone MA, Marks EC et al 1990 High-intensity strength training in nonagenarians. Effects on skeletal muscle. JAMA 263(22):3029–3034

Fiatarone MA, O'Neill EF et al 1994 Exercise training and nutritional supplementation for physical frailty in very elderly people. N Engl J Med 330(25):1769–1775

Folsom AR, Boland LL et al 2007 Frailty and risk of venous thromboembolism in older adults. J Gerontol A Biol Sci Med Sci 62(1):79–82

Fried LP, Tangen CM et al 2001 Frailty in older adults: evidence for a phenotype. J Gerontol A Biol Sci Med Sci 56(3):M146–156

Fried LP, Hadley EC et al 2005 From bedside to bench: research agenda for frailty. Sci Aging Knowl Environ 2005(31):pe24

Fried L, Walston JD et al 2009 Frailty. In: Halter J, Ouslander M, Tinetti M (eds) Hazzard's Geriatric Medicine and Gerontology, 6th edn. McGraw-Hill, New York, pp. 631–645

Gill TM, Baker DI et al 2002 A program to prevent functional decline in physically frail, elderly persons who live at home. N Engl J Med 347(14):1068–1074

Gruver AL, Hudson LL et al 2007 Immunosenescence of ageing. J Pathol 211(2):144–156

Harber MP, Konopka AR et al 2009 Aerobic exercise training improves whole muscle and single myofiber size and function in older women. Am J Physiol Regul Integr Physiol 297(5):R1452–R1459

Huang AJ, Brown JS et al 2007 Urinary incontinence in older community-dwelling women: the role of cognitive and physical function decline. Obstet Gynecol 109(4):909–916

Hubbard RE, Fallah N et al 2009 Impact of exercise in community-dwelling older adults. PLoS ONE [Electronic Resource] 4(7):e6174

Inouye SK, Studenski S et al 2007 Geriatric syndromes: clinical, research, and policy implications of a core geriatric concept. J Am Geriatr Soc 55(5):780–791

Jones DM, Song X et al 2004 Operationalizing a frailty index from a standardized comprehensive geriatric assessment. J Am Geriatr Soc 52(11):1929–1933

Kapasi ZF, Ouslander JG et al 2003 Effects of an exercise intervention on immunologic parameters in frail elderly nursing home residents. J Gerontol A Biol Sci Med Sci 58(7):636–643

Kenny AM, Boxer RS et al 2010 Dehydroepiandrosterone combined with exercise improves muscle strength and physical function in frail older women. J Am Geriatr Soc 58(9):1707–1714

Ko FC 2011 The clinical care of frail, older adults. Clin Geriatr Med 27(1):89–100

Latham NK, Anderson CS et al 2003 A randomized, controlled trial of quadriceps resistance exercise and vitamin D in frail older people: the Frailty Interventions Trial in Elderly Subjects (FITNESS). J Am Geriatr Soc 51(3):291–299

Latham NK, Bennett DA et al 2004 Systematic review of progressive resistance strength training in older adults. J Gerontol Ser A Biol Sci Med Sci 59(1):48–61

Layne JE, Nelson ME 1999 The effects of progressive resistance training on bone density: a review. Med Sci Sports Exerc 31(1):25–30

Lee Y, Park K 2008 Does physical activity moderate the association between depressive symptoms and disability in older adults? Int J Geriatr Psychiatr 23(3):249–256

Leng S, Chaves P et al 2002 Serum interleukin-6 and hemoglobin as physiological correlates in the geriatric syndrome of frailty: a pilot study. J Am Geriatr Soc 50(7):1268–1271

Leng SX, Cappola AR et al 2004 Serum levels of insulin-like growth factor-I (IGF-I) and dehydroepiandrosterone sulfate (DHEA-S), and their relationships with serum interleukin-6, in the geriatric syndrome of frailty. Aging Clin Exp Res 16(2):153–157

Leng SX, Xue Q-L et al 2007 Inflammation and frailty in older women. J Am Geriatr Soc 55(6):864–871

Li F, Harmer P et al 2005 Tai chi and fall reductions in older adults: a randomized controlled trial. J Gerontol A Biol Sci Med Sci 60(2):187–194

Lipsitz LA, Goldberger AL 1992 Loss of 'complexity' and aging. Potential applications of fractals and chaos theory to senescence. JAMA 267(13):1806–1809

Liu CJ, Latham NK 2009 Progressive resistance strength training for improving physical function in older adults. Cochrane Database Syst Rev 8(3):CD002759, doi: 10.1002/14651858.CD002759.pub2

Liu CK, Fielding RA 2011 Exercise as an intervention for frailty. Clin Geriatr Med 27(1):101–110

Liu-Ambrose T, Khan KM et al 2004 Resistance and agility training reduce fall risk in women aged 75 to 85 with low bone mass: a 6-month randomized, controlled trial. J Am Geriatr Soc 52(5):657–665

Manini T, Marko M et al 2007 Efficacy of resistance and task-specific exercise in older adults who modify tasks of everyday life. J Gerontol A Biol Sci Med Sci 62(6):616–623

Masel MC, Graham JE et al 2009 Frailty and health related quality of life in older Mexican Americans. Health Qual Life Outcomes 7:70

Metter EJ, Conwit R et al 1997 Age-associated loss of power and strength in the upper extremities in women and men. J Gerontol A Biol Sci Med Sci 52(5):B267–B276

Miller ME, Rejeski WJ et al 2000 Physical activity, functional limitations, and disability in older adults. J Am Geriatr Soc 48(10):1264–1272

Mitnitski AB, Mogilner AJ et al 2001 Accumulation of deficits as a proxy measure of aging. Scientific World J 1:323–336

Morley JE, Kaiser FE et al 1997 Testosterone and frailty. Clin Geriatr Med 13(4):685–695

Morley JE, Haren MT et al 2006 Frailty. Med Clin North Am 90(5):837–847

Nash CB 2008 Identifying frailty using the ICF: proof of concept. Thesis in fulfillment of degree of MSc in Rehabilitation Science, McGill University, Montreal, Canada

Poehlman ET, Toth MJ et al 1995 Sarcopenia in aging humans: the impact of menopause and disease. J Gerontol A Biol Sci Med Sci 50 Spec No: 73–77

Province MA, Hadley EC et al 1995 The effects of exercise on falls in elderly patients: a preplanned meta-analysis of the FICSIT Trials. Frailty and Injuries: Cooperative Studies of Intervention Techniques. JAMA 273(17):1341–1347

Rice CL, Cunningham DA et al 1989 Arm and leg composition determined by computed tomography in young and elderly men. Clin Physiol 9(3):207–220

Rockwood K 2005 Frailty and its definition: a worthy challenge. J Am Geriatr Soc 53(6):1069–1070

Rockwood K, Fox RA et al 1994 Frailty in elderly people: an evolving concept. CMAJ 150(4):489–495

Rockwood K, Stadnyk K et al 1999 A brief clinical instrument to classify frailty in elderly people. Lancet 353(9148):205–206

Sarkisian CA, Gruenewald TL et al 2008 Preliminary evidence for subdimensions of geriatric frailty: the MacArthur study of successful aging. J Am Geriatr Soc 56(12):2292–2297

Semba RD, Blaum CS et al 2006 Denture use, malnutrition, frailty, and mortality among older women living in the community. J Nutr Health Aging 10(2):161–167

Seynnes O, Fiatarone Singh MA et al 2004 Physiological and functional responses to low-moderate versus high-intensity progressive resistance training in frail elders. J Gerontol A Biol Sci Med Sci 59(5):503–509

Sternberg SA, Wershof Schwartz A et al 2011 The identification of frailty: a systematic literature review. J Am Geriatr Soc 59:2129–2138

Strawbridge WJ, Shema SJ et al 1998 Antecedents of frailty over three decades in an older cohort. J Gerontol B Psychol Sci Soc Sci 53(1):S9–16

Studenski S, Hayes RP et al 2004 Clinical global impression of change in physical frailty: development of a measure based on clinical judgment. J Am Geriatr Soc 52(9):1560–1566

Sugawara J, Miyachi M et al 2002 Age-related reductions in appendicular skeletal muscle mass: association with habitual aerobic exercise status. Clin Physiol Funct Imaging 22(3):169–172

Szanton SL, Seplaki CL et al 2010 Socioeconomic status is associated with frailty: the Women's Health and Aging Studies. J Epidemiol Commun Health 64(1):63–67

Theou O, Rockwood MR et al 2012 Disability and co-morbidity in relation to frailty: how much do they overlap? Arch Gerontol Geriatr 55(2):e1–8

Thorpe RJ, Weiss C et al 2009 Transitions among disability levels or death in African American and white older women. J Gerontol A Biol Sci Med Sci 64A(6):670–674

Tinetti ME, Williams CS 1997 Falls, injuries due to falls, and the risk of admission to a nursing home. N Engl J Med 337(18):1279–1284

Voukelatos A, Cumming RG et al 2007 A randomized, controlled trial of tai chi for the prevention of falls: the Central Sydney tai chi trial. J Am Geriatr Soc 55(8):1185–1191

Walston J, Hadley EC et al 2006 Research agenda for frailty in older adults: towards a better understanding of physiology and etiology: summary from the American Geriatrics Society/National Institute on Aging Research conference on frailty in older adults. J Am Geriatr Soc 54:991–1001

Weening-Dijksterhuis E, de Greef MH et al 2011 Frail institutionalized older persons: a comprehensive review on physical exercise, physical fitness, activities of daily living, and quality-of-life. Am J Phys Med Rehabil 90(2):156–168

Weiss CO 2011 Frailty and chronic diseases in older adults. Clin Geriatr Med 27(1):39–52

Wolf SL, Barnhart HX et al 1996 Reducing frailty and falls in older persons: an investigation of tai chi and computerized balance training. Atlanta FICSIT Group. Frailty and Injuries: Cooperative Studies of Intervention Techniques. J Am Geriatr Soc 44(5):489–497

Wolf SL, Sattin RW et al 2003 Intense tai chi exercise training and fall occurrences in older, transitionally frail adults: a randomized, controlled trial. J Am Geriatr Soc 51(12):1693–1701

Yao X, Li H et al 2011 Inflammation and immune system alterations in frailty. Clin Geriatr Med 27(1):79–87

Chapter 66

Evaluation of pain in older individuals

JOHN O. BARR

Chapter Contents

INTRODUCTION

Pain is the symptom that most commonly prompts individuals to seek healthcare, and it has come to be recognized as a 'fifth vital sign' (Molony et al., 2005). Over 80% of older adults have at least one chronic condition that results in some type of discomfort, including pain (Burke & Jerret, 1989). While arthritis is the most common cause of pain, other conditions that result in chronic pain for the elderly include cancer, compression fracture, degenerative disc disease, diabetic peripheral neuropathy, hip fracture, postherpetic or trigeminal neuralgia and stroke. Older individuals have noted the three most common sites of pain to be the back, leg/knee or hip, and other joints (Abdulla et al., 2013). In outpatient settings, older adults receive less adequate analgesia for moderate to severe acute pain (Moskovitz et al., 2011). During the last 2 years of life, pain is experienced by more than 25% of the elderly, with the prevalence increasing during the last 4 months of life (Smith et al., 2010). Across the continuum from acute postoperative to chronic persistent pain, older people experience less than optimal pain management. Unfortunately, older individuals frequently believe that pain is an inevitable consequence of aging that must simply be endured. Upon being questioned by a health professional, they may deny being in pain out of fear of medical procedures and related expenses, loss of autonomy and possible institutionalization.

The atypical presentation of pain in older persons complicates its clinical evaluation. The cardinal signs of inflammation, including pain, redness, elevated temperature and swelling, are less pronounced in the elderly. For example, acute myocardial infarction can occur without significant pain, while conditions such as appendicitis, bowel gangrene, peptic ulcers and pneumonia may result in only mild discomfort. Instead of producing pain, these conditions may contribute to other behavioral signs such as confusion and fatigue. Conversely, pain that is less common in the elderly, such as headache, can signal serious medical problems such as cerebrovascular accident and temporal arteritis (Papadakis et al., 2013). Inadequate assessment and undertreatment of pain are two primary problems for older individuals (Taylor et al., 2005).

EVALUATION OF PAIN

Key international organizations (e.g. World Health Organization, 2007), professional organizations (e.g. the American Geriatrics Society, 1998, 2000, 2009) and regulatory agencies (e.g. Joint Commission on Accreditation of Healthcare Organizations, 2013) have advocated for improved assessment and treatment of pain experienced by older people. Appropriate evaluation of pain involves the synthesis of information derived from the patient's history, subjective interview, objective physical examination and special tests (e.g. laboratory, imaging, electroneuromyography etc.). The evaluation should clarify the underlying basis for pain and guide therapeutic interventions or result in referral for other specialized healthcare services. Importantly, this evaluation provides baseline information needed to determine the effectiveness of treatment. Periodic re-evaluation allows assessment of the response to treatment, including adverse reactions. The evaluation of pain is unfortunately complicated by its very personal and subjective character. The manner in which an individual reports pain is related to a range of factors that include age, cognitive status, gender, personality, ethnic/cultural background, behavioral needs and past pain experiences.

The patient/client history should include information about current medical conditions and medications that are prescribed: over-the-counter and natural or home remedies. Past interventions that have been both successful and unsuccessful in controlling pain should also be noted. It may be possible to determine patient expectations for or biases against certain interventions, and also to gain further insight as to why a prior treatment was a success or a failure. For example, a previous lack of patient education may have contributed to poor adherence to a prior pain management strategy.

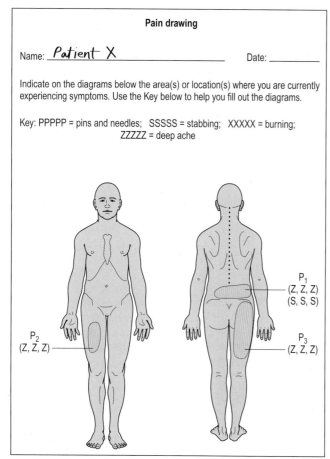

Pain drawing

Name: _Patient X_ _____   Date: _____

Indicate on the diagrams below the area(s) or location(s) where you are currently experiencing symptoms. Use the Key below to help you fill out the diagrams.

Key: PPPPP = pins and needles;   SSSSS = stabbing;   XXXXX = burning;
ZZZZZ = deep ache

P_1
(Z, Z, Z)
(S, S, S)

P_2
(Z, Z, Z)

P_3
(Z, Z, Z)

Figure 66.1 Body diagram completed by a patient to indicate location and quality of pain. (Pattern resulting from right L4–5 lumbar foraminal stenosis with neurogenic claudication.) *(Provided courtesy of Mark J. Levsen, Assistant Professor, Physical Therapy Department, St Ambrose University, Davenport, IA, USA.)*

Box 66.1 *Behaviors recommended to be described when assessing pain in older individuals who are nonverbal or cognitively impaired*

CHANGE IN BEHAVIOR
- Change in socialization, mood, or psychosocial function
- Change in activities of daily living or function
- Change in appetite
- Restlessness
- Agitation or aggressiveness
- Change in sleep pattern
- Change in ambulation

CHANGE IN BODY LANGUAGE
- Facial expression, grinding teeth or grimacing
- Change in body movement (includes stillness, decreased movement, guarding, holding body part, change in posture, limited range of motion, limping or increased muscle tension or tone)
- Unspecified

VOCALIZATION
- Moaning or groaning
- Crying or calling out
- Sighing or grunting
- Unspecified

Reproduced with kind permission from Molony et al., 2005.

---

and physical performance related to occupational and recreational pursuits. It should be recognized that some ADL assessment tools (e.g. the Katz Index of ADL or the Barthel Index) do not represent an adequate range of functional activities for community-active older people, while other tools require too high a level of functioning for some institutionalized cognitively impaired elderly individuals (e.g. the Physical Performance Test). Observational analysis of simulated ADL performance has been found to be sensitive and valid in assessing pain behavior in older people with chronic low back pain (Weiner et al., 1996). Importantly, functional limitations should be translated into treatment plan outcome goals.

PAIN ASSESSMENT TOOLS

A number of pain assessment tools have been developed over the years in the attempt to document clinical pain more objectively. The most basic tool for the assessment of pain intensity is the Verbal Descriptor Scale (VDS; also called the 'Verbal Rating Scale'). Patients are instructed to rate their pain intensity as being 'none', 'mild', 'moderate', 'severe', or 'unbearable'. This scale is preferred by individuals who find it easy to understand, resulting in low failure rates for their scoring. Lack of sensitivity in detecting changes based on the limited number of rating categories is the primary limitation of this type of scale. The Iowa Pain Thermometer (IPT) combines an expanded VDS and a pain thermometer (PT) (Taylor et al., 2005).

The Numeric Rating Scale (NRS; also call the Pain Estimate or PE) requires patients to rate the severity of

The individual should be given the opportunity to freely verbalize complaints of pain and related symptoms (e.g. aching, burning, fatigue, joint locking, joint warmth, paresthesia, stiffness etc.). The clinician should then direct specific questions concerning the onset, occurrence (e.g. at rest vs. activity), intensity (current vs. greatest and least during a specific time period), quality, distribution and duration of pain. Situations that aggravate and relieve pain should be identified (e.g. types of movement, postures, rest etc.). The patient can mark a body diagram to document the location(s) and quality of their pain (Fig. 66.1). Assessment of behavioral indicators of pain is especially useful for documenting the presence of pain in individuals with limited verbal or impaired cognitive abilities (Box 66.1).

The objective examination should focus on physical signs or impairments thought to be associated with a given pain problem (e.g. edema, gait parameters, joint tenderness, muscle strength and endurance, posture, pulmonary functions, range of motion, skin temperature, tissue healing, tolerance to palpation etc.). Typically, there are reduced levels of activity and functional independence, so it is important to evaluate physical function including activities of daily living (ADL)

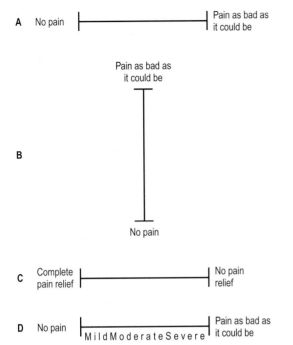

A   No pain   Pain as bad as it could be

B   Pain as bad as it could be ... No pain

C   Complete pain relief ... No pain relief

D   No pain   Mild Moderate Severe   Pain as bad as it could be

Figure 66.2 Simple pain rating scales. **(A)** Visual analogue pain rating scale (horizontal). **(B)** Visual analogue pain rating scale (vertical). **(C)** Visual analogue pain relief rating scale. **(D)** Graphic rating scale. *(Reproduced with permission from Barr, 2000.)*

their pain on a scale of 0 to 10, or 0 to 100 ('0' indicating no pain, and endpoints of '10' or '100' representing the worst possible pain that could ever be imagined). Understanding the definitions related to these endpoints is critical. If a patient mistakenly believes that a rating of '100' is to indicate 'the worst pain I've ever had', pain that is even more severe the next day could not be properly rated. The primary advantages of this approach are that it is easy to understand and that ratings can be done verbally.

The Visual Analogue Pain Scale (VAPS) employs a horizontal 10 cm line with 'no pain' at the left and 'pain as bad as it could be' at the right (Fig. 66.2). Patients mark one location on the line corresponding to the intensity of their pain. This scale may also be vertically oriented. An alternative format requires the rating of pain relief, employing scale anchors of 'complete pain relief' and 'no pain relief'. A major limitation of visual analogue scales is that they rely on vision and motor control, which may be limited in some older patients.

The Graphic Rating Scale (GRS) combines a visual analogue pain rating scale with word descriptors (e.g. mild, moderate, severe). It is important that the word descriptors be placed without spacing along the line between endpoint anchors in order to improve the distribution of patient responses.

Herr and colleagues have provided support for the use of the Faces Pain Scale (FPS) with both cognitively intact and cognitively impaired older individuals (Herr et al., 1998; Taylor et al., 2005). This scale consists of seven cartoon facial depictions arranged in order from least to most distressed (Fig. 66.3). The patient points to the face that best represents the intensity of their pain.

An ordinal pain intensity value ranging from 0 (face at left) to 6 (face at right) is then assigned by the clinician. In order to improve visualization by some older patients, it has been suggested that the height of the faces be increased to 4 cm, and facial markings be darkened and slightly separated.

The McGill Pain Questionnaire (MPQ) is the most widely recognized multidimensional tool for assessing pain in the general population. It includes a body diagram for locating sites of pain. Sensory, affective and evaluative qualities of pain are assessed using a pain rating index that is based on word descriptors. Pain intensity is measured with a five-category present pain intensity scale. A short form of the MPQ has reduced tool administration time from 15 minutes to 5 minutes or less (Melzack, 1987). Although this short form may be less fatiguing, complex word descriptors may present difficulty to some individuals based on their educational level, verbal intelligence and cognitive impairments.

Most of these pain rating scales have been criticized for focusing on the intensity of pain while excluding other important qualitative pain characteristics. It has been recommended that a comprehensive evaluation of pain should include both unidimensional (e.g. VDS, VAPS) and multidimensional (i.e. MPQ) measures as each assesses an important part of the overall pain experience (Gagliese & Melzack, 1997). The Philadelphia Pain Intensity Scale is a six-item scale that requires patients to assess pain at four points in time (i.e. over past few weeks, right now, at its worst and at its least) and to determine how much pain has interfered with daily activities (using integer ratings from '1' [not at all] to '5' [extremely]), and to note how many days a week that pain gets really bad (Parmelee, 1994). Alternatively, the 24-item Geriatric Pain Measure questionnaire assess pain intensity, patient disengagement and pain during ambulation, strenuous activities and other activities (Ferrell et al., 2000). For older individuals in acute pain, but unable to verbally communicate, the five item ALGOPLUS assesses characteristics related to the behaviors of facial expression (e.g. grimacing), look (e.g. inattentiveness, teary-eyed), vocalized complaints (e.g. groaning or screaming), body position (e.g. frozen posture) and atypical behaviours (e.g. agitation) (Rat et al., 2011). The presence of indicated characteristics for two or more of these behaviors has been determined to indicate that the patient is experiencing acute pain (with 87% sensitivity and 80% specificity).

The following is an overview of small number of studies that have critically assessed methods of rating pain used exclusively by older individuals. Goode and Barr (1993) found that a majority of community-active older people felt that the PE (i.e. NRS) was both easier to use and better described their recollected pain than the VAPS. However, participants committed very few errors when using the VAPS, thus helping to support the validity of its uses with older adults. Utilizing the FPS, NRS, VAPS and VDS with cognitively intact older individuals, almost half of whom were African Americans, Stuppy (1998) concluded that a majority preferred the FPS, which was also valid and reliable. Herr and Mobily (1993) determined that community-based elderly people preferred and

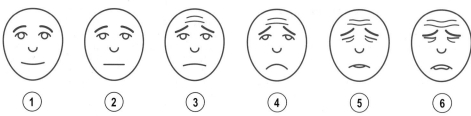

Figure 66.3 The faces pain scale. *(Reproduced with permission from Bieri et al., 1990.)*

found the VDS easier to use than the VAPS, the NRS or the PT. Using ambulatory geriatric clinic patients, Ferrell et al. (2000) reported that the GPM was both valid and reliable. Wynne et al. (2000) found that more than half of their cognitively impaired long-term care residents could utilize the FPS, VAS and VRS, but not the McGill word scale; lower cognitive function made completion of these scales more difficult. Examining cognitively impaired community elderly (mean Mini Mental State Exam score = 15.7), Krulewitch et al. (2000) determined that over 40% could complete the VAS, FPS and the Philadelphia Pain Intensity Scale. For those able to complete one or two scales, the greatest number completed the Philadelphia Scale. Taylor et al. (2005) reported that both cognitively intact and cognitively impaired older assisted living residents preferred the VDS and IPT over the NRS and FPS. Concurrent validity was support for all assessment tools, except for the FPS when used by the cognitively impaired group. Test–retest reliability was acceptable for the cognitively intact subjects using all these assessment tools, but was unacceptable for the cognitively impaired group for all tools except the VDS.

A number of practical suggestions for assessing pain experienced by older people have appeared in the literature (Herr & Mobily, 1991; Taylor et al., 2005). The health status of the patient/client, severity of pain and ability to cooperate should guide the number and complexity of evaluation sessions needed for adequate pain assessment. It is crucial to establish good rapport and to avoid being rushed during evaluation sessions, both increasingly difficult tasks in today's healthcare system. Impairments in vision, hearing, speech and mental processes should be taken into account and accommodated as these will have a direct impact on the use of specific pain assessment tools. Lighting should be adequate and larger print on evaluation tools may be needed. The patient must be able to successfully use a pain measurement tool, with supervision and even coaching if necessary. In the presence of cognitive impairment, time must be provided for patients to assimilate questions and to formulate their responses. A daily pain log or diary can be used by patients and caregivers to document pain intensity, medications, response to treatment and functional activities. Family members, friends and other healthcare workers can provide useful information about changes in behavior or functioning related to pain. Observational assessment, with inferences drawn from facial expression, body language and other nonverbal behaviors, can be used to identify pain in severely demented older people (see Box 66.1). The assessment of pain in older adults with cognitive impairment remains complex, and lacking in a gold standard for an assessment tool (Thuathail & Welford, 2011).

CONCLUSION

Appropriate evaluation of pain is critical to effective pain management for older individuals. Clinicians should utilize an individualized approach when evaluating pain, taking into account an array of age-related factors and patient/client preferences in the selection of pain assessment tools. Specific diagnoses associated with aging (e.g. dementias, including Alzheimer's disease) will require the development, validation and reliability testing of new pain assessment tools.

References

Abdulla A, Adams N, Bone M et al 2013 Guidance on the management of pain in older people. Age Aging 42:i1–i57

American Geriatrics Society Panel on Chronic Pain in Older Persons 1998 The management of chronic pain in older persons. J Am Geriatr Soc 46:635–651

American Geriatrics Society Panel on Persistent Pain in Older Persons 2002 Clinical practice guidelines: the management of persistent pain in older persons. J Am Geriatr Soc 50:S205–S224

American Geriatrics Society Panel on the Pharmacological Management of Persistent Pain in Older Persons 2009 Special article: Pharmacological management of persistent pain in older persons. J Am Geriatr Soc 57:1331–1346

Barr JO 2000 Conservative pain management for the older patient. In: Guccione AA (ed) Geriatric Physical Therapy, 2nd edn. Mosby, St Louis, MO

Bieri D, Reeve RA, Champion GD et al 1990 The Faces Pain Scale for the self-assessment of the severity of pain experienced by children: development, initial validation, and preliminary investigation for ratio scale properties. Pain 41:139–150

Burke SO, Jerret M 1989 Pain management across age groups. West J Nurs Res 11:164–178

Ferrell BA, Stein WM, Beck JC 2000 The Geriatric Pain Measure: validity, reliability and factor analysis. J Am Geriatr Soc 48(12): 1669–1673

Gagliese L, Melzack R 1997 Chronic pain in elderly people. Pain 70:3–14

Goode J, Barr JO 1993 Comparison of two methods of pain assessment by the elderly: pain estimate (PE) vs. visual analogue scale (VAS). Phys Ther 73:6S

Herr KA, Mobily PR 1991 Complexities of pain assessment in the elderly: clinical considerations. J Gerontol Nurs 17:12–19

Herr KA, Mobily PR 1993 Comparison of selected pain assessment tools for use with the elderly. Appl Nurs Res 6:39–46

Herr KA, Mobily PR, Kohout FJ et al 1998 Evaluation of the faces pain scale for use with elderly. Clin J Pain 14:29–38

Joint Commission on Accreditation of Healthcare Organizations 2013 Facts about pain management. www.jointcommission.org/assets/1/18/pain_management1.pdf

Krulewitch H, London MR, Skakel V et al 2000 Assessment of pain in cognitively impaired older adults: a comparison of pain assessment tools and their use by nonprofessional caregivers. J Am Geriatr Soc 48:1607–1611

Melzack R 1987 The short-form McGill Pain Questionnaire. Pain 30:191–197

Molony SL, Kobayashi M, Holleran EA et al 2005 Assessing pain as a fifth vital sign in long-term care facilities: recommendations from the field. J Gerontol Nurs 31(3):16–24

Moskovitz BL, Bensen CJ, Patel AA et al 2011 Analgesic treatment for moderate-to-severe acute pain in the United States: patients' perspectives in the Physicians Partnering Against Pain (P3) survey. J Opioid Manag 7(4):277–286

Papadakis M, McPhee SJ, Rabow MW 2013 Current Medical Diagnosis and Treatment. In: Lange, 52nd edn. McGraw-Hill, New York

Parmelee PA 1994 Assessment of pain in the elderly. In: Lawton MP, Teresi J (eds) Annual Review of Gerontology and Geriatrics. Springer, New York

Rat P, Jouve E, Pickering G et al 2011 Validation of an acute pain-behavior scale for older persons with inability to communicate verbally: Algoplus. Eur J Pain 15(198):e1–98

Smith AK, Cenzer IS, Knight SJ et al 2010 The epidemiology of pain during the last 2 years of life. Ann Intern Med 153(9):563–569

Stuppy D 1998 The Faces Pain Scale: reliability and validity with mature adults. Appl Nurs Res 11(2):84–89

Taylor JT, Harris J, Epps CD et al 2005 Psychometric evaluation of selected pain intensity scales for use with cognitively impaired and cognitively intact older adults. Rehabil Nurs 30(2):55–61

Thuathail N, Welford C 2011 Pain assessment tools for older people with cognitive impairment. Nurs Stand 26(6):39–46

Weiner D, Pieper C, McConnell E et al 1996 Pain measurement in elders with chronic low back pain: traditional and alternative approaches. Pain 67:461–467

World Health Organization 2007 WHO normative guideline on pain management: Report of a delphi study to determine the need for guidelines and to identify the number and topics for guidelines that should be developed by WHO. World Health Organization, Geneva

Wynne CF, Ling SM, Remsburg R 2000 Comparison of pain assessment instruments in cognitively intact and cognitively impaired nursing home residents. Geriatr Nurs 21(1):20–23

Special physical therapeutic intervention techniques

Chapter 67

Conservative interventions for pain control

JOHN O. BARR

CHAPTER CONTENTS

INTRODUCTION

The successful physical rehabilitation of older individuals requires that pain be eliminated or minimized to a level that allows the improvement of related impairments (e.g. weakness, low endurance, loss of joint range of motion [ROM], etc.), overcoming activity limitations (e.g. inability to ambulate independently, ability to sit for only brief periods, etc.) and the prevention of participation restrictions (e.g. inability to work at the community food bank or to travel to visit grandchildren, etc.). Analgesic medications are the most common treatment used for pain management in older adults. Fortunately, hazards associated with some popular medications used for pain control by the elderly are becoming increasingly well known. Factors related to proper pharmacological management of pain are discussed in Chapter 12.

Although Clinical Practice Guidelines established by the American Geriatrics Society have most recently emphasized pharmacologic interventions for persistent pain (American Geriatrics Society, 2009), non-pharmacologic (NP) approaches alone or in combination with medications have also been recognized as an integral part of care (American Geriatrics Society, 1998, 2002). Proper use of conservative interventions for pain control can lessen the need for medications and may allow postponement of elective surgery for some painful conditions that are common in older adults. Traditionally, conservative NP interventions have not been well utilized in the management of some diagnoses associated with pain in older individuals (e.g. osteoarthritis of the hip) (Shrier et al., 2006). Among the NP/non-surgical interventions rated at 89% or higher on strength of research in the Osteoarthritis Research Society International consensus guidelines for management of hip and knee osteoarthritis were: education, exercise, weight control, walking aides and referral to physical therapy for evaluation and instruction (Zhang et al., 2008). Interestingly, in a recent study of almost 600 community-dwelling older adults, NP approaches were used more frequently (68%) than pharmacological approaches (49%) to manage persistent pain (Stewart et al., 2013).

This chapter reviews evidence regarding the effectiveness of conservative interventions commonly used to control pain experienced by older people (i.e. individuals aged 55 years and more). Interventions discussed include assistive devices and orthotics, massage, electrical stimulation, thermal agents and exercise. Information from systematic reviews focused on diagnoses common for older people, and randomized control trials (RCTs) limited to older individuals are emphasized. Theoretical mechanisms of action for these interventions in controlling pain are outlined in Box 67.1 (Barr, 2000), which can be used to provide rationale for the selection and application of specific interventions.

ASSISTIVE AND ORTHOTIC DEVICES

Properly selected and fitted assistive or orthotic devices act to limit mechanical forces that would otherwise stimulate pain at a site of pathology, inflammation or trauma (see Box 67.1). Canes and walkers are among the most common assistive devices used by older individuals with pain. Hip joint contact forces can be reduced by more than 30% using a cane held in the hand opposite to the involved hip. Raised seats on toilets and chairs act to limit joint forces at the hips and knees during push-off from a seated position. However, assistive devices that are improperly fitted or used incorrectly can act to increase pain (Abdulla et al., 2013).

Impact-absorbing shoes may help to relieve foot, ankle, knee and hip pain from osteoarthritis (OA). Hodge et al. (1999) assessed foot orthotics (prefabricated, standard custom molded, custom with metatarsal bar, custom with metatarsal dome) for older patients with

---

Box 67.1 *Primary theoretical mechanisms of action for conservative interventions used to manage pain*

DECREASE ACTIVITY OF NOCICEPTORS OR THEIR SENSORY NEURONS

Limit mechanical stresses through:

- Use of assistive gait device (e.g. cane or walker) or orthosis (e.g. shoe insert, splint or brace)
- Minimizing effects of gravity via hydrotherapy or swimming
- Preventing acute edema formation with ice, compression and elevation
- Resorption of chronic edema via mild heat, massage, elevation, compression or electrical stimulation
- Elongation of connective tissue using vigorous heat (diathermy or ultrasound) and prolonged stretch
- Restoration of normal joint arthrokinematics via joint mobilization, stretching or strengthening exercise
- Application of ergonomic principles

Limit effects of depolarizing and sensitizing agents through:

- Enhanced local circulation with mild to moderate heat, massage, exercise or electrical stimulation
- Decreased local metabolic activity with cryotherapy (e.g. cold pack or ice massage)
- Decreased muscle spasm via heat, cold, massage, TENS or exercise

Create local anesthetic or anti-inflammatory effects through:

- Iontophoresis (e.g. with lidocaine [lignocaine] or dexamethasone)

- Phonophoresis (e.g. with hydrocortisone)
- Cryotherapy (e.g. cold pack or ice massage)
- TENS

INCREASE ACTIVITY OF MECHANORECEPTORS OR THEIR SENSORY NEURONS

Stimulate mechanoreceptors through:

- Passive and active joint range of motion (ROM) exercise
- Joint mobilization
- Comfortable massage (e.g. effleurage and petrissage)
- Voluntary (e.g. walking, swimming, bicycling) or electrically stimulated exercise

Directly stimulate large-diameter neurons from mechanoreceptors through:

- Comfortable low- to moderate-intensity TENS (e.g. conventional, pulse-burst or modulated TENS)

INCREASE DESCENDING OR SPINAL LEVEL INHIBITION WITHIN THE CENTRAL NERVOUS SYSTEM

Use of uncomfortable 'counterirritants' such as:

- Intense massage (e.g. vigorous kneading, strong friction, acupressure, connective tissue massage)
- Uncomfortable but tolerated TENS (e.g. strong low-rate, brief-intense or hyperstimulation TENS)
- Uncomfortable brief ice massage

TENS, transcutaneous electrical nerve stimulation
Adapted from Barr, 2000.

---

rheumatoid arthritis (RA). Pressure at the first and second metatarsal heads was significantly reduced by all orthoses tested. The standard custom molded and dome orthoses significantly decreased walking pain. However, only the dome orthosis significantly decreased pain during standing, and it was preferred by the majority of patients. A pilot study by Seligman and Dawson (2003) demonstrated that a combination of customized heel pads and soft orthotic inserts produced a significant decrease in heel pain from plantar fasciitis.

Knee pain from medial compartment OA may be decreased by the use of lateral heel wedges in shoes. These wedges shift more of the joint loading to the lateral side of the knee. With medial femorotibial osteoarthritis, Maillefert et al. (2001) found that, when compared with neutral insoles, laterally wedged insoles were associated with significantly decreased nonsteroidal anti-inflammatory drug (NSAID) consumption at 6 months. However, scores on Western Ontario & McMaster Universities Osteoarthritis (WOMAC) index subscales for pain, joint stiffness and physical function did not differ significantly for the two types of insoles. In a 2-year follow-up, Pham et al. (2004) found essentially the same outcomes, and no significant difference in the rates of joint space narrowing. Interestingly, using lateral wedges in combination with subtalar straps for 6 months, Toda and Tsukimura (2004) demonstrated significant decreases in both the femorotibial angle and pain but no significant changes with traditional insoles. Knee braces

incorporating a varus unloader increase femorotibial separation during walking and can be used for unicompartmental knee pain, but these have not been found to be effective for obese patients with knee OA (Buckwalter et al., 2001). Systematically reviewing brace and orthotic effectiveness in the treatment of knee OA, Brouwer et al. (2009) concluded that a brace or laterally wedged insoles have a 'silver' level of evidence for a small beneficial effect on pain; however, long-term adherence for either was low. Most recently, Shamliyan et al. (2012), as part of an Agency for Healthcare Research and Quality supported analysis, found orthotics to improve knee pain associated with OA.

Spinal orthoses can provide varying degrees of immobilization, plus important tactile cues, for patients with neck and back pain. While a soft cervical collar does little to immobilize, tactile cueing can help a patient with mild spondylosis to limit motion or improve alignment of the cervical spine. For a patient with RA and atlantoaxial subluxation, a rigid Philadelphia collar or a sternal–occipitoandibular immobilizer (SOMI) may be required.

Kyphosis related to spinal osteoporosis often causes chronic upper and middle back pain in older women. A cruciform anterior spinal hyperextension (CASH) orthosis or Jewett hyperextension orthosis can be used to limit spinal flexion. In contrast, an orthosis that limits extension, such as a Williams flexion orthosis, can be used to control pain from spinal stenosis. Compression fractures from spinal osteoporosis may call for a thoracic lumbosacral orthosis (TLSO). Pfeifer et al. (2004) evaluated the

'Spinomed', a lightweight perispinal metal orthosis, with an abdominal pad and shoulder straps. It was worn only 2 hours per day by women with osteoporotic vertebral fractures. At the end of 6 months, orthosis wearers demonstrated: a 38% decrease in 'average' pain; a 27% decrease in limits of daily living; an 11% decrease in kyphotic angle; a 25% decrease in sway; and an increase of 73% in back extension and 58% in abdominal flexor strength.

SPECIAL CONSIDERATIONS

When using assistive devices to limit forces on the lower extremities or spine, the clinician should be careful not to overload the patient's upper extremities. Adverse effects of orthotic use include skin breakdown due to pressure from orthotic components, psychological dependency and weakening of muscles whose action has been limited by the orthosis. Proper evaluation, selection, fit and short-term use of assistive devices and orthotics can help to prevent these problems.

MASSAGE

Massage is defined as the intentional and systematic manipulation of soft body tissues to enhance health and healing (Benjamin & Tappan, 2005). There are many varieties of massage, ranging from the comfortable and gentle superficial stroking of effleurage, to the invigorating kneading of petrissage, to uncomfortable forms of deep friction massage. Potential mechanisms underlying pain relief with these various forms of massage are noted in Box 67.1.

A limited number of studies on massage have been conducted exclusively with older individuals. Sansone and Schmitt (2000) had trained certified nursing assistants (CNAs) to provide 'tender touch' massage to older nursing home residents suffering from chronic pain and dementia over a period of 12 weeks. Patients experienced decreased pain and anxiety scores, and the CNAs reported improved ability to communicate with the residents. Mok and Woo (2004) determined that 10 minutes of nightly slow stroke back massage given to hospitalized patients with shoulder pain after cerebrovascular accident was associated with significantly decreased pain and anxiety that lasted for up to 3 days when compared with a control group.

SPECIAL CONSIDERATIONS

Massage is a safe intervention with a low risk of adverse effects. General contraindications for massage include skin infections, active inflammation and deep vein thrombosis. Specific contraindications for massage can be related to both the underlying pathology and the amount of force provided by a specific massage procedure. Contraindications would include, for example: superficial stroking over open wounds and areas of acute inflammation or infection; kneading massage to limbs at risk of deep vein thrombosis, with a nonconsolidated fracture, active cancer tumor, thrombophlebitis, or during anticoagulant therapy; and friction massage over a recently healed burn wound.

Vigorous massage strokes, such as deep effleurage or petrissage, should not be applied to fragile skin that is prone to tearing, as is encountered with many frail elderly individuals. Because of massage's influence in lowering heart rate and blood pressure, the clinician must be aware of other medical conditions (e.g. postural hypotension) that could be aggravated. Older individuals may require special positioning to receive massage based on underlying medical conditions (e.g. severe chronic obstructive pulmonary disease, preventing the use of a recumbent position) or deformity (e.g. severe kyphosis, limiting positioning in prone lying) (Benjamin & Tappan, 2005).

ELECTRICAL STIMULATION

Clinical electrical stimulation as done by rehabilitation professionals uses electrodes placed on the surface of the skin to stimulate nerves transcutaneously. More specifically, transcutaneous electrical nerve stimulation (TENS) involves the stimulation of cutaneous and peripheral nerves to control pain. At least six types, or 'modes', of TENS have been described in the literature: conventional (or 'high frequency'), strong low-rate (or 'acupuncture-like'), brief intense, pulse-burst, modulated and hyperstimulation (see Table 67.1) The potential mechanisms of action for these TENS modes are noted in Box 67.1.

Each mode of TENS involves specific electrical stimulator output characteristics that produce different perceptual-motor experiences related to the relief of pain (see Table 67.1). Placement of electrodes varies with the TENS mode used and can include positioning of a pair of electrodes: at the perimeter of the painful area (i.e. 'bracketing' the area); over a cutaneous or peripheral nerve proximal to the painful area; over a peripheral nerve to a muscle in the painful area; with one electrode over the site of pain and the other paraspinally over the related segmental nerve root; or at related acupuncture points.

The Philadelphia Panel (2001) found clinically important benefit for pain and patient global assessment, and noted good evidence to include TENS as an intervention for pain associated with knee OA. In contrast, based on analysis of the literature, Shamliyan et al. (2012) concluded the electrical stimulation actually worsened knee pain from OA.

The Cochrane Collaboration has published systematic reviews concerned with electrical stimulation for pain control, some of which have included older patients among their subjects. Osiri et al. (2000) assessed the effectiveness of TENS in treating knee OA. Pain relief from TENS and acupuncture-like TENS delivered over at least 4 weeks was significantly better than placebo treatment; knee stiffness was also significantly improved by TENS. Different TENS modes (high-rate and strong-burst) had significant benefit in pain relief over placebo. However, an update of this review could not confirm TENS to be effective for relief of pain associated with OA of the knee (Rutjes et al., 2009).

Two other applications of electrical stimulation have been systematically reviewed. Brosseau et al. (2010) evaluated the effectiveness of TENS for the treatment of RA of the hand. In comparison to a placebo, acupuncture-like TENS was found to be beneficial for reducing pain intensity and improving muscle power. Although conventional TENS had no clinical benefit in reducing

Table 67.1	**Common modes of transcutaneous electrical nerve stimulation (TENS) for pain**		
Mode Classification	TENS Unit Output Characteristics	Electrode Site Options	Desired Perceptual–Motor Experience
'Conventional'	Frequency: 10–100 Hz Intensity: low to medium	At perimeter of painful area; over nerve to region; or at segmentally related area	Comfortable paresthesia superimposed on painful area, or in segmentally related area
'Strong low-rate' (or 'acupuncture-like')	Frequency: 10 Hz Intensity: high	Over nerve related to muscle in or remote from painful area	Uncomfortable rhythmic muscle contractions at patient tolerance
'Brief-intense'	Frequency: 60–150 Hz Intensity: high	Over nerve related to muscle in or remote from painful area	Uncomfortable tetanic muscle contraction that fatigues, at patient tolerance
'Pulse-burst'	Frequency: high (60–100 Hz) modulated by low (0.5–4 Hz) Intensity: low to high	Over nerve related to muscle in or remote from painful area	Weak to strong intermittent tetanic muscle contraction and paresthesia
'Modulated'	Frequency, pulse duration, or amplitude modulated separately or together Intensity: low to high	Any of these listed sites	Weak to strong sensation, with or without muscle contraction; may minimize perceptual accommodation
'Hyperstimulation'	Frequency: 1–100 Hz Intensity: high, based on current density	Acupuncture points	Sharp burning sensation at tolerance; no muscle contraction

Adapted from Barr, 2000.

pain, it was seen to have more benefit for patient assessment of change in the disease process than acupuncture-like TENS. Price and Pandyan (2006) assessed the efficacy of common forms of surface electrical stimulation for preventing and treating poststroke shoulder pain. Evidence from the RCTs reviewed was not seen to either confirm or refute that electrical stimulation (including TENS) to the shoulder after stroke influenced reports of pain; however, passive lateral rotation of the shoulder appeared to benefit. No adverse effects were documented.

To date, only a small number of studies have examined the effect of TENS exclusively with older adults. Grant et al. (1999) compared acupuncture with TENS for chronic back pain. Both interventions significantly improved pain scores and decreased analgesic intake after 4 weeks of treatment and for up to 3 months after treatment. Barr et al. (2004) applied conventional TENS, high-intensity pulse-burst TENS, and sham TENS to assisted-living residents with chronic musculoskeletal pain. Pain was decreased significantly for both conventional and pulse-burst TENS, averaging 23% and 32% respectively. Not surprisingly, low-intensity conventional TENS was found to be more comfortable than high-intensity pulse-burst TENS. Defrin et al. (2005) treated patients with knee OA with either innocuous or noxious (hyperstimulation) intensities of interferential current (IFC) electrical stimulation. IFC to the knee produced significant decreases in chronic pain and morning stiffness, and significant increases in ROM and pain threshold. IFC was deemed to be very effective (with hyperstimulation being most effective in decreasing the intensity of knee pain). Most recently, Stewart et al. (2013) determined that fewer than 5% of

community-dwelling older adults used TENS to manage their persistent pain.

SPECIAL CONSIDERATIONS

The most common problem associated with TENS for a small number of patients is dermatitis at the electrode sites. Dry skin associated with aging and the use of alcohol-based skin care products can increase skin resistance to the flow of electrical current, which then requires higher intensity stimulation. This may cause discomfort and irritation to the skin. The use of additional electrode gel, slight moistening of an electrode's synthetic surface, and hydration of the skin with a nonalcohol-based cream can lower skin impedance and increase comfort for these patients. Regular use of alternate electrode sites can prevent the breakdown of fragile skin due to the cumulative effects of allergic, chemical, electrical and mechanical irritation. To prevent tearing of the skin during electrode removal, electrodes should be peeled off gently and slowly while holding down the underlying skin.

The primary contraindication for TENS in older adults is use near areas with implanted electrical devices, such as cardiac pacemakers that may be affected by the electrical field generated by the stimulator. All patients with cardiac pacemakers should be electrically monitored during initial trials and extended use of TENS. Carlson and colleagues have described a testing protocol to assess interference from a TENS unit for a patient with an implanted pacemaker (Carlson et al., 2009). If interference is noted, it is possible to have the cardiologist reprogram the pacemaker to a lower level of sensitivity.

In order to facilitate appropriate use and adherence, rehabilitation professionals should be familiar with the options available for TENS and unit components. TENS units that require no adjustment of complex controls may be best suited for a patient with cognitive limitations who needs to use TENS as part of a home program. Self-adhering electrodes or electrodes that are incorporated into a band with a Velcro closure may be the best option for an older adult with limited mobility or impaired hand dexterity.

THERMAL AGENTS

The thermal agents used in pain control include a variety of therapeutic cooling and heating modalities that have both direct and reflex effects, with theoretical mechanisms of action noted in Box 67.1. Thermal agents can target body tissues at various depths, ranging from the skin to the muscle/bone interface. The effective depths of penetration for common thermal agents are depicted in Table 67.2.

Superficial heating agents (e.g. hot packs, warm hydrotherapy, paraffin, fluidotherapy and infrared) or deep heating agents (e.g. short-wave and microwave diathermy, and ultrasound) can be used to increase blood flow, membrane permeability, tissue extensibility and joint ROM in ways that can contribute to decreasing pain. Heat and cold alter both peripheral and central nervous system excitability, and can thus serve as a means of modulating pain. Brief uncomfortable application of cold (e.g. brief ice massage) can be used as a 'counterirritant' to decrease pain (see Box 67.1 for the theoretical mechanisms of action).

The Philadelphia Panel (2001) determined in the general population that thermal agents were either of no benefit or lacked evidence to either include or exclude them as a therapeutic intervention for chronic low back pain, neck pain, shoulder pain and knee pain from OA or after surgery. However, ultrasound was found to have a clinically important benefit in managing pain associated with shoulder calcific tendonitis. Analysis by Shamliyan et al. (2012) found that ultrasound for knee OA improved pain, while diathermy and other forms of heat resulted in no improvements.

Only a couple of additional systematic reviews have been conducted for thermal agents. In contrast to the prior version of their review, Rutjes et al. (2010) found that therapeutic ultrasound administered over 2–8 weeks may be beneficial for decreasing pain and improving function in patients with knee OA. Welch et al. (2011) evaluated thermotherapy used for RA. While no significant effects on pain were determined for hot or ice packs, positive results for pain on non-resisted motion were seen with paraffin wax baths after four consecutive weeks of treatment. Assessing thermotherapy for treatment of OA, Brosseau et al. (2011) determined that, while ice massage had significant beneficial effect on knee ROM, strength and function, and cold packs decreased swelling, neither had a significant impact on pain.

Interventions that can afford pain relief for older people need not be technically complex. Robinson and Benton (2002) found that the use of warm blankets for elderly hospitalized patients produced reduced levels of

Table 67.2 **Depth of effective penetration into the body by common thermal agents**	
Thermal Agent	**Depth into Soft Tissues**
Cold pack	2 mm–4 cm
Hot pack	2–5 mm
Hydrotherapy (warm)	2–5 mm
Paraffin	2–5 mm
Fluidotherapy	2–5 mm
Infrared	
Nonluminous	2–5 mm
Luminous	5 mm–1 cm
Short-wave diathermy (27.12 MHz; subcutaneous fat, 2 cm thick)	1–3 cm
Microwave diathermy (2450 MHz; nondirect contact applicator; subcutaneous fat, 0.5 cm thick)	1–5 cm
Ultrasound	
3 MHz	1–2 cm
1 MHz	1–5 cm

Reproduced with permission from Barr, 2000.

discomfort (e.g. pain, being cold, or feeling anxious). Interestingly, Stewart et al. (2013) determined women to be nearly two times more likely than men to use thermal modalities for management of persistent pain.

SPECIAL CONSIDERATIONS

A range of precautions for thermal agents used with older adults have been noted in the professional literature. Contributing to an increased risk of thermal injury are factors such as: decreased hypothalamic thermoregulatory system reactivity; decreased autonomic and vasomotor responses; impairments in the circulatory system; loss of sweat glands; atrophy of skin and related reduction in circulation; decreased sensation of thirst; and decreased perception of thermal gradients. Medications can impair thermoregulatory control. For example, vasodilation of the skin may be hampered by diuretics that limit volume expansion. Anticholinergic drugs, dermatologic conditions and spinal cord lesions can impair sweating. Long-term use of steroids produces fragile capillaries easily damaged by thermal agents. Skin vasodilation from the heating of large body surface areas can produce hazardous demands on cardiac output. Cold agents may produce short-term increases in systolic and diastolic blood pressures, posing a risk for hypertensive patients. Cold agents may be associated with increases in mechanical stiffness of joints and cold intolerance for some patients.

Considerations for older patients when using thermal agents include (Barr, 2000):

1. Selecting an appropriate thermal agent for a given clinical condition. Deep heating of joints involved

with pathologies such as OA should be avoided because it may contribute to temperature-sensitive enzymatic lysis of joint cartilage. Superficial moist heating for less than 20 minutes has actually been shown to produce lowering of joint temperature. However, with arthritic knees, intra-articular temperature 3 hours after treatment was increased by superficial heat and decreased by superficial cold agents (Oosterveld & Rasker, 1994).

2. Lowering temperatures for heating agents and increasing temperatures for cooling agents. Hot and cold packs will need to be better insulated by using a greater thickness of toweling. If the patient can only be positioned comfortably by resting on top of these packs, additional layers of toweling must be used because of compression of the insulating layers.

3. Producing a slower rate of temperature change, particularly for ultrasound, which provides rapid deep temperature elevation. This can be accomplished by using a lower intensity, faster sound head movement and less overlap of sound head strokes.

4. Shortening treatment time. The traditional 30 minutes for superficial heating agents may need to be limited to no longer than 20 minutes. More conservative treatment durations for deep heating agents may be appropriate. For example, it may be necessary to perform ultrasound for 5 minutes for each $150\,cm^2$, as opposed to 5 minutes for an area two to three times the sound head area ($20-30\,cm^2$).

Although the above modifications may improve the safety of thermal agents used with older patients, further research is needed to determine whether the resultant treatment effects are increased or diminished.

EXERCISE

Exercise has been determined to be the most common NP strategy, reportedly used by 50% of older adults to manage persistent pain (Stewart et al., 2013). Exercise programs can range from low intensity (e.g. walking) to high intensity (e.g. strengthening or endurance exercises) and may include specific types of exercises, such as trunk extension and 'core' strengthening programs. Various forms of exercise may be employed to modulate pain either directly or indirectly, as depicted in Box 67.1. A direct effect on pain may be achieved by increasing input from joint mechanoreceptors through passive or active exercise. Indirect effects of exercise on pain may be related to: increased blood flow that disperses chemical depolarizing/sensitizing agents; decreased edema; inhibition or fatigue of muscle spasm; enhanced ROM, flexibility, strength or endurance, which may improve biomechanical factors; and relaxation and reduction in anxiety. Additionally, exercise is an important adjunct to other interventions (e.g. thermal agents, patient education, etc.) in attaining significant relief from chronic pain.

In the general population, the Philadelphia Panel (2001) determined that therapeutic exercise has clinically important benefits for: low back pain (i.e. postsurgical, subacute and chronic, but not for acute); knee pain (i.e. associated with OA; but not when done preoperatively for postsurgical pain); and chronic neck pain. Insufficient evidence was found relative to shoulder pain due to calcific tendonitis or non-specific shoulder pain. An analysis by Shamliyan et al. (2012) found that aerobic, strengthening, or proprioceptive exercises produced improvements in OA knee pain, but that tai chi resulted in no improvement in pain. Aerobic and aquatic exercise was also associated with improved function.

Systematic reviews by Fransen and McConnell (2009) found 'platinum level' evidence for land-based therapeutic exercise as having at least short-term benefit on pain and physical function associated with OA of the knee, but only a small effect on pain from hip OA. While no long-term effects were noted, a systematic review by Bartels et al. (2009) indicated that aquatic exercise appears to have beneficial short-term effects for hip and/or knee pain from OA.

A few specific RCTs warrant specific mention. Ferrell et al. (1997) assigned older adults with chronic musculoskeletal pain to 6 weeks of a supervised program of walking, a pain education program (i.e. demonstrations on heat, cold, massage, relaxation and distraction), or 'usual care' (i.e. continuation of already prescribed treatments, printed information about pain management, and weekly phone calls from a nurse educator). Pain improved significantly for patients in both intervention programs but not for those receiving usual care. Minor et al. (1989) compared 12 weeks of aerobic walking, aerobic aquatics, nonaerobic active ROM, and relaxation exercises for chronic RA and OA. Both the aerobic and the nonaerobic exercises demonstrated significant improvements in pain, and there was no significant difference between these groups. Baker et al. (2001) assessed the effectiveness of a 4-month progressive high-intensity home exercise program (HEP) on knee OA for community-dwelling elderly people (vs. nutrition education as a control group). Outcomes included significantly greater improvements for the HEP (vs. the control group) relative to pain, strength and improved function. The effectiveness of a 12-month community-based water exercise program was assessed by Lin et al. (2004) for sedentary community-dwelling elderly individuals (vs. monthly education combined with quarterly phone calls). Exercise participants had significantly better improvements in pain, physical function, ability to ascend/descend stairs, and both hip and knee ROM; however, differences were not significant for quadriceps strength and for ratings of psychological wellbeing. Callahan et al. (2008) studied more than 600 sedentary urban and rural 'PACE' program participants who had OA or RA, and trained for 1 hour twice weekly for 8 weeks using range of motion and low resistance exercises. At the end of training, the treatment group had significantly better outcomes than the control for pain, fatigue and self-efficacy for managing arthritis. These results were maintained at 6 months, without adverse events or exacerbation.

Tai chi has also been examined for its potential value in pain management with older adults. Evaluating the impact of a 12-week Sun-style tai chi exercise program for community-dwelling elderly women with knee OA,

Song et al. (2003) found that tai chi was associated with significantly less joint pain and stiffness, fewer difficulties in physical function, improved balance and increased abdominal muscle strength in comparison to a non-exercise control group. Brismee et al. (2007) assessed the effect of a 12 week Sun-style tai chi program for older adults with knee OA. Although the treated subjects had significantly better outcomes than the controls related to both maximum and overall knee pain, these effects were not sustained during a 6 week detraining period. In a systematic review concerned with use of tai chi in management of RA, Lee et al. (2007) concluded that its effectiveness in reducing pain had not been demonstrated.

Not all programs concerned with better pain management require the involvement of health professionals. Parker et al. (2011) assessed the impact of the Arthritis Foundation Self-Help Program (ASHP) on Hispanic, African American and non-Hispanic White older adults experiencing a range of non-cancer pain disorders. The program was conducted by a certified instructor for 2 hours, once each week, for 6 weeks. Program content included disease-specific information, stress management strategies, medication use, coping techniques and exercise alternatives. Surveyed in person prior to and by telephone 12 weeks after the program, all three groups reported significant reductions in pain intensity and increases in the number of days spent doing stretching, endurance and relaxation exercises.

While all the above-noted studies support the effectiveness of exercise in helping to control pain experienced by older adults, the effects of a specific period of training do have their limits. Reassessing patients with OA of the knee and hip who had participated in 12 weeks of exercise administered by a physical therapist, van Baar et al. (1999) found that a small to moderate effect on pain persisted at 6 months, but not at 9 months, post intervention. Rather than viewing exercise as a one-time rehabilitative intervention, appropriate exercises should be a regular component of a wellness program to ensure healthy aging and to compress morbidity.

SPECIAL PRECAUTIONS

Appropriate precautions should be followed when using exercise for pain management with older adults. During strenuous resistive exercise, a hypertensive patient who performs a Valsalva maneuver risks a dangerous elevation in blood pressure. Severe osteoporosis and degeneration of the alar ligaments in the cervical spine in patients with RA may pose limitations for even gentle ROM exercises. Excessive spinal flexion should be avoided as a component of exercise, or during activities of daily living, for individuals with osteopenia and osteoporosis who are at risk for vertebral fractures (Sinaki, 2013). Vigorous eccentric exercise in both young and old subjects induces muscle soreness 24–48 hours later. Although tissue repair rates are similar to those for younger subjects, older individuals show significantly greater muscle shortening following eccentric exercise. This may predispose the older individual to a greater risk of injury with additional exercise.

CONCLUSION

A range of conservative interventions can be successfully employed for pain control with older people. Based on studies conducted to date, the best support exists for the use of therapeutic exercise.

Practitioners who lack formal training in the use of these interventions, or do not have these interventions within their scope of practice, will need to refer patients to other members of the rehabilitation team who do. Historically, physical therapists have been educated in how to evaluate patients for and treat with the interventions discussed in this chapter. Increasingly, nurses and occupational therapists are being trained to use some of these interventions (e.g. heat/cold, massage and TENS). Healthcare professionals must be knowledgeable about the strength of evidence supporting the use of conservative interventions for pain control. However, based on the limited research available, it is often difficult to either accept or exclude selected interventions for use in pain management with older individuals. Improved research methodologies will need to be employed in order to better examine the effectiveness and efficacy of conservative interventions, singly and in combination, and combined with pharmacologic agents, to manage a wider range of painful conditions commonly experienced by older adults.

REFERENCES

Abdulla A, Adams N, Bone M et al 2013 Guidance on the management of pain in older people. Age Aging 42:i1–i57

American Geriatrics Society, Panel on Chronic Pain in Older Persons 1998 The management of chronic pain in older persons. J Am Geriatr Soc 46:635–651

American Geriatrics Society, Panel on Persistent Pain in Older Persons 2002 Clinical practice guidelines: the management of persistent pain in older persons. J Am Geriatr Soc 50:S205–S224

American Geriatrics Society, Panel on the Pharmacological Management of Persistent Pain in Older Persons 2009 Special article: Pharmacological management of persistent pain in older persons. J Am Geriatr Soc 57:1331–1346

Baker KR, Nelson ME, Felson DT et al 2001 The efficacy of home based progressive strength training in older adults with knee osteoarthritis: a randomized controlled trial. J Rheumatol 28(7):1655–1665

Barr JO 2000 Conservative pain management for the older patient. In: Guccione AA (ed) Geriatric Physical Therapy, 2nd edn. Mosby, St Louis, MO, pp. 351–375

Barr JO, Weissenbuehler SA, Cleary CK 2004 Effectiveness and comfort of transcutaneous electrical nerve stimulation for older persons with chronic pain. J Geriatr Phys Ther 27(3):93–99

Bartels EM, Lund H, Hagen K et al 2009 Aquatic exercise for the treatment of knee and hip osteoarthritis. Cochrane Database Syst Rev 4:CD005523

Benjamin PJ, Tappan FM 2005 Tappan's Handbook of Healing Massage Techniques – Classic, Holistic, and Emerging Methods. Pearson Prentice Hall, Upper Saddle River, NJ

Brismee JM, Paige RL, Chyu MC et al 2007 Group and home-based tai chi in elderly subjects with knee osteoarthritis: a randomized controlled trial. Clin Rehabil 21:99–111

Brosseau L, Yonge KA, Welch V et al 2010 Transcutaneous electrical nerve stimulation (TENS) for the treatment of rheumatoid arthritis in the hand. Cochrane Database Syst Rev 7:CD004377

Brosseau L, Yonge KA, Welch V et al 2011 Thermotherapy for treatment of osteoarthritis. Cochrane Database Syst Rev Issue 10:CD004522

Brouwer RW, Raaji TM, Jakma T et al 2009 Braces and orthoses for treating osteoarthritis of the knee. Cochrane Database Syst Rev. [Online] doi:http://dx.doi.org/10.1002/14651858.CD004020.pub2

Buckwalter J, Stanish W, Rosier R et al 2001 The increasing need for nonoperative treatment of patients with osteoarthritis. Clin Orthop Rel Res 385:35–45

Callahan LF, Mielenz T, Freburger J et al 2008 A randomized controlled trial of the People with Arthritis Can Exercise Program: symptoms, function, physical activity, and psychosocial outcomes. Arthritis Rheum 59(1):92–101

Carlson T, Andrell P, Ekre O et al 2009 Interference of transcutaneous electrical nerve stimulation with permanent ventricular stimulation: a new clinical problem? Europace 11:364–369

Defrin R, Ariel E, Peretz C 2005 Segmental noxious versus innocuous electrical stimulation for chronic pain relief and the effect of fading sensation during treatment. Pain 115(1–2):152–160

Ferrell B, Josephson K, Pollan A et al 1997 A randomized trial of walking versus physical methods for chronic pain management. Aging 9:99–105

Fransen M, McConnell S 2009 Exercise for osteoarthritis of the knee. Cochrane Database Syst Rev. [Online] doi:http://dx.doi.org/10.1002/14651858.CD004376.pub2/

Fransen M, McConnell S, Hernandez-Molina G et al 2009 Exercise of osteoarthritis of the hip. Cochrane Database Syst Rev. [Online] doi:http://dx.doi.org/10.1002/14651858.CD007912/full

Grant D, Bishop-Miller J, Winchester D et al 1999 A randomized comparative trial of acupuncture versus transcutaneous electrical nerve stimulation for chronic back pain in the elderly. Pain 82:9–13

Hodge M, Bach T, Carter G 1999 Orthotic management of plantar pressure and pain in rheumatoid arthritis. Clin Biomech 14:567–575

Lee MS, Pittler MH, Ernst E 2007 Tai chi for rheumatoid arthritis: systematic review. Rheumatology (Oxford) 46(11):1648–1651

Lin SY, Davey RC, Cochrane T 2004 Community rehabilitation for older adults with osteoarthritis of the lower limb: a controlled clinical trial. Clin Rehabil 18(1):92–101

Maillefert J, Hudry C, Baron G et al 2001 Laterally elevated wedged insoles in the treatment of medial knee osteoarthritis: a prospective randomized controlled study. Osteoarthritis Cartilage 9:738–745

Minor MA, Hewitt JE, Webel RR et al 1989 Efficacy of physical conditioning exercise in patients with rheumatoid arthritis and osteoarthritis. Arthritis Rheum 32:1396–1405

Mok K, Woo CP 2004 The effects of slow-stroke back massage on anxiety and shoulder pain in elderly stroke patients. Compl Ther Nurs Midwifery 10(4):209–216

Oosterveld FG, Rasker JJ 1994 Effects of local heat and cold treatment on surface and articular temperature of arthritic knees. Arthritis Rheum 37(11):1578–1582

Osiri M, Brosseau L, McGowan J et al 2000 Transcutaneous electrical nerve stimulation for knee osteoarthritis. Cochrane Database Syst Rev Issue 4:CD002823

Parker SJ, Vasquez R, Chen EK et al 2011 A comparison of the arthritis foundation self-help program across three race/ethnicity groups. Ethn Dis 21(4):444–450

Pfeifer M, Begerow B, Minne HW 2004 Effects of a new spinal orthosis on posture, trunk strength, and quality of life in women with postmenopausal osteoporosis. Am J Phys Med Rehabil 83:177–186

Pham T, Maillefert JF, Hudry C et al 2004 Laterally elevated wedged insoles in the treatment of medial knee osteoarthritis: a two-year prospective randomized controlled study. Osteoarthritis Cartilage 12(1):46–55

Philadelphia Panel 2001 Philadelphia Panel evidence-based clinical practice guidelines on selected rehabilitation interventions. Phys Ther 81:1629–1730

Price CIM, Pandyan AD 2006 Electrical stimulation for preventing and treating post stroke shoulder pain. Cochrane Database Syst Rev Issue 4:CD001698

Robinson S, Benton G 2002 Warmed blankets: an intervention to promote comfort for elderly hospitalized patients. Geriatr Nurs 23(6):320–323

Rutjes AW, Nuesch E, Sterchi R et al 2009 Transcutaneous electrical nerve stimulation for osteoarthritis of the knee. Cochrane Database Syst Rev Issue 4: 002823

Rutjes AW, Nuesch E, Sterchi R et al 2010 Therapeutic ultrasound for osteoarthritis of the knee or hip. Cochrane Database Syst Rev Issue 2:CD003132

Sansone P, Schmitt L 2000 Providing tender touch massage to elderly nursing home residents: a demonstration project. Geriatric Nurs 21(6):303–308

Seligman DA, Dawson DR 2003 Customized heel pads and soft orthotics to treat heel pain and plantar fasciitis. Arch Phys Med Rehabil 84(10):1564–1567

Shamliyan TA, Wang S-Y, Olson-Kellogg B et al 2012 Physical therapy interventions for knee pain secondary to osteoarthritis. Comparative Effectiveness Review No. 77. Effective Health Care Program, Agency for Healthcare Research and Quality publication no. 12(13)-EHC115-FH, Rockville, MD

Shrier I, Feldman DE, Gaudet MC et al 2006 Conservative non-pharmacological treatment options are not frequently used in the management of hip osteoarthritis. J Sci Med Sports May 9(1–2):81–86

Sinaki M 2013 Yoga spinal flexion positions and vertebral compression fracture in osteopenia or osteoporosis of spine: case series. Pain Pract 13(1):68–75

Song R, Lee EO, Lam P et al 2003 Effects of tai chi exercise on pain, balance, muscle strength, and perceived difficulties in physical functioning in older women with osteoarthritis: a randomized clinical trial. J Rheumatol 30(9):2039–2044

Stewart C, Leveille SG, Shmerling RH et al 2013 Management of persistent pain in older adults. J Am Geriatr Soc 60(11):2081–2086

Toda Y, Tsukimura N 2004 A six-month follow-up of a randomized trial comparing the efficacy of a lateral-wedge insole with subtalar strapping and an in-shoe lateral-wedge insole in patients with varus deformity osteoarthritis of the knee. Arthritis Rheum 50(10):3129–3136

van Baar M, Assendelft WJ, Dekker J 1999 Effectiveness of exercise therapy in patients with osteoarthritis of the hip or knee. Arthritis Rheum 12:1361–1369

Welch V, Brosseau L, Casimiro L et al 2011 Thermotherapy for treating rheumatoid arthritis. Cochrane Database Syst Rev. [Online] doi:http://dx.doi.org/10.1002/14651858.CD002826/pdf

Zhang W, Moskowitz RW, Nuki G et al 2008 OARSI recommendations for the management of hip and knee osteoarthritis, Part II: OARSI evidence-based, expert consensus guidelines. Osteoarthritis Cartilage 16:137–162

Chapter 68
Gait training

NICOLE L. EVANOSKY

CHAPTER CONTENTS

DEFINING THE PROBLEM

Gait training is one of the most frequently prescribed rehabilitation techniques for the older adult because gait is the most common of all human movements and, as such, any pathology that affects it requires immediate attention. Normal gait includes a complex sequence of limb motions that propel the body in a manner that is energy conserving, stable and shock absorbing. Rehabilitation therapists must be aware that gait in the healthy older adult includes a wide variety of 'normal', yet disruptions in the sequence of actions are easily identified (see Table 68.1). Typical changes in gait parameters with older adults include reduced gait speed, decreased stride length and increased double support time (Perry & Burnfield, 2010). In addition, executive function and visual deficits impact gait variability and fall risk in this population (van Iersel et al., 2008; Bock & Beurskens, 2011).

Gait changes due to aging, disease or disability become problematic when the individual suffers pain, has difficulty maintaining balance, lacks sufficient endurance, or has insufficient ability to ambulate to meet his/her activities of daily living (ADLs). Gait disorders are associated with falls in older adults. This is clinically relevant because falling is one of the leading causes of injury-related deaths among elderly people. For many older adults, the inability to ambulate safely results in loss of independence and frequently results in the need for institutional assistance (Quadri et al., 2005; Stevens, 2006).

GAIT ASSESSMENT

Gait analysis must be conducted in order to determine what gait deviations and/or problems are present. Gait is assessed in a variety of ways ranging from observation, to optical-motion analysis in a specialized gait lab. The 'gold standard' method for measurement parameters of human gait is considered to be the force-place and/or optical motion capture systems (Cliodhna et al.,

2011). Other gait assessment methods utilize measure of distance, stability and time (see Table 68.2). There are many valid and reliable gait assessment tools which are appropriate for use with the older adult. Observational gait analysis is routinely performed by clinicians and refers to the use of qualitative methods to assess gait deviations (Ranchos Los Amigos National Rehabilitation Center, 2001; McGinley et al., 2003). This analysis is portable and inexpensive, unlike some of the gait analysis systems which utilize force plates, gyroscopes, accelerometers and pressure sensitive insoles. In addition, the assessment of gait speed is important as it has been shown to be the single best predictor of disability and frailty among older adults (Studenski et al., 2011).

When assessing gait, the healthcare provider must consider that many specific pathologies (orthopedic, neurological, biomechanical, cardiopulmonary) may contribute to gait deviations and that the typical elderly client usually presents with multiple problems varying from acute to chronic in nature. Individual pathologies (i.e. stroke, Parkinson's disease, etc.) may result in a typical pattern of gait deviation but many elderly adults have one or more common gait deviations.

GAIT TRAINING

Findings from the results of gait analysis are used to design appropriate intervention. Gait difficulties may be attributed to impaired motor and postural control, abnormal joint range of motion, impaired sensation, vestibular hypofunction and/or pain. The challenge for the healthcare provider is to determine the relationship between impairments and deviations (Ranchos Los Amigos National Rehabilitation Center, 2001). A single impairment can result in multiple deviations. For example, decreased plantar flexor muscle function may result in excess knee flexion, excess dorsiflexion and lack of heel-off during single limb support. A single deviation may also be caused by multiple impairments. For example, excess plantar flexion may be caused by either a plantar flexion contracture or plantar flexion spasticity.

Table 68.1	**Normal versus pathological gait in elderly persons**	
Parameter	**Normal Aging Gait**	**Pathological Gait**
Speed	Decreased self-selected and fast speed, although ability remains to voluntarily increase speed from self-selected to fast speed	Significant decrease in free velocity (<0.85 m/s) with loss of ability to voluntarily increase speed from self-selected gait speed
Step/stride lengths	Smaller step and stride lengths but symmetrical	Significant decrease in step and stride length and/or nonsymmetrical steps
Step width	Averages 1 to 4 inches (2.5–10 cm)	Step width is greater than 4 inches (10 cm) or less than 1 inch; or too much or too little step width variability
Toe clearance	Small toe clearance	Either large toe clearance or tripping or both
Ankle–foot	Mild decrease in force at push-off and/or slight decreases in plantar flexion and dorsiflexion range of motion	Large toe clearance or tripping or both; forefoot or foot-flat contact during initial contact; excess plantarflexion or dorsiflexion
Knee	Range of motion from 5° of flexion during weight acceptance to 60° of flexion during swing limb advancement	Limited or excessive flexion, wobbling; extension thrust
Hip	15–20° of flexion during weight acceptance and 15–20° of apparent hyperextension at terminal stance	Limited flexion or extension; 'past retract' meaning a visible forward and then backward movement of the thigh during terminal swing; excessive abduction or adduction; excessive or limited internal or external rotation
Pelvis	5° of forward rotation during weight acceptance; and 5° of backward rotation at terminal stance and pre-swing; iliac crest on reference limb is higher or equal to the iliac crest on the opposite side during midstance	Limited or excess rotation forward or backward; pelvic drop; pelvic hiking
Trunk	Erect	Forward, backwards or sideways lean

Table 68.2	**Gait assessment and outcome measures**	
Measure	**Description**	**Findings**
Dynamic Gait Index (Shumway-Cook et al., 1997)	Eight elements are assessed on 0–3 scale where 3 = normal, 2 = mild impairment, 1 = moderate impairment, 0 = severely impaired. Items include: (1) 20 ft gait on level surface (pattern, speed, assistive device, balance) (2) Change in gait speed from comfortable to fast (3) Gait with horizontal head turns (4) Gait with vertical head turns (5) Gait and pivot turn (6) Step over obstacle (shoe box) (7) Step around obstacles (cones at 6 ft intervals) (8) Steps (using rail if necessary)	Scores of ≤19 are predictive of falls in older community living adults
Gait Abnormality Rating Scale (GARS) (Wolfson et al., 1990)	Gait is rated according to 16 elements on a 4-point scale ranging from 0 to 3 where 0 is normal. Items include: (1) Variability of stepping and arm movements (2) Guardedness in stepping and arm swing (3) Weaving (4) Waddling (5) Staggering (6) Lower extremity % time in swing (7) Lower extremity heel contact at heel strike (8) Lower extremity hip range of motion (9) Lower extremity knee range of motion (10) Elbow extension (range of motion) (11) Shoulder extension (range of motion) (12) Shoulder abduction (pathological increase) (13) Arm–heel strike synchrony (14) Head position (check for head held forward) (15) Shoulder position (check for elevation) (16) Trunk position (check for trunk flexion forward)	A higher GARS Score indicates a more impaired gait. GARS score >18 indicates patients who are at the greatest risk for falls

(Continued)

Measure	Description	Findings
	Table 68.2 (Continued)	
Gait Abnormality Rating Scale – Modified (GARS-M) (van Swearingen et al., 1996)	Gait is rated according to seven elements on a 4-point scale ranging from 0 to 3 where 0 is normal. GARS-M includes items 1, 2, 5, 7, 8, 11 and 13 from GARS (listed above)	A higher GARS-M score indicates a more impaired gait. GARS-M scores >8 indicates those who are at the highest risk for falls
Gait Speed (Guralnik et al., 2000; Steffen et al., 2002)	Instructions are 'to walk at your normal comfortable walking speed' and 'to walk as fast as you comfortably can' over an established distance (typical distances are 6 or 10 m). Note whether the distance measured included acceleration and deceleration. If preferred, measure the time to complete 3 consecutive stride lengths within a 9 m distance	Gait speed that is <0.8 m/s indicates a high risk for falls and/or disability
Performance Oriented Mobility Test (Tinetti, 1986)	Nine elements on the Balance test (maximum score = 16) plus 10-elements on the gait test (maximum score = 12) are assessed on either a 0, 1 or 0, 1, 2 scale with higher scores associated with better performance	Scores <19 indicate a high risk for falling, Scores of 19–24 indicate moderate risk for falling, Scores of 25–28 indicate a low risk for falling

Balance test items include:
(1) sitting balance (0, 1)
(2) arise from chair (0, 1, 2)
(3) attempts to arise from chair (0, 1, 2)
(4) immediate standing balance upon arising (0, 1, 2)
(5) standing balance, feet close together (0, 1, 2)
(6) standing balance with nudge to subject's sternum (0, 1, 2)
(7) standing balance, feet close together, eyes closed (0, 1)
(8) standing turn 360° continuity of steps (0, 1) and steadiness (0, 1)
(9) sitting down from standing (0, 1, 2)
Gait test items include:
(1) examine hesitancy at initiation of gait (0, 1)
(2) right swing foot step length (0, 1)
(3) right swing foot clearance (0, 1)
(4) left swing foot step length (0, 1)
(5) left swing foot clearance (0, 1)
(6) step symmetry (0, 1)
(7) step continuity (0, 1)
(8) path deviation, if any, over 10 foot course (0, 1, 2)
(9) trunk sway or walking aid, if any (0,1,2)
(10) walking stance – stride width (0,1)

Measure	Description	Findings
Timed 'Up & Go' (TUG) test (Podsiadlo & Richardson, 1991)	Using stopwatch, start timing at 'Go'. Start position is fully seated in the back of chair. Use chair with armrests. Time the period to rise from seated chair, walk 3 m, turn around, walk back to chair and sit. Document whether performed with or without use of arms (arms to be crossed over chest upon rising from chair) and whether assistive device was used	Young adults generally score <10 seconds; Older adults who take ≥13.5 seconds to perform the TUG are at greater risk for falls. Scores >30 seconds identifies individuals who will have significant difficulties in ADLs
Walk Tests (2 or 6 or 12 min) (Butland et al., 1982; Eng et al., 2002; Enright & Sherrill, 1998)	These tests estimate maximum oxygen consumption. Using standardized instructions, the patient is instructed to walk as far as possible in the time permitted. Prediction equations of the total distance walked during the first time 6 min walk for healthy adults (40–80 years): For men: Distance (m) = $(7.57 \times height_{cm}) - (5.02 \times age) - 1.76 \times weight_{kg}) - 309$ m For women: Distance (m) = $(2.11 \times height_{cm}) - (2.29 \times weight_{kg}) - (5.78 \times age) + 667$ m	Mean (SD) distances for healthy individuals aged 61 ± 12 years: 2 min test: 149 ± 35 m 6 min test: 413 ± 107 m 12 min test: 774 ± 229 m Mean (SD) distances for individuals with a diagnosis of stroke: 2 min test: 62.5 ± 8.5 m 6 min test: 267.7 ± 89.7 m 12 min test: 530.5 ± 184.9 m

Table 68.3	**Potential intervention strategies for common gait deviations**
Observed Deviation	**Strategy**
Difficulty rising from sitting	Scoot forward in chair, lean forward to rise Push from chair; strengthen triceps/latissimus dorsi Adapt chair height/firmness
Trunk forward lean (flexed posture)	Reduce hip flexor or other contractures, if present Strengthen hip extensors and ankle plantarflexors Provide feedback for normal posture Raise height of walker or cane, if needed
Trunk backward lean	Provide feedback for normal posture Strengthen hip flexors Practice disassociation of trunk muscles from pelvic motion
Trunk sideways lean	Strengthen hip abductors Correct leg length discrepancy
Trunk and pelvis decreased rotation	Practice trunk rotation exercise on mat, in sitting and standing Attempt 4-point gait drills Use PNF facilitation during gait Facilitate trunk rotation on upper body ergometer
Foot clearance	Strengthen and facilitate dorsiflexors Reduce lower extremity contractures, if any Assess appropriateness of ankle–foot orthosis (AFO)
Decreased pushoff at terminal stance	Strengthen plantarflexors Facilitate awareness of ankle push-off during gait
Decreased endurance	Adapt gait with appropriate assistive device to pattern that requires less energy (e.g. convert 4-point gait to swing-to pattern, use wheeled walker versus standard walker, etc.) Progress distances traveled and speed
Decreased balance	Assess need for assistive device Provide postural control training Assess and modify footwear Modify environment for safety (e.g. increase lighting, clear pathways, etc.)

Some suggested intervention strategies for common gait deviations of the elderly are included in Table 68.3.

Gait training may involve any combination of (1) mobility and transfer activities, (2) pregait mat and standing activities, (3) static and dynamic balance activities, (4) interventions during gait and (5) adaptation of assistive devices or environment in order to reduce gait deviations.

Mobility and transfer activities include rising-to-standing and returning-to-sitting. Compared to young adults, healthy older adults show similar patterns of rising from sitting, though they tend to minimize the forward body displacement during returning-to-sit. Frail elderly frequently demonstrate difficulty in initiating rising-to-standing and tend to perform a rapid descent when returning-to-sitting. Activities to facilitate safe chair rising and sitting should include using the upper extremities for assistance and facilitation awareness of body position relative to the chair. Floor-to-stand transfers are recommended for individuals who are tolerant of these high level activities.

Pregait exercises are designed primarily to improve trunk and extremity strength and control. Strength training should be directed toward improving lower extremity strength, particularly of ankle plantarflexors and dorsiflexors, quadriceps, hip abductors and hip extensors at an intensity sufficient to result in

improvement (70–80% of the one-repetition maximum). Upper extremity strengthening should be conducted to improve strength of the latissimus dorsi and triceps. Appropriate mat exercises include pelvic tilt movements, hip raising (bridging), trunk twisting, sitting push-ups (latissimus dorsi dips) and quadruped activities included rocking and arm/leg reaching. Pregait standing activities include weight shifting, arm raising, chair push-ups, toe raising, hip hiking and leg swinging, and a progression of drills from 4-point to swing-to to swing-through. Advanced standing activities include sideways and backwards ambulation. These pregait standing activities may be progressed from using the parallel bars to using an assistive device to free-standing movement. Normal postural alignment should be encouraged in all activities.

Static and dynamic balance activities for gait training may be performed in sitting and standing positions. Sitting activities include controlled reaching and leaning within the base of support, with movement side to side, forward and backward. Sitting postural control may be challenged by using external disturbances such as a gentle push. Standing balance may be enhanced with the use of weight shifting activities in which the patient is asked to move as far in all directions as he or she is comfortably able without needing to bend at the hips, or take a step. Controlled reaching, lifting and weight shift activities assist in training for standing balance. The

Table 68.4.	**Considerations for prescribing assistive devices for gait**	
Device	Objective	Considerations for Prescription
Cane – single-point – broad based – small-based – rolling quad	Enhances stability through weight redistribution; compensates for losses in vision and proprioception	Appropriate for individuals who need balance and stability assistance with minimal weight bearing shift (up to 25%) Coordination needed to use effectively; may not be appropriate for elderly with impairments in cognition or coordination Single point offers the least weight-bearing shift and broad base offers the most weight-bearing shift Rolling quad is effective for use in individuals with limited upper extremity strength or coordination
Crutches – axillary – Loftstrand	Permits significant weight bearing shift from legs to arms	Permits more weight-bearing shift (50% or greater) than a cane (up to complete non-weight-bearing on one leg) Less stable than a walker Requires good balance and upper body strength Inappropriate use of axillary crutches may result in brachial plexus injuries Loftstrand crutches permits hand use and reaching
Walkers – standard – rolling – hemi – platform – rollators	Offers greater stability and significant weight bearing shift from legs to arms	Provides more weight-bearing shift (50% or greater) than a cane but with more stability than crutches; difficult to maneuver on stairs Standard offers the greatest stability but may be difficult for older adult to maneuver; requires more attentional demand and has greater destabilizing effects compared to the rolling walker Rolling walker is less stable than standard but is easier to propel for those with upper body weakness; reduces energy costs by 5% compared to standard walkers Rollators have the advantages of a rolling walker with brakes and a seat Hemi walker allows a large base of support for individuals with one functional arm Platform walkers are heavy and increase energy cost but permit weight bearing shift through the humerus

level of difficulty may be increased by performing reaching, lifting and weight shift activities while standing on high-density foam. Sophisticated computerized force platform systems offer monitoring for various weight shifting and response activities, which in some cases might include responding to a moving floor. Evidence suggests that the older adult may demonstrate better balance during gait when wearing either a laced, firm, thin-soled walking or athletic shoe as opposed to walking barefoot or in a high-heel shoe (Menant et al., 2008).

Interventions during gait should focus on reducing deviations, improving gait efficiency and safety, and increasing endurance. Interventions during gait include assessment for assistive devices (a cane, walker, crutches, orthoses), feedback for movement control (manual, electrical stimulation, biofeedback, visual), practice of dynamic balance and progression from performing the standing activities listed above within the parallel bars to performing them outside of the bars. Treatment progression may advance from even surfaces to uneven surfaces (ramps, stairs, outdoors). Forward gait training may be progressed to sidestepping, turning, backwards stepping, reaching and carrying objects. Practice in stepping over obstacles and climbing stairs is relevant to improving the functional mobility of the client. Attentional demands may affect the gait of an older client, making training for gait safety during challenging or distracting situations appropriate (Ullmann & Williams, 2011). Utilizing dual task training methods, including visual distraction in gait training interventions can have beneficial carryover in situations requiring the older adult to attend to multiple factors (i.e. crossing the street in a timely fashion while looking for traffic) (Bock & Beurskens, 2011).

The prescription of an appropriate assistive device may help the client improve balance and mobility without loss of stability, as well as reduce lower limb loading (Bateni & Maki, 2005; Agree & Freedman, 2011). Advantages and disadvantages of various assistive devices for geriatric gait training are included in Table 68.4.

Most gait training programs focus on achieving mobility with stability prior to emphasizing increases in gait velocity. It is clinically relevant that self-selected gait speed is related to peak metabolic capacity (Fiser et al., 2010). With healthy aging, individuals have progressively smaller aerobic reserves. Gait disorders, as well as the use of assistive devices, add to the energy demands of walking. For these reasons, it is highly recommended that therapists monitor vital signs of older adults during gait training. Endurance training has been shown to improve gait and balance in older adults (Gmitter et al., 2009).

The use of technology is increasingly being used for gait training. Walking on a treadmill, with some body weight supported via a harness connected to an overhead support system, is a method of treating walking impairments post stroke. Results using this body-weight-support treadmill training have shown improvement in gait speed (Mulroy et al., 2010). Another technology for gait training includes the use of robotic gait orthoses that guide the patient's legs according to a pre-programmed physiological gait pattern. Both technologies are thought to enhance motor learning for locomotion by optimizing task-specific training (Mulroy et al., 2010); however, both are costly in terms of equipment and human resources.

CONCLUSION

Declining mobility is a common complaint among aging persons, and it is likely to lead to diminutions in the performance of ADLs and the quality of life. Gait training interventions include corrections of deviations during ambulation, as well as activities to improve the strength, mobility, balance and endurance needed for gait. Various pathologies may contribute to declining mobility and pathological gait in an elderly person, but significant improvements may be documented by using appropriate assessment tools and interventions.

REFERENCES

Agree EM, Freedman VA 2011 A quality-of-life scale for assistive technology: results of a pilot study of aging and technology. Phys Ther 91(12):1780–1788

Bateni H, Maki BE 2005 Assistive devices for balance and mobility: benefits, demands and adverse consequences. Arch Phys Med Rehabil 86:134–145

Bock O, Beurskens R 2011 Effects of a visual distracter task on the gait of elderly versus young persons. Curr Gerontol Geriatr Res. [Online] http://dx.doi.org/10.1155/2011/651718

Butland RJ, Pang J, Gross ER et al 1982 Two-, six-, and 12-minute walking tests in respiratory disease. Br Med J 284:1607–1608

Cliodhna NS, Garattini C, Greene BR et al 2011 Technology innovation enabling falls risk assessment in a community setting. Ageing Int 36:217–231

Eng JJ, Chu KS, Dawson AS et al 2002 Functional walk tests in individuals with stroke: relation to perceived exertion and myocardial exertion. Stroke 33:756–761

Enright PL, Sherrill DL 1998 Reference equations for the six-minute walk in healthy adults. Am J Respir Crit Care Med 158:1384–1387

Fiser WM, Hays NP, Rogers SC et al 2010 Energetics of walking in elderly people: factors related to gait speed. J Gerontol A Biol Sci Med Sci 65A(12):1332–1337

Gmitter JP, Mangione KK, Avers D 2009 Case report: an evidence-based approach to examination and intervention following hip fracture. J Geriatr Phys Ther 32(1):39–45

Guralnik JM, Ferrucci L, Pieper CF et al 2000 Lower extremity function and subsequent disability: consistency across studies, predictive models, and the value of gait speed alone compared to the short physical performance battery. J Gerontol 55:M221–M231

McGinley JL, Goldie PA, Greenwood KM et al 2003 Accuracy and reliability of observational gait analysis data: judgments of push-off in gait after stroke. Phys Ther 83:146–160

Menant JC, Steele JR, Menz HB et al 2008 Optimizing footwear for older people at risk for falls. J Rehabil Res Dev 45(8):1167–1181

Mulroy SJ, Klassen T, Grossen JK et al 2010 Gait parameters associated with responsiveness to treadmill training with body-weight support after stroke: an exploratory study. Phys Ther 90(2):209–223

Perry J, Burnfield J 2010 Gait Analysis: Normal and Pathological Function, 2nd edn. Slack Inc., Thoroughfare, NJ

Podsiadlo D, Richardson S 1991 The timed 'Up & Go': a test of basic functional mobility for frail elderly persons. J Am Geriatr Soc 39:142–148

Quadri P, Tettamanti M, Bernasconi S et al 2005 Lower limb function as predictor of falls and loss of mobility with social repercussions one year after discharge among elderly inpatients. Aging Clin Exp Res 17:82–89

Ranchos Los Amigos National Rehabilitation Center 2001 Observational Gait Analysis Handbook. Los Amigos Research and Education Institute, Inc, Downey CA

Shumway-Cook A, Baldwin M, Polissar NL et al 1997 Predicting the probability for falls in community-dwelling older adults. Phys Ther 77:812–819

Steffen TM, Hacker TA, Mollinger L 2002 Age- and gender-related test performance in community-dwelling elderly people: Six-Minute Walk Test, Berg Balance Scale, Timed Up & Go Test, and gait speeds. Phys Ther 82:128–137

Stevens JA 2006 Fatalities and injuries from falls among older adults – United States, 1993–2003 and 2001–2005. MMWR 50(6):1221–1224

Studenski S, Perera S, Patel K et al 2011 Gait speed and survival in older adults. JAMA 305(1):50–58

Tinetti ME 1986 Performance-oriented assessment of mobility problems in elderly patients. J Am Geriatr Soc 34:119–126

Ullmann G, Williams G 2011 The relationships among gait and mobility under single and dual task conditions in community-dwelling older adults. Aging Clin Exp Res 23(5–6):400–405

van Iersel MB, Kessels RP, Bloem BR et al 2008 Executive functions are associated with gait and balance in community-living elderly people. J Gerontol A Biol Sci Med Sci 63(12):1344–1349

van Swearingen JM, Paschal KA, Bonino P et al 1996 The modified Gait Abnormality Rating Scale for recognizing the risk of recurrent falls in community-dwelling elderly adults. Phys Ther 76:994–1002

Wolfson L, Whipple R, Amerman P et al 1990 Gait assessment in the elderly: a gait abnormality rating scale and its relations to falls. J Gerontol A Biol Sci Med Sci 45:M12–M19

Chapter 69

Orthotics

DAVID PATRICK

INTRODUCTION

An orthosis is a mechanical device applied to the body in order to support a body segment, correct anatomical alignment, protect a body part, or assist motion to improve body function (American Academy of Orthopedic Surgeons, 1985). In accomplishing these objectives, orthotic devices assist in promoting ambulation, reducing pain, preventing deformity and allowing greater activity. Orthotic devices are often indicated as a component of the rehabilitation process for a variety of diseases and conditions that affect the geriatric population. Successful orthotic intervention when working with aging individuals demands a practical balance between the objectives that are ideally desired and what the elderly individual will reasonably tolerate.

Orthotic devices accomplish their objectives by applying forces to the involved body segments. As a rule, the more aggressive the orthotic intervention, the greater the force generated (Edelstein, 1995). In general, elderly individuals are less tolerant of the resultant discomfort of aggressive orthotic intervention, and their skin and subcutaneous tissue are less tolerant of the external forces generated. This frequently results in the need to compromise between an ideal and an acceptable orthotic outcome and to choose more 'forgiving' orthoses in terms of comfort and tolerance – that is, less rigid orthotic devices. This discussion focuses on the lower extremity and spinal orthotic interventions, which are commonly associated with the geriatric population.

LOWER EXTREMITY ORTHOTIC SYSTEMS

SHOES

Proper distribution of forces in order to maintain the integrity of the skin of the foot is of primary importance. The shoe should fit properly and the volume of the shoe should appropriately accommodate the foot and any additions such as a foot orthotic or plastic ankle–foot orthosis (AFO). Generally, a sneaker or other athletic shoe with a removable inlay, or an extra-depth shoe with a removable inlay, is recommended. The inlay can be removed to accommodate fluctuating edema or the addition of an orthosis. In unilateral involvement the inlay can remain in the shoe on the uninvolved side, maintaining the fit on that side and balancing the patient in terms of height. It is recommended that the shoe have a soft upper (the portion of the shoe covering the dorsum of the foot) to reduce pressure in the presence of minor foot deformities such as bunions or hammer toes. Severe foot deformities may require a custom shoe made from a cast of the individual's foot.

FOOT ORTHOTICS

In general, flexible accommodative orthotics for the purpose of distributing forces to protect the skin and promote comfort are indicated. The bones of the foot of the geriatric patient are often functionally adapted and the joints may be restricted in terms of range of motion (ROM). Thus, attempting biomechanical correction may be inappropriate and may, thereby, contraindicate the use of rigid orthotic devices and necessitate careful consideration of the application of even semirigid devices.

ANKLE–FOOT ORTHOTICS (AFO)

AFOs are frequently utilized with the elderly to improve ambulation status and gait quality. AFOs are capable of controlling the foot and ankle directly and the knee indirectly. For example, by positioning the ankle in dorsiflexion, a knee flexion moment can be produced to control genu recurvatum. Also, positioning the ankle in plantar flexion can produce a knee extension moment to assist in stabilizing the knee. Neuromuscular conditions such as hemiparesis due to a cerebral vascular accident as well as musculoskeletal pathologies such as arthritis commonly result in foot and ankle dysfunctions in the geriatric population, which can be managed in part with AFOs.

A common challenge is deciding whether to use a plastic or a metal AFO system. The metal AFO has little skin contact except for the calf band and shoe which are the reaction points of the orthosis. This quality is a distinct advantage of the metal system for patients with fluctuating edema or poor skin integrity. In comparison, the total-contact nature of the plastic AFO results in a greater ability to control the foot and ankle. Additionally, the plastic AFO is lighter in weight, more cosmetically acceptable and has the practical advantage of easy interchange among shoes. Plastic AFOs would appear to be the orthosis of choice for geriatric patients whenever possible. One strategy to determine whether a metal AFO system is indicated for a particular patient is to consider the sensory status and volume stability (i.e. presence or absence of fluctuating edema) of the patient and the reliability of the patient or support person to monitor the skin integrity of the involved lower extremity. Negative findings in two of these categories would indicate consideration of a metal AFO instead of plastic orthosis.

A soft AFO such as a neoprene ankle sleeve may be appropriate for controlling minor discomfort from arthritis or to encourage ankle stability when a more rigid system cannot be tolerated. Such orthoses accomplish their goals remarkably well in some cases by retaining heat and providing proprioceptive and kinesthetic sensory input. Medial collapse of the foot/ankle complex from a pathology such as posterior tibialis tendon failure or lateral ankle instability/malalignment may be optimally managed with a specialty AFO such as an Arizona AFO or Richie Brace.

KNEE–ANKLE–FOOT ORTHOSES (KAFO)

Although AFOs are tolerated well by the geriatric population, the addition of a knee joint and a thigh cuff to form a KAFO system results in a much less acceptable orthotic intervention. A KAFO has the advantage of controlling the knee as well as the foot and ankle directly, and indirectly influences the hip joint. A KAFO is the orthosis of choice in the presence of severe genu recurvatum, or knee buckling, which cannot be managed with an AFO.

Historically, a knee that buckled during weight-bearing required the use of a locking type knee joint. This satisfied the need to stabilize the knee during the stance phase of gait. However, it prevented knee flexion at swing phase resulting in a less than desirable gait pattern that was energy consuming. As an alternative, stance control knee joints (Zissimopoulos et al., 2007) are now available. These joints lock the knee during the stance phase of gait but allow knee flexion during the swing phase. Some offer a limited degree of resisted knee flexion before locking which helps to normalize the gait pattern at initial stance.

Additionally, significant coronal plane instabilities at the knee (genu varum or valgum) are effectively managed by a KAFO. Less severe knee problems may be managed using a knee orthosis (KO), but the shortened lever arm (the shorter length of the orthosis) results in greater skin pressures, and the softer nature of the elderly patient's lower extremity (LE) musculature can create suspension problems as the KO tends to slide distally during use. One advantage of the KAFO is that the footplate serves to maintain the orthosis in its proper position.

HIP–KNEE–ANKLE–FOOT ORTHOSES (HKAFO)

The addition of a hip joint and pelvic band to a KAFO results in an orthosis that is difficult to don and doff, less comfortable than shorter ones and more cumbersome to wear. For the geriatric population, the hip joint and pelvic band are most commonly added when rotation control of the lower extremity is required.

HIP ORTHOSES

A hip orthosis is commonly used with the elderly to limit the extent of hip joint adduction and flexion following the dislocation of a hip arthroplasty (hip rotation is controlled to a lesser degree). Premanufactured systems are available that allow the limits of hip ROM to be adjusted as required to protect the hip adequately and simultaneously allow the patient to perform the activities of daily living (ADLs).

KNEE ORTHOSES

A postoperative knee orthosis is commonly used after a knee arthroplasty. The knee orthosis is usually designed to allow ROM adjustment in graduating increments, as desired. A soft knee orthosis with stays or hinges is commonly used to address arthritis-related pain and promote knee stability through a greater kinesthetic awareness. A knee orthosis with wraparound closure design is recommended for the elderly patient to facilitate donning and doffing. Some orthopedists order knee immobilizers postoperatively for their patients who have had total hip replacements. The rationale is that by preventing knee flexion, the operative hip flexion will be reduced, thereby mitigating risk for dislocation. This technique should be considered for individual patients only in the early postoperative period as it does impede mobility and may cause knee stiffness and hip pain because of the long lever arm.

Degenerative joint disease with related pain interfering with the ability to ambulate and climb stairs is a common pathology associated with aging. Osteoarthritis unloading knee braces (Briggs et al., 2009) are specifically designed to unload the involved knee compartment (often bone on bone) through application of a valgus or varus corrective force resulting in a reduction of pain and improvement in the ability to ambulate and perform ADLs. The objective of orthotic intervention is to manage the symptoms as opposed to resolve the underlying pathology in cases where, or at a time when, knee arthroplasty is not the preferred treatment. A variety of designs are available and careful consideration is required in selection to optimize the benefit for a particular individual.

FRACTURE ORTHOSES

Fracture orthoses are utilized with the geriatric population when surgical repair is contraindicated, or to reduce the amount of time the joints surrounding a fracture have to be immobilized in a cast. This reduces the potential negative effects of immobilization such as contractures and phlebitis. Additionally, lower extremity fracture orthoses may reduce the period of recumbency, thereby minimizing the risk of potentially life-threatening complications such as pneumonia. Fracture orthoses are tightened circumferentially around the involved area, and using the hydraulic effect of soft tissues (the noncompressibility of fluids) and gravity, they transmit forces that realign and support the fracture site while allowing motion in the surrounding joints. Fracture orthoses must be worn snugly; they are commonly used for the management of nondisplaced or minimally displaced fractures, especially those of the humerus, tibia, radius and ulna.

SPINAL ORTHOTIC SYSTEMS

Spinal orthotic intervention is particularly challenging when dealing with the elderly population. Older patients commonly present with a variety of pathologies involving the spine and soft tissues of the trunk that could well be treated by the application of a spinal orthosis. Tolerance to wearing such a device, however, is limited, particularly in the cases of the more rigid systems and those that cover an extensive body area.

Spinal orthoses accomplish their objectives through one or more of the following biomechanical principles:

1. Three-point pressure control
2. Indirect transfer of load by increasing intra-abdominal pressure
3. Correction of spinal alignment
4. Sensory feedback (kinesthetic reminder) (Edelstein, 1995).

Three-point pressure control (the design of the orthosis) determines which spinal motions are limited. The magnitude of control (the degree of limitation) is directly related to the rigidity of the orthosis and the degree of tightness with which it is worn. A rigid orthosis is capable of applying greater forces to the body to restrict motion than is a more flexible system. However, the geriatric patient is less tolerant of the resulting discomfort and potential breathing restriction, and the skin of the older patient is less capable of withstanding the forces generated without its integrity being compromised. The decision to use a rigid rather than a more flexible system should therefore be based on the degree to which spinal motion restriction is required. For example, a geriatric patient with an unstable fracture of the spine requires a rigid orthotic system to restrict motion in the involved spinal segment, whereas management of a stable compression fracture offers greater latitude to use a more flexible and lightweight device without compromising the patient's safety. It should be noted that a more rigid device is often preferred in terms of protecting the involved spinal segment, but the decision to use a more flexible system is based on the practical issue of orthotic tolerance and thus compliance with wearing the orthosis. The ideal orthosis serves no purpose at all if it is not worn and, particularly with the geriatric population, it is sometimes necessary to make practical decisions that involve relinquishing orthotic control to gain patient acceptance.

Soft and rigid spinal systems applied to the trunk typically incorporate a means of applying abdominal pressure, thereby increasing intra-abdominal pressure, which has been shown to reduce the load on the vertebrae and intervertebral discs. Some literature (Kulkarni & Ho, 2005) suggests that this may be the primary effect of the corsets and soft binders that are frequently used in geriatric applications.

The principle of correcting spinal alignment is seldom applied to the geriatric population because of restriction of spinal flexibility and poor tolerance of the required forces.

Flexible spinal orthoses serve to limit motion by acting as kinesthetic reminders to volitionally restrict movement as opposed to exerting three-point pressure control. Motion restriction accomplished through a flexible orthosis would obviously be better tolerated by the elderly.

CERVICAL ORTHOSES (CO)

Among cervical orthoses (COs), soft cervical collars are well tolerated and provide reasonable control of cervical flexion and extension. The Philadelphia, Aspen and Miami collars offer greater control than the soft cervical collar and are also reasonably well tolerated.

CERVICAL–THORACIC ORTHOSES (CTO)

When more definitive control of the cervical spine and upper thoracic region are required, a cervical orthosis with a thoracic extension (a cervical–thoracic orthosis, or CTO) is indicated. Rigid four-poster and sternal–occipital–mandibular immobilizer (SOMI) systems are difficult for the elderly to tolerate. The Minerva and Aspen CTOs tend to be better tolerated without sacrificing spinal control.

THORACO-LUMBO-SACRAL ORTHOSES (TLSO)

Thoraco-lumbo-sacral orthoses (TLSOs) are utilized to address spinal pathologies from approximately the T6 to the L3–4 region. An over-shoulder overlap may allow control of the T4–5 levels, and a cervical extension addition to the TLSO is recommended for more definitive control above the T6 level. TLSOs most effectively control from approximately the sixth thoracic to the third and fourth lumbar vertebral region and offer diminishing control of spinal segments farther away from this region. Rigid immobilization is typically accomplished using a 'body jacket' made of plastic with a soft foam interface (lining). Soft, high-density body jackets can incorporate high-density outer foam instead of plastic. Plastic stays (permanent or removable) or a plastic frame can be incorporated into the foam for additional restriction of motion if desired. These systems, when custom fabricated, offer excellent alternatives to the rigid body jacket. They tend to be much better tolerated by the elderly patient and offer moderately effective restriction of spinal motion (Lusardi & Nielsen, 2000).

The TLSO corset (semiflexible) or off-the-shelf semi-rigid TLSO (i.e. Ossur, Aspen types) is often used for patients whose acceptance of a more rigid spinal orthosis is questionable or for patients who require minimal restriction of spinal motion. Compression fractures are very common in the geriatric population and frequently it is appropriate to manage them with these types of orthoses. Rigid systems such as the Jewett, Taylor and Knight-Taylor are less frequently used for the elderly because they are difficult to tolerate. Osteoporosis which commonly accompanies aging can result in kyphosis and related compression fractures. The Spinomed IV (www.mediusa.com) is a specialty TLSO designed to address this pathology optimally in combination with a coordinated physical therapy program.

LUMBO-SACRAL ORTHOSES (LSO)

Utilized to address spinal pathologies from approximately L1 to L4–5, the lumbo-sacral orthosis (LSO) most effectively controls the L3–4 spinal level. As with the TLSO, a rigid system is used in the presence of spinal instability, whereas more flexible systems are preferred and better tolerated by the geriatric population and should be used whenever possible. Corsets are commonly used to manage soft-tissue injuries that result in back pain. The custom-made, soft, high-density LSO or off-the-shelf semi-rigid LSO with a compound closure system to optimize support (i.e. Ossur, Aspen types) are an excellent alternative to the rigid body jacket or corset, offering a balance between comfort and control. It should be noted that successful orthotic outcomes with the soft, high-density system appear to be more readily accomplished in patients with average to thin body types. Again, rigid LSO systems like the Chairback and Knight are poorly tolerated by geriatric patients.

CONCLUSION

The use of orthotics to support a body segment, correct anatomical alignment, protect a body area, or assist body movement is an important therapeutic consideration in geriatric rehabilitation. It is crucial to involve the patient in the choice of orthotic design whenever possible in order to attain a balance between objective ideals and patient adherence. Attention must be given to possible harmful effects of the orthotic device on the skin and the subcutaneous connective tissues of aged persons.

REFERENCES

American Academy of Orthopedic Surgeons 1985 Atlas of Orthotics: Biomechanical Principles and Application. Mosby, St Louis, MO

Briggs KK, Matheny AJ, Steadman R 2009 Patient evaluation of an unloader knee brace: a prospective cohort study. The Academy Today 5:2. Available at: www.oandp.org/AcademyTODAY/2009Mar/4.asp. Accessed February 2013

Edelstein JE 1995 Orthoses. In: Myers RS (ed) Saunders Manual of Physical Therapy Practice. WB Saunders, Philadelphia, PA

Kulkarni SS, Ho S 2005 Spinal orthotics. Available at: http://www.emedicine.com/pmr/topic173.htm. Accessed February 2013

Lusardi M, Nielsen CC 2000 Orthotics and Prosthetics in Rehabilitation. Butterworth–Heinemann, Boston, MA

Zissimopoulos A, Fatone S, Gard SA 2007 Biomechanical and energetic effects of a stance-control orthotic knee joint. J Rehabil Res Dev 44(4):503–514

Chapter 70

Prosthetics

DAVID PATRICK

CHAPTER CONTENTS

INTRODUCTION

The elderly make up the largest group of patients requiring lower extremity (LE) amputations. Review of the literature has determined that significant variation exists internationally in the incidence of LE amputation. The incidence of all forms of LE amputation ranges from 46.1–96 per million in the population of amputees with diabetes compared with 5.8–31 per million in the total population of amputees without diabetes (Moxey et al., 2011). Diabetes and its complications are identified as having the most profound influence while the role of ethnicity and social deprivation are also important factors. Globally, a wide variation also exists in the access to high-quality prosthetic and orthotic care for those in need, a major focus of the International Society for Prosthetics and Orthotics (ISPO). Differences in prosthetic and orthotic education have been identified worldwide ranging from no formal education to advanced university-based degrees, such as in the United States of America where the graduate Masters degree has been adopted as the entry level standard by the American Board for Certification. The advancement of global prosthetic and orthotic education utilizing creative educational models and concepts such as distance learning is being pursued in an effort to meet the needs of the underserved in developing countries and improving the standards and consistency of care throughout the world (Ferrendelli, 2012).

EVALUATING THE PATIENT

The physical therapy program starts with a comprehensive evaluation of the patient. This is particularly important with the elderly amputee, who commonly presents with a number of comorbid conditions that can impact his/her functional outcome. The following elements represent important considerations in evaluation and treatment of the geriatric amputee.

Age

Consider overall wellness and conditioning, functional abilities and motivation as being more important than chronological age.

Secondary Diagnosis

Investigate the presence of comorbid conditions. Elderly vascular amputees can demonstrate multiple secondary conditions in addition to the amputation. The presence of cardiac disease is common, as the same factors that increase the incidence of peripheral vascular disease (PVD) in diabetics also increase the incidence of atherosclerotic coronary artery disease. This leads to an increased death rate (there is an estimated 25–50% 3-year survival for a person with diabetes, with a major amputation) (Schofield et al., 2006) and an increase in the symptoms of angina, congestive heart failure (CHF) and arrhythmias.

Cognitive Status

Determine the patient's ability to understand and remember instructions. Provide instructions in writing that clearly state the wearing schedule of the shrinker, socks and prosthesis. Review the instructions with the patient frequently. Direct the patient to maintain a written diary of sock-ply use and color-code the various sock plys to assist the patient in maintaining proper socket fit.

Wheelchair

Recommend availability of a lightweight, easily transportable wheelchair for long-distance transportation, limited ambulation endurance, discontinued prosthetic use (because of skin breakdown) and prosthetic breakdown. Bilateral LE geriatric amputees commonly depend on wheelchairs or powered mobility as an option to walking with prostheses, particularly for long distances.

Transfers and Mobility

Train patients to change positions slowly to avoid episodes of syncope that could result in loss of balance.

Reduced proprioceptive feedback through the prosthetic extremity, and the predisposition of the elderly for postural hypotension, increase the risk of balance loss when changing positions.

Ambulation

Prioritize the maintenance of skin integrity, the prevention of falls and the control of energy expenditure. Assess the patient's ability to ambulate (post amputation) with an assistive device without a prosthesis.

Skin Integrity

The loss of elements of the connective tissue, the thinning of the dermis and alterations in the content of elastin and collagen represent characteristic skin changes that occur with aging and predispose the amputee to skin breakdown during prosthetic use (see Chapter 50, Skin Disorders). Particularly with the transtibial (below-knee) amputee, use a conservative, methodical progression of weight-bearing and ambulation distance and continue to monitor the skin of the residual limb (in the past, it was referred to as the stump) on a frequent basis. Consider shear-force-absorbing socket interfaces and prosthetic componentry to reduce forces on the residual limb.

Fall Prevention

Conservative advancement of assistive devices is recommended, prioritizing safety over progression. In the author's experience, the transfemoral (above-knee) geriatric amputee is less prone to skin breakdown than is the transtibial amputee, but the transfemoral amputee is at greater risk for falls.

Energy Expenditure

The geriatric amputee should not be encouraged to walk at a 'normal' walking speed. Allowing the patient to self-select ambulation velocity results in a more normal rate of metabolic energy expenditure, decreasing perceived exertion and potential cardiac difficulties. A slower self-selected walking velocity should be expected at higher amputation levels.

Prosthetic Donning and Doffing

Difficulty in donning and doffing the prosthetic may result from limitations in manual dexterity as well as visual dysfunction. Self-suspending systems, Velcro closures versus buckles, and oversized extensions on belts and socket inserts should be considered.

Range of Motion (ROM)

Adequate ROM is required for successful prosthetic outcome. Degenerative joint disease predisposes elderly amputees to contractures. Common areas of LE contractures include:

- the partial foot level: plantar flexors (due primarily to muscle imbalance)
- the transtibial level: knee flexors and hip flexors
- the transfemoral level: hip flexors, hip abductors, hip external rotators.

Strength and Endurance

Deconditioning, common with aging, may limit ability to participate in the rehabilitation program. Initiate a strengthening and endurance program as soon after surgery as possible.

Volume Containment

Controlling the volume of the residual limb is an important aspect of preparing it for definitive prosthetic fitting, reducing pain in the limb that is related to edema, and facilitating healing after the amputation surgery. Comorbid conditions such as renal failure and dialysis or CHF predispose the geriatric amputee to significant girth fluctuations. Shrinker socks are recommended instead of elastic wraps because of the relative ease of donning and the greater consistency of fit (they require less frequent reapplication and adjustment). A rigid dressing should be considered when protection of the residual limb is a priority. Premanufactured removeable rigid plastic shells (e.g. Flotector: APOPPS FLO-TECH-TOR products www.1800flo-tech.com/products.html) provide the dual benefits of protection of the residual limb from external trauma and positioning of the knee to prevent flexion contractures. Regular girth measurements of the residual limb are recommended to monitor the effectiveness of the volume-containment program.

Sensation

Sensory examination is important to accurate prediction of the amputee's ability to detect abnormal forces during prosthetic use and to detect soft-tissue trauma in the remaining limb. Vascular insufficiency and particularly diabetes may result in polyneuropathy involving the sensory nerve fibers, predisposing the elderly amputee to skin problems.

Condition of the Remaining LE

It is essential to examine the remaining LE for evidence of vascular insufficiency or sensory deficits that could lead to further amputation. Unilateral amputees with diabetes have more than a 40% risk over 4 years of having an amputation of the remaining LE (Johannesson et al., 2009). Polyneuropathy associated with diabetes may involve sensory, motor and autonomic nerve fibers. Motor deficits may cause atrophy of the foot intrinsics and muscle imbalances in the foot. These problems result in deformity that predisposes the skin to injury from fitting problems with shoes. Sensory deficits result in the lack of an appropriate avoidance response to abnormal forces. Autonomic involvement may result in dry skin which creates greater susceptibility to breakdown and infection. The importance of this evaluation cannot be overemphasized, as a peripheral neuropathy has been identified as the primary underlying cause of amputation in the elderly with diabetes. Patient education that emphasizes proper footwear and skin management is an essential component of the amputation prevention program. The incidence of LE amputations has been shown to be significantly reduced in specific at risk populations after the introduction of specialist diabetic foot clinics (Moxey et al., 2011).

PROSTHETIC PRESCRIPTION

Advances in the technology of prosthetic components have improved the possibility of successfully fitting the geriatric amputee with a prosthesis. Innovations in socket designs, lightweight components, improved suspensions and stable knee design options all contribute to improved prosthetic tolerance and better functional outcomes for elderly amputees. The application of advanced prosthetic componentry also results in increased expense, so judgments must be made about the relative costs and benefits of these components to each patient. In the US, the Lower Limb Prosthetics Medical Review Policy (LLPMRP: available from the US Department of Health and Human Services) developed by Medicare, structures financial sponsorship of the various prosthetic ankle, foot and knee components based on the patient's anticipated functional outcome. The LLPMRP should be considered by the prosthetics team in the process of prescribing prostheses for geriatric amputees as many third party payers follow this policy as a basis for financial sponsorship.

PREPARATORY VS. DEFINITIVE PROSTHESIS

A preparatory prosthesis is often recommended over a definitive prosthesis as the first prosthetic device for a geriatric amputee. The preparatory prosthesis includes basic components that are easily adjusted but is not finished cosmetically. The preparatory prosthesis allows earlier prosthetic fitting by avoiding the need to wait until shrinkage of the residual limb is complete (Edelstein, 1992). This may help to prevent secondary complications resulting from immobility that are potentially life-threatening to the elderly patient. The definitive prosthesis is the finished product, with all the appropriate components and cosmetic touches. The definitive prosthesis is fitted when the residual limb size stabilizes. The specific training and skills required for use of certain advanced componentry such as microprocessor knees has led to the debate of using high-tech componentry in the initial prosthesis and replacing only the socket of the prosthesis once the expected shrinkage of the residual limb occurs. The need for training can be reduced as the patient is not required to re-learn how to ambulate with different components. Gait performance, stability and safety may be improved through the earlier use of technology, and bad habits may be avoided in the initial gait training process.

ENDOSKELETAL VS. EXOSKELETAL DESIGN

The exoskeleton design has a hard, laminated plastic shell that provides the weight-bearing support. In contrast, the endoskeletal design consists of a tubular structure that constitutes the internal support to which the foot, ankle and knee assemblies are attached. The endoskeleton is covered with a pliable surface that is shaped and colored to match the opposite limb.

Endoskeletal prosthetic design is usually recommended for geriatric amputees because of the ease with which adjustments can be made and components interchanged, the reduced weight and the cosmetic benefits in transfemoral applications. Weight restrictions have been identified by the manufacturers of some endoskeletal components.

PROSTHETIC SOCKETS

At the level of the transtibial amputation, the patellar tendon-bearing (PTB) socket with a soft insert is commonly utilized. A patient with fragile skin or sensitivity in the residual limb may benefit from soft insert materials such as silicone that are designed to dissipate shock and shear forces. A flexible inner socket supported in a rigid outer frame may result in greater comfort for the elderly amputee by providing relief to pressure-sensitive structures. The flexible inner socket also facilitates necessary socket adjustments (American Academy of Orthotists and Prosthetists, 2004).

After a transfemoral amputation, a geriatric patient can be successfully fitted with either a quadrilateral or an ischial containment socket. A patient with a short residual limb, poor residual limb muscle tone, obesity, or a high activity level would be expected to achieve the greatest benefit from the ischial containment socket design. The elderly amputee may experience more comfort when sitting if he or she has chosen a flexible socket design that is capable of accommodating its shape to the supporting surface.

PROSTHETIC SUSPENSIONS

The following prosthetic suspensions are recommended for transtibial-level amputation:

- Supracondylar cuff with Velcro closure on strap.
- Supracondylar wedge self-suspension with tab extensions attached to medial and lateral insert wings.
- Sleeve suspension (determine if the patient has the hand dexterity to manage the sleeve).
- Silicone suction suspension (consider the patient's ability to manage the sleeve and the patient's skin's tolerance to silicone).
- Joint and corset (which may be necessary due to hypersensitivity, skin problems, or knee joint pathology that prohibits full weight-bearing through the residual limb).

For transfemoral-level amputation, the following prosthetic suspensions are suggested:

- Neoprene belt with Velcro closure.
- Hip joint and pelvic band with Velcro closure (indicated when hip stability or rotational control is required).
- Silicone suction.

PROSTHETIC FEET

The weight of the foot and function of the foot's keel in relationship to the patient's activity level are the two primary considerations for the geriatric amputee. The keel provides the inner rigidity of structure to control the function of the prosthetic foot.

SACH Feet

The solid ankle, cushion heel (SACH) feet are low cost and dependable. Geriatric lightweight versions are available. The rigid keel can interfere with the ability of the amputee to roll over the forefoot during the terminal stance phase.

Single-axis Feet

More readily plantar flex from heel strike to foot-flat during the early loading phase of gait. Single-axis feet are recommended for the geriatric transfemoral amputee using an unlocked knee when greater knee stability during the early stance phase of gait is desired.

Multiple-axis Feet

Accommodating to uneven surfaces, multiple-axis feet are recommended for geriatric patients with sensitive skin, who may benefit from the reduction in shear forces transmitted to the prosthetic socket–skin interface. Typically, this is a heavier prosthetic foot.

Elastic Keel Feet

The flexible nature of the elastic keel foot facilitates ambulation by allowing easier rollover at the terminal stance phase of gait. Lightweight designs are available. This prosthesis is appropriate for the moderately active individual.

Dynamic Response Feet

Typically more expensive, dynamic response feet are appropriate for an individual with a high activity level. They incorporate foot keels that bend in response to the patient's weight during rollover, then 'spring back', providing propulsion during the push-off phase of gait. Some dynamic response feet are available in a multiaxial design combining the benefits of ankle motion and push off during the gait cycle. Some also allow torsion motion or a torsion adaptor unit can be added, to improve comfort, reduce stress on the skin of the residual limb, or facilitate certain activities requiring torsional movement. Vertical shock absorbers are an integral component of some dynamic response designs.

Power Feet

Powered feet provide active toe lift in the swing phase to clear the ground minimizing the risk of tripping and reducing gait compensations. Additionally, the ankle angle is automatically adjusted to adapt to variations in ground surfaces increasing patient confidence and comfort walking on ramps and hills. Improvements have been cited in gait symmetry, safety and the ability to perform ADLs as well as reductions in mental fatigue and back and socket discomfort at both the transtibial and transfemoral levels.

PROSTHETIC KNEES

Insuring knee stability during stance phase is the highest priority for the geriatric transfemoral-level amputee. Lightweight versions of the various designs of prosthetic knees are available and are recommended for consideration for the elderly amputee.

Manual-locking Knees

Maximum knee stability during gait is important, and manual-locking knees provide it, but the resulting gait is the least cosmetic because the knee remains in extension during the swing phase. Manual-locking knees are appropriate when there is concern that the patient may not be able to control the prosthetic knee from buckling during weight bearing.

Weight-activated Friction Knees (Safety Knees)

Frequently used with geriatric patients, weight-activated friction knees provide inherent knee stability during the stance phase by locking in response to the patient's weight-bearing, then unlocking allowing the knee to bend during the swing phase, which provides a more natural gait appearance.

Polycentric Knees

Inherent alignment stability is provided by polycentric knees, but they are not commonly used by geriatric patients because of their greater weight and complexity.

Hydraulic or Pneumatic Swing-phase Controls

A very active individual might consider hydraulic or pneumatic swing-phase control knees which are designed to allow variation in gait velocity and cadence by adjusting the resistance to knee motion.

MICROPROCESSOR KNEES

The microprocessor knee (www.ossur.com, www.ottobockus.com) utilizes an onboard computer to control the prosthetic knee throughout the gait cycle. The microprocessor continually analyzes the motion and forces occurring at the knee and makes instantaneous adjustments allowing dynamic variation in swing phase while maximizing stability in stance phase and promoting more normal, energy-efficient movement patterns during gait on the variety of surfaces and obstacles encountered in one's environment. Knee flexion control in stance allows knee flexion to occur in the initial contact phase of gait providing shock absorption to reduce stress on the body and residual limb and promoting a more normal-appearing gait. This also allows the patient to bear weight through the prosthesis and 'ride the knee down' when sitting and descending ramps and stairs step over step. Stumble recovery recognizes if the knee is flexing too quickly and the user is in danger of collapse, instantaneously increasing resistance to provide the opportunity to recover and avoid a fall. Microprocessor knee technology is typically considered for the K3 and above functional level but the potential improvement in gait stability and safety warrant its consideration at times for the K2 ambulator. (For functional K level definitions, the reader is referred to the LLPMRP document mentioned in the Prosthetic Prescription portion of this chapter.)

POWER KNEE

The power knee is an active prosthetic knee which generates power to replace muscle activity to flex and extend the knee. The contribution of active power by the knee unit helps the user maintain walking speed with less energy and assists with upward movement required for ascending and resistance for descending stairs, curbs and inclines. Sensors and associated electronics process data and apply artificial intelligence to anticipate and control the movement and power of the knee during gait.

CONCLUSION

Amputations occur with increasing incidence as age rises. The conditions that most commonly necessitate amputation are PVD and complications of diabetes. Because of the high frequency of comorbid conditions in the elderly patient, a comprehensive examination and evaluation are requisite. A preparatory prosthesis is typically recommended for the geriatric patient because it allows early fitting and thus discourages the secondary complications of immobility. The various types of prosthetic components should be considered, including new advancements in technology, and then chosen to meet the individual patient's needs. The patient's date of birth is less important when considering a prosthesis than is overall wellness, fitness, functional ability and motivation.

REFERENCES

American Academy of Orthotists and Prosthetists 2004 Post-operative management of the lower extremity amputee. J Prosthet Orthot 16(suppl) no. 3

Edelstein JE 1992 Lower limb prosthetics. Top Geriatr Rehabil 8:1

Ferrendelli B 2012 International education: closing the gap. The O&P Edge. Available at: www.oandp.com/articles/2012-05_03.asp. Accessed February 2013

Johannesson A, Larsson GU, Ramstrand N et al 2009 Incidence of lower limb amputation in the diabetic and non-diabetic general population. Diabetes Care 32(2):275–280

Moxey PW, Gogalniceanu P, Hinchliffe RJ et al 2011 Lower extremity amputations – a review of global variability in incidence. Diabetic Med 28:1144–1153

Schofield CJ, Libby G, Brennan GM et al 2006 Mortality and hospitalization in patients after amputation. Diabetes Care 29(10):2252–2256

Chapter 71

Complementary therapies for the aging patient

CAROL M. DAVIS

INTRODUCTION

Alternative and complementary therapies, or holistic therapies, are becoming more common in the health-care of older individuals (Okoro et al., 2011; McLaughlin et al., 2012). First, let us define the terms we often read with this topic. 'Holistic' therapies emphasize the mind and the body working together to bring about the desired effect. For example, in tai chi, patients are told to bring their attention to a spot just below the umbilicus and drop their minds into their bodies like sand in an hourglass, and then lead their movement from that place. Mind and body working together, with the breath coordinated in a specific way, is the mark of a 'holistic' therapy.

The term 'alternative' refers to a therapy that is not known to be part of allopathic medicine, nor is it listed as a therapeutic measure in traditional 'gold standards' of care. The therapy is an *alternative* to standard care. An example would be when a patient turns to acupuncture for pain relief rather than taking acetaminophen. The term 'complementary' refers to a therapy that, again, is not part of standard allopathic regimens, but is used 'in addition to' standard care rather than replacing the care, so it 'complements' the care. This happens, for example, when physical therapists utilize John F. Barnes's method (sustained release) of myofascial release as a way of preparing a person's soft tissue for traditional exercise programs (Barnes, 1990, 2009). 'Integrative' therapy is a term used when traditional and holistic therapies are closely interwoven in care, *integrated* to the point that non-traditional and traditional methods flow together. As more holistic therapies become validated by the traditional gold standard randomized controlled trial, they are being integrated more smoothly into comprehensive care programs. Many hospitals have begun including wellness and prevention programs that integrate tai chi, yoga and Pilates as part of their outpatient clinics' group exercise programs.

Whether alternative, complementary or integrative is used, there is another, more profound, definition of holistic therapies that has to do with a theory about how they work. This author most commonly uses the term 'complementary' therapies when referring to those therapies that are not listed as standard for allopathic care, but integrate the mind and the body together in their action, thus are 'holistic'. The difference is that they have as their basic goal to unblock body energy that is not flowing freely, for whatever reason, and therefore the body/mind is hindered from healing itself, or self-regulating (Han, 2007).

Fundamental to this viewpoint is the belief that body and mind cannot be separated, and that all cells of the body vibrate naturally for their own healing. This natural vibration is facilitated by the flow of a vital energy (or *ch'i*), and this natural state of healing flow can be interrupted by injury, toxins or imbalances, causing the body energy or chi to become blocked, to not flow smoothly. When this happens, the body/mind becomes vulnerable to bacterial and viral invasion, endocrine imbalance (diabetes, depression) and loss of self-regulation that insures proper pH, body temperature and pituitary function. The goal is to restore the flow of chi so the body can once again heal itself, or self-regulate.

WHY COMPLEMENTARY THERAPIES LACK UNIVERSAL ACCEPTANCE

Controversy over the use of holistic therapies relates to the resistance of some practitioners to using any therapy that has not been proven efficacious by traditional randomized controlled trial (Harris, 2001). However, many alternative and complementary therapies arise from an Eastern philosophy in contrast to Western Cartesian and Newtonian thought. Traditional or mechanistic therapies, based on the physics of Isaac Newton, aim to 'fix what is broken'. Reliability and validity of traditional therapies are proven by randomized trials that can replicate the efficacy of an approach when the same outcome is observed within a variety of patients using the same process over and over.

Complementary therapies restore balance or homeostasis by removing blocks to the flow of bioelectric body energy. They do not lend themselves readily to validation by research methods that count on replication of the exact process. A subject's energy pattern and flow will change as it is impacted by the energy of the examiner. Thus, for example, a therapist placing her hands under the cranium of a patient to feel the craniosacral rhythm will impact that rhythm with her own energy that is emitted from her hands in the process. A second therapist attempting to validate the flow of the craniosacral rhythm at the feet will also be observing the flow of the patient and his energy flow. To then try to attempt interrater reliability between the two therapists with the patient's energy as that which is constant becomes an impossibility, as was shown by Rogers et al. (1998).

THE SCIENCE OF MECHANISTIC VS. HOLISTIC THERAPIES

Traditional mechanistic science or reductionism has its roots in the early 17th century. The philosopher René Descartes claimed that the best way to elevate and organize the search for truth would be to eliminate that which could not be observed with the five senses. All that could not be seen was to be ignored, and only that which could be measured and experienced was suitable in the scientific search for cause and effect. Later, Sir Isaac Newton developed the theory of gravity, outlined mathematical rules of physics and described the theories upon which contemporary science is based. From this foundation the randomized controlled trial has its base as a way of insuring the experimental variable is, indeed, causing the outcome, and not chance, or 'placebo' (Davis, 2009).

In the early 1900s, Einstein suggested another way of viewing reality based on his understanding of the behavior of subatomic particles. Subsequently, quantum physics and systems theory (from biology) formed the basis for the theoretical foundation of holism, a concept that attempts to describe the outcomes of alternative and complementary therapies (Davis, 2009). Holism as a concept is based on current knowledge of molecules, atoms and electron behavior, and states that it is no longer useful to regard humans solely as machines that can be fully understood simply by reducing the whole and analyzing the parts. The uniqueness and challenge of the human organism lies in how it is organized and how the parts interact and exchange information. Atoms, their electrons and other subatomic particles provide the basis of wave theory, bioelectromagnetism, energy and thus the flow of chi (Oschman, 2000; Davis, 2009).

Holism focuses on balance and integration of all interacting elements of the system. Information inherent in the organization of a system gets lost in the separation of the parts (Schwartz & Russek, 1997). The whole is more than simply the sum of the parts. For example, no matter how thoroughly one studies hydrogen and oxygen, one cannot understand water from that study. When two hydrogen atoms and one oxygen atom come together to form water, their electrons not only share orbits, but also they share information that results in formation of the new system, the new substance. Information sharing is the key to electron flow. All systems 'work' by way of electrons sharing information.

COMPLEMENTARY THERAPIES IN THE CARE OF AGING PATIENTS

A variety of complementary therapies have been found to be useful for all people, and particularly in caring for older people. Generally, each of these therapies aims to increase the flow of healthy bioelectric energy and, as a result, restore balance or homeostasis in the mind/body and restore information flow that facilitates the body's natural state of wholeness and healing (Davis, 2009).

THE MANUAL THERAPIES

These include myofascial release, craniosacral therapy, Rosen method, Rolfing, Hellerwork, Soma, neuromuscular therapy, osteopathic and chiropractic medicine. The manual therapies involve the use of hands directly on the body/mind surface, thereby stimulating bioelectromagnetic force. Research by Seto et al. (1992) and Rubik (1995) documents the measure of energy flow from the body and suggests that both mechanical and energy forces stimulate responses from the tissues.

MIND/BODY INTERVENTIONS

These include psychotherapies, support groups, meditation and imagery (Kim et al., 2012), hypnosis, dance (Granacher et al., 2012) and music therapy (Clark et al., 2012), art therapy, prayer, validation therapy, neurolinguistic psychology (Masin, 2012), biofeedback (Bottomley, 2009a; McClelland et al., 2012), yoga (Taylor, 2009; Roland et al., 2011) and tai chi (Bottomley, 2009b; Leung et al., 2011; Gillespie et al., 2012; Taylor et al., 2012). These mind/body interventions demonstrate how movement and verbal and nonverbal communication with the mind/body seem to open up new pathways for thought and, therefore, unblock energy flow. A growing body of literature examines the effects of tai chi on the ability to prevent falls in elderly people and on quality of life.

MOVEMENT AWARENESS TECHNIQUES

These include the Feldenkrais method (Stephens & Miller, 2009), the Alexander technique (Zuck, 2009), Pilates (Chapter 72) and the Trager approach (Stone, 1997). It is postulated that these movement awareness techniques help people recognize the way they move habitually. By practicing new ways of moving and identifying habitual postural holding patterns, energy trapped in tissue while maintaining habitual postures is freed.

TRADITIONAL CHINESE MEDICINE

These methods include acupuncture (LaRiccia & Galantino, 2009; Suzuki et al., 2012), acupressure and Qi Gong (Bottomley, 2009c). These approaches within the system of traditional Chinese medicine focus on enhancing the flow of chi along body pathways or meridians.

BIOELECTROMAGNETICS

Thermal applications of nonionizing radiation, such as radio-frequency hyperthermia lasers, low-energy laser (Reddy, 2009), radiofrequency surgery, radiofrequency diathermy and nonthermal applications of nonionizing radiation are used for bone repair and wound healing. Biomicroelectromagnetics is the term applied to the energy that seems to emanate from the hands of people who have proven to be healers (Rubik, 1995). Credible research exists on the effects of electromagnetic energy for wound healing and bone repair (Midura et al., 2005).

INFLUENCE OF THE MIND ON THE BODY

Mind/body medicine links traditional research methods with holistic healthcare practices. The influence of the mind on the body was first introduced by Herbert Benson's research on Tibetan monks who could control their autonomic nervous system (Wallace et al., 1971). These monks could lower their body temperature and respiration rates, and enter a wakeful hypometabolic physiological state at will. Ader and Cohen (1991) coined the term *psychoneuroimmunology*, wherein the mind affects the immune system via the autonomic nervous system and the 'fluid' nervous system, another name given to the neurotransmitters and neuropeptides. Pert (2002) articulated the physiological functioning of the fluid nervous system, which manifests through the effects of thought on neurotransmitters, neuropeptides and steroids in the body. This biochemistry differs from the flow of chi, but both concepts reinforce the theory that the mind and the body are inseparable, and that the mind communicates with every cell in the body.

Complementary therapies are energy-based therapies that require belief in the phenomenon of vital flow of energy in the body. We can observe energy at work in the body in many ways: electrocardiograms, electroencephalograms and electromyograms all measure the energy output from various organs. The piezoelectric effect enables osteoblastic activity that keeps our bones structurally intact. Biomicroelectropotentials, or the exchange of subtle energies in electromagnetic fields that emanate from the hands of healers, are being researched (Seto et al., 1992; Rubik, 1995).

TRADITIONAL THERAPIES APPLIED FROM A HOLISTIC APPROACH

In working with older people, massage, exercise and relaxation can be approached by practitioners in a conventional way, where the intention is a mechanical effect on a part (e.g. pushing fluid out of an edematous extremity), or a holistic effect, where the intention is to influence the flow of vital energy and bring about homeostasis (e.g. manual lymph drainage that 'energetically' opens up lymph passages in the central core of the body or the opposite side of the body from the edematous extremity so it can receive the fluid that is pushed out) (Funk, 2009).

Researchers confirm the importance of hope and faith in one's physician and practitioners. How this facilitates healing still remains unclear, but to ignore the positive effect of therapeutic presence is to neglect a powerful intervention (Greer, 1999). How practitioners are with their patients, not just what they do, is important. The exchange of energy with the intention to serve and facilitate healing is critical (DiBlasi et al., 2001).

Sustained Release Myofascial Release – the Role of Unrestricted Fascia in Conduction of Body Energy

James Oschman has stated (2012):

After some 40 years of basic and clinical research, Pischinger (2007) … identified the ground regulation system [of fascia] as the place where diseases and disorders begin and the place to focus both prevention and treatment.

A similar conclusion had already been reached by Andrew Tyler Still, the founder of osteopathy. Many of Still's insights have been incorporated into many modern complementary and alternative therapies:

The fascia (connective tissue surrounding nerves, muscles, bones, etc.) is the place to look for the cause of disease and the place to consult and begin the action of remedies in all diseases. (Still, 1899)

The involvement of the fascia in dysfunction and disease is pervasive. It is believed that, to some extent, the fascia will necessarily be involved in every type of human pathology. (Paoletti, 2006; Pischinger, 2007)

Recent research on the connection between fascia and breast cancer (Bissell, 2012) points to the realization that the extracellular matrix of fascia seems to communicate with the cell in ways that direct the cells' development. Bissell's research indicates that a cancer cell becomes a neoplastic tumor when it interacts with the surrounding cells of the connective tissue, the extracellular matrix of the fascia (Bissell, 2012).

Sustained release myofascial release has been shown to affect the ground substance of the fascia in profound ways structurally by elongating restrictions (LeBauer et al., 2008), relieving pain and improving fatigue (Cubick et al., 2011), and biochemically by stimulating the production of interleukins for vasodilation, and immune system response (Meltzer et al., 2010; Fernandez-Perez et al., 2013). This bioenergetic technique developed by Barnes (1990, 2009) is an effective manual therapy for older patients with diminished hydration of tissue, myofascial shortening and cross-linked collagen restrictions in their bodies. Other therapeutic approaches that use the term 'myofascial release' refer to a mechanistic impact on tissue by way of stretching and mechanically pressing on trigger points to try to influence the circulation to the area and the length of tissue mechanically, rather than focusing on using pressure and stretch to help 'melt' the type II gel matrix of the fascial web (Pollack, 2001). In contrast to using rapid mechanical strokes and short duration pressure, with Barnes' method of myofascial release the practitioner places his or her hands directly on the skin of the patient, and with slight pressure, separates the hands, eliminating the flexibility of the skin between the hands so that the tissue is taught, and then gently waits with this traction until the tissue responds energetically under the surface of the practitioner's hand. Within 90–120 seconds, the tissue begins to move in a flowing manner. This signals the beginning of the phase transition of polysaccharide ground substance from a solid to a more fluid gel as it releases and takes on fluid from the extracellular spaces (Pollack, 2001). The practitioner follows the flow of the tissue with his or her hands in order to increase the length of the tissue as the myofascia 'softens' underneath the hands. The cause of this softening of tissue is believed to be the effect of mechanical stress in gravity along with the therapist's energy causing a piezoelectric effect on the polyglycoid layer of the ground substance of the myofascia, which increases tissue length and results in a release of trapped energy. It has been demonstrated that mechanical force transforms the ground substance of the fascia, causing a flow of electrons in the fascial web by way of the piezoelectric effect. The result is the tissue under the therapist's hands seems to be 'melting' as it releases. Research by Wang et al. (2005) revealed that human cells send biochemical messages to each other as a result of tiny mechanical jabs. Actin filaments and microtubules in the fascia function as conduits for the spread of biochemical signals.

The patient then has more freedom to move, gains better posture and a relief of the pain caused by myofascial restriction (Barnes, 1990, 2009; Cubick et al., 2011). Fascial restrictions released in this way over time result in improved balance and strength and help to eliminate pain and poor posture. Outcome case studies on myofascial release demonstrate improvements in the quality of life of older people and the prevention of chronic musculoskeletal problems (Barnes, 1990, 2009; Cubick et al., 2011).

It is believed that complementary therapies have an effect on patients by way of the energy that emanates from the healer's hands (Seto et al., 1992; Oschman, 1997). The inadequacies of conventional medicine in overcoming chronic illness and autoimmune disease, and the growing tendency of patients and clients to seek out complementary therapies challenge healthcare professionals and researchers to know more about the science of subtle energy.

BENEFITS OF COMPLEMENTARY THERAPIES WITH OLDER PATIENTS

Alternative and complementary therapies are increasingly being used by older patients and physical therapists treating older patients because of their proven success in relieving pain and improving quality of life. As more research is done, we will be able to explain better how this takes place.

Most of our elderly patients have many chronic problems. Treating one problem with traditional healthcare may negatively impact other comorbid conditions. Traditional healthcare emphasizes the use of medications that often interact with one another. Complementary therapies aim to impact the whole of the patient to restore the flow of natural body energy.

Most older patients are dehydrated and experience postural problems that exacerbate pain and pathology. Complementary therapies along with proper hydration and exercise can restore balance and improve posture. Holistic therapies stress empathic communication between therapist and patient, and involve the patient in goal-setting and problem-solving. Older patients appreciate being treated in humanistic and caring ways that are emphasized in holistic therapies. Finally, many of the complementary therapies are pleasurable; older people enjoy the socialization of tai chi and yoga classes, for example.

CONCLUSION

Complementary, alternative, integrative therapies are holistic approaches to healthcare, many of which have been used successfully for centuries around the world in other cultures. A growing body of research evidence suggests that holistic therapies have much to offer for older patients in rehabilitation, and as approaches that help to prevent the usual changes with aging and promote wellness. As more healthcare professionals use and research these therapies, two major advantages will emerge: patients will be better served for their chronic problems that are not well treated allopathically, and we will come to better understand the impact of subatomic vibration or quantum physics at work in human biophysiological functioning.

REFERENCES

Ader R, Cohen N 1991 The influence of conditioning on immune responses. In: Ader R, Felten DL, Cohen N (eds) Psychoneuroimmunology, 2nd edn. Academic Press, San Diego, CA, pp. 611–646

Barnes JF 1990 Myofascial Release/The Search for Excellence. Rehabilitation Services, Paoli, PA

Barnes JF 2009 Myofascial release: the missing link in traditional treatment. In: Davis CM (ed) Complementary Therapies in Rehabilitation: Evidence for Efficacy in Therapy, Prevention and Wellness, 3rd edn. Slack, Thorofare, NJ, pp. 89–112

Bissell M 2012 Ted talks. Ted Global, July 2012

Bottomley J 2009a Biofeedback: connecting the body and mind. In: Davis CM (ed) Complementary Therapies in Rehabilitation: Evidence for Efficacy in Therapy, Prevention and Wellness, 3rd edn. Slack, Thorofare, NJ, pp. 159–182

Bottomley J 2009b T'ai chi: choreography of body and mind. In: Davis CM (ed) Complementary Therapies in Rehabilitation: Evidence for Efficacy in Therapy, Prevention and Wellness, 3rd edn. Slack, Thorofare, NJ, pp. 137–158

Bottomley J 2009c Qi Gong for health and healing. In: Davis CM (ed) Complementary Therapies in Rehabilitation: Evidence for Efficacy in Therapy, Prevention and Wellness, 3rd edn. Slack, Thorofare, NJ, pp. 279–304

Clark IN, Taylor NF, Baker F 2012 Music interventions and physical activity in older adults: a systematic literature review and meta-analysis. J Rehabil Med 44(9):710–719

Cubick EE, Quesada VY, Schumer AD et al 2011 Does sustained release myofascial release improve function and decrease pain in a patient with rheumatoid arthritis and collagenous colitis? Intern J Ther Massage Body Work 4(3):25–33

Davis CM 2009 Quantum physics and systems theory – the science behind complementary and alternative therapies. In: Davis CM (ed) Complementary Therapies in Rehabilitation: Evidence for Efficacy in Therapy, Prevention and Wellness, 3rd edn. Slack, Thorofare, NJ, pp. 31–40

DiBlasi Z, Harkness E, Ernst E et al 2001 Influence of context effects on health outcomes: a systematic review. Lancet 357(9358):757–762

Fernandez-Perez A, Peralta-Ramirez I, Pilat A et al 2013 Can myofascial techniques modify immunological parameters? J Altern Complement Ther 19(1):24–28

Funk B 2009 Complete decongestive therapy. In: Davis CM (ed) Complementary Therapies in Rehabilitation: Evidence for Efficacy in Therapy, Prevention and Wellness, 3rd edn. Slack, Thorofare, NJ, pp. 113–126

Gillespie LD, Robertson MC, Gillespie WJ et al 2012 Interventions for preventing falls in older people living in the community. Cochrane Database Syst Rev(9):CD007146, doi: 10.1002/14651858.CD007146.pub3

Granacher U, Muehlbauer T, Bridenbaugh SA et al 2012 Effects of salsa dance training on balance and strength performance in older adults. Gerontology 58(4):305–312

Greer S 1999 Mind–body research in psychooncology. Adv Mind–Body Med 15:236–281

Han J-X 2007 Acupuncture principle of tonifying qi and regulating blood, supporting the root and fostering the source on aging and senile diseases. Chin J Integr Med 13(3):166–167

Harris S 2001 Challenging myths in physical therapy. Phys Ther 81:1181–1182

Kim BH, Newton RA, Sachs ML et al 2012 Effect of guided relaxation and imagery on falls self-efficacy: a randomized controlled trial. J Am Geriatr Soc 60(6):1109–1114

LaRiccia PJ, Galantino ML 2009 Acupuncture theory and acupuncture-like therapeutics in physical therapy. In: Davis CM (ed) Complementary Therapies in Rehabilitation: Evidence for Efficacy in Therapy, Prevention and Wellness, 3rd edn. Slack, Thorofare, NJ, pp. 331–346

LeBauer A, Brtalik R, Stowe K 2008 The effect of myofascial release (MFR) on an adult with idiopathic scoliosis. J Bodyw Mov Ther 12:356–363

Leung DP, Chan CK, Tsang HW et al 2011 Tai chi as an intervention to improve balance and reduce falls in older adults: a systematic and meta-analytical review. Altern Ther Health Med 17(1):40–48

McClelland J, Zeni J, Haley RM et al 2012 Functional and biomechanical outcomes after using biofeedback for retraining symmetrical movement patterns after total knee arthroplasty. J Orthop Sports Phys Ther 42(2):135–144

McLaughlin D, Adams J, Sibbritt D et al 2012 Sex differences in the use of complementary and alternative medicine in older men and women. Australas J Ageing 2:78–82

Masin H 2012 Communicating to establish rapport and reduce negativity using neurolinguistic psychology. In: Davis CM (ed) Patient Practitioner Interaction: An Experiential Manual for Developing the Art of Health Care, 5th edn. Slack, Thorofare,, NJ, pp. 127–142

Meltzer KR, Thanh V, Cao BA et al 2010 In vitro modeling of repetitive motion injury and myofascial release. J Bodyw Mov Ther 14(2):162–171

Midura RJ, Ibiwoye MO, Powell KA et al 2005 Pulsed electromagnetic field treatments enhance the healing of fibular osteotomies. J Orthop Res 23(5):1035–1046

Okoro CA, Zhao G, Li C et al 2011 Use of complementary and alternative medicine among USA adults with functional limitations: for treatment or general use? Complement Ther Med 4:208–215

Oschman JL 1997 What is healing energy? Part 3: Silent pulses. J Bodyw Mov Ther 1(3):179–189

Oschman JL 2000 Energy Medicine: The Scientific Basis. Churchill Livingstone, Edinburgh

Oschman JL 2012 Personal correspondence with Carol Davis regarding the ground substance of fascia as the seat of all human pathology. 16 July 2012

Paoletti S 2006 The Fasciae: Dysfunctions and Treatment. Eastland Press, Seattle, WA

Pert C 2002 The wisdom of the receptors: neuropeptides, the emotions and body–mind. Adv Mind–Body Med 18(1):30–35

Pischinger A 2007 The Extracellular Matrix and Ground Regulation – Basis for a Holistic Biological Medicine. North Atlantic Books, Berkeley, CA

Pollack G 2001 Cells, Gels and the Engines of Life. Ebner and Sons, Seattle, WA, pp. 126–127

Reddy GK 2009 Biomedical applications of low-energy lasers. In: Davis CM (ed) Complementary Therapies in Rehabilitation: Evidence for Efficacy in Therapy, Prevention and Wellness, 3rd edn. Slack, Thorofare, NJ, pp. 383–397

Rogers JS, Witt PL, Gross MT et al 1998 Simultaneous palpation of the craniosacral rate at the head and feet: intrarater and interrater reliability. Phys Ther 78:1175–1185

Roland KP, Jakobi JM, Jones GR 2011 Does yoga engender fitness in older adults? A critical review. J Aging Phys Act 19(1):62–79

Rubik B 1995 Energy medicine and the unifying concept of information. Altern Ther Health Med 1:34–39

Schwartz GE, Russek LG 1997 Dynamical energy systems and modern physics: fostering the science and spirit of complementary and alternative medicine. Altern Ther Health Med 3(3):46–56

Seto A, Kusaka C, Nakazato S et al 1992 Detection of extraordinary large bio-magnetic field strength from human hand. Acupuncture Electro-Therapeut Res Int J 17:75–94

Stephens J, Miller TM 2009 Feldenkrais method in rehabilitation. Using functional integration and awareness through movement to explore new possibilities. In: Davis CM (ed) Complementary Therapies in Rehabilitation: Evidence for Efficacy in Therapy, Prevention and Wellness, 3rd edn. Slack, Thorofare, NJ, pp. 227–244

Still AT 1899 Philosophy of Osteopathy. AT Still, Kirksville, MO

Stone A 1997 The Trager approach. In: Davis CM (ed) Complementary Therapies in Rehabilitation: Holistic Approaches for Prevention and Wellness. Slack, Thorofare, NJ, pp. 199–212

Suzuki M, Muro S, Ando Y et al 2012 A randomized, placebo-controlled trial of acupuncture in patients with chronic obstructive pulmonary disease (COPD): the COPD–Acupuncture Trial (CAT). Arch Intern Med 172(11):878–886

Taylor D, Hale L, Schluter P et al 2012 Effectiveness of tai chi as a community-based fall prevention intervention: a randomized controlled trial. J Am Geriatr Soc 60(5):841–848

Taylor MF 2009 Yoga therapeutics: an ancient practice in a 21st century setting. In: Davis CM (ed) Complementary Therapies in Rehabilitation: Evidence for Efficacy in Therapy, Prevention and Wellness, 3rd edn. Slack, Thorofare, NJ, pp. 183–206

Wallace RK, Benson H, Wilson AF 1971 A wakeful hypometabolic physiologic state. Am J Physiol 221(3):795–799

Wang Y, Botvinick E, Zhao U et al 2005 Visualizing the mechanical activation of src. Nature 434:1040–1045

Zuck D 2009 The Alexander technique. In: Davis CM (ed) Complementary Therapies in Rehabilitation: Evidence for Efficacy in Therapy, Prevention and Wellness, 3rd edn. Slack, Thorofare, NJ, pp. 207–226

Chapter 72

Safe Pilates for bone health

SHERRI R. BETZ

CHAPTER CONTENTS

INTRODUCTION

Baby boomers are flocking to Pilates and yoga classes! They appear to be seeking a more gentle form of exercise that focuses on posture, balance, flexibility and relaxation. It is those in the 30–60-year-old age range who mostly comprise the population seeking Pilates classes (von Sperling de Souza & Brum Vieira, 2006). Imagine a deconditioned 60-year-old woman with decreased bone density, mild thoracic kyphosis and slightly decreased balance attending a Pilates class for the first time. What exercises would she be expected to do? Does the instructor have any information as it pertains to dealing with osteoporosis or teaching exercise safely to an older adult? These are all very important questions for the baby boomer to ask if they are to participate safely in this style of exercise.

PILATES BACKGROUND

If you take a look at Joseph Pilates' original method of exercise as outlined in *Return to Life* you would see that the first three exercises are: Hundred, Rollup and Rollover. All three are contraindicated for someone with osteoporosis (Sinaki, 2013). At first glance, the knowledgeable practitioner would advise their patient or client to completely avoid the Pilates exercise method. However, the guiding principles of Joseph Pilates' original work focused on breathing, whole body health and whole body commitment. The vast majority of Pilates' work was developed in the early 1900s (Pilates & Miller, 2003). He and his wife, Clara, developed the Contrology exercise method, and in 1934 Joseph wrote a small book exposing his controversial theories about health and fitness, called *Your Health* (Pilates, 1934). *Return to Life* followed soon after as a low-cost, home exercise program of 34 mat exercises originally called 'Contrology'. Many practitioners believe that Pilates mat classes or programs should always follow this strict regimen or sequence of exercises, as set forth in *Return to Life*.

PILATES INTERPRETATIONS

Without important modifications, many clients coping with pathological conditions would be unable to participate safely in Pilates exercise programs. If the Pilates method is seen as a philosophy or a system of precise movements coupled with specific breathing patterns, the method can be easily modified for any type of client. The essential movement elements of Pilates are breathing, alignment and control. There are several styles and interpretations of Pilates, some being very true to the original exercises, some that do not believe in modifications and others that use Pilates as a form of rehabilitation. The Pilates Method Alliance (PMA), the non-profit professional association for Pilates teachers, archives these lists of exercises but the PMA believes that Pilates should evolve along with the advances in scientific research. Bone health experts believe it is imperative that traditional Pilates be modified for the older adult and especially for the osteoporotic client. For this reason, this chapter will focus on Polestar Pilates, a rehabilitation-based Pilates approach as compared to the historical or traditional Pilates method (Anderson & Spector, 2000).

WHY PILATES FOR OLDER ADULTS AND BONE HEALTH?

At least 60% (20/34) of Pilates mat exercises involve spine flexion. Joseph's idea about spinal health stemmed from his theory that the spine should be flat 'like a newborn baby' (Pilates & Miller, 2003). We know that older adults tend toward thoracic kyphosis even without the presence of osteoporosis. Kyphosis increases with age, with the most rapid increases occurring between ages 50 and 60 years (Ball et al., 2009).

If Pilates is seen as a system of balanced muscle development, then the Pilates teacher should consider selecting the specific Pilates exercises that would bring the client's body back into balance. For instance, in a client

511

with a forward head and increased thoracic kyphosis, we would select Pilates exercises that involve thoracic extension and avoid exercises that involve thoracic flexion. Our fitness culture is extremely attracted to abdominal exercises with a flexed spine position in an effort to flatten the abdominals. Ironically, the best way to facilitate core control is with exercises or postures performed in a neutral spine (Rydeard et al., 2006).

One of the important movement principles in Polestar Pilates is axial elongation. Joseph Pilates never used this term in his original work but it is analogous to a concept he described called 'centering'. Axial elongation is the idea of lengthening the spine and the extremities away from center from head to coccyx, from shoulder girdle to hand/fingers and from pelvic girdle to feet/toes. This action appears to facilitate core control, activating the small or local joint stabilizers throughout each joint system (Smith & Smith, 2005). Levin adapted this concept for the musculoskeletal system which is a good model for describing musculoskeletal control (Hutson & Ellis, 2006).

The concept of loading and unloading is important in postural training and bone health. Bones and joints need both compression and decompression to stimulate bone formation and synovial fluid to keep tissues healthy. Constant compression has a detrimental effect on bone and joint tissues, as does non-weight-bearing (Jortikka et al., 1997). Unloading may create a tensile force in the vertebral bodies that is beneficial for bone. Unloading may also decrease shear and compression between vertebral segments. Core control occurs with the concept of axial elongation so that deep stabilizers of the spine are triggered with the idea of lifting the ribcage off the pelvis and the head away from the torso.

PILATES AS COMPARED TO OTHER FORMS OF EXERCISE

Pilates is an ideal transition from water-based to land-based exercise. Older adults often love aquatic classes, but they may not be the best choice for the older adult with osteoporosis. Bravo et al. (1997) studied 70 postmenopausal women with low BMD, ages 50–70 years, exercising in waist-high water for 60 minutes, including 40 minutes of jumping and muscular exercises designed to promote bone accretion, strength and endurance. Bravo saw a significant decrease in spine BMD and no change in the femoral neck after 12 months of vigorous water exercises three times weekly. Also, cyclists appear to have lower bone mineral density as compared to runners and age-matched controls even with higher calcium intake in several studies of healthy males. If Pilates were placed in a bone-building exercise spectrum graded from most to least effective, it might look as shown in Box 72.1.

BALANCE

Traditional Pilates mat classes generally do not contain standing balance activities and there are no original Pilates mat exercises that incorporate single leg stance. There are only three traditional apparatus exercises

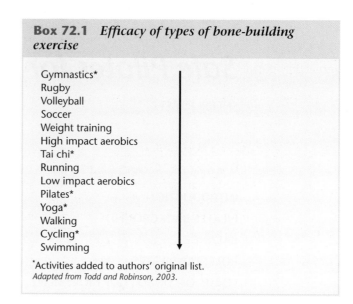

Box 72.1 *Efficacy of types of bone-building exercise*

Gymnastics*
Rugby
Volleyball
Soccer
Weight training
High impact aerobics
Tai chi*
Running
Low impact aerobics
Pilates*
Yoga*
Walking
Cycling*
Swimming

*Activities added to authors' original list.
Adapted from Todd and Robinson, 2003.

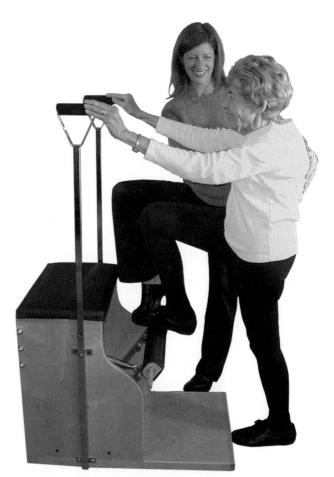

Figure 72.1 Pilates Chair: Standing Leg Pumps.

(see Fig. 72.1) that involve single leg balance: Forward and Sideward Lunge on the Chair and the dismount for Control Balance on the Reformer. However, many Pilates apparatus exercises are taught in upright stance with emphasis on lower extremity and torso organization. Dynamic weight-shifting activities with a special focus in sidestepping should be added to a Pilates program for the geriatric client. Training should include arm reaching and neuromuscular patterning to facilitate proper protective postural responses. Since falls are the leading cause of injury-related death and hospitalization in people age 75 years and older (Lord et al., 2003), balance activities should be included in Pilates classes.

PILATES IMPROVES BALANCE

Roller et al. (2012) conducted a randomized controlled trial with 72 subjects ranging in age from 65 to 95 years who were known fallers or at risk for falls. Subjects participated once weekly for 45 minutes in a Pilates Reformer Class lasting 10 weeks. Outcome measures showed significant improvements on the Activities-specific Balance Confidence (ABC) scores, the Timed Up and Go (TUG), the Berg Balance Scale, the 10-Meter Walk Test and the Adaptation Test (ADT) on the Smart Balance Master™ (NeuroCom International, Clackamas, OR). AROM significantly increased for straight leg raise, hip extension and ankle dorsiflexion. Sensory Organization Test™ (SOT; NeuroCom International) composite equilibrium scores increased significantly in both exercise and control groups by 6.5/100 points suggesting improved postural stability or learning effect. The control group demonstrated significant change on the SOT only.

POLESTAR PILATES

Polestar Pilates advocates working in bare feet to exercise the intrinsic muscles of the foot, decrease dependence on shoes and promote increased awareness of the feet.

Generally, the balance progression in Polestar Pilates is to work sequentially from:

- Supine
- Side-lying
- Prone
- Quadruped
- Kneeling
- Standing
- Single leg standing
- Standing on unstable surfaces.

The Polestar Pilates Functional Outcome Measure (FMOM) is a Pilates-based assessment tool designed to establish a baseline of function in order to select appropriate exercises for developing a Pilates program (Betz et al., 2013). This measurement is designed to assess quality of movement that exceeds basic ADL. Polestar Pilates' unique principles of movement are integrated into the individual test sections of Posture, Functional Tasks and Pilates' Movements (Anderson & Spector, 2000). The tests identify faulty movement patterns that may be contributing to pathology or pain.

One principle of Pilates is to obtain correct alignment before starting strengthening exercises (Smith & Smith, 2005). For example: prepare the spine for back extensor strengthening by having the client lay over the Baby Arc or Ladder Barrel in a supine position. The client then molds the thoracic spine into increased extension

with the assistance of the rounded shape of the barrel and gravity prior to performing a prone thoracic extension exercise. This is a great example of applying the principles of neuromuscular re-education by using the Pilates apparatus to assist the client into greater range of motion or into better alignment before asking the client to perform an exercise or movement against gravity without assistance. The proprioceptive system can then experience the joint and body position with the assistance of the apparatus to allow for carryover into function.

FOCUS ON QUALITY OF MOVEMENT

Briggs et al. (2007) studied paraspinal muscle control in people with vertebral compression fractures (VCF) and postulated that better neuromuscular control might lead to decreased fracture risk. The Pilates focus on body awareness, initiation of movement and 'the how' of moving through an exercise appears to be excellent for older adults who would benefit from heightened awareness and control. One of the main differences in traditional fitness programs and the Pilates approach is the 'just do it' versus 'how are you doing it' approach to each part of this exercise. The underlying philosophy of Pilates is that all movements are performed in the best alignment possible. Movements are modified or discontinued if they cannot be performed in biomechanically correct alignment.

Pilates is missing the upright dynamic, fast movement activities that are essential for fall prevention. Dynamic weight-shifting activities with a special focus in sidestepping should be added to a Pilates program for the geriatric client. Warden et al. (2005) found that a sideways fall increased the hip fracture risk 3- to 5-fold, and up to 30-fold with direct impact to the greater trochanter. Training should include sidestepping and arm reaching and neuromuscular patterning can be facilitated to utilize proper protective postural responses.

FRACTURE PREVENTION

SPINE

Sinaki and Mikkelsen (1984) conducted a hallmark study in 1984 dividing 59 postmenopausal women who had osteoporosis and one known VCF into four groups. Group 1 performed only extension exercises (similar to Pilates mat exercise – Double Leg Kick); Group 2 performed only flexion exercises (curl-ups in hook-lying position with feet on the floor; similar to the Pilates Hundred or Roll-Ups); Group 3 performed both extension and flexion exercises; and Group 4 did no exercises. All groups received biomechanical counseling and fracture prevention tips such as avoiding lifting greater than 10 pounds and to bend their knees when lifting. The results after 1 year showed there were 16% additional VCFs in Group 1, 89% in Group 2, 53% in Group 3 and 67% in Group 4.

Subsequent research papers have affirmed this risk of compression fracture with osteoporosis (Bassey, 2001; Keller et al., 2003).

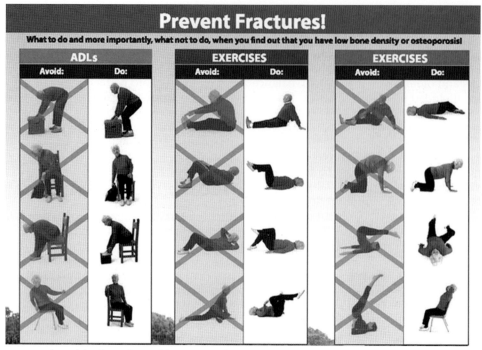

Figure 72.2 Fracture prevention advice for patients with osteoporosis. *(From Do It Right and Prevent Fractures, courtesy of American Bone Health.)*

Spinal flexion causes excessive compression force on the anterior surface of the vertebral bodies, which consist mostly of trabecular bone. In those with low bone density of the spine, the weakened bone cannot withstand such force and fractures may occur, especially with extreme positions of spinal flexion as found in yoga and Pilates movements (Sinaki, 2013). Compression forces on the vertebrae may also be excessive during spinal side-bending and rotation; however, there is no specific research to support or reject this potential risk. It may be prudent to avoid side-bending and rotation to endrange, and especially when combined with flexion. The posterior surface of the vertebral bodies, the pars interarticularis, the pedicals and the lamina all have a higher composition of cortical bone and are at less risk for fracture. These areas do get compressed as the spine moves into extension, but the movement is much less risky than with flexion because of the vertebral bony composition and strength of cortical bone.

Stronger back extensor musculature correlates to a reduction in fracture risk in the vertebral bodies as well as an improvement in quality of life (Hongo et al., 2007). Also significantly fewer refractures occurred in patients who engage in back-extensor-strengthening exercises after vertebroplasty (Fig. 72.3A) (Huntoon et al., 2008). A study looking at community-based group exercise for older adults showed that back extension exercises prevent the natural progression of kyphosis (Ball et al., 2009).

Modified Pilates programs can emphasize body awareness, transfers and transitions from one mat exercise to the other in a mat class, and can help a great deal with carryover into daily life.

When persons with low bone density or newly healed fractures are ready to start a strengthening program,

modified Pilates is an option. But safety is paramount because the risk of a new VCF within a year is five-fold (Lindsay et al., 2001). Powlowsky et al. (2009) showed stability of kyphosis and physical performance gains from a 1-year group exercise program that contained many exercises that are similar to ones often taught in Pilates mat classes.

The *Do It Right and Prevent Fractures* booklet was developed by American Bone Health to be placed in the hands of patients who receive a diagnosis of osteoporosis. The booklet is designed to be placed in doctor's offices and bone densitometry centers so that patients have helpful information about fracture prevention and proper movements and exercises (see Fig. 72.2).

HIP

Hip fractures mostly occur due to falls. Focus on balance and alignment is of paramount importance in any osteoporosis, bone health or older adult exercise program. The pigeon pose, a deep external rotation hip stretch, may be too aggressive for older persons but a safer alternative is shown in Figure 72.3. Decreased hip mobility does not directly lead to hip fractures but hip stiffness can contribute to decreased reaction times and therefore may lead to greater risk of falling.

Weight-bearing exercise with a focus on leg strengthening has repeatedly been shown to increase bone density in the hip (Fig. 72.3B). Ironically, walking programs have been shown to maintain bone density but do not appear to build bone (Todd & Robinson, 2003). The best effects on bone are achieved through dynamic, brief, intense bouts of exercise such as jumping, soccer, volleyball or gymnastics. If Pilates teachers can increase the resistance and keep the repetitions low to bring muscles

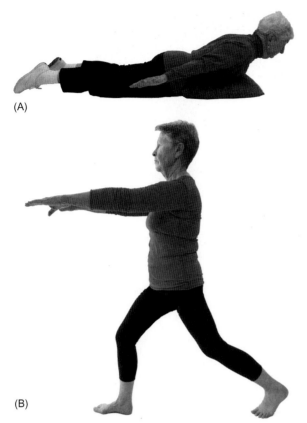

(A)

(B)

Figure 72.3 (A) Modified Double Leg Stretch; **(B)** Marriage Proposal Lunge.

to fatigue within 8–12 repetitions, the bone benefits may improve. Evidence has shown that humans lose 1% of their leg muscle strength and 0.5% of their bone mineral density per year after the age of 50 (Gourlay et al., 2012).

WRIST

Wrist fractures are due to falls, mostly in postmenopausal women between the ages of 50 and 60 years. Upper body strength does not decrease at nearly the rate of lower body strength as a person ages. The wrist builds bone differently than the femur, which depends upon weight-bearing to stimulate bone-building. Interesting studies of NASA astronauts upon return from space travel showed greater losses of bone mineral density from lower body bone than upper body bone due to the diminished weight-bearing in space (Carmeliet et al., 2001).

Balance and standing training is essential for fall prevention, which in turn may decrease wrist fractures due to falls. Gymnasts have 24% larger bone mineral content and 34% larger bone mineral density at the ultra-distal radius than the control group, indicating that weight-bearing and dynamic impact may have a positive effect on bone mineral density (Bareither et al., 2008). Pilates weight-bearing exercises like Quadruped and Leg Pull Front are excellent for training the upper body in a functional position. If weight-bearing is not tolerated then modifications like blocks, small free weights on the ground or special gloves can be used.

SCREENING FOR FRACTURES

Some easy red flags to identify persons at risk for fracture are:

- Height loss: loss of 6 cm or 2.4 inches of height is strongly predictive of vertebral compression fracture (Siminoski et al., 2005)
- Previous fracture
- Family history (70% contributing factor)
- Occiput to wall distance – indicates the presence of kyphosis. Greater than 7 cm occiput to wall distance is strongly predictive of fracture (Antonelli-Incalze et al., 2007).

THE PILATES BONE-BUILDING PROGRAM

GENERAL PRINCIPLES

Throughout the program emphasize body awareness, axial elongation, and – always – alignment. Clinical pearls for Pilates programs for older persons are enumerated in Box 72.2. Exercises that are contraindicated are shown in Box 72.3. Focus especially on the abdominals – but without using 'crunches' or abdominal exercises using the head as the lever to challenge the abdominals in a flexed spine position, which places compressive forces on the vertebral bodies of the spine and may increase fracture risk. The 90/90 supine tabletop position and the Hundred with the head down can safely challenge the abdominal wall in a neutral spine position.

CONCLUSION

In summary, in order to maximize the bone health benefits of Pilates for older adults, it is of paramount importance to build a program around posture, balance and leg strength. Thoracic extension mobility and strength, and hip extension mobility and strength are essential elements to assess and improve in the older adult with or without osteoporosis.

REFERENCES

Anderson BA, Spector A 2000 Introduction to Pilates-based rehabilitation. Orthop PT Clinic North Am 9(3):395–410

Antonelli-Incalze R, Pedone C, Cesari M 2007 Relationship between the occiput wall distance and physical performance in the elderly: a cross sectional study. Aging Clin Exp Res 19(3):207–212

Ball JM, Cagle P, Johnson BE et al 2009 Spinal extension exercises prevent natural progression of kyphosis. Osteopor Int 20(3):481–489

Bareither ML, Grabiner MD, Troy KL 2008 Habitual site-specific upper extremity loading is associated with increased bone mineral of the ultradistal radius in young women. J Women's Health 17(10):1577–1581

Bassey EJ 2001 Exercise for prevention of osteoporotic fracture. Age Aging 30(Suppl 4):29–31

Betz SR, Stolze L, Anderson BA 2013 FMOM: Functional Movement Outcome Measure. Polestar Pilates Comprehensive Manuals. Polestar Education, Miami, FL

Bravo G, Gauthier P, Roy PM et al 1997 A weight-bearing water-based exercise program for osteopenic women: its impact on bone, function, fitness and well-being. Arch Phys Med Rehab 78(12):1375–1380

Briggs AM, Greig AM, Bennell KL et al 2007 Paraspinal muscle control in people with osteoporotic vertebral fracture. Eur Spine J 16(8):1137–1144

Carmeliet G, Vico L, Bouillon R 2001 Space flight: a challenge for normal bone homeostasis. Crit Rev Eukaryot Gen Expr 11(1-3):131–144

Gourlay ML, Fine JP, Preisser JS et al 2012 Bone density testing interval and transition to osteoporosis in older women. N Engl J Med 366(3):225–233

Hongo M, Itoi E, Sinaki M et al 2007 Effect of low-intensity back exercise on quality of life and back extensor strength in patients with osteoporosis: a randomized controlled trial. Osteoporos Int 18(10):1389–1395

Huntoon EA, Schmidt CK, Sinaki M 2008 Significantly fewer refractures after vertebroplasty in patients who engage in back-extensor-strengthening exercises. Mayo Clin Proc 83(1):54–57

Hutson M, Ellis Ret al (eds) 2006 Textbook of Musculoskeletal MedicineOxford University Press, Oxford

Jortikka MO, Inkinen RI, Tammi MI et al 1997 Immobilisation causes longlasting matrix changes both in the immobilised and contralateral joint cartilage. Ann Rheum Dis 56:255–260

Keller TS et al 2003 Prediction of spinal deformity. Spine 28(5):455–462

Lindsay R, Sliverman SL, Cooper C et al 2001 Risk of new vertebral fracture in the year following a fracture. JAMA 285(3):320–323

Lord SR, March LM, Cameron ID et al 2003 Differing risk factors for falls in nursing home and intermediate-care residents who can and cannot stand unaided. J Am Geriatric Soc 51(11):1645–1650

Pilates JH 1934 Your Health: A Corrective System of Exercising That Revolutionizes the Entire Field of Physical Education. Republished 1998 by Presentation Dynamics Inc., Incline Village, NV

Pilates JH, Miller WR 2003 Return to Life Through Contrology. (Originally published 1945.) Pilates Method Alliance, Inc., Miami, FL

Powlowsky SB, Hamel KA, Katzman WB 2009 Stability of kyphosis, strength, and physical performance gains 1 year after group exercise program in community-dwelling hyperkyphotic older women. Arch Phys Med Rehab 90(2):358–361

Roller M, Ickes DM, Shrier G et al 2012 Pilates-based exercise for fall risk reduction in older fallers: a randomized controlled trial. Platform Presentation at PMA Conference: Research Forum Las Vegas

Rydeard R, Leger A, Smith D 2006 Pilates-based therapeutic exercise: effect on subjects with nonspecific chronic low back pain and functional disability: a randomized controlled trial. J Orthop Sports Phys Ther 36(7):472–484

Siminoski K, Jiang G, Adachi JD et al 2005 Accuracy of height loss during prospective monitoring for detection of incidental vertebral fractures. Osteoporos Int 16:403–410

Sinaki M 2012 Exercise for patients with osteoporosis: management of vertebral compression fractures and trunk strengthening for fall prevention. Phys Med Rehab 4(11):882–888

Sinaki M 2013 Yoga spinal flexion positions and vertebral compression fracture in osteopenia or osteoporosis of spine: case series. Pain Practice 13(1):68–75

Sinaki M, Mikkelsen BA 1984 Postmenopausal spinal osteoporosis: flexion versus extension exercises. Arch Phys Med Rehab 65:593–596

Smith K, Smith E 2005 Integrating Pilates-based core strengthening into older adult fitness programs: implications for practice. Top Geriatr Rehabil 21(1):57–67

Todd JA, Robinson RJ 2003 Osteoporosis and exercise (Review). Postgrad Med J 79:320–323

von Sperling de Souza M, Brum Vieira C 2006 Who are the people looking for the Pilates method? J Bodywork Movement Ther 10:328–334

Warden SJ, Fuchs RK, Castillo AB et al 2005 Does exercise during growth influence osteoporotic fracture risk later in life? J Musculoskelet Neuronal Interact 5:344–346

FURTHER READING

Pilates JH, 1998 Your Health: A Corrective System of Exercising that Revolutionizes the Entire Field of Physical Education. (Originally published 1934.) Presentation Dynamics Inc., Incline Village, NV

Pilates JH, Miller WR, 2003. Return to Life Through Contrology. (Originally published 1945.) Pilates Method Alliance, Inc., Miami

Chapter 73

Aquatic therapy

BETH E. KAUFFMAN • BENJAMIN W. KAUFFMAN

CHAPTER CONTENTS

INTRODUCTION

Aquatic physical therapy may be one of the most dynamic modalities used in the treatment of the older adult. For many reasons, it is underutilized in today's healthcare settings. Throughout history, aquatic therapy has been used for healing, strengthening and relaxation. The Native Americans used hot springs for healing purposes. The Greeks and Romans used the 'baths' for relaxation. Franklin Delano Roosevelt along with many others with polio and postpolio syndrome used and acknowledged the benefits of water. The aquatic setting for physical therapy can be utilized in many different ways, including gait training, improved cardiovascular efficiency, strengthening, balance, improved neuromuscular coordination, reduction of muscle spasms or tightness in joints, and edema control and wound care in specialized hydrotherapy settings.

PROPERTIES OF WATER

Part of the reason why therapy in water is so advantageous is because of the density of water. Hydrostatic pressure is an important concept in aquatic therapy; it is the static force of the water pressing against a person or object. Also, this force creates the upward thrust that we experience known as buoyancy. It is important to note that buoyancy has a direct effect on therapeutic exercise. For example, as the patient performs standing hip abduction, the limb is assisted by buoyancy. During the limb's return to neutral, increased hip adductor force is required to overcome buoyancy. Therefore, buoyancy can be assistive and resistive at the same time (Atkinson, 2005). A person's body mass index (BMI), adipose tissue vs. muscle mass, is the primary determining factor in the degree to which a person sinks or floats. Muscle mass has a greater density than water, causing it to sink. Adipose tissue is less dense, causing it to float. Each individual's unique level of buoyancy requires appropriate flotation devices or weights, depending upon the desired effects of treatment. Buoyancy allows the body to be unloaded. The greater the depth of submersion, the less the effect of gravity on body weight. A basic breakdown of buoyancy and the unloading of gravity on a patient goes as follows: waist deep 50%, chest deep 75%, neck deep 90% of body weight (Atkinson, 2005). The exact percentage of unloading may vary by gender and mass. Hydrostatic pressure increases the efficiency of the heart by helping in venous return. It also applies compression to joints, muscles and soft tissue, facilitating reduction of swelling and adding lymphatic drainage (Jamison, 2005).

Hydrodynamics, another important concept in aquatic therapy, is the force created when moving through water, causing resistance in front of the object. By changing the shape or surface area of an object, one can increase or decrease the hydrodynamic resistance (Brody & Geigle, 2009). By increasing the speed of movement, the resistance of the water becomes greater. In other words, the harder you push, the harder water pushes back. Water itself will not create a greater force of resistance than that which the individual is able to perform. This concept makes exercise in water a safe alternative to resistance training on land. Equipment, such as webbed gloves or water paddles, can be added to increase resistance. In some aquatic pools, the use of jets can add an increased level of resistance, or could be used for massage post exercise. It should be noted that an increase in water turbulence, even by a small amount, can significantly increase resistance depending on the activity (Atkinson, 2005). At other times the turbulence created by the therapist will create an increased balance challenge or facilitate the forward movement of the patient. This is important to remember when performing a group aquatic session.

A therapist or group leader should be cognizant that light refraction occurs when light passes from air to water, causing a perception of bending. This is caused by the reduction in the speed at which light is traveling upon entering the water. This bending may cause a visual disturbance to the patient's balance mechanism (Atkinson, 2005).

SPECIAL CONSIDERATIONS IN THE AGING ADULT

The aquatic therapy setting may be more beneficial to people who have a history of being comfortable in the water. They do not need to be swimmers; however, that is advantageous with advanced activities. It is possible for people with a fear of water or who have previously had a bad experience to benefit from aquatic therapy. Patience and encouragement are important with every individual, but for those with a fear of water, it is imperative. Flotation devices may need to be used by the patient to increase their confidence.

A complete initial examination and evaluation by a physical therapist is essential for assessing each individual's needs, which must be performed prior to entering the water. This requisite is to screen individuals who may not be candidates for aquatic therapy and to establish goals of care (Larsen et al., 2002; Geigle & Norton, 2005). It is important to note that some patients may need assistance changing into their bathing suits, or entering and exiting the water. Some may require full assistance throughout the entire treatment session with the clinician in the water assisting. Being in the water with the patient is advantageous but not always necessary, depending on the activity or performance level. Some aging adults may not have been in a bathing suit for many years and may feel uncomfortable or self-conscious. It is recommended that, prior to entering the pool for the first time, the patient understands what is going to happen during the session.

Water temperatures for the older adult that facilitate therapeutic benefits range from 93–95°F or 34–35°C (Larsen et al., 2002). Depending on the patient, the diagnosis and indications, the ideal water temperature may differ. A temperature less than 90°F (32.2°C) is often too cool for many older patients, because their speed of movement is typically slower, and they will not be generating as much additional body heat. Maintaining a thermoneutral water environment is important to allow for a therapeutic exercise environment. This is when the body neither gains nor loses temperature while in the water (33.5–34.5°C) (Larsen et al., 2002). Sustained exercise at temperatures greater than 95°F is too hot with respect to cardiovascular and thermoregulatory systems. Greater than 100°F is dangerous for persons with heart conditions and is considered unsafe for exercise.

The amount of work being performed by the patient is deceiving, on account of the buoyancy and resistance of the water. Thus, it is important to monitor the patient during exercise to determine exertion and fatigue levels. On land, it is common to use heart rate and oxygen saturation for monitoring a person's level of fitness or stress on the body. However, in water, these are not the most accurate or good determiners of exertion. When comparing the cardiac response of deep water running (up to the neck) with shallow water running (up to the xiphoid process), heart rate is 10 beats per minute slower in the deeper water (Robertson et al., 2001). This is due to the hydrostatic pressure adding in venous return and other possible hemodynamic changes. It is suggested that one use a Perceived Exertion Scale, physical observation, as well as a Talk Test: shortness of breath while trying to talk will provide indications of the patient's exertion level. Skin coloration changes may include paleness, redness, blotchiness and/or excessive sweating. These are warning signs of overexertion or overheating. When submerged in water, it is difficult for the body to thermoregulate due to the radiant and conduction temperature gain or loss in water. Simply communicating with the patient about their general feeling may provide clues as to how the patient is tolerating the level of exercise, temperature and overall intervention.

Dehydration is an important concern with the older adult. Hydration should be included in a comprehensive aquatic therapy program. Patients should be encouraged to drink 8 oz (240 ml) of water at least 1 hour before entering the pool. They should be reminded that drinking or eating large amounts prior to entering the water might cause cramping. Patients exercising in the water do sweat, and they may not realize it. Water should be available before, during and after each session. It is important to encourage patients to void prior to aquatic sessions. The hydrostatic pressure on the abdomen stimulates the internal organs and facilitates kidney function and lymph return, which may increase the need to void (Atkinson, 2005).

It is important to assess skin integrity prior to entering the water. An open wound is contraindicated for the aquatic setting, except when it is specifically being used as a wound care modality. A person's skin may be sensitive to pool chemicals; thus, chlorine or bromine as well as pH levels need to be observed and maintained. Usually, smaller indoor pools use bromine as the sanitizing agent; larger or outdoor pools typically use chlorine. Chlorine is harder on the skin; it tends to dry it out more rapidly. Ideally, pool pH should be 7.4–7.6: higher or lower may cause skin irritation. Having the patient shower prior to and after aquatic sessions assists with the maintenance of chemical levels as well as protecting the patient's skin. Aqua shoes may also be worn to protect feet and maintain skin integrity, especially in people with diabetes. Shoes aid in traction, increasing confidence and avoidance of falls secondary to slipping.

There are many considerations to remember when deciding if aquatic therapy is appropriate for a particular patient (Morris, 2005). In addition to medical screening and the above-mentioned concerns, there are contraindications (Hayes, 2012) for aquatic therapy, including:

1. active bleeding or open wounds
2. significant bowel or bladder incontinence
3. acute inflammatory conditions, i.e. fracture or neurological trauma
4. significant cardiac or respiratory instability
5. any unstable medical condition
6. fever or infection.

EVIDENCE FOR AQUATIC THERAPY

Exercise, rehabilitation and training in water is effective for elite athletes and people in mid- to late life with a variety of diagnoses (Binkley et al., 2002; Pechter et al., 2003; Brody & Geigle, 2009). After 12 weeks of low-intensity aquatic exercise by people with mild to moderate renal failure, Pechter et al. (2003) reported beneficial effects in all cardiopulmonary functional measurements and significant changes in resting blood pressure, proteinuria, lipid peroxidation and serum glutathione. Similarly, oxygen uptake was significantly improved in hypertensive elderly inner city females after 10 weeks of a water exercise program. Also, heart rate response to submaximal walking in the water declined significantly as did systolic blood pressure (Binkley et al., 2002). Significant gains in peak torque measurements have been reported after 12 weeks of graded aquatic exercise (Kendrick et al., 2002).

BALANCE

The following research supports the use for aquatics to improve balance, which will decrease fall risk in different populations. After 6 weeks of water exercise, subjects with a primary diagnosis of early to mid-stage Parkinson disease, demonstrated a significant improvement on the Berg Balance Scale and Step test (Jacobs et al., 2012). Some of this improvement may be attributed to increased tactile sensation from the water that improved body awareness and position sense. (Jacobs et al., 2012; Sato et al., 2012) After 5–6 weeks of water exercise by individuals in the eighth and ninth decades of life, significant improvements have been shown on balance measurements on the Berg Balance Scale (Douris et al., 2003). A combination of aquatic exercise and patient education produced significant findings in fall prevention in persons with hip osteoarthritis. Statistical analysis included the Berg Balance Scale, 6 minute walk test, 30 second chair stand, ABC questionnaire and the Timed Up and Go (Arnold & Faulkner, 2010).

OSTEOARTHRITIS

Benefits of aquatic exercise for persons with hip and knee osteoarthritis have been noted in several research studies. A study of 6 weeks of aquatic exercise resulted in less pain and joint stiffness, improved physical function, quality of life and hip muscle strength in 71 subjects with symptomatic hip or knee osteoarthritis (Hinman et al., 2007). In a study of 64 subjects with knee osteoarthritis, aquatic exercises performed for 18 weeks demonstrated significant pain reduction when compared to a land-based program, noting that both land and aquatic groups improved with therapy intervention (Silva et al., 2008).

CONCLUSION

Aquatic therapy is an excellent choice of exercise medium for many aging individuals and unfortunately is under-utilized. It is important for clinicians working in the realm of aquatic therapy to attend continuing education courses, and to learn proper techniques that will most benefit their patients. Care should always be aimed at meeting mutually agreed upon needs and goals. Aquatic therapy adds an excellent modality to meet goals as well as to enhance health and wellbeing.

REFERENCES

Arnold C, Faulkner R 2010 The effect of aquatic exercise and education on lowering fall risk in older adults with hip osteoarthritis. J Aging Phys Act 18:245–260

Atkinson K 2005 Hydrotherapy in orthopaedics. In: Atkinson K, Coutts F, Hassenkamp AM (eds) Physiotherapy in Orthopaedics, 2nd edn. Elsevier, Oxford, pp. 312–351

Binkley H, Kendrick ZV, Doerr E et al 2002 Effects of water exercise on cardiovascular responses of hypertension elderly inner-city women. J Aquatic Phys Ther 10(1):28–33

Brody L, Geigle P 2009 Aquatic Exercise for Rehabilitation and Training. Human Kinetics, Champaign, Il, pp. 1–368

Douris P, Southard V, Varga C et al 2003 The effect of land and aquatic exercise on balance scores in older adults. J Geriatr Phys Ther 26(1):3–6

Geigle P, Norton C 2005 Medical screening for aquatic physical therapy. J Aquatic Phys Ther 13(2):6–10

Hayes K 2012 Manual for Physical Agents, 6th edn. Pearson Education Inc., Upper Saddle River, NJ

Hinman R, Heywood S, Day A 2007 Aquatic physical therapy for hip and knee osteoarthritis: results of a single-blind randomized controlled trial. Phys Ther 87(1):32–43

Jacobs M, Fasano J, Seyboth M et al 2012 The effect of an aquatic exercise program on balance in individuals with Parkinson disease. J Aquatic Phys Ther 19:4–15

Jamison L 2005 Aquatic therapy for the patient with lymphedema. J Aquatic Phys Ther 13(1):9–12

Kendrick ZV, Binkley H, McGettigan J et al 2002 Effects of water exercise on improving muscular strength and endurance in suburban and inner-city older adults. J Aquatic Phys Ther 10(1):21–28

Larsen J, Pryce M, Harrison J et al 2002 Guideline for physiotherapists working in and/or managing hydrotherapy pools. Austral Physiother Assoc

Morris DM 2005 The 'go' or 'no go' decision in aquatic physical therapy. J Aquatic Phys Ther 13(2):4

Pechter U, Ots M, Mesikepp S et al 2003 Beneficial effects of water-based exercise in patients with chronic kidney disease. Int J Rehabil Res 26(2):153–156

Robertson JM, Brewster EA, Factora KI 2001 Comparison of heart rates during water running in deep and shallow water at the same rating of perceived exertion. J Aquatic Phys Ther 9(1):21–26

Sato D, Yamashiro K, Onishi K et al 2012 The effect of water immersion on short-latency somatosensory evoked potentials in human. Biomedical Central (BMC) Neuroscience 13:13

Silva L, Valim V, Pessanha A et al 2008 Hydrotherapy versus conventional land-based exercise for the management of patients with osteoarthritis of the knee: a randomized clinical trial. Phys Ther 88(1):12–21

Social and government implications, ethics and dying

Chapter 74

Legal considerations

RON SCOTT

CHAPTER CONTENTS

INTRODUCTION

Rehabilitation professionals who treat geriatric patients face potential malpractice liability exposure for their conduct, and for that of their extenders and support professionals acting within the scope of their employment. According to the CNA's Physical Therapy Liability monograph, malpractice claims against physical therapists in 'aging services facilities' accounted for the third highest paid indemnity, averaging $88 537 per incident (CNA, 2012: 12).

The United States of America is the most highly litigious society in human history. In 2012, more than 15 million lawsuits were filed in state courts alone – one for every 12 American adults (Legal Reform Now!, 2012). Although only a small proportion of these legal cases involved healthcare malpractice, the risk of liability exposure in healthcare practice generally, and in geriatric rehabilitation practice in particular, is significant. Geriatric rehabilitation professionals must strike a careful balance between providing optimal quality patient care (a prospect made more difficult in the current cost containment-focused fiscal austerity and managed care environments) and minimizing their own healthcare malpractice liability risk exposure incident to practice (Scott, 2009).

Medical malpractice lawsuits have attracted significant public and legislative attention, in part because of rising insurance and healthcare costs. The average payment for malpractice claims for physicians and other licensed providers was $250 000 in 2011, with only one in five cases brought resulting in a settlement or judgment against defendant–healthcare professionals (Stobbe, 2011).

In geriatric rehabilitation, professional practice that complies with legal and ethical standards includes knowledge by health professionals of, and compliance with, such laws as the Patient Self-Determination Act, state-specific statutory reporting requirements for suspected elder abuse, and a seeming myriad of other important mandates. Because nearly two-thirds of the population between the ages of 55 and 64 and 17% of those aged 65 or over are employed, rehabilitation healthcare professionals must be cognizant of laws protective of the employment rights of their geriatric clients, including the Age Discrimination in Employment Act, the Americans with Disabilities Act and the Family and Medical Leave Act (US Bureau of the Census, 2012).

HEALTHCARE MALPRACTICE

PROFESSIONAL NEGLIGENCE

Healthcare malpractice is defined as physical and/or mental injury incurred by a patient in the course of healthcare examination, intervention or consultation, coupled with a recognized legal basis for imposing civil liability on a healthcare provider for the harm suffered by the patient. Traditionally, the only basis for imposing healthcare malpractice liability was professional negligence, or substandard care.

In a professional negligence lawsuit brought by a patient against a healthcare professional, the patient must normally prove four core elements by a preponderance, or greater weight, of evidence. These four elements are:

- that the defendant–healthcare professional owed a special duty of care to the plaintiff–patient;
- that, in the course of healthcare delivery, the healthcare professional breached, or violated, the high legal duty owed, by failing to meet at least minimally acceptable care standards;
- that the breach of duty by the healthcare provider caused injury to the patient; and
- that the patient sustained the kind of injuries for which a judge or jury may legally order compensation in the form of a money damages judgment, designed to make the patient as 'whole' as possible.

In addition to being legally responsible for his or her own conduct, a healthcare professional providing geriatric rehabilitation services is also normally vicariously, or indirectly, responsible for the conduct of extenders and supportive personnel acting under the supervision of the licensed or certified primary professional. Healthcare professionals must clearly communicate orders to extenders and support personnel to whom care tasks are delegated, and establish competency standards and actually assess the competency of supportive personnel on an ongoing basis.

ADDITIONAL LEGAL BASES FOR MALPRACTICE

Other legal bases for imposing healthcare malpractice liability, in addition to professional negligence, include:

* intentional care-related misconduct, including battery (injurious or otherwise offensive physical contact with a patient) and sexual battery (physical contact intended to arouse or gratify a healthcare provider's illicit sexual desires);
* strict product liability, for patient injury caused by dangerously defective treatment-related products or equipment, such as durable medical equipment supplied to a geriatric client; and
* breach of contract liability, for failure to fulfill a therapeutic promise made to a patient.

Geriatric rehabilitation professionals and clinic and agency managers are advised to develop, educate staff about and enforce formal risk management policies and procedures designed to minimize healthcare malpractice liability exposure of professional employees and organizations. Legal counsel should be consulted proactively for advice on developing and implementing such initiatives (Scott, 2009).

Consider the following hypothetical example:

A home health physical therapist is charged by a geriatric patient with sexual battery. In this case, involving myofascial release, there was, in fact, no therapist misconduct; the patient was simply confused about the nature of the therapeutic touch involved in the procedure and honestly believed it to be improperly applied by the therapist to her torso.

What risk management measures should the physical therapist and agency have undertaken to prevent this kind of allegation?

The agency and its professional and support staff should have developed and practiced under a professional–patient relations policy that requires:

1. Patient understanding of and informed consent for intensive hands-on therapy, such as myofascial release and massage.
2. Notification by the treating healthcare provider to the patient of the right to have a same-gender chaperone present during treatment (such a policy obligates the employer to make available a chaperone upon the patient's request).
3. Respect by providers for patient autonomy and modesty, including appropriate patient draping procedures prior to and during treatment.

In this scenario, the physical therapist faces primary liability exposure for his or her conduct, and the employing agency possible vicarious liability for the physical therapist–employee's conduct within the scope of his or her employment.

PATIENT INFORMED CONSENT

In any healthcare delivery setting, adult patients with full mental capacity have the right to give informed consent before evaluation or intervention. The duty to make relevant information disclosure and obtain patient informed consent to treatment is premised on respect for patient autonomy, or self-determination. Although the exact disclosure requirements for patient informed consent may vary from state to state, the following elements are commonly included:

* disclosure of the patient's diagnosis and relevant information about a proposed intervention or interventions;
* disclosure of serious risks of possible harm or complications associated with a proposed intervention that would be material to the patient's decision about whether to accept or refuse the intervention;
* discussion about the expected benefits, or goals, associated with, the proposed intervention(s); and
* disclosure of reasonable alternatives to a proposed intervention, and their material risks and benefits.

After the above disclosure elements are discussed with the patient, the provider is additionally obligated to solicit and satisfactorily answer the patient's questions (in a language that the patient understands) and formally ask for the patient's consent to proceed before doing so.

It may not be necessary to individually document in patients' records each patient's informed consent for routine care. An agency, institution or group may elect instead to memorialize an informed consent policy in a policy and procedures manual; orient providers upon employment of their informed consent obligations; monitor informed consent processes on an ongoing basis; and reinforce the duty to obtain patients' informed consent with providers on a regularly recurring basis during in-service education.

Managed care 'gag clause' employment provisions requiring providers to refrain from discussing with the patient care options that are not offered by patients' insurance plans are in conflict with the principles of respect for patient autonomy and the informed consent requirement for disclosure of reasonable alternatives to proposed care options, and are therefore unethical and, in many jurisdictions, expressly illegal (Scott, 2009).

REPORTING SUSPECTED ELDER ABUSE

Geriatric rehabilitation professionals have a legal duty to act reasonably to identify elder abuse or neglect involving their patients, and to take appropriate action to prevent further abuse. This may include reporting suspected elder abuse to social service departments or agencies or to law enforcement agencies, as appropriate (Joshi & Flaherty, 2005).

Elder abuse may be less often recognized and reported by healthcare professionals than spousal or child abuse. Most state laws on reporting abuse provide for qualified immunity from defamation or other bases of liability for persons making good faith reports of suspected abuse involving child, spousal or elder victims.

Signs and symptoms of possible elder abuse may be present in a geriatric client and in the client's abuser, who may be present with the client during examination or treatment. Signs and symptoms in the geriatric client may include, among others: unexplained or untreated injuries; reticence; poor hygiene; malnutrition and dehydration; and dirty or inappropriate dress for ambient conditions. Indices of possible elder abuse in abusers, who may be caregivers or family members, include, among others: aggression toward or verbal abuse of the geriatric patient; speaking for the client during an examination or treatment; and indifference to instructions or suggestions in the elder patient's best interests, offered by the provider (Scott, 2009).

Consider the following case:

Mr Doe is an 83-year-old patient who is status post-right cerebrovascular accident, with mild left upper limb hemiparesis. He has just been referred as an outpatient to ABC Rehab, Inc. His examining physical therapist notices the following about Mr Doe:

1. He is accompanied by his 51-year-old daughter, Sue, who does most of the talking for the patient.
2. He has scratches and petechiae on the dorsal forearms.
3. He is dressed in a Navy pea-coat, food-stained long-sleeved shirt and wool trousers, despite it being June and 78°F (25°C).

How should the physical therapist proceed, based on the above information?

Based on the presentation above, Mr Doe may be a victim of elder abuse and/or neglect. The physical therapist should annotate pertinent objective examination findings in Mr Doe's health record and consult with a supervisor or professional colleague about this patient. The therapist may also, as an exercise of professional judgment, report his or her suspicion to the facility's social service department for follow-up. Whether or not a report to a social service department is made at this time, the physical therapist should closely monitor Mr Doe for any further indicators of possible abuse.

PATIENT SELF-DETERMINATION ACT

The Patient Self-Determination Act (PSDA) of 1990 is a federal statute that memorializes a patient's right to control routine and extraordinary treatment-related decisions. The PSDA, like the law of patient informed consent, is premised on respect for patient autonomy.

The PSDA does not create any new substantive patient rights; it simply requires healthcare facilities – including hospitals and long-term care facilities – to provide patients with written information about their rights under state law to make advance directives; to ask patients about any advance directives that they might have in effect; and to honor any advance directives executed by patients under their care.

Advance directives are legal instruments that memorialize patients' desires regarding care options in the event of such patients' incapacitation. They are of two basic types: living wills, which spell out patients' wishes concerning the scope of permissible healthcare interventions in the event of patient incapacity; and durable powers of attorney for healthcare decision-making, which empower third parties to act on behalf of incapacitated patients. Patient health records should prominently include information about existing patient advance directives.

HEALTH INSURANCE PORTABILITY AND ACCOUNTABILITY ACT

The Health Insurance Portability and Accountability Act (HIPAA) became effective in 2003. The intentions of this federal statute are: to make health insurance more portable, especially as people change jobs; to prevent healthcare fraud and abuse; and to safeguard the privacy of patient protected health information (PHI). Its Privacy Rule requires all 'covered entities' (healthcare practitioners, healthcare plans and healthcare clearinghouses [electronic billing services], among others, including covered entities' business associates) to protect patients' PHI from unauthorized disclosure, including demographic data and any other information that may potentially identify a particular individual patient. HIPAA was augmented with the Health Information Technology for Economic and Clinical Health Act (HITECH, 2009), which increased penalties for HIPAA noncompliance to up to $1 million. The confidentiality protections in HIPAA's Privacy Rule have reportedly caused some problems for providers and adult protective services that address issues of elder abuse (Dyer et al., 2005).

EMPLOYMENT PROTECTION FOR OLDER WORKERS

There are three federal statutes that serve primarily to protect the employment interests of older workers. These are the Age Discrimination in Employment Act, the Americans with Disabilities Act, and the Family and Medical Leave Act (Scott, 2009).

The Age Discrimination in Employment Act (ADEA) of 1967 prohibits employer discrimination against workers aged 40 years or older. The broad prohibition of discrimination against older workers encompasses nearly all aspects of the employment relationship, from recruitment, selection and retention to promotions and training and to employee benefits. Under case law developed after implementation of the ADEA, employers may discharge older workers from employment if such workers contractually waive their ADEA rights in exchange for monetary compensation.

The Americans with Disabilities Act (ADA) of 1990 offers significant protection from discrimination to older workers and patients. Under Title I of the ADA, business organizations having 12 or more workers are prohibited from discriminating against physically or mentally disabled employees, and must provide reasonable accommodation for employees' disabilities that affect their ability to carry out essential functions of their jobs. In 2008, Title I of the ADA was amended to strengthen protections for disabled workers by broadening the definition of disability and expanding the definition of 'impairment'. Title III of the ADA protects the rights of disabled consumers to equal access to public accommodation, including privately owned healthcare facilities.

The Family and Medical Leave Act (FLMA) of 1993 requires employers having 20 or more full-time employees to allow employees to take up to 12 weeks per year of unpaid, job-protected leave for personal or family illness or for adoption or childbirth. Unlike the ADEA and the ADA, which are enforced by the federal Equal Employment Opportunity Commission, the FLMA is administered by the federal Department of Labor.

Consider the following scenario:

A 68-year-old rehabilitation client informs an occupational therapist during the patient history interview of circumstances that might constitute employment discrimination (age-related discharge) related to the client's disability. *What should the therapist do?*

Even though the therapist is generally familiar with employment laws, the therapist should not attempt to advise the client about possible legal options. Instead, the therapist should inform the client of the right to seek legal advice with an attorney of choice or through the public service county bar association's legal referral service, which is available in every county and parish in the US at no cost or for a low charge for 'initial' legal advice.

CONCLUSION

Geriatric rehabilitation professionals must be cognizant of key laws and legal requirements affecting their practice and their clients' civil rights. Under managed care, the rehabilitation milieu has become extremely business-like and impersonal, making malpractice avoidance more difficult. Clinicians and managers must simultaneously strive for optimal quality patient care and effective clinical liability risk management in order to survive and thrive.

Knowledge of laws respecting patient autonomy, including the PSDA concerning patients' advance directives, and of employment protection benefiting elderly clients, enables geriatric rehabilitation professionals to better serve their clients. Legal advice, however, should be given to clients only by attorneys.

The information presented in this chapter is intended as legal information only and not as specific legal advice for any health professional. Individual legal advice can be given only by a person's personal or institutional attorney, based on the distinct laws of the particular jurisdiction (state or federal law, as applicable).

REFERENCES

Bureau of the Census 2012 Aging in the United States: Past, Present and Future. US Bureau of the Census, Washington, DC

CNA 2012 Physical therapy liability. CNA, Chicago, IL

Dyer C, Heisler C, Hill C et al 2005 Community approaches to elder abuse. Clin Geriatr Med 21:429–447

HITECH 2009 Health Information Technology for Economic and Clinical Health Act, Title XIII of Division A and Title IV of Division B of the American Recovery and Reinvestment Act of 2009 (ARRA), Pub. L. No. 111-5, 123 Stat. 226 (17 Feb. 2009), codified at 42 U.S.C. §§300jj et seq.; §§17901 et seq

Joshi S, Flaherty J 2005 Elder abuse and neglect in long term care. Clin Geriatr Med 21:333–354

Legal Reform Now! 2012. Available at: www.legalreform-now.org. Accessed December 2012

Scott RW 2009 Promoting legal and ethical awareness: a primer for health professional and patients. Elsevier-Mosby, St Louis, MO

Stobbe M 2011 Medical malpractice suits: only one in five pay. Christian Science Monitor, 19 August 2011 (csmonitor.com)

Chapter 75

Ethics

MARY ANN WHARTON

CHAPTER CONTENTS

INTRODUCTION

Decisions regarding moral choices, what is right vs. what is wrong, are difficult, and frequently complicate treatment interventions and service delivery in geriatric rehabilitation. These moral decisions are often made more limited by factors such as ageism, societal attitudes and available reimbursement for healthcare services. This is especially true in the current healthcare delivery system, which intermingles patient care with technology, a reimbursement-driven environment and a societal mandate to conserve healthcare dollars. An understanding of the concept of professionalism and of ethical principles and theory can provide a framework for analyzing the values involved in moral decision-making in geriatrics. However, these principles and theories alone are not adequate to provide practitioners with answers for judgments and actions. Practitioners must be able to uncover the context in which ethical situations arise and the underlying narratives of those involved in order to analyze and respond to the ethical concerns when dealing with vulnerable older adults.

PROFESSIONALISM, ETHICS AND GERIATRIC PHYSICAL THERAPY PRACTICE

It has been said that every clinical decision involving a patient has a moral or ethical dimension. The physical therapist's response to this ethical circumstance requires that the therapist possesses the moral courage to formulate a reply to the ethical situation and implement a decision that will benefit the patient. The ability to act ethically on behalf of a patient's needs is inherent in the notion of professionalism. In our society, a professional is regarded as possessing more than a body of knowledge and technical expertise. A true professional is expected to perform a valuable service to society. In exchange for autonomy to make decisions on behalf of vulnerable patients and on behalf of society, a professional is expected to abide by high ethical standards. In essence, they are expected to exercise professional expertise responsibly, and to make accountable decisions that are in the patient's and society's best interests (Swisher, 2005). The American Physical Therapy Association (APTA), recognizing the intimate relationship between professionalism and ethics, has adopted a consensus document that identifies the core values of professionalism in physical therapy practice. These core values can be viewed as guiding principles for the ethical treatment of patients, especially those older individuals who are entrusted to our care. The core values are accountability, altruism, compassion and caring, excellence, integrity, professional duty and social responsibility (APTA, 2003).

ETHICS AND MORALITY

Morality is defined by Purtilo as guidelines that are designed to preserve the fabric of society. Ethics, on the other hand, can be viewed as 'a systematic reflection on and analysis of morality' (Purtilo & Doherty, 2011). As such, ethics is based on principles that provide a conceptual framework within which it is possible to place perceptions of ethical cases and problems. These principles allow the imposition of some sense of artificial order on a story, and they affect people's response to it. Ethical concepts are tied to society's customs, manners, traditions and institutions. In essence, these concepts define how members of a society deal with the world.

Professional ethics that arise in the context of healthcare provide guidelines that are ultimately no different from those that arise from religious, philosophical, cultural and other societal sources (Purtilo & Doherty, 2011). Ethical situations in geriatrics are similar to ethical situations in other aspects of healthcare, but the context in which situations arise may be more complex. Therefore, similar reasoning processes can be utilized as a basis to answer questions of morality when dealing with older individuals.

ETHICAL PRINCIPLES

Ethical principles serve as one tool for solving complex ethical problems. Ethical theories provide a sense of order. They can help to simplify a complicated case for initial problem-solving, and that simplification in itself can be useful in ordering and focusing a wide range of disparate intuitions.

The foundational principles of biomedical ethics that govern geriatric rehabilitation professionals include the following ethical duties and rights:

- beneficence – the duty to do the best possible
- nonmaleficence – the minimal duty to do no intentional malicious harm
- justice – the allocation of time and resources
- autonomy – the ethical right of self-determination.

AUTONOMY

Respect for patient autonomy is an ethical principle that requires further understanding and definition. According to the ethical principle of autonomy, the patient has the right to actively negotiate his or her own healthcare decisions. In geriatrics, issues of autonomy may revolve around questions of individual capacity and competency to make decisions. Healthcare providers must recognize that questions of patient competency are determined legally and are not to be presumed by the professional or by family members or caregivers.

In general, the decision-making capacities of older individuals with cognitive deficits must be respected as long as possible. For patients with dementia, determination of capacity and competency is especially problematic. However, the respect for autonomy must be balanced with the notion of protection of that individual from potential harm. The tension between autonomy and protection may direct caregivers to make decisions that are in conflict with patient wishes. Ethically, the rights of the individual to express a choice regarding his or her care should be made in light of several observations, including the severity of the dementia, the presence or absence of actual mental illness, the physical and functional state of the individual and the availability of family and community resources (Brindle & Holmes, 2005).

When caregivers judge an individual to be incapable of making or contributing to decisions about his or her life, they may conclude that their perspective of beneficence or nonmaleficence overrules the patient's autonomy. The risk is that the caregivers may force a decision that is contrary to the older person's preference or choice. On the other hand, caregivers may be tempted to err on the side of giving undue weight to patient autonomy and allow a risky, unsound or unsafe decision. The goal in all situations is to strike a balance between autonomy and beneficence in order to effect the best possible choice (Jensen et al., 2012).

A concern specific to the autonomy of the older patient may be the reliance of the professional on family members or caregivers to make decisions for that individual even when the older patient is legally competent to make the decision himself or herself. In these situations, in which the older client is legally competent, the moral and legal appropriateness of consulting such individuals must be determined by the patient. This is an especially difficult issue for caregivers when the patient is ill, recovering from surgery or pathological insult, or taking certain medications, all of which can negatively affect the patient's judgment.

One factor that may influence the ability of older individuals to make autonomous healthcare choices is their own beliefs or expectations regarding healthcare. In these situations, understanding the context of the situation rather than applying ethical principles is critical. Specific factors to consider might include whether they view healthcare as a right or a privilege. They must also analyze whether they believe that they are a passive recipient of healthcare vs. the more current concept that stresses an individual's responsibility to actively participate in the rehabilitation process. Informed consent, which provides the legal basis for autonomy, requires patient education according to the 'reasonable man standard'. Specifically, this standard obliges the healthcare professional to provide information in terms understandable to a reasonable individual of like circumstances. Informed consent is recognized as one way to achieve patient adherence.

An additional factor to consider with respect to ethics and patient autonomy is the issue of paternalism. Paternalism may be defined as coercion, or interference with another person's freedom of action. The healthcare professional justifies paternalism by reasons related to the welfare and happiness of the individual being coerced. In the ethics of healthcare, paternalism stems from the principle that the practitioner should act to bring about the maximum benefit for the patient, even at the expense of the patient's autonomy. It is rooted in the healthcare provider's knowledge and professional understanding coupled with the duty of beneficence and the healthcare provider's desire to bring about the best outcome. In its extreme, paternalism can result in a violation of autonomy, which is not considered acceptable in this society. On the other hand, contemporary healthcare may accept gentle paternalism, which combines with informed consent to achieve patient adherence. In geriatrics, healthcare professionals need to respect autonomy and provide competent care in a way that is not forced or coerced but collaborative.

The issues of patient autonomy and paternalism may also be complicated by Medicare and other insurance regulations that require specified treatment times and frequencies. Thus, the ill or depressed patient may be coerced into going to rehabilitation in order to protect Medicare payment benefits, which may be suspended if the patient fails to attend the regulated number of daily hours or treatment days per week, depending upon the treatment setting – rehabilitation unit or skilled nursing facility respectively. Some medical providers maintain the attitude that the patient may not refuse the required care, which is paternalistic.

Even though these foundational ethical principles are still widely used as a tool for solving ethical problems, they do not always address the complex issues presented in today's healthcare environment. Beneficence, nonmaleficence and autonomy focus primarily at the individual level and do not answer questions that arise at the institutional and societal levels. Ethical malfunctioning at institutional and societal levels has the potential to leave more discomfort. Justice may come closer to addressing these problems.

FIDELITY, VERACITY AND CONFIDENTIALITY

Secondary ethical duties inherent in healthcare include the following:

- Faithfulness, or the fidelity/fiduciary relationship: entails meeting a patient's reasonable expectations.
- Truth-telling, or veracity and honesty: obligates a healthcare provider not only to the patient but also to other sources such as the reimbursement source (this is a frequent source of conflict).
- Confidentiality, or the patient's expectation that the healthcare provider will honor personal information as private: requires that a healthcare provider only shares sensitive information with those who have a legitimate right to know. The legal basis for confidentiality exists in the constitutional concept of the right to privacy.

VIRTUE ETHICS AND THE ETHICS OF CARE

Traditional bioethical principles may have limited value in guiding ethical decisions that must be made daily when caring for geriatric patients in today's complex healthcare environment. Virtue ethics is another theory that may provide the physical therapist with additional insight into ethical care. Virtue ethicists look at character rather than rules for moral guidance in patient care decisions. Grounding oneself in virtue provides a foundation for acting in a certain way when interpreting and applying ethical principles. Therefore, virtue ethics is considered as a theory of being that focuses on the character of the moral agent rather than on the acts of that agent. For example, a virtue ethicist would look at the patience of the therapist treating the older individual, rather than judge the lack of productivity that resulted from the therapist taking additional time to address the complex concerns of an older patient. A virtue is defined as a good habit that balances excesses and deficiencies. As agents, physical therapy practitioners may apply virtue ethics to geriatric care by developing trusting relationships with patients, being compassionate, and developing a deep awareness of the lives and wishes of the patient. Compassion is considered a cardinal virtue of physical therapists treating geriatric patients, and moral and ethical actions are guided by that compassion. Respect for human dignity is another important virtue to consider when dealing with older individuals. Respect involves more than good manners. It acknowledges both personal and inherent dignity. Personal dignity refers to privacy or breach of patient confidence. The concept that every human has inherent dignity represents the deeper virtue or aspect of respect. Vulnerable older adults, including those with diminished cognitive capacity, are worthy of the type of respect that supersedes good manners and leads us to assume our role as moral agents (Pellegrino & Thomasma, 1993; Nalette, 2001; Jonsen et al., 2006).

Regardless of the ethical theory, when physical therapists deliberate an ethical concern or attempt to determine a solution to an ethical situation, the goal should be to provide a caring response. In spite of competing loyalties, the primary loyalty must be to the patient, and the caring response must lead to a conclusion with purposeful action. Purtilo states that care means 'seeking the deepest understanding of what that other person really needs. Care is what you pay attention to. And that's important within the health professional–patient relationship' (Ries, 2003). Ethically, it means going beyond evidence-based practice that simply looks at the results of research studies and, instead, incorporates the essence of true evidence-based practice, which includes client-centered goals in patient care. This may involve helping the patient to understand how your knowledge and expertise may benefit them, and empowering older patients to make decisions that are in their best interests. It means listening to the older individual's story, and respecting their ideas, concerns and perspectives as you jointly develop a meaningful plan of care (Ries, 2003).

CODES OF ETHICS

One hallmark of a profession is its adoption and enforcement of a code of ethics. An underlying assumption is that a code of ethics articulates the values of that profession and holds members of the discipline accountable for adhering to ethical standards. The purpose of a code is to make positive statements of ethical values and to educate professionals about the ethical dimensions of practice. Perhaps more importantly, a code of ethics is meant to educate the public through statements of what can be expected from members of that profession. As such, a code of ethics is an official statement by the profession that is intended to promote public trust. It serves as a guide for professionals to solve moral problems. However, it is not a substitute for good moral judgment or personal commitment.

The World Confederation of Physical Therapy (WCPT) has adopted ethical principles that are recognized as prototypes for member organizations to develop their own code of ethics or code of conduct (see Box 75.1). The ethical principles articulated by WCPT can offer ethical guidance for physical therapists providing care for geriatric patients. Specifically, the *first principle* states that physical therapists respect the rights and dignity of all individuals. This principle directs practitioners to respect patients regardless of age, gender, race, nationality, religion, ethnic origin, creed, color, sexual orientation, disability, health status or politics. It implies the patient/client's right to the highest quality services, make an informed decision, have access to their physical therapy data, and confidentiality. The *second principle* requires that physical therapists comply with laws and regulations that govern the practice of physical therapy in the country in which they work. It specifies that physical therapists have a right to advocate for patient/client access to those who have a capacity to benefit from services. In addition to licensing laws, this principle implies that therapists in the United States of America who treat older individuals have knowledge of the legal implications of informed consent. It also implies that therapists understand the regulations related to Medicare reimbursement. The *third principle* states that physical therapists accept responsibility for the exercise of sound judgment. Inherent in this principle is the notion of professional independence and autonomy and the idea that a therapist is qualified to make judgments regarding the physical therapy plan of care. Implied is that the therapist is working within the scope of the profession, is competent based on knowledge and skill, has made an appropriate assessment and determined a diagnosis, and will implement the plan of care based on the assessment and diagnosis. This principle also addresses the fact that physical therapists must not delegate to another health professional or support worker any activity that requires the unique skill, knowledge and judgment of the physical therapist, that the therapist should encourage consultation with referring practitioners when the recommended treatment program is not appropriate, and states that physical therapists have the right to expect cooperation from colleagues. The *fourth principle* directs physical therapists to provide honest, competent and accountable professional services.

This principle directs therapists to ensure that behaviour and conduct is professional at all times, to deliver timely patient/client-specific physical therapy interventions in line with the individual's goals, and to ensure that patients/clients understand the nature of the service being provided, including costs. It directs therapists to keep adequate client records and to disclose those records only to individuals who have a legitimate right to access the information contained in the documentation. Finally, this principle requires physical therapists to undertake a continuous, planned, personal development program in order to maintain and enhance professional knowledge and skills. Included in this principle is the notion that ethical practice takes precedence over business practices in the provision of physical therapy services. The *fifth principle* states that physical therapists must be committed to providing quality services. As stated, this principle requires physical therapists to be aware of current standards of practice, and to participate in continuing professional development to enhance basic knowledge, to support research and keep up to date with best evidence and implement it in their practice, and to support quality education in academic and clinical settings. The *sixth principle* identifies the physical therapist's entitlement to just and fair remuneration for services rendered. The *seventh principle* directs therapists to provide accurate information to patients, other agencies and the community regarding physical therapy services. This principle recommends that physical therapists participate in public education programs to provide information about the profession, and to provide truthful information to inform the public and referring professionals about the profession. It permits advertising, provided that therapists do not use false, fraudulent, misleading, deceptive, unfair, or sensational statements. The *eighth principle* expects physical therapists to contribute to the planning and development of services that address the health needs of the community. This principle obliges therapists to work toward achieving justice in the provision of healthcare for all people, and may be particularly applicable in view of the needs and access to care provided for geriatric clients under the current constraints imposed by healthcare regulations and financing in the US healthcare delivery system (WCPT, 2011).

The APTA's code of ethics for the physical therapist, 2009 revision, is markedly similar to the principles adopted by the WCPT. This code of ethics contains eight principles that provide broad guidance for ethical decisions and that are each linked to specific core values. The code is built on the five roles of the physical therapist, including patient/client management, consultation, education, research and administration. It incorporates the core values of the profession, and addresses the therapist's ethical obligations at the individual, organizational and societal realms of practice. *Principle 1* directs physical therapists to respect the inherent dignity and rights of all individuals, while *Principle 2* requires physical therapists to be trustworthy and compassionate in addressing the rights and needs of patients/clients. *Principle 3* addresses accountability for making sound professional judgments that are in the patient's best interest and that are informed by professional standards, practitioner experience, current evidence and patient values. It guides therapists to make judgments within their scope of practice, and to communicate, collaborate and refer to other healthcare professionals when necessary. It further directs therapists to not engage in conflicts of interest that interfere with professional judgment, and requires therapists to provide appropriate direction of and communication with other physical therapists and support personnel. *Principle 4* addresses integrity in all professional relationships, and includes reference to not exploiting persons in situations where there is a supervisory relationship. It also mandates reporting of misconduct, illegal or unethical acts to relevant authorities, including suspected cases of abuse of vulnerable individuals. *Principle 5* directs physical therapists to fulfil legal and professional obligations; *Principle 6* requires therapists to enhance expertise through lifelong acquisition and refinement of knowledge, skills, abilities and professional behaviors. Promotion of organizational behaviors and business practices that benefit individual patients/clients and society are mandated under *Principle 7*. This includes the obligation to promote practice environments that support autonomous and accountable professional judgments; seeking reasonable and deserved remuneration for physical therapy services, and refraining from employment arrangements that prevent physical therapists from fulfilling professional obligations to patients/clients. Finally, *Principle 8* directs physical therapists to participate in efforts to meet the health needs of people locally, nationally, or globally (APTA, 2009a). Similarly, APTA adopted eight associated standards of ethical conduct for the physical therapist assistant. These standards direct physical therapist assistants to respect the dignity and rights of all individuals; provide trustworthy and compassionate care in addressing the rights and needs of patients/clients; make sound decisions in collaboration with the physical therapist and within the boundaries established by laws and regulations; demonstrate integrity in relationships; fulfil legal and ethical obligations including compliance with applicable laws and regulations and supporting the supervisory role of the physical therapist to ensure quality care and promote patient/client safety; enhance competence through lifelong acquisition and refinement of knowledge, skills and abilities; support organizational behaviors and business practices that benefit patient/clients and society; and participate in efforts to meet the health needs of people locally, nationally or globally (APTA, 2009b). Physical therapists and physical therapist assistants who provide care for older individuals are responsible for maintaining the standards of ethical conduct when providing patient care, regardless of association membership.

WCPT's ethical principles and the code of ethics for physical therapists and standards of ethical conduct for the physical therapist assistant adopted by APTA provide valuable resources to assist physical therapists and physical therapist assistants who provide care to geriatric patients in making ethical decisions. In addition to the ethical theories and principles, they articulate principles that help to direct responsible, ethical and caring practice. However, it must be recognized that these resources are tools to be used as guidelines for solving ethical dilemmas. They cannot address every situation or provide exhaustive advice to guide ethical decision-making. Moreover, the guidance is typically limited to the principles that address respect, trustworthiness, compassion/caring, autonomy and accountability. They do not take into account the complex issues associated with providing ethical care for older patients. For example, the principles that discuss respectful and trustworthy care give general guidance about allowing patients and surrogates to make informed decisions about care, but fail to provide guidance for situations in which a patient exhibits diminished cognitive ability and subsequent inability to participate in sound decision-making. These principles also lack guidance for situations that affect a patient's life circumstances including acceptance or refusal of care, safety and discharge decisions. Finally, the principles provide no specific guidance on how to resolve situations in which surrogates are conflicted about decisions regarding care of an elderly individual with dementia, or when the professional judgments of caregivers responsible for making surrogate decisions that are in the best interest of the patient conflict with institutional or societal constraints (Jensen et al., 2012).

ETHICAL MINDFULNESS

It is in the context of real-life cases where codes take on meaning. In these situations, reflective processes are critical for thoughtful moral judgment (Pozgar, 2010). Clinicians need to engage in reflective practice in order to understand the underlying ethical implications of a given situation. In order to do this, clinicians need to listen more attentively, recognize bias and judgment, and act with compassion based on insight. Ethical mindfulness requires the integration of phenomenological inquiry skills in clinical reasoning and decision-making frameworks. Phenomenological, mindful, conscious inquiry skills allow one to more fully grapple with the relationships that are part of the situation, rather than rely strictly on ethical principles and codes. Clinicians can use narratives or stories to assist in seeing the ethical dimensions, issues, questions and concerns that are part of the challenges in the situation at hand. Trigger questions can be used in this process of ethical engagement that provide an analytical and interpretive view that allows one to think more deeply about the situation. The following are examples of questions that the clinician can ask. What are the relevant ethical principles and how do they relate to one another? How has the story been cast? What are the important ethical moments? Who is telling the story and what is being left out? What is ethically at stake? How does this story lead us to ethical mindfulness? Reflecting on these and similar questions will assist the mindful clinician to more fully understand the context and circumstances that frame the situation and allow the clinician to make a more informed and meaningful ethical decision (Jensen et al., 2012).

SOURCES OF CONFLICTS IN GERIATRIC REHABILITATION

Several broad sources of ethical conflicts are recognized in geriatric rehabilitation, including personal vs. professional beliefs, an interdisciplinary team's perception and conflicts, and organizational and societal conflicts.

In dealing with older patients, a healthcare professional must recognize that occasionally a conflict exists between personal feelings about a patient or situation and professional duties. The professional must know how to weigh personal values against professional obligations and responsibilities. Additionally, expectations of team members involved in the care of geriatric patients may differ or not be clearly understood. Conflicts may develop regarding the role and responsibility of each professional. It is important that each individual in the team clarifies the promises implicit in the commitment to work in an interdisciplinary team. Finally, current healthcare reflects rapid changes in delivery and service models, especially as managed care principles have come to predominate in organizations. Conflict often exists between the healthcare professional's obligation to the patient and obligations to the organization. Our society expresses a wide variety of opinions about the attitude that should be taken toward elders. Recent dilemmas involve the allocation of healthcare resources, especially the financing of care and reimbursement for services. Therapists must look at each case on an individual basis and at the same time consider that case in the context of societal issues.

ETHICAL DECISION-MAKING

Purtilo and Doherty (2011) have identified the following six-step process as a tool that can be used to address ethical problems:

1. Gather relevant information.
2. Identify the type of ethical problem.
3. Use ethics theories or approaches to analyze the problem.
4. Explore the practical alternatives.
5. Complete the action.
6. Evaluate the process and outcome.

SPECIAL TECHNIQUES TO PROMOTE ETHICAL DECISION-MAKING IN GERIATRIC CARE

A variety of techniques can be used to promote ethical decision-making in geriatric care. Included in these techniques are value histories, use of ethics committees and team conferences.

A value history is a summary of a patient's values and beliefs. The information is obtained prior to the onset of a cognitive impairment that impedes the exercise of autonomous judgment. It can be constructed with the help of family members or significant others. This tool helps to preserve respect for the individual patient and his or her autonomy.

Groups of individuals in an institution may be identified as an ethics committee. Such committees have the authority to facilitate the resolution of ethical dilemmas in healthcare. They can develop policy and guidelines, provide consultation and case review, offer theological reflection and educate others in the institution regarding matters of morality. Membership varies and is often determined by the purpose of the committee. Generally, membership includes attorneys, clergy, ethicists, medical practitioners and community representatives. Specific limits of authority vary, depending on the policy developed by the institution. One model specifies optional consultation with the committee, leaving compliance with their recommendations to the discretion of the professionals involved in the case. Another model specifies mandatory review of certain decisions, for example those regarding life support measures, but continues to allow professionals to retain their authority in the final decision. A third model dictates mandatory review by the ethics committee and mandatory compliance with its conclusions (Lucke, 2007).

The interdisciplinary team may be used for additional input when ethical issues about patients must be addressed. In order to effectively consider issues of morality and value as they affect geriatric patient care, both patients and appropriate family members and caregivers should be included in the team.

Finally, any time an ethical concern arises, the clinicians should also determine whether legal remedies, such as durable power of attorney or guardianship, apply. Legal remedies are beyond the scope of this chapter, and are addressed in Chapter 74.

SPECIAL AREAS OF ETHICAL CONCERN IN GERIATRIC REHABILITATION

DISCHARGE PLANNING

Complex ethical concerns can be identified with respect to discharge planning in geriatric rehabilitation. Typically, discharge involves transition from a hospital to a site of continuing care. It can also be viewed as a transition from illness to rehabilitation and health. Ethical conflicts can be identified in relation to patient autonomy and involvement in the decision-making process. Additionally, ethical concerns may be identified with respect to discharge plans as they impact on the interests of multiple parties, including the patient, the family, the healthcare providers, the institutions, the reimbursement sources, the referral sources and society itself. Specific concerns arise in the context of the current US healthcare delivery systems. The system typically accessed by employed, middle-income Americans is based on prospective payment systems with defined lengths of stay and managed care principles designed to control the expenditure of healthcare dollars. Healthcare providers caring for patients funded through this system may experience pressure to advocate discharge plans that put financial considerations ahead of decisions that are in the patient's best interest and safety. As the healthcare delivery systems designed for the unemployed, uninsured and largely minority Americans, the military medical care system, and the veterans administration healthcare system adopt managed care principles in an effort to conserve healthcare dollars, healthcare practitioners working in these delivery systems may experience similar pressures (Torrens, 2002).

One variable in discharge planning may be that the healthcare providers' prescription for long-term care may not show sufficient respect for individual autonomy. Typically, an individual's ability to participate in any decision-making process is determined, at least in part, by performance on mental status examinations. These examinations, although considered to be reliable in judging mental capacity, are of limited value in judging capacity to make complex decisions related to discharge. Of primary importance is that such examinations fail to account for an elderly individual's ability to function in the community, based on social ability and the strength of support networks, in spite of the fact that both these factors are strong predictors of success in community living. An ethical decision related to discharge that truly accounts for patient autonomy should include some prediction of the individual's ability to address the challenges of independent living.

If the individual with dementia wishes to be discharged to their own home, that option should be considered in view of the individual's age, physical dependency, cognitive impairment and competency to perform physical, mental and functional tasks. An attempt must be made to determine whether the individual who wishes to return home has adequate insight into his or her level of dependency in order to address safety issues. In order to facilitate successful discharge home, an assessment must be made of whether that individual's needs could be met through a holistic flexible care plan that utilizes community teams and ongoing assessment and observation (Brindle & Holmes, 2005).

Another factor that complicates the ethics of discharge plans is that every decision affects the rights of many people and must account for competing obligations. It is widely recognized that the elderly individual has the moral and legal right to decide autonomously what is appropriate. However, the impact of that decision on the rights, duties and obligations of family members must also be considered. Specifically, the patient's goal must be accommodated to the family's ability and willingness to help, if such support is part of the proposed discharge plan. Bioethics has historically largely ignored the rights of families. Although families are traditionally obliged to care for each other in ways not expected from friends, neighbors and strangers, the burden of care associated with prolonged life of individuals with chronic and debilitating injuries is an important factor for consideration. Therefore, the obligation to care for family members must be balanced against the obligation of the family member to care for their own physical and emotional needs (Haddad, 2000). While the rights of family members must be factored into discharge plans, they must not have more influence on the plan than the rights of the older patient. One current temptation is to consult and address the needs of family members while virtually ignoring the decision-making

right and ability of the older individual, even when that individual is capable of involvement in the process.

A significant discharge challenge may be encountered when a frail, but cognitively-capable elderly client chooses to live at risk. In this situation, the frail older adult is deemed capable of understanding the information relevant to making a decision about his or her living situation, appreciates the reasonable and foreseeable consequences of a decision, and still makes a decision that the healthcare team deems risky. When confronted with this type of ethical situation, the clinician should consider use of mindful reflection and narrative, in light of the ethical principles of autonomy, nonmaleficence and beneficence, empowerment, advocacy, as well as applicable principles in codes of ethics, to navigate the totality of the ethical concerns. Consideration must be given to the risk of harm to the patient as well as to others, and an attempt must be made to achieve a balance between respect for individual freedom and the welfare of all. Considerations should also include the degree of risk versus the probability of harm and the amount of risk the individual is willing to assume. Clinicians must avoid ageist viewpoints and take care to avoid questioning the rights and behaviors of older adults in ways that would never be acceptable when dealing with younger adults. A question that should be asked when an older adult wants to live at risk is whether there would be the same degree of worry if the patient were 25 or 55. The clinician should also consider why it is more concerning that a competent 85-year-old at risk for falling wants to say at home than it is for a 16-year-old wanting to drive a car or a 25-year-old wanting to rock climb. The end result of the ethical decision making process may be that the clinicians respect the individual's choice, and set up a plan to support that decision in spite of their personal concerns and fears for the older individual's safety. Ultimately, the clinician may come to terms with the fact that there is no challenge, possibility of triumph, or real aliveness without risk (Baker et al., 2007).

From an administrative standpoint, discharge involves balancing the good of the patient against other goods, including the needs of the hospital and of society. Conflicts may arise between the financial interests of the institutions and society and the welfare of the patients. These are especially evident when financial considerations are viewed in light of the mission of the institution and its administrative obligations to the staff and the community. The code of ethics of the American College of Hospital Administrators specifically addresses such conflicts of interest by stating that the welfare of the individual must prevail. The code, however, is silent on issues of conflicts in administrative obligations. Therefore, an underlying motivation in effecting the discharge or transfer of a patient from an institution may be the administrative obligation to insure that the institution remains viable. This obligation may be seen to supersede the obligations of the institution to the community, the medical staff and even the patient. As a result, the needs of individual patients may play a relatively minor role in ethical frameworks espoused by some administrators. Rather, in this context, a patient's needs are balanced against the needs and interests of others. This may pose an ethical dilemma for those care-givers directly involved in effecting an appropriate discharge plan for an individual patient (Spielman, 1988).

Discharge plans that involve placement in long-term care are often among the most difficult. The health delivery system provides the older individual with little opportunity to choose either the site of care or its details. Such decisions are often made by discharge planners or social workers who have little opportunity to consult with the individual patient. Frequently, the discharge plan is determined without discussing the circumstances with the patient, family or caregiver, and is based on the physician's judgment that the older patient 'needs 24 hour care'. Additionally, the patient is rarely informed that the primary purpose of the discharge planner is to facilitate prompt discharge while automatically following rules for referral to post-acute care settings. The older individual is expected to make a critical life decision with inadequate time and information and may be being advised by professionals who have not fully disclosed the constraints imposed on them by their jobs. Furthermore, little consideration is given to the individual's right to make an informed, autonomous decision to return home when that decision is considered risky or hazardous by the physician or healthcare team. This is often the result not only of the healthcare professionals' desire to do what they know is best for the patient, but also of the fear of litigation resulting from the adverse outcome of a risky discharge decision (Kane, 1994).

Recurrent ethical conflicts may revolve around discharge orders that violate the conscience of those caring for the patient but do not necessarily violate the law. An example of a recurring theme seen in geriatric care would be situations in which discharge is planned for patients who are medically ready, but a discharge location that meets the patient's and family's need is not available. In these situations, the therapist and discharge planner recognize that the geriatric patient's needs may be in conflict with the discharge order. In this case, it may be argued that hospitals are held to a higher standard than a patient's medical status alone. Discharge must not be effected until there is adequate care and support in the home or an appropriate healthcare facility. The institution must not discharge a patient under adverse conditions, whether of medical status or social support. On the other hand, patients have no right to prolong their stay simply because they are comfortable or the desired discharge destination is not available. Patient autonomy is not absolute in this example, and questions of distributive justice must be considered, and patient's rights must be balanced against institutional policies. The institution might argue that the patient is entitled to be discharged to a facility as long as it meets minimally acceptable criteria, and has no right to demand discharge to the best possible facility. Such a discharge would serve the principle of justice as this same standard would apply to all patients. On the other hand, consistency offers only a minimal standard of justice. It does not take into consideration the impersonality of the institution in enforcing its own regulations. In attempting to do the right thing in these cases, the therapist and discharge planner

are continually presented with a hopeless choice and an unfair set of circumstances. There are no easy answers at the individual case level. In these types of situations, practitioners may look to preventive ethics, which focuses on the overall problem rather than the individual case. The right thing to do, then, becomes the mandate to change conditions so that a more equitable, ethical solution may be effected for future cases (Moody, 2004).

ETHICS AND LONG-TERM CARE

Long-term care, in current health services delivery, refers to a broad range of services that are available to assist an individual who has functional impairments. These services can include personal care, social support and health-related services. Settings for the provision of long-term care include an individual's home as well as a variety of institutional setting. The same ethical issues described above arise in the care of any older person receiving long-term care.

As noted previously, a primary ethical concern in decisions about long-term care involves the admission process itself. Frequently, decisions are made with little respect for patient autonomy. An individual may be denied the right to choose what is perceived as a risk-laden choice (to remain at home), and that may be a violation of his or her autonomy. In order to preserve autonomy and allow a patient to return home, he or she must understand the risks and consequences and must also understand that the decision should not have an adverse impact on the rights of others.

Another consideration in long-term care is the issue of privacy and dignity. Providers of geriatric rehabilitation services must be cognizant of individual dignity when assisting with personal care services such as bathing and toileting. In institutional settings, sensitivity to issues of privacy and dignity must be heightened, as the environment, by its nature, is not conducive to either. Examples of situations that may lead to violation of these rights include multiple occupancy rooms, responsiveness to call buttons and the use of first names without permission from the patient.

Rehabilitation in long-term care may evoke ethical dilemmas unique to that setting. By definition, rehabilitation implies fostering maximum patient independence in functional tasks. Geriatric patients seek long-term care precisely because they are dependent to some degree. An ethical challenge exists between respecting a patient's autonomy and complying with his or her request for help and encouraging independence. In a broader sense, a similar challenge may exist in decisions related to protecting a patient from risky situations such as falls or adverse health events. Healthcare providers must determine when a person needing care should be allowed to consciously choose a course that professionals consider risky in order to maximize values vs. allowing a patient to be unattended and potentially unsafe.

The lack of patient autonomy in long-term care living environments may be the result of the caregivers' and administrators' roles, their job descriptions, the physical environment and the regulations that govern these institutions. Administrators and staff may be trained to be task-oriented, which provides little opportunity to consider autonomy or even clients' involvement in daily decisions about their own care. The physical environment is often one of little space for storage of clothing and personal possessions, minimal security for personal items and limited privacy. Care plans and routines dominate the timing and the content of daily activities. Regulations, although designed to protect the welfare and safety of residents, frequently discourage residents' participation in decision-making and often allow for little freedom of choice. Examples include restrictions on what residents can keep in their rooms, requirements about supervision and the charting of patient activity, and safety requirements. Conversely, some regulations may enhance patient autonomy, such as those that mandate the availability of consumer information, enforce privacy regulations and place limits on the use of restraints (Kane, 1994).

The Center for Advocacy for the Rights and Interests of the Elderly (CARIE) developed a curriculum for guiding and improving ethical decision-making in long-term care. The program is based on the premise that long-term care involves the overall wellbeing of the resident, including the emotional, spiritual, psychological and social wellbeing, as well as the physical health of the resident. It takes into account the relationships that exist with family members, friends and staff that may be supported and strengthened by including them in the resident's care. The program recognizes that long-term care residents have physical dependencies and often suffer from dementing illnesses, and recognizes that the experience of dependency is magnified by the variety of ways in which a resident relies upon facility staff. The Center's model recognizes that traditional bioethics is inadequate to address the ethical issues confronting staff and residents in long-term care. The resulting curriculum, *Promises to Keep: Creating an Ethical Culture in Long-Term Care*, represents an ethics education curriculum that proposes commitment to the resident as the ethical basis of the long-term care admission. The program identified five themes: health, safety, pain and suffering, respect for personhood, and life story. These themes are coupled to commitments to preserve and promote the resident's health, protect the resident's safety, palliate the pain and suffering, practice respect and care for the attributes of personhood, and provide opportunity and support for the continuation and completion of the resident's life story. In this model, health is concerned with maximizing functional ability rather than curing disease, and safety addresses the resident's interaction with the external environment. Spiritual and emotional pain is deemed to be as important as physical pain. Life story is viewed as a continuation of that person's being, and involves honoring, encouraging and supporting in the resident the qualities that are associated with personhood including self-awareness, intentionality, decision-making, agency, emotions, relationships and creativity. CARIE developed a five-step process called IDEAS, which provides a framework for working through care dilemmas to reach ethical solutions. The steps are: (i) identify the ultimate issues, stakeholders and other decision points; (ii) develop a resident narrative; (iii) explore all conceivable responses to the issue; (iv) assess each response in light of the provider's commitments to the residents; and (v) select a course of action and create an implementation plan. This program contributes to care providers' ability to identify ethical dilemmas and provides a process for examining and sensitively resolving problems that are unique to long-term care (Mathes et al., 2004).

RESTRAINTS

The use of restraints in the care of the elderly poses several ethical and legal questions that must be addressed by healthcare providers. A restraint is defined as any device that restricts freedom of movement. The rationale for restraint use with the elderly is frequently cited as prevention of injury to self or others, but often the underlying motivation is fear of institutional liability.

When considering the use of restraints to control a patient for safety or because of behavior, the rehabilitation professional must be cognizant of the fact that the literature reports little scientific basis to support the efficacy of restraints in safeguarding patients from harm (Hieleman, 1991; Moss & LaPuma, 1991). In fact, adverse effects cited in relation to restraint use include such consequences as reduced functional capacity secondary to immobilization, as well as physiological changes including contractures, decreased muscle mass and strength, loss of bone integrity, decubitus ulcers and adverse psychological response to stress. It should also be noted that, with respect to geriatric rehabilitation, the use of restraints is inconsistent with and frequently in conflict with the goals of rehabilitation (Hieleman, 1991).

Hieleman (1991) identifies several issues that must be addressed when weighing the option of using restraints:

- informed consent
- risk vs. benefit analysis
- determination of competency
- the resident's rights and empowerment
- risk reduction.

It should be noted that the use of restraints without the patient's informed consent may be legally restricted. The Omnibus Budget Reconciliation Act (OBRA) of 1987 strongly implies that nursing facilities must obtain informed consent for whatever approach is taken to effect resident safety. Also, the Fourteenth Amendment to the US Constitution guarantees freedom from harm and unnecessary restraints (Moss & LaPuma, 1991).

It may be ethically permissible to override the refusal of a competent patient to apply a mechanical restraint if that individual is jeopardizing the safety and welfare of others. In such cases, the ethical principle of preventing harm to others supersedes the patient's right to refuse, and the negative rights of an individual to be free from interference ends as the autonomy of others is violated. In this case, the professional must balance professional responsibility to an individual patient with societal and legal obligations to protect public health (Moss & LaPuma, 1991).

If restraints are used as a punitive measure, there is no ethical justification for their application. Such a practice would be defined as abusive.

When the use of restraints is consistent with treatment goals, their application may be ethically indicated. One example is when a restraint such as wrist cuffs is applied to prevent interference with a life-sustaining treatment such as a nasogastric tube. In such cases, it should be emphasized, the treatment goal is to restore the patient to health (Moss & LaPuma, 1991).

MANAGED CARE

Part of the tradition of health professionals' service toward society's common good is based on the notion of altruism, or selfless concern for the welfare of the patient. Patients are viewed not as customers, but as individuals who are vulnerable and require the intervention of the healthcare provider. In turn, physical therapists promise to meet the health needs of the patient under the ethical principles of do no harm and provide benefit, while fostering autonomy and justice. In essence, the healthcare professional is a trustee who works for the good of the client and knows the limits of his or her expertise. However, in the current healthcare delivery system that embraces managed care principles, this concept may be challenged, especially when treating older patients who come to us with complex medical and social problems that require our professional expertise and interventions (Nalette, 2001). As such, managed healthcare poses special challenges in geriatric rehabilitation and ethics. One consideration is the managed care organization, structure and function itself. In the managed care structure, there are multiple actors with incompatible interests. For example, the rehabilitation provider has a fiduciary responsibility to patients, but may also be an employee of or contractor with the organization. The organization itself may have legal and financial obligations to shareholders to maintain low costs, yet an ethical obligation to patients to provide quality care.

Another current source of ethical conflict is the morality of market-driven healthcare, which has the potential to threaten professionalism. The introduction of market-driven practices into healthcare may divide professional loyalties between providing the best treatments in order to improve the patient's quality of life and keeping expenses to a minimum by limiting services, increasing efficiency and lessening the amount of time spent with each patient. The result may be that the professional must choose between the best interests of the patient and economic survival. Frequently, reimbursement drives the care.

The integrity of the patient–provider relationship may also be threatened in the current healthcare delivery climate. Focus on the patient is the primary concern of healthcare. Managed care, however, may threaten this relationship through policies that deny access to care, restrict the professional's ability to perform tests, and withhold or limit treatment. Such policies create conflicting loyalties and undermine the trust between provider and patient. The provider may be in the dual and potentially conflicting positions of being guardian of society's resources and being a primary advocate for the individual patient. With respect to geriatric patients, it can be stated that, ethically, the profession may not be able to afford to rehabilitate someone who is about to die, in which case rehabilitation would not be effective anyway. On the other hand, it is imperative that the professional never withholds treatment just because a person is old. The difficulty lies in determining who is ready to die and who may benefit, and how much, from rehabilitation efforts or from palliative care rehabilitation plans to make the dying process more humanistic.

Managed care may impact on the ethical principle of patient autonomy, and it potentially threatens the patient's freedom of choice. When healthcare coverage is provided as an employee or retirement benefit, the employee's choice may be even more restricted. In order to take advantage of healthcare coverage as a benefit, the employee or retiree is often forced to accept a plan that limits service access and does not meet healthcare needs. A person has the responsibility of understanding the terms of his or her own healthcare plan.

One more factor related to patient autonomy is the perceived right to have all treatment choices funded. It is paramount to acknowledge that autonomy does not guarantee funding. Rather, some balance must be achieved between conserving society's healthcare dollars and paying for individual healthcare needs. Providers and elderly patients must recognize that autonomy also entails responsibility. It obliges individuals to use resources wisely, to assist in conserving resources and to live a healthy lifestyle.

In 2000 and 2001, the American College of Physicians and the Harvard Pilgrim Health Care Ethics Program convened a group of patients, physicians, managed care representatives and medical ethicists. The purpose of the meeting was to develop a statement of ethics for managed care. The statement that they developed offers guidance on preserving the patient–client relationship, patient rights and responsibilities, confidentiality and privacy, resource allocation and stewardship, the obligation of health plans to foster an ethical environment for the delivery of care, and the clinician's responsibility to individual patients, the community and public health. The statement identifies four ethical principles to address the ethical challenges posed by limitations realized in association with managed care and that recognizes that healthcare resources should be distributed justly. *Principle I* addresses the relationships that are critical in the delivery of health services. It states that health plans, purchasers, clinicians and patients should be characterized by respect, truthfulness, consistency, fairness and compassion. *Principle II* states that health plans, purchasers, clinicians and the public share responsibility for the appropriate stewardship of healthcare resources. One tenet of this principle is that a clinician's first and primary duty is to promote the good of the patient while honoring the responsibility to practice effective and efficient healthcare that utilizes healthcare resources responsibly. It also states that health plans should engage purchasers in discussions about the health coverage that can reasonably be met, and that health plans should work with purchasers to insure that benefit packages are consistent with the healthcare needs and cultural norms of the purchasers' constituents. Contracts must not only contain costs, but should enhance efforts to improve quality care. *Principle III* states that all parties should foster an ethical environment for the delivery of effective and efficient quality healthcare. Financial incentives should enhance the provision of quality care and support professional ethical obligations. *Principle IV* states that patients should be well informed about care and treatment options and the financial and benefit issues that affect the provision of care (Povar et al., 2004).

ELDER ABUSE

Abuse of the elderly may take many forms, from causing actual physical harm or mental anguish to denial of needed medical and social services to financial exploitation. Abusive behavior toward the elderly may come from family members, caregivers or healthcare providers themselves. Often, the abuse may not be overt or intentional, but may stem from personal and professional values, including the desire to protect the elderly patient at the expense of his or her right to make autonomous choices.

One ethical consideration that must be acknowledged when healthcare providers become aware of actual abuse is the need to maintain a balance between sensitivity to patient trust and the need to abide by regulatory statutes that mandate reporting. This is especially important if knowledge of the abusive situation was gained through confidential disclosure of information.

As recognized previously, components of elder abuse must be acknowledged in discharge planning, use of restraints and denial of services enforced through regulations and managed care.

CONCLUSION

Ethical concerns and sources of conflict abound in regard to the rehabilitation of the geriatric patient. It is imperative that the healthcare practitioner who works with elders should be sensitive to these issues, understand the underlying ethical principles and incorporate moral values into the decision-making process. In addition to traditional bioethics principles and codes of ethics, clinicians should be mindful of reflective practice, and incorporate care and compassion, and avoid ageism when making decisions that impact on the lives of older adults, their families and society.

REFERENCES

American Physical Therapy Association (APTA) 2003 Professionalism in physical therapy. Available at: www.apta.org/uploadedFiles/APTAorg/About_Us/Policies/Judicial_Legal/ProfessionalismCoreValues.pdf. Accessed March 2014

American Physical Therapy Association (APTA) 2009a APTA Code of Ethics for the Physical Therapist. Available at: www.apta.org/uploadedFiles/APTAorg/About_Us/Policies/Ethics/CodeofEthics.pdf. Accessed March 2014

American Physical Therapy Association (APTA) 2009b APTA Standards of Ethical Conduct for the Physical Therapist Assistant. Available at: www.apta.org/uploadedFiles/APTAorg/About_Us/Policies/Ethics/StandardsEthicalConductPTA.pdf. Accessed March 2014

Baker K, Campton T, Gillis M et al 2007 Whose life is it anyway? Supporting clients to live at risk. Gerontol Nurs Assoc Perspect 31:19–24

Brindle N, Holmes J 2005 Capacity and coercion: dilemmas in the discharge of older people with dementia from general hospital settings. Age Ageing 34:16–20

Haddad A 2000 Acute care decisions: Ethics in action. RN 63(21–22):24

Hieleman F 1991 Restraint reduction in nursing facilities: the issues involved in decision-making. Geritopics 14:26–27

Jensen GM, Randall AD, Wharton MA 2012 Cognitive impairment in older adults. Top Geriatr Rehab 28:163–170

Jonsen AR, Siegler M, Winsslade W 2006 Clinical Ethics: A Practical Approach to Ethical Decisions in Clinical Medicine, 6th edn. McGraw-Hill, New York

Kane RA 1994 Ethics and long-term care. Clin Geriatr Med 10:489–499

Lucke KT 2007 Ethical considerations. In: Linton AD, Lach HW (eds) Matteson & McConnell's Gerontological Nursing Concepts and Practice, 3rd edn. Saunders Elsevier, St Louis, MO

Mathes M, Reifsnyder J, Gibney M 2004 Commitment, relationship, voice: cornerstones for an ethics of long-term care. Ethics Law Aging Rev 10:3–24

Moody HR 2004 Hospital discharge planning: carrying out orders? J Gerontol Social Work 43:107–118

Moss RJ, LaPuma J 1991 The ethics of mechanical restraints. Hastings Cent Rep 21:22–25

Nalette E 2001 Physical therapy: ethics and the geriatric patient. J Geriatr Phys Ther 24(3):3–7

Pellegrino ED, Thomasma DC 1993 The Virtues in Medical Practice. Oxford University Press, New York

Povar GJ, Blumen H, Daniel J et al 2004 Academia and clinic: Ethics in practice. Managed care and the changing healthcare environment: Medicine as a Profession Managed Care Ethics Working Group Statement. Ann Intern Med 141:131–136

Pozgar G 2010 Legal and Ethical Issues for Health Professionals, 2nd edn. Jones & Bartlett Learning, Sudbury, MA

Purtilo RB, Doherty RF 2011 Ethical Dimensions in the Health Professions, 5th edn. Elsevier Saunders, Philadelphia, PA

Ries E 2003 The art and architecture of caring. PT Mag 11(4):36–43

Spielman BJ 1988 Financially motivated transfers and discharges: administrators' ethics and public expectations. J Med Humanities Bioeth 9:32–43

Swisher LL 2005 Ethics in geriatric physical therapy. An independent home study course for individual continuing education. APTA Section on Geriatrics, Alexandria, VA

Torrens PR 2002 Overview of the organization of health services in the United States. In: Williams SJ, Torrens PR (eds) Introduction to Health Services, 6th edn. Delmar Publishers, Albany, NY

World Confederation for Physical Therapy (WCPT) 2011 WCPT Ethical Principles. Available at: www.wcpt.org/sites/wcpt.org/files/files/Ethical_principles_Sept2011.pdf. Accessed March 2013

Chapter 76

Generational conflict and healthcare for older persons

TIMOTHY L. KAUFFMAN • ADRIAN SCHOO

CHAPTER CONTENTS

INTRODUCTION

The conflict between the older generation and the younger generation is an age-old problem. The issue is particularly poignant in societies and nations that do not venerate their seniors. An important world population demographic was the subject of an editorial in which T.F. Williams, former Director of the National Institute of Ageing in the United States of America, was quoted as saying, 'Of all human beings who have ever lived on the earth and have reached age 65 years, the majority are alive today' (Williams, 1987). 'This statement holds significant implications for the society in general and especially for healthcare providers and their aged patients' (Kauffman, 1988). By now, everyone has heard the demographic litany about the increasingly aging population and the rising costs of caring for the elderly. The problem that we, as a civilization, face is how to handle this growing dilemma, both fiscally and ethically.

PARTISAN POLITICS

A member of the US House of Representatives addressed a group of physical therapists at the 1996 Combined Sections Meeting of the American Physical Therapy Association. He presented a scenario in which a family had a choice between healthcare for a terminally ill mother or more money for the discretionary use of the younger family members through tax savings derived from reduced healthcare benefits for Medicare patients and pensioners. The Congressman insisted that we must cut the healthcare benefits, even though it is 'cold hearted' because we must offer hope and a future (which is being 'warm-hearted') to our children and grandchildren. This simplistic either/or verbiage is the source of an increasingly intense generational conflict that pits one generation against another.

These political confrontations persist. The Patient and Affordable Care Act (derisively called Obamacare) became law in the US in 2010 and zero congressional members of one of the political parties voted for the bill. They believe expanding healthcare will add costs to the system and burden employers and younger workers. A major battle was waged during the 2012 US presidential election, with each party accusing the other of cutting Medicare and one party pledged to repeal Obamacare. 'Medicare, in particular, is the largest driver of future debt' (GOP, 2012) and the 'fiscal cliff' crisis – averted at the last hour of 2012 – would have imposed cuts in Medicare services and to providers.

Demographically, the world's population has been divided in generational cohorts: traditional (born pre 1946); baby boomers (born 1946–1964); generation X (born 1965–1980); generation Y (born 1981–1995); and 1996 to present are called millennials, which may also include generation Y. Generational conflict pits one age cohort against the other, although this issue is not a requisite of the 21st century. In fact, an aging workforce may be beneficial for individuals, employers and society by integrating them with younger workers (Guest & Shacklock, 2005).

David Willetts, a Conservative Member of Parliament (at the time of this writing) in the United Kingdom published a book entitled the *The Pinch: How the Baby Boomers Took Their Children's Future – And Why They Should Give It Back*. He argues that the 'Boomers' have accumulated wealth and benefited from the welfare state at the expense of younger generations. As 'Boomers' retire, the younger generations will be pinched with higher health and social care costs for their elders while at the same time they did not benefit from low housing costs and good work pensions as the Boomers did (Willetts, 2010).

Dollars, euros, yen and the other monetary units drive this conflict, aided by partisan politics and sensationalism.

Political concerns about healthcare costs and wealth distribution are heard around the world, especially in countries with aging populations. This is part of the demographic that is manipulated in the conflict of 'us against them', especially because older people use more healthcare and social security/pensioner dollars/euros. Also the eurozone crisis stemming from increasing government debts in Greece, France, Ireland, Spain and Portugal has fanned the flames of generational conflict. Böcking (2012) wrote, 'older people are living at the expense of the young, and it's high time the next generation took to the streets to confront their parents'.

GLOBAL DEMOGRAPHICS

The world has known many ages, like the Stone Age or the Bronze Age, but today we are embarking on the 'Age of Age', which brings many positives but also, significant challenges for individuals, families, agencies, cultures and governments. According to the World Health Organization, every second of time, 2 persons somewhere on earth will celebrate a 60th birthday, which amounts to 58 million new 60-year-old persons yearly. It is estimated that persons 60 years old or older account for 11.5% of the world's population and this will increase to 21.8% by 2050. The number of people living into the ninth decade of life will increase nearly 300% between 2012 and 2050. Life expectancy at birth is over 80 years in 30 countries, an increase from 19 countries only 5 years ago. Based on multiple sources, projections for percent of population aged 80, sex ratios, life expectancy at birth and at age 60 are shown in Table 76.1 (UNFPA and HelpAge, 2012).

Europe was the first region in the world in which the demographic transformation resulting from increased life expectancy was manifested. It has the highest proportion of old people in the world. Of 35 European countries in 2010, Germany has the highest population aged over 64 years (20.7%), followed by Italy (20.2%), Greece (18.9%) and Sweden (18.1%) (eurostat, 2010). In Australia the median age was estimated to be 36.6 years in 2005 and is predicted to reach 43.6 in 2050, and the percentage of

people over 65 years of age from 12.3% in 2000 to 23.9% in 2050 (Guest & Shacklock, 2005). Japan has the world's oldest population, with 31.6% of people being over the age of 59 years. In 2011 there were 316 600 centenarians and this is projected to explode to 3.2 million by 2050. In juxtaposition to life expectancy is life span, that is, the maximum number of years a member of a species has lived. In 1798 the oldest human in recorded data was 103, and in 1898 it was 110 years. The record increased in 1990 to 115 and later to 122.45 years in 1997 (UNFPA and HelpAge, 2012).

A key factor in increased life expectancy is that fertility has decreased worldwide from 5 children per woman in 1950–55 to 2.5 children in 2010–15 (UNFPA and HelpAge, 2012). The fertility rate (children per woman) in Japan dropped from 2.13 in 1970 to 1.37 in 2009; with sustainability or replacement rate being 2.1 children per woman (Er, 2010). Germany has the highest percentage of aging population in Europe but the number of persons living there despite immigration has decreased from 82.4 million in 2003 to 82 million in 2008. The fertility rate is 1.4 children per woman (Karsch & Hossmann, 2010). This demographic is not often presented in the popular press or in political rhetoric that adds to the generational conflict.

These demographics portend dire challenges to societies and governments as the trends, if continued, suggest that most persons born since 2000 will live to age 100 years or more (Christiansen et al., 2009). But not all aging researchers agree with this demographic. From a biological perspective, Carnes et al. (2013) argue that the genetics of persons born today are not much changed from our prehistoric ancestors. At that time deaths resulted from acute diseases and the harshness of hunting and gathering. Today's demographics are due to changes in civilization such as healthcare delaying mortality and conveniences like grocery stores obviating the need to hunt wild animals. The catabolic effects of aging can be delayed but not stopped because there is no biological dictate that humans live beyond the age of grandparent caregivers. The genetics of aging are too complex to establish a single or several genome manipulations to allow most persons to reach

Table 76.1	**Worldwide aging and life expectancy**							
	Percentage Population Aged 80+		Sex Ratio: Men per 100 Women 2012		Life Expectancy at Birth (year) 2010–2015		Life Expectancy at Age 60 (year) 2010–2015	
	2012	2050	60+	80+	Men	Women	Men	Women
Africa	1.6	4.3	84	61	67	72	18	22
Asia	0.7	3.3	98	74	73	78	18	22
Europe	4.4	9.3	72	49	73	80	20	24
Caribbean	2.0	6.3	86	71	70	75	20	23
Central America	1.4	4.8	87	67	74	79	21	23
South America	1.6	5.7	80	63	71	78	20	23
North America	3.9	8.0	81	57	76	82	22	25
Oceania*	2.9	6.3	88	67	75	80	22	25

*Includes Australia and New Zealand.

100 years of age. Predictions are important but can be wrong; only time will tell.

HEALTHCARE FOR OLDER PERSONS

In light of the demographics, how will governments be able to continue the old age pension and healthcare programs for younger generations? Financial security is important for governments and those who are governed. It is notable that in 2011–12, 33% of persons aged 60 years and above were employed worldwide yet 47% had 'cash worries', including health costs. Internationally, 44% of persons 60 years and older rated their health status as 'fair' and 22% were 'bad or very bad' and rising healthcare and medication costs are a source of stress and anxiety (UNFPA and HelpAge, 2012). Retirement income and health status are related and used to promote generational conflict; however, the purpose in this chapter is not to expound on social security or pension plans, but instead on how people can access healthcare.

Many of the world's countries provide universal healthcare through taxation and most also allow for private insurance, which shortens waiting lists for care. Most of the countries have seen the costs go up partially due to the aging demographics shown above. In the United Kingdom, total government healthcare costs increased from 58.26 billion pounds in 2001–2 to 109.43 billion pounds in 2008–9. The National Health Service (NHS) has a core principle 'to provide a universal service for all based on clinical need, not on ability to pay' (Boyle, 2011). In collaboration, the European Union Insurance Card allows all cardholders access to state-provided healthcare when travelling in any of the 27 members of the European Union. The card is free and the cost for care is aligned with the costs in home countries, which is free in some.

Brazil, Argentina, Saudi Arabia, Russia, Australia and New Zealand have similar systems which are working well but also face the demography of aging. In Japan, long-term care costs are expected to increase from 1.4% of gross domestic product in 2006 to 4% in 2050 (Colombo et al., 2011). A trend in Japan, as in many countries, is to provide more care at home rather than in hospitals or long-term care facilities (UNFPA and HelpAge, 2012).

UNITED STATES OF AMERICA AND MEDICARE

In the US, the rehabilitation of geriatric patients takes place largely within the Medicare and Medicaid programs, which are nearly universal socialized medical systems. As the population ages, the systems have become an increasingly partisan political battleground, with a moderate to high level of distrust, frustration and confusion among the various players on the field, including the beneficiaries and their advocates, lobbyists and families; the care providers, both individuals and institutions; the insurance companies; and the politicians and regulatory bureaucrats.

There is some justification for this sociopolitical quagmire because the Medicare and Medicaid (low-income seniors and run by state governments) systems are large, changing and expensive. In 2012 over 50.7 million people were covered by the Medicare system,

costing $574.2 billion in benefits. Government income for the year was $536.9 billion. The Medicare Part A (Hospital Insurance, HI) Trust Fund was enhanced by the Affordable Care Act innovations but is projected to be exhausted by 2026 if no changes are made. Medicare Part B for outpatient services 'is adequately funded for the next 10 years' but average annual costs have increased 6.1% for the past 5 years. Total Medicare expenditures for 2012 amounted to 3.6% of Gross Domestic Product (GDP). The average benefit cost in 2012 per enrollee was $5227 Part A and $5097 Part B (Trustees, 2013).

MEDICARE PARTS A AND B: THE CONFUSION

As stated above, Medicare Part A is a hospital insurance; however, services under the HI trust fund may be rendered in a hospital, rehabilitation unit, hospice system, skilled nursing facility or home healthcare situation. In contrast, coverage under Medicare Part B may take place in an outpatient setting in the hospital, a patient's home, an extended care facility, a skilled nursing facility, rehabilitation agency, comprehensive outpatient rehabilitation facility (CORF) or other outpatient treatment center. Thus, the strict nomenclature of inpatient versus outpatient care is not fully appropriate. This continuum of healthcare under the Medicare system is shown in Figure 76.1. From the rehabilitation perspective, there should be no difference in the sophistication of the level of care rendered to a patient, whether it falls under Part A or Part B. The differentiation arises only from the sociomedical factors that necessitate inpatient rather than outpatient care.

HOME HEALTH SERVICES

Geriatric rehabilitation taking place in the home is largely a result of legislative and regulatory decisions made in the 1980s. At that time, the prospective payment system (PPS) with diagnosis-related groups (DRGs) was enacted, which encouraged hospitals to discharge people as quickly

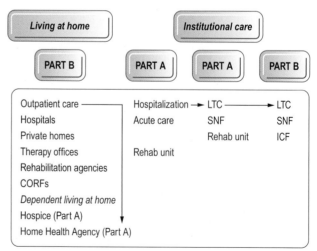

Figure 76.1 Continuum of healthcare settings for the geriatric patient. LTC, long-term care; SNF, skilled nursing facility; ICF, intermediate care facility; CORFs, comprehensive outpatient rehabilitation facilities.

as possible. The concept behind this PPS was that the efficient hospitals would benefit and the inefficient hospitals would suffer financial demise. However, as the late Senator John Heinz reported, the DRG system encouraged patients to leave hospitals 'sicker and quicker'.

As a result, the home healthcare industry grew so rapidly that, by the late 1990s, it had become a major concern for budget watchers because of the increase in home healthcare costs. In 2013 a prospective payment system will go into effect for home health agencies and is expected to reduce costs to Medicare by 0.01 % (CMS. gov, 2012).

Home health services are usually covered under Medicare Part A, provided certain criteria are met. As stated above, the patient must have an appropriate diagnosis, and there should be a reasonable expectation that the patient will recover from the condition. Obviously, in the geriatric setting, the functional declines are not always clearly attributable to an acute episode and this creates some ambiguity about medical necessity.

A person who requires skilled rehabilitative services must be determined to be confined to home in order to receive home healthcare. Also, the physician must certify that the patient is confined to home. If the patient is able to leave home, it should be achievable only with considerable and taxing effort. The patient may leave home for short durations to obtain medical care such as outpatient dialysis, chemotherapy, radiation or for an occasional trip to a barber or a walk or drive around the block.

Further, the patient is considered housebound if he or she has a condition or illness that restricts the ability to leave home except with assistance from another person or requires special transportation, or leaving home is contraindicated. Any condition such as a stroke that may cause the loss of the use of the upper extremities so that the patient is unable to open doors or use handrails will fit the criteria of being housebound. Post-hospital care with resultant asthenia or weakness, pain or other medical conditions that restrict activities also qualify the patient for home healthcare. For example, a person with atherosclerotic cardiovascular disease may have cardiac risk with physical activity and should not be leaving home. Additionally, a psychiatric problem in which a patient refuses to leave home or a circumstance in which it is unsafe to leave a person unattended may qualify the person as housebound.

The patient is not confined to home if he or she has the ability to obtain healthcare in an outpatient setting. The aged person who does not often travel from home because of feebleness and insecurity brought on by advanced age would not be considered to be housebound for the purposes of receiving home health services unless he or she meets one of the above conditions.

PARADIGM SHIFT

The German artist Bernd Stolz has nicely illustrated the weight (or burden) of the young and the old resting upon the shoulders of healthy, young, working adults (Fig. 76.2). The question to be answered is, must the generational difference be viewed as an either/or situation? The answer is no. What if the headlines in the newspapers

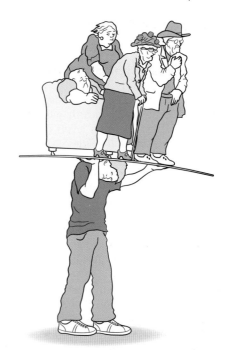

Figure 76.2 The weight of the young and the old resting upon the shoulders of healthy, young, working adults *(Bernd Stoltz, 1996.)*

reported that nearly 100% of education costs go to persons under the age of 30 years? Should pensioners in the UK or any other country stop paying community charges and other taxes that benefit younger persons? Public education (kindergarten to high school) in the US is funded largely by real estate taxes on property owners. 'Investing in young people's education will improve well-being and quality of life as they age' (UNFPA and HelpAge, 2012).

In the US the majority of expenses for state and local governments are for education and criminal justice. For example, the California 2013–14 budget has 62% designated for these services (California Budget, 2013), mostly benefitting persons under the age of 30 years. When the debate about the costs for healthcare and social care for the elderly are couched in terms of generational conflict, these data on spending levels are not included. Also, a major omission is the fact that healthcare costs add jobs and contribute not only to the wellbeing of individuals and their families but also to the GDP.

Harbingers of doom aside, not all the information is catastrophic. First, although the population of the world is aging, the morbidity of the aging population is being compressed into a shorter time period (UNFPA and HelpAge, 2012). This means that people are living longer and healthier lives. Adding years to life does not automatically mean adding excessive cost to the system. This presents a promising scenario for counteracting the costs of an aging society for future decades and centuries if morbidity is compressed. Other trends may reduce health costs, such as the increased use of advanced directives and do-not-resuscitate orders. Also, there is a shift from hospitals to home as place of death. Emphasis in all societies should be directed toward controlling infectious and communicable diseases as well as reducing/preventing disability. It is estimated that 46% of persons worldwide have disabilities

(UNFPA and HelpAge, 2012). Life-long healthy habits such as proper nutrition, adequate exercise and not smoking must be taught at a young age and practiced.

The challenge for the generations is to be smart and to work together proactively for mutual benefit. Keeping aging populations healthy and out of hospitals must lower the tax burden. Great public health gains are obtained from increasing and maintaining levels of physical activity of people who are sedentary (Fries, 2012) or becoming increasingly sedentary as they age, particularly in rural areas where active commuting is limited and leisure-time related infrastructure and clubs are sparse. Although incidental and unstructured forms of physical activity such as walking do not require expensive infrastructure and can reduce health risk factors (Strath et al., 2007), occupational physical activity and associated contacts and active commuting are more likely to be meaningful and therefore maintained

Part-time work or job-sharing between younger and older workers provides opportunities for building active, strong and resilient communities. Older people are likely to be willing to support younger colleagues (e.g. during maternity leave), share their experiences and act as mentors. Also, older people are more likely to be involved in voluntary work that benefits the community. It has been estimated that in Australia in 1997 the monetary value of all volunteering was about $41 billion, which is equal to the amount of money the government spent in that year on aged care services. Voluntary work can be very meaningful and can reduce the tax burden by keeping aging people active and engaged, for example by caring for their older peers (Healy, 2004).

Although Australia has a comparable aging problem, as demonstrated under global demographics earlier in this chapter, and there are also other similarities between North America and Australia (e.g. Medicare), there are also marked differences (e.g. social safety net for the disadvantaged) that did not lead to the young versus old debate that the US experienced. In Australia there appears to be a greater acceptance that successful transition to an era with more older people is a responsibility of young and old. Responsible behavior for younger people is to respect their older fellow citizens and to encourage them to remain physically and socially active in the community, and for older people to support their younger as well as older peers and to be engaged in the community. Maintaining good health and wellbeing seems a worthy investment that goes beyond generational differences and that is a responsibility for all.

THE ROLE OF HEALTHCARE PROVIDERS

Healthcare providers are very much involved in the entire process. We are involved as caregivers with our patients and our families. We are involved as researchers, hoping to find better ways of providing the best possible care within the social structures and financial constraints of each country, and we share that information through this text and many others. We are involved as citizens, hoping that our governments will listen to our needs and the needs of our patients. We, as healthcare providers, are the future elderly ourselves. We can look forward to

living longer and healthier lives than past generations. For these reasons, it is crucial that we voice our concerns, needs and ideas for our future. We are seeking the wisdom and ability to amalgamate our personal interests with our professional interests and the interests of our societies. However, Binstock (1986), past president of the Gerontological Society of America, reminds us of an enduring and universal truth: 'Politics, not research, will resolve value conflicts regarding the nature and extent of hardship and what actions, if any, governments should undertake to alleviate hardships.' The political climate in the US in the second decade of the 21st century supports Binstock's contention, although it seems not to apply as well to other aging countries. Maybe we need to remind our politicians wherever and whenever they frame policy as a generational conflict that 'When, due to financial restrictions, resources are allocated in a hard and pitiless manner, society's response to its vulnerable old and ill members becomes an even greater sign of its humaneness' (Allert et al., 1994).

NO EASY ANSWERS

The determination to remain independent despite the travails of age-related pathology and the fear of becoming a burden on family and society is an attitude that correlates with the compression of morbidity. This phenomenon of aging has forced society to consider issues such as advance directives (living wills) and do-not-resuscitate orders which resulted in declines of high-intensity medical interventions such as cardiopulmonary resuscitation, invasive tests and minor surgery. Requiring consent to treatment may reduce undesired and costly medical and surgical interventions. Palliative care must be maintained out of human decency, and this requires physical therapy for comfort and for pain control. At this time, there is very little support for the highly emotional subjects of euthanasia (deliberate acts that lead directly to death) or assisted suicide (the provision to a knowing patient of medical means to cause self-death). Civilization must continue to wrestle with these issues, especially as we enter this age of aging.

CONCLUSION

The issues of generational conflict are not new, and they need not be magnified. The biblical story of Abraham and Isaac serves as a concluding comment. Abraham, a centenarian, was tempted by God to sacrifice his only son, Isaac, who was then only a lad. Abraham instructed his servants to wait for him and Isaac and stated, 'We will return.' Seeing the wood, fire and knife, Isaac asked, 'Where is the lamb?' Abraham answered, 'God will provide himself a lamb' [Genesis 22:1–13, King James Version]. The important message is that Abraham never lost sight of what he needed to do, which was to obey God and sacrifice his son, the next generation. In this story, a desirable solution to Abraham's dilemma was reached. As this world ages, the solution will be found by young people and old people working together for the common good. We, as healthcare providers, must be participants in that solution.

REFERENCES

Allert G, Sponholz C, Baitsch H 1994 Chronic disease and the meaning of old age. Hastings Cent Rep 24:11–13

Binstock R 1986 Perspectives on measuring hardship: concepts, dimensions, and implications. Gerontologist 26:60

Böcking D 2012 Euro crisis morphs into generational conflict. Spiegel online. Available at: www.schpiegel.de/international/Europe/commentary_why_the_euro_crisis_is_also_a_generational_conflict_a_849165_druck.html. Accessed January 2013

Boyle S 2011 United Kingdom (England) Health Systems in Transition. European Observatory on Health Systems and Policies, Copenhagen, Denmark, p 1–514

California Budget 2013 Available at: www.ebudget.ca.gov/. Accessed January 2013

Carnes BA, Olshansky SJ, Hayflick L 2013 Can human biology allow most of us to become centenarians? J Gerontol A Biol Sci Med Sci 68(2):136–142

Christiansen K, Doblhammer G, Rau R et al 2009 Ageing populations: the challenges ahead. Lancet 374:1196–1208

CMS.gov 2012 Available at: www.cms.gov/Center/Provider_Type/home_health_agency_hha_center.html?redirect=/center/Hospice.asp. Accessed January 2013

Colombo F, Llena-Nozal A, Mercier J et al 2011 Help Wanted? In: Providing and Paying for Long-Term Care. OECD Publishing, Paris, pp. 61–84

Er LP 2010 Challenges and prospect for Japan's ageing population: no easy choices in ageing and politics consequences for Asia and Europe. Konradadenauer-Stiftung, Singapore, pp. 139–156

eurostat 2010 Available at: http://eppa.eurostat.ec.europa.eu/statistics_explained/index.php/Population_structure_and_aging. Accessed January 2013

Fries JF, 2012 The theory and practice of active aging. Curr Gerontol Geriatr Res article ID 420637

GOP 2012 Restoring the American Dream: economy and jobs. Available at: www.gop.com/2012-republican-platform_Restoring/#6. Accessed January 2013

Guest R, Shacklock K 2005 The impending shift to an older mix of workers: perspectives from the management and economics literatures. Int J Org Behav 10:713–728

Healy J 2004 The Benefits of an Ageing Population. The Australian Institute, Bruce, ACT

Karsch M, Hossmann I 2010 Consequences of the demographic change in Germany. Konradadenauer-Stiftung, Singapore, pp. 139–156

Kauffman T 1988 Physiotherapy as the world ages. Physio Theory Pract 4:61–62

Strath S, Swartz A, Parker S et al 2007 Walking and metabolic syndrome in older adults. J Phys Act Health 4:397–410

Trustees 2013 Annual Report of the Boards of Trustees of the Federal Hospital Insurance and the Federal Supplementary Medical Insurance Trust Funds. Available at: www.cms.gov/Research-Statistics-Data-and-Systems/Statistics-Trends-and-Reports/ReportsTrustFunds/. Accessed January 2014

UNFPA and HelpAge 2012 Ageing in the Twenty-First Century: A Celebration and a Challenge. United Nations Population Fund New York and Help Age International, London

Willetts D 2010 The Pinch: How the Baby Boomers Took Their Children's Future—and Why They Should Give It Back. Atlantic Books, London

Williams TF 1987 The future of aging. Arch Phys Med Rehabil 68:335–338

Chapter 77

The end of life

TIMOTHY L. KAUFFMAN

INTRODUCTION

Death and Dying
Death is a finite moment
  known only to God
Dying is a process that
  everyone does differently and uniquely.
Death is a victory
  A gift from Jesus on the cross
Dying is a plethora of emotions
  frustration
  inconsistent days
    some joyful
    some angry
    some, maybe many, in pain
    or some days when you just sense
    an overall loss of wellness
Death is the final goodbye to life on earth
  as we know it
Dying is the goodbyes to people, events, yes, even things
  close to you.
The hardest and most overwhelming goodbye to me is
  leaving my children
    Their careers I'll not see develop and flourish
    Their weddings I'll never participate in
    The grandchildren I'll never hold or spoil and of
      course other immediate family, friends, colleagues,
      places
  I've traveled, forests, waterfalls, lakes, flowers, mountains,
    rustic roads, parks, oceans, my cats, Tabitha and
Magnum, my stuffed animals, and more and more.
Death is our greatest victory
  propelling us to a peace beyond our own understanding.
Dying is the vehicle that transports us, not always a smooth
  and tranquil ride but at journey's end remains the promise
  of a safe arrival.
LYNN PHILLIPPI, WRITTEN AT LINEN & LACE B&B, JUNE 26, 1997

Struggling with her own medical problems and shortly before her own death, Lynn Phillippi composed these words. She wrote the chapter on 'Stiffness' in the first edition of this book. As Lynn noted, death is but a finite moment, and each person's death is different and unique. As healthcare providers to geriatric patients, we are faced with the reality of patients dying, but the process and timing of that moment are not always simple or clearly delineated.

But the dying process is often protracted, filled with repetitive losses and rebounds as the progressive decline and downward spiral transpire, so rehabilitation shifts to palliative care to meet the changing needs of increasingly frail and debilitated patients (Rome et al., 2011). In these commonly occurring cases, the purposes of care are to assist the patient and other caregivers with quality of life issues such as pain control (Dalacorte et al., 2011), positioning, mobility, handling and toileting, and to provide dignity to a human being and his or her family.

THE END OF LIFE

When does the end of life start – after the second stroke or when a terminal illness is diagnosed, or when a person is admitted to an extended care facility or when a doctor says so…? In an abstract way, the end of life may start at the time of birth, and luck, choice and genetics determine how long the involution will be. Most healthcare providers in the field of geriatrics recognize when a patient is approaching the end of life; but most also realize that some patients will 'hang on' for days, months or even years. Therefore, to withdraw rehabilitation services too early or to deny those services may approach neglect or abuse, especially if rehabilitation specialists are not consulted.

Admittedly, constraints such as patient potential exist, but the decision should be arrived at by the family, care providers, physicians and rehabilitation specialists with due consideration given to pathology, family and patient desires, availability of services and financial realities. Included among the family's and patient's desires are sociological differences, for the end of life is surrounded by a variety of habits, beliefs, customs and values. Culture and religion are crucial considerations that influence the provision of healthcare to people as they approach death.

PALLIATIVE CARE

When a patient has little or no potential or refuses rehabilitative care, then respect, dignity and physical as well as emotional comfort must be given freely by all ethical people who come into contact with this human being. At such a time, rehabilitation for the purpose of restoring or recovering function is obviously not appropriate; however, palliative care is. 'Palliative care is to relieve the suffering of patients and their families' at the time when life is ending (Rome et al., 2011). Often, care is directed toward the dying patient's family as much as it is given to the patient. For example, the family might need help in accepting the harsh and sad reality of the impending expiration.

In palliative care, an interdisciplinary team including nurses, social workers, physical therapists, pastoral counselors, family therapists and physicians usually provides the better services. Family members are crucial members of this team. The desired outcome is a 'good death', which is defined as 'one that is free from avoidable distress and suffering for the patients, families and caregivers: in general accord with the patients' and families' wishes; and reasonably consistent with clinical, cultural and ethical standards' (Field & Cassel, 1997).

Scarre (2012) suggests that there is no such thing as a 'good death'. This has led to an increased interest in wishing to hasten death (Monforte-Royo et al., 2012).

Emanuel and associates (2001) developed the 'needs at the end-of-life screening tool' (NEST), which is concerned with four areas: (i) needs that are social, financial, caregiving and access to care; (ii) existential needs that are spiritual, purpose, distress and settledness; (iii) symptoms that are physical and mental; and (iv) therapeutic needs that are relationship, information and goals of care (Emanuel et al., 2001). These categories of care may be helpful for all members of the team and may enable a 'good death' (Della-Santina & Bernstein, 2004).

Emanuel et al. (2004) reported that talking in a structured interview with terminally ill patients and their caregivers caused little or no stress in nearly 90% of their subjects and that nearly 50% found it to be helpful. These researchers found the interview to be helpful, especially for ethnic minorities and persons who were anxious. Over 50% of dying patients who were having difficulty in coming to closure with family and friends reported that the discussion was helpful.

Appropriate services from a physical or occupational therapist may help with proper positioning or mobility in bed, with sitting and with assisting to toilet. Speech therapy may be helpful for teaching swallowing, mouth care and communication modifications. Perhaps at this stage of life, the end, the ability to communicate at any level is a most crucial need, especially for the sake of family and intimate friends.

Palliative care is not something that is done only at the end of life. Efforts to moderate the intensity of pain and minimize functional limitations and impairment should have been made prior to clinical recognition that the patient has poor rehabilitative potential and is approaching the end of life. So rehabilitative and palliative care are not mutually exclusive but are on a continuum, with the emphasis on curative recovery of function lost lying at one end of the spectrum and on comfort and moderating the intensity of pain lying at the other, when restoration is unlikely or impossible.

This concept of the continuum of rehabilitation/palliation fits well within the parameters of the Guide to Physical Therapist Practice (1997), especially with the roles of the physical therapist in consultation and communication. The interventions of coordination and communication are particularly pertinent, as they can be used to coordinate care of the patient with family, significant others, caregivers and other professionals. This involves instruction in proper procedures and techniques but holds quality of life issues and palliation as the focus. In 205 the American Physical Therapy Association (APTA) validated the purpose of physical therapy care at the end of life in the hospice setting (Emerging PT Practice: No. 13).

THE ROLE OF REHABILITATION

Because each individual patient and family approaches the dying process with a different set of medical, spiritual and physical needs, the role of rehabilitation must be varied. In the early stages, mobility is an important treatment consideration, and thus typical gait, balance and therapeutic strengthening exercises may be appropriate. The use of assistive devices for balance, safety, pain reduction and joint protection may enable the patient to maintain a sense of independence and involvement in life's activities. Joint protection with the use of an orthotic or splint may enhance functional capacity and, as a patient becomes more confined to bed, it may be used to prevent painful and disfiguring contractures, swelling or skin breakdown.

Therapeutic exercise to maintain breathing capacity and exercise tolerance is useful. The inability to breathe is frightening and can usually be controlled until the very last days or hours of life. Exercise tolerance should be aimed at sitting up on the bedside or in an easy chair or wheelchair. The world looks better from an upright posture, and the patient may be able to eat or at least sit at a meal with family and friends. Breathing and eating may be easier in the upright position.

Adaptive equipment for eating, dressing and bathing may help to maintain independence and a sense of self-worth. A wheelchair is most useful for transport and to conserve energy; however, it can cause injury or at least pain and fatigue if it is ill-fitted. Pressure ulcers can occur, and edema may result in dependent extremities. A poorly fitted wheelchair or prolonged sitting encourages kyphosis of the spine, which can cause back pain, reduce chest expansion for breathing and compress the abdomen, making eating more difficult.

Pain management for the terminally ill patient usually involves medication, especially narcotics. Some patients and their families choose not to use these types of medications because of their beliefs or because of the lightheadedness or drowsiness that results. The physical modalities of the various heat or cold applications and electrical stimulation are beneficial, although realistic expectations are requisite. The effects of the portable and easily used transcutaneous electrical nerve stimulator (TENS) are less potent and not identical to the effects of a dose of morphine, but they are of value. The physical modalities are described in more detail in Chapter 67, 'Conservative interventions for pain control'.

Range of motion exercises help to control pain and to prevent contractures, stiffness and tissue breakdown. These can often be taught to family members; that way, they have an opportunity to participate in the care of their loved one rather than being just bystanders. Further, these exercises require physical contact, which is an important human need that may be lost to the dying patient because of medical interventions or simply because family members do not know whether or not handling will cause harm. Gentle massage is therapeutic too, both physically and emotionally.

Complementary and alternative therapies such as acupuncture, music therapy, homeopathy, healing touch, imagery and relaxation techniques may be helpful. Dying persons who inquire about these interventions should not be left with a sense of hopelessness even if efficacy has not been firmly established (Dalacorte et al., 2011).

EMOTIONS

When providing healthcare, be it curative or palliative, it is vital to remember that patients and their families have real emotions that must be considered. Bereavement is a process that starts before death and continues after it. The family and intimate friends are facing a loss, sometimes one that they are not ready to accept, and denial is a common coping mechanism. Denial may be used by the patient, too, and that can impede the more important acts of completing one's life work, settling one's affairs and saying goodbyes. When working with a patient and family members at a time when all of them may be in various stages of denial, it is necessary to be honest, but not brutally so. Empathy and honesty help, especially when they come from all members of the healthcare team and from clergy (Rome et al., 2011).

Anger and frustration are also commonly encountered in a dying patient and may be directed at family members, at God, or at some or all of the medical care providers. Fear and guilt may also be present, for death is an unknown. Several of the world's major religions have taught the concept of sin, and the dying person may have a sense of guilt about the commissions or omissions of life, and may regret the inability to do something about them in the last remaining days.

Again, empathy, honesty and dignity are important. At the end of life, a person should feel that he or she is okay and is valued by the medical providers as a human being until death and then as a memory.

Many patients and families are most appreciative of anything that can be done to provide additional comfort, dignity and worth. Therein lies the inner strength

to continue to work with patients and their families as life completes its journey.

HOSPICE CARE

The hospice concept developed in the 1960s in the UK; in the US, it is now a Medicare Part A program, which usually starts when a patient is determined by a physician to have less than 6 months left to live. A wide variety of physical capabilities and needs are found among hospice patients. In the early stages of hospice care, rehabilitation services may indeed be curative and, in the end, only palliative. The blending of one phase into the other is usually gradual, but the consultation and care provided by rehabilitation specialists as members of the hospice team will maintain the quality of life at its optimal level (Della-Santina & Bernstein, 2004; APTA, 2005).

IMPENDING DEATH

Certain signs indicate that death will occur soon. In the final days the patient may become increasingly somnolent and diaphoretic, and intake of fluids and food may nearly cease. Parenteral nutrition is not advocated at this time; however, oral care and the use of lip salve and ice chips is palliative (The Merck Manual of Geriatrics, 2011). The toes and fingers as well as the nose and ears may become cyanotic as the circulation and oxygen perfusion decline. The death rattle, a frequent cause of distress for family members, results from bronchial congestion or palatal relaxation. If desired, clergy should be consulted, and the family can be present and hold hands or touch or rub the loved one to say final goodbyes. Peace, dignity and respect must prevail.

CONCLUSION

As Lynn Phillippi wrote, 'Death is the final goodbye to life on earth'. It is an individual experience inherent in life. Knowing what stops life allows a better understanding of what life is. Healthcare providers to aging and dying patients participate in this universal college frequently. Rehabilitative services, curative and palliative, enhance the quality of life for the dying patient and for the patient's family.

The following words were written as I sat at the funeral of a patient I had treated, off and on, for 8 years, both curatively and palliatively.

The Meaning of Life
What is the meaning of life?
The answer is unclear;
And it is not the same for all.
Part of the answer is in death
When it is not.
Death begets life
For it is the aging, the passage
of time that nourishes the young;
Without someone before us,
there can be none behind us.
Life is not easy.

It is filled with problems,
  heartaches, sadness. Yet
  there is joy abundant.
Sometimes it is hard to find. Accept
the bad, for it is life, too. But search
and focus on the good,
  the beauty.
It passes every day.

Those who precede us and those
  who pass through life with us
  are ALWAYS present.
They live with us forever
  in our thoughts,
  our actions,
  our lives.

In life, there is no absolute beginning
  and no absolute ending;
  there is only conception and there is death
  which mark these times.
But what preceded and followed these events,
  both conception and death?
Are the lives of loved ones
  both giving and receiving love;
  sharing learning and living.
We are our parents, our spouses,
  our children, our grandparents, and
  grandchildren,
  and others who enter our lives
  sharing, learning, living, loving.

The meaning of life is the here and now,
  which are built upon what preceded and
  provide for what follows.

The meaning of life is to experience it,
  the good and the bad,
But most important is to focus
  on the beauty of its experiences.

TIM KAUFFMAN, MARCH 1993

REFERENCES

American Physical Therapy Association (APTA) 2005 Hospice Care: Emerging PT Practice, No. 13, Rehabilitation. Oncology 23(2):24–26

Dalacorte R, Rigo J, Dalacorte A 2011 Pain management in the elderly at the end of life. North Am J Med Sci 3:348–354

Della-Santina C, Bernstein R 2004 Whole patient assessment, goal planning, and inflection points: their role in achieving quality end-of-life care. Clin Geriatr Med 20:595–620

Emanuel L, Alpert H, Emanuel E 2001 Concise screening questions for clinical assessments of terminal care: the needs near the end-of-life screening tool. J Palliat Med 4:465–474

Emanuel E, Fairclough D, Wolfe P et al 2004 Talking with terminally ill patients and their caregivers about death, dying, and bereavement. Arch Intern Med 164:1999–2004

Field M, Cassel C 1997 Approaching Death: Improving Care at the End of Life. National Academy Press, Washington, DC

Guide to Physical Therapist Practice 1997 Phys Ther 77(11):1162–1650

The Merck Manual of Geriatrics (Beers MH, Berkow R, eds) 2011 3rd edn. [Online]. Merck & Co. Inc., Whitehouse Station, NJ. (Accessed at www.merckmanuals.com/professional/geriatrics.html December 2013)

Monforte-Royo C, Vilavicencio-Chavez C, Tomas-Sabado J et al 2012 What lies behind the wish to hasten death? A systematic review and meta-ethnography from the perspective of patients. PLOS ONE Published online 14 May 2012, doi: 10.1371

Rome R, Luminais H, Bourgeois D et al 2011 Role of palliative care at the end of life. Ochsner J 11:348–352

Scarre G 2012 Can there be a good death? J Eval Clin Pract 18:1082–1086

Chapter 78

Entry-level competencies for health professionals who work with older adults

JOHN O. BARR • JENNIFER NITZ • RITA A. WONG

CHAPTER CONTENTS

OVERVIEW AND INTRODUCTION

COMPETENCIES

IMPLEMENTATION

REFERENCES

OVERVIEW AND INTRODUCTION

In most Western countries, individuals wanting to practice physical therapy must complete a course of study intended to prepare them to meet standards of practice in physical therapy and to behave in accordance with the codes of conduct for healthcare practitioners established in that country. Designated groups in each country establish and enforce these standards. These standards of practice are generally written broadly to capture the overarching scope of practice of the profession and the knowledge, skills and behaviors necessary for safe, effective, ethical and patient-centered professional practice. Competencies specific for practice with older adults are generally not separately identified in national standards for physical therapist practice. Rather, standards of practice include statements that practitioners are competent to practice across all categories of patients pertinent to the profession, including older adults. It is clear from these standards that all major categories of patients/clients (including older adults) need to be included in entry-level professional education processes, but this does not help the educator or clinician determine what knowledge and skills are most important.

In April, 2008, the Institute of Medicine's Committee on the Future Health Care Workforce for Older Americans released its 312 page report *Retooling for an Aging America: Building the Health Care Workforce* (IOM, 2008). This report called for fundamental reform in the way that the healthcare workforce in the United States of America is both trained and used in the care of older adults. A key recommendation of this report was that licensure, certification and maintenance of certification for healthcare professionals should include demonstration of competence in the care of older adults.

Responding to this report in June of 2008, the American Geriatrics Society convened 21 organizations representing professionals involved with care of older adults, a group that subsequently became the Partnership for Health in Aging (PHA), which has since grown to 36

organizations. An initial PHA workgroup was comprised of representatives from disciplines having consensus-based, endorsed and/or validated geriatric competencies (i.e. Medicine, Nursing, Pharmacy and Social Work). This workgroup: identified the need for a set of core competencies related to care of older adults by health professionals at completion of their entry-level professional degrees, and that were relevant and capable of being endorsed by all health professional disciplines; and determined competency criteria. By May of, 2009, the workgroup was expanded to include 10 disciplines (adding Dentistry, Nutrition, Occupational Therapy, Physical Therapy, Physician Assistants and Psychology).

Meeting through a regular series of conference calls that employed an iterative process, the workgroup developed a comprehensive matrix of 73 competencies in eight domains. After common themes and areas of overlap were identified, the resulting 23 competencies in six domains were approved by the workgroup, and these were circulated to 28 professional organizations for review and comment. Subsequent feedback was reviewed and final wording for the competencies was based on workgroup member consensus. The final competencies were returned to the 28 professional organizations, their official endorsement was attained, and *Multidisciplinary Competencies in the Care of Older Adults at the Completion of the Entry-level Health Professional Degree* was published online in September, 2010 (Partnership for Health in Aging, 2010).

COMPETENCIES

The multidisciplinary competencies and their domains are presented in Box 78.1.

IMPLEMENTATION

As noted by the PHA, these competencies are intentionally broad, in order to provide a baseline for training in any health profession involved in the care of older adults

Box 78.1 *Multidisciplinary competencies and their domains*

DOMAIN 1: HEALTH PROMOTION AND SAFETY

1. Advocate to older adults and their caregivers interventions and behaviors that promote physical and mental health, nutrition, function, safety, social interactions, independence and quality of life.
2. Identify and inform older adults and their caregivers about evidence-based approaches to screening, immunizations, health promotion and disease prevention.
3. Assess specific risks and barriers to older adult safety, including falls, elder mistreatment and other risks in community, home and care environments.
4. Recognize the principles and practices of safe, appropriate and effective medication use in older adults.
5. Apply knowledge of the indications and contraindications for, risks of and alternatives to the use of physical and pharmacological restraints with older adults.

DOMAIN 2: EVALUATION AND ASSESSMENT

1. Define the purpose and components of an interdisciplinary, comprehensive geriatric assessment and the roles individual disciplines play in conducting and interpreting a comprehensive geriatric assessment.
2. Apply knowledge of the biological, physical, cognitive, psychological and social changes commonly associated with aging.
3. Choose, administer and interpret a validated and reliable tool/instrument appropriate for use with a given older adult to assess: (a) cognition, (b) mood, (c) physical function, (d) nutrition and (e) pain.
4. Demonstrate knowledge of the signs and symptoms of delirium and whom to notify if an older adult exhibits these signs and symptoms.
5. Develop verbal and nonverbal communication strategies to overcome potential sensory, language and cognitive limitations in older adults.

DOMAIN 3: CARE PLANNING AND COORDINATION ACROSS THE CARE SPECTRUM (INCLUDING END-OF-LIFE CARE)

1. Develop treatment plans based on best evidence and on person-centered and directed care goals.
2. Evaluate clinical situations where standard treatment recommendations, based on best evidence, should be modified with regard to older adults' preferences and treatment/care goals, life expectancy, co-morbid conditions, and/or functional status.

3. Develop advanced care plans based on older adults' preferences and treatment/care goals, and their physical, psychological, social and spiritual needs.
4. Recognize the need for continuity of treatment and communication across the spectrum of services and during transitions between care settings, utilizing information technology where appropriate and available.

DOMAIN 4: INTERDISCIPLINARY AND TEAM CARE

1. Distinguish among, refer to and/or consult with any of the multiple healthcare professionals who work with older adults, to achieve positive outcomes.
2. Communicate and collaborate with older adults, their caregivers, healthcare professionals and direct-care workers to incorporate discipline-specific information into overall team care planning and implementation.

DOMAIN 5: CAREGIVER SUPPORT

1. Assess caregiver knowledge and expectations of the impact of advanced age and disease on health needs, risks and the unique manifestations and treatment of health conditions.
2. Assist caregivers to identify, access and utilize specialized products, professional services and support groups that can assist with caregiving responsibilities and reduce caregiver burden.
3. Know how to access and explain the availability and effectiveness of resources for older adults and caregivers that help them meet personal goals, maximize function, maintain independence and live in their preferred and/or least restrictive environment.
4. Evaluate the continued appropriateness of care plans and services based on older adults' and caregivers' changes in age, health status and function; assist caregivers in altering plans and actions as needed.

DOMAIN 6: HEALTHCARE SYSTEMS AND BENEFITS

1. Serve as an advocate for older adults and caregivers within various healthcare systems and settings.
2. Know how to access, and share with older adults and their caregivers, information about the healthcare benefits of programs such as Medicare, Medicaid, Veterans' Services, Social Security and other public programs.
3. Provide information to older adults and their caregivers about the continuum of long-term care services and supports – such as community resources, home care, assisted living facilities, hospitals, nursing facilities, sub-acute care facilities and hospice care.

(Partnership for Health in Aging, 2012). In their application, these competencies must take into account the unique characteristics and needs of older adults, and ensure person-centered care that supports the rights, autonomy and dignity of older adults. Further, individual preferences, ethnic backgrounds, culture, spiritual beliefs and levels of health literacy of older adults and their caregivers must be considered. Finally, the strengths, deficits and adaptive strategies exhibited by older adults and their caregivers in coping with late-life issues and challenges must be recognized. It is anticipated that there will be variations in the application of these competencies by each health profession, including variations in the depth of knowledge or level of involvement with a given competency. Each profession will need to determine how these competencies will be utilized by their entry-level professional education programs, and be employed by their accrediting, licensing and credentialing organizations.

At this juncture, of the healthcare professions in the US, the physical therapy profession has developed more discipline-specific competencies based on this multidisciplinary competency model (Section on Geriatrics, 2011 [note that the Section on Geriatrics became the Academy of Geriatric Physical Therapy in 2014]).

In reviewing the competency standards and codes of practice of Australian physiotherapists (Australian Physiotherapy Council, 2006), New Zealand physiotherapists (Physiotherapy Board of New Zealand, 2009), United Kingdom physiotherapists (Van der Gaag, 2012) and the Core Standards for Physiotherapy Practice in Europe (European Region of World Confederation for Physical Therapy, 2008), very little difference was found to those developed and covered in the domains presented for the US. However, these standards and codes embrace patients/clients of all ages and do not specifically focus on older adults.

To date, PHA workgroup members have presented the competencies at professional society conferences, disseminated them to members of their professional organizations and aging/geriatrics/gerontology special interest groups, published them in organizational newsletters, and distributed them to various committees and organizations responsible for education, certification and accreditation requirements. The PHA envisions these efforts to be the first steps in utilizing these multidisciplinary competencies to enhance geriatrics education for all healthcare professionals. The demand for quality healthcare for older adults, both in the US and worldwide, will not be met through the preparation of specialists alone, but through the improved competence of all health professionals during their entry-level professional education.

References

Australian Physiotherapy Council 2006 Australian Standards for Physiotherapy. www.physiocouncil.com.au/files/the-australian-standards-for-physiotherapy

European Region of World Confederation for Physical Therapy 2008 European Core Standards of Physiotherapy Practice. www.physio-europe.org/download.php?document=71&downloadarea=6

Institute of Medicine 2008 Retooling for an aging America: building the health care workforce. The National Academic Press, Washington, DC

Partnership for Health in Aging 2010 Multidisciplinary competencies in the care of older adults at the completion of the entry-level health professional degree. American Geriatrics Society. www.americangeriatrics.org/files/documents/health_care_pros/PHA_Multidisc_Competencies.pdf

Partnership for Health in Aging 2012 Considerations for implementation. www.americangeriatrics.org/about_us/partnership_for_health_in_aging/multidisciplinary_competencies/considerations_for_implementation.pdf

Physiotherapy Board of New Zealand 2009 Physiotherapy Competencies for Physiotherapy Practice in New Zealand. www.physioboard.org.nz/docs/PHYSIO_Competencies_09_for_web.pdf

Section on Geriatrics, American Physical Therapy Association 2011 Essential Competencies in the Care of Older Adults at the Completion of the Entry-level Physical Therapist Professional Program of Study. www.geriatricspt.org/pdfs/Section-On-Geriatrics-Essential-Competencies-2011

Van der Gaag 2012 Standards of Proficiency – Physiotherapists. Health and Care Professions Council. http://www.csp.org.uk/professional-union/professionalism/regulation/hcpc-standards

The rehabilitation team

UNIT CONTENTS

Chapter 79

Caregivers: valuing unpaid care

CHERYL L. ANDERSON

CHAPTER CONTENTS

INTRODUCTION

INFORMAL NETWORKS

THE MULTIPLE ROLES OF THE
CAREGIVER

THE STAGES OF CAREGIVING

CAREGIVER RECOGNITION

REFERENCES

INTRODUCTION

The focus of most medical care and concern in dealing with frail elderly patients is on their medical treatments. However, this is a small fraction of the overall care most chronically ill older adults receive. Over 90% of all care to the elderly and disabled is provided by an informal network of family, friends and faith-based organizations (Family Caregiver Alliance, 2011). This invisible network of support sustains most older adults throughout their lives.

In 2009, 61 million Americans were unpaid caregivers during the previous year (Andrus, 2011). This number rose to 65.7 million in 2012 (National Alliance for Caregiving, 2012). At any one time, 43.5 million family caregivers are providing care to older adults in some capacity. The value of this unpaid care is well over $450 billion each year, representing a significant rise from $375 billion in 2007 (Andrus, 2011; National Alliance for Caregiving, 2012). Families provide the bulk of unpaid care to older adults.

Almost two-thirds of all caregivers are women, caring for an adult who is at least 50 years old. The voluntary work is not without hardship. Caregivers surveyed reported paying more than $5000 of their own money to provide care to another (Andrus, 2011). Further, almost 70% of caregivers need to adjust their working schedules to accommodate their caregiving roles (Andrus, 2011). This change in ability to work results in decreased wages, lost retirement savings and potentially the loss of a job.

According to Coughlin (2010) unpaid caregivers will likely be the largest single source of long-term care to the nation's older citizens in future years. This source of care is often unrecognized and undervalued by healthcare providers.

Almost half of all caregivers are employed full time outside the home (Scharlach et al., 2007). These caregivers are more likely to use caregiver support services and hire paid caregivers to fill in possible gaps. This type of caregiving also leads to fragmentation of services and may prove a frustrating mix for an older adult with dementia (Levine et al., 2009).

The age of a caregiver offers important information into who provides care and to whom. Table 79.1 provides a visual comparison of the age of caregivers and the percentage of care delivered (National Alliance for Caregiving, 2012). While those 49 years of age and younger provide most care, 24% of care is provided by those older than 65.

Table 79.2 is derived from the National Alliance for Caregiving and AARP (2012). Care to adults older than 75 years accounted for 44% of all care.

While there are informal care needs across all demographic groups, 80% of all healthcare dollars spent on caregiving and supporting caregivers is devoted to older adults (Kaye et al., 2010). The increase in governmental support and transition away from skilled nursing and long-term care facilities will result in a rise in federal and state dollars devoted toward keeping informal and family networks in place. Current health policy shifts costs from expensive settings like skilled nursing facilities (SNFs) to more home-like settings with a focus on the individual and their family.

INFORMAL NETWORKS

As primary elements of the invisible elder caregiver network, family members are faced with determining living

Table 79.1 Age of informal caregivers	
Age of Caregivers	**Percentage of Care Delivered**
18–49 years	51% of all care
50–64 years	25% of all care
65+ years	24% of all care

Table 79.2 Recipients of informal care	
Percentage of Care Delivered	**Age of Recipient**
44% of care delivered	Age 75 and older
56% of care delivered	Under age 75
28% of care delivered	Under age 50

Table 79.3 **Trends in caregiver living arrangements, 2004–2009**		
	2009	2004
Lives alone	43%	47%
Lives with spouse	27%	26%
Lives with grown children	13%	11%
Lives with someone else	1%	1%

Source: National Alliance for Caregiving and AARP, 2012.

Table 79.4 **Faith-based care**	
Essential Aspect	**Purpose**
Assessment	Provides information for determining effective ministry
Networking	Determine avenues and resources that may be most effective to meet the needs of an older adult
Nurturing	Provide a direct response to the care needs of individual older adults
Advocacy	Accept responsibility to speak for older adults in basic needs, economic concerns, healthcare, housing and legal assistance
Ministry	Provide prayer and fellowship in time of need

Source: Heasty and Lakatos, 1998.

arrangements, and bear responsibility for most elder care decisions (Kane et al., 2006). Financial considerations, including a desire to preserve wealth, often results in elders receiving care at home (Chandra et al., 2006). Most care recipients receive care in their own home, while 20% receive care in the home of their caregiver (usually a child) (Gallup, 2011).

Table 79.3 examines living arrangements for caregivers and older adults. The table compares findings from 2004 and 2009, revealing that fewer older adults live alone; more are living with a spouse or with grown children.

Friends are the second group of informal caregivers. Lifelong acquaintances or neighbors often find their simple acts of kindness turn into ongoing, often reluctant caregiver roles. Shoveling snow may turn into routine home maintenance, transportation, medical advocacy and serving as a communication conduit with the family. It is difficult for these Good Samaritans to limit or terminate their services.

Egging et al. (2011) studied the phenomenon of friends and neighbor-caregivers for older adults. Nine percent of those providing care to an older adult are considered friends, while another 9% are neighbors living within walking distance of the older adult's home. Friends and neighbors tend to provide a lower level of care delivery than family members. However, they report a high level of stress and feelings of guilt if they plan to be away or need to disrupt their care routines (Egging et al., 2011). This important group of caregivers needs to be recognized in any policy discussion that centers on informal networks of caregiving.

The third variable, faith-based care, has less of a role than family and friends. Faith is important to many older adults. About 35% of all religious memberships are made up of older adults. Half or more of clergy are elderly (Heasty & Lakatos, 1998). Faith-based caregiving provides a level of spiritual and physical care that is comforting for many older adults. Table 79.4 provides information on faith-based elder care.

The integration of medical care delivery in faith-based organizations is characterized by the rising trend of parish nursing, particularly in the United States of America. More than 15 000 registered nurses report involvement in parish nursing (Nursing World, 2012), and faith community nursing (FCN) is now recognized as a specialty practice for registered nurses.

Parish nurses do not generally provide medical care to older adults beyond screenings offered at no charge at church or during home visits. Parish nurses attempt

to coordinate services for older adults and work with families to help find resources. The varied roles of a parish nurse include: serving as health advisor, screener and educator; visiting a church member at home, in the hospital, or in a care facility; making referrals to community resources and providing assistance in receiving services; and developing support groups (Nursing World, 2012).

The informal caregiver network is faced with multiple conflicting issues. In the case of spouses, friends and some faith providers, the caregiver is often at least as old as the person requiring help (National Alliance for Caregiving, 2012). These people are often ill-equipped to deal with comorbid conditions of aging elders. This informal network begins to fail when chronic illnesses progress and difficult behaviors arise causing a frail older adult to wear out their caregivers and begin to outlive their own assets. Such is the testament for many admissions to skilled nursing facilities and the growing need for Medicaid dollars to pay for this care (Kaye et al., 2010).

As part of the clinical team treating frail older adults, physical and occupational therapists must be cognizant of each elder patient's care network. Therapists need to monitor and assess the wellbeing of the caregivers for their older patients. Often the overwhelming burden of caregiving places a risk on the caregiver becoming a patient, too.

Caregivers and care recipients share a unique relationship with complex emotions, experiences and memories. This relationship and responsibility places caregivers at high risk for developing disorders such as anxiety and depression, which may contribute to hostility toward, and even abuse of, the difficult or demented elder. Furthermore, the risk for caregivers developing their own physically debilitating symptoms increases with increased caregiver burden (Alzheimer's Association, 2011).

DEMOGRAPHICS OF CAREGIVING

Ethnicity

The graying demographic is found in all industrialized nations. Like the rest of the world, the US is faced with cultural differences in caregiving for older adults.

Rates of caregiving do vary according to ethnicity. Among Americans who provide informal care to others, 72% are white, 13% black, 12% Hispanic and 2% are Asian-Americans (National Alliance for Caregiving, 2012). Asian-Americans constitute the fastest growing minority group, and have the highest longevity (Young et al., 2002).

LGBT

In a 2010 study of caregiving characteristics among the lesbian–gay–bisexual–transsexual (LGBT) community, caregiving was nearly equal between genders. In this group, 22% of women and 20% of men report providing care to another adult on an ongoing basis. However, LGBT men report far more hours in caregiving than do men in the general population. LBGT men provide an average of 41 hours of care per week compared to 29 hours per week for men generally (Metlife, 2010).

SOCIETAL VIEWPOINTS

Societal pressures and the stigma of placing relatives or friends in skilled nursing or long-term care facilities place great pressure on informal caregivers to provide care to elders in home and community settings. There is a general belief that all senior citizens desire to grow old and eventually die in their life-long home. This, like most stereotypes, is not accurate for all persons (Smith & Feng, 2010).

When family caregivers turn to professionals for recommendations, the results are varied. Kane et al. (2006) pointed out that many professionals will direct families toward the type of care that the professional is most familiar with. The actual recommendation may have little to do with what would be the best option for the elder patient.

Families are increasingly faced with caregiver concerns for their elderly relatives. About 3.4% of the American public resides in a skilled nursing facility at any one time; another 3–4% reside in assisted living facilities, while 5–8% receive care through home and community based services (HCBS) (University of Maryland, 2005; AHCA, 2012).

The 1999 passage of the National Family Caregiver Support Program acknowledged the prominent public policy issue associated with aging, long-term care and informal caregivers (Administration on Aging n.d.). This legislation laid the groundwork for HCBS programs that focused funding needs on the frail elders, but ignored the needs of the caregivers.

HCBS put a face on the invisible caregiver network. The mission of HCBS is to keep elderly in their own homes and communities for as long as possible. HCBS are designed to decrease institutionalization. This legislation was the main force credited with the closure of nursing homes in favor of community alternatives.

A positive outcome of HCBS type care is monetary support for caregivers. Funding is now available to pay people who provide care, including families (Brown & Finkelstein, 2011). There are restrictions on who may be paid for what services, e.g. a spouse cannot be paid for providing ADL support, while a daughter may

be reimbursed. Many caregivers would provide care whether paid or not.

Families face difficult pressures. With child-bearing occurring later in life, many dual-income, middle-age couples have school-age children at home. Further, these couples often have their own 70+ -age parents and their 90+ -age grandparents to worry about (Finkelstein et al., 2012). The stress of caregiving for the elderly falls squarely on the busiest of people in American society.

Current baby boomers are the major informal caregivers in the US. However, as this population ages, these same people may move into a role of requiring care. Finkelstein (2012) investigated the association between current caregiver status and planning for one's own long-term care needs. The study found that, while caregivers are more likely to anticipate needing services in the future, they are not currently taking specific planning actions. Further, baby boomer caregivers expect that they will receive their own future elder care in their own homes, rather than in institutions.

CLINICIANS' VIEWPOINTS

Elder-care clinicians recognize families as decision makers and short-term caregivers following acute incidents. However, the incidence of multiple comorbidities in elder family members increases responsibilities beyond most expectations.

Minnesota has examined this phenomenon. The 2005 report to the legislature completed by the Department of Human Services found that one in four adults in Minnesota were involved in some level of caregiving for older relatives. The dollar value of informal care far outweighs other sources of funding spent caring for Minnesota elders. This longitudinal study found that $6.84 billion was spent in 2004 for all care provided to Minnesota seniors. Medicare accounted for 7% of expenditures; Medicaid and other state programs 13%; out-of-pocket 11%; private insurance 1%; with 67% provided through informal care (MN DHS, 2005; Blumenstock, 2006).

COGNITION AS THE DECISION DRIVER

One of the most difficult issues for all caregivers is cognitive decline in their elder patients, notably, Alzheimer's disease (Alzheimer's Association, 2011). Families often find themselves trying to sort through a dizzying array of services and placements provided by mismatched and awkward systems.

THE MULTIPLE ROLES OF THE CAREGIVER

Caregivers have many roles to perform in supporting aging patients. Some have no idea how to help older adults reach maximal rehabilitation potential. A caregiver, for example, may view exercise as too hard, time consuming, or unnecessary. These caregivers may also do things that the older adult may be able to do independently.

Physical and occupational therapists involved with older adults and their caregivers need to patiently discuss rehabilitation plans and goals with both parties. The caregiver needs to know the value of therapy and improved independence for the older adult. The therapist may need to be direct in pointing out the harm of too much assistance from the caregiver in achieving meaningful functional gains for the older adult.

The following are descriptions of several of the roles that a caregiver may assume.

MEDICAL ADVOCATE

Advocating for appropriate medical care is one of the first roles that an informal caregiver assumes. Caregivers begin this process through their role in patient transport, including bringing frail older adults to appointments, assisting in providing an oral history and accurately conveying the current abilities of their loved ones. Caregivers may even bear the burden for care-related decisions, including treatments implemented and even end-of-life decision making (Finkelstein et al., 2012).

Caregivers become increasingly responsible for making medical decisions as their elder patients' physical and cognitive status deteriorate. For these reasons, it is very important for caregivers to fully understand the nature of chronic, debilitating conditions and treatment approaches, benefits, limitations, side-effects and alternatives. Since caregiving may be anywhere from 2 to 20 or more years, this is a long-term partnership that requires mutual respect between caregiver and patient.

Difficulties and disagreements often arise as caregivers assume this role. Children or others may have power of attorney or be legally appointed healthcare guardians; however, daily care decisions may be made by others, including onsite caregivers.

CLINICAL PARTNER

In order for a frail older adult to achieve optimal rehabilitation potential, the caregiver needs to be seen as a clinical partner. Caregivers need to have realistic expectations about what benefits can be realized and how they contribute to their success or failure. If the caregiver does not fully understand and support the treatment plan, an older adult's progress may suffer.

Therapists must effectively communicate with caregivers to ensure that care regimens comport with the needs and abilities of older adults and their caregivers. Overzealous treatment programs or too many exercises may result in failure for all involved. Focus on function, mobility and recognition of what life is like in the home setting will help each therapist to realistically assist the caregiver to be a clinical partner.

PERSONAL CARE ATTENDANT

One of the most difficult tasks for caregivers is providing ADL support. Bathing and grooming may be delegated to caregivers who are ill-equipped to deal with another's personal needs. Incontinence problems are disdainful to deal with, and are often a leading driver toward institutionalization. Feeding assistance and meal preparation are also burdensome tasks for many caregivers.

Forty-six percent of family caregivers perform medical tasks, while 96% provide ADL support (Gallup, 2011). Personal hygiene, grooming and transport in and out of bed are the tasks most often performed. Instrumental activities of daily living (IADL) center around providing vehicle transportation and grocery shopping (Gallup, 2011).

GUARDIAN

Caregivers often take on the responsibility of preventing harm to a frail, older adult. 'Parenting the parent' is a term often used to describe this phenomenon. Guardian duties involve graded responsibility, depending on the cognitive and physical abilities of the elder patient.

Therapists should assist families in accessing alternate sources of care and respite. Community resources may be utilized to relieve some of this burden; elder visiting networks may also provide necessary companionship for home-bound elders.

CHIEF COOK AND BOTTLE WASHER

A sudden acute illness causes most people to rush to the aid of ill or injured persons, bringing in food and offering household help. Unfortunately, the rush quickly turns to a trickle with a few or just one left to fill in the gaps of services required to run a home. For a married couple, it is the spouse that takes on most duties the two previously shared (National Alliance for Caregiving, 2012). In the case of a widow or widower, children step-in as long as possible, often supported by life-long family friends, including the faith-based community. Recognizing the long-term nature of this role early may help caregivers to plan in advance how this role is to be filled. Most communities have services that may be accessed for meals, house maintenance and yard work. Relinquishing these tasks to formal, paid or unpaid community providers may help manage caregivers' burdens.

THE STAGES OF CAREGIVING

Caregiving may be viewed as a linear process beginning from the insidious start of dependency through greater involvement to the eventual demise of the elder. Pfeiffer (2005) identified seven distinct states of caregiving, as outlined below:

Stage 1 Coping with initial impact
Stage 2 Deciding whether a family member can take on a caregiver role
Stage 3 At-home care giving
Stage 4 Considering residential placement
Stage 5 Caregiving during residential placement
Stage 6 Death of the patient – grief and relief
Stage 7 Resuming life – healing and renewal.

These seven stages are important for therapists and caregivers to understand. Though Pfeiffer applied much of this research to Alzheimer's patients, it is an applicable model for caregivers in varied settings. Each stage describes a new responsibility for caregivers and legitimizes the multiple, conflicting emotions felt at each stage. Keep in mind that not all people will neatly progress through stages, nor do staging systems always accurately describe the process for all.

CAREGIVER RECOGNITION

Caregivers need to be recognized as an integral component of successful patient rehabilitation and achievement of optimal quality of life. Therapists need to fully understand the breadth and depth of the care delivery system, noting particularly that most care is delivered outside the medical arena. Health professionals must analyze each patient and their networks individually, before determining how best to integrate rehab programs.

Each patient is an individual, as are their caregivers. No system, no matter how well developed or planned, can precisely address individual needs. In the drive to do the right thing, empathy toward the caregivers needs to become a core value for health professionals treating elder patients.

REFERENCES

Administration on Aging (n.d.) National Family Support Giver Program. OAA Title IIIE. Available at: www.aoa.gov/aoa_programs/hcltc/caregiver/index.aspx. Accessed December 2013

AHCA (American Health Care Association) 2012 Trends in nursing facility characteristics. American Health Care Association Reimbursement and Research Department. Available at: www.ahcancal.org/research_data/trends_statistics/Documents/Trend_PVNF_FINALRPT_December2012.pdf. Accessed December 2013

Alzheimer's Association 2011 Alzheimer's disease facts and figures. Alzheimer's Dement 7(2):3–34

Andrus D 2011 Value of unpaid caregivers. AARP report. Available at: www.advisorone.com/2011/07/22/aarp-value-of-unpaid-caregivers-worth-450-billion. Accessed December 2013

Blumenstock C 2006 Baby boomers are reinventing long term care. Nurs Homes: Long Term Care Manage 55(11):22–54

Brown J, Finkelstein A 2011 Insuring long term care in the United States. Natl Bur Econ Res 25(4):119–142

Chandra A, Smith LA, Paul DP 2006 What do consumers and healthcare provides in West Virginia think of long term care? Hosp Top 84(3):33–38

Coughlin J 2010 Estimating the impact of caregiving and employment on well being. Outcomes Insights Health Manage 2(1):41085. Available at: www.healthways.com/success/library.aspx?id=615. Accessed December 2013

Egging S, de Boer AH, Stevens NL 2011 Caring friends and neighbors as informal caregivers of older adults. Dutch J Gerontol 42(6):243–255

Family Caregiver Alliance 2011 The State of the States in Family Caregiver Support: A 50-State Survey. Family Caregiver Alliance, Washington, DC

Finkelstein E, Reid M, Kleppinger A et al 2012 Are baby boomers who care for their older parents planning for their own future long term care needs? J Aging Soc Policy 24(1):29–45

Gallup 2011 Most Caregivers Look after Elderly Parent. Gallup Healthways Wellbeing Survey. Available at: www.gallup.com/poll/148682/caregivers-look-elderly-parent-invest-lot-time.aspx. Accessed January 2014

Heasty D, Lakatos R 1998 Faith Based Caregiving. All for Seniors. Striped Rock Publications. Available at: www.stripedrock.org/all_for_seniors/pdf/articles/FaithBased_Caregiving.pdf. Accessed December 2013

Kane RL, Bershadsky B, Bershadsky J 2006 Who recommends long term care matters? Gerontologist 46(4):474–482

Kaye S, Harrington C, LaPlante M 2010 Long term care: who gets it, who provides it, who pays, and how much? Health Aff 29(1):11–21

Levine C, Halper D, Peist A et al 2009 Bridging troubled waters: family caregivers, transitions, and long term care. Health Aff 29(1):116–124

Metlife 2010 Still out, still aging. Study of lesbian, gay, bisexual, and transgender baby boomers. Available at: www.metlife.com/assets/cao/mmi/publications/studies/2010/mmi-still-out-still-aging.pdf. Accessed December 2013

MN DHS (Minnesota Department of Human Services) 2005 Financing long-term care for Minnesota's baby boomers. A report to the Minnesota Legislature. [Online] Available at: www.dhs.state.mn.us/main/groups/aging/documents/pub/dhs_id_025734.hcsp. Accessed December 2013

National Alliance for Caregiving and AARP 2012 Caregiving in the US. National Alliance for Caregiving, Washington, DC. Available at: www.caregiver.org/caregiver/jsp/content_node.jsp?nodeid=439. Accessed December 2013

Nursing World 2012 Parish nursing. Available at: www.nursingworld.org/MainMenuCategories/ANAMarketplace/ANAPeriodicals/OJIN/TableofContents/Volume82003/No2May2003/CarePlanning forBaby-Boomers.html. Accessed January 2014

Pfeiffer EA 2005 Caring for the caregiver. Available at: http://www.medscape.com/viewarticle/465785_22

Scharlach AE, Gustavson K, Santo TD 2007 Assistance received by employed caregivers and their care recipients: who helps care recipients when caregivers work full time? Gerontologist 47(6):752–756

Smith DB, Feng Z 2010 The accumulated challenges of long term care. Health Aff 29(1):29–34

University of Maryland 2005 Partnership for long-term care. [Online] Available at: www.hhp.umd.edu/AGING/index.html. Accessed 2007

Young H, McCormick W, Vitaliano P 2002 Evolving values in community-based long term care services for Japanese Americans. Adv Nurs Sci 25(2):40–56

Chapter 80

Interdisciplinary geriatric assessment

CHRISTI STEWART • MICHAEL L. MORAN • TIMOTHY L. KAUFFMAN

CHAPTER CONTENTS

INTRODUCTION

Many approaches to the care of the geriatric patient have been lumped under the rubric of 'geriatric assessment'. Indeed, in terms of process and outcome, geriatric assessment is one of the most widely studied aspects of geriatric healthcare. By 2013, there were thousands of published reports on geriatric assessment and numerous meta-analyses had been performed.

The American Geriatrics Society (AGS) Core Writing Group of the Task Force on the Future of Geriatric Medicine has outlined a series of core attributes and competencies for geriatric medicine (Besdine et al., 2005). These include 'coordinated care that includes communication among providers' and 'interdisciplinary team care with shared responsibility for patient care processes and outcomes'. The goal of this chapter is to examine the philosophical underpinnings of the interdisciplinary approach to geriatric medicine and to examine some of the models of how geriatric assessment has been operationalized and to point out some of the weaknesses and future directions of research for this model of healthcare.

PHILOSOPHICAL UNDERPINNINGS OF GERIATRIC ASSESSMENT

SECONDARY AGING MUST BE DISTINGUISHED FROM PRIMARY AGING

Physiologists often divide aging into two categories – primary or physiological aging and secondary or pathological aging. Primary aging includes those physiological changes that can be ascribed solely to the passage of time. Several theories have been set forth to explain the changes caused by primary aging. These include denaturation of proteins through cross-linking, cumulative damage from free radicals, a programmed decline in immune function and an internal biological clock that is genetically determined. This last theory gained credibility from cross-species studies that related longevity to the number of cell doublings that could occur in cell culture. The number of cell doublings proved to be species-specific and varied directly with the longevity of the species. (See Chapter 1 for additional information about theories of aging.)

Secondary aging involves those decrements in function that can be ascribed to disease processes. Primary and secondary aging are sometimes difficult to distinguish from each other. For example, it was once thought that there was a substantive decline in cardiac output that was age related and due to primary aging. However, it has been discovered that the aging heart has no significant alteration of heart rate, stroke volume, or cardiac output (Sebastian & Pfeifer, 2007).

Likewise, in the era before autopsy studies had been done upon people with dementia, it was believed that dementia was simply a primary process of the senium rather than secondary aging. Autopsy series later disclosed that cognitive losses could be explained by specific pathologies such as multiple strokes or the senile plaques and neurofibrillary tangles of Alzheimer's disease. It is now known that, even though the speed of effortful mental processing slows with aging due to cortical atrophy, in the absence of disease, cognition remains well preserved (Weaver et al., 2006).

How do these principles relate to geriatric assessment? It is the role of geriatric assessment to tease out the effects of secondary aging and to reverse them through specific treatments, to ameliorate them through interventions that may improve, although not cure, the underlying condition or to assist the patient to function better by enlisting support services or altering the patient's environment to make that environment more conducive to the patient's needs.

COEXISTENCE OF MULTIPLE DISEASES AND THE CASCADE OF ILLNESS

When clinicians are first trained in medicine, they are commonly taught to think in terms of the 'chief complaint'. This approach proves to be much too restrictive in the practice of geriatric medicine. Here, the most common scenario is one of multiple, coexisting pathologies that are all conspiring to harm the patient's functional ability and that the patients themselves may find difficult to describe from a symptomatic perspective.

An example of the cascade effect of multiple problems might be the patient who presents with delirium. Such a change in mental status is a final common pathway for many medical and psychiatric conditions. In this example, the pathology might be traced back as follows: the patient has some moderate renal insufficiency and prostatic hypertrophy. The prostatic hypertrophy leads to urinary retention, which further worsens renal function, which leads to azotemia and anorexia, which leads to reduced fluid and nutritional intake, which leads to even further worsening of renal function and a relentless downward spiral. This example of the interrelationship of organ system function demonstrates a cascade of illness that affects many organs.

A challenge of geriatric assessment is to trace the cascade of events back to find key points in each patient's unique pathophysiology where treatment or addition of medical or support services may halt or reverse the downward spiral. Because of the complexity of this process, an interdisciplinary approach is often most successful. The National Institute of Aging defines a comprehensive geriatric assessment as a multidisciplinary evaluation in which the multiple problems of older persons are uncovered, described and explained, if possible, and where the resources and strengths of the person are catalogued, needs for services assessed and coordinated care plan developed to focus interventions on the person's problems.

AS ANY COHORT AGES, VARIABILITY INCREASES

Given the overlap of physiological and pathological aging, and the intrinsic difficulty of teasing one process apart from others for any given organ system, it is impossible to predict the physiological function of any individual based on age alone. One may speak of chronological age vs. physiological age. To speak of a young 80-year-old or an old 65-year-old does not sound like an oxymoron to the geriatric practitioner.

What can be predicted is that, as people age, they become less and less like each other. No two persons age identically. Some encounter diseases, others suffer traumatic injuries and others cope with both. Genetics and lifestyle choices add to the variability of aging individuals. With this complicated picture of aging in mind, the ACOVE (Assessing Care of the Vulnerable Elderly) guidelines developed in 2007 define the vulnerable elderly as anyone over 75 years old, and anyone aged 65–74 years old who is at greater risk of death or functional decline over a 2-year period. These guidelines also recommend that any vulnerable elderly person should receive the elements of a comprehensive geriatric assessment within 3 months (Wenger et al., 2007).

The increasing diversity that comes with age has a direct effect on geriatric assessment. For geriatric assessment to work well, it is crucial that both diagnostic and therapeutic approaches be individualized for each patient. Attempting a 'cookbook' approach to the solution of clinical problems in such a diverse group could easily lead to iatrogenic harm. The recent trend toward the creation and application of clinical pathways or protocols in the treatment of specific conditions must proceed carefully and contain greater flexibility when dealing with issues in geriatric medicine.

Again, the interdisciplinary approach, because of its greater clinical diversity, can better account for the pluralism of this unique population.

DIMINISHED HOMEOSTATIC RESERVE BLOCKS RECOVERY

Perhaps the best definition of aging is 'increasing susceptibility to the forces of mortality due to decreased homeostatic reserve'. Homeostasis concerns the body's ability to maintain itself in a steady state and to get itself back on track whenever there is perturbation from that steady state. Ability to maintain a constant temperature, constant blood pressure and constant blood glucose level are all examples of homeostasis.

When homeostatic reserves are constrained, there is diminished likelihood of survival with any extreme stress. A key principle in geriatric assessment is to recognize that homeostatic reserves are diminished and that patients are more sensitive to both the disease processes and the iatrogenic effects of intervention. This should lead to a more conservative and individualized approach in the application of therapeutic maneuvers and drug therapies.

These issues are especially important in geriatric rehabilitation. A common scenario is the elderly patient who has suffered a hip fracture and requires surgical repair. With postoperative pain and analgesia, the patient often suffers such setbacks as postoperative delirium, fever, anemia from blood loss, atelectasis and hypoxemia. Thus, the rehabilitation measures may be delayed for several days by intercurrent illness. While at bedrest, the older patient may be losing in the order of 11–12% of their muscle strength per week (English & Paddon-Jones, 2010) and 1–2% of aerobic capacity daily. Given that up to 70% of geriatric patients have poor muscle mass (sarcopenia) at baseline (Fiatarone, 2009), these losses become highly significant and make rehabilitation and recovery all the more difficult.

In this setting, the patient might not cope well physically or psychologically with the arduous exercise demands of rehabilitation. The twice-daily treatments of up to 4 hours imposed by government regulations for Medicare reimbursed rehabilitation may be too rigorous for some of these more frail individuals. Sometimes, rehabilitation must occur at a more gradual pace and in the long-term care setting.

DISEASES PRESENT IN AN ATYPICAL FASHION

Among geriatric patients, the common presentations of illness are often replaced by the less specific and more global findings of increased confusion, weakness, anorexia and tendency to fall. One sees such phenomena as 'silent myocardial infarction', 'afebrile pneumonia' and 'depression without sadness'. The first manifestation of urosepsis might be falling, or the presenting symptom of a myocardial infarction might be increased agitation. In geriatric assessment, the clinician must cast a wider net in attempting to make diagnoses.

Other diseases typically present only in the elderly or much more frequently in the elderly, and the index of suspicion for these problems must remain higher. These disorders include such entities as polymyalgia rheumatica, temporal arteritis and Parkinson's disease.

DISEASES ARE UNDERREPORTED

Geriatric patients commonly underreport their problems. Sometimes, cognitive impairment gets in the way of an accurate relating of historical information. Occasionally patients assume that their concerns, such as pain or incontinence, are a normal part of the aging process. They may also be fearful that their symptoms indicate a more ominous diagnosis, such as cancer, with unpleasant and costly treatment options. Older persons can also be concerned that their medical problems will lead to a loss of independence, and their reports may under-represent the impact these problems have on their overall functioning. At other times, depression may lead to a sense of hopelessness about the possibility of getting help.

Self-report questionnaires and structured assessment tools to measure cognition, affect and function can yield quite useful information if they are administered carefully by a trained individual and in a nonthreatening manner. These tools add additional important information to the historical database and are often included in a comprehensive geriatric assessment.

THE PROCESS OF GERIATRIC ASSESSMENT

To maximize benefit, the process of geriatric assessment involves an interdisciplinary approach. The most consistent team members that form the traditional core of this assessment process are the geriatrician or geriatric nurse practitioner, nurse and social worker. Ancillary team members have included the occupational therapist, physical therapist, psychiatrist or psychologist, nutritionist, speech therapist, exercise physiologist, recreational therapist and respiratory therapist. One of the very first outpatient assessment programs even employed an architect because of the frequency with which changes in the patient's home environment were being recommended.

The process of a comprehensive geriatric assessment involves making a diagnosis, weighing diagnostic and therapeutic options, monitoring health outcomes, prognostication, long-term care planning, maximizing function and wellbeing, and reduction of poor outcomes. It is a multidisciplinary, multidimensional assessment designed to evaluate functional ability, physical health, cognition and mental health, and socioenvironmental circumstances (Elsawy & Higgins, 2011). It can also include assessment of nutrition, hearing and vision, urinary and fecal continence, gait and falls risk, osteoporosis and polypharmacy.

The key components of a comprehensive geriatric assessment involve an initial determination of goals of the assessment by patients and family members, which can often help to elucidate concerns regarding functional or cognitive incapacities and socioeconomic weaknesses. Then data are collected through collateral interviews with caregivers and family members and with patients to help with objective evidence to support and explain those concerns and help with diagnosis. Various cognitive and psychological testing is also done with patients at this time. In order to coordinate and implement the various recommendations of the separate professionals involved in the interdisciplinary approach, a team conference is typically held after the initial assessment. The care plan is crafted with input from the various team members. Often, a family conference is then held with the patient and all involved family members and caregivers. The purpose of this conference is to communicate with and educate the patient and caregivers, to make official recommendations, and to answer questions. It also provides yet another opportunity to assess for caregiver burden and to move to alleviate it if it is clinically significant.

Follow up remains essential to ensuring the success of the recommendations made at the initial visit. The follow up plan for patients will depend on the initial presentation, complexity of medical conditions and setting in which the initial assessment was performed. However, it is critical to assure there is a follow up plan so that patients and families can review test results with the provider, monitor response to therapy and revise the treatment plan if necessary. It is also important to ensure follow-up and accurate relay of information with appropriate specialists, such as neurologists, psychiatrists, physical and occupational therapists and community resources.

The interdisciplinary model of geriatric assessment has been applied to a variety of settings (Gill, 2010). The most common have been adult medical–surgical hospital wards, outpatient clinics, inpatient geropsychiatry units, nursing homes, rehabilitation hospitals and patient homes. There are also more complex models that involve many team members and are found in the inpatient and consultation models. In terms of traditionally measured outcomes (such as mortality, functional status, frequencies of hospitalization and nursing home placement), research study results are mixed. Because of the mixed models of geriatric assessment and differing sites of practice, meta-analyses and generalizations about the value of geriatric assessment are difficult. Nevertheless, some reviewers (Jouanny, 2005) have felt that the data are convincing in terms of reduction in mortality, lowered rates of nursing home placement and lowered levels of caregiver burden.

The Case Study of Mrs A (see Case Study), an example of the geriatric team in action, may help to illustrate many of the principles of geriatric assessment. This 85-year-old patient was suffering primarily from an illness (polymyalgia rheumatica) that is found exclusively in the elderly population. In the absence of any symptoms suggesting cranial arteritis, many clinicians would institute an empiric trial of corticosteroid therapy without doing a temporal artery biopsy and gauge the response to therapy. A dramatic response, as was seen in this case, helps to confirm the diagnosis.

The next most important problems, those of the cognitive impairment and dysphoria, reveal how multiple coexisting pathologies can conspire to create dysfunction.

The suddenness of the onset of the patient's delusions and cognitive decline suggested either a vascular process or a reaction to the anticholinergic effects of amitriptyline. The low cobalamin level is also a common finding and could also be contributing to the cognitive loss. In many instances of geriatric assessment the caregiver becomes as much a client as the patient. Predictable respite is one effective means of reducing caregiver stress, and referral of the patient to an adult daycare program is an ideal way to provide predictable respite. In this case, when alleviated of some of the caregiving burden, the daughter could once again enjoy her relationship with her mother.

The perception on the part of family members that the patient was functioning much better cognitively even though objective improvement could not be measured represents another phenomenon deserving of mention. Significant disparity between 'perceived' and 'measured' improvement often exists.

The benefits of the comprehensive geriatric assessment can also be demonstrated through this case report. These include an opportunity to gather family/caregiver input and allowing those persons to feel heard in the difficult times as well as in the success of the treatment plan. It also allows the chance for interdisciplinary interaction and discussion regarding a patient, and provides an overall assessment, education and treatment plan to be identified in a short period of time, and provides support to a patient's primary care provider to allow comprehensive follow-up and continuation of the treatment plan through that provider.

DIRECTIONS FOR FUTURE RESEARCH

The technology of geriatric assessment has been under attack because it is viewed as labor-intensive and inadequately reimbursed. Were the data of research studies more conclusive with regard to outcomes, it would be easier to advocate the widespread application of interdisciplinary geriatric assessment. The main challenge in the light of what has been learned seems to be selective application of this interdisciplinary approach, targeting those subjects and contexts in which geriatric assessment is determined to be cost-effective.

Other areas of active research in this field include investigation into the optimal place to perform geriatric assessment. Some intriguing studies suggest that the optimal site may be in the patient's own home (Nikolaus & Bach, 2003). Other important questions also have to be answered. Do data that have been collected largely through interview reflect what the patient is actually able to perform? Do data on functional status, which are often garnered by physical therapy and occupational therapy in a laboratory setting, correlate well with what the patient can do in his or her own home?

CASE STUDY

MRS A

Mrs A was an 85-year-old widowed woman who was living with and being cared for by her 54-year-old daughter. She was referred by her daughter for outpatient geriatric assessment. The patient had been suffering from gradual and progressive memory loss for the preceding 3 years. Three weeks previously, she had become more apathetic and withdrawn, and had ceased to be able to climb the stairs because of arthritic complaints. On intake, she was being treated with amitriptyline 25 mg at night for depression.

On further questioning it was learned that the patient was becoming delusional, believing that people on the television screen were real. Her functional status a month earlier had been much better and her incontinence was new. She complained of a feeling of profound weakness. The social worker learned that the daughter was extremely resentful that the caregiving burden had fallen to her and was not being shared by her two siblings. She felt guilty about her resentment, and this made her caregiving even more difficult.

Medical workup disclosed moderate degenerative joint changes, moderate hearing loss and dysphoric mood. The patient made seven depressive responses on the Geriatric Depression Scale and scored 20/30 on the Folstein Mini-Mental Examination. She remembered zero out of three objects on early recall. Mobility testing showed profound weakness, with difficulty arising from the examination chair and broadening of the support base. Screening laboratory tests showed a mild anemia with a hemoglobin of 11.3 g/dl and a mean corpuscular volume (MCV) of 81. The serum cobalamin level was low normal at 200 pg/ml. The sedimentation rate was markedly elevated at 110 mm/h. Other blood parameters were normal. A magnetic resonance imaging (MRI) scan showed periventricular hyperintensity and multiple lacunae. Soon after the initial assessment, the patient was begun on 15 mg of prednisone daily for a presumptive diagnosis of polymyalgia rheumatica. In addition, she was begun on cobalamin injections. The amitriptyline was discontinued.

When the patient was returned to the clinic for a family conference, her mobility had improved dramatically, as had her pain symptoms. The incontinence had resolved because the patient was now mobile enough to get to the bathroom. The delusions had also disappeared, but the patient remained dysphoric. The family was educated and counseled about the spectrum of the patient's problems. It was pointed out that her cognitive loss might not be due to Alzheimer's disease, as she had been told previously, and that the prognosis was uncertain. It was decided to continue to monitor the patient's mood for another month and to consider treating her with one of the newer selective serotonin uptake inhibitors if her mood remained depressed. The patient was referred to an adult daycare program. She began to attend 3 days per week.

Six months later, the patient was being maintained on 5 mg of prednisone daily. Her mobility remained good and the sedimentation rate was 26 mm/h. The patient had been started on sertraline 50 mg daily, and her mood had improved. The hemoglobin had risen to 13.0 g/dl. She was still occasionally delusional and the score on the Mini-Mental examination had not improved. The patient's daughter, however, was feeling greatly relieved, and she perceived her mother to be functioning at a much higher level of cognition, even though this could not be objectively demonstrated. The daughter was planning to have her mother enter a 1-week respite program while the family went on a week-long vacation.

The development of critical pathways, or clinical algorithms, is a process that is being repeated at virtually every acute care hospital in an effort to standardize care and reduce costs. As healthcare systems become globalized to include the entire continuum, these pathways must become more extended. They will cease to be disease- or organ-specific and, rather, will evolve into a 'syndromic' approach. To work effectively, these pathways must take into account the various principles of geriatric assessment that have been under discussion. The effects of the application of such pathways on outcomes have been positive (Smyth, 2001; Endo et al., 2004).

Many other important questions about the approach to treating the geriatric patient must be addressed. Some of these are the following: How stable are people's advance directives and how can we improve the process of prognostication and helping people to develop plans for end of life? Do these plans change when patients are more immediately confronted with life-threatening situations and the issues are more immediate and less abstract than when the directive was originally formulated? How valuable are exercise prescriptions in later life? What are some of the long-term effects of nutrition on health? Are there ways to ameliorate the effects of bedrest deconditioning and the development of delirium that so often add to the morbidity of hospitalization of geriatric patients? Is there a role for anticipatory conditioning prior to elective hospitalizations or procedures (so-called prehabilitation)?

CONCLUSION

It remains for the upcoming generation of researchers and practitioners to improve the knowledge base and give good health and meaning to the later stages of people's lives. Not enough students are entering this important field, yet it can be among the most rewarding and challenging of endeavors.

To recapitulate the previous clinical scenario of the 85-year-old woman with both physical and cognitive impairments, recall that the patient's subjective improvement vastly surpassed what could be measured objectively. When a patient is marginally compensated and just barely able to get by, then slight improvements in condition are often perceived as dramatic, even when the degree of improvement can scarcely be measured by our crude assessment tools. This magnified effect of intervention on the patient's and family's perceptions of health and well-being can be one of the most gratifying aspects of serving a frail geriatric population.

It is hoped that the information in this book will help to enable accomplishment of the AGS Task Force goals for geriatric medicine. They include: (i) 'continuity and seamlessness across all sites and providers' and (ii) 'appropriateness of care within the context of the goals of the individual patient and the values of society'. But to achieve this, new models must be developed for healthcare delivery, especially in the United States of America, which is largely determined by the Medicare system. In this system, benefits are not uniform and obstacles exist within the fee-for-service model that encourages payment for units of care but not for case/disease management (Besdine et al., 2005).

Acknowledgment

David C. Martin and Margaret Basiliadis wrote this chapter in the first edition.

REFERENCES

Besdine R, Boult C, Brangman 2005 Caring for older Americans: the future of geriatric medicine. J Am Geriatr Soc 53(Suppl 6):S245–S256
Elsawy B, Higgins K 2011 The geriatric assessment. Am Fam Phys 83(1):48–56
Endo H, Nippon R, Igakkai Z 2004 Comprehensive geriatric medicine. Jap J Geriatr 41(4):375–377
English K, Paddon-Jones D 2010 Protecting muscle mass and function in older adults during bedrest. Curr Opin Clin Nutr Metab Care 13(1):34–39
Fiatarone S 2009 Methodology and baseline characteristics for the SHIP study. J Gerontol A Biol Sci Med Sci 64(5):568–574
Gill TM 2010 Assessment. In: Pacala JT, Sullivan GM (eds) Geriatrics Review Syllabus: A Core Curriculum in Geriatric Medicine, 7th edn. American Geriatrics Society, New York, ch 6
Jouanny P 2005 Pharmacological treatment in severe dementia. Psychol Neuropsychiat Vieill 3(Suppl 1):S51–S55
Nikolaus T, Bach M 2003 Preventing falls in community dwelling frail older people using a home intervention team (HIT): results from the randomized falls-HIT trial. J Am Geriatr Soc 51(3):300–305
Reuben DB, Rosen S 2009 Principles of geriatric assessment. In: Halter JB, Ouslander JG, Tinetti M (eds) Hazzard's Geriatric Medicine and Gerontology, 6th edn. McGraw-Hill, New York, ch 11
Sebastian JL, Pfeifer KJ 2007 Cardiac disorders. In: Duthie Jr EH, Katz PR, Malone ML (eds) Practice of Geriatrics, 4th edn. Elsevier Saunders, Philadelphia, PA, ch 31
Smyth C 2001 Creating order out of chaos: models of GNP practice with hospitalized older adults. Clin Excellence Nurse Pract Int J NPACE 5(2):88–95
Weaver CJ, Maruff P, Collie A et al 2006 Mild memory impairment in healthy older adults is distinct from normal aging. Brain Cognition 60(2):146–155
Wenger N, Roth C, Shekelle P 2007 Introduction to the Assessing Care of Vulnerable Elders-3 Quality Indicator Measurement Set. J Am Geriatr Soc 55(s2):s247–s252

Chapter 81

Gerontological and geriatric nursing

BRENDA L. HAGE

Chapter Contents

INTRODUCTION

The nursing profession has a long history of providing healthcare to sick older people. Initially, geriatric nursing focused on physical care, comfort measures and palliation. The care was often given almost entirely by nurses and their assistants in nursing homes or in people's own homes. As knowledge, technology, public policy and societal expectations changed, the scope, types of geriatric services and quality of nursing care also changed. The establishment of the first formal standards for nursing care for older adults, adopted in 1970 by the American Nurses Association (ANA), was a landmark initiative for nurses in geriatrics. It provided a link to nursing science, which is defined by the ANA as the deliberate problem-solving process, grounded in the biopsychosocial sciences, of diagnosing and treating actual or potential health problems (American Nurses Association, 1970).

As these practice standards were reviewed and modified over time, patient-centered care, family participation and nursing services related to the prevention of disease and disability and the promotion of good health for older adults were articulated more explicitly as major components of geriatric nursing practice. This paved the way for the use of the term 'gerontological nursing' to refer to a domain in the continuum of the science and practice of nursing that is devoted to the complex care of older people and their families and to balancing the effects of normal aging and pathology. Today, the term 'geriatric nursing' indicates specialized clinical care for the health problems of the elderly in various interdisciplinary patient-care settings. Nurses with advanced training who practice in this area are known as primary care or acute care adult/gerontologic nurse practitioners or gerontologic clinical nurse specialists.

An overall goal for gerontological and geriatric nursing is to provide humanistic healthcare to older adults and their families by paying careful attention to individual circumstances, needs and goals. Preventing impairment, restoring function and maintaining an enduring state of health and wellbeing are embedded in these goals. A key strategy that is used to meet these goals is the application of the nursing process that consists of assessment, planning, intervention and evaluation within the context of healthcare issues presented by the elder and their family.

Gerontological and geriatric nurses have critical roles in the collaboration of the healthcare team, as they must be involved in planning, implementing and evaluating patient care. The nurses' roles and functions include nursing management and other therapeutic activities for direct patient care, case management, patient and family health education and counseling, administration, advocacy, public policy development and education and research.

DIRECT PATIENT CARE

To ensure seamless care, continuous leadership and accountability are necessary. Professional nurses act on these responsibilities in acute care units, ambulatory care clinics, long-term care facilities, homecare agencies and other sites where the need for geriatric care can be fulfilled.

At least three different types of nursing expertise, using different levels of critical thinking and clinical decision-making skills, are available to older patients to assist them in meeting their healthcare needs:

1. Registered nurses have clinical, technical and humanistic skill in one-to-one interaction so they can strengthen and support the biopsychosocial processes of recovery, rehabilitation, healing, preventing disease and disability, and death with dignity. Nurses functioning in this role practice in acute care settings, skilled nursing facilities, home health settings and hospices, and a smaller number practice in ambulatory care

clinics or doctors' offices. Licensed vocational or practical nurses may also work in these settings under the supervision of the registered nurse.

2. Advanced practice nursing roles in gerontological nursing primarily include clinical specialists and nurse practitioners. These master's degree or doctorally prepared nurses function in a variety of roles to support this challenging patient population:

A. Gerontologic clinical nurse specialists have expertise in working with complex nursing care problems and draw from their advanced skills in direct clinical care, critical analysis and decision-making, teaching, counseling, and coordination and follow-up of interdisciplinary care plans. They practice in acute and long-term care settings and may be consultants to community clinics and home-based geriatric care programs. They also have roles in organizational leadership, research, evaluation of program outcomes and coordination of quality improvement activities.

B. Gerontologic nurse practitioners have expertise in performing comprehensive physical examination and assessments, ordering and interpreting laboratory and diagnostic testing, differential medical diagnosis, and developing pharmacologic and non-pharmacologic management plans, and outcome evaluations for medical problems, in partnership with other team members. Primary care nurse practitioners provide services in ambulatory clinics, long-term care facilities, and adult day health programs while acute care nurse practitioners see patients in mostly inpatient settings. Crossover may occur between these settings and the primary care and acute nurse practitioner roles (National Organization of Nurse Practitioner Faculties, 2012).

THE NURSING PROCESS

The nursing process guides the registered nurse to individualize, contextualize and prioritize problem areas. The steps consist of assessment, nursing diagnosis, planning, intervention and evaluation.

STEP 1: ASSESSMENT

Biopsychosocial data about geriatric patients is collected by means of interviews, record reviews, direct observations and other approaches, as time allows, building a composite picture of the multiple and often competing needs of the geriatric patient and the informal caregiver. For example, the federally mandated multidisciplinary assessment called the Minimum Data Set is used in nursing homes by long-term care nurses to record assessment data as part of the team approach to care planning and treatment (Burke & Walsh, 1997). The Care Dependency Scale offers a framework for assessing the care needs of institutionalized patients for nursing care (Dijkstra et al., 2012).

STEP 2: DIAGNOSIS

Data from nursing assessments are necessary to identify problems in the order of clinical significance at a specific time and according to the urgent need for nursing interventions. The information may include general and specific data on the presenting problems as defined by the patient and the caregiver, medical diagnoses, prescribed medical treatments, status of physical and mental functions, alternate healthcare resources, patient goals and expectations, safety risks, self-care abilities for recovery, including the ability to perform activities of daily living, and other information that a nurse considers clinically relevant to the case or situation. Identifying nursing diagnoses and prioritizing these problem areas are the major intended process outcomes.

Since 1973, the North American Nursing Diagnosis Association (NANDA) has continued to develop a taxonomy of nursing diagnoses, and currently there are approximately 130 approved classifications of patient care problems in nine categories. In 1987, the Center for Nursing Classification and Clinical Effectiveness at the College of Nursing, University of Iowa (USA) developed taxonomies for classifying and organizing nursing interventions and nursing outcomes through the use of the Nursing Intervention Classification (NIC) (McCloskey Dochterman & Bulacheck, 2004). This was followed by the development of Nursing Outcomes Classification (NOC) coding systems in 1992 (Moorhead et al., 2004). The NIC/NOC codes are linked to the NANDA diagnoses and serve to document the effectiveness of nursing interventions and outcomes. Refinement of the NIC/NOC classification systems has been ongoing. The use of nursing taxonomies facilitates the capture of nursing data useful for evaluation, quality improvement and research activities.

STEP 3: PLANNING

The nursing care plan incorporates specific nursing interventions and activities to treat specific nursing diagnoses or deal with problem areas such as changes in food intake, impaired capacity for personal care, risk for accidental injuries due to general weakness and mild dementia, grief unrelated to the health problem and other needs of the geriatric patient and the caregiver. Included in the plan are nursing actions to ensure the continuity of all prescribed medical treatments and other intervention modalities for the geriatric patient. Clinical judgment is an important nursing skill in this process because it enables an accurate identification of the nursing diagnosis.

STEP 4: IMPLEMENTATION

The process of implementation utilizes the collective efforts of members of the nursing staff, including auxiliary nursing personnel, and directs them so that the nursing care plan can be carried out. Safe and compassionate approaches that are clinically and technically appropriate are used to achieve the desired clinical outcomes. Nursing actions may include activities such as checking vital signs, changing the position of an immobilized elderly patient, orienting an elder with a memory deficit to time, place and activity, interviewing a family caregiver prior to home care, consulting other healthcare professionals, advocating for an elder to obtain a local community resource, and other actions aimed at resolving a nursing problem or reducing the impact of a nursing diagnosis.

STEP 5: EVALUATION

A patient's physical, verbal and behavioral responses, informal caregivers' reports, and observations by healthcare providers from other disciplines are important aspects of the feedback mechanism that helps the nursing staff to maintain a dynamic, flexible care plan. Critical analysis of information obtained while nursing interventions are in progress may be used to modify nursing interventions, redirect patient and family participation in the overall treatment and management plan, reexamine the healthcare team's understanding of the clinical problem, determine cost benefits, realign leadership and support the standards of quality patient care.

CASE MANAGEMENT

The nurse case manager follows a group of elderly patients and informal caregivers. As a rule, frailty, multiple chronic illnesses, unstable functional status, complex psychosocial and financial situations, and other multilayered clinical issues trigger the need for this type of professional nurse. Advanced skills in clinical decision-making, communication, resource identification, referral, management, systems analysis, and cost analysis are essential for effective case management. The role of a nurse case manager involves consulting with healthcare providers; meeting with patients, family members and other support systems; advocating for need-specific health and social services; planning for discharge; ensuring safe termination of services; facilitating shared decision-making; and recording appropriate documentation. Case managers may also negotiate a change of health benefit with third party payers to ensure that the older patient's needs are being optimally addressed. As healthcare delivery systems change, the number of nurse case managers for older people is expected to increase, particularly in community-based programs such as home-based services, adult day health programs, and respite and hospice services. For example, in the home health arena, the nurse is the ideal team leader; in that role, the nurse can coordinate the case and facilitate the completion of required documentation by interdisciplinary care providers, institutions, physicians in group or private practice, and payers. With the growing trend toward managed care, the nurse in such a role might be called a case manager. Other administrative functions may also be a part of the geriatric nurse case manager's responsibility in the practice sites mentioned earlier.

HEALTH EDUCATION AND COUNSELING FOR PATIENTS AND FAMILIES

A major focus of the teaching and counseling done by gerontological and geriatric nurses relates to the implementation of treatment and management prescribed by healthcare providers in acute care, home care, or community care. Teaching patients before they are discharged to home or another site of care helps to prepare the patient and the family. Education in ways of preventing disease, disability and complications of existing chronic health conditions becomes increasingly necessary as the shift to community care expands. Teaching and counseling by these nurses take place across the continuum of care of the elderly. This function may be combined with direct patient care and case management functions.

ADMINISTRATION

Professional roles for administrative nurses include director of nursing services in a skilled-nursing facility and administrator in a variety of settings, such as home care, adult day health, respite care, hospice and other community care programs for older adults. Some nurse entrepreneurs take on the challenge of administering small board-and-care (i.e. personal care) homes. The legislative mandates of Medicare and Medicaid, regulations, and the standards of care, to name a few, are complex bodies of information that the geriatric nurse administrator is able to translate into practice in order to support quality standards of care and ensure fiscal responsibility.

ADVOCACY AND PUBLIC POLICY DEVELOPMENT

Although nurse activism is found among all types of practitioners of nursing, some nurses in gerontology and geriatrics build careers in advocacy dedicated to shaping and changing public policy. Their expertise in the legislative process and their analyses of public policies may be applied to issues related to healthcare access for the aging population and other relevant concerns. They find employment in governmental agencies, in the offices of public officials, with advocacy organizations, or with other entities oriented toward public policy issues and aging.

EDUCATION AND RESEARCH

With the increasing number of education programs in gerontological and geriatric nursing being taught in colleges and universities, the need for faculty members with doctoral and master's degrees in gerontology and geriatrics will continue to grow. Clinical nurse specialists, nurse practitioners and nursing educators predominate in the faculties of many nursing schools across the country. Gerontological and geriatric nurses with doctoral degrees typically have teaching and research responsibilities. Advanced practice nurse faculty members who are clinical nurse specialists or nurse practitioners are also required to maintain clinical practice in order to maintain role competency. Faculty members with research doctorates are prepared to function as principal investigators in research projects and clinical trials and to establish research programs in gerontological and geriatric nursing science. Knowledge generation is an important commitment of these nurse researchers. Some of the domains of nursing research are sleep disturbances, agitation, family caregiving, falling behavior, sensory disabilities, use of technology to support aging in place and self-care deficits. The body of knowledge produced by their studies contributes to improving healthcare for older people and to advancing the science of aging. In addition, these researchers create opportunities for other nurses to experience the research process as assistants, graduate students or participants in the study. Nurses with the practice doctorate (DNP) use this evidence-based nursing knowledge in practice change projects to improve nursing practice (American Association of Colleges of Nursing, 2006).

CONCLUSION

Gerontological and geriatric nurses have a variety of roles and functions. With the trend toward downsizing and the shift to managed care programs, these roles and functions are being fused and structured in different ways. New personnel who deliver direct bedside care but have limited formal education and training are being introduced into the clinical arena. The challenge to nursing, in particular to nurses in gerontology and geriatrics, is to maintain the standards of healthcare for older adults, especially those who are disempowered by chronic disability, socioeconomic status, racial or cultural factors, environmental situations, low health literacy or technological illiteracy and lack of technology access. Also, the aging of the baby boomers, a social and historical phenomenon, is already shifting the focus of healthcare from the curative model to the chronic care model. The high incidence of chronic disease in this population requires new approaches to assisting older adults in the development of self-management skills needed to effectively deal with these problems. It is clear that new expertise and more advance-practice nurses will be needed in this specialty.

REFERENCES

American Association of Colleges of Nursing 2006 The essentials of doctoral education for advanced nursing practice. AACN, Washington, DC

American Nurses Association 1970 Statement on gerontologic nursing practice. ANA, Washington, DC

Burke M, Walsh M et al (eds) 1997 Gerontologic Nursing: Holistic Care of the Older Adult. Mosby Year Book, St Louis, MO

Dijkstra A, Yont GH, Korhan EA et al 2012 The Care Dependency Scale for measuring basic human needs: an international comparison. Journal of Advanced Practice Nursing 68(10):2341–2348

McCloskey Dochterman J, Bulacheck GM et al (eds) 2004 Nursing Intervention Classification (NIC), 4th edn. Mosby, Philadelphia, PA

Moorhead S, Johnson M, Maas M et al (eds) 2004 Nursing Outcomes Classification (NOC), 3rd edn. Mosby, Philadelphia, PA

National Organization of Nurse Practitioner Faculties 2012 Statement on Acute Care and Primary Care Certified Nurse Practitioner Practice. Washington, DC

Chapter 82

Geriatric occupational therapy

MOLLY MIKA

INTRODUCTION

Occupation may be defined as any meaningful and purposeful activity or series of activities in which an individual engages. According to the occupational therapy practice framework of the American Occupational Therapy Association (AOTA), areas of occupation include activities of daily living (eating, dressing, toileting, etc.), instrumental activities of daily living (homemaking, meal preparation, money management, etc.), education, work, play, leisure and social participation (AOTA, 2002). Disease, dysfunction and loss associated with advanced age threaten the older adult's satisfactory engagement in occupations. Occupational therapy (OT) practitioners, consisting of both occupational therapists and occupational therapy assistants, therapeutically use meaningful and purposeful activities to insure and enhance an individual's participation in chosen occupations.

OT practitioners serve older adults in various settings, including a variety of inpatient settings such as acute care hospitals, rehabilitation centers, skilled nursing facilities and psychiatric centers. Community-based OT may be provided in outpatient settings, clients' homes or in adult daycare and senior centers. OT professionals may fulfill the roles of direct service provider, administrator, consultant, educator and researcher.

OCCUPATIONAL THERAPY ASSESSMENT

In order to provide effective, efficient therapeutic intervention, occupational therapists conduct a thorough twofold assessment of their clients. The therapist conducts an occupational profile (a client-centered interview) designed to gather pertinent information regarding the individual's occupational history and preferences, the various contexts in which the client engages in occupation, and the client's values, beliefs and goals regarding his or her current functional performance (AOTA, 2002).

Additionally, the OT clinician conducts an analysis of the client's occupational performance (AOTA, 2002). He or she observes the older adult engaging in a valued occupation, such as eating, dressing, moving in bed or preparing a meal, to identify the client's functional strengths and limitations. The clinician then performs standardized and/or nonstandardized tests to specifically pinpoint impairments, such as decreased strength or decreased ability to initiate a task.

Occupational therapists and the interdisciplinary team members share their assessment findings with one another in order to develop a comprehensive treatment plan. In some settings, such as hospitals and home healthcare, interdisciplinary team members contribute their findings to a joint team evaluation. Using the Functional Independence Measure (FIM) or the Katz Activities of Daily Living Scale in hospitals across the United States of America for example, enables healthcare providers to establish a baseline level of performance for each client and provides all team members with a method of tracking a client's progress in primary areas of daily functioning (Uniform Data System for Medical Rehabilitation, 1993; The Merck Manual of Geriatrics, 2011). While the FIM tool may be entirely conducted by any treatment team member, occupational therapists are often responsible for completing the self-care and transfers portion of the assessment.

Through joint and discipline-specific evaluation, the occupational therapist and the treatment team members, in collaboration with the older adult, prepare for the client's discharge either home or to the next level of service.

OCCUPATIONAL THERAPY INTERVENTION

Upon completion of the OT assessment, the OT practitioner begins intervention planning and implementation. Practitioners may employ a combination of interventions, including the therapeutic use of self, the therapeutic use of occupations and activities, education

CASE STUDY

ARLENE

Arlene's physician referred her to home healthcare services including nursing, physical therapy and OT. The physician's orders for OT included training in activities of daily living, transfers, instrumental activities of daily living (homemaking), increasing left upper extremity active range of motion (ROM) and left upper extremity strengthening.

Arlene, an 83-year-old female, recently fractured her left distal humerus, her dominant extremity, when she fell trying to get to the bathroom one night. While the doctor performed no surgery or casting to Arlene's left arm, he had immobilized it with a simple sling for 6 weeks. He has removed the sling and has ordered therapeutic services through a home health agency. Arlene has diabetes and experiences atrial fibrillation. Her right middle finger was surgically amputated 12 months ago. Arlene has type II diabetes and undergoes kidney dialysis three times per week.

OCCUPATIONAL PROFILE

Arlene resides in a two-story home with her husband and adult son. Her husband uses compressed oxygen 24 hours per day and her son works full time in a warehouse. Prior to her fall and subsequent left humeral fracture Arlene slept in her bedroom and used the bathroom on the second floor of her home. Arlene currently does not access her second story because she cannot use the single handrail when descending the stairs because of left upper extremity pain and ROM limitations. She sleeps in a rented hospital bed on the first floor. As there is no bathroom on the first floor, Arlene toilets using a portable commode and sponge bathes in the kitchen. She relies on her son to empty the commode and for assistance with bathing and dressing. Arlene reports significant limitations when attempting her favorite occupations, cooking and baking.

Arlene reports that she longs to sleep in her bed upstairs as well as use the second-story bathroom. She also wishes to prepare a simple lunch for herself and her husband without the assistance of her son.

Arlene uses a straight cane when ambulating throughout her home and requires supervision to do so as her compromised endurance and dynamic standing balance put her at risk of future falls.

ANALYSIS OF OCCUPATIONAL PERFORMANCE

The occupational therapist observed Arlene's performance in functional mobility (transferring to and from the bed, the commode, a kitchen chair and a reclining chair) and in self-care (item retrieval required for grooming in the kitchen and hand washing). Arlene required minimal assistance (a helper contributed approximately 25% of the effort necessary for Arlene to engage in the tasks) with transfers and moderate assistance (a helper contributed approximately 50% of the effort necessary for Arlene to engage in the tasks) with most

self-care tasks. The therapist also assessed Arlene's left upper extremity status and function, including pain and edema (excess swelling that had accumulated in Arlene's hand as a result of sustained immobilization and now interfered with her mobility) evaluation, active/passive ROM and muscle strength measurement. Moderate edema of Arlene's left hand and wrist was noted. She experienced moderate pain during gentle passive ROM of her shoulder and elbow and had significant active and passive ROM and strength limitations throughout her left upper extremity. Additionally, the therapist assessed Arlene's home in order to make recommendations to insure the client's safety and to optimize her future occupational performance. The occupational therapist noted obstacles such as clear oxygen tubing strewn on the floor in multiple rooms.

The occupational therapist, in collaboration with Arlene, set the following long-term goals:

1. Arlene will perform all self-care with supervision only within 5 weeks.
2. Arlene will prepare a simple lunch for her husband independently within 5 weeks.

The occupational therapist set corresponding short-term goals for each long-term goal. For example, in order to meet long-term goal number 1, Arlene would first meet the following short-term goal:

Arlene will comb her hair using her left hand with minimal assistance within 2 weeks.

OCCUPATIONAL THERAPY INTERVENTION

Arlene's occupational therapist used a variety of intervention approaches to insure Arlene's goal accomplishment:

Prevention: As Arlene's humeral fracture resulted from a fall, the occupational therapist educated her and her family in fall prevention. To increase visibility, yellow duct tape was applied to the clear oxygen tubing at 6-inch intervals. Additional lighting in hallways, especially for night use, was also recommended.

Restoration: The occupational therapist instructed Arlene in left upper extremity active assistive ROM exercises. Additionally, she engaged Arlene in therapeutic activities and occupations designed to increase shoulder, elbow, wrist and finger strength and ROM. For example, Arlene used her right hand to assist the left hand in pressing out a graham cracker pie crust and later cleaned the table using her left upper extremity, stretching to reach a bit further with each swipe of the dishcloth.

Modify: The occupational therapist introduced Arlene to adaptive dressing equipment, a sock aid and shoe horn to assist her with lower extremity dressing. Arlene is not expected to fully regain the function of her left upper extremity, but would still like to don her socks and shoes independently.

---

and consultation with either individuals or groups (AOTA, 2002).

Additionally, based on the etiology of the client's deficits, practitioners use a combination of the following treatment approaches: create/promote, establish/restore, maintain, modify and prevent. (This approach is used when a client's pathological condition, Alzheimer's or Parkinson's disease for example, is progressive in nature.

In these situations, the absence of OT intervention would result in significant decline in a client's functional performance, thereby increasing his or her burden of care.)

The Case Study of Arlene (see Case Study) illustrates how OT might be applied in geriatrics.

An OT consultant, hired by the manager of a high-rise apartment building for independent seniors, uses the create/promote approach when instituting a work simplification and energy conservation program in the setting so that seniors might not become overly fatigued when shopping or preparing meals. The create/promote approach targets the well population with the aim of enhancing quality of life through participation in occupation.

An OT practitioner uses the establish/restore approach to intervention when he/she facilitates a patient's functional skills that were lost as a result of a particular condition. An OT practitioner teaching a stroke survivor how to use a spoon again uses the establish/restore approach to intervention.

Occupational therapists work with families whose loved ones have dementia. A client with dementia is forgetful and will progressively decline in functional performance. Graff et al. (2007) have shown in a randomized trial that OT significantly improves quality of life for dementia patients and their caregivers. When using the modify approach to treatment, OT practitioners alter tasks or environments to insure the client's success in functional performance. Finally, OT practitioners concern themselves with preventing further disability among their clients. Older adults recovering from lower extremity joint replacement, for instance, would benefit from a fall prevention program.

CONCLUSION

OT practitioners work closely with a number of different healthcare professionals in caring for geriatric clients. They use therapeutic occupation and activities as their primary modality in meeting their patients' needs. Finally, regardless of the setting, occupational therapists and assistants, upon completion of a thorough assessment, insure clients participate as fully as possible by employing a variety of treatment approaches including creation/promotion, restoration/establishment, maintenance, modification and prevention.

NOTE

Text updated by Tim Kauffman.

REFERENCES

AOTA (American Occupational Therapy Association) 2002 Occupational therapy practice framework: domain and process. Am J Occup Ther 56:609–639

Graff M, Vernooij-Dassen M, Thijssen M et al 2007 Effects of community occupational therapy on quality of life, mood, and health status in dementia patients and their caregivers: a randomized controlled trial. J Gerontol A Biol Sci Med Sci 62:1002–1009

The Merck Manual of Geriatrics (Beers MH, Berkow R, eds) 2011 3rd edn. [Online]. Merck & Co. Inc., Whitehouse Station, NJ. (Accessed at www.merckmanuals.com/professional/geriatrics.html December 2013)

Uniform Data System for Medical Rehabilitation 1993 Guide for the Uniform Data Set for Medical Rehabilitation (Adult FIM). UB Foundation Activities, Buffalo, NY

Chapter 83

Geriatric physical therapy

WILLIAM H. STAPLES

CHAPTER CONTENTS

INTRODUCTION

NEED FOR TRAINED PROFESSIONALS

REFERRALS TO A PHYSICAL
THERAPIST

MULTIPLE CONDITIONS

ASSESSMENT OF THE GERIATRIC
PATIENT

GOAL-SETTING AND INTERVENTIONS

CONCLUSION

REFERENCES

INTRODUCTION

This chapter is designed to introduce the reader to current physical therapy practice and its importance in the rehabilitation process. Physical therapy is an integral part of the rehabilitation process of the older adult. As the population ages, the role of physical therapists will be pivotal in the recovery of geriatric clients who have experienced disease or illness.

The American Physical Therapy Association's (APTA) *Guide to Physical Therapist Practice* provides the following definition: 'Physical therapy is a dynamic profession with an established theoretical base and widespread clinical applications in the restoration, maintenance, and promotion of optimal physical function' (APTA, 2003). The World Confederation for Physical Therapy (WCPT), which is a non-profit organization comprising 106 member organizations, states that it is the sole international organization representing over 350000 physical therapists worldwide and that it is dedicated to furthering the physical therapy profession and improving global health (WCPT, 2012).

The primary goal of geriatric physical therapy is to prevent, maintain or rehabilitate impairments, improve activity limitations and decrease participation restrictions that are accomplished with the application of evidence-based scientific principles. Prevention of functional loss should be of primary concern for all healthcare providers. Preventative care and education are much less costly to provide to avert injury or illness as opposed to treating the sequelae of a health-related problem. The rehabilitative process should be geared to assist the older person to achieve the highest level of function possible within their environment. Physical therapy focuses on functional mobility while maintaining safety, enabling the older adult to enjoy a longer life by living it more independently and with less pain. The Academy of Geriatric Physical Therapy (AGPT, 2014) section of the APTA mission is to 'further our members ability to provide best practice physical therapy

and to advocate for optimal aging' (AGPT, 2014). This includes being 'advocates for the health, wellness, fitness, and physical function needs of the aging adult' (AGPT, 2014). The WCPT has a subgroup called the International Association of Physical Therapists Working with Older People (IPTOP, 2012), whose goal is to serve as the international resource for physical therapists working with the elderly. IPTOP states that 'The prime purpose of physical therapists working with older people is to maintain and/or restore function, activity and independence. This requires a person-centered, collaborative, inter-professional approach to a wide range of conditions affecting this population' (IPTOP, 2012).

Physical therapists are healthcare professionals involved in the examination and evaluation of individuals with neuromuscular, musculoskeletal, cardiopulmonary and integumentary disorders. The physical therapist can then determine a physical therapy diagnosis and develop an individualized intervention plan to achieve short- and long-term goals for improved function. Physical therapists do not limit their skills to treating people who are ill. A significant portion of time is spent working on health promotion and prevention of primary and secondary problems to avert an initial injury or secondary impairment that would lead to subsequent loss of movement and function.

A physical therapist in the United States of America is a graduate of a college or university accredited by the Commission on Accreditation in Physical Therapy Education (CAPTE), and has passed a licensing examination that is conducted by the Federation of State Boards of Physical Therapy (FSBPT) and is regulated by each state. The physical therapist assistant holds an Associates Degree from a college program also accredited by CAPTE. Physical therapist assistants are licensed in most US states through examination. They are not permitted to perform evaluations, but can perform many of the treatment activities under the supervision of a physical therapist. Supervision requirements vary from state to state.

The WCPT currently recommends a minimum of 4 years of university level studies to achieve professional recognition and that the first professional qualification should be completion of a curriculum that qualifies the physical therapist for practice as an independent autonomous professional. WCPT (2012) expects that any program, irrespective of its length and mode of delivery, should deliver a curriculum that will enable physical therapists to attain the knowledge, skills and attributes described in the guidelines for physical therapist professional entry level education.

The APTA had set forth a goal that by the year 2020 physical therapy will be provided by physical therapists who are doctors of physical therapy. As of 2012, all but one of the more than 200 CAPTE accredited physical therapist education programs offered a Doctor of Physical Therapy (DPT) degree. To maintain or be granted accreditation, programs will be required to award the DPT degree by 2015 and will have until 2017 to come into compliance with this decision (CAPTE, 2013).

Geriatric physical therapy can be practiced in a variety of settings, including acute care hospitals, rehabilitation centers, skilled nursing facilities, continuing care communities, home healthcare agencies and outpatient clinics. In addition to prevention, geriatric physical therapy is committed to combating, minimizing and forestalling the accumulative disabling effects of physical illness in association with the aging process. This is performed by hastening convalescence and reducing institutionalization, education of the patient and caregivers, contributing to the comfort and wellbeing of the patient, and assisting the individual to return to optimal living within their capabilities. Geriatric physical therapy has been recognized as an area of specialization that requires a specific set of advanced skills and knowledge that address the aging process. Specialists in geriatric physical therapy understand the differences between 'normal' aging and pathological changes that commonly occur in the older adult. Assisting the geriatric client can be an arduous task due to multisystem involvement and multiple comorbidities. Special considerations such as psychosocial issues, reimbursement, environmental, frailty, nutritional, pharmacological and cultural factors must be accounted for in a successful rehabilitation process. The American Board of Physical Therapy Specialties first recognized individuals as board-certified Geriatric Clinical Specialists (GCS) in 1992. To become a GCS one must be a licensed physical therapist, spend a prescribed number of hours in direct patient care with the elderly and pass a rigorous written examination (ABPTS, 2013). The WCPT (2012) supports the specialization process.

NEED FOR TRAINED PROFESSIONALS

As the world's older population grows, the US and other nations will require a well-trained workforce of healthcare providers with expert knowledge in geriatric care. Compared with younger adults, older Americans use a disproportionately larger share of healthcare services. Longer life spans and greater prevalence of chronic illnesses, such as diabetes, arthritis, hypertension and kidney disease, in older adults has placed a greater demand on the healthcare system (Thorpe et al., 2010). The average healthcare expense in 2002 was $11 089 per year for elderly people but only $3352 per year for working-age people (ages 19–64) (Agency for Healthcare Research and Quality, 2010). The Kaiser Family Foundation (2012) estimated that healthcare costs for chronic disease treatment account for more than 75% of US national health expenditures. Healthcare professionals who are trained in geriatric care can help to maintain the health and quality of life of older adults. The complex needs of older patients often require a team of healthcare providers with aging-related expertise to work together to assess the patient's physical and mental wellbeing and to coordinate care in a variety of environments. These teams need to work cooperatively with informal caregivers, such as family and friends, who play a crucial role in helping the older patient maintain health and independence.

Older patients who receive specialized geriatric care tend to do better than those who receive usual care. Cohen et al. (2002) found that patients who received inpatient and outpatient care in geriatric units experienced large reductions in functional decline and improvements in mental health at no additional cost. In another study, older patients cared for by nurses trained in geriatrics had fewer readmissions to the hospital and were less likely to be transferred from nursing facilities to a hospital for inappropriate reasons (Kovner et al., 2002). Bardach and Rowles (2012) found that this need for trained geriatric specialists remains substantiated. This need should provide incentive for physical therapists to enter the geriatric field to assist in filling this gap.

REFERRALS TO A PHYSICAL THERAPIST

There are many reasons to seek out the knowledge and skills of a physical therapist. Box 83.1 is a useful, but not an entirely inclusive, list of possible indications for a physical therapy referral. Physical therapists understand a vast array of problems that affect physical function and general health. They utilize screening to enable

---

Box 83.1 *Possible indications for geriatric physical therapy referral*

- Recent fall or history of falls
- Deficits in strength or range of motion
- Loss of mobility or ambulation requiring an assistive device
- Musculoskeletal pain
- Difficulty with transfers
- Orthotic or prosthetic needs
- Open wound
- Neurologic disorder
- Dizziness or balance deficits
- Decreased endurance for ADLs
- Bedbound status
- Need for adaptive equipment to enhance safety and function
- Incontinence
- Frailty

them to refer to other appropriate healthcare practioners if the therapist is serving as a portal to the healthcare system. Physical therapy is a rapidly evolving profession. In most US states an individual can have direct access to a physical therapist for evaluation and treatment without first seeing a physician for a referral. The APTA (2013) has the vision statement: 'Transforming society by optimizing movement to improve the human experience'. One of the guiding principles in this new vision statement is identity, for which:

The physical therapy profession will define and promote the movement system as the foundation for optimizing movement to improve the health of society. Recognition and validation of the movement system is essential to understand the structure, function, and potential of the human body. The physical therapist will be responsible for evaluating and managing an individual's movement system across the lifespan to promote optimal development; diagnose impairments, activity limitations, and participation restrictions; and provide interventions targeted at preventing or ameliorating activity limitations and participation restrictions. The movement system is the core of physical therapist practice, education, and research.

APTA, 2013

Many older people do seek out a physician as the traditional first stop in the healthcare process, with subsequent referral for physical therapy, although this may be underutilized. Johnson et al. (1994) determined that almost one-half of the patients that were hospitalized and found to be deficient in ambulatory or transfer skills compared to status at admission did not receive physical therapy services. Interestingly, those patients who received physical therapy in the hospital were significantly more likely to receive it in the post-acute period. It is possible to infer that elderly medical patients develop functional disabilities during hospitalization that are not appropriately recognized. Routine physical screening of all elderly patients should be performed by nursing staff to determine if there has been any loss in physical performance. Freburger et al. (2003) found that even after controlling for diagnosis, illness severity and physical therapy supply, referrals to physical therapy were much less likely from primary care physicians in comparison to orthopedic surgeons. This lack of referrals affects the quality of care received and may eventually result in an increased cost if a treatable condition worsens. Delays in care can also lead to decreased functional outcomes and frustration for clients and patients.

In a hospital, the physician is traditionally in charge of the patient as he/she has admitting privileges. The therapist may very well be an employee who is assigned the case through a scheduling rotation or based on their specific skills (e.g. GCS) and does not usually have the authority to seek older persons in need of services without a referral from the physician. The physician has traditionally served as the 'gatekeeper' to the healthcare system.

Outside the hospital, a great number of states do allow direct access, although the majority of therapists still receive referrals from a physician, physician's assistant or nurse practioner. Direct access varies considerably in terms of legal, practice and reimbursement models. Some limitations or barriers to receiving physical therapy services are due to legal issues, but other reasons include such factors as lack of public and healthcare provider education. Additionally, most secondary payers such as the federal government and private insurance carriers limit reimbursement without a physician referral.

Interestingly, Miller et al. (2005) found that more than 66% of physician orders or referrals to physical therapy for geriatric clientele specified only 'evaluate and treat', or 'P.T. Consult'. This finding does indicate some degree of confidence from physicians in the expertise and decision-making skills of physical therapists.

MULTIPLE CONDITIONS

A physical therapist has a great deal to consider when assessing the geriatric client. Conditions of normal aging such as loss of eyesight and hearing can make assessment and intervention more difficult. Decline in physical reserve (homeostasis) may transform mild problems into those that are life-threatening. More than 50% of older adults have three or more comorbidities, including chronic diseases (Anderson, 2010). Older adults with multiple health problems have higher rates of death, disability, adverse effects, institutionalization, use of resources and a poorer quality of life (Boyd & Fortin, 2011). A comprehensive review of systems and a biopsychosocial or patient-centered approach must be utilized when assessing and planning intervention for these clients. Health is best understood in terms of a combination of biological, psychological and social factors rather than purely in biological terms. This concept was first put forth by Dr George Engel (1977). Physical therapists must not only understand internal factors such as physical abilities, cognition and pharmacological interaction, but also how external factors such as environment, financial resources and social support will affect the therapeutic relationship and eventual outcome.

Not all older adults' problems can be classified into specific disease categories. The term 'geriatric syndrome' (Inouye et al., 2007) has been utilized to categorize many of the most common health interrelated problems in older adults. Geriatric syndromes include falls, incontinence, delirium and functional decline, and represent a state of impaired health (Inouye et al., 2007). These complex syndromes are multifactorial and associated with poor outcomes, frailty, dependence and significant morbidity. A change in health status may be precipitated by one of the inter-related conditions. For instance, a urinary tract infection may lead to delirium which may then cause a fall that results in a fractured hip which will affect physical function for weeks, months or the remainder of one's life. We can explore this inter-relatedness in considering a specific case (see Case Study), which to the professional who lacks specific geriatric training may appear as a 'simple' case.

MRS S

Mrs S is an 82-year-old retired school teacher who lives alone in a two-story walk-up apartment. She had fallen at home, fracturing the left femoral head. After a 5-day hospitalization for a left hemiarthroplasty, followed by a 2-week stay at a skilled nursing facility she was referred to a home health agency. The physical therapist is scheduled to open this case the day after her Mrs S returns home.

Box 83.2 *Tests and measures provided by physical therapists*

- Aerobic capacity/endurance
- Anthropometric characteristics
- Arousal, attention and cognition
- Assistive and adaptive devices
- Circulation (arterial, venous, lymphatic)
- Cranial and peripheral nerve integrity
- Environmental, home and work (job/school/play) barriers
- Ergonomics and body mechanics
- Gait, locomotion and balance
- Integumentary integrity
- Joint integrity and mobility
- Motor function (motor control and motor learning)
- Muscle performance (including strength, power and endurance)
- Neuromotor development and sensory integration
- Orthotic, protective and supportive devices
- Pain
- Posture
- Prosthetic requirements
- Range of motion (including muscle length)
- Reflex integrity
- Self-care and home management (including activities of daily living and instrumental activities of daily living)
- Sensory integrity
- Ventilation and respiration/gas exchange
- Work (job/school/play), community and leisure integration or reintegration (including instrumental activities of daily living)

Source: APTA, 2003.

ASSESSMENT OF THE GERIATRIC PATIENT

Evaluation of clients, whether referred or by direct access, must include an inclusive history as well as a physical examination using various tests and measures (see Box 83.2). The examination should also include a systems review for screening purposes to rule out any pathological conditions that need to be referred to other health professionals. The therapist then evaluates the data collected and makes clinical judgments based on this information to establish a physical therapy diagnosis. The geriatric physical therapist is able to interpret the data gathered into categories, syndromes or clusters to determine the appropriate intervention strategies. This can be quite a challenge in older adults because they present with more complex problems. The aging process has taken some toll on the body and multiple pathologies may exist that may exaggerate, or hide underlying conditions. The experienced therapist will attempt to determine, where possible, which problems are age-related and which are due to pathology. The educated therapist will utilize evidence-based practice during the clinical decision making process when determining which functional tests will be administered.

Returning to our case study, the examination of Mrs S reveals that she has had several recent falls, and has a history of osteoarthritis, hypertension and atherosclerotic heart disease. She was taking Lasix-K (furosemide) and Lopressor (metoprolol) for hypertension, ibuprofen for long-term arthritis pain and Boniva (ibandronate) prior to the hospitalization and has resumed them again. She has been prescribed Vicodin (hydrocodone) for hip pain since surgery. Tests and measures reveal left hip strength of 3+/5; a mild kyphosis; independent gait with a rolling walker, weight bearing as tolerated at approximately 85%, limited due to pain 3/10 on a Numeric Rating Scale (NRS); difficulty with activities of daily living (ADLs); decreased balance (Berg Balance Scale 1989), score of 38/56; limited endurance as she is only able to ambulate 80 feet in 2 minutes before requiring a rest period; and she is hard of hearing. Vital signs at rest: blood pressure (BP) 140/82, heart rate (HR) 74, respiratory rate (RR) 20, rating of perceived exertion (RPE) 1/10. Vital signs after gait: BP 148/86, HR 86, RR 28, RPE 8/10. She has not been on a regular exercise program.

The physical therapist must now analyze this data. There are a myriad of factors that will need to be considered before progressing to the next steps of goal-setting and selection of interventions. The geriatric therapist has to screen for a possible lower extremity, deep vein thrombosis (DVT) because of recent surgery and recognize that some non-steroidal anti-inflammatory drugs (NSAIDs) may cause an increase in blood clots. According to the US Food and Drug Administration (US FDA, 2011), long-term use of NSAIDs may increase the risk of blood clots, heart attack and stroke.

The geriatric therapist must understand the Wells Criteria (Wells et al., 2003). The Wells Criteria is a clinical assessment of probability, or clinical prediction rule, for those with suspected DVT, and can be useful to determine which medical tests to perform. The physician will need to be contacted if the likelihood is high that a blood clot may be present. Additionally, people who take NSAIDs for a long time are at risk for developing stomach ulcers and bleeding (US FDA, 2011). The risk of stomach ulcers and bleeding also rises with increased dose and duration of NSAIDs use. Bleeding and ulceration can occur at any time, and with no symptoms, and the educated therapist would know to observe for this possibility.

Knowing that the best predictor of a fall is a previous fall, the therapist must try to determine the underlying cause of her falls (Tromp et al., 2001). The Berg Balance Scale (Berg et al., 1989) was chosen by the therapist because the therapist thought the patient would not achieve the ceiling score. Importantly, this test can be used to show specific activities that the patient has difficulty completing. The patient is not allowed to use an assistive device for this test, so the therapist must

Box 83.3 *The Berg Balance Scale (Berg et al., 1989)*

TEST

14-item scale

For each item, a 5-point scale, ranging from 0 to 4. Score of 0 indicates the lowest level of function and score of 4 indicates the highest level of function. Total possible score = 56.

Score >45 = less likely to fall, not predictive of frequency (Bogle Thorbahn & Newton, 1996).

MINIMAL DETECTABLE CHANGE (MDC)

A change of **4 points** is needed to be 95% confident that true change has occurred if a patient scores within 45–56 initially, **5 points** if they score within 35–44, **7 points** if they score within 25–34 and, finally, **5 points** if their initial score is within 0–24 on the Berg Balance Scale (Donoghue & Stokes, 2009).

Table 83.1 **Case study evaluation and interventions**

Evaluation Findings	Interventions
Decreased hip strength	Progressive resistance exercise 80% 1 rep max, 8–12 reps without pain
Decreased balance	Balance exercise at kitchen counter or heavy chair, progress with less upper extremity support, single leg support
History of falls	External: loose rugs, cords, pets Internal: check BP sit to stand and provide education
Diminished gait status	Gait training with appropriate assistive device including stair climbing. May need to order cane or quad cane
Decreased endurance	Increased ambulatory distance, while monitoring vital signs/RPE, home exercise program. Monitor through use of target heart rate or perceived exertion
Other needs	Raised toilet seat, grab bars for bathroom, adequate banisters in stairwell, assistance for shopping or meal preparation

determine proper guarding techniques. In Mrs S, the Berg Balance Score (see Box 83.3) indicates that she is at risk for falling.

The therapist must also determine whether the cause of previous falls is external (environmental, such as loose carpeting) or internal (possibly orthostatic hypotension caused by taking Lasix and Lopressor as an anti-hypertensive medication). Is she able to get in and out of her apartment independently in case of emergency or to be able to shop for food? Will she require a call alert, home health aide, provision of meals on wheels or other services? These factors must be accounted for in order to insure a successful rehabilitation process.

GOAL-SETTING AND INTERVENTIONS

Improved function must be the priority focus of interventions provided by the geriatric physical therapist. Functional goals are established with the patient, and sometimes with family or caregiver, in order to determine the appropriate treatment interventions. The skills of the therapist are utilized to provide appropriate treatment strategies and techniques. For this study, the long-term goal of return to being an independent functioning, community-dwelling individual was determined. To meet this long-term goal, several short-term goals were set. These included:

- Safe and independent gait with full weight-bearing left lower extremity with a progression to a cane and stair climbing as appropriate.
- Increase lower extremity strength to 4/5 to enable progression to cane.
- Increase Berg score to 46/56 to decrease risk of falls, and showing detectable change.
- Independent with ADLs to decrease outside care and expense.
- Increase endurance and ambulatory velocity to 200 feet in 2 minutes with a perceived exertion level not to exceed a 5 on a 0/10 scale or a 13 on the 0/20 RPE.

The therapist must monitor and continually assess the client's progress in the short-term goals in order to update them and progress toward the long-term goal. Modification of the interventions must be made if

outcomes are not being successfully achieved. Since this patient is taking a beta-blocker, which blunts the cardiac response to exercise, the traditional target heart using the Karvonen formula (ACSM, 2009) or Tanaka method (Tanaka et al., 2001) to calculate the intensity of exercise cannot be effectively utilized. The RPE must be used to monitor physical stress in lieu of heart rate and blood pressure.

Additionally, the therapist must provide preventative and wellness education to this client regarding the importance of regular exercise, osteoporosis and posture. The final goal would to promote optimal aging, a term described by Brummel-Smith (2007) as 'The capacity to function across many domains – physical, functional, cognitive, emotional, social, and spiritual – to one's satisfaction and in spite of one's medical conditions' (Brummel-Smith, 2007).

In our case study, in order to achieve the long-term functional goal, interventions are planned to improve Mrs S's impairments. These interventions will be tailored to meet this individual's needs and tolerance (see Table 83.1).

Finally, along with the noted interventions, the physical therapist must identify the need for additional services. Referrals may be made to occupational therapy for intensive ADL training and to social services in order to arrange meals on wheels. Geriatric patients, in particular, benefit from a team approach. The elderly are commonly affected by a variety of interacting problems that can be better solved with input from several points of view. It is essential that members of the team communicate with each other in order to achieve a positive outcome. The case study in this chapter has tried to validate the need for more specific training in geriatric physical therapy to better address the needs of this population.

CONCLUSION

The geriatric population is a unique group to work with because of the aging and disease processes that interact to produce a wide variation in each individual. Physical therapists, as healthcare providers, are also health educators and health promoters and will continue to play an ever-more important role in the provision of healthcare services. Time should be spent to teach, counsel and modify the behaviors of individuals which, if left unattended, would lead to dysfunction. Some of the concerns that can affect the older adult, such as nutritional concerns, psychosocial problems and limited finances, may fall outside the immediate practice of physical therapists, but must be addressed in order to maximize therapeutic outcomes. The geriatric practitioner must also understand reimbursement issues to better serve their clientele. Rather than working in a vacuum, communication and teamwork must be utilized for the best overall care of the patient or client. Geriatric rehabilitation offers a huge challenge to the talent and creativity of each therapist. As the geriatric population continues to grow, so will the challenges.

REFERENCES

ABPTS (American Board of Physical Therapy Specialties) 2013 Home Page. Available at: www.abpts.org/home.aspx. Accessed January 2013

ACSM's Guidelines for Exercise Testing and Prescription 2009, 8th edn. Lippincott Williams & Wilkins, Baltimore, MD

Agency for Healthcare Research and Quality 2010 The high concentration of US health care expenditures. Research in Action Issue 19. [Online] Available at: www.ahrq.gov/research/ria19/expendria.htm. Accessed December 2012

AGPT (Academy of Geriatric Physical Therapy) 2014. Mission statement. [Online] Available at: www.geriatricspt.org. Accessed February 2014

Anderson G 2010 Chronic care: making the case for ongoing care. Robert Wood Johnson Foundation. [Online] Available at: www.rwjf.org/files/research/50968chronic.carechartbook.pdf. Accessed December 2012

APTA (American Physical Therapy Association) 2003 Guide to Physical Therapist Practice, 2nd edn. APTA, Alexandria, VA

APTA (American Physical Therapy Association) 2013 Vision Statement for the Physical Therapy Profession. [Online] Available at: www.apta.org. Accessed December 2013

Bardach SH, Rowles GD 2012 Geriatric education in the health professions: are we making progress? Gerontologist 52:607–618

Berg KO, Wood-Dauphinee SL, Williams JT et al 1989 Measuring balance in the elderly: preliminary development of an instrument. Physiother Canada 41:304–311

Bogle Thorbahn LD, Newton RD 1996 Elderly persons use of the Berg Balance Test to predict falls in elderly persons. Phys Ther 76:576–583

Boyd CM, Fortin M 2011 Future of multimorbidity research: how should understanding of multimorbidity inform health system design? Publ Health Rev 32:451–474

Brummel-Smith K 2007 Optimal aging, Part I: demographics and definitions. Ann Long Term Care 15:26–28

CAPTE (Commission on Accreditation in Physical Therapy Education) 2013 Home Page. Available at: www.capteonline.org/home.aspx. Accessed January 2013

Cohen HJ, Feussner JR, Weinberger M et al 2002 A controlled trial of inpatient and outpatient geriatric evaluation and management. N Engl J Med 346:905–912

Donoghue D, Stokes EK 2009 Physiotherapy Research and Older People (PROP) group. How much change is true change? The minimum detectable change of the Berg Balance Scale in elderly people. J Rehabil Med 41(5):343–346

Engel GL 1977 The need for a new medical model: a challenge for biomedicine. Science 196:129–136

Freburger JK, Holmes GM, Carey TS 2003 Physician referrals to physical therapy for the treatment of musculoskeletal conditions. Arch Phys Med Rehabil 84:1839–1849

Inouye SK, Studenski S, Tinetti ME et al 2007 Geriatric syndromes: clinical, research, and policy implications of a core geriatric concept. J Am Geriatr Soc 55:780–791

IPTOP (International Association of Physical Therapists Working with Older People) 2012 About IPTOP. [Online] Available at: www.wcpt.org/iptop/about. Accessed December 2012

Johnson JH, Sager MA, Hirn G et al 1994 Referral patterns to physical therapy in elderly hospitalized for acute medical illness. Phys Occup Ther Geriatr 12:1–12

Kaiser Family Foundation 2012 US health care costs. [Online] Available at: www.kaiseredu.org/Issue-Modules/US-Health-Care-Costs/Background-Brief.aspx#. Accessed December 2012

Kovner CT, Mezey M, Harrington C 2002 Who cares for older adults? Workforce implications of an aging society. Health Aff 21:78–89

Miller EW, Ross K, Grant S et al 2005 Geriatric referral patterns for physical therapy: a descriptive analysis. J Geriatric Phys Ther 28:20–27

Tanaka H, Monahan KD, Seals DR 2001 Age-predicted maximal heart rate revisited. J Am Coll Cardiol 37:153–156

Thorpe K, Ogden L, Galactionova K 2010 Chronic conditions account for rise in Medicare spending from 1987 to 2006. Health Aff 29:718–724

Tromp AM, Pluijm SMF, Smit JH et al 2001 Fall-risk screening test: a prospective study on predictors for falls in community-dwelling elderly. J Clin Epidemiol 54:837–844

US FDA (US Food and Drug Administration) 2011 Medication guide for non-steroidal anti-inflammatory drugs (NSAIDs). Available at: www.fda.gov/downloads/Drugs/DrugSafety/ucm089822.pdf. Accessed December 2012

WCPT (World Confederation for Physical Therapy) 2012 Home Page. www.wcpt.org/. Accessed 23 December 2012

Wells PS, Anderson DR, Rodger M et al 2003 Evaluation of D-Dimer in the diagnosis of suspected deep-vein thrombosis. N Engl J Med 349:1227–1235

Chapter 84

Providing social services to the older client

JAMES SIBERSKI

INTRODUCTION

Today's older adults are confronted with numerous challenges as they age (Lemme, 2006). The onslaught of baby boomers will change how one ages. In addition to normal age-related changes and the still undefined boomer changes, frequently there are disease states that must also be addressed in order to age successfully. The social service provider plays an important role in assisting older adults to adjust to age-related changes through adaptive changes and devices, and adjust to the disease state through the rehabilitative process.

As a member of the rehabilitative team, the social service provider performs a key role. In order to succeed, the team needs specific information from the social worker or geriatric care manager. Initially, this individual completes a comprehensive social work assessment and social history providing important data that will be incorporated into the rehabilitative care plan and enable the older client to achieve his or her goals. While various forms are available (see Form 84.1) for completing this task, in many settings the format is dictated by the agency or department. As a result of education and training, professional social service providers are efficient at completing an assessment, taking a social history, determining needs and strengths, and developing discipline-specific goals. In assessing the elderly, additional considerations must be entertained in order to facilitate the return of the older client to an appropriate placement at the completion of rehabilitation.

ADDITIONAL CONSIDERATIONS IN ASSESSMENT

Additional considerations, which include baby boomers, goal incongruence, cure verses care, client and family perceptions, personality, activities and diversity issues, can either assist or detract from the success of the rehabilitative process.

BABY BOOMERS

All 78 million boomers have experienced every stage of life in their own way; if there was a mold, they broke it, and there is no reason to believe that their older years will be any different (Frey, 2010). Complicating the situation is the diversity of the boomers – Catholics, Jews, Protestants, etc. and African Americans, Native Americans, Hispanic Americans, etc. Social service workers should be aware that they will soon be faced with tremendous diversity and with demands from boomers for services that previously did not exist. Consider their need for social connectivity, i.e. the internet, including its availability in senior living/nursing facilities; social differences, i.e. taste in music and clothing preferences; sex, i.e. different expectations for sexual freedom in nursing facilities; waking and dining time preferences; and support groups for their emotional wants (Feldman, 2012), all of which will place additional stress on the social service provider. It will be necessary for social histories to be specific for: past and current drug use; sexual preferences; desirable leisure activities; and how that boomer views rehabilitation. This will create an interesting challenge for the social service provider in goal incongruence, cure vs. care, client and family perceptions, personality, activities and diversity issues.

GOAL INCONGRUENCE

In the rehabilitative process, the team often determines that the appropriate placement is a structured living arrangement while the older client believes that the appropriate living arrangement is their home. This goal incongruence between team and client is not restricted to just placement but can include driving, employment, financial management and other issues of autonomy. Unresolved goal incongruence hinders the rehabilitative process. In addressing this issue, the social worker should capitalize on the client's motivation to go home

Room #: _____ Admission date: _____

Name: _____

Address:_____

_____

Phone: _____

Rehab. DX: _____

Employment status:_____

Income source(s):_____

Age: _____ DOB: _____

Hospital admitted from: _____

Insurance info.: _____

Physician: _____

Other DX: _____

Employer: _____

Work phone: _____

FAMILY/CAREGIVER

Marital status: S/M/D/W/Sep.   Spouse name: _____

Others in household: Name: _____ Age: _____

Other contact: Name: _____

Address:_____

Name: _____

Empl.: _____

Phone: _____

Phone: _____

HOME/ENVIRONMENT

Type of home: Own: _____ Rent: _____ No. of floors: _____ No. of steps: _____

Primary entry: _____ No. of steps: _____ Handrails: _____

Bedroom location: _____ Bath location: _____ Handrails: _____

Mental status and emotional reaction: _____

Alert? _____ Oriented? _____ Depressed? _____

Equipment at home: _____ Anticipated equipment needs: _____

Home health agency? _____ Other community services? _____

Patient family goals: _____

Plan: _____ Comments: _____

Social worker: _____ Date: _____

Form 84.1 Social work assessment form.

by communicating that several steps are necessary for attaining this goal. By graphically demonstrating the intervening steps toward the goal (see Fig. 84.1), the social worker utilizes the client's motivation to achieve the rehabilitative team's goal as well as his or her own personal goal. In Figure 84.1, several possible steps are identified in a rehabilitation process to capitalize on a patient's motivation to return to their own home. Step one is attending therapy until X% of function is gained. Step two is learning to use adaptive devices. Step three is discussing the required supports and home adaptations with the social worker and family. Step four is placement in a personal care home for a period of 6 months in order to demonstrate the ability to do X. Step five is to return home. While returning home may not even be an attainable goal, the social worker should avoid making this an issue so as not to detract from the rehabilitative process.

CURE VS. CARE

The social service assessment should address the older client's desire for care or for cure. The rehabilitative team needs to be aware that older clients need care. Care is the opportunity for such things as intimate touch by

the physical therapist, occupational therapist, nurse or physician. Care also gives purpose to the day. The older client needs to go to the outpatient clinic on Monday; to cardiac rehabilitation on Tuesday; to the pharmacy on Wednesday, etc. The older client's regular interaction with the social worker or home health aide is an opportunity to socialize and to feel valued by the provider. In contrast, cure, by eliminating therapy or treatment, creates a loss. Recognizing this situation, the rehabilitative team can then plan around the loss so that the client will not be excessively concerned.

CLIENT, FAMILY AND OTHERS' VIEWS OF REHABILITATION

The social service provider needs to assess both the client's and the family's view of the expected outcomes of rehabilitation. If the prevailing view is that the rehabilitative plan will not help or that the client is doomed to fail, the client's potential for success is seriously impaired. The social worker must provide education, appropriate for reading and comprehension level, and perhaps even involve other team members in the education process.

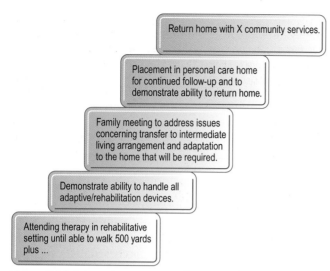

Figure 84.1 Intervening steps towards return to home.

PERSONALITY

Knowledge of the client's personality in their youth is beneficial in determining possible issues and appropriate team approaches prior to therapy (Hoyer & Roodin, 2009). Someone who was guarded at age 40 tends to be more guarded, if not suspicious, as they age, especially when under stress. Since an overly friendly approach would increase suspicion and hinder therapy, the social worker should employ a passive friendly approach. This would entail briefly discussing the rehabilitation process and then pulling back and letting the client ponder the information. Next, could be one or two more short visits by the social worker asking if there are any questions or concerns, followed by gently asking the client what are their thoughts and when might they be ready to start the rehabilitation process? This process can take a bit more time but yield more positive results. If someone had always demanded perfection, and with therapy, could not expect 100% return to function, the social worker would also need to address pertinent limitations.

ACTIVITIES

An assessment of the older individual's activities and activity style enables one to get a good understanding of the severity of the client's condition and its impact on the client's life. The passionate reader, who after completing therapy has 50% mobility, may be satisfied, whereas the passionate walker would be upset. The social worker needs to address this situation by first discovering the needs met by walking, e.g. stress reduction, and then by providing either alternative methods to meet the needs or by modifying the walking pattern, e.g. a slower pace, a shorter distance, or a different frequency, which might require the involvement of other members of the team. A bright light at the end of the rehabilitation tunnel will motivate the older person to work harder and ultimately experience better results from rehabilitation.

DIVERSITY

Social service providers need to be cognizant of ethnic diversity and cultures. African Americans, Pacific Asian Americans, American Indians and Hispanic Americans all have different belief systems. The older American Indian will approach rehabilitation differently from the African American. The manner in which the team approaches, addresses and instructs the client is important to the outcome of therapy (Quadagno, 2005). The social worker should educate the team as to how to address diverse populations as well as their cultural beliefs in terms of medical care, and in fact, if they are even accepting of traditional medical care.

THE GERIATRIC CARE MANAGER

A Geriatric Care Manager (GCM), as defined by the National Association of Professional Geriatric Care Managers, is a health and human services professional, such as a gerontologist, social worker, counselor or nurse, with a specialized body of knowledge and experience related to aging and elder care issues. The GCM assists older adults and persons with disabilities in attaining their maximum functional potential. They strive to respect the autonomy of the individual and to deliver care coordination and support services with sensitivity, in order to preserve the dignity and the respect of the individual. This includes end of life care and the client's right to choose his or her wishes for rehabilitation or end of life care. A program spreading across the United States of America is Physician Orders for Life Sustaining Treatment (POLST), which ensures the client's wishes are communicated and honored as to what kind of medical treatment the client wants toward the end of their life (McDonnell, 2013). Additionally, the GCM is an experienced guide and resource for families of older adults and others with chronic needs. As time progresses and as baby boomers age, the rehabilitative team will work hand in hand with this newly emerging professional. Clinical journals, business publications and weekly news magazines frequently discuss the current concept of care management for older individuals. The GCM can be quite helpful to the social worker in terms of assessment and understanding the older person in need of rehabilitation.

When discharge approaches, the social worker and the rehabilitation team need to consider post-rehabilitation requirements and needs of the client and family. Those requirements and needs include the home, durable medical equipment, home health and community services.

THE HOME

A home visit by members of the rehabilitation team allows family members to be interviewed in a familiar, non-threatening setting. It allows therapists to evaluate for barriers and adaptations that may be needed. Occasionally, a home may be dangerous or inappropriate for a patient's return. Extreme clutter, filth, lack of utilities, or disrepair may require community intervention.

The social worker will have to refer these rare situations to the Protective Service Unit of the Area Agency on Aging or some other appropriate agency. A first-hand view of the home environment helps the social worker prepare the family for the patient's return and also helps to coordinate community services for the patient's return home.

DURABLE MEDICAL EQUIPMENT

Most rehabilitation patients require the use of assistive devices, if only for a short time. Ordering durable medical equipment (DME) in a managed care climate requires knowledge of preferred provider relations and limits of coverage. Patients and families rely on social workers for this knowledge.

Basic items such as canes, walkers and wheelchairs are covered by most insurance carriers for appropriate patients. Larger items such as lifts, continuous passive-motion units and even hospital beds are less readily available and may not be covered at all. Items like lift chairs or stair glides are rarely, if ever, covered by insurance. Some DME suppliers have previously used lift chairs and stair glides, as well as other items available at reduced cost.

Some patients injured under workers' compensation or automobile plans may be covered for special items. Each individual has to be reviewed separately.

Some rehabilitation facilities or agencies for the disabled may employ an equipment adaptor. This professional person modifies and customizes medical equipment to individual needs. This can be a very helpful service for the geriatric patient.

HOME HEALTH

Medicare and most major insurance plans cover rehabilitative and nursing services in the home after the patient has been discharged from a facility if a skilled service (a PT or a RN) is ordered by a physician. In some cases, a nurse's aide may be covered for personal care, such as bathing. As with DME, many carriers are now requiring the use of preferred providers for home health services.

It should be noted that rural areas are often underserved by home health rehabilitative services. This can delay the initiation of care in the home.

Many people are under the impression that Medicare or other insurances provide for private nurses or aides in a patient's home. Medicare has never covered this service and most other plans have long since discontinued such benefits. There are many agencies that offer this help for a fee.

COMMUNITY SERVICES

The following are useful community services that have traditionally helped older people to remain at home; however, as public funds for these programs have dwindled, agencies have initiated fee-for-service arrangements. This has resulted in shorter waiting lists and faster start-up for services. Of course, it has also resulted in increased costs to the older consumer.

An *Area Agency on Aging (AAA)* is a local, public agency funded by federal and state monies; the agencies were created to provide support for older people in their homes. Some of the services offered include homemakers, personal care aides, friendly visitors, meals on wheels and so forth. A means test determines eligibility, and the services are generally limited to one or two hours a week. Some AAA offer personal attendant care or Title XX (Lamp II or Options) programs designed to help the most physically challenged individuals stay at home. Agencies on Aging are generally run by county governments. Phone numbers and addresses can be found in the blue pages of the telephone book or on the internet.

Chore services may be available through AAA or another public agency. This useful program can help to build ramps, attach handrails, or provide other minor adaptations. All materials are purchased by the individual receiving the service. Contact the AAA for more information.

Perhaps the best known service is *meals on wheels* (MOW), which provides a full meal for the homebound individual on 5 days a week or more. There is generally a fee charged for this service.

Adequate *transportation* services are the most common need of the elderly, especially for the geriatric rehabilitation patient. Most communities offer some type of subsidized transportation for eligible individuals. These programs function as a cross between a bus and a taxi. The vehicles, usually modified vans, travel specified routes but require advance notification of appointments. Vans equipped with wheelchair lifts are available, but extra notice may have to be given. Ambulance transport for routine medical appointments is rarely covered by insurance and is very expensive. Many ambulance providers offer a wheelchair van service at more reasonable rates.

PLACEMENT

Despite the best efforts and the fervent hopes of all, the goal of returning home may not be possible for all patients. Inadequate progress in therapy or insufficient support at home may make nursing home placement the only appropriate course of action. The social worker has to be sensitive to feelings of guilt, abandonment and hopelessness as he or she guides the patient and family through the application process. Furthermore, if the realities of modern healthcare make the first choice of a facility unachievable, the social worker must be frank and straightforward in dealing with placement issues. At all times, lines of communication must be kept open to make the patient's transition as smooth as possible.

CONCLUSION

While the social assessment and history provide a good basis for the rehabilitative process, it is important to be cognizant of the older person's special needs. Assessing and evaluating these additional considerations enhances the social worker or social service provider's opportunity for positive outcomes from the rehabilitative effort. The social worker's counseling skills, knowledge of community resources and ability to provide education throughout the rehabilitation process helps the client and family cope with the process and reach their rehabilitation goals. Social workers need to pay close attention to the research and developments surrounding the baby boomers in terms of rehabilitation expectations. This information will develop in the near future and should be sought out by social service providers as it is made available.

REFERENCES

Feldman BE 2012 Ten anticipated psychosocial needs of baby boomers. Long-Term Living 61(2):32–33

Frey WH 2010 Baby boomers and the new demographics of America's seniors. Generations 34(3):28–37

Hoyer JW, Roodin P 2009 Adult Development and Aging, 5th edn. McGraw–Hill, New York

Lemme HB 2006 Development in Adulthood, 4th edn. Allyn & Bacon, Boston, MD

McDonnell A 2013 Managing Geriatric Health Care. Jones & Bartlett Publishers, Sudbury, MA

Quadagno J 2005 Aging and the Life Course: An Introduction to Social Gerontology, 3rd edn. McGraw–Hill, New York

RESOURCES

NIH SeniorHealth

http://nihseniorhealth.gov/
   Health and wellness information for older adults from the National Institutes of Health.

BenefitsCheckUp

www.benefitscheckup.org/
   Takes 15–20 minutes to fill out information and assess what federal, state and local resources the client is entitled to.

National Association of Professional Geriatric Care Managers

www.caremanager.org/

National Alliance for Caregiving

Suite 642, 4720 Montgomery Lane
Bethesda, MD 20814
(301) 718-8444
www.caregiving.org

National Association for Home Care

228 7th Street, NE
Washington, DC 20003
(202) 547-7424
www.nahc.org

National Council on the Aging

Suite 200, 409 3rd Street, SW
Washington, DC 20024
(202) 479-1200
www.ncoa.org

National Family Caregivers Association

Suite 500, 10400 Connecticut Avenue
Kensington, MD 20895
(800) 896-3650
www.nfacares.org

Index

Note: Page numbers followed by "*b*", "*f*" and "*t*" refer to boxes, figures and tables, respectively.